BREAST CANCER

BREAST CANCER

Prognosis, Treatment, and Prevention

Second Edition

Edited by
Jorge R. Pasqualini
Hormones and Cancer Research Unit
Institut de Puériculture et de Périnatalogie
Paris, France

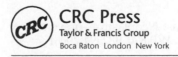

CRC Press is an imprint of the
Taylor & Francis Group, an **informa** business

CRC Press
Taylor & Francis Group
6000 Broken Sound Parkway NW, Suite 300
Boca Raton, FL 33487-2742

First issued in paperback 2019

ISBN-13: 978-1-4200-5872-7 (hbk)
ISBN-13: 978-0-367-38749-5 (pbk)

Library of Congress Cataloging-in-Publication Data

Breast cancer : prognosis, treatment, and prevention / edited by Jorge R. Pasqualini. — 2nd ed.
p. ; cm.
Includes bibliographical references and index.
ISBN-13: 978-1-4200-5872-7 (hardcover : alk. paper)
ISBN-10: 1-4200-5872-X (hardcover : alk. paper) 1. Breast—Cancer.
I. Pasqualini, Jorge R.
[DNLM: 1. Breast Neoplasms. 2. Breast Neoplasms—prevention & control. 3. Breast Neoplasms—therapy. WP 870 B82394 2008]
RC280.B8B672288 2008
616.99'449—dc22 2007045873

Visit the Taylor & Francis Web site at
http://www.taylorandfrancis.com

and the CRC Press Web site at
http://www.crcpress.com

Preface

Since the first edition of *Breast Cancer: Prognosis, Treatment and Prevention* was published there has been a tremendous amount of new information related to the basic and clinical applications of this disease which can affect 1 of 8 people in the USA and 1 of 12 in European countries.

This second edition of the book: *Breast Cancer: Prognosis, Treatment and Prevention* contains recent and very new information on the process of breast carcinogenesis, new prognostic factors and methods of prevention, the role of the breast as an intracrine organ, the enzymatic control in the bioformation and transformation of different hormones in the breast tissue, and the recent advances in the hormonal and non-hormonal treatment of breast cancer.

This second edition was made possible through spontaneous and strong support from the contributors to the first edition, as well as the enthusiastic response from new invited authors.

The 25 chapters of this book examine many aspects of breast cancer, including: basic information on breast pathogenesis; prognostic factors; the mechanisms of estrogens formation and its control; breast cancer and pregnancy; the cellular origin of the disease; role of hormone receptors; action of anti-hormones and anti-growth factors; apoptosis; aromatase inhibitors; the role of androgens; chemoprevention (SERMs); action of LHRH analogs; the role of Vitamin D; insulin-like growth factor; the control of proliferation; importance of lignans and isoflavones; breast cancer and body size; anti-angiogenic therapy; cytotoxic therapy for the treatment of metastatic breast cancer and locally advanced breast cancer, BRCA1, BRCA2 and hereditary breast cancer.

Briefly, this book provides very recent updated information on a wide range of breast cancer aspects and should be useful for oncologists, endocrinologists, gynecologists, general clinicians, biologists, physiologists, and graduate students.

I would like to express my deep thanks to all the authors for their valuable contribution to their chapters as well as to Ms. Sandra Beberman and her colleagues of Informa Healthcare.

Jorge R. Pasqualini

Contents

Contributors

Herman Adlercreutz Folkhälsan Research Center and Division of Clinical Chemistry, Biomedicum, University of Helsinki, Helsinki, Finland

Gregor M. Balaburski Fox Chase Cancer Center, Philadelphia, Pennsylvania, U.S.A.

Franco Berrino Dipartimento di Medicina Preventiva e Predittiva, Fondazione IRCCS Istituto Nazionale dei Tumori, Milano, Italy

Betsy A. Bove Clinical Molecular Genetics, Department of Pathology, Fox Chase Cancer Center, Philadelphia, Pennsylvania, U.S.A.

Angela M. H. Brodie University of Maryland School of Medicine, Baltimore, Maryland, U.S.A.

Francesca Cacciamani Division of Medical Oncology, S. Filippo Neri Hospital, Rome, Italy

Carlo Campagnoli S.C. Ginecologia Endocrinologica, Ospedale Ginecologico Sant'Anna, Torino, Italy

Angelo Casa Breast Center, Departments of Medicine and Molecular and Cellular Biology, Baylor College of Medicine, Houston, Texas, U.S.A.

Gérard S. Chetrite AP-HP, CHU Bicêtre, INSERM U693, Faculté de Médecine Paris-Sud, Le Kremlin-Bicêtre, France

Robert B. Clarke Breast Biology Group, Division of Cancer Studies, University of Manchester, Christie Hospital, Manchester, U.K.

Robert Clarke Department of Oncology and Department of Physiology and Biophysics, Lombardi Comprehensive Cancer Center, Georgetown University Medical Center, Washington D.C., U.S.A.

Aurélie Courtin INSERM U673, Hôpital Saint Antoine, Paris, France

Robert Dearth Breast Center, Departments of Medicine and Molecular and Cellular Biology, Baylor College of Medicine, Houston, Texas, U.S.A.

Jörg B. Engel Frauenklinik der Julius Maximilians-Universität Würzburg, Germany

Suzanne A. W. Fuqua Lester and Sue Smith Breast Center, Baylor College of Medicine, Houston, Texas, U.S.A.

Giampietro Gasparini Division of Medical Oncology, S. Filippo Neri Hospital, Rome, Italy

J. M. W. Gee Tenovus Centre for Cancer Research, Welsh School of Pharmacy, Cardiff University, Wales, U.K.

Anne Gompel Université Paris Descartes, Unité de Gynécologie Endocrinienne, APHP, Hôtel Dieu de Paris, and INSERM U673, Hôpital Saint Antoine, Paris, France

Paul E. Goss Massachusetts General Hospital Cancer Center and Harvard Medical School, Boston, Massachusetts, U.S.A.

S. E. Hiscox Tenovus Centre for Cancer Research, Welsh School of Pharmacy, Cardiff University, Wales, U.K.

Anthony Howell CRUK Department of Medical Oncology, Division of Cancer Studies, University of Manchester, Christie Hospital, Manchester, U.K.

Sacha J. Howell CRUK Department of Medical Oncology, Division of Cancer Studies, University of Manchester, Christie Hospital, Manchester, U.K.

I. R. Hutcheson Tenovus Centre for Cancer Research, Welsh School of Pharmacy, Cardiff University, Wales, U.K.

H. E. Jones Tenovus Centre for Cancer Research, Welsh School of Pharmacy, Cardiff University, Wales, U.K.

V. Craig Jordan Fox Chase Cancer Center, Philadelphia, Pennsylvania, U.S.A.

Helenius J. Kloosterboer KC2, Oss, The Netherlands

Fernand Labrie Laboratory of Molecular Endocrinology and Oncology, Laval University Hospital Research Center (CRCHUL) and Laval University, Québec City, Québec, Canada

Adrian V. Lee Breast Center, Departments of Medicine and Molecular and Cellular Biology, Baylor College of Medicine, Houston, Texas, U.S.A.

Beate Litzenburger Breast Center, Departments of Medicine and Molecular and Cellular Biology, Baylor College of Medicine, Houston, Texas, U.S.A.

Marie Löf Department of Medical Epidemiology and Biostatistics, Karolinska Institutet, Stockholm, Sweden

Raffaele Longo Division of Medical Oncology, S. Filippo Neri Hospital, Rome, Italy

Mads Melbye Department of Epidemiology Research, Statens Serum Institute, Copenhagen, Denmark

Mark Messina Department of Nutrition, School of Public Health, Loma Linda University, Loma Linda, California, U.S.A.

Robert I. Nicholson Tenovus Centre for Cancer Research, Welsh School of Pharmacy, Cardiff University, Wales, U.K.

Patrizia Pasanisi Dipartimento di Medicina Preventiva e Predittiva, Fondazione IRCCS Istituto Nazionale dei Tumori, Milano, Italy

Jorge R. Pasqualini Hormones and Cancer Research Unit, Institut de Puériculture et de Périnatalogie, Paris, France

Christine M. Pellegrino Department of Oncology, Montefiore Medical Center, Albert Einstein College of Medicine, Bronx, New York, U.S.A.

Clementina Peris S.C. Ginecologia Endocrinologica, Ospedale Ginecologico Sant'Anna, Torino, Italy

Michèle Pujos-Gautraud Saint Emilion, France

Jean-Pierre Raynaud Université Pierre et Marie Curie, Paris, France

Rebecca B. Riggins Department of Oncology, Lombardi Comprehensive Cancer Center, Georgetown University Medical Center, Washington D.C., U.S.A.

Jose Russo Breast Cancer Research Laboratory, Fox Chase Cancer Center, Philadelphia, Pennsylvania, U.S.A.

Irma H. Russo Breast Cancer Research Laboratory, Fox Chase Cancer Center, Philadelphia, Pennsylvania, U.S.A.

Paula D. Ryan Massachusetts General Hospital Cancer Center and Harvard Medical School, Boston, Massachusetts, U.S.A.

Roberta Sarmiento Division of Medical Oncology, S. Filippo Neri Hospital, Rome, Italy

Andrew V. Schally Miller School of Medicine, University of Miami, and Department of Veterans Affairs Medical Center, Miami, Florida, U.S.A.

Rachel Schiff Lester and Sue Smith Breast Center, Baylor College of Medicine, Houston, Texas, U.S.A.

Willem G. E. J. Schoonen Research and Development, Organon, a part of Schering-Plough Corporation, Oss, The Netherlands

Jennifer Selever Lester and Sue Smith Breast Center, Baylor College of Medicine, Houston, Texas, U.S.A.

Ayesha N. Shajahan Department of Oncology, Lombardi Comprehensive Cancer Center, Georgetown University Medical Center, Washington D.C., U.S.A.

Andrew H. Sims Breast Biology Group, Division of Cancer Studies, University of Manchester, Christie Hospital, Manchester, U.K.

Joseph A. Sparano Department of Oncology, Montefiore Medical Center, Albert Einstein College of Medicine, Bronx, New York, U.S.A.

K. Taylor Tenovus Centre for Cancer Research, Welsh School of Pharmacy, Cardiff University, Wales, U.K.

Francesco Torino Division of Medical Oncology, S. Filippo Neri Hospital, Rome, Italy

Herman A. M. Verheul Research and Development, Organon, a part of Schering-Plough Corporation, Oss, The Netherlands

Elisabete Weiderpass Department of Medical Epidemiology and Biostatistics, Karolinska Institutet, Stockholm, Sweden; Cancer Registry of Norway, Oslo, Norway; and Samfundet Folkhälsan (NGO), Helsingfors, Finland

JoEllen Welsh Department of Biomedical Sciences and Gen*NY*Sis Center for Excellence in Cancer Genomics, University at Albany, Rensselaer, New York, U.S.A.

Jan Wohlfahrt Department of Epidemiology Research, Statens Serum Institute, Copenhagen, Denmark

Ling Yang Clinical Trial Service Unit & Epidemiological Studies Unit, University of Oxford, Oxford, U.K.; Department of Medical Epidemiology and Biostatistics, Karolinska Institutet, Stockholm, Sweden; and Samfundet Folkhälsan (NGO), Helsingfors, Finland

1

Breast Architecture and the Pathogenesis of Cancer

JOSE RUSSO and IRMA H. RUSSO
Breast Cancer Research Laboratory, Fox Chase Cancer Center, Philadelphia, Pennsylvania, U.S.A.

INTRODUCTION

An important concept that has emerged from the study of breast development is that the terminal ductal lobular unit or TDLU, which had been identified as the site of origin of the most common breast malignancy, the ductal carcinoma, corresponds to a specific stage of development of the mammary parenchyma, the lobules type 1 (Lob 1) (Russo et al., 1991; Wellings, 1980; Wellings et al., 1975). This observation is supported by comparative studies of normal and cancer-bearing breasts obtained at autopsy. It was found that the nontumoral parenchyma in cancer-associated breasts contained a significantly higher number of hyperplastic terminal ducts, atypical Lob 1, and ductal carcinomas in situ originated in Lob 1 than those breasts of women free of breast cancer. Lob 1 is affected by preneoplastic as well as by neoplastic processes (Russo et al., 1991; Russo and Russo, 1997). The finding that Lob 1, which are undifferentiated structures, originate in the most undifferentiated and aggressive neoplasm acquires relevance in the light that these structures are more numerous in the breast of nulliparous women, who are, in turn, at a higher risk of developing breast cancer (Russo et al., 1992; Russo and Russo, 1997). The Lob 1 found in the breast of nulliparous women never went through the process of differentiation, whereas the same structures, when found in the breast of postmenopausal parous women did (Russo et al., 1992).

More differentiated lobular structures have been found to be affected by neoplastic lesions as well, although they originate tumors whose malignancy is inversely related to the degree of differentiation of the parent structure, i.e., lobules type 2 (Lob 2) originate lobular carcinomas in situ, whereas lobules type 3 (Lob 3) give rise to more benign breast lesions, such as hyperplastic lobules, cysts, fibroadenomas, and adenomas, and lobules type 4 (Lob 4) to lactating adenomas (Russo et al., 1991). It was concluded from these observations that each specific compartment of the breast gives origin to a specific type of lesion and also provides the basis for a new biological concept that the differentiation of the breast determines the susceptibility to neoplastic transformation.

SUPPORTING EVIDENCE FOR THE STEM CELL CONCEPT IN BREAST CANCER

The relationship of lobular differentiation, cell proliferation, and hormone responsiveness of the mammary epithelium is just beginning to be unraveled. Of interest is the fact that the content of estrogen receptor-alpha (ERα) and progestrone receptor (PgR) in the lobular structures of the breast is directly proportional to the rate of cell proliferation (Russo et al., 1999). These three parameters are maximal in the undifferentiated Lob 1, decreasing progressively in Lob 2, Lob 3, and Lob 4. The determination of the rate of cell proliferation, expressed as the percentage of cells that stain positively with Ki67 antibody, has revealed that proliferating cells are predominantly found in the epithelium lining ducts and lobules, and less frequently in the myoepithelium and in the intralobular and interlobular stroma. Ki67 positive cells are most frequently found in Lob 1. The percentage of positive cells is reduced by threefold in Lob 2 and by more than tenfold in Lob 3 (Russo and Russo, 1997; Russo et al., 1999). ERα and PgR positive cells are found exclusively in the epithelium; the myoepithelium and the stroma are totally devoid of steroid receptor–containing cells. The highest number of cells positive for both receptors is found in Lob 1, decreasing progressively in Lob 2 and Lob 3 (Russo et al., 1999).

The content of ERα and PgR in the normal breast tissue varies with the degree of lobular development, in a linear relationship with the rate of cell proliferation of the same structures. The utilization of a double-labeling immunocytochemical technique for staining in the same tissue section of those cells containing steroid hormone receptors and those that are proliferating, i.e., Ki67 positive, allowed us to determine that the expression of the receptors occurs in cells other than the proliferating cells, confirming results reported by other authors (Clarke et al., 1997). Immunocytochemical stains for ERα, PgR, and Ki67 in human breast tissues were compared vis-à-vis with the in vivo incorporation of ^{3}H-thymidine into cells that were synthesizing DNA in the mammary glands of young virgin Sprague-Dawley rats. The analysis of the rat mammary gland confirmed that maximal proliferative activity occurs in the terminal end buds (TEBs), as previously reported (Russo and Russo, 1980). It also revealed that the TEBs, alveolar buds (ABs), and lobules of the virgin rat mammary gland contain receptors for both estrogen and progesterone, and that the number of cells positive for both receptors was higher in the epithelium of TEB, progressively declining in the more differentiated AB and lobules. The higher concentration of ERα and PgR in the immature mammary gland of rodents and other species has been reported by other authors (Haslam, 1987). Similar to what has been observed in humans, the rat mammary gland contains steroid hormone receptor positive cells only in the ductal and lobular epithelium, but no positive cells were found in the stroma. These findings contrast with results obtained by cytosolic determination that reported that a high percentage of receptors were located in the mammary stroma. The findings that proliferating cells are different from those that are ERα and PgR positive support data that indicate that estrogen controls cell proliferation by an indirect mechanism. This phenomenon has been demonstrated using supernatants of estrogen-treated ERα positive cells that stimulate the growth of ER negative cell lines in culture. The same phenomenon has been shown in vivo in nude mice bearing ER negative breast tumor xenografts. ER positive cells treated with antiestrogens secrete TGF-β to inhibit the proliferation of ER negative cells (Clarke et al., 1992; Knabbe et al., 1987). Our studies have shown that the proliferative activity and the percentage of ERα and PgR positive cells are highest in Lob l in comparison with the various lobular structures composing the normal breast. These findings provide a mechanistic explanation for the higher susceptibility of these structures to be transformed by chemical carcinogens in vitro (Russo et al., 1988, 1993), supporting as well the observations that Lob l are the site of origin of ductal carcinomas (Russo et al., 1991).

The relationship between ER positive and ER negative breast cancers is not clear (Habel and Stamford, 1993; Harlan et al., 1993). It has been suggested that ER negative breast cancers result from either the loss of the ability of the cells to synthesize ER during clinical evolution of ER positive cancers, or that ER positive and ER negative cancers are different entities (Habel and Stamford, 1993; Moolgavkar et al., 1980). Our data allowed us to postulate that Lob l contain at least three cell types, ERα positive cells that do not proliferate, ERα negative cells that are capable of proliferating, and a small proportion of ERα positive cells that can also proliferate (Russo et al., 1999). Therefore, estrogen might stimulate ERα positive cells to produce a growth factor that, in turn, stimulates neighboring ERα negative cells capable of proliferating. In the same fashion, the small proportion of cells that are ERα positive and can proliferate could be the source of ERα positive tumors. The possibility exists, as well, that the ERα negative cells convert to ERα-positive cells. The conversion of ERα negative to ERα positive cells has been reported (Kodama et al., 1985). The findings that proliferating cells in the human breast are different from those that contain steroid hormone receptors explain much of the in vitro data (Foster and Wimalasena, 1996; Wang et al., 1997; Levenson and Jordan, 1994; Weisz and Bresciani, 1993). Of interest are the observations that while the ERα positive MCF-7 cells respond to estrogen treatment with increased cell proliferation, and that the enhanced expression of the receptor by transfection also increases the proliferative response to estrogen (Foster and Wimalasena, 1996; Zajchowski et al., 1993), ERα negative cells, such as MDA-MB-468 and others, when transfected with ERα, exhibit inhibition of cell growth under the same type of treatment (Levenson and Jordan, 1994; Weisz and Bresciani, 1993). Although the negative effect of estrogen on those ERα negative cells transfected with the receptor has been interpreted as an interference with the transcription factor used to maintain estrogen-independent growth (Pilat et al., 1996), there is no definitive explanation for their lack of survival. These data can be explained in light of the present work, in which proliferating and ERα positive cells are two separate populations. Furthermore, we have observed that when Lob l of normal breast tissue are placed in culture they lose the ERα positive cells, indicating that only proliferating cells, that are also ERα negative, can survive, and become stem cells. These observations are supported by the fact that MCF-10F, a spontaneously immortalized human breast epithelial cell line derived from breast tissues containing Lob l and Lob 2, is ERα negative (Calaf et al., 1994). Recently we have shown that estradiol-7β (E_2), the predominant circulating ovarian steroid, is carcinogenic in human breast epithelial cells and that this process is a nonreceptor mechanism (Russo et al., 2003, 2006c; Fernandez et al., 2006). The induction of complete transformation of the ER-negative human breast epithelial cell (MCF-10F) in vitro confirms the carcinogenicity of E_2, supporting the concept that this hormone could act as an initiator of breast cancer in women. This model provides a unique system for understanding the genomic changes that intervene for leading normal cells to tumorigenesis and for testing the functional role of specific genomic events taking place during neoplastic transformation (Russo et al., 2006c).

BREAST ARCHITECTURE AS A DETERMINING FACTOR IN THE SUSCEPTIBILITY TO CANCER

The breast of women that underwent reduction mammoplasty (RM) contains the three types of lobules studied that follow the same morphological characteristics described previously (Russo et al., 1992). The three lobular structures are in general surrounded by a loose stroma that demarcates them from the interlobular stroma that may have a different ratio of connective and fat tissue. All the lobules were very well demarcated and no fibrous tissue was observed (Table 1). Quantitation of the three lobular structures in the overall population of breast tissue studied indicated that Lob 1 represented 22.5% of the structures, whereas Lob 2 were 37.3%, and Lob 3 38.4% of the total number of structures. The differences are statistically significant. The separation of the breast samples, based on the pregnancy history of the host, such as nulliparity and parity, showed a different pattern of lobular development. The breast of nulliparous women contained a significantly higher number of Lob 1 and Lob 2, with 45.9% and 47.2%, respectively and a highly significantly lower number of Lob 3 (6.9%) (Table 1). In the breast of parous women, the pattern was inverse, being the Lob 2 and Lob 3 the most abundant, 35.5% and 47.9%, respectively whereas, Lob 1 comprised only 16.9% of the total.

The breast tissue of women with familial breast cancer (verified to be either BRCA+, or carriers of genetic abnormalities) (Table 2) was obtained from prophylactic mastectomies. The average age of these women was 37.0 ± 2.9 years of age (Table 2). The whole mount, as well as the histological appearance of the lobular structures, was different from that observed in the breast tissue of women that underwent RM. Eight of 17 breast samples presented a well-demarcated lobular structure, but all of them had a moderate or marked fibrous of the intralobular stroma (Table 3). Ductal hyperplasia (mild to severe) in the Lob 1 or Lob 2 was observed in seven cases, carcinoma insitu (solid, cribriform, and papillary)

Table 1 Lobular Architecture of the Breast Tissue from Reduction Mammoplasty (RM)

Group	No. of cases	Age X ± SD	Lob 1 X ± SD (%)	Lob 2 X ± SD (%)	Lob 3 X ± SD (%)
RM (all)	33	29.4 ± 8.2	22.5 ± 23.7	37.3 ± 28.6	38.4 ± 34.2
RM (nulliparous.)	9	22.9 ± 6.7	45.9 ± 27.4	47.2 ± 22.0	6.9 ± 7.0
RM (parous)	24	31.9 ± 2.3	16.9 ± 8.3	35.5 ± 3.1	47.9 ± 33.4

Abbreviation: X ± SD, mean ± standard deviation.

Table 2 Lobular Architecture of the Breast Tissue from Prophylactic Mastectomy for Familial Breast Cancer (FAM)

Group	No. of cases	Age X ± SD	Lob 1 X ± SD (%)	Lob 2 X ± SD (%)	Lob 3 X ± SD (%)
FAM (all)	17	37.0 ± 2.9	47.9 ± 37.3	39.9 ± 31.3	9.91 ± 4.41
FAM (nulliparous)	8	37.6 ± 3.2	51.3 ± 34.4	39.9 ± 26.2	8.83 ± 8.39
FAM (parous)	9	36.5 ± 2.6	44.0 ± 42.00	40.0 ± 38.1	16.10 ± 9.9

Abbreviation: X ± SD, mean ± standard deviation.

Table 3 Profile of the Lobular Structures in the Breast Tissues Obtained from Reduction Mammoplasty (RM), Prophylactic Mastectomy for Familial Breast Cancer (FAM), and Modified Radical Mastectomy (MRM) for Invasive Cancer

				Fibrosis		
Group	No. of cases	Well-defined lobules (%)	Not well-defined lobules (%)	None	Mild to moderate	Marked
RM	33	33 (100)	0 (0)	33 (100)	0	0
FAM	17	8 (47)	9 (53)	0	3 (17.6)	14 (82.4)
MRM	43	40 (93)	3 (7.0)	1 (2.3)	39 (90.3)	3.0 (7.4)

Table 4 Type of Lesions Found in the Breast Tissue Studied from Reduction Mammoplasty (RM), Prophylactic Mastectomy for Familial Breast Cancer (FAM), and Modified Radical Mastectomy (MRM)

			Ductal hyperplasia		Ductal carcinoma in situ	
Group	Number of cases	Number of lobules counted	Number	%	Number	%
RM	33	31,220	0	0	0	0
FAM	17	3,162	7	41.2	1	5.9
MRM	43	2,901	27	63	5	11.4

in one case, and invasive carcinomas was observed in nine cases (Table 4).

The distribution of Lob 1, Lob 2, and Lob 3 in the breast tissue derived from women with BRCA+, or being carriers of genetic abnormalities by linked analysis was 47.9%, 39.9%, and 9.9%, respectively (Table 2). This pattern was significantly different from that observed in the RM group I, containing a higher percentage of Lob 1 ($p < 0.0008$) whereas Lob 3 were significantly lower ($p < 0.00004$) (Table 2).

The separation of the breast samples, based on the pregnancy history of the host, such as nulliparity and parity, indicated that in both subgroups the percentage of Lob 1 was significantly higher than Lob 3 (Table 2), and that the differences between nulliparous and parous observed in the control or RM group (Table 1) were not present in the breast tissue derived from women with familial breast cancer (Table 2). Lob 1 represents 51.3% and 44.0% in the nulliparous and parous women, respectively. This indicates a reversion of the pattern observed in the parous in which the Lob 1 are less frequent. In the familial cases, the comparison of the nulliparous from the RM group with those of the prophylactic mastectomy for familial breast cancer (FAM) group is not statistically different. Instead, the parous breast tissue of the RM group was significantly different from those of the FAM group (Tables 1 and 2). To determine if the breast tissue of those with BRCA+ was different from those designated to be carriers but in which no BRCA was determined yet, these two groups (BRCA+ and carriers) were separated and it was found that the percentage of lobular structures were not significantly different.

The age of women from the RM group was different from thosc of the FAM group; the average age was 29.4 years for the first group and 37.0 years for the second group. This difference is significant. In order to determine if age may be contributory to the differences observed, the data were retabulated for the RM group for the women with matching age to those of FAM group, and it was found that the difference between both groups still persists, indicating that the familial factor could in itself be a deterrent in the pattern of architectural development of the breast.

The architectural pattern of the breast tissue obtained from modified radical mastectomy (MRM) were from 43 breast samples. The average age for this group is 35.4 years with no significant difference between the age for the nulliparous and parous women (Table 5). Quantitation of the three lobular structures in the overall population of breast tissue studied indicated that Lob 1 represented 74.25% of the structures, whereas Lob 2 were 22.3% and Lob 3 3.4% of the total number of structures. The differences are statistically significant. The separation of the breast samples, based on the pregnancy history of the host, such as nulliparity and parity, showed no different pattern of lobular development. The breast of nulliparous women contained a significantly higher number of Lob 1 and Lob 2, with 80.0% and 16.8%, respectively, and a highly significantly lower number of Lob 3 (1.7%) (Table 5). In the breast of parous women, the pattern was similar, Lob 1 and Lob 2 being the most abundant, 70.4% and 25.4%, respectively, whereas, Lob 3 comprised only 3.8% of the total. The differences between nulliparous and parous were not statistically significant (Table 5).

The histological appearance of the lobular structures was not as different from that observed in the breast tissue of women who underwent RM, but when compared with the FAM group, 92.8% of the lobular structures were well

Table 5 Lobular Architecture of the Breast Tissue from Modified Radical Mastectomy (MRM)

Group	Number of cases	Age X ± SD	Lob 1 X ± SD (%)	Lob 2 X ± SD (%)	Lob 3 X ± SD (%)
MRM (all)	43	35.4 ± 3.9	74.3 ± 25.8	22.3 ± 22.1	3.35 ± 10.0
MRM (nulliparous)	7	36.0 ± 3.6	80.0 ± 19.0	16.8 ± 15.0	1.74 ± 4.6
MRM (parous)	36	35.2 ± 4.3	70.4 ± 26.4	25.4 ± 22.7	3.80 ± 12.48

Abbreviation: X ± SD, mean ± standard deviation.

defined as opposed to only 47.0% in the FAM group, as 4 out of 43 breast samples were marked fibrous with the intralobular stroma (Table 2), which was significantly lower than the FAM group in which most of the lobules presented were marked intralobular fibrous. Ductal hyperplasia in Lob 1 or Lob 2, on the other hand, was observed in 62.9% of the cases and carcinoma in situ in 11.4% of the cases. Invasive carcinomas were observed in 88.6% of the cases (Table 4). The age of the women from the MRM group was not different from those of the FAM group.

Altogether these results show that the breast of parous women from the FAM and the MRM group exhibited a different architectural pattern from those of parous women of the RM group, which can be considered the normal or control population (Russo et al., 2003, 2006a,b; Fernandez et al., 2006). The observation that Lob 1 of the breast of both nulliparous and parous women of the FAM and MRM group are the most frequent structure is in agreement with the knowledge that the cancer in the breast starts in Lob 1 (Russo and Russo, 1994a,b; Russo et al., 1991; Wellings et al., 1975). The greater proportion of Lob 1 found in the breast of nulliparous and parous women of the FAM and MRM groups suggest that these breasts were at higher risk of developing malignancies because each Lob 1 is the target of carcinogenic insult (Russo et al., 1991; Wellings et al., 1975).

It has been postulated that BRCA1 and/or BRCA2 may serve to control cell proliferation and differentiation during developmental stages characterized by rapid growth (Rajan et al., 1997). This model predicts that individuals possessing germline mutations in BRCA1 and/or BRCA2 may be particularly susceptible to early events in mammary carcinogenesis during pregnancy (Rajan et al., 1997). How BRCA1 and/or BRCA2 control breast differentiation is unknown. In both sporadic and familial breast cancer, the pattern of lobular development is very similar. In rodents as well as in the breast tissue of women that underwent plastic surgery for cosmetic reasons, parity is associated with lobular differentiation (Russo et al., 1991; Russo and Russo, 1978). In both cases, lobular differentiation makes the mammary tissue refractory to neoplastic transformation by chemical carcinogens (Hu et al., 1997a). Moreover, the relation of the differentiation effect induced by pregnancy and the induced protection against breast cancer in women who have undergone this first full-term pregnancy early in life (Lambe et al., 1994) is an indication that the same operational events are modified in both familial and sporadic cases of breast cancer.

ROLE OF THE STROMA IN THE PATHOGENESIS OF BREAST CANCER

In addition to the overall architectural differences described above, the breast tissues from women with hereditary breast cancer present histological differences in the intralobular stroma (Table 3). The intralobular stroma at difference of the more dense collagenized interlobular stroma is a dynamic compartment of the breast composed of loosely arranged connective tissue, containing cells such as fibroblasts, blood vessels, and inflammatory cells such as lymphocytes, mast cells, and macrophages (Eyden et al., 1986; Ozzello, 1970). The intralobular stroma contrasts with the interlobular stroma that has fewer cells separated by larger quantities of more compact collagen. The role of intralobular stroma during breast development from adolescence to premenopausal maturity, pregnancy and lactation, and involution and postmenopausal changes has been implicated; however, how the interaction with the epithelial cells takes place is unknown. Most of our understanding of the interaction between epithelial and stroma in the breast is from the experiments of Sakakura et al. (1979). The intralobular stroma of the Lob 1 of the breast of women with familial breast cancer has lost the loosely arranged connective tissue for a denser stroma that erases its demarcation from the intralobular stroma. The intralobular stroma of the breast tissue from the FAM group was more fibrotic and dense. These findings suggest either that in the breast cancer families, the development of the breast parenchyma has failed to respond to the normal physiological stimuli that determine the formation of lobular structures indicative of differentiation, or that the involution pattern of Lob 3 after pregnancy is more rapid in these women than in those in the control. It is noteworthy that early pregnancies influence breast cancer risk by altering the structure of the mammary parenchyma (Russo et al., 1991, 1992).

It has been hypothesized that late pregnancies could likewise influence breast cancer risk via alterations in the mammary parenchyma, by delaying or interrupting the normal process of involution of glandular tissue of the breast (Henson and Tarone, 1994). It has been observed that BRCA1 in mice is induced during puberty and pregnancy and following treatment of ovariectomized animals with 17β-estradiol and progesterone. Therefore, it is not surprising that in the human breast, alteration of this gene may explain the altered morphological pattern observed. The findings that the intralobular stroma is more fibrotic in the FAM group than in the MRM and RM groups may in part explain the increased mammographic density in women with familial breast cancer. Although the intralobular stroma is only a small component of all the factors that determine the mammographic pattern, the mammographic breast density reflects proliferation of breast stroma through collagen formation and fibrosis. The factors that determine breast densities depend on the interplay of hormones, such as estrogen and growth factors such as epidermal growth factor, transforming growth factor, and insulin growth factors I and II. How all these factors and the genes related to familial breast cancer interrelate in the biology of the intralobular stroma is not known (Marquis et al., 1995; Pankow et al., 1997; Wilkinson et al., 1977; Wolfe et al., 1980; Saftlas et al., 1989).

The development of mammary ductal structures involves a complex interplay between epithelium and mesenchyme (Sakakura et al., 1976, 1979; Oza and Boyd, 1993; Russo J, et al., 2001a,b; Propper, 1972; Cunha et al., 1992; Kratochwil and Schwartz, 1976). The branching of the mammary ducts depends on circulating hormones for stimulation and synchronization with reproductive events, but is also influenced by local factors to provide signals that influence glandular growth, differentiation, and morphogenesis. The matrix-degrading metaloproteinase stromelysin-1, stromelysin-3, and gelatinase A are expressed during ductal branching morphogenesis of the murine mammary gland (Faulkin and DeOme, 1960), whereas the role of metalloproteinases in the branching pattern of the mammary gland and its relation with BRCA1 require further investigation. On the basis of these data it is possible to postulate that the breast tissue from women with hereditary breast cancer is affected by an alteration of the interaction between the epithelium and the stroma, resulting in a modified interaction between the stroma parenchyma as described here.

GLAND ARCHITECTURE IN THE SPORADIC AND FAMILIAL BREAST CANCER

As indicated in Table 2, BRCA1 or related genes associated with familial breast cancer play a role in the lobular pattern of the breast mainly by altering the pattern of involution after pregnancy, with the consistent increase in the Lob 1 compared with the control population (Table 1). However, the fact that familial breast cancer patients have an even larger proportion of Lob 1 in their unaffected breast points toward other genes that control the process and may be equally affected in both groups (Russo et al., 2001b). More specific to the role of familial breast cancer genes is the alteration in the epithelial stroma relationship by increasing the percentage of lobular structures with marked intralobular fibrosis (Table 3). These observations indicate that more studies in this direction must be attended. Genetic influences are responsible for at least 5% of the breast cancer cases; they also seem to influence the pattern of breast development and differentiation, as evidenced by the study of prophylactic mastectomy specimens obtained from women with familial breast and breast/ovarian cancer, or proven to be carriers of the BRCA1 gene, as determined by linkage analysis. The study of prophylactic mastectomy specimens obtained from both nulliparous and parous women revealed that the morphology and architecture of the breast were similar in these two groups of women (Russo et al., 2001b). Their breast tissues were predominately composed of Lob 1, and only a few specimens contained Lob 2 and Lob 3, in frank contrast with the predominance of Lob 3 found in parous women without familial history of breast cancer (Russo et al., 1992, 1994, 2001b). The developmental pattern of the breast of parous women of the familial breast cancer group was similar to that of nulliparous women of the same group and less developed than the breast of parous women without history of familial breast cancer. The breast of women belonging to the familial breast cancer group also presented differences in the branching pattern of the ductal epithelium, an observation suggesting that the genes that control lobular development might have been affected in those women belonging to families with a history of breast and breast/ovarian cancer (Russo et al., 1992, 1994a,b, 2001b). Supporting evidence to this fact is the poor milk production reported in carriers of the BRCA1 mutation compared with female relatives without mutation (Jernstrom et al., 1998) and the poor differentiation of the mammary gland of mice with BRCA1 mutations (Xu et al., 1999).

INFLUENCE OF PARITY IN BREAST DEVELOPMENT AND CANCER RISK

Despite their architectural similarity, there are important differences between the Lob 1 of the nulliparous woman and the regressed Lob 1 of the parous woman. Lob 1 of nulliparous women have a very active intralobular stroma, whereas those of the parous woman are more hyalinized and indicative of a regressed structure. Another important difference is the higher proliferative activity in Lob 1 of nulliparous than in parous women. The cells of both Lob 1 and Lob 3 in the parous breast are predominantly in the G0 phase or resting phase, while in Lob 1 of the nulliparous breast, proliferating cells predominate and the fraction of cells in G0 is quite low. Thus, parity, in addition to exerting an important influence on the lobular composition of the breast, profoundly influences its proliferative activity (Russo et al., 1992; Russo and Russo, 1997).

These biological differences that are influenced by the pattern of breast development may provide some explanation for the increased susceptibility of the breast of nulliparous women to develop breast cancer. It is hypothesized that unlike parous women, the Lob 1 found in the breast of nulliparous women never went through the process of differentiation, seldom reaching the Lob 3, and never the Lob 4, stages (Russo et al., 1992; 1994a,b; Russo and Russo, 1997). Although the lobules of parous women regress at menopause to Lob 1, they are permanently genetically imprinted by the differentiation process in some way that protects them from neoplastic transformation, even though these changes are no longer morphologically observable (Russo et al., 2006a,b; Balogh et al., 2006). Thus, they are biologically different from the Lob 1 of nulliparous women. Thus, the hypothesis is that parous women who develop breast cancer may do so because they have a defective response to the differentiating influence of the hormones of pregnancy (Russo et al., 1991; Russo and Russo, 1993, 1994a,b, 1997). Among the genes that have been proposed as mediating the favorable influence of pregnancy are inhibin (Russo and Russo, 1993, 1994a,b), mammary-derived growth factor inhibitor (Hu et al., 1997b; Huynh et al., 1995), or a serine protease inhibitor (serpin)-like gene (Russo et al., 1991).

Developmental differences might provide not only an explanation for the protective effect induced by pregnancy but also a new paradigm to assess other differences between the Lob 1 of parous and nulliparous women, such as their ability to metabolize estrogens or repair genotoxic damage. Such differences exist, and they have been shown to modulate the response of the rodent mammary gland to chemically induced carcinogenesis. It has been postulated (Russo et al., 2001b) that unresponsive lobules that fail to undergo differentiation under the stimulus of pregnancy and lactation are responsible for cancer development despite the parity history. It stands to reason that having more of these lobules increases the risk of breast cancer. In fact, the extent of age-related menopausal involution of the Lob 1 appears to influence the risk of breast cancer and may modify other breast cancer risk factors, including parity. This early observation postulated by us (Russo et al., 1992, 1994a,b, 2001b) has been confirmed in a recent report (Milanese et al., 2006) focused on breast biopsy specimens from 8736 women with benign breast disease. Milanese et al. (2006) have evaluated not only Lob 1 or TDLU but also the atrophic or involuted structures resulting from the normal process of aging in the human breast. The extent of involution of the terminal duct lobular units or Lob 1 was characterized as complete ($\geq$75% of the lobules involuted), partial (1–74% involuted) or none (0% involuted). The relative risk (RR) of breast cancer was estimated on the basis of standardized incidence ratios by dividing the observed numbers of incident breast cancers by expected values of population-based incident breast cancers from the Iowa Surveillance, Epidemiology, and End Results (SEER) registry. The following findings were noted: (1) Greater degrees of involution were positively associated with advancing age and inversely associated with parity. (2) Overall, the risk of breast cancer was significantly higher for women with no involution than for those with partial or complete involution (RRs 1.88, 1.47, and 0.91, respectively. This particular finding is of great interest because it confirms the previous observations of Russo et al. (Russo et al., 2001), indicating that Lob 1 are a marker of risk. (3) The degree of involution modified the risk of developing breast cancer in women who had atypia in their breast biopsies (RR 7.79, 4.06, and 1.49 for women with none, partial, and complete involution, respectively) as well as for those with proliferative disease without atypia (RR 2.94 and 1.11 for those with no and complete involution, respectively). (4) There was an interaction with family history as well: Women with a weak or no family history of breast cancer who had complete involution had a risk for breast cancer that was fivefold lower than the risk of those with a strong family history and no involution (RR 0.59 vs. 2.77, respectively). These data also confirm the previous observations of Russo et al. (2001b). (5). Among nulliparous women and those whose age at first birth was over 30 years, the absence of involution significantly increased the risk of breast cancer (RR 2.41 vs. 2.74, respectively). In contrast, for both groups there was no excess risk if involution was complete.

Altogether the study of Milanese et al. (2006) provides a powerful confirmation of the risk of Lob 1 or TDLU in the breast (Russo et al. 1992, 1994a,b, 2001b) and provides an additional morphological parameter like atrophic or involution of Lob 1 or TDLU as an indication of protection. However, this conclusion must be taken with reservation because in a recent finding by Harvey et al. (2004) postmenopausal women who had received hormonal replacement therapy showed an increase in breast density associated with a significant increase in the number of Lob 1 or TDLU, indicating that reactivation of the so-called involuted Lob 1 or TDLU can increase the risk of breast cancer in a woman.

REFERENCES

Balogh GA, Heulings R, Mailo DA, Russo PA, Sheriff F, Russo IH, Moral R, Russo J. Genomic signature induced by pregnancy in the human breast. Int J Oncol 2006; 28:399–410.

Calaf G, Tahin Q, Alvarado ME, Estrada S, Cox T, Russo J. Hormone receptors and cathepsin D levels in human breast epithelial cells transformed by chemical carcinogens. Breast Cancer Res Treat 1994; 29:169–177.

Clarke R, Dickson RB, Lipton ME. Hormonal aspects of breast cancer. Growth factors, drugs and stromal interactions. Crit Rev Oncol Hematol 1992; 12:1–23.

Clarke RB, Howell A, Anderson E. Estrogen sensitivity of normal human breast tissue in vivo and implanted into athymic nude mice: analysis of the relationship between estrogen-induced proliferation and progesterone receptor expression. Breast Cancer Res Treat 1997; 45:121–183.

Cunha GR, Young P, Hamamoto S, Guzman R, Nandi S. Developmental response of adult mammary epithelial cells to various fetal and neonatal mesenchymes. Epithelial Cell Biol 1992; 1:105–118.

Eyden B, Watson RJ, Harris M, Howell A. Intralobular stromal fibroblasts in the resting human mammary gland: ultrastructural properties and intercellular relationship. J Submicrosc Cytol 1986; 18:397–408.

Faulkin JL, DeOme KB. Regulation of growth and spacing of gland elements in the mammary fat pad of the C3H mouse. J Natl Cancer Inst 1960; 24:953–969.

Fernandez SV, Lareef MH, Russo IH., Balsara BR, Testa JR, Russo J. Estrogen and its metabolites 4-Hydroxy-estradiol induce mutations in TP53 and LOH in chromosome 13q12.3 near BRCA2 in human breast epithelial cells. Int J Cancer 2006; 118:1862–1868.

Foster JS, Wimalasena J. Estrogen regulates activity of cyclin-dependent kinases and retinoblastoma protein phosphorylation in breast cancer cells. Mol Endocrinol 1996; 10:488–498.

Habel LA, Stamford JL. Hormone receptors and breast cancer. Epidemiol Rev 1993; 15:209–219.

Harlan LC, Coates RJ, Block G. Estrogen receptor status and dieting intakes in breast cancer patients. Epidemiology 1993; 4:25–31.

Harvey JA, Santen RJ, Petroni GR, Bovbjerg V, Smolkin MA, Sheriff F, Russo J. Histologic changes in the breast with menopausal hormone therapy use: correlation with breast density, ER, PgR, and proliferation indices. Menopause 2008; 15:67–73.

Haslam S. Role of sex steroid hormones in normal mammary gland function. In: Neville MC, Daniel CW, eds. The Mammary Gland: Development, Regulation and Function. New York: Plenum Press, 1987: 499–533.

Henson DE, Tarone RE. On the possible role of involution in the natural history of breast cancer. Cancer 1994; 71:2154–2156.

Hu YF, Russo IH, Zalipsky U, Lynch HT, Russo J. Environmental chemical carcinogens induce transformation of breast epithelial cells from women with familial history of breast cancer. In vitro Cell Dev Biol Anim 1997a; 33:495–498.

Hu YF, Russo IH, Xiang A, Russo J. Mammary derived growth inhibitor (MDGI) cloned from human breast epithelial cells is expressed in fully differentiated lobular structures. Int J Oncol 1997b; 11:5.

Huynh HT, Larsson C, Narod S, Pollak M. Tumor suppressor activity of the gene encoding mammary-derived growth inhibitor. Cancer Res 1995; 55:2225.

Jernstrom H, Johannsson O, Borg A, Ivarsson H, Olsson H. BRCA1-positive patients are small for gestational age compared with their unaffected relatives. Eur J Cancer 1998; 34(3):368–371.

Knabbe C, Lippman ME, Wakefield LM, Flanders KC, Kasid A, Derynck R, Dickson RB. Evidence that transforming growth factor β is a hormonally regulated negative growth factor in human breast cancer cells. Cell 1987; 48:417–428.

Kodama P, Green GL, Salmon SE. Relation of estrogen receptor expression to clonal growth and antiestrogen effects on human breast cancer cells. Cancer Res 1985; 45:2720–2724.

Kratochwil K, Schwartz P. Tissue interaction in androgen response of embryonic mammary rudiment of mouse: identification of target tissue of testosterone. Proc Natl Acad Sci U S A 1976; 73:4041–4044.

Lambe M, Hsieh CC, Trichopoulos D, Ekbom A, Pavia M, Adami Ho. Transient increase in the risk of breast cancer after giving birth. N Engl J Med 1994; 331:5–9.

Levenson AS, Jordan VC. Transfection of human estrogen receptor (ER) cDNA into ER negative mammalian cell lines. J Steroid Biochem Mol Biol 1994; 51:229–239.

Marquis ST, Rajan JV, Wynshaw-Boris A, Xu J, Yin GY, Abel KJ, Weber BL, Chodosh LA. The developmental pattern of BRCA1 expression implies a role in differentiation of the breast and other tissues. Nature Genet 1995; 11:17–26.

Milanese TR, Hartmann LC, Sellers TA, Frost MH, Vierkant RA, Maloney SD, Pankratz VS, Degnim AC, Vachon CM, Reynolds CA, Thompson RA, Melton LJ, Goode EL, Visscher DW. Age-related lobular involution and risk of breast cancer. J Natl Cancer Inst 2006; 98(22):1600–1607.

Moolgavkar SH, Day NE, Stevens RG. Two-stage model for carcinogenesis: epidemiology of breast cancer in females. J Natl Cancer Inst 1980; 65:559–569.

Oza AM, Boyd NF. Mammographic parenchymal patterns: a marker of breast cancer risk. Epidemiol Rev 1993; 15:196–208.

Ozzello L. Epithelial-stromal junction of normal and dysplastic mammary glands. Cancer 1970; 25:586–600.

Pankow JE, Vachon CM, Kuni CC, King RA, Arnett DK, Grabrick DM, Rich SS, Anderson VE, Sellers TA. Genetic analysis of mammographic breast density in adult women: evidence of a gene effect. J Natl Cancer Inst 1997; 89:549–556.

Pilat MJ, Christman JK, Brooks SC. Characterization of the estrogen receptor transfected MCF-10A breast cell line 139B6. Breast Cancer Res Treat 1996; 37:253–266.

Propper A. Role du mesenchyme dans la differenciation de la glande mammaire chez l'embryon de lapin. Bull Soc Zool Fr 1972; 97:505–512.

Rajan JV, Marquis ST, Gardner HP, Chodosh LA. Developmental expression of BRCA2 co-localizes with BRCA1 and is associated with proliferation and differentiation in multiple tissues. Dev Biol 1997; 184:385–401.

Russo J, Ao X, Grill C, Russo IH. Pattern of distribution for estrogen receptor a and progesterone receptor in relation to proliferating cells in the mammary gland. Breast Cancer Res Treat 1999; 53:217–227.

Russo J, Balogh GA, Chen J, Fernandez SV, Fernbaugh R, Heulings R, Mailo DA, Moral R, Russo PA, Sheriff F, Vanegas J, Wang R, Russo IH. The concept of stem cell in the mammary gland and its implication in morphogenesis, cancer and prevention. Front Biosci 2006a; 11:151–172.

Russo J, Balogh GA, Heulings R, Mailo DA, Moral R, Russo PA, Sheriff F, Vanegas J, Russo IH. Molecular basis of pregnancy induced breast cancer protection. Eur J Cancer Prev 2006b; 15:306–342.

Russo J, Calaf G, Russo IH. A critical approach to the malignant transformation of human breast epithelial cells. Crit Rev Oncog 1993; 4:403–417.

Russo J, Fernandez SV, Russo PA, Fernbaugh R, Sheriff FS, Lareef HM, Garber J, Russo IH. 17 beta estradiol induces transformation and tumorigenesis in human breast epithelial cells. FASEB J 2006c; 20:1622–1634.

Russo J, Gusterson BA, Rogers AE, Russo IH, Wellings SR, van Zwieten MJ. Comparative study of human and rat mammary tumorigenesis. Lab Invest 1991; 62:1–32.

Russo J, Hu Y-F, Silva ID, Russo IH. Cancer risk related to mammary gland structure and development. Microsc Res Tech 2001a; 52:204–223.

Russo J, Lareef MH, Balogh G, Guo S, Russo IH. Estrogen and its metabolites are carcinogenic in human breast epithelial cells. J Steroid Biochem Mol Biol 2003; 87:1–25.

Russo J, Lynch H, Russo IH. Mammary gland architecture as a determining factor in the susceptibility of the human breast to cancer. Breast J 2001b; 7:278–291.

Russo J, Reina D, Frederick J, Russo IH. Expression of phenotypical changes by human breast epithelial cells treated with carcinogens in vitro. Cancer Res 1988; 48:2837–2857.

Russo J, Rivera R, Russo IH. Influence of age and parity on the development of the human breast. Breast Cancer Res Treat 1992; 23:211–218.

Russo J, Romero AL, Russo IH. Architectural pattern of the normal and cancerous breast under the influence of parity. Cancer Epidemiol Biomarkers Prev 1994; 3:219–224.

Russo IH, Russo J. Developmental stage of the rat mammary gland as determinant of its susceptibility to 7,12-dimethylbenz(anthracene). J Natl Cancer Inst 1978; 61:1439–1449.

Russo J, Russo IH. Influence of differentiation and cell kinetics on the susceptibility of the rat mammary gland to carcinogenesis. Cancer Res 1980; 40:2677–2687.

Russo J, Russo IH. Development pattern of human breast and susceptibility to carcinogenesis. Eur J Cancer Prev 1993; 3(suppl 2):85.

Russo J, Russo IH. Toward a physiological approach to breast cancer prevention. Cancer Epidemiol Biomarkers Prev 1994a; 3:353–364.

Russo IH, Russo J. Role of hCG and inhibin in breast cancer. Int J Oncol 1994b; 4:297.

Russo J, Russo IH. Role of differentiation in the pathogenesis and prevention of breast cancer. Endocr Relat Cancer 1997; 4:7–21.

Saftlas AF, Wolfe JN, Hoover RN, Brinton LA, Schairer C, Salane M, Szklo M. Mammographic parenchymal patterns as indicators of breast cancer risk. Am J Epidemiol 1989; 129:518–526.

Sakakura T, Nishizuka Y, Dawe C. Mesenchyme-dependent morphogenesis and epithelium specific cytodifferentiation in mouse mammary gland. Science 1976; 194:1439–1441.

Sakakura T, Sakagami Y, Nishizuka Y. Persistence of responsiveness of adult mouse mammary gland to induction by embryonic mesenchyme. Dev Biol 1979; 72:201–210.

Wang W, Smith R, Burghardt R, Safe SH. 17β estradiol-mediated growth inhibition of MDA-MB 468 cells stably transfected with the estrogen receptor: cell cycle effects. Mol Cell Endocrinol 1997; 133:49–62.

Weisz A, Bresciani F. Estrogen regulation of proto-oncogenes coding for nuclear proteins. Crit Rev Oncogen 1993; 4:361–388.

Wellings SR. Development of human breast cancer. Adv Cancer Res 1980; 31:287–299.

Wellings SR, Jensen HM, Marcum RG. An atlas of subgross pathology of 16 human breasts with special reference to possible precancerous lesions. J Natl Cancer Inst 1975; 55:231–275.

Wilkinson E, Clopton C, Gordonson J, Green R, Hill A, Pike MC. Mammographic parenchymal pattern and the risk of breast cancer. J Natl Cancer Inst 1977; 59:1397–1400.

Wolfe JN, Albert S, Belle S, Salane M. Familial influences on breast parenchymal patterns. Cancer 1980; 46:2433–2437.

Xu X, Wagner KU, Larson D, Weaver Z, Li C, Reid T, Henniqhausen L, Wynshaw-Boris A, Deng CX. Conditional mutation of BRCA1 in mammary epithelial cells results in blunted ductal morphogenesis and tumour formation. Nat Genet 1999; 22:37–43.

Zajchowski DA, Sager K, Webster L. Estrogen inhibits the growth of estrogen receptor negative, but not estrogen receptor positive, human mammary epithelial cells expressing a recombinant estrogen receptor. Cancer Res 1993; 53:5004–5011.

2

The Enzymatic Systems in the Formation and Transformation of Estrogens in Normal and Cancerous Human Breast: Control and Potential Clinical Applications

JORGE R. PASQUALINI

Hormones and Cancer Research Unit, Institut de Puériculture et de Périnatalogie, Paris, France

GÉRARD S. CHETRITE

AP-HP, CHU Bicêtre, INSERM U693, Faculté de Médecine Paris-Sud, Le Kremlin-Bicêtre, France

INTRODUCTION

In latter years the intratumoral formation and transformation of estrogens and other hormones, as a result of the activity of the various enzymes involved, attracted particular attention for their role play in the development and pathogenesis of hormone-dependent breast cancer. These enzymatic activities are more intense in the breast carcinoma tissue than in the normal breast, particularly in postmenopausal patients where the ovary has ceased to produce hormones and in whom, in addition, the tissular concentrations of estrogens are various times higher than the circulating plasma levels.

The enzymatic process concerns the aromatase, which transforms androgens into estrogens; the sulfatase, which hydrolyzes the biologically inactive sulfates to form the active hormone; 17β-hydroxysteroid dehydrogenases (17β-HSDs), which are involved in the interconversion estradiol (E_2)/estrone (E_1) or testosterone/androstenedione; hydroxylases, which transform estrogens into mitotic and antimitotic derivatives; sulfotransferases and glucuronidases, which convert, respectively, into the biologically inactive sulfates and glucuronidates. It is also important to consider the metabolic transformations of progesterone and their role in normal and cancerous breast. Concerning aromatase, the application of antiaromatase substances is extensively used as the first-line treatment of breast cancer, with very positive results (for details see chapters 10 and 11). In this chapter, we summarize the recent developments of the mechanism of these enzymatic processes, their control, use of the enzymatic expression as a prognostic factor in breast cancer patients, as well as possible clinical applications. To indicate the evolutionary findings in the different sections, we recall previous basic and important pioneer studies.

EVOLUTION OF THE BREAST FROM NORMAL TO CANCEROUS

The evolution of the breast cell from normal to cancerous is a long process (probably decades) where the mechanism of the initial transformation is still unknown. A series of recent studies using new molecular technology concludes that breast cancer is a heterogeneous disease including a wide variety of pathological entities.

Table 1 Main Factors Involved in Low-grade and High-grade Breast Cancer Tumors

	Proliferation	Apoptosis	Receptor		p53	ErbB-2	Lymphocystic infiltration
			ER	PR			
Low-grade tumors	Low	Low	+	+	Wild type	−	−
High-grade tumors	High	High	−	−	Mutant	+	+

Most breast cancers (about 95%), whether in pre- or postmenopausal women, are initially hormone dependent, where the hormone E_2 plays a crucial role in their development and progression (Segaloff, 1978; Henderson and Canellos, 1990; Hulka and Stark, 1995; Henderson and Feigelson, 2000; Yager and Davidson, 2006). The hormone and estrogen receptor (ER) complex can mediate activation of the proto-oncogenes and oncogenes (e.g., c-myc, c-fos) histones and other nuclear proteins, as well as various target genes. Besides this classic genomic mechanism of estrogen, there is evidence that E_2 also exerts rapid, nongenomic actions initiated by binding to cytoplasmic or membrane receptors, implicated ERs, ER-related proteins, or G-protein-coupled receptors such as GPR30, which activate in particular the production of the second messengers (cAMP, Ca^{2+}, or nitric oxide) and the growth factor kinase signaling pathways, mitogen-activated protein kinase (MAPK), and phosphatidylinositol-3-kinase (PI3K)/Akt (Levin, 2005; Rai et al., 2005). Despite the importance of E_2 in breast carcinogenesis there is at present no proof of a "direct effect" of the hormone in the initiation of this process.

After a period which may last several years, the tumor becomes hormone independent by a mechanism which, though not fully elucidated, is under scrutiny. One explanation for the progression toward hormone independence could be the presence of ER mutants (Raam et al., 1988; Fuqua et al., 1991, 1992; Schiff and Fuqua, 2002). In hormone-dependent cells the interaction of the hormone with the receptor molecule is the basic step for eliciting a hormone response. As the cancer cell evolves, mutations, deletions, and truncations appear in the receptor gene (McGuire et al., 1992; Castles et al., 1993), the ER becomes "nonfunctional" and, despite the estrogen binding, the cell fails to respond to the hormone. A non-functional ER might explain why 35% to 40% of patients with ER-positive tumors do not respond to antiestrogen therapy (Litherland and Jackson, 1988). The possibility that ER mutants could be involved in the transformation of breast cancer from hormone dependency to hormone independency requires further study. However, it is interesting that these mutants are found in ER-negative breast tissue (Herynk and Fuqua, 2004). Komagata et al. (2006) suggest that the naturally occurring human ERα mutants with amino acid changes may modulate the responsiveness to estrogens and antiestrogens. Very interesting clinical results were obtained during treatment by selective estrogen receptor modulators (SERMs), such as tamoxifen, droloxifene, toremifene, raloxifene, or by fulvestrant, a new type of pure ER antagonist that downregulates the ER. Unfortunately, development of endocrine-resistant breast cancer cells over time can also be explained by the fact that SERMs activate nongenomic activity of E_2, in particular via cooperation with the EGF receptor/MAPK pathway, and contribute to SERMs resistance (Osborne et al., 2005; Fan et al., 2007).

Another attractive aspect in the evolution of breast cancer from hormone dependency to independency involves coactivators and corepressors in the activity and control of various enzymes that act in the formation and transformation of estrogens during this process (Pasqualini and Chetrite, 1996).

Two distinct major pathways can be considered in the evolution of breast cancer, one showing positive ER and progesterone receptor (PR) with 16q loss and a low grade of invasive carcinoma, the other with overexpressed Her-2/neu (c-erbB-2), negative ER and PR, and a high grade of invasive carcinoma. Table 1 indicates the main factors and characteristics of low- and high-grade tumors. Figure 1 schematizes the progression of normal mammary cells toward a hormone-independent carcinoma. In terms of therapeutic options, patients with triple-negative breast cancer (15% of all breast cancer), defined by a lack of ER, PR and ErbB-2 receptor expression, lead to high rates of local and systemic relapse since no specific treatment, hormonal or by biological target therapies (e.g., signal transduction inhibitors, such as monoclonal antibody against Her-2/neu (e.g., trastuzumab: herceptin®) or small molecule receptor tyrosine kinase inhibitors) is available.

With new methodology in molecular genetics, proteomic analysis, and immunohistochemistry, the concept of different steps in the evolution of breast cancer has introduced interesting data detailed in various studies concerning DNA amplification (Lage et al., 2003), tissue microdissection (Emmert-Buck et al., 2001), genoma, and transcriptional analysis (Ma et al., 2003).

There is growing evidence that local and specific peritumoral microenvironments, created by mammary stromal cells and extracellular matrix components, have an important pathophysiological role in tumorigenesis (Schäffler et al., 2007; Celis et al., 2005). Since epithelial breast cancer cells are surrounded by large amounts of adipose tissue, adipose stromal fibroblasts and (pre)-adipocytes particularly, can produce local estrogens as they express high levels of aromatase (Amin et al., 2006). Further, some soluble secreted factors such as adipokines (e.g., leptin, adiponectin, tumor necrosis factor-α, interleukin-6) have crucial endocrine,

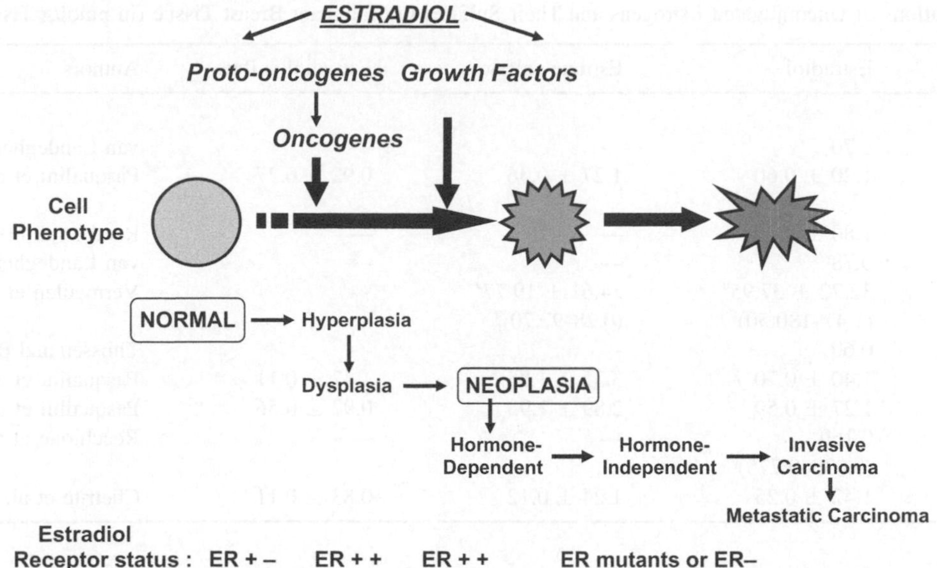

Figure 1 Evolutive transformation of the breast cell from normal to carcinogen. Estradiol plays important roles in the development and progression of breast cancers by acting with its receptor (ER) via (1) nuclear genomic action as a transcription factor or a coactivator; (2) extranuclear (plasmatic membrane), rapid and nongenomic action as activator of growth factor pathways and protein kinases cascades (MAPK and PI3K/Akt). Prognosis of the disease evolution is very good in the period when the breast cancer is hormone dependent, but very poor when the cancer becomes hormone independent. *Abbreviations*: ER+, estrogen receptor positive (detectable and functional); ER mutants, estrogen receptor detectable but nonfunctional; ER–, estrogen receptor negative (not detectable).

paracrine, and/or autocrine functions implicated in the tumor-stromal interaction, by modulating proliferation, apoptose, metabolism, and angiogenesis of breast cancer cells (Tworoger et al., 2007; Garofalo et al., 2006; Yamaguchi et al., 2005). Epidemiological studies suggest that increase of adipose tissue mass and obesity can influence both breast cancer risk and tumor behavior. This way represents new therapeutic targets for the prevention and treatment of breast cancer. For example, some glitazones (rosiglitazone, pioglitazone) that activate peroxisome proliferator-activated receptor-γ implicated in the upregulation of adiponectin expression, an antiproliferative adipokine of breast cancer cells, are under evaluation (Rubin et al., 2000; Yee et al., 2007).

Simpson et al. (2005) questioned whether the designations "ductal" and "lobular" were still appropriate. They considered that the majority of neoplastic breast diseases arise from the terminal duct lobular unit whereby this terminology is not intended to reflect the microanatomical site of origin but rather a difference in cell morphology (Reis-Filho and Lakhani, 2003; Simpson et al., 2003).

Progesterone is another major though controversial player in mammary gland biology. This ovarian steroidal hormone also acts in conjunction with estrogens through its specific receptor PR in the normal epithelium to regulate breast development. The effects of these hormones on the proliferative activity of the breast, indispensable for its normal growth and development, have been and still remain the subject of heated controversy (for reviews see Russo and Russo, 2002, 2008; Pasqualini et al., 1998; Pasqualini, 2007).

The remaining 5% of breast cancers, denoted BRCA-1 or BRCA-2, are hereditary breast cancers (for details see Bove et al., 2002; Bove, 2007).

CONCENTRATION OF ESTROGENS IN NORMAL AND CANCEROUS BREAST

As breast cancer tissue is very active in the biosynthesis of estrogens, especially in postmenopausal patients (Pasqualini and Chetrite, 2005a), and concentration levels are significantly higher in relation to normal breast (Chetrite et al., 2000), it was interesting to summarize the values obtained in different studies in both the breast tissue and the plasma concentration of various estrogens.

In the Breast Tissue

Information on estrogen levels in breast tissue is very limited. Table 2 summarizes the tissular concentration values of E_2, E_1, and their sulfates obtained by different authors in the breast tumors of pre- and postmenopausal patients. All the data agree that higher levels of E_2 were found in particular in the postmenopausal patients. Analyzing the tissue-plasma ratio, it is observed that for E_1, E_2, and estradiol sulfate there is a significant tissue to plasma gradient, which increases in postmenopausal patients where, for instance, E_2 increases to 23 from a ratio of 5 in premenopausal patients (Pasqualini et al., 1996a). In a study of 90 breast cancer patients (pre- and postmenopausal), Miyoshi et al. (2004) found a

Table 2 Concentrations of Unconjugated Estrogens and Their Sulfates in Malignant Breast Tissue (in pmol/g Tissue)

Estrone	Estradiol	Estrone sulfate	Estradiol sulfate	Authors
Premenopausal				
1.04	0.70	—	—	van Landeghem et al. (1985)
1.40 ± 0.08	1.20 ± 0.60	1.27 ± 0.36	0.92 ± 0.27	Pasqualini et al. (1994a)
Postmenopausal				
1.14 ± 0.22	1.80 ± 0.29	—	—	Reed et al. (1983)
0.60	0.78	—	—	van Landeghem et al. (1985)
25.18 ± 51.10[a]	32.72 ± 37.95[a]	14.61 ± 19.77[a]	—	Vermeulen et al. (1986)
(0.37–248)[a]	(1.47–180.50)[a]	(0.28–97.70)[a]		
0.25	0.60	—	—	Thijssen and Blankenstein (1989)
1.00 ± 0.15	1.40 ± 0.70	3.35 ± 1.85	1.47 ± 0.11	Pasqualini et al. (1996a)
1.06 ± 0.43	1.27 ± 0.59	2.89 ± 1.93	0.97 ± 0.56	Pasqualini et al. (1994a)
-	0.169	—	—	Recchione et al. (1995)
	(0.033–0.775)			
1.20 ± 0.28	1.42 ± 0.25	1.24 ± 0.12	0.83 ± 0.11	Chetrite et al. (2000)

[a]In pmol/g protein.

Table 3 Plasma E_2 Levels and Risk of Breast Cancer

Breast cancer patients/controls	RR (95% CI) by category of circulating E_2[a]		Authors
	1	4	
Premenopausal women			
285/555	1.0	1.0 (0.7–1.5)	Kaaks et al. (2005a,b)
185/368 (follicular phase)	1.0	2.1 (1.1–4.1)	Eliassen et al. (2006)
175/349 (luteal phase)	1.0	1.0 (0.5–1.9)	Eliassen et al. (2006)
Postmenopausal women			
663/1765	1.0	1.8 (1.3–2.4)	EHBCCG (2002)[b]
322/643	1.0	2.1 (1.5–3.2)	Missmer et al. (2004)
297/563	1.0	1.7 (1.0–2.8)	Zeleniuch-Jacquotte et al. (2004)
677/1309	1.0	1.7 (1.2–2.4)	Kaaks et al. (2005a,b)

[a]Estradiol (E_2) values presented in quartiles (4).
[b]The Endogenous Hormone and Breast Cancer Collaborate Group.
Source: From Hankinson and Eliassen (2007).

correlation between intratumoral E_2 and the PR content in ER-positive, but not with ER-negative, tumors and suggested that patients with E_2-high tumors showed a significantly better prognosis than those with E_2-low tumors.

In the Plasma

A series of studies carried out between 1971 and 1996 clearly show that for premenopausal breast cancer patients, compared with controls, there are no significant differences in the plasma concentrations of E_1, E_2, or estrone sulfate (E_1S) (for a review see Pasqualini, 2004). A study including 663 postmenopausal breast cancer patients and 1765 controls, circulating estrogen levels were found to be positively associated with breast cancer risk (Key et al., 2002). Another study demonstrated an increase of plasma E_2 levels in postmenopausal patients (Manjer et al., 2003; Missmer et al., 2004; Zeleniuch-Jacquotte et al., 2004; Kaaks et al., 2005a,b) (Table 3). However, there were no significant differences in premenopausal patients with the exception of an evaluation carried out during the follicular phase (Eliassen et al., 2006). It is interesting to mention that in postmenopausal patients, a positive association of estrogen plasma levels and ER+/PR+ tumors was found, whereas a weak or no association was noted in ER+/PR− or ER−/PR− tumors (Missmer et al., 2004). It was demonstrated that plasma estrogens, but not androgens or sex hormone–binding globulin, were strongly and significantly associated with risk of breast hyperplasia in postmenopausal women, suggesting that estrogens can be important in the pathological process toward breast cancer.

Circulating androgens are important precursors of estrogens, as summarized in Figure 2 showing the concentration values of various androgens and estrogens in breast cancer patients.

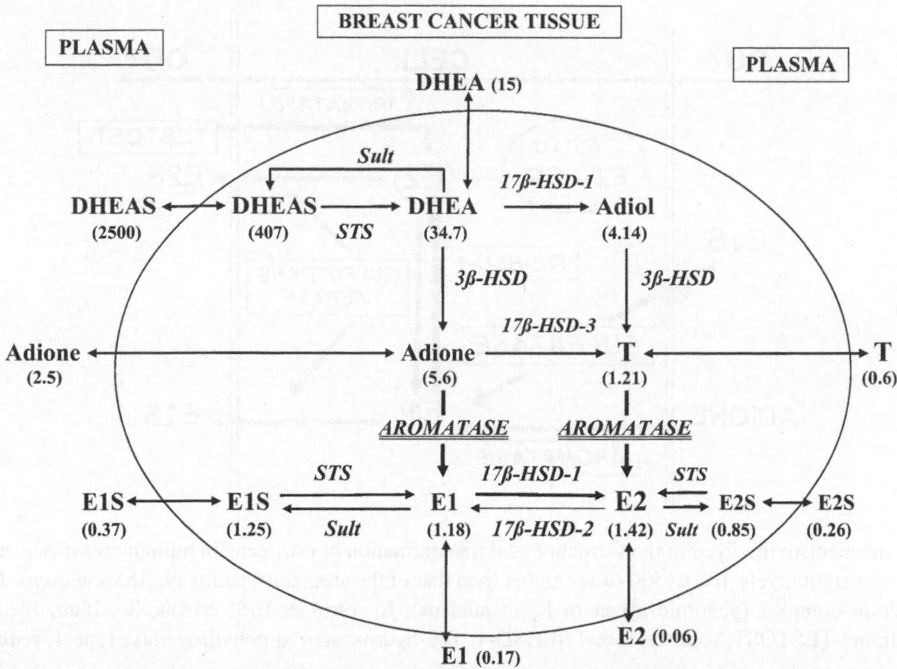

Figure 2 Enzymatic mechanism involved in the formation of estrogens in human breast cancer tissue of postmenopausal patients. Plasmatic steroid concentrations (indicated in brackets) were expressed in pmol/mL and tissular steroid concentrations in pmol/g tissue. *Abbreviations*: DHEA, dehydroepiandrosterone; DHEAS, dehydroepiandrosterone sulfate; Adiol, androstenediol (androst-5-ene-3β,17β-diol). This androgen has a high affinity for the estrogen receptor and exerts estrogenic effect; Adione, androstenedione; T, testosterone; E_1S, estrone sulfate; E_1, estrone; E_2, estradiol; STS, steroid sulfatase; SULT, sulfotransferase; 17β-HSD, 17β-hydroxysteroid dehydrogenase; 3β-HSD, 3β-hydroxysteroid dehydrogenase. Tissular concentrations of DHEAS and DHEA quoted from van Landeghem et al. (1985). Tissular concentrations of Adiol, Adione, and T quoted from Thijssen et al. (1993). Plasmatic concentrations of DHEAS, DHEA, Adione, and T quoted from Simpson et al. (2005). Plasmatic and tissular concentrations of E_1, E_2, E_1S, and E_2S quoted from Pasqualini et al. (1996a) and Chetrite et al. (2000).

ENZYMATIC PROCESS INVOLVED IN THE BIOFORMATION AND TRANSFORMATION OF ESTROGENS IN NORMAL AND CANCEROUS BREAST AND ITS CONTROL

As a great variety of enzymes are involved in the formation and metabolic transformation of estrogens in breast tissue, these pathways and the mechanistic controls are summarized here. Figures 3 and 4 schematize the main conversions of estrogens in the human breast.

Hydroxylated Metabolic Pathway of Estrogens in the Breast

It is well documented that breast tissues have the capacity to convert estrogens (particularly E_2 and E_1) to C_2, C_4, and C_{16} hydroxylated derivatives. The role of these compounds has become very attractive in the search for knowledge of the biological response of estrogens in the normal or cancerous human breast. E_1 and E_2 are substrates of cytochromes P450 CYP1A1/1A2 and CYP1B1, which generate predominantly 2- and 4-hydroxy-catecholestrogens (4-OH-CE) (Lee et al., 2003; Dawling et al., 2004).

C_2-Hydroxy Derivatives

Early studies in human breast cancer tissue demonstrate the conversion of E_1 or E_2 to 2-hydroxy-estrogens (2-OH-Es), then by the action of a catechol-*O*-methyltransferase to the 2-methoxy-E_1 or 2-methoxy-E_2 (Assicot et al., 1977). 2-OH-Es generate stable DNA adducts, and after transformation to methoxy derivatives possess antiproliferative and antiangiogenic properties (Lottering et al., 1992; Zhu and Conney, 1998; Lippert et al., 2003). As the antiproliferative effect can be obtained in negative ER cell lines, it is suggested that the biological response of 2-methoxy-E_2 is mediated by another pathway than the classical ER; for instance, it was demonstrated that 2-methoxy-E_2 activity takes place independent of ER α or β (Lakhani et al., 2003).

Liu and Zhu (2004) demonstrated that 2-methoxy-E_2 has a consistent antiproliferative effect on the ER-negative breast cancer cells and has both mitogenic and antiproliferative activity in the ER-positive cells. In another study it was shown that a combination of tamoxifen and 2-methoxy-E_2 can have an additive inhibitory effect on the proliferation of ER-positive and ER-negative breast cancer cell lines (Seeger et al., 2003, 2004). Vijayanathan et al. (2006)

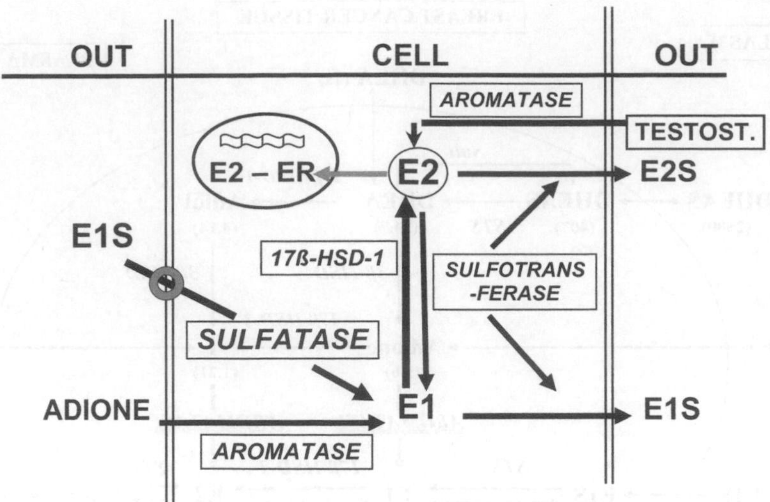

Figure 3 Enzymatic mechanism involved in the formation and transformation of estrogens in human breast cancer, intracrine concept. The sulfatase pathway is quantitatively 100 to 500 times higher than that of the aromatase pathway. *Abbreviations*: E_2, estradiol; E_2-ER, estradiol-estrogen receptor complex (genomic effect of E_2 in nucleus); E_1, estrone; E_1S, estrone-3-sulfate; E_2S, estradiol-3-sulfate; ADIONE, androstenedione; TESTOST, testosterone; 17β-HSD-1, 17β-hydroxysteroid dehydrogenase type 1, reductive activity.

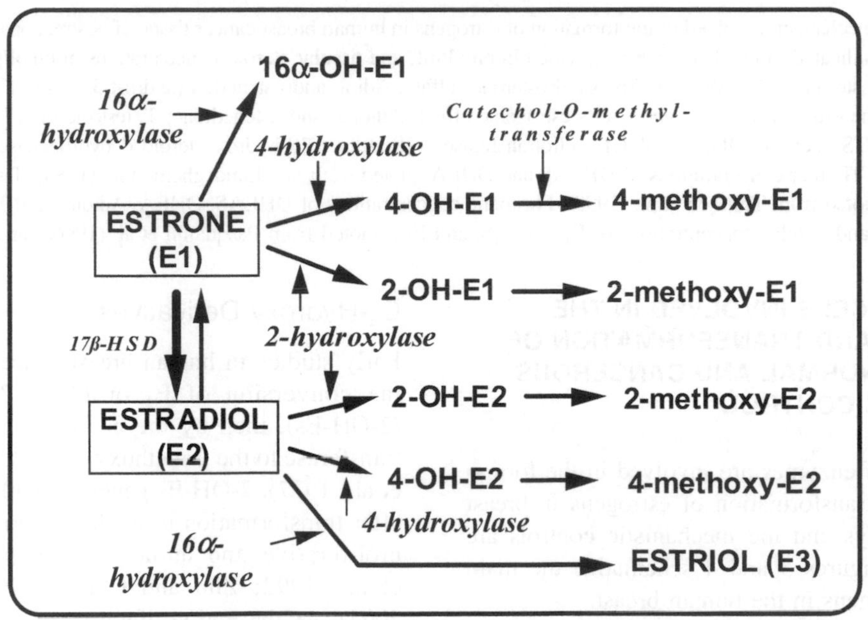

Figure 4 Hydroxyl pathways of estrogens in human breast cancer. *Abbreviations*: 2-OH-E_1, 2-hydroxy-estrone; 2-OH-E_2, 2-hydroxy-estradiol; 4-OH-E_1, 4-hydroxy-estrone; 4-OH-E_2, 4-hydroxy-estradiol; 16α-OH-E_1, 16α-hydroxy-estrone; 17β-HSD, 17β-hydroxysteroid dehydrogenase.

provided evidence for the nongenomic action of 2-methoxy-E_2 in ER-positive breast cancer cells. These authors found that with E_2, 2-methoxy-E_2 can suppress E_2-induced cell growth, whereas it acts as an estrogen in the absence of E_2.

It is of interest to mention that 2-methoxy-E_2 can inhibit oocyte maturation and early embryonic development (Lattanzi et al., 2003).

Recently, a new derivative, 2-methoxy-E_2-3,17-*O*, *O-bis*-sulfamate (STX140), shows very efficient antitumor activities (cell cycle arrest and apoptosis) *in vitro* and *in vivo* in both wild-type and multidrug-resistant MCF-7 breast cancer cells and tumors (Newman et al., 2008).

C_4-Hydroxy Derivatives

In opposition to 2-hydroxy-estrogens, the 4-hydroxy derivatives (4-OH-Es) possess estrogenic properties and exert a stimulatory effect on the growth of breast cancer cells (Schütze et al., 1993; Mueck et al., 2002). 4-OH-Es are particularly carcinogenic because they form unstable DNA adducts and induce tumor formation in animal models (Liehr et al., 1986; Newbold and Liehr, 2000). Elevated 4-hydroxy enzyme activity was found in breast cancer specimens (Liehr and Ricci, 1996) as well as high concentrations of 4-hydroxy estrogens (Castagnetta et al., 1992). Liehr and Ricci (1996) suggested that 4-hydroxylation of estrogens could be a marker for human mammary tumors. Paquette et al. (2005) showed that the accumulation of 4-OH-E_2 in breast tumors could enhance the invasiveness of breast cancer cells.

The inactivation of 4-OH-CE can be caused by the formation of glucuronides. Thibaudeau et al. (2006) demonstrated that the genetic variants of uridine-diphosphate-glucuronosyltransferase (UGT), UGT1A8, UGT1A9, and UGT2B7 enzymes, are involved in the inactivation of 4-OH-CE in breast cancer.

Cheng et al. (2005) suggest that catecholestrogen–metabolizing gene profiles are involved in the initiation of breast cancer by estrogens and that exposure to estrogens confers a high risk of breast cancer, causing a double strand break of DNA. In the control of 2- and 4-hydroxyestradiol catecholestrogens and the conversion to the inactive methoxy derivatives by catechol-*O*-methyltransferase (COMT), van Duursen et al. (2004) observed that phytochemicals with a catechol structure have the capacity to reduce COMT activity in mammary tissues and consequently reduce the inactivation of potentially mutagenic E_2 metabolites thereby increasing the risk of DNA damage. Rogan et al. (2003) found that the ratio of 2-catechol/4-catecholestrogens was higher in the normal breast tissues, but 4-catecholestrogens were three times higher than 2-catecholestrogens in the cancerous breast tissues, suggesting that some catecholestrogen metabolites and conjugates could serve as biomarker to predict the risk of breast cancer.

C_{16}-Hydroxy Derivatives

16α-OH-E_1 has estrogenic activity that, based on the increased uterine weight of ovariectomized rats, is more potent than that of E_2 itself (Fishman and Martucci, 1980). It was suggested that 16α-OH-E_1 could be implicated in carcinogenesis; for instance, a comparison of the E_2 metabolism of murine mammary epithelial cells revealed that 16-hydroxylation was significantly elevated in high-risk animals (Telang et al., 1991; Suto et al., 1992). It was demonstrated that in MCF-7 cells, 16-OH-E_1 is capable of accelerating cell cycle kinetics and stimulating the expression of cell cycle regulatory proteins (Lewis et al., 2001). Using MCF-7 and T-47D breast cancer cells, it was observed that the mitogenic potencies of 16α-OH-E_1 and 16α-OH-E_2 were comparable to or greater than E_2 (Gupta et al., 1998). High levels of 16-OH-E_1 were found in the tumoral tissue of breast cancer patients (Castagnetta et al., 2002).

Sulfatase Activity and Its Control

Estrogen (or other steroid hormones) sulfates are implicated in the regulation of various physiological or pathophysiological processes in normal and malignant tissues, including during pregnancy, prodrug processing, cell-signaling pathways, neurotransmission and memorization, immune response, inherited skin disorder (e.g., X-linked ichthyosis), and hormone-dependent cancers (e.g., breast, endometrium, prostate). E_1S and dehydroepiandrosterone sulfate (DHEA-S) are important intermediates and storage forms of hormones in human steroidogenesis. Their desulfation by the enzyme provides the corresponding hydroxysteroids as precursors for the intracellular active estrogens and androgens.

For many years, endocrine therapy in breast cancer has mainly utilized SERMs, compounds which block the ER activity. Treatment with the antiestrogen tamoxifen (Nolvadex®, tamoxifen citrate) to millions of women with breast cancer has had a significantly beneficial effect, resulting in both freedom from symptoms of the disease and reduction in mortality. More recently, another endocrine therapy has been explored using different antienzyme agents involved in the biosynthesis of E_2 to inhibit the tissular concentration and production of this hormone. At present, the positive effect of antiaromatase compounds as first-line treatment of breast cancer patients is well documented (Brodie et al., 1986; Brodie, 2002, 2008; Brodie and Pasqualini, 2007; Miller and Pasqualini, 2005; de Jong et al., 1997; Ryan and Goss, 2008). However, as in human breast cancer, E_1S is quantitatively the most important precursor of E_2 (Pasqualini et al., 1996a; Santner et al., 1984), new possibilities can be opened to block E_2 originated through this conjugate via the "sulfatase pathway" (Nussbaumer and Billich, 2005).

Steroid sulfatase (STS) is a member of a subset of six enzymes (classes A, B, C, D, E, and F) in the human genome named arylsulfatases for their capability to cleave various nonphysiological arylsulfates. These enzymes are expressed in various target organs, such as endometrium, liver, bone, brain, prostate, adipocytes, white blood cells, and are prevalent in the placenta and breast carcinoma tissues (Fujikawa et al., 1997; Dooley et al., 2000; Hughes et al., 2001; Nussbaumer and Billich, 2004). For details in structure, function and enzymatic characteristics of the STSs, see Pasqualini and Chetrite (2002).

E_1 sulfatase activity is significantly higher in the cancerous tissue in relation to the normal tissue (Chetrite et al., 2000) and is also higher in the breast tissue of postmenopausal, related to premenopausal, patients (Pasqualini et al., 1996a). It is notable that in the breast tissue, sulfatase activity is in equilibrium with the formation of the steroid sulfate by the sulfotransferase activity, which is also present in the breast.

Using immunohistochemical analysis, Selcer et al. (2007) found strong positive staining against the STS antibody. High levels were shown in the ER/PR-positive tumors. Normal human breast also showed moderate levels and ER/PR-negative breast cancer showed weak immunoreactivity. In another study, Yamamoto et al. (2003) found 59% positive immunohistochemical analysis of E_1 sulfatase in 83 samples of breast cancer tissues. STS activity was found in mammary myoepithelial cells, suggesting that they can have an important role in hormonal regulation within mammary tissue (Tobacman et al., 2002).

An intriguing question is the site where the sulfatase acts in the breast cells; when these are incubated with labeled estrogen sulfates, only unconjugated estrogens are detected inside the cell, suggesting that the sulfatase (as well as the sulfotransferase) is present inside the cell but that its activity is exerted in the cell membrane. This hypothetical mechanism was described previously (Pasqualini and Chetrite, 1996). A similar process was also demonstrated for the sulfotransferase activity in the Ishikawa human endometrial adenocarcinoma cells (Chetrite and Pasqualini, 1997). Hernandez-Guzman et al. (2003) described the association of STS with the membrane of the endoplasmic reticulum by X-ray crystallography at 2.60-Å resolution. In this connection, it is interesting to mention that Pizzagalli et al. (2003) found the organic anion transporting polypeptide OATP-B (SLCZ1A9) to be the most functionally relevant steroid sulfate carrier present and is able to account for delivery of both estrogen sulfate and DHEA-S to normal and tumoral breast tissues.

Control of Sulfatase Activity in the Breast

Inhibition by antiestrogens, various progestins, and tibolone and its metabolites

In early studies it was reported that the antiestrogens tamoxifen and its more active metabolite 4-hydroxytamoxifen, as well as ICI 164,384, are inhibitors of sulfatase activity in breast cancer cells, probably through a noncompetitive mechanism (Pasqualini and Gelly, 1988; Pasqualini et al., 1990).

A series of progestins including the progesterone derivative, medrogestone; the retroprogesterone, dihydrogesterone; the 19-nor-testosterone derivatives, norethisterone and norelgestromin; the 17α-hydroxy-nor-progesterone, nomegestrol acetate; the 19-nor-progesterone derivative, promegestone and danazol provoke a significant decrease of E_2 formation when physiological concentrations of E_1S are added in breast cancer cells (Pasqualini et al., 1992a,b, 2003; Nguyen et al., 1993; Chetrite et al., 1996, 1999a; Shields-Botella et al., 2005). It was also demonstrated that dydrogesterone (Duphaston®) and its 20-dihydro derivative are potent inhibitors of E_1 sulfatase in MCF-7 breast cancer cells (Chetrite et al., 2004).

Using total breast cancer tissues from postmenopausal patients, it was shown that nomegestrol acetate or medrogestone can block the sulfatase activity. The effect was significantly more active in breast carcinoma than in the area of the breast considered as normal (Chetrite et al., 2005, 2008a,b).

Further studies explored the effect of tibolone on sulfatase activity. Tibolone (Org OD-14, active substance of Livial®) is a synthetic steroid with a 19-nor-testosterone derivative structure. This activity of the compound is tissue specific, with weak estrogenic, progestagenic, and androgenic properties, and is extensively used to prevent climacteric symptoms and postmenopausal bone loss (Bjarnason et al., 1996). Tibolone and its main metabolites Org 4094, Org 30126 (the 3α- and 3β-hydroxy derivatives) and its 4-en isomer Org OM-38 are potent sulfatase inhibitors at low concentration in hormone-dependent breast cancer cells (Chetrite et al., 1997; Raobaikady et al., 2005) and in breast tumoral tissues (Chetrite et al., 2008b). Table 4 shows the relative inhibitory effects of various progestins, tibolone, and its metabolites, as well as of E_2, in T-47D breast cancer cells.

Inhibition of E_1 sulfatase by other steroidal compounds

Generally steroidal sulfatase inhibitors are substrate or product based, and show reversible inhibition. However,

Table 4 Comparative Effect of Various Progestins, Tibolone and Its Metabolites, and of Estradiol on Estrone Sulfatase Inhibitors in T-47D Breast Cancer Cells

Compounds	Inhibition (%)
Progesterone	22
Promegestone	30
20α-Dihydrogesterone	32
Nomegestrol acetate	45
Medroxyprogesterone acetate	47
Medrogestone	54
Norethisterone	63
4-en Isomer of tibolone	69
Norelgestromin	74
3α-Hydroxy tibolone	77
3β-Hydroxy tibolone	79
Tibolone	82
Estradiol	86

The T-47D cells were incubated with physiological concentrations of $[^3H]$-estrone-sulfate (5×10^{-9} M) without or with addition of the various compounds (at a concentration of 5×10^{-7} M). Control value of the conversion of estrone sulfate to estradiol was considered as 100%. *Source*: From Chetrite et al. (1996, 1997, 1999a), Pasqualini et al. (1992a,b, 2003), Pasqualini and Chetrite (2001).

the prototype of the potent irreversible inhibitor structure, estrone-3-*O*-sulfamate (EMATE), features the arylsulfamate moiety (Nussbaumer and Billich, 2004).

As STS can accept substrates, not only with an aromatic A-ring (E_1S) but also with an alicyclic A-ring (DHEAS or cholesterol sulfate), it is competitively inhibited by a number of natural steroids and steroid sulfates (MacIndoe et al., 1988; Payne, 1972; Townsley et al., 1970). Carlström et al. (1984) have shown a significant decrease in the concentration of circulating steroids as a consequence of the therapeutic application of danazol, an anabolic steroid with a blocking isoxazol group at position 2,3 of the steroidal skeleton. This compound is also active in breast cancer cells (Nguyen et al., 1993). E_1 phosphate and DHEA-phosphate are also potent inhibitors of estrogen sulfatase activity (Anderson et al., 1995).

EMATE is a potent synthesized sulfatase inhibitor, as at the concentration of 10^{-7} M the inhibition of E_1 sulfatase is 99% in MCF-7 cells (Howarth et al., 1994). This inhibition is described as time and concentration dependent and is classified as an active site–directed irreversible inhibitor (Purohit et al., 1995). Unfortunately, the potent estrogenic activity of this compound precludes its use in clinical applications (Elger et al., 1995). However, a new 2-substituted analogue of EMATE, 2-difluoromethylestrone 3-*O*-sulfamate has an IC50 of 100 pM and is 90 times more potent sulfatase inhibitor than EMATE in placental microsomal preparations (Reed et al., 2004). STX213, a new second generation of STS inhibitor with D-ring modified, was developed and presented an activity 18 times more intense than EMATE and 3 times more than the nonsteroidal inhibitor 667 COUMATE (STX64) (Foster et al., 2006).

Most new STS inhibitor derivatives correspond to modifications concerning A-ring, D-ring, and/or C-17 side chain, most on a steroid sulfamate base. Leese et al. (2005a,b) screen A-ring or D-ring substituted estrogen-3-*O*-sulfamates for general antitumor activity. Among antiproliferative and antiangiogenesis activities, some of these compounds (e.g., sulfamoylated derivatives of the 2-methoxy-E_2) show potent antisulfatase activity, such as 2-methoxy-3-*O*-sulfamoyl estrone (2-MeOEMATE). The introduction of a 17α-benzyl substituent to such 2-substituted estrogen sulfamates enhances STS inhibition.

Ishida et al. (2007a,b) described a potent and selective STS inhibitor (KW-2581, a 17β-(*N*-alkylcarbamoyl)-estra-1,3,5(10)trien-3-*O*-sulfamate derivative) with antitumor effects in breast cancer models in vitro and in vivo. The inhibition is irreversible, and this compound is without estrogenicity. In MCF-7 cells transfected with the STS gene, KW-2581 inhibited the growth of cells stimulated by E_1S but also Adiols (androstenediol, androst-5-ene-3β,17β-diol) and DHEAS. The STS activity of ZR-75-1 cells is inhibited with an IC50 of 13 nM, a potency equal to that of the nonsteroidal STS inhibitor, 667 COUMATE. KW-2581 inhibited the E_1S-stimulated growth of ZR-75-1 cells with an IC50 of 0.18 nM, but failed to inhibit the growth stimulated by E_2.

In other studies, Boivin et al. (2000) and Poirier and Boivin (1998) attempted to develop sulfatase inhibitors without residue estrogenic activity by synthesizing a series of E_2 derivatives bearing an alkyl, a phenyl, a benzyl, substituted or not, or an alkan amide side chain at position 17α. These authors showed that sulfatase inhibitors act by a reversible mechanism and that the hydrophobic group at the 17α position increased the inhibitory activity, while steric factors contributed to the opposite effect. The most potent inhibitor is a 17α-benzyl-substituted E_2 derivative with an IC50 value of 22 nM. When these 17α-substituents were added to the 3-*O*-sulfamate E_2 structure, the combined inhibitory effect was more potent. The IC50 value is 0.15 nM (Ciobanu et al., 1999). Recently, a more potent derivative has been synthesized, 3β-sulfamoyloxy-17α-*t*-butylbenzyl-5-androsten-17β-ol, showing nonestrogenic and nonandrogenic activity (Ciobanu et al., 2003a,b).

New irreversible inhibitor compounds described an E_1 formate type (Schreiner and Billich, 2004) or steroidal 2′,3′,-oxathiazine structures, able to inhibit the growth of MCF-7 cells induced by E_1S (Peters et al., 2003). An E_2 derivative bearing a boronic acid group at the 3-position and a benzyl group at the 17-position was a potent reversible, noncompetitive STS inhibitor with a K_i of 250 nM (Ahmed et al., 2006).

Inhibition of E_1 sulfatase by nonsteroidal compounds

Nonsteroidal sulfatase inhibitors generally mimick some target elements of steroidal skeleton (cycles and/or side chains), and hence can support some steroidal activities, such as estrogenicity.

Anderson et al. (1997) show that the basic structure for the binding of inhibitors does not include the steroid nucleus. These authors determined that the nonsteroidal phosphate compound, *n*-lauroyl tyramine phosphate, is a good inhibitor, and suggested that sulfatase can differentiate the phosphoryl group from the sulfuryl group with respect to catalysis only and not to binding.

A new interesting family of compounds has been synthesized with a coumarin sulfamate structure, COUMATE (4-methylcoumarin-7-*O*-sulfamate) and 667 COUMATE (its tricyclic derivative) (Purohit et al., 1998; Malini et al., 2000). These nonsteroidal sulfatase inhibitors, which mimick the CD rings of EMATE, are active in vitro and in vivo, are nonestrogenic and possess, in vitro, an IC50 value of approximately 1 nM. However, the most potent inhibitor in vivo does not correspond to the better compound in vitro. Recently, a phase I clinical trial of 667 COUMATE (STX64) was tested as a STS inhibitor in postmenopausal women with breast cancer (Stanway et al., 2006).

Compounds based on cyclic esters of 4-[(aminosulfonyl)-oxy]-benzoate are also potent sulfatase inhibitors. The effects are stronger than 667 COUMATE and EMATE (Patel et al. 2003, 2004).

In another study, Billich et al. (2000) proposed a new class of nonsteroidal irreversible inhibitors with substituted chromenone sulfamates. These compounds are exempt of estrogenic activity and can block E_1S and DHEAS-stimulated growth of MCF-7 cells. Recently, new potent reversible sulfatase inhibitors of this type of compound, 2-(1-adamantyl)-4-(thio)chromenone-6-carboxylic acids and 6-[2-(adamantylidene)-hydroxybenzoxazole]-*O*-sulfamate, were reported by these authors (Billich et al., 2004; Horvath et al., 2004).

New nonsteroidal compounds, corresponding to a 1-(*p*-sulfamoyloxyphenyl)-5-(*p*-*t*-butylbenzyl)-5 alkanol series, have been proposed by Ciobanu et al. (2002). The best inhibitors are the undecanol derivatives in the sulfamate series (IC50 value, 0.4 nM).

An interesting new class of sulfatase inhibitors, sulfamoyloxy-substituted 2-phenylindoles and sulfamoyloxy-substituted stilbenes, shows a dual mode of action as these compounds block gene expression by inhibition of E_1 sulfatase and by antiestrogenic action (Golob et al., 2002; Walter et al., 2004a,b).

Recently, two new potent classes of nonsteroidal STS inhibitors without estrogenicity have been reported: BENZOMATE (benzophenone-4,4′,-*O,O*-bis-sulfamate) and related analogues (Hejaz et al., 2004), and some biphenyl-4-*O*-sulfamate derivatives (e.g., 2′,4′,-dicyanobiphenyl-4-*O*-sulfamate) (Okada et al., 2003; Saito et al., 2004).

New concept strategies attempt to combine dual activities (or more) on a single molecule to obtain a wider therapeutic efficacy. Thus, the drug design favored a sulfamate-based structure (Winum et al., 2005), and some new synthesized compounds show antisulfatase and antiaromatase activities (Wood et al., 2005; Numazawa et al., 2005, 2006; Woo et al., 2007), antisulfatase and antiestrogen activities (Rasmussen et al., 2007), antisulfatase and anti-17β-HSD-1 activities (Ciobanu and Poirier, 2006), antisulfatase and antiangiogenic activities (Chander et al., 2007), or antisulfatase and anticarbonic anhydrases (anti-CAs) activities; CA isoforms, particularly II, IX, and XII are highly overexpressed in tumors and generally absent in the normal tissues (Lloyd et al., 2005a,b).

Inhibition of E_1 sulfatase by E_2 and other estrogens

An interesting and paradoxical effect of E_2 was demonstrated in MCF-7 and T-47D breast cancer cells in that it can block its own bioformation by inhibiting, in a dose-dependent manner, the conversion of E_1S to E_2 in the range of concentrations from 5×10^{-10} to 5×10^{-5} M (Pasqualini and Chetrite, 2001), (see Table 4). Similarly, exposure to E_2 (10^{-8} M) was associated with 70% reduction in E_1 sulfatase activity in the MCF-7 cells after six days incubation (Tobacman et al., 2002). These authors found, in comparative studies using mammary myoepithelial cells, a 9% stimulatory effect of E_2 on the sulfatase activity as well as a markedly greater sulfatase activity than in the MCF-7 cells. They suggest that this activity is consistent with a functional role in converting the abundant circulating sulfated steroids into active unsulfated hormones that are then available to the luminal epithelial cells.

In more recent studies using the total breast tissue, a similar inhibitory effect of E_2 on sulfatase activity was demonstrated. E_2 activity was significantly higher in cancerous than in normal tissue (Chetrite et al., 2007a). Comparative studies show that in breast cancer cells the inhibitory effect on sulfatase activity is significantly higher for the unconjugated E_1 or E_2 than for their respective sulfates (Bhattacharyya and Tobacman, 2007).

mRNA Expression of Estrogen Sulfatase

Early studies demonstrated that mRNA sulfatase expression is correlated with the enzyme activity (Pasqualini et al., 1994b). Using immunohistochemistry, E_1 sulfatase mRNA expression was detected in microdissected carcinoma cells but not in stromal cells (Suzuki et al., 2003a,b). YM Chong (personal communication, 2007) found that in ER-positive breast cancer patients, estrogen sulfatase correlated with the enzyme activity in the adjacent noncancerous tissue, suggesting that ER-positive tumor cells may be able to induce mRNA sulfatase expression in adjacent normal cells.

Information concerning control of mRNA sulfatase is limited. Previous studies in this laboratory found that the progestin promegestone (R-5020) can inhibit E_1 sulfatase mRNA in MCF-7 and T-47D breast cancer cells (Pasqualini et al., 1994b, 1996b). The effect is correlated with a decrease of enzymatic activity. Tobacman et al. (2002) observed that in mammary myoepithelial cells, the levels of mRNA sulfatase were slightly lower compared with those in MCF-7 cells.

It was observed that medroxyprogesterone acetate (MPA), levonorgestrel (LNG), norethindrone (NET), and dienogest (DNG) can stimulate the mRNA sulfatase expression in MCF-7 cells, whereas DNG, NET, and LNG, in the presence of E_2, have no effect (Xu et al., 2007). These controversial effects of progestins agree with the concept that the biological response of the different progestins is a function of their structure, receptor affinity, metabolic transformations, experimental conditions, target

Table 5 Relative Binding Affinities of Progesterone and Synthetic Progestins to Steroid Receptors and Serum-Binding Proteins

Progestin	PR	AR	ER	GR	MR	SHBG	CBG
Progesterone	50	0	0	10	100	0	36
Dydrogesterone	75	0	–	–	–	–	–
Chlormadinone acetate	67	5	0	8	0	0	0
Cyproterone acetate	90	6	0	6	8	0	0
Medroxyprogesterone acetate	115	5	0	29	160	0	0
Megestrol acetate	65	5	0	30	0	0	0
Nomegestrol	125	6	0	6	0	0	0
Promegestone (R-5020)	100	0	0	5	53	0	0
Drospirenone	35	65	0	6	230	0	0
Norethisterone	75	15	0	0	0	16	0
Levonorgestrel	150	45	0	1	75	50	0
Norgestimate	15	0	0	1	0	0	0
3-Keto-desogestrel	150	20	0	14	0	15	0
Gestodene	90	85	0	27	290	40	0
Dienogest	5	10	0	1	0	0	0

Abbreviations: PR, progesterone receptor (promegestone = 100%); AR, androgen receptor (metribolone = 100%); ER, estrogen receptor (estradiol-17β = 100%); GR, glucocorticoid receptor (dexamethasone = 100%); MR, mineralocorticoid receptor (aldosterone = 100%); SHBG, sex hormone–binding globulin (dihydrotestosterone = 100%); CBG, corticosteroid-binding globulin (cortisol = 100%).
Source: From De Lignières et al. (1995), Neumann and Duesterberg (1998), Kuhl (2001).

tissue, and dose. An important aspect of the biological action of progestins can be the result of binding to various receptors or serum-binding proteins (Table 5).

Correlation of Sulfatase Activity and Proliferation

As estrogen sulfatase is one of the major routes in the biosynthesis of E_2 in the breast tissue itself, it was consequently of interest to explore a possible correlation between the effect of the tumor growth and cell proliferation by antisulfatase agents. Nakata et al. (2003) showed that the antisulfatase compound-9 (*p*-O-sulfamoyl)-*N*-tetradecanoyl tyramine, which has no estrogenic activity, can block tumor growth in female nude mice obtained by transplantation with MCS-2 cells, a human breast cancer cell line overexpressed with sulfatase (Fig. 5). Saito et al. (2004) used another antisulfatase compound with no estrogenic activity, 2′,4′-dicyanobiphenyl-4-*O*-sulfamate (TZS-8478), and observed a suppression of the E_1S-stimulated proliferation of MCF-7 cells, as well as a reduction in the growth of nitrosomethylurea-induced breast tumors stimulated by E_1S.

A further series of studies showed that the antisulfatase agent 2-methoxy-3-sulfamoyloxy-17α-benzylestra-1,3,5

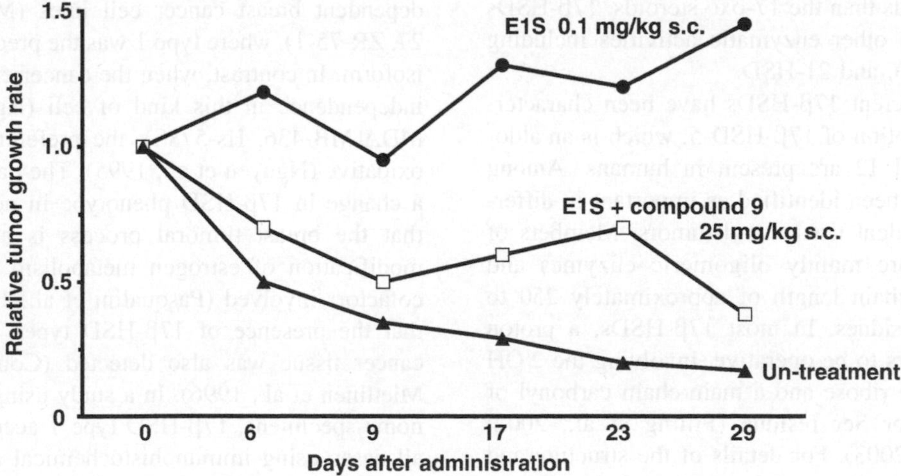

Figure 5 Antitumor activity of sulfatase inhibitor (compound 9) against sulfatase overexpressed human breast cancer MCS-2 cells transplanted in female nude mice. Sulfatase inhibitor compound 9 corresponds to [(p-*O*-sulfamoyl)-*N*-tetradecanoyl tyramine] structure. *Source*: From Nakata et al. (2003).

(10)-trien-17β-ol can block the uterine growth provoked by the sulfatase inhibitors 3-sulfamoyloxy-17α-*p*-*t*-butylbenzyl (or benzyl) estra-1,3,5(10)-trien-17β-ols and EMATE. These antisulfatase agents have estrogenic properties and can induce uterine growth stimulation (Ciobanu et al., 2003a,b).

James et al. (2001) observed that the STS Clone 20 cell line, obtained from MCF-7/2 cells treated with retroviral vectors containing the STS genes, exhibit a significant increase in the proportion of proliferating tumors in nude ovariectomized mice supplemented with estradiol sulfate, which, surprisingly, appears to be more effective than E_2 itself administered in similar concentrations. These authors suggest that the intratumoral sulfatase activity can support estrogen-dependent tumorigenity in an experimental model and may contribute to the acceleration of human breast tumor growth. Walter et al. (2004a) prepared 2-phenylindole with lipophilic side chains in the 1- or 5-position and found that these sulfatase inhibitors are potent antiproliferative agents of the MCF-7 breast cancer cells. Golob et al. (2002) synthesized a number of sulfamoyloxy-substituted 2-phenylindoles with side chains at the indol nitrogen. These compounds have a double effect: they are antisulfatase agents and also present antiestrogenic activity, and consequently they inhibit growth proliferation of estrogen-sensitive breast cancer cells.

17β-HSDs in the Breast

The 17β-HSD family of enzymes (EC 1.1.1.62) is mainly involved in the interconversion of hydroxyl/keto structures at the C17 position of estrogens and androgens and can regulate steroid hormone responses as the binding to the respective receptor has a much higher affinity for the 17β-hydroxy steroids than the 17-oxo steroids. 17β-HSDs can be involved in other enzymatic activities including 3α-HSDs, 20α-HSD, and 21-HSD.

To date, 14 different 17β-HSDs have been characterized, with the exception of 17β-HSD-5, which is an aldo-keto reductase, and 12 are present in humans. Among these, several have been identified as important in different hormone-dependent tissues and tumors. Members of the HSD family are mainly oligomeric enzymes and display a subunit chain length of approximately 250 to 350 amino acid residues. In most 17β-HSDs, a proton relay system appears to be operative, involving the 2′OH of the nicotinamide ribose and a main-chain carbonyl of a conserved Asn or Ser residue (Filling et al., 2002; Oppermann et al., 2003). For details of the structure and function of HSDs, see Pasqualini and Chetrite (2002) and Lukacik et al. (2006).

The 17β-HSD types 1, 3, 5, and 7 are reductive enzymes, NADPH dependent, and facilitate binding of the steroid to the receptor, whereas types 2, 4, 6, 8, 9, 10, 11, and 14 are preferentially oxidative enzymes, NAD+ dependent and transform the steroid with very low affinity to bind the receptor (Peltoketo et al., 1999; Labrie et al., 2000).

In the Normal Human Breast

Both 17β-HSD types 1 and 2 are present in the epithelium of normal breast tissue. However, it was observed that the oxidative 17β-HSD activity (E_2 to E_1) is the preferential direction (Speirs et al., 1998; Miettinen et al., 1999; Vihko et al., 2001) and that this activity is more intense during the secretory phase of the menstrual cycle (Pollow et al., 1977).

Miettinen et al. (1999) using normal HME epithelial cells confirmed that the main 17β-HSD enzyme corresponds to type 2. Gompel et al. (1986) obtained interesting data showing that the progestin, promegestone (R-5020) can stimulate 17β-HSD type 2 in normal breast epithelial cells.

In Human Breast Cancer

Of the 14 different 17β-HSDs characterized, 2 are preferential: type 1 (conversion of E_1 to E_2) and type 2 (conversion of E_2 to E_1) in breast cancer tissues, and various studies indicate a greater activity of type 1 than type 2. In their early studies, McNeill et al. (1986) demonstrated that after isotopic infusion of estrogens to postmenopausal breast cancer patients, the reductive direction was greater than the oxidative. However, in vitro studies by other authors using human tumor homogenates found a predominant oxidative 17β-HSD activity. It should be noted that the enzymatic activity can be influenced by the experimental conditions, including the nature and concentration of cofactors (e.g., NADPH or NADP), pH, and type of cancer tissue.

Interesting data was obtained using hormone-dependent breast cancer cell lines (MCF-7, T-47D, R-27, ZR-75-1), where type 1 was the predominant reductive isoform. In contrast, when the cancer evolves to hormone independence in this kind of cell (e.g., MDA-MB-231, MDA-MB-436, Hs-578S), the preferential orientation is oxidative (Nguyen et al., 1995). The data is suggestive of a change in 17β-HSD phenotype in neoplastic cells and that the breast tumoral process is accompanied by a modification of estrogen metabolism as well as of the cofactors involved (Pasqualini et al., 1995). It is notable that the presence of 17β-HSD types 2 and 4 in breast cancer tissue was also detected (Couture et al., 1993; Miettinen et al., 1996). In a study using 794 breast carcinoma specimens, 17β-HSD type 1 accounted for 20% of all cases using immunohistochemical analysis, and 16% using in situ hybridization (Oduwole et al., 2004). Song et al. (2006) found that 17β-HSD types 7 and 12, but not type 1, are commonly expressed in human breast cancer, and suggested that the increased coexpression of 17β-HSD type 12 and ERβ in breast cancer cells, compared with their expression in adjacent nonmalignant tissue, may play an important role in the progression of breast cancer. Jansson et al. (2006a) suggested that the proliferative response to altered 17β-HSD type 2 expression in human breast cancer cells is dependent on endogenous expression of 17β-HSD type 1 and of the ERs.

Control of 17β-Hydroxysteroid Dehydrogenase Activity and Its mRNA Messenger in the Breast

The control of 17β-HSD type 1 (transformation of E_1 to E_2) has long been known as a potentially attractive target for tissue specificity in the modulation of E_2 levels, particularly in cancerous breast tissue.

Control by progestins, tibolone and its metabolites, and antiestrogens

In early studies, Fournier et al. (1985) observed that tumors from breast cancer patients treated with the progestin, lynestrenol, displayed a higher oxydative 17β-HSD activity than those from untreated patients and that this activity was also function of the ER and PR status of the tumor. The data from studies using the progestin, MPA, are contradictory, where some showed a stimulation of 17β-HSD type 1 in MCF-7 cells (Coldham and James, 1990) while others observed an inhibition of this enzyme in the hormone-dependent ZR-75-1 cells (Couture et al., 1993). A series of experiments carried out in this laboratory demonstrated that various progestins, including promegestone (R-5020), danazol (Nguyen et al., 1995), medrogestone (Prothil®) (Chetrite et al., 1999b), or nomegestrol acetate (Chetrite et al., 1996), are inhibitory agents of 17β-HSD in different hormone-dependent breast cancer cells. This relative effect is indicated in Table 6.

Tibolone (Org OD14), a 19-nor-testosterone derivative with specific estrogenic, androgenic, and progestagenic properties, significantly decreases the reductive activity in hormone-dependent T-47D and MCF-7 cells. A similar effect was also observed with the 3α-hydroxy and 3β-hydroxy tibolone metabolites, as well as with the 4-en isomer (Chetrite et al., 1999d) (Table 6).

Table 6 Comparative Effect of Various Progestins, Tibolone and Its Metabolites, on 17β-Hydroxysteroid Dehydrogenase Type 1 in T-47D Breast Cancer Cells

Compounds	Inhibition (%)
Medrogestone	53
3β-Hydroxy tibolone	45
Tibolone	37
3α-Hydroxy tibolone	31
Nomegestrol acetate	30
Danazol	20
Promegestone (R-5020)	10

The T-47D cells were incubated with physiological concentrations of $[^3H]$-estrone (5×10^{-9} M) without (control) or with addition of the various compounds at a concentration of 5×10^{-7} M. Control value of the conversion of estrone sulfate to estradiol was considered as 100%.
Source: From Chetrite and Pasqualini (2001), Chetrite et al. (1996, 1999b,d).

Control of 17β-HSD by other compounds

In several studies it was demonstrated that E_1 and E_2 C-16 derivatives are potent inhibitors of 17β-HSD type 1 (Tremblay and Poirier, 1998; Tremblay et al., 2001; Qiu et al., 2002). Among these compounds, E_2 16β-benzyl was the best inhibitor of the series (Poirier et al., 2005). Husen et al. (2006) transferred a plasmid expressing human 17β-HSD type 1 to mice MCF-7 cells and observed that the size of the produced tumor was reduced by 86% using a new inhibitor of 17β-HSD type 1, the Solvay compound B10720511. Other studies demonstrated that various pyrimidone derivatives are potent inhibitory agents of 17β-HSD type 1 (Messinger et al., 2006). Sawicki et al. (1999) showed that equilin at 10 μM using a transient assay inhibited 17β-HSD type 1 by 96%. *m*-Pyridylmethylamidomethyl derivatives are also attractive compounds for inactivation of 17β-HSD type 1 (Purohit et al., 2006). Compounds with modifications of positions 3 and 6 of E_2 were also active inhibitors of 17β-HSD type 1 (Tremblay et al., 2005). Brozic et al. (2006) found that cinnamic acids are potent inhibitors of 17β-HSD type 5, the most active being α-methylcinnamic acid.

It may be remarked that different factors, such as insulin-like growth factors, retinoic acid, cytokines, interleukin 6, as well as tumor necrosis factor-α, have important roles in the control of 17β-HSDs. Brooks and Thompson (2005) observed that mammalian lignans enterolactone and enterodiol can inhibit 17β-HSD type 1 in MCF-7 cells, and suggested that this effect is in relation to the cell proliferation.

Role of Sulfotransferase in the Breast

Sulfotransferases (SULTs) are divided into two broad classes of enzymes: (1) membrane-bound SULTs, located in the Golgi apparatus, affecting structural and functional aspects of peptides, proteins, glycosaminoglycans, and lipids, and (2) cytosolic SULTs implicated in the metabolism of drug, xenobiotic, and endobiotic substrates. The focus of this part concerns the role of the human cytosolic SULT isoforms present in the breast (for a review see Pasqualini and Chetrite, 2005b).

Functions of Cytosolic SULTs

The super gene family of cytosolic SULTs belongs to an important class of conjugation enzymes implicated in (1)

the detoxification of relatively small hydrophobic molecules as drugs and xenobiotics and (2) modulation of the activity of physiologically important endobiotics, such as steroids, thyroid hormones, bile acids, and neurotransmitters (catecholamines, dopamine). The other major similar class of enzymes is the UGTs, which forms glucuroconjugates from practically the same substrates as for SULTs. The difference between these two enzymatic systems seems to correspond at two different pathways, thus SULTs system is a high-affinity, low-capacity pathway, whereas UGTs system is considered as a low-affinity, high-capacity pathway (Burchell and Coughtrie, 1997; see sec. "Glucuronidases in the Breast"). Another interesting observation is that SULTs are more greatly expressed in human fetus than UGTs and can represent the mean detoxifying enzymatic system before birth (Pasqualini and Kincl, 1986; Coughtrie, 2002). However, some human SULT isoforms can also bioactivate a broad range of potential mammary carcinogens, including iodothyronines, hydroxylated aromatic amines, or phenolic xenobiotics, such as polycyclic aromatic hydrocarbons (PAH), by forming highly reactive electrophiles, which can interact with DNA and form PAH-DNA adducts with mutagenic and carcinogenic potential (Glatt, 2002; Kester et al., 2000, 2002; Tang et al., 2003).

SULT enzymes catalyze the transfer of a sulfuryl group, donated by the cosubstrate 3′-phosphoadenosine-5′-phosphosulfate (PAPS), to an acceptor substrate that may be a hydroxyl or an amine group in a process called sulfonation or sulfurylation. Thus, SULTs can sulfonate a great range of substrates, including aromatic structures (phenols, estrogens, PAH), hydroxy steroids (DHEA), arylamines and *N*-hydroxy-arylamines or *N*-heterocyclic amines, primary and secondary alcohols, iodothyronines. Members of the SULTs enzyme family have considerable overlap in both amino acid sequence identity and substrate specificity (Glatt, 2000, 2001; Coughtrie, 2002; Gamage et al., 2006), thus the binding sites of some SULT isoforms are flexible and can adopt various conformations (Gamage et al., 2005).

Classification of Cytosolic Sulfotransferase Superfamily

Recently, an attempt to unify many various and confusing nomenclatures of the cytosolic SULT superfamily have been proposed. Briefly, this nomenclature system was based on the identity of the amino acid sequence: if 45% of the sequence is common, these SULTs belong to the same family (Arabic number) as SULT1, SULT2, SULT4; the subfamily members (alphabetical category) share at least 60% identity (e.g., SULT1A, SULT1B, etc.). Isoforms within a subfamily are identified using Arabic numbers following the subfamily designation (e.g., SULT1A1). For more complete information on the sulfotransferase nomenclature, at the protein and genetic level (allelic variants, allozymes, suballele, pseudogenes, cDNA, etc.) see Blanchard et al. (2004).

Cytosolic SULT in Human

To date, three families of human SULTs have been characterized: SULT1, which includes eight subfamilies and distinct isoforms, A1, A2, A3, A4, B1, C2, C4, E1; SULT2 family includes two subfamilies, A1 and B1 (with two isoforms -v1 and -v2); and SULT4 family has one subfamily, A1 (with two isoforms -v1 and -v2). Collectively, the human SULT family accounts for at least 13 distinct members.

The SULT1A subfamily members are referred to as "phenol SULTs" as all the isoforms can catalyze the sulfonation of phenolic molecules. The SULT1B subfamily is involved in the sulfonation of thyroid hormones. The SULT1C subfamily appears to be implicated in the sulfonation of procarcinogens. The SULT1E subfamily is identified specifically as estrogen sulfotransferase (EST) and sulfonates the 3-hydroxy group of endogenous (E_1, E_2) or synthetic and xenobiotic estrogens [diethylstilbestrol, 17α-ethinylestradiol (EE_2)], and some SERM molecules (tamoxifen, raloxifene).

The SULT2 family (hydroxysteroid SULTs) is implicated in the sulfonation of 3β-hydroxysteroids of non-aromatic A cycle, including DHEA (SULT2A subfamily), cholesterol, pregnenolone, androsterone, and other steroids (SULT2B subfamily).

The SULT4 family is predominantly localized in the brain, but recent microarray data seem to indicate a wider tissue distribution. However, no endogenous or xenobiotic substrates have yet been attributed. Table 7 indicates the common name, chromosomal location, and mean substrates for each human cytosolic SULTs.

Cytosolic SULT in Breast

In breast tissue, steroid hormones are the main physiological compounds of concern for cytosolic SULTs: estrogens (E_1 and E_2), androgens (dehydroepiandrosterone), progestagens (pregnenolone). What is the metabolic role of these sulfoconjugates? Besides the classic first step of the detoxifying process forming more water-soluble molecules to aid their excretion, in most cases formation of sulfonate conjugates involves loss of biological activity of the unconjugated steroid hormone parent. As for estrogen metabolism, estrogen sulfates are unable to have genomic action because they do not bind to the ER. Through this process, sulfonation reduces the exposure of target tissues to estrogens; however, estrogen sulfates can also represent a local hormone reservoir that can liberate the active hormone after hydrolysis by the sulfatase. In fact, many

Table 7 The Human Cytosolic SULT Superfamilies

SULT	Common name	Gene	Chromosome	nb amino acids	Substrate preference (endogenous)	Sequence identities with SULT1A1
SULT1 (phenol) family						
SULT1A1	P-PST/-1 TS-PST H-PST HAST1/2	*STP* *STP1*	16q11.2-12.1	295	Phenols Estrogens	
SULT1A2	ST1A2 HAST4 TS-PST2	*STP2*	16q11.2-12.1	295	Phenols	95.6%
SULT1A3	M-PST TL-PST HAST3 hEST/1	*STM* *HAST*	16q11.2	295	Phenols Catecholamines Estrogens	92.9%
SULT1A4		*SULT1A4*	16q12.1		Not known	99.99% homology with SULT1A3
SULT1B1	ST1B2	*SULT1B2*	4q11.13	296	Thyroid hormones	53.4
SULT1C2	HAST5 SULT1C1	*SULT1C1*	2q11.2	296	Phenols	52.2
SULT1C4	hSULT1C	*SULT1C2*	2q11.2	302	Not known	53.2
SULT1E1	hEST/-1	*STE*	4q13.2	294	estrogens (high affinity)	50.1
SULT2 (hydroxysteroid) family						
SULT2A1	DHEA-ST HST	*STD*	19q13.3	285	3β-hydroxysteroid DHEA	34.6
SULT2B1-v1	hSULT2B1a	*SULT2B1*	19q13.3	350	DHEA, pregnenolone	36.3
SULT2B1-v2	hSULT2B1b			365	DHEA, cholesterol	36.9
SULT4 (brain specific) family						
SULT4A1-v1	hBR-STL	*SULT4A1*	22q13.1-13.2	284	Not known	34.2

steroids (e.g., DHEA, estrogens) are transported in the circulation as sulfoconjugated forms and possess a half-life considerably longer than their free parent; thus, the half-life of E_1S is 10 to 12 hours instead of 20 to 30 minutes for E_1. This observation reinforces the concept of intracrine mechanism in breast, particularly after the menopause, when ovaries are nonfunctional and the incidence of breast cancer is higher. James et al. (2001) have shown that the addition of estradiol sulfate strongly supports the growth of estrogen-dependent tumors in an in vivo model using ovariectomized nude mice bearing STS-transduced human breast cancer cells.

SULTs associated with STS assume the dynamic steady-state equilibrium of estrogen sulfates in breast tissues (normal and cancerous).

SULTs and estrogens

SULT1E1, originally named estrogen sulfotransferase (EST), has a significantly higher affinity for the sulfation of E_2 (K_m value of 4 nM) and EE_2 (Schrag et al., 2004) than for other potent estrogens, such as diethylstilbestrol and equine estrogens. Consequently, the ability of SULT1E1 to sulfate estrogens at physiological concentrations is important in regulating their activation of ER in target tissues of estrogens. The human SULT1E1 enzyme contains 294 amino acids and was first cloned by Weinshilboum's group (Aksoy et al., 1994). The native enzyme is a dimer of 35 kDa subunits, and kinetic studies indicate that two E_2 are bound per subunit (Zhang et al., 1998). Human endometrial Ishikawa adenocarcinoma cells demonstrate high levels of EST activity (Hata et al., 1987; Chetrite and Pasqualini, 1997). The SULT1E1 enzyme is important in the inactivation of E_2 during the luteal phase of the menstrual cycle.

Pedersen et al. (2002) obtained the crystal structure of the human SULT1E1–PAPS complex. Specifically, the authors observed that the side chain nitrogen of the catalytic Lys (47) interacts with the side chain hydroxyl of Ser (137) and not with the bridging oxygen between the 5′-phosphate and sulfate groups of the PAPS molecule as is seen in the PAP-bound structures.

SULT1E1 is not the only enzyme to sulfate estrogens, but it is distinguishable from the other enzymes involved by the very high affinity for E_2 (e.g., Zhang et al., 1998). Members of the SULT1A family, particularly SULT1A1, are able to sulfate estrogens at micromolar concentrations (e.g., Falany et al., 1994). SULT1E1 is present mainly in the normal breast cell. However, in the breast carcinoma cell lines, E_1 and E_2 could be sulfoconjugated by the action of SULT1A1, SULT1A3, or SULT2A1, and SULT1E appears to be expressed at low levels in breast cancer cells (Falany and Falany, 1996a).

Another important aspect of the metabolic transformation of estrogens is its conversion to catecholestrogens by hydroxylations in C-2 and C-4. These catecholestrogens can undergo further metabolism to form quinones that interact with DNA and could be involved in carcinogenesis, and the sulfonation of catecholestrogens could impede this process. Adjei and Weinshilboum (2002) show that of all SULTs, EST has the lowest K_m values, with 0.31, 0.18, 0.27, and 0.22 μM for 4-OH-E_1, 4-OH-E_2, 2-OH-E_1, and 2-OH-E_2, respectively.

SULTs in normal breast

High levels of EST were detected in a normal breast cell line, the Huma 7 obtained from reductive mammoplasty (Wild et al., 1991). These authors observed that EST activity in this cell line far exceeded than that in either MCF-7 or ZR-75-1 breast cancer cells. In one study, after 24-hour incubation, the normal cell sulfated 50% of estrogens compared with less than 10% in the malignant cells. The data were confirmed by Anderson and Howell (1995) using two normal breast epithelial cells: the MTSV 1-7 and the MRSV 4-4 produced by Simian virus 40 immortalization cells obtained from human milk. In these normal breast cells, SULT1E1 has the affinity for E_2 sulfation in the nanomolar concentration range. Consequently, SULT1E1 may be active in altering the levels of unconjugated estrogens in the cell and thus cellular responsiveness to estrogens, as estrogens in the nanomolar concentration range interact with the ER. Estrogen-dependent breast cells with high SULT1E1 levels grow more slowly than cells with low or no detectable EST. Metabolic evidence indicates that this is due to the ability of SULT1E1 to render estrogens physiologically inactive via sulfoconjugation (Falany and Falany, 1996a,b; Qian et al., 1998, 2001).

SULTs in cancerous breast

There are some discrepancies in the various reports of SULT activities in breast cancer: some authors found significant amounts of phenol sulfotransferase, but only trace levels of hydroxysteroid and EST activities in several hormone-dependent breast cancer cells (Falany et al., 1993; Falany and Falany, 1996a). However, others report EST and hydroxysteroid activities in MCF-7 and ZR-75 cells and in mammary tumors. An interesting observation was made by Falany and Falany (1996a) who felt that human SULT1E1 is not detectable in most breast cancer cell lines and suggested that the sulfoconjugated activity in these cells is mainly due to the SULT1A1, an enzyme that is more efficient with estrogens at micromolar than at nanomolar concentrations. SULT1A1 has an affinity for estrogen sulfation approximately 300-fold lower than that of human SULT1E1 (Falany et al., 1993, 1994). Comparative studies using normal human mammary epithelial (HME) and MCF-7 breast cancer cells showed that after incubation with 20-nM E_2, the level of sulfated E_2 detected in the medium of HME was 10 times that found in the medium of MCF-7 cells (Falany and Falany, 1996a). The data indicate that HME cells secreted E_2 sulfate into the medium at a significantly higher rate than did MCF-7 breast cancer cells. As estrogen sulfates do not bind to the ER, factors that modify EST levels and consequently affect estrogen metabolism may be important in controlling hormone-dependent cellular growth. The data suggest that in normal breast tissue, estrogen stimulation of growth and differentiation is carefully controlled, contrasting markedly with the abnormal proliferation of breast cancer cells (Zajchowski et al., 1993). Normal HME cells possess endogenous SULT1E1 at physiological levels and are not present in MCF-7 and some other breast cancer cells (e.g., T47-D, BT-20, ZR75-1, and MDA-MB-231; Falany et al., 1993; Falany and Falany, 1996a). These authors suggested that in the breast cancer cells, E_2 or E_1 is sulfated by the SULT1A1, an enzyme that only acts preferentially at micromolar concentrations of estrogens. The loss of SULT1E1 expression during the process of breast cancer oncogenesis may be critical because this enzyme inactivates E_2, suggesting that the inability of the breast cell to block E_2 could be an important mechanism in contributing to abnormal growth of these cells through the presence of this hormone. To explore the possibility that SULT1E1 disappears during the process of tumorigenesis, Falany and Falany (1996a, 1997) transfected MCF-7 cells with a SULT1E1-expression vector and observed that after incubation of 20 nM of E_2, sulfation occurs significantly more rapidly with the transfected MCF-7 cells than in control cells, thereby rendering E_2 physiologically inactive. In addition, SULT1E1/MCF-7 cells require a higher concentration of E_2 to stimulate growth than do the MCF-7 control cells. This observation was confirmed by Qian et al. (1998), who evaluated the physiological significance of SULT1E1 expression by cDNA transfection using MCF-7 cells and observed that in these transformed cells the response to physiological concentrations of E_2 (10 nM) is reduced by up to 70%, as determined in an estrogen-responsive reporter gene assay.

The physiological importance of SULT1E1 was also largely demonstrated in other estrogen-responsive tissue such as the endometrium. Falany et al. (1994) reported that SULT1E1 is present at significant levels in human endometrial tissues during the secretory phase of the cycle, but this enzyme was not detectable during the proliferative phase.

It is well known that estrogens play an important role in regulating the proliferation of breast tumors via the induction or suppression of growth regulatory factors (Molis et al., 1995). As an interesting effect, estrogens inhibit expression of the potent growth factor repressor, transforming growth factor (TGF-β1) (Cho et al., 1994; Eckert and Katzenellenbogen, 1982; Knabbe et al., 1987). Also, it was observed that MCF-7 cells expressing SULT1E1 activity did not show a decrease in ER-α levels, an increase in PR, or a decrease in transforming growth factor-β expression upon exposure to 100 pM or 1 nM of E_2, which is suggested due to the rapid sulfation and inactivation of the unconjugated E_2 by SULT1E1 (Falany et al., 2002).

In conclusion, knowledge of the expression and regulation of the different SULTs is of extreme importance in understanding the changes in the normal breast cell during the process of carcinogenesis as well as the hormonal implication in this mechanism.

Control of SULT Activities in Normal and Cancerous Breast

Comparative studies of the quantitative evaluation of SULT activity in various breast cancer cells show significantly higher levels in the hormone-dependent (e.g., MCF-7, T47-D) than in the hormone-independent (e.g., MDA-MB-231) cells (Chetrite et al. 1999c). However, a high SULT activity was found with the hormone-independent MDA-MB-468 mammary cancer cells (Pasqualini, 1992). The control of the formation of estrogen sulfoconjugates represents an important mechanism to modulate the biological effect of the hormone in breast tissue as it is well established that estrogen sulfates are biologically inactive. Here we summarize the action of various substances that may inhibit or stimulate SULTs in breast tissue.

Control by progestins and tibolone and its metabolites

Different progestins have been tested on the effect of the SULT activities in breast cancer cells. Medrogestone, a synthetic pregnane derivative that is used in the treatment of pathological deficiency of the natural progesterone, has a biphasic effect on SULT activity in MCF-7 and T47-D breast cancer cells. At a low concentration (5×10^{-8} mol/L) it stimulates the formation of estrogen sulfates, whereas at a high concentration (5×10^{-5} mol/L) the SULT activity is not modified in the MCF-7 cells or inhibited in T47-D cells. Other progestins, such as promegestone (R-5020) and nomegestrol acetate, at a low concentration can also increase SULT activity in breast cancer cells (Chetrite et al., 1998, 1999a, 2003). In relation to these findings, it is interesting to mention that the natural progesterone can induce SULT1E1 activity in the Ishikawa human endometrial adenocarcinoma cells, as well as in the excretory endometrial tissue (Clarke et al., 1982; Falany and Falany, 1996b; Tseng and Liu, 1981) (Table 8).

Table 8 Comparative Effect of Various Progestins, Tibolone and Its Metabolites, on Sulfotransferase Activity in T-47D Breast Cancer Cells

Compounds	Stimulation (%)
Promegestone (R-5020)	31
Tibolone	41
Nomegestrol acetate	42
Medrogestone	85
3β-Hydroxy tibolone	102

T-47D cells were incubated with physiological concentrations of [^{3}H]-estrone (5×10^{-9} M) without or with the various compounds (at a concentration of 5×10^{-7} M). Control value of the conversion of estrone to the estrogen sulfate was considered as 100%.
Source: From Chetrite et al. (1998, 1999a,c, 2003).

Tibolone is largely metabolized in three main derivatives: the 3α- and 3β-hydroxy, which are estrogenic, and the 4-en isomer, which is progestagenic. These compounds also provoke a dual effect on SULT activity in breast cancer cells: stimulatory at low doses (5×10^{-8} mol/L) and inhibitory at high doses (5×10^{-5} mol/L). The 3β-hydroxy derivative is the most potent compound in the stimulatory effect of the SULT activity in both the MCF-7 and T-47D breast cancer cells (Chetrite et al., 1999c) (Table 8).

SULT activity, hormone replacement therapy, and SERMs

A series of studies demonstrated the role of SULT activity in the bioavailability of therapeutic agents in target human tissues. Specific expression of SULT isoforms in target tissues can regulate the tissue-specific activity of HRT agents such as tibolone or SERM compounds such as raloxifene used in the treatment of osteoporosis, or tamoxifen and its active metabolite 4-OH-tamoxifen used in the treatment and prevention of breast cancer (Vos et al., 2002; Falany et al., 2004, 2006; Falany and Falany, 2007; Yasuda et al., 2005). Tibolone and its metabolites are rapidly sulfated mainly by SULT2A1 and SULT1E1. Tibolone and the 4-en isomer are sulfated at the 17β-OH group by SULT2A1, and this binding is known to be resistant to hydrolysis by sulfatase. Thus, regeneration of active forms of HRT agents could be abolished. The 3α- and 3β-hydroxy metabolites can form both 3- and 17-monosulfates by the SULT1E1 isoform as well as disulfates by the SULT2A1 isoform. Only the 3β-monosulfate seems able to be hydrolyzed and represents a more important therapeutic metabolite, so the hormonal effect of tibolone depends greatly on the

SULT isoforms expressed in a given tissue, as well as the level of sulfatase activity. Raloxifene can form monosulfates by at least seven SULT isoforms, but is essentially sulfonated by SULT2A1 and SULT1E1. SULT1E1 isoform can produce disulfate and two monosulfate forms: one identical to the monosulfate synthetized by SULT2A1 and the other corresponding to the low abundance, which is resistant to hydrolysis.

Similarly, celecoxib, a specific cyclooxygenase-2 (COX-2) inhibitor, can switch on the formation of E_2-3-S by SULT2A1 to E_2-17-S in a concentration-dependent manner. The ability of celecoxib to alter the E_2 sulfonation position by encouraging production of E_2-17-S, a resistant form to sulfatase hydrolysis (Pasqualini and Kincl, 1986), may explain why celecoxib was effective in breast cancer treatment (Wang and James, 2005).

Modulation of SULT activity by phytoestrogens

Epidemiological studies have suggested that dietary phytoestrogens (e.g., soya products, tea, fruit, etc.), rich in flavonoids, isoflavonoids, and other phenolic compounds, can protect against hormone-dependent breast cancer. One of the mechanisms implicated for this chemoprotective effect is the ability of phytoestrogens to inhibit human cytosolic SULTs as the sulfation process is a key step in the metabolic activation of some dietary or environmental procarcinogens and promutagens in mammary tissues (Banoglu, 2000; Kirk et al., 2001; Pai et al., 2001).

Quercetin and resveratrol are dietary flavonoids with potent inhibitory effects of the human SULT1A1 (Eaton et al., 1996; Walle et al., 1995). Otake et al. (2000) observed that quercetin and resveratrol are substrates for SULT1E1 in the normal HME cells, with K_m values similar to their K_i values for inhibition of E_2 sulfation. Quercetin is 25 times more potent in inhibiting SULT1E1 in the HME cells than in inhibiting SULT1A1 activity in the intact human hepatoma cell line Hep G2, which has SULT1A1 expression levels similar to the human liver (Shwed et al., 1992).

Inhibition of SULT1E1 by quercetin resulted in elevated E_2 levels in the normal breast cell, which can have a potentially harmful effect. However, it is interesting to note that in the HME cells, SULT1E1 could catalyze the bioactivation of the cooked food mutagen and procarcinogen *N*-hydroxy-2-amino-1-methyl-6-phenylimidazol (4,5-b)pyridine (*N*-OH-PhIP) and its subsequent binding to genomic DNA (Lewis et al., 1998). In breast cancer cell lines (MCF-7, ZR-75-1), resveratrol suppresses *O*-acetyltransferase and SULT activities (Dubuisson et al., 2002).

However, another group (Harris et al. 2004) observed that flavonoids and dietary isoflavones (including genistein, daidzen) act as substrates and/or inhibitors of SULT1A1, SULT1E1, and in a lesser proportion SULT1A3. Genistein and equol were potent mixed inhibitors of SULT1E1 with IC50 values of 500 nM and 400 nM, respectively. Genistein and daidzen were also potent inhibitors of SULT1A1 with IC50 values of 500 nM and 600 nM, respectively. As circulating levels of isoflavones may approach 1 μM in individuals consuming some dietary supplements, the activity of both SULT1A1 and SULT1E1 may be inhibited by concentrations of flavonoids that can occur in vivo. SULT1A3 is particularly implicated in the sulfonation of these flavonoids at high concentrations (greater than 1 μM). These data suggest that high doses of dietary isoflavonoids may lead to elevated levels of active estrogens in target tissues including the mammary gland.

Parabens (*p*-hydroxybenzoate esters) are a group of preservatives widely used in cosmetics, food, and pharmaceutical products, which can exhibit estrogenic effects in animal models. Prusakiewicz et al. (2007) demonstrate an inhibitory effect of the EST activity present in skin cytosol. Butylparaben, the most potent inhibitor, has an IC50 value of 37 μM. The authors suggest that SULTs inhibition by parabens could stimulate or prolong estrogen signaling cascades by elevating the levels of E_2 and E_1. Thus, the skin antiaging benefits of many topical cosmetics could be derived from the estrogenicity of the preservatives (parabens) present in the formulations.

Regulation of SULT activity and pathophysiology of breast cancer

As the apparent affinities of SULT1E1 for estrogens are in the same order as those of K_d for the ER (nanomolar concentrations), it was postulated that SULT1E1 can compete with ER for E_2 binding and abolish the steroid action after processing of ligand-charged ER (Anderson and Howell, 1995; Hobkirk, 1993; Hobkirk et al., 1985; Roy, 1992; Saunders et al., 1989). In support of this hypothesis, it is interesting to remark that a significant sequence homology was observed between the ligand domain of the ER and the putative estrogen-binding domain deduced from bovine placental SULT1E1 cDNA (Nash et al., 1988). Previous studies in this laboratory demonstrated that low doses of medrogestone, as well as tibolone and its metabolites, can block the sulfatase activity in the conversion of E_1S to E_2. As these compounds also stimulate SULT1E activity in the same concentration range, this dual effect can contribute to decreasing estrogenic stimulation by encouraging excretion of estrogens to the sulfate form. If a similar action can operate in vivo, this represents a new possibility to block E_2, with interesting clinical applications. The mechanism implicated for the different dose-response effects observed with medrogestone or tibolone and its metabolites remains to be elucidated. However, there are a substantial number of examples where a hormone or antihormone produced an opposite effect according to its concentration.

SULT Expression and Its Control in Breast Cancer

SULT1E1 is the only sulfotransferase that displays affinity for 17β-E_2 in a physiological (nanomolar) concentration range (Zhang et al., 1998). Other SULTs, including SULT1A1, SULT1A3, and SULT2A1 are able to sulfate estrogens in vitro, however. For example, cells transfected with the cDNA coding for the enzyme originally named placental hEST1 (Bernier et al., 1994a,b; Luu-The et al., 1996), but now identified as SULT1A3, were able to transform E_1 to E_1S at nanomolar concentrations.

Using reverse transcriptase–polymerase chain reaction amplification (RT-PCR), the expression of hEST1, which now corresponds to SULT1A3 mRNA, was detected in the hormone-dependent MCF-7 and T47-D, as well as in hormone-independent MDA-MB-231 and MDA-MB-468, human breast cancer cells. An interesting correlation of the relative SULT activity and the SULT1A3 mRNA expression was found in various breast cancer cells studied (Chetrite et al., 1998).

Qian et al. (1998) demonstrated that restoration of SULT1E1 expression in MCF-7 cells by cDNA transfection could significantly attenuate the response on both gene activity and DNA synthesis, and cell numbers were used as markers of estrogen-stimulated cell growth and proliferation. These authors suggest that loss or down-regulation of SULT1E1 expression may enhance the growth-stimulating effect of estrogens and contribute to the process of tumor initiation.

It is interesting to mention that some groups report that in human breast cancer cell lines and tumors a positive correlation between the expression of SULT1E1 and that of ER. Patients whose tumors presented no SULT activity failed to respond to adrenalectomy and had a poor prognosis (Pewnim et al. 1982; Adams et al. 1989; Luu-The et al. 1996).

SULTs expression and progestins

A study on the effects of the progestin promegestone (R-5020) on hEST1, now named SULT1A3, mRNA and the formation of estrogen sulfates in the T-47D and MCF-7 cells showed that at low doses of R-5020 there was a significant increase of mRNA levels in these breast cancer cell lines. This was accompanied by an increased formation of estrogen sulfates in these cell lines following the treatment. However, at high doses of this progestin, an inhibitory effect was observed on SULT1A3 mRNA and the formation of estrogen sulfates (Chetrite et al., 1998).

Pharmacogenetics and SULTs

Single-nucleotide polymorphisms (SNPs) in SULTs can have functional consequences on the translated protein (variation of enzymatic activity), and pharmacogenetic studies confirm the impact of this polymorphism on breast cancer risk and on response to therapeutic agents. The isoform SULT1A1 has been implicated in clinical genetic variations of sulfation, as the *SULT1A1*2* allele encoding the His 213 variant allozyme (low activity), instead of a common Arg (high activity), can be a risk factor for breast cancer (Zheng et al., 2001) as well as a factor associated with survival in patients treated with tamoxifen (Nowell et al., 2002; Nowell and Falany, 2006). These results were confirmed by Tang et al. (2003); however, Langsenlehner et al. (2004) showed in a case-control study that the SULT1A1 Arg-213-His polymorphism is not a general risk factor for breast cancer, but may be associated with the presence of lymph node metastases.

The process of carcinogenesis is accompanied by multiple alterations of gene expression, and it is a challenge to find and underline determinant variations in the proteasome. Aust et al. (2005) observed by semiquantitative RT-PCR a possible modification in the SULT enzyme pattern between malignant and nonmalignant breast tissues. Substantial expression of the major isoforms of SULT1 and 2 subfamily was observed in tumoral and normal breast tissue. Significantly, expression of SULT1C1 is increased in tumoral tissue and the SULT1A2 mRNA is unspliced between exons 7 and 8 in normal tissue. These observations suggest an important role of SULT-mediated biotransformation in the breast.

It is interesting to note that pharmacogenetic variations in SULT1E1 gene may contribute to individual differences in lifetime estrogen exposure as well as variation in the metabolism (Adjei et al., 2003).

Conclusions

The intracellular metabolism of estrogens within breast cancer cells is important for the bioformation and activity of E_2 as well as to stimulate breast cancer cell growth (Pasqualini and Chetrite, 2007a). Cellular levels of E_2 are the result of a balance between (1) its synthesis via the sulfatase pathway and the aromatase pathway and (2) its transformation via SULT (SULT1A1, SULT1A3, SULT1E1, SULT2A1), which convert E_2 to the biologically inactive estradiol sulfate. What is the site of SULT action in breast cancer cells? Most studies indicate that SULT activity is highest in the cytosol (Adams and Phillips, 1990; Evans et al., 1993; Rozhin et al., 1986); however, in all breast cancers studied, very little or no estrogen sulfates could be localized inside the cells after incubation with E_1 or E_2. In addition, when these cells were incubated with estrogen sulfates, only unconjugated estrogens were detected inside the cell. The data suggest that both SULT and sulfatase are present inside the cell (at the cytosol and the endoplasmic reticulum, respectively), but that sulfated estrogens are rapidly exported from the cells. These compounds are substrates for several members of the organic anion transporters (OATP-B, -D, -E) that are responsible for the uptake of such molecules, the solute carrier proteins (SLC), and for members of the efflux pump families: multidrug resistance protein (MRP) or breast cancer resistance protein (BCRP), the ATP binding cassette (ABC) protein, that transport them out of cells, which may well explain these findings (Keppler et al., 2000; Leslie et al., 2001; Pizzagalli et al., 2003; Imai et al., 2003; Nozawa et al., 2005). The inhibition of E_1S transporter provides the basis for a novel strategy for breast cancer treatment.

The finding that some progestins (e.g., promegestone, nomegestrol acetate, medrogestone), as well as tibolone and its metabolites at physiological concentrations, can stimulate sulfotranferase activity in hormone-dependent breast cancer cells is an important point in the physiopathology of this disease as it is well known that estrogen sulfates do not bind to the ER.

Aromatases and Antiaromatases

The aromatase cytochrome P450 catalyzes aromatization of androgens to estrogens; biochemical and immunocytochemical studies have revealed the presence of this enzyme in the adipose stromal cells of breast cancer tissues, although levels of aromatase activity are relatively low in the breast (normal or cancerous) (Pasqualini et al., 1996a; Chetrite et al., 2000). This local production of estrogens in situ can contribute to the pathogenesis of estrogen-dependent breast cancers.

Aromatase inhibition by antiaromatase agents has been largely developed in the treatment of breast cancer patients, with very positive results (for details see chapters 10 and 11). These most useful aromatase inhibitors (AIs) include steroidal compounds exemestane (Aromasin®) and 4-hydroxy-androstenedione (formestane, Lentaron®), and nonsteroidal compounds aminoglutethimide, anastrozole (Arimidex®), letrozole (Femara®), and vorozole (Rivizor®). In contrast to steroidal AIs, which irreversibly inactivate the aromatase enzyme complex, nonsteroidal AIs reversibly interact with the heme moiety of the cytochrome P450 subunit, thus excluding both ligand and oxygen interaction with the enzyme complex and inhibiting steroidal aromatization. A series of reviews on the biological effects and therapeutic applications of these compounds in breast cancer has been published in latter years (Bhatnagar et al., 1996; Brodie et al., 2002; Miller and Pasqualini, 2005; Brodie and Pasqualini, 2007). Table 9 shows an interesting comparative study of the relative potency of different antiaromatases applied mostly in clinical treatments using breast cancer homogenates, mammary fibroblasts in culture, and placental microsomes (Miller and Jackson, 2003).

Recent studies demonstrated that coumarin derivatives (Chen et al., 2004), estrogen-3-sulfamates (Numazawa et al., 2006), and methylated flavones (Hong and Chen, 2006) can act as potent antiaromatase agents. It is intriguing to note that in MCF-7aro cells (a cell line stably transected with the aromatase gene) E_2 very significantly inhibits aromatase activity (Pasqualini and Chetrite, 2006a). Similarly, it was demonstrated that the natural androgens, androstenedione and testosterone, are antiaromatase agents in the MCF-7aro breast cancer cells (Pasqualini and Chetrite, 2006b). Other studies showed that 20α-dihydroprogesterone, a main metabolite of this hormone in normal breast tissue, is a potent antiaromatase agent (Pasqualini and Chetrite, 2007b, see details in section below). In conclusion, new antiaromatase agents can provide novel, most attractive therapeutic applications for the treatment of breast cancer patients.

Glucuronidases in the Breast

In the last years it was demonstrated that E_2 in breast tissue can be inactivated and eliminated through the formation of glucuronides by the action of the UGTs. UGTs is a family of enzymes that catalyze the formation of water-soluble metabolites through the transfer of glucuronic acid from the cofactor UDP-glucuronic acid to target

Table 9 Inhibition of Aromatase Activity by Different Antiaromatase Compounds Used in Clinical Therapy for Breast Cancer Patients

	Breast cancer homogenates		Mammary fibroblast cultures		Placental microsomes	
Antiaromatase compound	Relative potency	IC50 (nm)	Relative potency	IC50 (nm)	Relative potency	IC50 (nm)
Letrozole	1800	2.5	10.000	0.8	250	12
Anastrozole	450	10.0	570	14.0	250	12
Examestane	300	15.0	1600	5.0	60	50
Formestane	150	30.0	180	45.0	60	50
Aminoglutethimide	1	4500.0	1	8000.0	1	3000

IC50, 50% inhibitory concentration.
Source: From Miller and Jackson (2003).

substrates, including steroids, bile acids, dietary constituents, bilirubin, and carcinogen agents (Tukey and Strassburg, 2000). At present 15 different UGTs have been identified, which have been shown to glucuronidate more than 350 substances (Tukey and Strassburg, 2000; Guillemette et al., 2004; Thibaudeau et al., 2006).

The UGT family of enzymes includes two subclasses, UGT1 and UGT2. The UGT1A enzyme, mainly expressed in the liver and gastrointestinal tract, glucuronidates a range of substrates including bilirubin (Tukey and Strassburg, 2000). The UGT2B enzyme, expressed not only in the liver but also in the breast and prostate, is responsible for the formation of the majority of steroid glucuronidates. It was proposed that UGT2B enzymes are involved in the regulation of steroid signaling through targeted inactivation of steroids (Mackenzie et al., 1996). UGTs for estrogens were characterized in MCF-7 breast cancer cells (Hum et al., 1999). Some members of the UGT family (UGT1A8, UGT1A9, and UGT2B7 variants) are also involved in inactivation of the carcinogen 4-OH-E_2 in breast tissue (Thibaudeau et al., 2006).

An interesting UGT is the UGT2B15, which is highly expressed in various steroid target tissues, including the breast, prostate, liver, placenta, adipose tissue, and uterus (Levesque et al., 1997). The UGT2B15 is highly homologous to the androgen-specific UGT2B17 (Beaulieu et al., 1996). UGT2B15 glucuronidates a wide range of steroids, including estrogens, catecholestrogens, and various androgens such as testosterone, 5α-dihydrotestosterone, 5α-androstane-3α, and 17β-diol (Green et al., 1994).

As indicated in section "Concentration of Estrogens in Normal and Cancerous Breast", estrogen concentrations in breast tumor tissue are several times higher than serum estrogen levels. This local production of estrogens could be controlled by the action of antiaromatases (see sec. "Aromatases and Antiaromatases" and chapters 10 and 11), anti-sulfatase agents (see sec. "Sulfatase Activity and Its Control"), inhibition of 17β-hydroxysteroid dehydrogenase type 1 (see sec. "17β-HSDs in the Breast"), or by the stimulation of SULTs (see sec. "Role of Sulfotransferase in the Breast"). In early studies it was demonstrated that human breast cancer cell lines can convert E_2 into E_2 glucuronides (Adams et al., 1999), and more recently it was observed that plasma E_2 levels vary depending on the identity of the polymorphic variants of UGT2B15 found in breast cancer patients (Sparks et al., 2004).

In a recent study, Harrington et al. (2006) found that E_2 can stimulate UGT2B15 activity in ER-positive breast cancer cells, which represents a new mechanism in the control of E_2 levels in breast cancer. This increase of UGT2B15 can affect other hormone signaling pathways, as described by Green et al. (1994), who found that it can glucuronidate the potent androgen 5α-dihydrotestosterone.

The stimulatory effect of E_2 on UGT activity in breast cancer can be related to previous studies that demonstrated that E_2 can also control its own bioformation in breast tissue by blocking sulfatase (Pasqualini and Chetrite, 2001) or aromatase (Pasqualini and Chetrite, 2006a) activities.

PROGESTERONE TRANSFORMATION IN THE BREAST

In combination with E_2, progesterone plays a capital role in normal breast development as well as in the menstrual cycle, pregnancy, and lactation (Pike et al., 1993) (for a review see Pasqualini and Kincl, 1986; Pasqualini, 2005).

Progesterone is extensively metabolized in various organs. These transformations are important not only in blocking the biological effect of the hormone but also by the fact that the metabolic products can play a major role in the biological responses. Using gas chromatography mass spectrometry and chemical derivatives, at least 10 different progesterone metabolites were characterized in both normal and cancerous breast tissues (Wiebe et al., 2000). Two main classes of metabolites were reported: (1) those which retain the double bond and (2) those which are 5α-pregnanes by the action of a 5α-reductase; these transformations are summarized in Figure 6.

Most progesterone metabolites are found in both normal and cancerous breast tissues, but there are significant quantitative differences: in the normal breast, conversion to 4-ene derivatives greatly exceeds conversion to 5α-pregnane derivatives, whereas in the tumor tissue the latter are predominant (Wiebe et al., 2005; Wiebe, 2006). These authors suggested that breast carcinoma is accompanied by changes of in situ progesterone metabolism, resulting in increased concentrations of cancer-promoting 5α-pregnanes and a decrease of cancer-inhibiting 4-ene-pregnanes. A possible therapeutic regimen might involve decreasing 5α-pregnanes and increasing 3α-pregnanes by blocking 5α-reductase, as well as blocking the binding of 5α-pregnanes to the receptor. These metabolic differences of progesterone in normal and cancerous breast cells can have important physiological actions. It was demonstrated that 20α-dihydroprogesterone, the main transformation of the hormone in the normal breast cells, can block aromatase activity in MCF-aro breast cancer cells (Pasqualini and Chetrite, 2007b) suggesting that this progesterone metabolite could be involved in the control of E_2 availability in normal breast cells, which in turn suggests a role in breast carcinogenesis.

The presence of the membrane 5α-pregnane-3,20-dione (5α-P) receptors was detected in MCF-7 hormone-dependent breast cancer cells and in the nontumorigenic

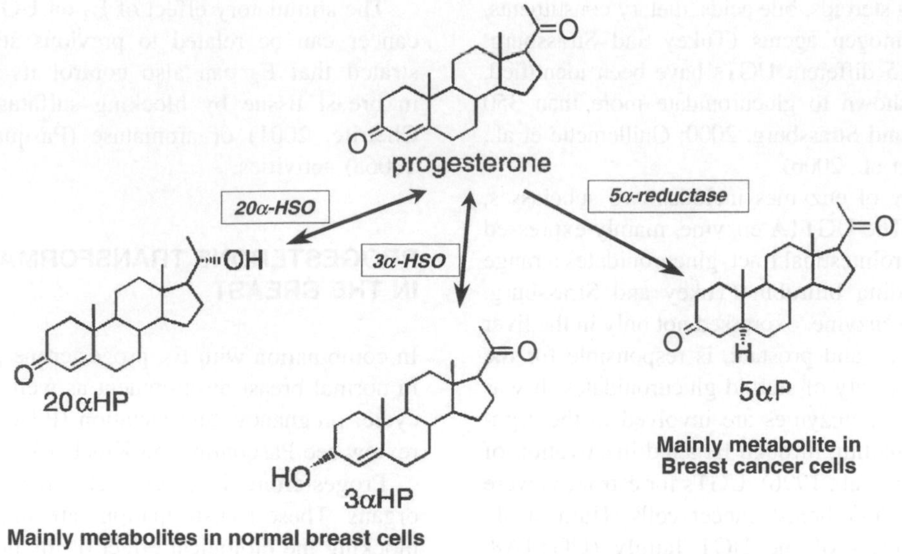

Figure 6 Transformation of progesterone in human breast cells (normal and tumoral). P is directly metabolized in two pathways: (1) to the 4-pregnene structures, 3α-hydroxy-4-pregnen-20-one (3α-dihydroprogesterone; 3α-HP) and 20α-dihydroprogesterone (20α-HP), by the reversible actions of 3α-hydroxysteroid oxidoreductase (3α-HSO) and 20α-HSO, respectively; (2) to the 5α-pregnane structure, 5α-pregnane-3,20-dione (5α-dihydroprogesterone; 5α-P), by the irreversible action of 5α-reductase. In normal tissue, the ratio of 4-pregnenes:5α-pregnanes is high because of high 3α-HSO and 20α-HSO activities/expression and low 5α-reductase activity/expression. In breast tumor tissue and tumorigenic cell lines, the ratio is reversed in favor of the 5α-pregnanes because of altered P-metabolizing enzyme activities/expression. The evidence suggests that the promotion of breast cancer is related to changes in in situ concentrations of cancer-inhibiting and cancer-promoting P metabolites. *Abbreviation*: P, progesterone. *Source*: From Wiebe (2006).

breast cell line MCF-10A. Exposure of MCF-7 cells to E_2 or 5α-P resulted in significant dose-dependent increases of 5α-P levels but, conversely, treatment with 3α-hydroxy-P or 20α-hydroxy-P resulted in significant dose-dependent decreases of 5α-P receptors (Pawlak et al., 2005). Pawlak and Wiebe (2007) also show that in MCF-7 cells treatment with the mitogenic 5α-P provoked an increase in ER, whereas, in opposition, treatment with the anti-mitogenics 3α-hydroxy-P or 20α-hydroxy-P resulted in decreased ER. The clinical applications of these progesterone metabolites in breast cancer patients is to be explored.

ENZYMATIC PROGNOSTIC FACTORS IN BREAST CANCER

Various studies carried out in latter years have shown that enzymes and their mRNA can be involved as interesting prognostic factors for breast cancer. This section covers the data concerning enzymes implicated in the formation and transformation of estrogens in breast cancer.

17β-Hydroxysteroid Dehydrogenases

Gunnarsson et al. (2001, 2003, 2005) investigated the expression of 17β-HSD types 1 and 2 and the correlation to recurrence-free survival. They found that high levels of 17β-HSD-1 were associated with decreased survival in ER-positive breast cancer. Vihko et al. (2006) confirmed these findings and observed that the survival rate was significantly worse in patients with breast cancer expressing 17β-HSD type 1 mRNA and that the disease-free interval was also shorter for these patients than in the other cases (Fig. 7). Another 17β-HSD, type 5, enzyme is an aldo-keto reductase expressed mainly in the mammary gland and prostate where it is involved in the formation of testosterone (Penning et al., 2001). It was found that patients with tumors expressing high levels of 17β-HSD-5 had a worse prognosis than those in the group with either low or no expression (Oduwole et al., 2004). Miyoshi et al. (2003) found a nonsignificant trend toward a decrease in five-year disease-free survival in breast cancer patients having high levels of 17β-HSD type 1 expression.

In ER-positive patients treated with tamoxifen, Gunnarsson et al. (2005) found a significantly higher risk for late relapse in those with high expression of 17β-HSD type 1, as well as a statistically significant positive correlation between recurrence-free survival and expression of 17β-HSD type 2.

An interesting 17β-HSD enzyme is the type 14, which is involved in the oxidative process, conversion of E_2 to E_1, or testosterone to androstenedione. Jansson et al.

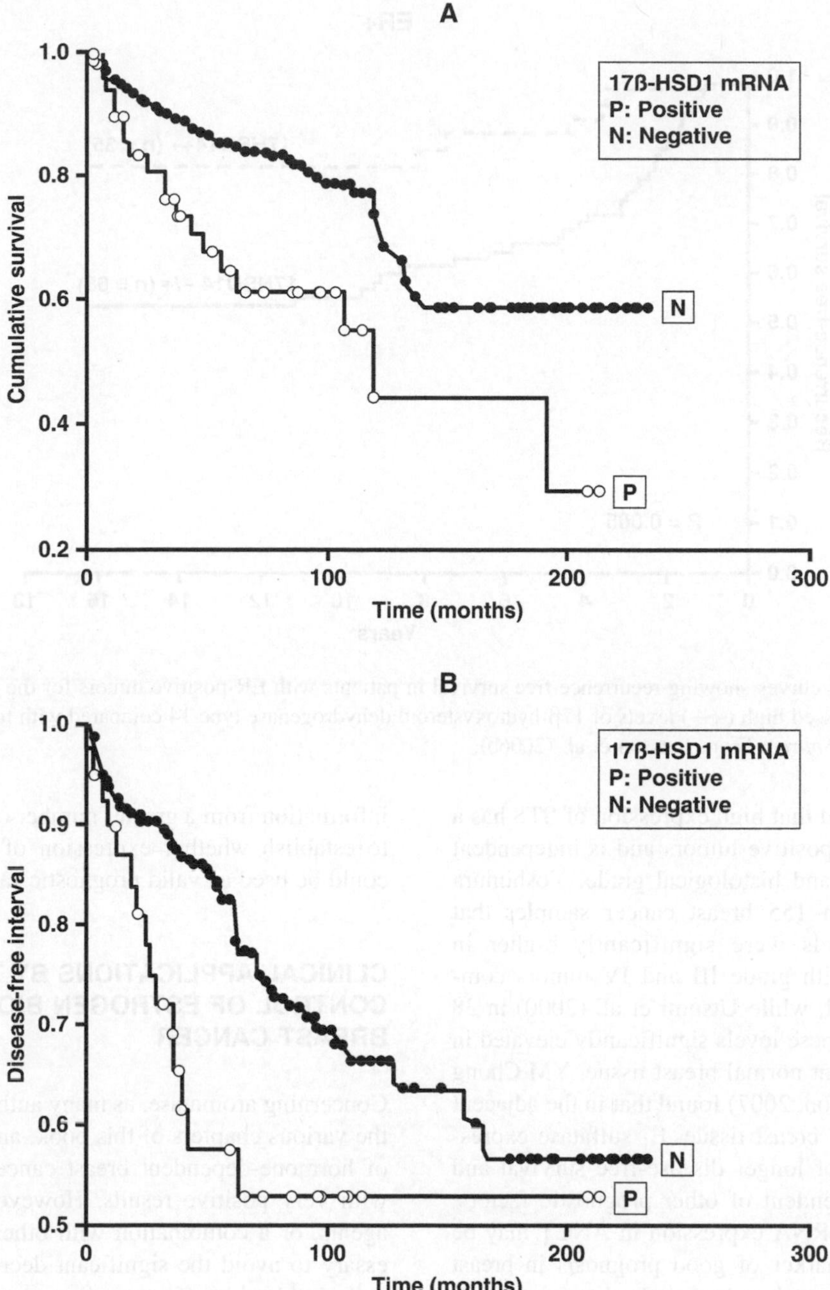

Figure 7 (A) Kaplan-Meier curve showing the survival of patients with breast carcinoma in relation to 17β-hydroxysteroid dehydrogenase-1 (17β-HSD1). Patients with tumors expressing 17β-HSD1 mRNA had a significantly worse prognosis ($p = 0.0010$, log rank). (B) Kaplan-Meier curve showing the disease-free interval of breast carcinoma patients in relation to 17β-HSD1. Patients with 17β-HSD1 mRNA expressing tumors had a significantly shorter disease-free interval than the other patients. *Source*: Data from Oduwole et al. (2004).

(2006b) found that patients with ER-positive breast cancer and high levels of 17β-HSD-14 expression had a significantly better prognosis for recurrence-free survival than patients with low levels (Fig. 8) as well as specific survival from breast cancer.

Sulfatase and Sulfotransferase

Many studies have explored the possibility of using STS mRNA expression as a prognostic factor to predict breast cancer. Miyoshi et al. (2003) studied 181 cases of invasive

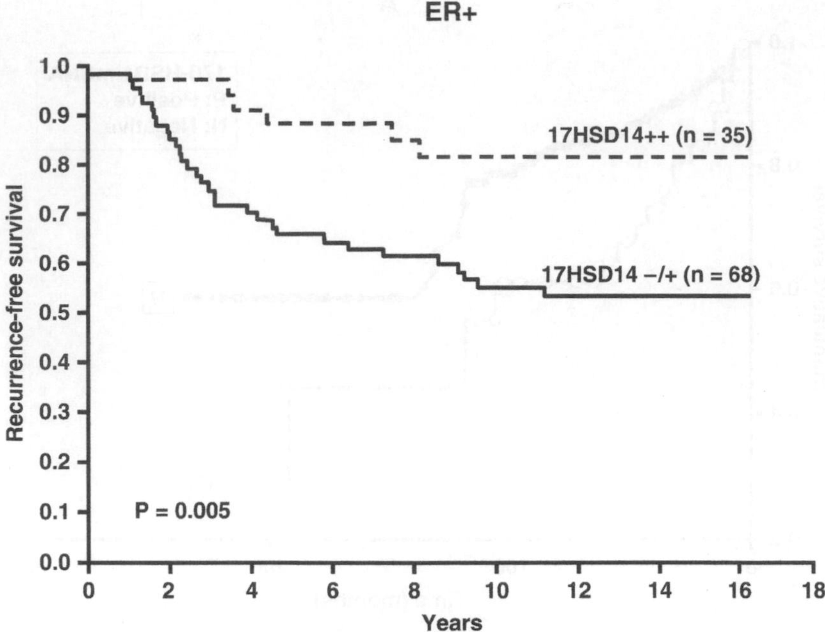

Figure 8 Kaplan-Meier curves showing recurrence-free survival in patients with ER-positive tumors for the whole follow-up period after diagnosis that expressed high (++) levels of 17β-hydroxysteroid dehydrogenase type 14 compared with tumors with intermediate (+) and low (–) levels. *Source*: From Jansson et al. (2006b).

breast cancer and found that high expression of STS has a poor prognosis in ER-positive tumors and is independent of lymph node status and histological grade. Yoshimura et al. (2004) noted in 155 breast cancer samples that sulfatase mRNA levels were significantly higher in those from patients with grade III and IV tumors compared to grade I and II, while Utsumi et al. (2000) in 38 tumor samples found these levels significantly elevated in relation to nonmalignant normal breast tissue. YM Chong (personal communication, 2007) found that in the adjacent noncancerous (ANCT) breast tissue, E_1 sulfatase expression was a predictor of longer disease-free survival and overall survival independent of other prognostic factors, suggesting that STS mRNA expression in ANCT may be used as a surrogate marker of good prognosis in breast cancer; however, these authors conclude that tumor STS expression has no significant prognostic value. Suzuki et al. (2003a,b) suggest that STS immunoreactivity is significantly associated with levels of mRNA and enzymatic activity and is positively correlated with tumor size, risk of recurrence, and worse prognosis (Fig. 9). These authors also explored the prognostic value of sulfotransferase (EST) and found that its reactivity correlated with tumor size or lymph node status and was strongly associated with a decreased risk of recurrence and/or improved prognosis. These findings suggest that EST and STS play an important role in the regulation of in situ estrogen production, and EST can be a prognostic factor in breast carcinoma (Sasano et al., 2006). In conclusion, further information from a greater number of patients is necessary to establish whether expression of STS or EST mRNA could be used as valid prognostic factors in breast cancer.

CLINICAL APPLICATIONS BY THE ENZYMATIC CONTROL OF ESTROGEN BIOFORMATION IN BREAST CANCER

Concerning aromatase, as many authors have confirmed in the various chapters of this book, antiaromatase treatment of hormone-dependent breast cancer is extensively used with very positive results. However, new antiaromatase agents, or a combination with other substances, are necessary to avoid the significant decrease of estrogens and undesirable side effects such as osteoporosis, as well as to preserve resistance due to antiaromatase treatment. AIs have been shown to have increased efficacy, compared with tamoxifen, for disease-free survival and reduction of contralateral breast cancer incidence, but not for increasing overall survival (Coombes et al., 2004; ATAC Trialists' Group, 2005). One attractive possibility and an important target is to discover a molecule to block aromatase activity in the mammary gland only.

With regard to clinical applications in breast cancer treatment to inhibit or stimulate the other enzymes involved in the formation or transformation of E_2 in breast tissue, data is very limited. At present, as STS is quantitatively the most important precursor of E_2 in breast

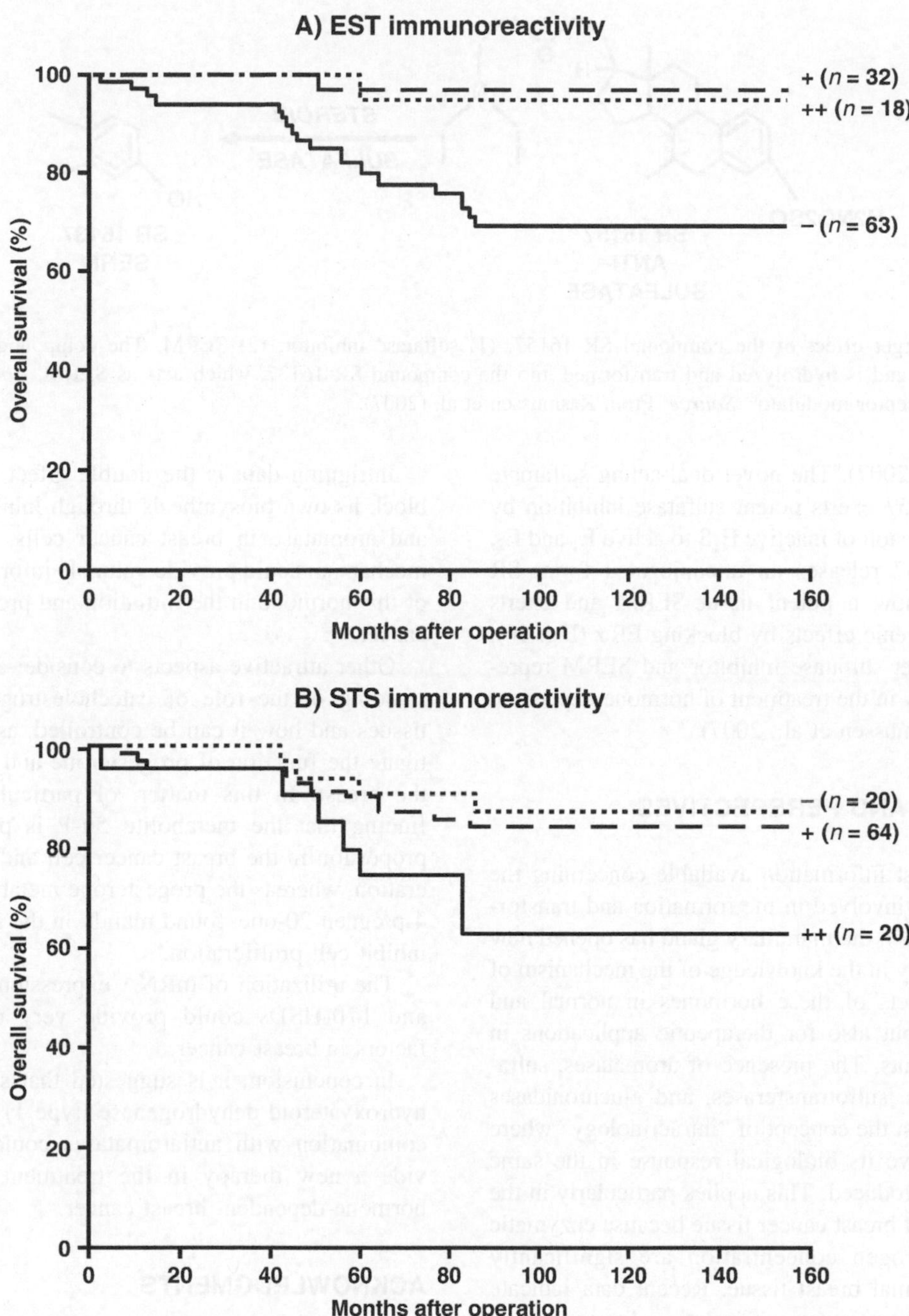

Figure 9 Overall (A and B) survival of 113 patients with breast carcinoma according to EST or STS immunoreactivity (Kaplan-Meier method). In (A), EST immunoreactivity was associated with an improved overall survival. In (B), STS immunoreactivity was associated with overall survival. *Source*: From Suzuki et al. (2003b).

cancer tissue (see sec. "Sulfatase Activity and Its Control"), an antisulfatase inhibitor, the STX64 (667 COUMATE) was explored in phase I of postmenopausal breast cancer patients, nine of whom received 5 mg and five 20 mg of STX64. This compound inhibits sulfatase activity in peripheral blood lymphocytes and tumor tissues and causes a notable decrease in serum concentration of estrogens and androstenediol, an androgen with estrogenic properties which is derived mainly from DHEA-S (Stanway et al., 2006).

Further interesting data in breast cancer therapy concerns the compound SR-16157 (SRI International, Menlo Park, California, U.S.) whose use provides a dual effect: it exerts an inhibition on STS while also acting as an antiestrogen agent and is in addition highly effective as a growth inhibitor, being 10 times more potent than tamoxifen

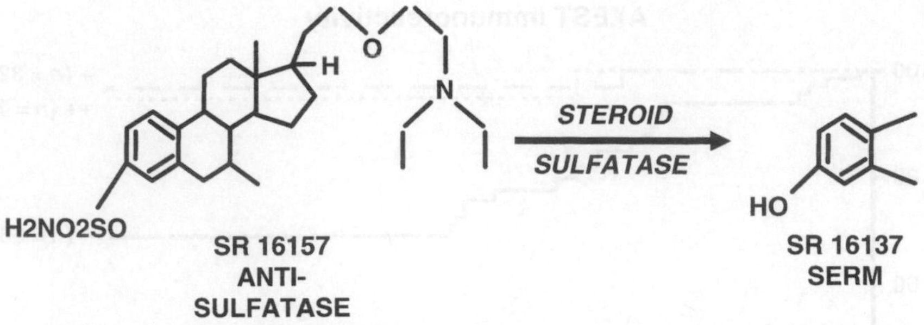

Figure 10 Dual target effect of the compound SR 16157: (1) sulfatase inhibitor, (2) SERM. The compound SR 16157 exerts antisulfatase activity and is hydrolyzed and transformed into the compound SR 16137, which acts as SERM. *Abbreviation*: SERM, selective estrogen receptor modulator. *Source*: From Rasmussen et al. (2007).

(Rasmussen et al., 2007). The novel dual-acting sulfamate compound SR 16157 exerts potent sulfatase inhibition by blocking the conversion of inactive E_1S to active E_1 and E_2. Moreover, SR16157 releases an unconjugated form, SR 16137, which is now a potent tissue-SERM and exerts profound antiestrogenic effects by blocking ERα (Fig. 10). Use of a dual-target sulfatase inhibitor and SERM represents a new strategy in the treatment of hormone-dependent breast cancer (Rasmussen et al., 2007).

CONCLUSIONS AND PERSPECTIVES

The recent and vast information available concerning the enzymatic systems involved in the formation and transformation of estrogens in the mammary gland has opened new possibilities not only in the knowledge of the mechanism of the biological effects of these hormones in normal and cancerous breast, but also for therapeutic applications in breast cancer patients. The presence of aromatases, sulfatases, hydroxylases, sulfotransferases, and glucuronidases extends to the breast the concept of "intracrinology" where a hormone can have its biological response in the same organ where it is produced. This applies particularly in the hormone-dependent breast cancer tissue because enzymatic activities and estrogen concentration are significantly higher than in normal breast tissue. Recent data indicate in postmenopausal patients a correlation between high levels of plasma estrogens and breast cancer risk, and it will be interesting to explore whether this increase in plasmatic estrogens is the consequent of the tumoral production and secretion of these hormones.

The discovery of antiaromatase agents was a major advance as these are presently extensively used in the treatment of breast cancer, with positive benefits as confirmed in other chapters of this book. However, as estrone sulfatase is quantitatively the most important pathway in E_2 bioformation in breast cancer tissues, there are new possibilities for the potential use of combined antisulfatase and 17β-hydroxysteroid dehydrogenase (type I) agents.

Intriguing data is the double effect of E_2, which can block its own biosynthesis through inhibition of sulfatase and aromatase in breast cancer cells, so exploring this mechanism could provide valuable information on the role of this hormone in the initiation and progression of breast cancer.

Other attractive aspects to consider are a better understanding of the role of catecholestrogens in the breast tissues and how it can be controlled, as well as to investigate the function of progesterone and its metabolites in the breast. In this matter, of particular interest is the finding that the metabolite 5α-P is present in a great proportion in the breast cancer cell and stimulates proliferation, whereas the progesterone metabolite 3α-hydroxy-4-pregnen-20-one, found mainly in the normal breast, can inhibit cell proliferation.

The utilization of mRNA expression of both sulfatase and 17β-HSDs could provide very useful prognostic factors in breast cancer.

In conclusion, it is suggested that sulfatase and 17β-hydroxysteroid dehydrogenase (type 1) inhibitors used in combination with antiaromatases could potentially provide a new therapy in the treatment of patients with hormone-dependent breast cancer.

ACKNOWLEDGMENTS

The authors express deep thanks to Ms Sandra MacDonald for efficient assistance in the preparation of this chapter.

REFERENCES

Adams JB, Phillips NS. Properties of estrogen and hydroxysteroid sulphotransferases in human mammary cancer. J Steroid Biochem 1990; 36:695–701.

Adams JB, Phillips NS, Pewnim T. Expression of hydroxysteroid sulphotransferase is related to estrogen receptor status in human mammary cancer. J Steroid Biochem 1989; 33:637–642.

Adams JB, Phillips NS, Young CE. Formation of glucuronides of estradiol-17β by human mammary cancer cells. J Steroid Biochem Mol Biol 1999; 33:1023–1025.

Adjei AA, Thomae BA, Prondzinski JL, Eckloff BW, Wieben ED, Weinshilboum RM. Human estrogen sulfotransferase (SULT1E1) pharmacogemics: gene resequencing and functional genomics. Br J Pharmacol 2003; 139:1373–1382.

Adjei AA, Weinshilboum RM. Human estrogen sulfotransferase (SULT1E1) pharmacogemics: gene resequencing and functional genomics. Biochem Biophys Res Commun 2002; 292:402–408.

Ahmed V, Liu Y, Silvestro C, Taylor SD. Boronic acids as inhibitors of steroid sulfatase. Bioorg Med Chem 2006; 14:8564–8573.

Aksoy IA, Wood R, Weinshilboum R. Human liver estrogen sulfotransferase: identification by cDNA cloning and expression. Biochem Biophys Rec Commun 1994; 200:1621–1629.

Amin SA, Huang C-C, Reierstad S, Lin Z, Arbieva Z, Wiley E, Saborian H, Haynes B, Cotterill H, Dowsett M, Bulun SE. Paracrine-stimulated gene expression profile favors estradiol production in breast tumors. Mol Cell Endocrinol 2006; 253:44–55.

Anderson C, Freeman J, Lucas LH, Farley M, Dalhoumi H, Widlanski TS. Estrone sulfatase: Probing structural requirements for substrate and inhibitor recognition. Biochemistry 1997; 36:2586–2594.

Anderson CJ, Lucas LJH, Widlanski TS. Molecular recognition in biological systems: phosphate esters vs sulfate esters and the mechanism of action of steroid sulfatase. J Am Chem Soc 1995; 117:3889–3890.

Anderson E, Howell A. Oestrogen sulphotransferases in malignant and normal human breast tissue. Endocr Relat Cancer 1995; 2:227–233.

Assicot M, Contesso G, Bohuon C. Catechol-o-methyltransferase in human breast cancer. Eur J Cancer 1977; 13:961–966.

ATAC Trialists' Group. Results of the ATAC (Arimidex, Tamoxifen, alone or in combination) trial after completion of 5 years adjuvant treatment for breast cancer. Lancet 2005; 365:60–62.

Aust S, Obrist P, Klimpfinger M, Tucek G, Jager W, Thalhammer T. Altered expression of the hormone- and xenobiotic-metabolizing sulfotransferase enzymes 1A2 and 1C1 in malignant breast tissue. Int J Oncol 2005; 26:1079–1085.

Banoglu E. Current status of the cytosolic sulfotransferases in the metabolic activation of promutagens and procarcinogens. Curr Drug Metab 2000; 1:1–30.

Beaulieu M, Levesque E, Hum DW, Belanger A. Isolation and characterization of a novel cDNA encoding human UDP-glucuronosyltransferase on C19 steroids. J Biol Chem 1996; 271:22855–22862.

Bernier F, Leblanc G, Labrie F, Luu-The V. Structure of human estrogen and aryl sulfotransferase gene. J Biol Chem 1994a; 269:28200–28205.

Bernier F, Lopez-Solache I, Labrie F, Luu-The V. Cloning and expression of cDNA encoding human placental estrogen sulfotransferase. Mol Cell Endocrinol 1994b; 99:R11–R15.

Bhatnagar AS, Batzl C, Häusler A, Schieweck K, Lang M, Trunet PF. Pharmacology of nonsteroidal aromatase inhibitors. In: Pasqualini JR, Katzenellenbogen BS, eds. Hormone Dependent Cancer. New York, Basel: Marcel Dekker Inc., 1996:155–168.

Bhattacharyya S, Tobacman JK. Steroid sulfatase, arylsulfatases A and B, galactose-6-sulfatase, and iduronate sulfatase in mammary cells and effects of sulfated and non-sulfated estrogens on sulfatase estrogens on sulfatase activity. J Steroid Biochem Mol Biol 2007; 103:20–34.

Billich A, Meingassner JG, Nussbaumer P, Desrayaud S, Lam C, Winiski A, Schreiner E. 6-[2-(Adamantylidene)-hydrobenzoxazole]-*O*-sulfamate, a steroid sulfatase inhibitor for the treatment of androgen- and estrogen-dependent diseases. J Steroid Biochem Mol Biol 2004; 92:29–37.

Billich A, Nussbaumer P, Lehr P. Stimulation of MCF-7 breast cancer cell proliferation by estrone sulfate and dehydroepiandrosterone sulfate: inhibition by novel non-steroidal steroid sulfatase inhibitors. J Steroid Biochem Mol Biol 2000; 73:225–235.

Bjarnason NH, Bjarnason K, Haarbo J, Christiansen C. Tibolone: prevention of bone loss in late postmenopausal women. J Clin Endocrinol Metab 1996; 81:2419–2422.

Blanchard RL, Freimuth RR, Buck J, Weiushilboum RM, Coughtrie MWH. A proposed nomenclature for the cytosolic sulfotransferase (SULT) superfamily. Pharmacogenetics 2004, 14:199–211.

Boivin RP, Luu-The V, Lachance R, Labrie F, Poirier D. Structure-activity relationships of 17alpha-derivates of estradiol as inhibitors of steroid-sulfatase. J Med Chem 2000; 43:4465–4478.

Bove BA. BRCA1, BRCA2, and hereditary breast cancer. In: Pasqualini JR, ed. Breast Cancer Prognosis, Treatment, and Prevention. 2nd ed. New York, London, Boca Raton, Singapore: Informa Healthcare, 2008:523–582.

Bove BA, Dunbrack RL, Godwin AK. BRCA1, BRCA2, and hereditary breast cancer. In: Pasqualini JR, ed. Breast Cancer: Prognosis, Treatment, and Prevention. 1st ed. New York, Basel: Marcel Dekker, Inc., 2002:555–624.

Brodie AMH. Aromatase inhibitors and their application to the treatment of breast cancer. In: Pasqualini JR, ed. Breast Cancer: Prognosis, Treatment and Prevention. New York: Marcel Dekker, Inc., 2002:251–269.

Brodie AMH. Aromatase inhibitors and their application to the treatment of breast cancer. In: Pasqualini JR, ed. Breast Cancer Prognosis, Treatment, and Prevention. 2nd ed. New York, London, Boca Raton, Singapore: Informa Healthcare, 2008:157–168.

Brodie AMH, Pasqualini JR, eds. Proceeding of the VIII International Aromatase Conference "AROMATASE 2006" Philadelphia. J Steroid Biochem Mol Biol 2007; 106:1–186.

Brodie AMH, Wing LY, Dowsett M, Coombes RC. Aromatase inhibitors and treatment of breast cancer. J Steroid Biochem Mol Biol 1986; 24:91–97.

Brooks JD, Thompson LU. Mammalian lignans and genistein decrease the activities of aromatase and 17β-hydroxysteroid dehydrogenase in MCF-7 cells. J Steroid Biochem Mol Biol 2005; 94:461–467.

Brozic P, Golob B, Gomboc N, Rizner TL, Gobec S. Cinnamic acids as new inhibitors of 17beta-hydroxysteroid dehydrogenase type 5 (AKR1C3). Mol Cell Endocrinol 2006; 248:233–235.

Burchell B, Coughtrie MW. Genetic and environmntal factors associated with variation of human xenobiotic glucuronidation and sulfatation. Environ Health Perspect 1997; 105 (suppl 4):739–747.

Carlström K, Döberl A, Pousette A, Rannavik G, Wilking N. Inhibition of steroid sulfatase activity by danazol. Acta Obstet Gynecol Scand Suppl 1984; 123:107–111.

Castagnetta L, Granata OM, Arcuri F, Polito LM, Rosati F, Cartini GP. Gas chromatography/mass spectrometry of catechol estrogens. Steroids 1992; 57:437–443.

Castagnetta LA, Granata OM, Traina A, Ravazzolo B, Amoroso M, Miele M, Bellavia V, Agostara B, Carruba G. Tissue content of hydroxyestrogens in relation to survival of breast cancer patients. Clin Cancer Res 2002; 8:3146–3155.

Castles CG, Fuqua SAW, Klotz DM, Hill SM. Expression of a constitutively active estrogen receptor variant in the estrogen receptor-negative BT-20 human breast cancer cell line. Cancer Res 1993; 53:5934–5939.

Celis JE, Moreira JM, Cabezon T, Gromov P, Friis E, Rank F, Gromova L Identification of extracellular and intracellular signaling components of the mammary adipose tissue and its interstitial fluid in high risk breast cancer patients: toward dissecting the molecular circuitry of epithelial-adipocyte stromal cell interactions. Mol Cell Proteomics 2005; 4:492–522.

Chander SK, Foster PA, Leese MP, Newman SP, Potter BV, Purohit A, Reed MJ. In vivo inhibition of angiogenesis by sulphamoylated derivatives of 2-methoxyoestradiol. Br J Cancer 2007; 96:1368–1376.

Chen S, Cho M, Kalsberg K, Zhou D, Yuan -C. Biochemical and biological characterization of a novel anti-aromatase coumarin derivate. J Biol Chem 2004; 79:48071–48078.

Cheng TC, Chen ST, Huang CS, Fu YP, Yu JC, Cheng CW, Wu PE, Shen CY. Breast cancer risk associated with genotype polymorphism of the catechol estrogen-metabolizing genes: A multiple study on cancer susceptibility. Int J Cancer 2005; 113:345–353.

Chetrite G, Cortes-Prieto J, Philippe JC, Wright F, Pasqualini JR. Comparaison of estrogen concentrations, estrone sulfatase and aromatase activities in normal, and in cancerous, human breast tissues. J Steroid Biochem Mol Biol 2000; 72:23–27.

Chetrite G, Cortes-Prieto J-C, Philippe J-C, Pasqualini JR. Estradiol inhibits the estrone sulfatase activity in normal and cancerous human breast tissues. J Steroid Biochem Mol Biol 2007; 104:289–292.

Chetrite G, Cortes-Prieto J, Pasqualini JR. Medrogestrone is an anti-sulfate agent in the total human breast cancer tissue. 2008a (in preparation).

Chetrite G, Cortes-Prieto J, Pasqualini JR. Tibolone and its metabolites are anti-sulfatase agents in the total human breast cancer tissue. 2008b (in preparation).

Chetrite G, Ebert C, Wright F, Philippe J-C, Pasqualini JR. Control of sulfatase and sulfotransferase activities by medrogestone in the hormone-dependent MCF-7 and T-47D human breast cancer cells lines. J Steroid Biochem Mol Biol 1999a; 70:39–45.

Chetrite G, Ebert C, Wright F, Philippe J-C, Pasqualini JR. Effect of Medrogesterone on 17β-hydroxysteroid dehydrogenase activity in the hormone-dependent MCF-7 and T-47D breast cancer cell lines. J Steroid Biochem Mol Biol 1999b; 68:51–56.

Chetrite G, Kloosterboer HJ, Pasqualini JR. Effect of Tibolone (Org OD14) and its metabolites on estrone sulphatase activity in MCF-7 and T-47D mammary cancer cells. Anticancer Res 1997; 17:135–140.

Chetrite G, Kloosterboer H J, Philippe J-P, Pasqualini JR. Effect of Org OD14 (Livial R) and its metabolites on human estrogen sulphotransferase activity in the hormone-dependent MCF-7 and T-47D, and the hormone-independent MDA-MB-231, breast cancer cells lines. Anticancer Res 1999c; 19:269–276.

Chetrite G, Kloosterboer HJ, Philippe J-P, Pasqualini JR. Effect of Org OD14 (Livial R) and its metabolites on 17β-hydroxysteroid dehydrogenase activity in hormone-dependent MCF-7 and T-47D breast cancer cells. Anticancer Res 1999d; 19:261–268.

Chetrite G, Le Nestour E, Pasqualini JR. Human estrogen sulfotransferase (hEST1) activities and its mRNA in various breast cancer cell lines. Effect of the progestin, promegestone (R-5020). J Steroid Biochem Mol Biol 1998; 66: 295–302.

Chetrite G, Paris J, Botella J, Pasqualini JR. Effect of nomegestrol actetate on estrone sulfatase and 17β-hydroxysteroid dehydrogenase activities in human breast cancer cells. J Steroid Biochem Mol Biol 1996; 58:525–531.

Chetrite GS, Paris J, Shields-Botella J, Philippe J-C, Pasqualini JR. Effect of nomegestrol acetate on human estrogen sulfotransferase activity in the hormone-dependent MCF-7 and T-47D breast cancer cell lines. Anticancer Res 2003; 3:4651–4655.

Chetrite G, Pasqualini JR. Steroid sulphotransferase and 17β-hydroxysteroid dehydrogenase activities in Ishikawa human endometrial adenocarcinoma cells. J Steroid Biochem Mol Biol 1997; 61:27–34.

Chetrite G, Pasqualini JR. The selective estrogen enzyme modulator (SEEM) in breast cancer. J Steroid Biochem Mol Biol 2001; 76:95–104.

Chetrite GS, Thole HH, Philippe J-C, Pasqualini JR. Dydrogesterone (Duphaston®) and its 20-dihydro-derivate as selective estrogen enzyme modulators in human breast cancer cell lines. Effect on sulfatase and on 17β-hydroxysteroid dehydrogenase (17β-HSD) activity. Anticancer Res 2004; 24:1433–1438.

Chetrite G, Thomas JL, Shields-Botella J, Philippe J-C, Cortes-Prieto J, Philippe JC, Pasqualini JR. Control of sulfatase activity by nomegestrol acetate in the normal and cancerous human breast tissues. Anticancer Res 2005; 25:2827–2830.

Cho H, Aronica SM, Katzenellenbogen BS. Regulation of progesterone receptor gene expression in MCF-7 breast cancer cells: a comparaison of the effects of cyclic adenosine 3′,5′-monophosphate, estradiol, insuline-like growth factor-I, and serum factors. Endocrinology 1994; 134:658–664.

Ciobanu LC, Boivin RP, Luu-The V, Labrie F, Poirier D. Potent inhibition of steroid sulfatase activity by 3-*O*-sulfamate 17α-benzyl (or 4′tert-butylbenzyl)estra-1,3,5(10)-trienes: combinaison of two substituents at positions C3 and C17α of estradiol. J Med Chem 1999; 42:2280–2286.

Ciobanu LC, Boivin RP, Luu-The V, Poirier D. 3Beta-sulfamate derivatives of C19 and C21 steroids bearing a t-butylbenzyl or a benzyl group: synthesis and evaluation as non-estrogenic and non-androgenic steroid sulfatase inhibitors. J Enzyme Inhib Med Chem 2003a; 18:15–26.

Ciobanu LC, Luu-The V, Martel C, Labrie F, Poirier D. Inhibition of estrone sulfate-induced uterine growth by potent nonestrogenic steroidal inhibitors of steroid sulfatase. Cancer Res 2003b; 63:6442–6446.

Ciobanu LC, Luu-The V, Poirier D. Nonsteroidal compounds designed to mimic potent steroid sulfatase inhibitors. J Steroid Biochem Mol Biol 2002; 80:339–353.

Ciobanu LC, Poirier D. Synthesis of libraries of 16beta-aminopropyl estradiol derivates for targeting two key steroidogenic enzymes. Chem Med Chem 2006; 1:1249–1259.

Clarke CL, Adams JB, Wren BG. Induction of oestrogen sulfotransferase activity in the human endometrium by progesterone in organ culture. J Clin Endocrinol Metab 1982; 55:70–75.

Coldham NG, James VHT. A possible mechanism for increased breast cell proliferation by progestins through increased reductive 17β-hydroxysteroid dehydrogenase activity. Int J Cancer 1990; 45:174–178.

Coombes RC, Hall E, Gibson LJ. A randomized trial of exemestane after two to three year of tamoxifen therapy in postmenopausal women with primary breast cancer. N Engl J Med 2004; 350:1081–1092.

Coughtrie MW. Sulfation through the looking glass—recent advances in sulfotransferase research for the curious. Pharmacogenomics J 2002; 2:297–308.

Couture P, Theriault C, Simard J, Labrie F. Androgen receptor-mediated stimulation of 17β-hydroxysteroid dehydrogenase activity by dihydrotestosterone and medroxyprogesterone acetate in ZR-75-1 human breast cancer cells. Endocrinology 1993; 132:179–185.

Dawling S, Hachey DL, Roodi N, Parl FF. In vitro model of mammary estrogen metabolism: structural and kinetic differences between catechol estrogens 2-and 4-hydroxyestradiol. Chem Res Toxicol 2004; 17:1258–1264.

de Jong PC, van de Ven J, Nortier HWR, Maitimu-Smeele I, Donker TH, Thijssen JHH, Slee PHTJ, Blankenstein RA. Inhibition of breast cancer tissue aromatase activity and estrogen concentrations by the third-generation aromatase inhibitor Vorozole. Cancer Res 1997; 57:2109–2111.

De Lignières B, Dennerstein L, Backstrom T. Influence of route of administration on progesterone metabolism. Maturitas 1995; 21:251–257.

Dooley TP, Haldeman-Cahill R, Joiner J, Wilborn TW. Expression profiling of human sulfotransferase and sulfatase gene superfamilies in epithelial tissues and cultured cells. Biochem Biophys Res Commun 2000; 277:236–245.

Dubuisson JG, Dyess Dl Gaubatz JW. Resveratrol modulates human mammary epihelial cell O-acetyltransferase, sulfotransferase, and kinase activation of the heterocyclic amine carcinogen N-hydroxy-PhIP. Cancer Lett 2002; 182:27–32.

Eaton EA, Walle UK, Lewis AJ, Hudson T, Wilson AA, Walle T. Flavonoids, potent inhibitors of the human P-form phenolsulfotransferase: potential role in drug metabolism and chemoprevention. Drug Metab Dispos 1996; 24:232–237.

Eckert Rl, Katzenellenbogen BS. Effects of estrogens and antiestrogens on estrogen receptor dynamics and the induction of progesterone receptor in MCF-7 human breast cancer cells. Cancer Res 1982; 42:139–144.

Elger W, Schwarz S, Hedden A, Reddersen G, Schneder B. Sulfamates of various estrogens are prodrugs with increased systemic and reduced hepatic estrogenicity at oral application. J Steroid Biochem Mol Biol 1995; 55:395–403.

Eliassen AH, Missmer SA, Tworoger SS, Speigelman D, Barbieri RL, Dowsett M, Hankinson SE. Endogenous steroid hormone concentrations and risk of breast cancer among premenopausal women. J Natl Cancer Inst 2006; 98: 1406–1415.

Emmert-Buck MR, Bonner RF, Smith PD, Chauqui RS, Zuang Z, Golstein SR, Weiss RA, Liotta LA. Laser capture microdissection. Science 2001; 274:998–1001.

Evans T, Rowlands M, Silva M, Law M, Coombes R. Prognostic significance of aromatase and estrone sulfatase enzymes in human breast cancer. J Steroid Biochem Mol Biol 1993; 44:583–587.

Falany JL, Falany CN. Expression of cytosolic sulfotransferases in normal mammary epithelial cells and breast cancer cell lines. Cancer Res 1996a; 56:1551–1555.

Falany JL, Falany CN. Regulation of oestrogen sulfotransferase in human endometrial adenocarcinoma cells by progesterone. Endocrinology 1996b; 137:1395–1401.

Falany JL, Falany CN. Regulation of estrogen activity by sulfation in human MCF-7 human breast cancer cells. Oncol Res 1997; 9:589–596.

Falany JL, Falany CN. Interactions of the human cytosolic sulfotransferases and steroid sulfatase in the metabolism of tibolone and raloxifene. J Steroid Biochem Mol Biol 2007; 107:202–210.

Falany JL, Lawing L, Falany CN. Identification and characterization of cytosolic sulfotransferase activities in MCF-7 human breast carcinoma cells. J Steroid Biochem Mol Biol 1993; 46:481–487.

Falany JL, Macrina N, Falany CN. Regulation of MCF-7 breast cancer cell growth by 17β-estradiol sulfation. Breast Cancer Res Treat 2002; 74:167–176.

Falany JL, Macrina N, Falany CN. Sulfatation of tibolone and tibolone metabolites by expressed human cytisolic sulfotransferases. J Steroid Biochem Mol Biol 2004; 8:383–392.

Falany JL, Pillof DE, Leyh TS, Falany CN. Sulfatation of raloxifene and 4-hydroxytamoxifen by cytosolic sulfotransferases. Drug Metab Dispos 2006; 34:361–368.

Falany CN, Wheeler J, Oh TS, Falany JL. Steroid sulfation by expressed human cytosolic sulfotransferases. J Steroid Biochem Mol Biol 1994; 48:369–375.

Fan P, Wang J, Santen RJ, Yue W. Long-term treatment with tamoxifen facilitates translocation of estrogen receptor α out of the nucleus and enhances its interaction with EGFR in MCF-7 breast cancer cells. Cancer Res 2007; 67: 1352–1360.

Filling C, Brendt KD, Benach J, Knapp S, Prozorovski T, Nordling E, Ladenstein R, Jornvall H, Oppermann U. Critical residues for structure and catalysis in short-chain dehydrogenases/reductases. J Biol Chem 2002; 277: 25677–25684.

Fishman J, Martucci C. Biological properties of 16α-hydroxyestrone: implications in estrogen physiology and pathophysiology. J Clin Endocrinol Metab 1980; 51:611–615.

Foster PA, Newman SP, Chander SK, Stengel C, Jhalli R, Woo LL, Potter BV, Reed MJ, Purohit A. In vivo efficacy of STX213, a second-generation steroid sulfatase inhibitor, for hormone-dependent breast cancer therapy. Clin Cancer Res 2006; 12:5543–5549.

Fournier S, Brihmat F, Durand JC, Sterkers N, Martin Pm, Kutten F, Mauvais-Jarvis P. Estradiol 17β-hydroxysteroid dehydrogenases, a marker of breast cancer hormone dependency. Cancer Res 1985; 45:2895–2899.

Fujikawa H, Okura F, Kuwano Y, Sekizawa A, Chiba H, Shimodaira K, Saito T, Yanaihara T. Steroid sulfatase activity in osteoblast cells. Biochem Biophys Res Commun 1997; 231:42–47.

Fuqua SAW, Fitzgerald SD, Chamness GC, Tandon AK, McDonnell DP, Nawaz Z, O'Malley BW, McGuire WL. Variant human breast tumor estrogen receptor with constitutive transcriptional activity. Cancer Res 1991; 51:105–109.

Fuqua SAW, Greene GL, McGuire WL. Inhibition of estrogen receptor action by a naturally occurring variant in human breast tumors. Cancer Res 1992; 52:483–486.

Gamage N, Barnett A, Hempel N, Duggleby RG, Windmill KF, Martin JL, McManus ME. Human sulfotransferases and their role in chemical metabolism. Toxicol Sci 2006; 90:5–22.

Gamage NU, Tsvetanov S, Duggleby RG, McManus ME, Martin JL. The structure of human SULT1A1 crystallized with estradiol. An insight into active site plasticity and substrate inhibition with multi-ring substrates. J Biol Chem 2005; 280:41482–41486.

Garofalo C, Koda M, Cascio S, Sulkowska M, Kanczuga-Koda L, Golaszewska J, Russo A, Sulkowska S, Sumacz E. Encreased expression of leptin and the leptin receptor as a marker of breast cancer progression: possible role of obesity-related stimuli. Clin Cancer Res 2006; 12:1447–1453.

Glatt H. Sulfotransferases in the bioactivation of xenobiotics. Chem Biol Interact 2000; 129:141–170.

Glatt H. Sulphotransferases. In: Ioannides C, ed. Enzymes Systems that Metabolise Drugs and Other Xenobiotics. Wiley, Chichester 2002:353–439.

Glatt H, Boeing H, Engelke CE, Ma L, Kuhlow A, Pabel U, Pomplun D, Teubner W, Meinl W. Human cytosolic sulphotransferases: genetics, characteristics, toxicological aspects. Mutat Res 2001; 482:27–40.

Golob T, Liebl R, von Angerer E. Sulfamoyloxy-substitued 2-phenylindoles: antiestrogen-based of steroid sulfatase in human breast cancer cells. Bioorg Med Chem 2002; 10:3941–3953.

Gompel A, Malet C, Spritzer P, Lalardrie J-P, Kuttenn F, Mauvais-Jarvis P. Progestin effect on cell proliferation and 17β-hydroxysteroid dehydrogenase activity in normal human breast cells in culture. J Clin Endocrinol Metab 1986; 63:1174–1180.

Green MD, Oturu EM, Tephly TR. Stable expression of a human liver UDP-glucuronosyltransferase (UGT2B15) with activity toward steroid and xenobiotic substrates. Drug Metab Dispos 1994; 22:799–805.

Guillemette C, Berlanger A, Lepine J. Metabolic inactivation of estrogens in breast tissue by UDP-glucuronosyltransferase enzymes: an overview. Breast Cancer Res 2004; 6:246–254.

Gunnarsson C, Hellqvist E, Stal O, and the South East Breast Cancer Group. 17β-Hydroxysteroid dehydrogenases involved in local oestrogen synthesis have prognostic significance in breast cancer. Br J Cancer 2005; 92:547–552.

Gunnarsson C, Kirschner K, Hellqvist E. Expression of 17β-hydroxysteroid dehydrogenases and correlation to prognosis in postmenopausal breast cancer patients. Breast Cancer Res Treat 2003; 82:459 (abstr).

Gunnarsson C, Olson BM, Stal O. Members of the souththeast Sweden Breast Cancer Group Anormal expression of 17β-hydroxysteroid dehydrogenase in breast cancer predicts late recurrence. Cancer Res 2001; 61:8448–8451.

Gupta M, McDougal A, Safe S. Estrogenic and antiestrogenic activities of 17β and 2-hydroxy metabolites of 17β-estradiol in MCF-7 and T47D human breast cancer cells. J Steroid Biochem Mol Biol 1998; 67:413–419.

Hankinson SE, Eliassen AE. Endogenous estrogen, testosterone, and progesterone levels in relation to breast cancer risk. J Steroid Biochem Mol Biol 2007; 106:24–30.

Harrington WR, Sengupta S, Katzenellenbogen BS. Estrogen regulation of the glucuronidation enzyme UGT2B15 in estrogen receptor-positive breast cancer cells. Endocrinology 2006; 147:3843–3850.

Harris RM, Wood DM, Bottomley L, Blagg S, Owen K, Hughes PJ, Waring RH, Kirk CJ. Phytoestrogens are potent inhibitors of estrogen sulfation: implications for breast cancer risk and treatment. J Clin Endocrinol Metab 2004; 89: 1779–1789.

Hata H, Holinka CF, Pahuja SL, Hochberg RB, Kuramoto H, Gurpide E. Estradiol metabolism in Ishikawa endometrial cancer cells. J Steroid Biochem Mol Biol 1987; 26: 699–704.

Hejaz HA, Woo LW, Purohit A, Reed MJ, Potter BVL. Synthesis in vitro and in vivo activity of benzophenone-based inhibitors of steroid sulfatase. Bioorg Med Chem Lett 2004; 12:2759–2772.

Henderson IC, Canellos GP. Cancer of the breast: the past decade. N Engl J Med 1990; 302:17–30.

Henderson BE, Feigelson HS. Hormonal carcinogenesis. Carcinogenesis 2000; 21:427–433.

Hernandez-Guzman FG, Higashiyama T, Pangborn W, Osawa Y, Ghosh D. Structure of human estrone sulfatase suggests function roles of membrane association. J Biol Chem 2003; 278:22989–29997.

Herynk MH, Fuqua SAW. Estogen receptor mutations in human disease. Endocr Rev 2004; 25:869–898.

Hobkirk R, Girard LR, Durham NJ, Khalil MW. Behavior of mouse placental and uterine estrogen sulfotransferase during chromatography and other procedures. Biochim Biophys Acta 1985; 828:123–129.

Hobkirk R. Steroid sulfatation—current contents. Trends Endocrinol Metab 1993; 4:69–74.

Hong Y, Chen S. Aromatase inhibitors: structural features and biochemical characterization. Ann N Y Acad Sci 2006; 1089:237–251.

Horvath A, Nussbaumer P, Wolff B, Billich A. 2-(1-adamantyl)-4(thio)chromenone-6-carboxylic acids: potent reversible inhibitors of human steroid sulfatase. J Med Chem 2004; 47:4268–4276.

Howarth NM, Purohit A, Reed MJ, Potter BVL. Estrone sulfamates: potent inhibitors of estrone sulfatase with therapeutic potential. J Med Chem 1994; 37:219–221.

Hughes PJ, Twist LE, Durham J, Choudhry MA, Drayson M, Chandraratna R, Michell Rh, KirK CJ, Brown G. Up-regulation of steroid sulphatase activity in HL60 promyelocytic cells by retinoids and 1alpha, 25-dihydroxyvitamin D3. Biochem J 2001; 355:361–371.

Hulka BA, Stark AT. Breast cancer: cause and prevention. Lancet 1995; 346:883–887.

Hum DW, Belanger A, Levesque E, Barbier O, Beaulieu M, Albert C, Vallee M, Guillemette C, Tchernof A, Turgeon D, Dubois S. Characterization of UDP-glucuronosyltransferases active on steroid hormones. J Steroid Biochem Mol Biol 1999; 69:413–423.

Husen B, Huhtinen K, Poutanen M, Kangas L, Messinger J, Thole H. Evaluaton of inhibitors for 17β-hydroxysteroid deshydrogenase type 1 in vivo in immunodeficient mice inoculated with MCF-7 cells stably expressing the recombinant human enzyme. Mol Cell Endocrinol 2006; 248:109–113.

Imai Y, Asada S, Tsukahara S, Ishikawa E, Tsuruo T, Sugimoto Y. Breast cancer resistance protein exports sulfated estrogens but not free estrogens. Mol Pharmacol 2003; 64: 610–618.

Ishida H, Nakata T, Sato N, Li PK, Kuwabara T, Akinaga S. Inhibition of steroid sulfatase activity and cell proliferation in ZR-75-1 and BT-474 human breast cancer cells by KW-2581 in vitro and in vivo. Breast Cancer Res Treat 2007a; 104:211–219.

Ishida H, Nakata T, Suzuki M, Shiotsu Y, Tanaka H, Sato N, Terasaki Y, Takebayashi M, Anazawa H, Murakata C, Li PK, Kuwabara T, Akinaga S. A novel steroidal selective steroid sulfatase inhibitor KW-2581 inhibits sulfated-estrogen dependent growth of breast cancer cells in vitro and in animal models. Breast Cancer Res Treat 2007b; 106:215–227.

James MR, Skaar TC, Lee RY, MacPherson A, Zwiebel JA, Ahluwalia BS, Ampy F, Clarke R. Constitutive expression of the steroid sulfatase gene supports the growth of MCF-7 human breast cancer cells in vitro and in vivo. Endocrinology 2001; 142:1497–1505.

Jansson AK, Gunnarsson C, Cohen M, Sivik T, Stal O. 17β-Hydroxysteroid dehydrogenase 14 affects estradiol levels in breast cancer cells and is a prognostic marker in estrogen receptor-positive breast cancer. Cancer Res 2006b; 66:11471–11477.

Jansson A, Gunnarsson C, Stal O. Proliferative responses to altered 17beta-hydroxysteroid dehydrogenase (17HSD) type 2 expression in human breast cancer cells are dependent on endogenous expression of 17HSD type 1 and the oestradiol receptors. Endocr Relat Cancer 2006a; 13: 875–884.

Kaaks R, Berrino F, Key T, Rinaldi S, Dossus L, Biessy G, Secreto G. Serum sex steroids in premenopausal women and breast cancer risk within the European Prospective Investigation into Cancer and Nutrition (EPIC). J Natl Cancer Inst 2005a; 97:755–765.

Kaaks R, Rinaldi S, Key TJ, Berrino F, Peeters PHM, Biessy C, Dossus L, Lukanova A, Bingham S, Khaw KT, Allen NE, Bueno-de-Mesquita HB, van Gils CH, Grobbee D, Boeing H, Lahmann PH, Nagel G, Chang-Claude J, Clavel-Chapelon F, Fournier A, Thiébaut A, González CA, Quirós JR, Tormo MJ, Ardanaz E, Amiano P, Krogh V, Palli D, Panico S, Tumino R, Vineis P, Trichopoulou A, Kalapothaki V, Trichopoulos D, Ferrari P, Norat T, Saracci R, Riboli E. Postmenopausal serum androgens, oestrogens and breast cancer risk: the European prospective investigation into cancer and nutition. Endocr Relat Cancer 2005b; 12:1071–1082.

Keppler D, Kamisako T, Leier I, Cui Y, Nies AT, Tsujii H, Konig J. Localisation, substrate specificity, and drug resistance conferred by conjugate export pumps of the MRP family. Adv Enzyme Regul 2000; 40:339–349.

Kester MH, Bulduk S, Tibboel D, Meinl W, Glatt H, Falany CN, Coughtrie MW, Bergman A, Safe SH, Kuiper GG, Schuur AG, Brouwer A, Visser T J. Potent inhibition of estrogen sulfotransferase by hydroxylated PCB metabolites: a novel pathway explaining the estrogenic activity of PCBs. Endocrinology 2000; 141:1897–1900.

Kester MH, Bulduk S, van Toor H, Tibboel D, Meinl W, Glatt H, Falany CN, Coughtrie MW, Schuur AG, Brouwer A, Visser TJ. Potent inhibition of estrogen sulfotransferase by hydroxylated metabolites of polyhalogenated aromatic hydrocarbons reveals alternative mechanism for estrogenic activity of endocrine disrupters. J Clin Endocrinol Metab 2002; 87:1142–1150.

Key T, Appelby P, Barnes I, Reeves G, and the Endogenous Hormones and Breast Cancer Collaborative Group. Endogenous sex hormones and breast cancer in postmenopausal women: reanalysis of nine prospective studies. J Natl Cancer Inst 2002; 94:606–616.

Kirk CJ, Harris RM, Wood DM, Waring RH, Hughes PJ. Do dietary phytoestrogens influence susceptibility to hormone-dependent cancer by disrupting the metabolism of endogenous oestrogens? Biochem Soc Trans 2001; 29:209–216.

Knabbe C, Lippman ME, Wakefield LM, Flanders KC, Kasid A, Derynck R, Dickson RB. Evidence that transformation growth factor-beta is a hormonally regulated negative growth factor in human breast cancer cells. Cell 1987; 48:417–428.

Komagata S, Nakajima M, Tsuchiya Y, Katoh M, Kizu R, Kyo S, Yokoi T. Decreased responsiveness of naturally occuring mutants of human estrogen receptor ato estogens and antiestrogens. J Steroid Biochem Mol Biol 2006; 100: 79–86.

Kuhl H. Pharmacology of progestins. Basic aspects-progesterone derivatives. Menopause Rev 2001; 6:9–16.

Labrie F, Luu-The V, Lin SX, Simard J, Labrie C, El-Alfy M, Pelletier G, Belanger A. Intracrinology: role of the family of 17beta-hydroxysteroid deshydrogenase in human physiology and disease. J Mol Endocrinol 2000; 25:1–16.

Lage JM, Leamon JH, Pejovic T, Haman S, Lacey M, Dillon D, Segraves R, Vossbrink B, Gonzalez A, Albertson, DG, Costa G, Lizardi PM. Whole genome analysis of genetic alterations in small DNA samples using hyperbranched stand displacement amplification and array-CGH. Genome Res 2003; 13:294–307.

Lakhani NJ, Sarlkar MA, Venitz J, Figg WD. 2-Methoxyestradiol, a promising anticancer agent. 2-Methoxyestradiol, a promising anticancer agent. Pharmacotherapy 2003; 23:165–172.

Langsenlehner U, Krippl P, Renner W, Yazdani-Biuki B, Eder T, Wolf G, Wascher TC, Paulweber B, Weitzer W, Samonigg H. Genetic variants of the sulfotransferase 1A1 and breast cancer risk. Breast Cancer Res Treat 2004; 87:19–22.

Lattanzi ML, Santos CB, Mudry MD, Baranao JL. Exposure of bovine oocytes to endogenous metabolite 2-methoxyestradiol during in vitro maturaton inhibits early embryonic development. Biol Reprod 2003; 69:1793–1780.

Lee AJ, Cai MX, Thomas PE, Conney AH, Zhu BT. Characterization of the oxidative metabolite of 17β -estradiol and estrone formed by 15 selectively expressed human cytochrome p-450 isoforms. Endocrinology 2003; 98: 3382–3398.

Leese MP, Hejaz HA, Mahon MF, Newman SP, Purohit A, Reed MJ, Potter BV. A-ring-substituted estrogen-3-O-sulfamates: potent multitargeted anticancer agents. J Med Chem 2005a; 48:5243–5256.

Leese MP, Leblond B, Newman SP, Purohit A, Reed MJ, Potter BV. Anti-cancer activities of novel D-ring modified 2-substituted estrogen-3-0-sulfamates. J Steroid Biochem Mol Biol 2005b; 94:239–251.

Leslie EM, Mao Q, Oleschuk CJ, Deeley RG, Cole SP. Modulation of multidrug resistance protein 1 (MRP1/ABCC1) transport and atpase activities by interaction with dietary flavonoids. Mol Pharmacol 2001; 59:1171–1180.

Levesque E, Beaulieu M, Green MD, Tephly TR, Belanger A, Hum DW. Isolation and characterization of UGT2B15 (Y85): a UDP-glucuronosyltransferase encoded by a polymorphic gene. Pharmacogenetics 1997; 7:317–325.

Levin ER. Integration of the extranuclear and nuclear action of estrogen. Mol Endocrinol 2005; 19:1951–1959.

Lewis JS, Thomas TJ, Klinge CM, Gallo MA, Thomas T. Regulation of cell cycle and cyclins by 16alpha-hydroxyestrone in MCF-7 breast cancer cells. J Mol Endocrinol 2001; 27:293–307.

Lewis AJ, Walle UK, King RS, Kadlubar FF, Fanaly CN, Walle T. Bioactivation of the cooked food mutagen N-hydroxy-2-amino-1-methyl-6-phenylimidazol [4,5-b]pyridine by estrogen sulfotransferase in cultured human mammary epithelial cells. Carcinogenesis 1998; 19:2049–2053.

Liehr JG, Fang WF, Sirbasku DA, Ari-Ulubelen A. Carcinogenicity of catechol estrogens in Syrian hamsters. J Steroid Biochem Mol Biol 1986; 24:353–356.

Liehr JG, Ricci MJ. 4-Hydroxylaton of estrogens as marker of human mammary tumors. Proc Natl Acad Sci U S A 1996; 93:3294–3296.

Lippert C, Seeger H, Mueck O. The effect of endogenous estradiol metabolites on the proliferation of human breast cancer cells. Life Sci 2003; 72:877–883.

Litherland S, Jackson IM. Antiestrogens in the management of hormone-dependent cancer. Cancer Treat Rev 1988; 15:183–194.

Liu ZJ, Zhu BT. Concentration-dependent mitogenic and antiproliferative actions of 2-methoxyestradiol in estrogen receptor-positive human breast cancer cells. J Steroid Biochem Mol Biol 2004; 88:265–275.

Lloyd MD, Pederick RL, Natesh R, Woo LW, Purohit A, Reed MJ, Acharrya KR, Foster PA. Crystal structure of human carbonic anhydrase II at 1.95A resolution in complex with 667-coumate, a novel anti-cancer agent. Biochem J 2005a; 385:715–720.

Lloyd MD, Thiyagarajan N, Ho YT, Woo LW, Sutcliffe OB, Purohit A, Reed MJ, Acharya KR, Potter BV. First cristal structures of human carbonic anhydrase II in complex with dual aromatase-steroid sulfatase inhibitors. Biochemistry 2005b; 44:6858–6866.

Lottering ML, Haag M, Seegers JC. Effects of 17β-estradiol metabolites on cell cycle events in MCF-7 and HeLa cells. Cancer Res 1992; 52:5926–5932.

Lukacik P, Kavanagh KL, Oppermann U. Structure and function of human 17β-hydroxysteroid dehydrogenases. Mol Cell Endocrinol 2006; 248:61–71.

Luu-The V, Bernier F, Dufort I. Steroid sulfotransferases. J Endocrinol 1996; 50:S87–S97.

Ma XJ, Salunga R, Tuggle JT, Gaudet J, Enright E, McQuary P, Payette T, Pistone M, Stecker K, Zhang BM, Zuou YX, Varnholt H, Smith B, Gadd M, Chatfield E, Kessler J, Baer TM, Erlander MG, Sgrol DC. Gene expression profiles of human breast cancer progression. Proc Natl Acad Sci U S A 2003; 100:5974–5979.

MacIndoe JH, Woods G, Jeffries L, Hinkhouse M. The hydrolysis of estrone sulfate and dehydroepiandrosterone sulfate by MCF-7 human breast cancer cells. Endocrinology 1988; 123:1281–1287.

MacKenzie PI, Mojarrabi B, Meech R, Hansen A. Steroid UDP glucuronosyltransferases: characterisation and regulation. J Endocrinol 1996; 150(suppl):S79–S86.

Malini B, Purohit A, Ganeshapillai D, Woo LWL, Potter BVL, Reed MJ. Inhibition of steroid sulphatase activity by tricyclic coumarin sulphamates. J Steroid Biochem Mol Biol 2000; 75:253–258.

Manjer J, Johansson R, Berglund G, Janzon L, Kaaks R, Agren A, Lenner P. Postmenopausal breast cancer risk in relation to sex steroid hormones, prolactin and SHBG (Sweden). Cancer Causes Control 2003; 14:599–607.

McGuire WL, Chamness GC, Fuqua SAW. Abnormal estrogen receptor in clinical breast cancer. J Steroid Biochem Mol Biol 1992; 43:243–247.

McNeill JM, Reed MJ, Beranek PA, Newton CJ, Ghilchik MW, James VHT. The effect of epidermal growth factor, transforming growth factor and breast tumor homogenates on the activity of oestradiol 17β-hydroxysteroid deshydrogenase in cultured adipose tissue. Cancer Lett 1986; 31:213–219.

Messinger J, Hirvela L, Husen B, Kangas L, Koskimies P, Pentikäinen O, Saarenketo P, Thole H. New inhibitors of 17β-hydroxysteroid deshydrogenase type 1. Mol Cell Endocrinol 2006; 248:192–198.

Miettinen MM, Mustonen M, Poutanen M, Isomaa V, Vihko RK. Human 17β-hydroxysteroid dehydrogenase type 1 and type 2 isoenzymes have opposite activities in cultured cells and characteristic cell- and tissue-specific expression. Biochem J 1996; 314:839–845.

Miettinen MM, Mustonen M, Poutanen M, Isomaa V, Wickman M, Söderqvist G, Vihko R, Vihko P. 17β-hydroxysteroid dehydrogenases in normal human mammary epithelial cells and breast tissue. Breast Cancer Res Treat 1999; 57: 175–182.

Miller WR, Jackson J. The therapeutic potential of aromatase inhibitors. Expert Opin Investig Drugs 2003; 12:337–351.

Miller W, Pasqualini JR, eds. Proceeding of the VII International Aromatase Conference "AROMATASE 2004" Edinburg, Scotland, UK. J Steroid Biochem Mol Biol 2005; 95:1–188.

Missmer SA, Eliassen AH, Barbieri RL, Hankinson SE. Endogenous estrogen, androgen, and progesterone concentrations and breast cancer among postmenopausal women. J Natl Cancer Inst 2004; 96:1856–1865.

Miyoshi Y, Akazawa K, Kamigaki S, Ueda S, Yanagisawa T, Inoue T, Yamamura J, Taguchi T, Tamaki Y, Noguchi S. Prognostic significance of intra-tumoral estradiol level in breast cancer patients. Cancer Lett 2004; 216:115–121.

Miyoshi Y, Ando A, Hasegawa S, Ishitobi M, Taguchi T, Tamaki Y, Noguchi S. High expression of steroid sulfatase mRNA predicts poor prognosis in patients with estrogen receptor-positive breast cancer. Clin Cancer Res 2003; 9:2288–2293.

Molis TG, Spriggs LL, Jupiter Y, Hill SM. Melatonin modulation of estrogen regulated proteins, growth factors, and proto-oncogenes in human breast cancer. J Pineal Res 1995; 18:93–103.

Mueck AO, Seeger H, Lippert TH. Estradiol metabolism and malignant disease. Maturitas 2002; 43:1–10.

Nakata T, Takashima S, Shiotsu Y, Murakata C, Ishida H, Akinaga S, Li P-K, Sasano H, Suzuki T, Saeki T. Role of steroid sulfatase in local formation of estrogen in post-menopausal breast cancer patients. J Steroid Biochem Mol Biol 2003; 86:455–460.

Nash AR, Glenn WK, Moore SS, Kerr J, Thompson AR, Thompson E OP. Oestrogen sufotransferase: molecular cloning and sequencing of cDNA for the bovine placenta enzyme. Aust J Biol Sci 1988; 41:507–516.

Neumann F, Duesterberg D. Entwicklung auf dem Gebeit der Gestagene. Reproduktionsmedizin 1998; 14:257–264.

Newbold RR, Lierh JG. Induction of uterine adeno-carcinoma in CD-1 mice by catechol estrogens. Cancer Res 2000; 60:235–237.

Newman SP, Foster PA, Stengel C, Day JM, Ho YT, Judde JG, Lassalle M, Prevost G, Leese MP, Potter BV, Reed MJ, Purohit A. STX140 is efficacious in vitro and in vivo in taxane-resistant breast carcinoma cells. Clin Cancer Res 2008; 14:597–606.

Nguyen BL, Chetrite G, Pasqualini JR. Transformation of estrone and estradiol in hormone-dependent and hormone independent human breast cancer cells. Effects of the antiestrogen ICI 164,384, danazol, and promegestone (R-5020). Breast Cancer Res Treat 1995; 34:139–146.

Nguyen B-L, Ferme I, Chetrite G, Pasqualini JR. Action of danazol on the conversion of estrone dulfate to estradiol and on the sulfatase activity in the MCF-7, T-47D and MDA-MB-231 human mammary cancer cells. J Steroid Biochem Mol Biol 1993; 46:17–23.

Nowell S, Falany CN. Pharmacogenetics of human cytosolic sulfotransferases. Oncogene 2006; 25:1673–1678.

Nowell S, Sweeney C, Winters M, Stone A, Lang NP, Hutchins LF, Kadlubar FF, Ambrosone CB. Association between sulfotransferase 1A1 genotype and survival of breast cancer patients receiving tamoxifen therapy. J Natl Cancer Inst 2002; 94:1635–1640.

Nozawa T, Suzuki M, Yabuuchi H, Irokawa M, Tsuji A, Tamai I. Suppression of cell proliferation by inhibition of estrone-3-sulfate transporter in estrogen-dependent breast cancer cells. Pharm Res 2005; 22:1634–1641.

Numazawa M, Ando M, Watari Y, Tominaga T, Hayata Y, Yoshimura A. Structure-activity relationships of 2-, 4-, or 6-substituted estrogens as aromatase inhibitors. J Steroid Biochem Mol Biol 2005; 96:51–58.

Numazawa M, Tominaga T, Watari Y, Tada Y. Inhibition of estrone sulfatase by aromatase inhibitor-based estrogen 3-sulfamates. Steroids 2006; 71:371–379.

Nussbaumer P, Billich A. Steroid sulfatase inhibitors. Med Res Rev 2004; 24:529–576.

Nussbaumer P, Billich A. Steroid sulfatase inhibitors: their potential in the therapy of breast cancer. Curr Med Chem Anticancer Agents 2005; 5:507–528.

Oduwole OO, Li Y, Isomaa VV, Mantyniemi A, Pulkka AE, Soini Y, Vihko PT. 17β-Hydroxysteroid dehydrogenase type 1 is an indepedent prognostic marker in breast cancer. Cancer Res 2004; 64:7604–7609.

Okada M, Nakagawa T, Iwashita S, Takegawa S, Fujii T, Koizumi N. Devclpment of novel steroid sulfatase inhibitors. I. Synthesis and biological evaluation of biphenyl-4-O-sulfamates. J Steroid Biochem Mol Biol 2003; 87:141–148.

Oppermann U, Filling C, Hult M, Shafqat N, Wu X, Lindh M, Shafqat J, Nordling E, Kallberg Y, Persson B, Jornvall H. Short chain dehydrogenases/reductases (SDR): the 2002 update. Chem Biol Interact 2003; 143–144:247–253.

Osborne CK, Shou J, Massarweh S, Shiff R. Crosstalk between estrogen receptor and growth factor receptor as a cause for endocrine therapy resistance in breast cancer. Clin Cancer Res 2005; 11:865S–870S.

Otake Y, Nolan AL, Walle UK, Walle T. Quercetin and resveratrol potently reduce estrogen sulfotransferase activity in normal human mammary epithelial cells. J Steroid Biochem Mol Biol 2000; 73:265–270.

Pai TG, Suiko M, Sakakibara Y, Liu M. Sulfatation of flavonoids and other phenolic dietary compounds by the human cytosolic sulfotransferases. Biochem Biophys Res Commun 2001; 285:1175–1179.

Paquette B, Bisson M, Baptiste C, Therriault H, Lemay R, Cantin AM. Invasiveness of breast cancer cells

MDA-MB-231 through extracellular matrix is increased by the estradiol metabolite 4-hydroxyestradiol. Int J Cancer 2005; 113:706–711.

Pasqualini JR. Steroid sulphotransferase activity in the human hormone-independent MDA-MB-468 mammary cancer cells. Eur J Cancer 1992; 28A:758–762.

Pasqualini JR. The selective estrogen enzyme modulators in breast cancer: a review. Biochim Biophys Acta 2004; 1654:123–143.

Pasqualini JR. Enzymes involved in the formation and transformation of steroid hormones in the fetal and placental compartments. European Progestin Club JSBMB 2005. J Steroid Biochem Mol Biol 2005; 96:401–415.

Pasqualini JR. Progestins and breast cancer. Gynecol Endocrinol 2007; 23(suppl 1):32–41.

Pasqualini JR, Caubel P, Friedman J, Philippe J-C, Chetrite GS. Norelgestromin as selective estrogene enzyme modulator in human breast cancer cell lines. Effect on sulfatase activity in comparison to medroxyprogesterone acetate. J Steroid Biochem Mol Biol 2003; 84:193–198.

Pasqualini JR, Chetrite G. Activity, regulation and expression of sulfatase, sulfotransferase, and 17β-hydroxysteroid dehydrogenase in Breast Cancer. In: Pasqualini JR, Katzenellenbogen BS, eds. Hormone-Dependent Cancer. New York, Basel, Hong Kong: Marcel Dekker, Inc., 1996:25–80.

Pasqualini JR, Chetrite G. Paradoxical effect of estradiol: it can block its own bioformation in human breast cancer cells. J Steroid Biochem Mol Biol 2001; 78:21–24.

Pasqualini JR, Chetrite GS. Selective estrogen enzyme modulators (SEEM). In: Pasqualini JR, ed. Breast Cancer: Prognosis, Treatment and Prevention. New York: Marcel Dekker, Inc., 2002:187–249.

Pasqualini JR, Chetrite GS. Recent insight on the control of enzymes involved in estrogen formation and transformation in human breast cancer. J Steroid Biochem Mol Biol 2005a; 93:221–236.

Pasqualini JR, Chetrite GS. Estrogen sulfotransferase and breast cancer. In: Pacifici GM, Coughtrie MWH, eds. Human Cytosolic Sulfotransferase. London: Taylor & Francis, 2005b:135–157.

Pasqualini JR, Chetrite G. Estradiol is an anti-aromatase agent in human breast cancer cells. J Steroid Biochem Mol Biol 2006a; 98:12–17.

Pasqualini JR, Chetrite G. Androstenedione and testosterone inhibits aromatase activity in human breast cancer cells. 29th Annual San Antonio Symposium, San Antonio, US, December 14–17, 2006. Breast Cancer Res Treat 2006b; 100(suppl 1):S249.

Pasqualini JR, Chetrite GS. Correlation of estrogen sulfotransferase activity and proliferation in normal and carcinomatous human breast. A hypothesis. Anticancer Res 2007a; 27:3219–3226.

Pasqualini JR, Chetrite G. The anti-aromatase effect of the natural metabolites of progesterone: 20α-dihydroprogesterone and 5α-dihydroprogesterone on MCF-7 aro breast cancer cells (abstract). 30th San Antonio Breast Cancer Symposium, December 13–16, 2007. Breast Cancer Res Treat 2007b; 106(suppl 1):9202 (abstr 4105).

Pasqualini JR, Chetrite G, Blacker M-C, Feinstein C, Delalonde L, Talbi M, Maloche C. Concentrations of estrone, estradiol, estrone sulfate and evaluation of sulfatase and aromatase activities in pre- and post-menopausal breast cancer patients. J Clin Endocrinol Metab 1996a; 81: 1460–1464.

Pasqualini JR, Chetrite GS, Le Nestour E. Control and expression of oestrone sulphatase activities in human breast cancer. Fifth International Congress on Hormones and Cancer (Quebec, Canada, September 1995). J Endocrinol 1996b; 150:S99–S105.

Pasqualini JR, Chetrite G, Nguyen B-L, Blacker C, Feinstein M-C, Maloche C, Talbi M, Delalonde L. Control of estrone sulfatase activity and its expression in human breast cancer. In: Motta M, Serio M, eds. Sex Hormones and Antihormones in Endocrine Dependent Pathology: Basic and Clinical Aspects [International Congress Series (Excerpta Medica)]. Amsterdam: Elsevier Science B.V., 1994a: 257–265.

Pasqualini JR, Chetrite G, Nguyen B-L, Maloche C, Delalonde L, Talbi M, Feinstein M-C, Blacker C, Botella J, Paris J. Estrone sulfate-sulfatase and 17β-hydroxysteroid dehydrogenase activities: a hypothesis for their role in the evolution of human breast cancer from hormone-dependence to hormone-independence. J Steroid Biochem Mol Biol 1995; 53:407–412.

Pasqualini JR, Gelly C. Effect of tamoxifen and tamoxifen derivatives on the conversion of estrone-sulfate to estradiol in the MCF-7 and R-27 mammary cancer cell lines. Cancer Lett 1988; 40:115–121.

Pasqualini JR, Giambiagi N, Gelly C, Chetrite GS. Antioestrogen action in mammary cancer and in fetal cells. J Steroid Biochem Mol Biol 1990; 37:343–348.

Pasqualini JR, Kincl FA, eds. Hormones and the Fetus. Vol I. Oxford: Pergamon Press, 1986:73–172.

Pasqualini JR, Maloche C, Maroni M, Chetrite G. Effect of the progestagen promegestone (R-5020) on mRNA of the oestrone sulphatase in the MCF-7 human mammary cancer cells. Anticancer Res 1994b; 14:1589–1593.

Pasqualini JR, Paris J, Sitruk-Ware R, Chetrite G, Botella J. Progestins and breast cancer. J Steroid Biochem Mol Biol 1998; 65:225–235.

Pasqualini JR, Schatz B, Varin C, Nguyen BL. Recent data on estrogen sulfatases and sulfotransferases activities in human breast cancer. J Steroid Biochem Mol Biol 1992a; 41: 323–329.

Pasqualini JR, Varin C, Nguyen BL. Effect of the progestagen R5020 (promegestone) and of progesterone on the uptake and on the transformation of estrone sulfate in the MCF-7 and T-47D human mammary cancer cells: correlation with progesterone receptor levels. Cancer Lett 1992b; 66:55–60.

Patel CK, Owen CP, Ahmed S. The design, synthesis, and in vitro biochemical evaluation of a series of 4-[(aminosulfonyl)oxy]benzoate as novel and potent inhibitors of estrone sulfatase. Biochem Biophys Res Commun 2003; 307: 778–781.

Patel CK, Owen CP, Ahmed S. Inhibition of estrone sulfatase (ES) by alkyl and cycloalkyl ester derivates of

4-[(aminosulfonyl)oxyl] benzoic acid. Bioorg Med Chem Lett 2004; 14:605–609.

Payne AH. Gonadal steroid sulfates and sulfatase. V. Human testicular steroid sulfatase: patial characterization and possible regulation by free steroids. Biochim Biophys Acta 1972; 258:473–483.

Pawlak KJ, Wiebe JP. Regulatory of estrogen receptor levels in MCF-7 cells by progesterone metbolites. J Steroid Biochem Mol Biol 2007; 106:3–5.

Pawlak KJ, Zhang G, Wiebe JP. Membrane 5α-pregnane-3,20-dione (5αP) receptors in MCF-7 and MCF-10A breast cancer cells are up-related by estradiol and 5αP and down-regulated by progesterone metabolites, 3α-dihydroprogesterone and 20α-dihydroprogesterone, with associated changes in cell proliferation and detachment. J Steroid Biochem Mol Biol 2005; 97:278–288.

Pedersen LC, Petrochenko E, Shevtsov S, Negishi M. Crystal structure of the human estrogen sulfotransferase-PAPS complex: evidence for catalytic role of Ser137 in the sulfuryl transfer reaction. J Biol Chem 2002; 277: 17928–17932.

Peltoketo H, Luu-The V, Simard J, Adamski J. 17β-Hydroxysteroid dehydrogenase (HSD)/17-ketosteroid reductase (KSR); Nomenclature and main characteristics of the 17HSD/KSR enzymes. J Mol Endocrinol 1999; 23:1–11.

Penning TM, Burczynski ME, Jez JM, et al. Structure-function aspects and inhibitor design of type 5 17β-hydroxysteroid dehydrogenase (AKR1C3). Mol Cell Endocrinol 2001; 171:137–149.

Peters RH, Chao WR, Sato K, Shigeno K, Zaveri NT, Tanable M. Steroidal oxathiazine inhibitors of estrone sulfatase. Steroids 2003; 68:97–110.

Pewnim T, Adams JB, Ho KP. Estrogen sulfurylation as an alternative indicator of hormone dependence in human breast cancer. Steroids 1982; 39:47–52.

Pike MC, Spicer DV, Dahmoush L, Press MF. Estrogens, progestogens, normal breast cell proliferation, and breast cancer risk. Epidemiol Rev 1993; 15:17–35.

Pizzagalli F, Varga Z, Huber RD, Folkers G, Meier PJ, St Pierre MV. Identification of steroid sulfate transport process in the human mammary gland. J Clin Endocrinol Metab 2003; 88:3902–3912.

Poirier D, Boivin RP. 17α-Alkyl- or 17α-substituted benzyl-17β-estradiols: a new family of estrone-sulfatase inhibitors. Bioorg Med Chem Lett 1998; 8:1891–1896.

Poirier D, Chang HJ, Azzi A, Boivin RP, Lin S-X. Estrone and estradiol C-16 derivatives as inhitors of type 1 17β-hydroxysteroid deshydrogenase. Mol Endocrinol 2005; 248:236–238.

Pollow K, Boquoi E, Baumann J, Schmidt-Gollwitzer M, Pollow B. Comparison of the in vitro conversion of estradiol-17β to estrone of normal and neoplastic human breast tissue. Mol Cell Endocrinol 1977; 6:333–348.

Prusakiewicz JJ, Harville HM, Zhang Y, Ackermann C, Voorman RL. Parabens inhibit human skin estrogen sulfotransferase activity: possible link to paraben estrogenic effects. Toxicology 2007; 232:148–256.

Purohit A, Tutill HJ, Day JM, Chander SK, Lawrence HR, Allan GM, Fisher DS, Vicker N, Newman SP, Potter BVL, Reed MJ. The regulation and inhibition of 17β-hydroxysteroid deshydrogenase in breast cancer. Mol Cell Endocrinol 2006; 248:199–203.

Purohit A, Vernon KA, Hummelinck AEW, Woo LWL, Hejaz HAM, Potter BVL, Reed MJ. The development of A-ring modified analogues of oestrone-3-*O*-sulphamate as potent steroid sulphatase inhibitors with reduce oestrogenecity. J Steroid Biochem Mol Biol 1998; 64:269–276.

Purohit A, Williams GJ, Howarth NM, Potter BVL, Reed MJ. Inactivation of steroid sulfatase by an active site-directed inhibitor, estrone-3-*O*-sulfamate. Biochemistry 1995; 34:11508–11514.

Qian Y, Deng C, Song W-C. Expression of estrogen sulfotransferase in MCF-7 cells by cDNA transfection suppresses the estrogen response: potential role of the enzyme in regulating estrogen-dependent growth of breast epithelial cells. J Pharmacol Exp Ther 1998; 286:555–560.

Qian Y-M, Sun XJ, Tong MH, Li XP, Richa J, Song W-C. Targeted disruption of the mouse estrogen sulfotransferase gene riveals a role of estrogen metabolism in intracrine and paracrine estrogen regulation. Endocrinology 2001; 142:5342–5350.

Qiu W, Campbell LR, Gangloff A, Dupuis P, Boivin RP, Tremblay MR, Poirier D, Lin SX. A concerted, rational design of type 1 17β-hydroxysteroid dehydrogenase inhibitors: estradiol-adenosine hybrids with high affinity. FASEB J 2002; 16:1829–1831.

Raam S, Robert N, Pappas CA, Tamura H. Defective estrogen receptors in human mammary cancers: their significance in defining hormone dependence. J Natl Cancer Inst 1988; 80:756–761.

Rai D, Frolova A, Frasor J, Carpenter AE, Katzenellenbogen BS. Distinctive actions of membrane-targeted versus nuclear localized estrogen receptors in breast cancer cells. Mol Endocrinol 2005; 19:1606–1617.

Raobaikady B, Day JM, Purohit A, Potter BV, Reed MJ. The nature of inhibition of steroid sulphatase activity by tibolone and its metabolites. J Steroid Biochem Mol Biol 2005; 94:229–237.

Rasmussen LM, Zaveri NT, Stenvang J, Peters RH, Lykkesfeldt AE. A novel dual-target steroid sulfatase inhibitor and antiestrogen: SR 16157, a promising agent for the therapy of breast cancer. Breast Cancer Res Treat 2007; 106:191–203.

Recchione C, Venturelli E, Manzari A, Cavalleri A, Martinetti A, Secreto G. Testosterone dihydotestosterone and oestradiol levels in postmenopausal breast cancer tissues. J Steroid Biochem Mol Biol 1995; 52:541–546.

Reed MJ, Cheng RW, Noel CT, Dudley HAF, James VHT. Plasma levels of estrone, estrone sulfate, and estradiol and the percentage of unbound estradiol in postmenopausal women with and without breast disease. Cancer Res 1983; 43:3940–3943.

Reed JE, Woo LW, Robinson JJ, Leblond B, Leese MP, Purohit A, Reed MJ, Potter BVL. 2-Difluoromethyloestrone 3-*O*-sulfamate, a highly potent steroid sulphatase inhibitor. Biochem Biophys Res Commun 2004; 317:169–175.

Reis-Filho JS, Lakhani SR. The diagnosis and management of pre-invasive breast disease: genetic alterations in pre-invasive lesions. Breast Cancer Res 2003; 5:313–319.

Rogan EG, Badawi AF, Devanesan PD, Meza JL, Edney JA, West WW, Higginbotham SM, Cavalieri E.M. Relative imbalances in estrogen metabolism and conjugation in breast tissue of women with carcinoma: potential biomarkers of susceptibility to cancer. Carcinogenesis 2003; 24:697–702.

Roy AK. Regulation of steroid hormone action in target cells by specific hormone-inactivating enzymes. Proc Soc Exp Biol Med 1992; 199:265–272.

Rozhin J, Corombos JD, Horwitz JP, Brooks SC. Endocrine steroid sulfotransferases: steroid alcohol sulfotransferase from human breast carcinoma cell line MCF-7. J Steroid Biochem 1986; 25:973–979.

Rubin GL, Zhao Y, Kalus AM, Simpson ER. Rubin GL, Zhao Y, Kalus AM, Simpson ER. Peroxisome proliferator-activated receptor gamma ligands inhibit estrogen biosynthesis in human breast adipose tissue: possible implications for breast cancer therapy. Cancer Res 2000; 60:1604–1608.

Russo J, Russo I. Mechanism involved in carcinogenesis of the breast in breast cancer cells. In: Pasqualini JR, ed. Breast Cancer: Prognosis, Treatment and Prevention. New York: Marcel Dekker, Inc, 2002:1–18.

Russo J, Russo I. Breast architecture and pathologenesis of Cancer. In: Pasqualini JR, ed. Breast Cancer Prognosis, Treatment, and Prevention. 2nd ed. New York, London, Boca Raton, Singapore: Informa Healthcare, 2008:1–9.

Ryan PD, Goss PE. Aromatase inhibition in Breast Cancer: Update of clinical applications. In: Pasqualini JR, ed. Breast Cancer Prognosis, Treatment, and Prevention. 2nd ed. New York, London, Boca Raton, Singapore: Informa Healthcare, 2008:169–180.

Saito T, Kinoshita S, Fujii T, Banhoh K, Fuse S, Yamauchi Y, Koizumi N, Horiuchi T. Development of a novel steroid sulfatase inhibitors II. TZS-8478 potently inhibits the growth of breast tumors in postmenopausal breast cancer model rats. J Steroid Biochem Mol Biol 2004; 88:167–173.

Santner SJ, Feil PD, Santen RJ. In situ estrogen production via estrone sulfatase pathway in breast tumors: relative importance versus the aromatase pathway. J Clin Endocrinol Metab 1984; 59:29–33.

Sasano H, Suzuki T, Nakata T, Moriya T. New development in intracrinology of breast carcinoma. Breast Cancer 2006; 13:129–136.

Saunders DE, Lozon MM, Corombos JD, Brooks SC. Role of porcine endometrial estrogen sulfotransferase in progesterone mediated downregulation of estrogen receptor. J Steroid Biochem Mol Biol 1989; 32:749–757.

Sawicki MW, Erman M, Puranen T, Vihko P, Ghosh D. Structure of the ternary complex of human 17b-hydroxysteroid dehydrogenase type 1 with 3-hydroxyestra-1,3,5,7-tetraen-17-one (equilin) and NADP(+). Proc Natl Acad Sci U S A 1999; 96:846–851.

Schäffler A, Schölmerich J, Buechler C. Mechanisms of disease: adipokines and breast cancer—endocrine and paracrine mechanisms that connect adiposity and breast cancer. Nat Clin Pract Endocrinol Metab 2007; 3:345–354.

Schiff R, Fuqua SAW. The importance of the estrogen receptor in breast cancer. In: Pasqualini JR, ed. Breast Cancer: Prognosis, Treatment and Prevention. New York: Marcel Dekker, Inc, 2002:149–186.

Schrag ML, Cui D, Rushmore TH, Shou M, Ma B, Rodrigues AD. Sulfotransferase 1E1 is a low K-M isoform mediating the 3-*O*-sulfatation of ethinyl estradiol. Drug Metab Dispos 2004; 32:1299–1303.

Schreiner EP, Billich A. Estrone formate: a novel type of irreversible inhibitor of human steroid sulfatase. Bioorg Med Chem Lett 2004; 14:4999–5002.

Schütze N, Vollmer G, Tiemann M, Geiger M, Knuppen R. Catecholestogens are MCF-7 cell estrogen receptor agonists. J Steroid Biochem Mol Biol 1993; 46:781–789.

Seeger H, Diesing D, Guckel B, Wallwiener D, Mueck AO, Huober J. Effect of tamoxifen and 2-methoxyestradiol alone and in combination on human breast cancer cell proliferation. J Steroid Biochem Mol Biol 2003; 84: 255–257.

Seeger H, Huober J, Wallweiner D, Mueck AO. Inhibition of human breast cancer cell proliferation with estradiol metabolites is as effective as with tamoxifen. Horm Metab Res 2004; 36:277–280.

Segaloff A. Hormones and mammary carcinogenis In: McGuire WL, ed. Breast Cancer 2: Advances in Research and Treatment. New York: Plenum Press, 1978:1–22.

Selcer KW, DiFrancesca H, Chandra AB, Li P-K. Immunohistochemical analysis of steroid sulfatase in human tissues. J Steroid Biochem Mol Biol 2007; 105:115–123.

Shields-Botella J, Chetrite G, Meschi S, Pasqualini JR. Effect of nomegestrol acetate on estrogens biosynthesis and transformation in the MCF-7 and T47-D breast cancer cells. J Steroid Biochem Mol Biol 2005; 93:327–335.

Shwed JA, Walle UK, Walle T. Hep G2 cell line as a human model for sulphate conjugation of drugs. Xenobiotica 1992; 22:973–982.

Simpson PT, Gale T, Fulford LG, Reis-Filho JS, Lakhani SR. The diagnosis and management of pre-invasive breast disease: pathology of atypical lobular hyperplasia and lobular carcinoma in situ. Breast Cancer Res 2003; 5:258–262.

Simpson ER, Jones M, Misso M, Hewitt K, Hill R, Maffei C, Carani C, Boon WC. Estrogen, a fundamental player in energy homeotasis. J Steroid Biochem Mol Biol 2005; 95:3–8.

Song D, Liu G, Luu-The V, Zhao D, Wang L, Zhang H, Xueling G, Li S, Desy L, Labrie F, Pelletier G. Expression of aromatase and 17b-hydroxysteroid dehydrogenase Type 1, 7, and 12 in breast cancer. An immunocytochemical study. J Steroid Biochem Mol Biol 2006; 101:136–144.

Sparks R, Ulrich CM, Bigler J, Tworoger SS, Yasui Y, Rajan KB, Porter P, Stanczyk FZ, Ballard-Barbash R, Yuan X, Lin MG, McVarish L, Aiello EJ, McTiernan A. UDP-glucuronosyltransferase and sulfotransferase polymorphisms, sex hormone concentrations, and tumor receptor status in breast cancer patients. Breast Cancer Res 2004; 6:R488–R498.

Speirs V, Green AR, Atkins L. Activity and gene expression of 17β-hydroxysteroid dehydrogenases type 1 in primary cultures of epithelial and stromal cells derived from normal and tumurous human breast tissue: the role of IL-8. J Steroid Biochem Mol Biol 1998; 67:267–274.

Stanway SJ, Purohit A, Woo L, Sufi S, Vigushin D, Ward R, Wilson RH, Stanczyk FZ, Dobbs N, Kulinskaya E, Elliot M, Pottter BVL, Reed MJ, Coombes RC. Phase 1 study of STX 64 (667 Coumate) in breast cancer patients: the first study of a steroid sulfatase inhibitor. Clin Cancer Res 2006; 12:1585–1592.

Suto A, Bradlow HL, Wong GY, Osborne MP, Telang NT. Persitent estrogen responsiveness of ras oncogene-transformed mouse mammary epthelial cells. Steroids 1992; 57:262–268.

Suzuki T, Miki Y, Nakata T, Shiotsu Y, Akinaga S, Inoue K, Ishida T, Kimura M, Moriya T, Sasano H. Steroid sulfatase and estrogen sulfotransferase in normal human tissue and breast carcinoma. J Steroid Biochem Mol Biol 2003a; 86:449–454.

Suzuki T, Nakata T, Miki Y, Kaneko C, Moriya T, Ishida T, Akinaga S, Hirakawa G, Kimura M, Sasano H. Estrogen sulfotransferase and steroid sulfatase in human breast carcinoma. Cancer Res 2003b; 63:2763–2770.

Tang D, Rundle A, Mooney L, Cho S, Schnabel F, Estabrook A, Kelly A, Levine R, Hibshoosh H, Perera F. Sulfotransferase 1A1 (SULTA1) polymorphism, PAH-DNA adduct levels in breast tissue and breast cancer risk in a case-control study. Breast Cancer Res Treat 2003; 78:217–222.

Telang NT, Narayanan R, Bradlow HL, Wong GY, Osborne MP. Coordinated expression of intermediate biomarkers for tumorigenic transformation in RAS-transfected mouse mammary epithelial cells. Breast Cancer Res Treat 1991; 18:155–163.

Thibaudeau J, Lepine J, Tojcic J, Duguay Y, Pelletier G, Plante M, Brisson M, Tetu B, Jacob S, Perusse L, Belanger A, Guillemette C. Characterization of common UGT1A8, UGT1A8, and UGT2B7 variants with different capacities to inactive mutagenic 4-hydroxylated metabolites of estradiol and estrone. Cancer Res 2006; 66:125–133.

Thijssen JH, Blankenstein MA. Endogenous oestrogens and androgens in normal and malignant endometrial and mammary tissues. Eur J Cancer Clin Oncol 1989; 25:1953–1959.

Thijssen JH, Daroszewski J, Milewicz A, Blankenstein MA. Local aromatase activity in human breast tissues. J Steroid Biochem Mol Biol 1993; 44:577–582.

Tobacman JK, Hinkhouse M, Khalkhali-Ellis Z. Steroid sulfatase activity and expression in mammary myoepithelial cells. J Steroid Biochem Mol Biol 2002; 81:65–68.

Townsley JD, Scheel EJ, Rubin EJ. Inhibition of steroid-3-sulfatase by endogenous steroids. A possible mechanism controling placental estrogen synthesis from conjugated precursors. J Clin Endocrinol Metab 1970; 311:670–678.

Tremblay MR, Boivin RP, Luu-The V, Poirier D. Inhibitors of type 1 17β-hydroxysteroid dehydrogenase with reduced estrogenicactivity: modifications of the positions 3 and 6 of estradiol. J Enzyme Inhib Med Chem 2005; 20:153–163.

Tremblay MR, Lin SX, Poirier D. Chemical synthesis of 16beta-propylaminoacyl derivatives of estradiol and their inhibitory potency on type 1 17beta-hydroxysteroid dehydrogenase and binding affinity on steroid receptors. Steroids 2001; 66:821–831.

Tremblay MR, Poirier D. Overview of a rational approch to design type I 17β-hydroxysteroid dehydrogenase inhibitors without estrogenic activity: chemical synthesis and biological evaluation. J Steroid Biochem Mol Biol 1998; 66:179–191.

Tseng L, Liu HC. Stimulation arylsulfotransferase activity by progestins in human endometrium in vitro. J Clin Endocrinol Metab 1981; 53:418–421.

Tukey RH, Strassburg CP. Human UDP-glucuronosyltransferases: metabolism, expression, and disease. Annu Rev Pharmacol Toxicol 2000; 40:581–616.

Tworoger SS, Eliassen AE, Kelesidis T, Colditz GA, Willet WC, Mantzoros C, Hankinson SE. Plasma adiponectin concentrations and risk of incident breast cancer. J Clin Endocrinol Metab 2007; 92:1510–1516.

Utsumi T, Yoshimura N, Takeuchi S, Maruta M, Maeda K, Harada N. Elevated steroid sulfatase expression in breast cancers. J Steroid Biochem Mol Biol 2000; 73:141–145.

van Duursen MB, Sanderson JT, de Jong PC, Kraaij M, van den Berg M. Phytochemicals inhibit catechol-O-methyltransferase activity in cytosolic fractions from healthy human mammary tissues: implications for catechol estrogen-induced DNA damage. Toxicol Sci 2004; 81:316–324.

van Landeghem AAJ, Poortman J, Nabuurs M, Thijssen JHH. Endogenous concentration and subcellular distribution of androgens in normal and malignant human breast tissue. Cancer Res 1985; 45:2907–2912.

Vermeulen A, Deslypere JP, Paridaens R, Leclercq G, Roy F, Heuson JC. Aromatase, 17β-hydroxysteroid deshydrogenase and intratissular sex hormone concentrations in cancerous and normal glandular breast tissue in postmenopausal women. Eur J Cancer Clin Oncol 1986; 22:515–525.

Vihko P, Herrala A, Härkönen P, Isomaa V, Kaija H, Kurkela R, Pulkka A. Control of cell proliferation by steroids: the role of 17HSDs. Mol Cell Endocrinol 2006; 248:141–148.

Vihko P, Isomaa V, Ghosh D. Structure and function of 17beta-hydroxysteroid dehydrogenase type 1 and type 2. Mol Cell Endocrinol 2001; 171:71–76.

Vijayanathan V, Venkiteswaran S, Nair SK, Verma A, Thomas TJ, Zhu BT, Thomas T. Physiologic levels of 2-methoxyestradiol interfere with nongenomic signaling of 17beta-estradiol in human breast cancer cells. Clin Cancer Res 2006; 12:2038–2048.

Vos RM, Krebbers SF, Verhoeven CH, Delbressine LP. The in vivo human metabolism of tibolone. Drug Metab Dispos 2002; 30:106–112.

Walle T, Eaton EA, Walle UK. Quercetin, a potent and specific inhibitor of the human P-form phenolsulfotransferase. Biochem Pharmacol 1995; 50:731–734.

Walter G, Liebl R, von Angerer E. 2-Phenylindole sulfamates: inhibitors of steroid sulfatase with antiproliferative activity in MCF-7 breast cancer cells. J Steroid Biochem Mol Biol 2004a; 88:409–420.

Walter G, Liebl R, von Angerer E. Stilbene-based inhibitors of estrone sulfatase with a dual mode of action in human breast cancer cells. Arch Pharm (Weinheim) 2004b; 337:634–644.

Wang LQ, James MO. Sulfotransferase 2AI forms estradiol-17-sulfate and celecoxib switches the dominant product from estradiol-3-sulfate to estradiol-17-sulfate. J Steroid Biochem Mol Biol 2005; 96:367–374.

Wiebe JP. Progesterone metabolites in breast cancer. Endocr Relat Cancer 2006; 13:717–738.
Wiebe JP, Lewis MJ, Cialacu V, Pawlak KJ, Zhang G. The role of progesterone metabolites in breast cancer: potential for new diagnostics and therapeutics. J Steroid Biochem Mol Biol 2005; 93:201–208.
Wiebe JP, Muzia D, Hu J, Szwajcer D, Hill SA, Seachrist JL. The 4-pregnene and 5α-pregnane progesterone metabolites formed in non-tumorous and tumorous breast tissue have opposite effects on breast cells proliferation and adhesion. Cancer Res 2000; 60:936–943.
Wild MJ, Rudland PS, Back DJ. Metabolism of the oral contraceptive steroids ethynylestradiol and norgestimate by normal (Huma 7) and malignant (MCF-7 and ZR 75-1) human breast cells in culture. J Steroid Biochem Mol Biol 1991; 39:535–543.
Winum JY, Scozzafava A, Montero JL, Supuran CT. Sulfamates and their therapeutic potential. Med Res Rev 2005; 25: 186–228.
Woo LWL, Bubert C, Sutcliffe OB, Smith A, Chander SK, Mahon MF, Purohit A, Reed MJ, Potter BVL. Dual aromatase-steroid sulfatase inhibitors. J Med Chem 2007; 50:3540–3560.
Wood PM, Woo LW, Humphreys A, Chander SK, Purohit A, Reed MJ, Potter BV. A letrozole-based dual aromatase-sulphatase inhibitor with in vivo activity. J Steroid Biochem Mol Biol 2005; 94:123–130.
Xu B, Kitawaki J, Koshiba H, Ishihara H, Kiyomizu M, Teramoto M, Kitaoka Y, Honjo H. Differential effects of progestogens, by type and regimen, on estrogen-metabolizing enzymes in human breast cancer cells. Maturitas 2007; 56:142–152.
Yager JD, Davidson MD. Estrogen carcinogenesis in breast cancer. N Engl J Med 2006; 354:270–282.
Yamaguchi Y, Takei H, Suemasu K, Kobayashi Y, Kurosumi M, Harada N and Hayashi S-I. Tumor-stromal interaction through the estrogen-signaling pathway in human breast cancer. Cancer Res 2005; 65:4653–6462.
Yamamoto Y, Yamashita J, Toi M, Muta M, Nagai S, Hanai N, Furuya A, Osawa Y, Saji S, Ogawa M. Immunohistochemical analyssis of estrone sulfatase and aromatase in human breast cancer tissues. Oncol Rep 2003; 10:791–796.
Yasuda S, Suiko M, Liu MC. Oral contraceptives as substrates and inhibitors for human cytosolic SULTs. J Biochem (Tokyo) 2005; 137:401–406.
Yee LD, Williams N, Wen P, Young DC, Lester J, Johnson MV, Farrar WB, Walker MJ, Povoski SP, Suster S, Eng C. Pilot study of rosiglitazone therapy in women with breast cancer: effects of short-term therapy on tumor tissue and serum markers. Clin Cancer Res 2007; 13:246–252.
Yoshimura N, Harada N, Bukholm I, Karesen R, Borresen-Dale AL, Kristensen VN. Intratumoural mRNA expression of genes from the oestradiol metabolic pathway and clinical and histopathological parameters of breast cancer. Breast Cancer Res 2004; 6:R46–R55.
Zajchowski DA, Sager R, Webster L. Estrogen inhibits the growth of estrogen receptor-negative, but not estrogen receptor-positive, human mammary epithelial cells expressing a recombinant estrogen receptor. Cancer Res 1993; 53:5004–5011.
Zeleniuch-Jacquotte A, Shore RE, Koenig KL, Akhmedkhanov A, Afanasyeva Y, Kato I, Kim MY. Postmenopausal levels of oestrogen, androgen, and SHBG and breast cancer: long-term results of a prospective study. Br J Cancer 2004; 90:153–159.
Zhang HP, Varlamova O, Vargas FM, Falany CN, Leyh TS, Varmalova O. Sulfuryl transfer: the catalytic mechanism of human estrogen sulfotransferase. J Biol Chem 1998; 273:10888–10892.
Zheng W, Xie D, Cerhan JR, Sellers TA, Wen W, Folsom AR. Sulfotransferase 1A1 polymorphism, endogenous estogen exposure, well-done meat intake, and breast cancer rsik. Cancer Epidemiol Biomarkers Prev 2001; 10:89–94.
Zhu BT, Conney AH. Is 2-methoxyestradiol an endogenous estrogen metabolite that inhibits mammary carcinogenis. Cancer Res 1998; 58:2269–2277.

3

Pregnancy and Breast Cancer

JAN WOHLFAHRT and MADS MELBYE
Department of Epidemiology Research, Statens Serum Institute, Copenhagen, Denmark

INTRODUCTION

For many years it has been known that women have a lower risk of breast cancer following childbirth compared with before childbirth, and that the younger the woman is at first childbirth, the larger is the risk reduction after childbirth. (Kelsey et al., 1993). The reduction is not only seen immediately after birth or in the reproductive years, but is a long-term effect probably present throughout life. However, there is also evidence that in the first few years after giving birth, the woman experiences a short-term increased risk of breast cancer (Lambe et al., 1994). The mechanisms behind this dual effect of pregnancy are still unclear. The dominating explanation for these findings has been that the elevated level of endogenous hormones during pregnancy, and on the one hand induces a long-term reduction by stimulating a terminal differentiation of breast cells making them less prone to any carcinogenic process, on the other hand induces a short-term increased risk by stimulating growth in already existing occult tumors (Miller, 1993).

This review is not intended to be a complete discussion of the association between pregnancy and breast cancer risk. It focuses on epidemiological aspects of the topics dealt with within our research group. Only when suited for this perspective will endocrinological and clinical aspects be included.

THE LONG-TERM EFFECT

Age at Birth

Since MacMahon and colleagues in 1970 showed that age at first childbirth was related to breast cancer risk, many subsequent studies have confirmed that age at first childbirth is important for a woman's risk of breast cancer (Kelsey et al., 1993; MacMahon et al., 1970). The dominating explanation has been that a birth through endogenous hormones in the final phase of pregnancy stimulates a final differentiation of breast cells, thereby making the cells less prone to carcinogenic stimuli and thus to malignant development (Miller, 1993). Evidently, an early childbirth induces an early differentiation and thereby a lower risk. However, also subsequent births reduce the maternal breast cancer risk. Figure 1 shows the effect of age at first birth and multiparity in three Nordic countries with register-based information from studies in the Danish cohort (Wohlfahrt et al., 1999b), Norway (Albrektsen et al., 1994), and Sweden (Lambe et al., 1996b).

The effect of age at first birth is very similar and shows that compared with women with a first childbirth at age 20 to 24, a woman with a first childbirth at 30 years of age or older has around 30% higher breast cancer risk. This underlines the importance of the first childbirth. Also the effect of subsequent births is similar in these studies

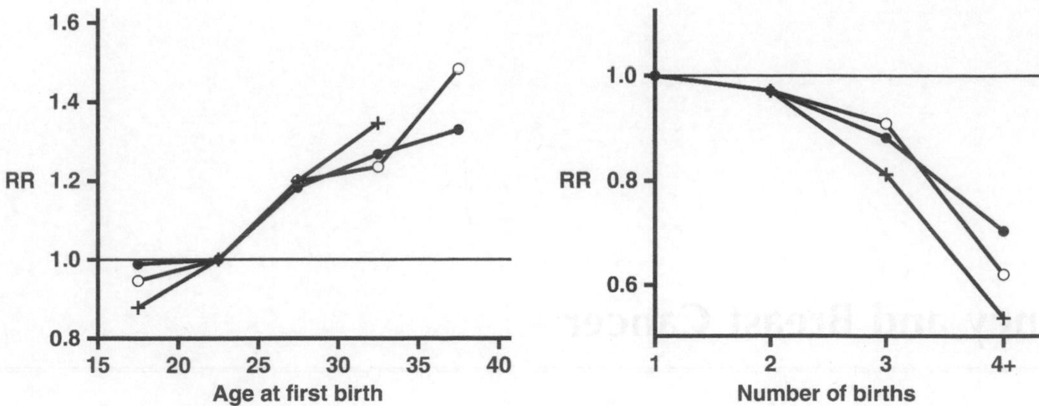

Figure 1 Relative risk of breast cancer according to age at first birth (*left*) (reference = 20–24 years) and number of births (*right*) (reference = uniparous) in three Nordic countries. (•) Denmark: (Wohlfahrt et al., 1999b), (+) Norway: (Albrektsen et al., 1994), (o) Sweden: (Lambe et al., 1996b). The 4+ estimates for Norway and Sweden is an inverse variance–weighted estimate of estimates from groups of women with higher parity.

and shows that compared with women with one childbirth, women with four births or more have around 30% lower breast cancer risk. With these relatively large effects of later births, it is natural to speculate whether the age at later births likewise is of importance and if so, whether the effect is of the same magnitude as the first birth.

Table 1 presents summarized results from studies on the independent effect of age at childbirths subsequent to the first where it was possible to extract a trend estimate. The largest study is from the Danish cohort where it was observed that the risk of breast cancer increased by 9% (5–12%) per five-year increase in age at first birth (Wohlfahrt and Melbye, 2001). However, age at subsequent births also affected the breast cancer risk. Thus, the breast cancer risk increased by 7% (4–11%), 5% (0–11%), and 14% (4–26%) per five-year increase in age at second, third, and fourth birth, respectively. Comparing the effects of first to fourth birth, they were found to be equal with a general increase of 8% (6–9%) per five-year increase in age at first to fourth birth. A study from the United States, including 9891 cases, also observed an effect of age at any birth, although with a stronger effect of age at first birth compared with subsequent births (Chie et al., 2000). They reported that breast cancer risk increased by 7% (1–13%) per five-year increase in age at first birth, and 2% (0–5%) per five-year increase in age at subsequent births.

Summarizing the results from the studies presented in Table 1 by an inverse variance–weighted regression, the increase in risk by five-year increase in age at first and subsequent births was 11% and 5%. Although the two largest studies differed in the estimation of the relative importance of the age at births subsequent to the first, they agree on the importance of age at all births, thereby suggesting a similar mechanism behind the risk reduction after any birth.

Table 1 Studies on the Relative Increase in Maternal Breast Cancer Risk per Five-Year Increase in Age at First Birth and per Five-Year Increase in Age at Subsequent Births

Study	Design	Cases	First birth RR (%) (95% CI)	Subsequent births RR (%) (95% CI)
Trichopoulos et al., 1983	Hospital case control	4,225	19% (12–26%)	5% (2–8%)
Rosner et al., 1994[a]	Cohort	2,249	9% —	2% —
Decarli et al., 1996[b]	Hospital case control	2,569	25% (15–37%)	4% (−4–11%)
Robertson et al., 1997	Population case control	624	24% (5–51%)	5% (−10–22%)
Chie et al., 2000	Population case control	9,891	7% (1–13%)	2% (0–5%)
Wohlfahrt and Melbye, 2001[c]	Cohort	13,049	9% (5–12%)	7% (5–9%)
Summary[d]	—	—	11% (9–13%)	5% (4–6%)

[a]Estimate for premenopausal women.
[b]Estimate for subsequent births is an inverse variance–weighted estimate of parity-specific estimates.
[c]Estimate for subsequent births is not presented in the paper but calculated for this review.
[d]Summary measures are based on inverse weighted estimation with Rosner et al. (1994) weighted as Decarli et al. (1996).
Abbreviation: RR, risk ratio.

Obviously, early timing of births is related to relatively lower breast cancer risk, but this does not indicate whether the risk reduction occurs after births at any age. MacMahon noted in his review on the etiology of human breast cancer from 1973 that the risk reduction after first birth only was seen in women younger than 30 years at birth (MacMahon et al., 1973). This has led to the idea that the period as nulliparous before first birth is a specially vulnerable time window (Russo and Russo, 1997). However, investigations in the Danish cohort revealed that exactly the same pattern could be seen for subsequent births, i.e. subsequent births before the age of 30 are associated with a risk reduction (Wohlfahrt and Melbye, 2001). These risk-reducing effects of young age at subsequent births are illustrated in Figure 2, where the relative risk of breast cancer after second, third, and fourth birth is compared with the risk among women with one birth less. These findings again underline the seemingly similar effect of first and subsequent births, and that it would be more reasonable to assume that the life period before 30 years of age is the vulnerable time period in life, but only in the sense that a woman in that period can change her lifetime risk of breast cancer by having childbirths.

MacMahon furthermore noted in his review from 1973 that the effect of age at first birth seemed to persist even in women older than 75 years (MacMahon et al., 1973). Subsequent studies have observed a stronger effect of age at first birth (and a lesser/no effect of multiparity) on breast cancer risk in younger women compared with older women (Velentgas and Daling, 1994). However, in the Danish cohort study the same effect of age at (any) birth in

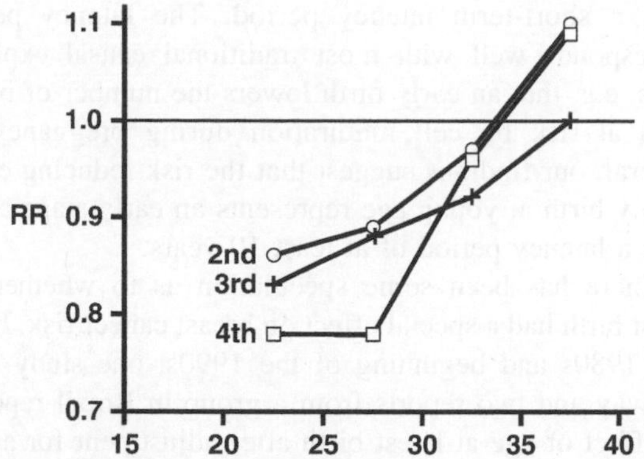

Figure 2 Relative risk of breast cancer more than 10 years after second, third, fourth birth compared with women with one birth less according to age at birth in the Danish cohort. *Source*: Wohlfahrt and Melbye, 2001.

women below 50 years and women 50 years or older was observed.

Besides attained age, an even more etiology-revealing time stratification appears to be time since birth. Thus, when stratifying the effect of age at birth by time since birth, the effect was restricted to more than 10 years after birth [7% (6–9%)], whereas there was no effect the first 10 years after birth [2% (2–5%)]. Performing approximate calculation of the effect of age at first birth by time since first birth in other studies (without this being necessarily the specific purpose of these studies) revealed, to some degree, the same pattern (Fig. 3). Thus, according to our findings the effect of age at birth is a long-term effect, but

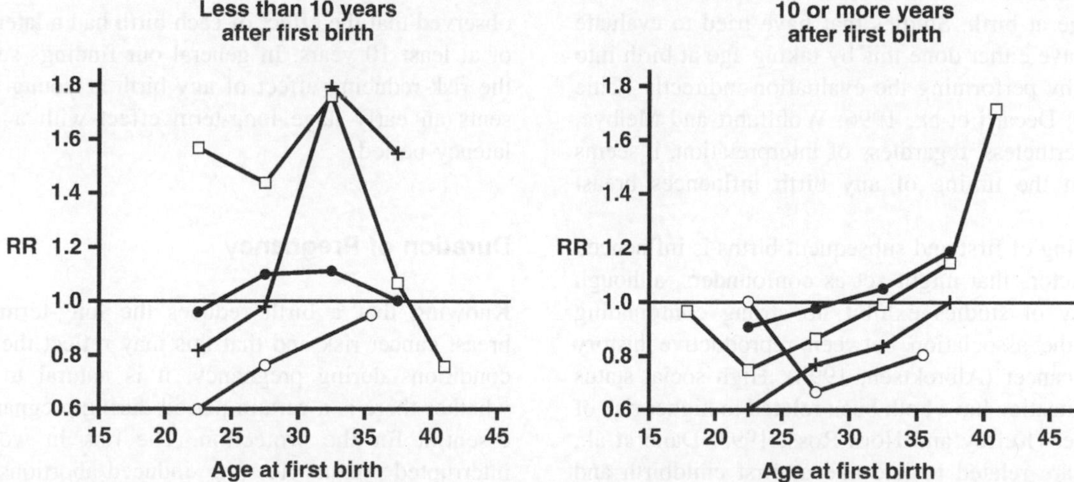

Figure 3 Studies on cancer risk in uniparous compared with nulliparous according to age at first birth the first 10 years after birth (*left*) and 10 or more years after birth (*right*). (o): (Cummings et al., 1997) table 4. Estimates for the time intervals 0 to 5 and 6 to 11 years are combined as a weighted average, as are the periods 12 to 17 and ≥18. (□): (Lambe et al., 1994) data from first and last result rows in table 3 in the parallel method paper (Hsieh and Lan, 1996). The estimate for age at first birth less than 20 years in the period less than 10 years after first birth (OR = 3.47 (0.63–19.02), $n = 3$) is not included. (•): Wohlfahrt and Melbye, (2001, table 2) (estimation includes multiparous). (+): Hsieh et al. (1994, first and last result rows in table 3). The RR estimate of 2.26 for 30 to 34 years at first birth during the first 10 years after birth is substituted by 1.8 for graphical convenience.

with a short-term latency period. The latency period corresponds well with most traditional causal explanations, e.g. that an early birth lowers the number of breast cells at risk by cell maturation during pregnancy. In general, our findings suggest that the risk-reducing effect of any birth at young age represents an early-stage effect with a latency period of at least 10 years.

There has been some speculation as to whether the latest birth had a special effect on breast cancer risk. In the late 1980s and beginning of the 1990s, one study from Norway and two reports from a group in Brazil reported an effect of age at latest birth after adjustment for age at first birth (Kvale and Heuch, 1987; Kalache et al., 1993; Albrektsen et al., 1994). In the Danish cohort, a strong effect of age at latest birth was observed when adjustment was restricted to age at first birth. However, after adjustment for the effects of age at first and subsequent births, there was no independent effect of age at latest birth (Wohlfahrt and Melbye, 2001). Likewise, two other studies found no effect of latest birth after adjustment for births subsequent to the first (Chie et al., 2000; Hsieh et al., 1996). Therefore, in addition to the lack of a biological rationale for an effect of age at latest birth, the study from the Danish cohort supports the idea that these findings are artifacts representing the effects of age at first and subsequent births.

An alternative way to interpret the importance of the timing of pregnancies is that young age at birth is essential combined with shortness of interbirth intervals. In other words, early timing of subsequent births might be important due to short interbirth time intervals. An effect of interbirth intervals is very difficult to separate from the effect of age at birth. Studies that have tried to evaluate the effect have either done this by taking age at birth into account or by performing the evaluation indirectly (Chie et al., 2000; Decarli et al., 1996; Wohlfahrt and Melbye, 2001). Nevertheless, regardless of interpretation, it seems evident that the timing of any birth influences breast cancer risk.

Late timing of first and subsequent births is influenced by many factors that might act as confounders, although the majority of studies exhibit no strong confounding effects on the association between reproductive history and breast cancer (Albrektsen, 1998). High social status and high education have both been related to higher risk of breast cancer (Kelsey and Horn-Ross, 1993; Dano et al., 2003) and are related to late age at first childbirth and probably number and timing of subsequent births, although this is less obvious in modern society. However, the association between high socioeconomic status and breast cancer is primarily thought to reflect the association between reproductive history and breast cancer and not the opposite (Kelsey and Horn-Ross, 1993). Thus, in a recent Nordic study it was found that the association between education and breast cancer risk could be explained by reproductive and anthropometric factors, with parity and age at first childbirth explaining 50% of the association (Braaten et al., 2004). Furthermore, if the risk reduction after a birth simply was a marker of the maternal socioeconomic situation, one should expect an apparent risk reduction immediately after birth and not only some years after birth. Also subfertility influences the number and timing of births and may therefore act as a confounder. Subfertility is related to old age at childbirth and can be related to a special level of endogenous hormones. However, several studies have found no enhanced risk in subfertile women (Klip et al., 2000). Early timing of menarche and late menopause are both risk factors and may also influence the number and timing of births. However, in modern society, the influence of early menarche on reproductive history is probably small, and late menopause is, if anything, associated with high parity. Breastfeeding is associated with high parity and low breast cancer risk. However, results from the Collaborative Group on Hormonal Factors in Breast Cancer reveal that the protective effect of births cannot be explained by subsequent breastfeeding (Collaborative Group on Hormonal Factors in Breast Cancer, 2002b).

In conclusion, it is generally accepted that a first birth before 30 years of age reduces breast cancer risk, and that subsequent births further reduce the risk. The importance of age at subsequent births is less known. Using the Danish cohort, we found that the long-term risk reduction after birth depends on the age at birth in a similar way for first and subsequent births, i.e. any birth at early age has a similar, long-term reducing effect. We furthermore observed that the effect of each birth had a latency period of at least 10 years. In general our findings suggest that the risk-reducing effect of any birth at young age represents an early-stage long-term effect with a short-term latency period.

Duration of Pregnancy

Knowing that a birth reduces the long-term maternal breast cancer risk and that this may reflect the hormonal conditions during pregnancy, it is natural to speculate whether there is a certain period during pregnancy that is essential for the protection. The risk in women with interrupted pregnancies (e.g. induced abortions) and preterm births can give an epidemiological indication of whether women "missing" specific periods of pregnancy have a different risk profile, thereby revealing these missing periods as essential.

The association between induced abortion and breast cancer has been much debated, not only because of the etiological importance, but also because of the sensitive nature of induced abortion. A meta-analysis based on a selection of case-control studies found a significantly increased risk of 1.3 (1.2–1.4) in women with a history of induced abortion (Brind et al., 1996). However, the use of case-control studies raises concern about the potential problem of differential misclassification. Even after its legalization, abortion remains a sensitive issue. It is therefore likely that women with breast cancer may be more willing to report induced abortions than healthy women. This bias can be avoided in cohort studies with exposure information collected before the diagnosis of breast cancer. This is evident in the large collaborative reanalysis of data from 53 epidemiological studies where the relative risk of breast cancer in women with and in women without history of induced abortion was 1.11 (se = 0.025) in studies with retrospective information on induced abortion, but only 0.93 (se = 0.020) in studies with prospective data (Beral et al., 2004). By far the largest study is the Danish cohort with 10,247 breast cancer cases (Melbye et al., 1997). In this study the relative risk between women with and without a history of induced abortion was 1.00 (0.94–1.06).

The overall lack of effect of induced abortion suggests that a pregnancy termination in first trimester (where almost all induced abortions are performed) is not related to an enhanced risk. However, a very small proportion of induced abortions are performed in the second trimester, and if these could be identified, an investigation of the effect of second trimester could be performed. Unfortunately almost all the studies do not report the breast cancer risk according to the duration of pregnancy before the induced abortion. In a case control study from 1994, Daling et al. found no clear pattern according to gestational age, 1 to 8 weeks: 1.4 (1.0–1.8), 9 to 12 weeks: 1.9 (1.3–2.9), ≥13 weeks: 1.4 (0.7–2.8) (Daling et al., 1994). But in a study from 1996, they observed an opposite association, 1 to 8 weeks: 1.4 (1.1–1.8), ≥9 weeks: 1.1 (0.8–1.4). Likewise in a Dutch case-control study, no clear pattern was seen, 1 to 8 weeks: 2.1 (1.1–4.2), >8 weeks: 1.6 (0.8–3.5) (Rookus and van Leeuwen, 1995). The studies were based on self-reported information. In the Danish cohort, the information on gestational age was available from the National Registry of Induced Abortions (Melbye et al., 1997). A significant increase in risk was observed according to gestational age among women with induced abortion in the study from 1997, <7 weeks: 0.81 (0.58−1.13), 7 to 8 weeks: 1.01 (0.89−1.14), 9 to 10 weeks: 1(ref), 11 to 12 weeks: 1.12 (0.95−1.31), 13 to 14 weeks: 1.13 (0.51−2.53), 15 to 18 weeks: 1.23 (0.76−2.00), >18 weeks: 1.89 (1.11–3.22). However, in an updated analysis in the Danish cohort, including pregnancies and breast cancer cases up to the end of 2000, the overall finding of no association was confirmed, but an association between the gestational age of latest induced abortion and breast cancer risk was no longer observed (unpublished data).

Another way to evaluate the impact of pregnancy duration on breast cancer risk is to study the risk of breast cancer in women with preterm births. Besides an early study from 1983 that found no effect (Polednak and Janerich, 1983), all studies on this subject have been published since 1998 (Table 2).

In a very small cohort study from Finland (Smith et al., 2000) and in a study from the Unites States (Troisi et al., 1998), there was no association between gestational age and breast cancer risk, however in the latter no measure size was presented and all types of pregnancies were included. In a Swedish study Hiseh et al. (1999) found an enhanced risk in women with a history of premature delivery (risk ratio = 1.17 (0.98–1.40)). Interestingly, they only observed the effect more than 10 years after the birth and in women older than 40 years, clearly stressing the long-term nature of the effect. In the Danish cohort, the relative risk associated with preterm births is 1.21 (0.96–1.51) (Table 2). Summarizing the results in Table 2, the risk of breast cancer is 1.15 (1.01–1.32) in women with

Table 2 Studies on the Relative Risk of Maternal Breast Cancer in Women with a History of Preterm Birth Compared with Women with no History of Preterm Birth and Extremely Preterm Birth Compared with no Extremely Preterm Birth

Study	Design	Cases: all (preterm)[a]	<37 wk vs. ≥37 wk RR (95%)	<32 vs. ≥32 wk RR (95%)
Polednak and Janerich, 1983[b]	Case control	314 (12)	0.81 (0.45–1.38)	0.33 (0.06–1.00)
Hsieh et al., 1999	Population case control	2318 (—)	1.17 (0.98–1.40)	—
Melbye et al., 1999[c]	Cohort	1363 (81)	1.21 (0.96–1.51)	1.72 (1.14–2.59)
Smith et al., 2000	Cohort	40 (—)	0.31 (0.04–2.29)	—
Summary			1.15 (1.01–1.32)	

[a]Number of extremely preterm births was 1 (Polednak and Janerich, 1983) and 20 (Melbye et al., 1999).
[b]Used 31 and 37 weeks as cutpoints.
[c]The estimate for "<37 weeks vs. ≥37 weeks" is not presented in the paper, but is calculated for this review.
Abbreviation: RR, risk ratio.

Table 3 Adjusted[a] Relative Risk of Breast Cancer in 474,156 Parous Women According to Gestational Age at Delivery (Melbye et al., 1999)

Gestational age (weeks)	Number of cases	Person years ($\times 10^3$)	RR (95% CI)
<29	7	9	2.11 (1.00–4.45)
29–31	13	17	2.08 (1.20–3.60)
32–33	11	26	1.12 (0.62–2.04)
34–35	22	58	1.08 (0.71–1.66)
36–37	82	214	1.04 (0.83–1.32)
38–39	350	949	1.02 (0.89–1.17)
40	552	1526	1 (reference)[b]
>40	326	985	1.03 (0.90–1.18)

[a]Adjusted for age, calendar period, parity, and age at first birth.
[b]Reference category for the adjusted relative risk.
Abbreviation: RR, risk ratio.

preterm births compared with term births. In the Danish cohort, a significant association between a further categorized gestational age and breast cancer was observed (Table 3). Thus, a clearly higher risk was observed in women with extremely preterm birth compared with other women, RR = 1.72 (1.14–2.59) (Table 2).

The association with extremely preterm, as well as preterm, birth could be due to confounding. Smoking during pregnancy and high pre-pregnancy body weight have been linked to preterm birth as well as low social class and low educational level (Schieve et al., 2000; Slattery and Morrison, 2002). However, there is no association between smoking and breast cancer (Collaborative Group on Hormonal Factors in Breast Cancer, 2002a), and low socioeconomic status is associated with low breast cancer risk (Kelsey and Horn-Ross, 1993; Dano et al., 2003). The association between high body mass and premenopausal breast cancer is, if anything, inverse (Friedenreich, 2001), and confounding by body weight among the relatively young cases in the two studies is therefore not likely. However, as high body mass is associated with postmenopausal breast cancer, future studies on postmenopausal generations should take this into account.

The lack of association with pregnancy duration in induced abortions and the slightly increased risk in women with a preterm birth suggest that only a full-term birth induces a reduced risk (assuming an approximate average of 10–20% risk reduction after a full-term birth). In other words, the finding suggests that the risk reduction after a birth is due to factors occurring late in pregnancy. Combined with the even higher relative risk in women with an extremely preterm birth, this is a novel support for Russo and Russo's hypothesis that only a full-term pregnancy allows complete differentiation of breast cells, thereby reducing the breast cancer risk, whereas an extremely preterm delivery hinders the late protective effect of differentiation, thereby increasing the subsequent breast cancer risk. On the contrary, neither the finding on induced abortion nor preterm birth corresponds with the alternative hypothesis that the reduced risk after a birth is due to temporary removal of normal hormonal stimulation while the woman is pregnant. In that case, the risk change after a pregnancy should to a higher degree be proportional to duration of pregnancy.

In conclusion, using the Danish cohort with register-based information on induced abortions, it was shown that induced abortion is not associated with subsequent breast cancer risk. Breast cancer risk is not associated with gestational age in pregnancies with short duration (induced abortions), whereas women with a term birth had a lower risk compared with women with an extremely preterm birth. Taken together, this suggests that the risk reduction after a birth is due to factors occurring late in pregnancy, and the finding is therefore a novel support for Russo and Russo's hypothesis.

Subtype at Diagnosis

One way to study the differential effect of reproductive history on end-stage disease is to evaluate the association between reproductive history of the women and the tumor presentation. At diagnosis, the disease is defined by subtype and stage. There is no clear distinction between subtype and stage (e.g., receptor status), but the interpretation of an association with reproductive history differs. Thus, in the following associations with subtype (receptor status, histological subtype, and location) and with stages (tumor size and nodal status) will be discussed in two separate sections. The comparisons of the effect of reproductive history on different subtypes and stages in different studies can be complicated by the many categories of age at birth and multiparity. Therefore, in the following, the differences in effect for age at first birth (multiparity) between subtypes/stages in selected studies are illustrated by the ratio between the relative increase in risk per five years (per birth) in a subtype/stage compared with another.

If the long-term influence of reproductive history is thought to act through estrogens, one should expect that reproductive history primarily affects the incidence of estrogen receptor (ER)-positive tumors. Results from case-control studies and the Danish cohort are summarized in Table 4. Most previous studies have found nulliparity and late age at first birth to be associated with estrogen receptor positive tumors only, whereas studies on the effect of additional births have revealed fewer differences by receptor status. However, the number of cases in previous studies with known receptor status has been limited. In the Danish cohort the association between reproductive history and the incidence of ER-positive tumors was not statistically different from the association with the incidence of ER-negative tumors. However, especially late age at first birth tended to be more strongly

Table 4 Case-Control[a] and Cohort Studies on the Association Between Reproductive History and the Incidence of ER+ and ER− Breast Tumors

Study[a]	Design	Number of cases ER+, ER−	Age at first birth[b]: $RR_{ER+, per 5 yr}$/ $RR_{ER-, per 5 yr}$	Multiparity[b]: $RR_{ER+, per birth}$/ $RR_{ER-, per birth}$	Nulliparity[b]: $RR_{ER+, (p = 1 + vs. 0)}$/ $RR_{ER-, (p = 1 + vs. 0)}$
McTiernan et al., 1986	Population case control	143 + 97	1.24 (0.94–1.64)	1.00 (0.52–1.94)	—
Hislop et al., 1986	Population case control	345 + 167	0.89 (0.69–1.15)	0.56 (0.34–0.90)	—
Hildreth et al., 1983	Hospital case control	104 + 44	1.46 (0.93–2.31)	—	0.24 (0.06–0.94)
Stanford et al., 1987	Population case control	204 + 254	0.92 (0.77–1.11)	0.81 (0.71–0.93)	0.90 (0.48–1.67)
Cooper et al., 1989	Population case control	238 + 119	1.12 (0.81–1.54)	0.93 (0.64–1.36)	—
Yoo et al., 1997	Hospital case control	291 + 167	1.07 (0.79–1.46)	1.04 (0.81–1.35)	—
Wohlfahrt et al., 1999c	Cohort	4134 + 1910	1.08 (1.00–1.17)	1.00 (0.94–1.06)	0.87 (0.74–1.03)
Summary			1.06 (1.00–1.13)	0.96 (0.91–1.01)	0.86 (0.73–1.00)

[a]Additional case studies are reviewed in Stanford et al. (1986).
[b]The trend ratio is estimated as described in the statistical appendix.
Abbreviations: ER+, estrogen receptor positive; ER−, estrogen receptor negative; RR, risk ratio.

related to the risk of receptor-positive tumors. Thus, the ratio between the increase in risk per five-year increase in age at first birth was 1.08 for ER-positive compared with ER-negative tumors. Summarizing the results from Table 4, the trend ratio between increase in risk per five-year increase in age at first birth was 1.06 for ER-positive compared with ER-negative tumors. The ratio of the decrease in risk per birth was 0.96.

In recent years it has been debated whether particularly tumors being both progesterone and ER-positive are more hormonally sensitive. Studies on the combinations of both progesterone and ER status have, however, been conflicting (Britton et al., 2002; Huang et al., 2000) and in the Danish cohort no association between reproductive history and progesterone receptor status was observed (Wohlfahrt et al., 1999a).

It has been discussed whether estrogen status reflects different types of breast cancer or rather different stages in the neoplastic process, with receptor positive tumors gradually becoming receptor-negative (Habel and Stanford, 1993). If ER status reflects different types of breast cancer, a stronger association between the incidence of receptor positive tumors and both nulliparity and late age at first birth (i.e. high risk of being nulliparous at the initiation of a tumor) would be compatible with the hypothesis that the higher level of estrogen in nulliparous women can stimulate initiation and promotion of breast tumors.

While there have been many studies on the effect of reproductive history according to receptor status, the studies on the effect according to histological subtype have been limited. The two main subtypes of breast cancer are ductal carcinoma and lobular carcinoma, representing 80% and 9% of breast cancer cases in the Danish cohort, respectively (Wohlfahrt et al., 1999c). In the Danish cohort, reproductive history was associated with the incidence of both ductal and lobular carcinomas, but the association with lobular carcinomas was significantly stronger than the association with ductal carcinomas (Wohlfahrt et al., 1999c). Studies presenting estimates of the relative risk of lobular and ductal carcinomas according to reproductive history are presented in Table 5.

In summary, the ratio of the increase in risk by each five-year postponement of first birth for lobular compared with ductal carcinomas is 1.12. The ratio of the decrease in risk by a birth for lobular compared with ductal carcinomas is 1.07. The stronger association for lobular tumors probably reflects higher hormonal sensitivity in the cells from which lobular carcinomas originate. Thus, a strong association limited to the ER-positive lobular carcinomas was observed in the Danish cohort (Wohlfahrt et al., 1999c). This does not imply that the difference according to histology can be explained by difference in receptor status, but suggests that the difference depends on hormonal sensitivity. Furthermore, recent studies on the use of hormone replacement therapy (HRT) reveal that the risk associated with use of HRT similarly was particular to lobular tumors (Chen et al., 2002; Li et al., 2000).

Only two studies (Stalsberg et al., 1989; Wohlfahrt et al., 1999c) have systematically investigated the effect of reproductive history on less prevalent subtypes of breast cancer, i.e. mucinous (1%), medullar (2%), papillary (<1%), and tubular (2%) carcinomas. Most of these subtypes are not significantly related to reproductive history. The lack of association may, however, be due to low statistical power because of the small number of these types. This is further supported by the fact that the associations between reproductive history and the less prevalent subtypes were statistically similar to the (statistically significant) association between reproductive history and the incidence of ductal carcinomas (Wohlfahrt et al., 1999c). The only exception is that parous status is significantly strongly associated with the incidence of mucinous carcinoma compared with the incidence of ductal carcinomas, which cannot be explained by differences according to

Table 5 Studies[a] on the Association Between Reproductive History and the Incidence of Ductal and Lobular Carcinoma

Study[a]	Design	Cases: ductal + lobular	Age at first birth[b]: $RR_{lobular, per 5 yr}$/ $RR_{ductal, per 5 yr}$	Multiparity[b]: $RR_{lobular, per birth}$/ $RR_{ductal, per birth}$	Nulliparity[b]: $RR_{lobular, (p = 1 + vs. 0)}$/ $RR_{ductal, (p = 1 + vs. 0)}$
LiVolsi et al., 1982	Case control	284 + 32	1.14 (0.63–2.07)	—	2.00 (0.71–5.67)
Stalsberg et al., 1989[c]	Cases	1924 + 303	1.47 (1.14–1.90)	1.00 (0.64–1.57)	0.75 (0.52–1.08)
Wohlfahrt et al., 1999c[d]	Cohort	8669 + 963	1.12 (1.02–1.23)	1.07 (0.98–1.17)	1.20 (0.96–1.50)
Hinkula et al., 2001[e]	Cohort	1.017 + 123	1.11 (0.86–1.41)	1.25 (1.04–1.49)	—
Li et al., 2003	Population case control	656 + 196	0.99 (0.84–1.17)	0.97 (0.83–1.14)	0.82 (0.43–1.54)
Summary			1.12 (1.04–1.20)	1.07 (1.00–1.15)	1.06 (0.88–1.26)

[a]Only the largest case study, the case-control studies, and cohort studies where it is possible to estimate a trend ratio are presented.
[b]The trend ratios are estimated as described in the statistical appendix.
[c]Information on population from external source.
[d]The study by Ewertz and Duffy (1998) (with $RR_{lobular, per 5 yr}/RR_{ductal, per 5 yr} = 1.16$) is not included as cases are included in Wohlfahrt et al. (1999c).
[e]The study only includes women with five or more births.
Abbreviation: RR, risk ratio.

receptor status or tumor size. The incidence of mucinous carcinomas in parous women is 36% (24–53%) of the incidence in nulliparous women. The finding is in line with (Stalsberg et al., 1989) who observed the incidence of mucinous carcinomas in gravi women to be only 30% of the incidence in nulligravi women.

The incidence of left-sided breast cancer is generally observed to be slightly higher than that of right-sided breast cancers (Weiss et al., 1996b). One explanation has been that there is a higher amount of susceptible cells in the left breast, as the left breast is generally larger (Ekbom et al., 1994) although the evidence is weak (Weiss et al., 1996b). Two studies have suggested that reproductive history is also associated with the left-sided dominance. Thus, two case studies report a relation between nulliparity and the left-right ratio. According to the study by Ekbom et al. (1994) ($n = 11{,}274$), nulliparous women under 45 years had a right-sided dominance, whereas Senie et al. (1980) ($n = 980$) found a left-sided dominance in parous women over 40 years. It was speculated that the observed inverse ratio in the Swedish study was due to an interaction between parous status and an inverse hemodynamic asymmetry of the breasts in early fetal life. However, in the Danish cohort no difference in left-right ratio according to parous status was observed (Wohlfahrt et al., 1999c) ($n = 10{,}241$). Furthermore, performing a formal comparison of the incidence of tumors in the left and right breast, no difference was observed in the association with reproductive history and the incidence of left versus right-sided breast cancer, neither overall nor in women under or over 45 years of age. Results from the Danish cohort therefore do not support the hypothesis that a left-side dominance is associated with reproductive history.

Only the Danish cohort has focused on the association between reproductive risk factors and the risk of breast cancer according to the localization of the tumor in the breast. The incidence of tumors in the four noncentral parts of the breast (upper lateral, lower lateral, upper medial, lower medial) was statistically similarly related to either parous status, number of births, or age at birth. However, parous status and age at first birth were to a much greater extent related to the incidence of centrally located tumors compared with tumors located noncentrally, and the number of additional births was not associated with the incidence of centrally located tumors. These special associations for centrally located tumors were not related to Paget's disease of the nipple or a special proportion of lobular or receptor positive tumors in this area of the breast. However, some of the effect can be explained by the fact that central tumors on average are larger at diagnosis.

In general, the studies from the Danish cohort reveal that reproductive history is associated with the incidence of most traditional subtypes of breast cancer. In other words, the risk-reducing effect of a pregnancy appears to have a general effect on most breast cells. However, the association was more pronounced in tumors with higher hormonal sensitivity, i.e. ER-positive tumors and lobular tumors. To investigate the possible mechanisms behind this finding, the later developed statistical model (as described earlier) can be applied (Wohlfahrt and Melbye, 2001). Thus, Table 6 illustrates the effect of first to fourth birth according to age at birth (more than 10 years after birth) on the incidence of ER-positive and ER-negative tumors. Generally (with some exceptions), the results in Table 6 reveal that the smaller effect of age at (first) birth primarily is due to a smaller long-term risk reduction after a birth at young age. A natural interpretation of this is that

Table 6 Effect[a,b] of First to Fourth Birth ≥10 Years After Birth According to Age at Birth on the Risk of Being Diagnosed with an ER+ Tumor and ER− Tumor

		ER− RR (95% CI)	ER+ RR (95% CI)
Age at first birth	<30	0.91 (0.76–1.08)	0.88 (0.79–0.99)
	≥30	1.02 (0.80–1.29)	0.99 (0.85–1.15)
Age at second birth	<30	1.05 (0.92–1.21)	0.82 (0.75–0.90)
	≥30	1.04 (0.87–1.23)	0.98 (0.88–1.10)
Age at third birth	<30	0.71 (0.61–0.83)	0.85 (0.77–0.94)
	≥30	0.77 (0.65–0.92)	0.99 (0.89–1.11)
Age at fourth birth	<30	1.02 (0.62–1.68)	0.98 (0.70–1.39)
	≥30	1.08 (0.78–1.50)	1.16 (0.96–1.42)

[a]The estimates are based on DBCG data, the method described in Wohlfahrt and Melbye (2001) and the ER definition described in Wohlfahrt et al. (1999c).
[b]The reference group is women with one birth less.
Abbreviations: ER+, estrogen receptor positive; ER−, estrogen receptor negative; DBCG, Danish Breast Cancer Cooperative Group; RR, risk ratio; CI, confidence interval.

the risk-reducing effect occurring late in pregnancy to some degree is hormonally mediated (probably through estrogens) and therefore to a relatively larger degree affects hormonally sensitive breast cells.

In conclusion, using clinical information from the national registry of the Danish Breast Cancer Cooperative Group (DBCG), we concluded that the risk-reducing effect following a birth is observed for most subtypes of breast cancer and in that sense is a general effect. However, the risk reduction following births at an early age is apparently relatively larger for estrogen-sensitive tumors compared with nonsensitive tumors. This suggests that the effect, to some degree, is hormonally mediated.

Stage at Diagnosis

Only few studies have investigated the effect of reproductive history according to stage at diagnosis, which potentially can reveal whether reproductive history also has a late-stage impact on breast cancer incidence.

In the Danish cohort, age at first birth and nulliparity were more strongly associated with the incidence of large tumors than with the incidence of small tumors. In contrast, the effect of increasing number of births was less pronounced on the incidence of large compared with small tumors (Wohlfahrt et al., 1999b). Case-control and cohort studies on this subject are presented in Table 7. The stage definition differs, and it is therefore difficult to directly compare the results. Nevertheless a strikingly similar pattern is revealed when calculating the ratio between the increase in risk per five-year increase in age at first birth and the increase in risk per birth in "late-stage" versus "early-stage" breast cancer. Age at birth is clearly more strongly associated with late-stage breast cancer, with a 1.00 to 1.15 ratio of the increase in risk per five-year increase in age at first birth for "late-stage" breast cancer (Brinton et al., 1983: >1 cm; Weiss et al., 1996a: regional + distant; Wohlfahrt et al., 1999b: 2 to 5 cm; Hinkula et al., 2001: regional) compared with "early-stage" breast cancer (Brinton et al., 1983: ≤1 cm; Weiss et al., 1996a; Hinkula et al., 2001: local; Wohlfahrt et al., 1999b: ≤2 cm). On the other hand, the ratio of the effect of multiparity was 1.06 to 1.18. In two studies, the effect on more extreme late-stage groups was also investigated (Wohlfahrt et al., 1999b: >5 cm; Hinkula et al., 2001:

Table 7 Studies on the Association Between Reproductive History and Breast Cancer Risk According to Stage at Diagnosis

Study	Design	Stage	Cases	Age at first birth: $RR_{late,\ per\ 5\ yr}/RR_{early,\ per\ 5\ yr}$	Multiparity: $RR_{late,\ per\ birth}/RR_{early,\ per\ birth}$	Nulliparity: $RR_{late,\ (p\ =\ 1+\ vs.\ 0)}/RR_{early,\ (p\ =\ 1+\ vs.\ 0)}$
Brinton et al., 1983	Case control	≤1 cm	210	1	—	1
		>1 cm	788	1.01 (0.81–1.25)	—	1.32 (0.80–2.19)
Weiss et al., 1996a	Population case control	Local	784	1	1	1
		Regional, distant	604	1.00 (0.86–1.31)	1.18 (1.00–1.39)	1.36 (0.88–2.12)
Wohlfahrt et al., 1999b[a]	Cohort	≤2 cm	5595	1	1	1
		2–5 cm	3678	1.10 (1.03–1.16)	1.06 (1.01–1.11)	0.74 (0.65–0.84)
		>5 cm	707	1.23 (1.11–1.36)	1.13 (1.04–1.24)	0.57 (0.46–0.71)
Hinkula et al., 2001[b]	Cohort	Local	738	1	1	—
		Regional	552	1.15 (0.99–1.33)	1.10 (0.98–1.22)	—
		Distant	101	1.84 (1.34–2.52)	1.04 (0.85–1.28)	—

[a]Same pattern was seen according to nodal status.
[b]The study only includes women with five or more births.
Abbreviation: RR, risk ratio.

distant). Comparing these more extreme "late-stage" groups with "early-stage" breast cancer, the differences for age at first birth were even stronger. Thus, the ratio of the increase in risk per five-year increase in age at first birth was 1.23 to 1.84 and the ratio of the decrease in risk per birth was 1.04 to 1.13.

In the Danish cohort, the differences in the effect of reproductive history were observed, both when defining late-stage by tumor size and by nodal status (Wohlfahrt et al., 1999b). As these characteristics are correlated, it is difficult to determine whether differences according to one classification simply may be an effect of differences according to the other correlated classification. Using data from the Danish cohort, a statistical model was developed based on the new concept of multivariate competing risks to separate effects according to different tumor characteristics at diagnosis (Wohlfahrt et al., 1999a). These analyses revealed that the strong association with risk of late stage breast cancer was just as much expressed when characterizing stage by nodal status instead of size of the tumor.

Another stage marker with even more interpretational complications is ductal carcinoma in situ of the breast (DCIS) versus invasive breast cancer. Table 8 presents results from case-control and cohort studies with DCIS cases and invasive cases.

The differences in the effects of age at first birth and multiparity on DCIS compared with invasive breast cancer are small, suggesting little or no effect of reproductive history on the progression from DCIS to invasive breast cancer. In the Danish cohort, the ratio of the increase per five years in age at first birth for the incidence of DCIS compared with invasive cancer was 1.06. The ratio of the decrease in risk per birth for DCIS compared with invasive cancer was 1.03. Due to the extensive information from a clinical database (DBCG) used in the Danish cohort, it was furthermore possible to divide DCIS cases according to stage markers. The association with late DCIS (>10 mm, comedo type, grade II + III) was stronger compared with early DCIS (Wohlfahrt et al., 2004). The observed pattern for DCIS lesions is comparable with the stage differences observed for invasive cancer (Wohlfahrt et al., 1999b).

The observed differences in the effect of reproductive history by stage for both invasive tumors and CIS lesions can be ascribed to differences in progression rates and/or to differences in detection rates as illustrated in Figure 4.

Obviously, a large tumor at some point must have been small. Under the assumption that certain tumors grow more rapidly than others, they will stay in the category of small tumors for a shorter time before moving on to medium and eventually large tumors. Thus, according to one interpretation, nulliparous women and women with a late age at first childbirth, who were particularly at high risk of being diagnosed with large tumors, may have tumors with a rapid growth potential and in that sense have a late-stage impact on breast cancer risk. This interpretation is in line with the hypothesis that tumors initiated in undifferentiated breast cells are more aggressive (Olsson, 1989). However, a study from the USA revealed no association between reproductive history and two measures of tumor cell proliferation (Oestreicher et al., 2004).

An alternative explanation would be that associations exist between reproductive factors and the probability of early tumor detection. For example, differences in detection rates might arise if breast self-examination is more difficult

Table 8 Studies on the Association Between Reproductive History and the Risk of DCIS and Invasive Breast Cancer[a]

Study[a]	Design	Cases: DCIS + invasive	Age at 1st birth[b]: $RR_{DCIS, per 5 yr}/RR_{invasive, per 5 yr}$	Multiparity[b]: $RR_{DCIS, per birth}/RR_{invasive, per birth}$	Nulliparity[b]: $RR_{DCIS, (p = 1+ vs. 0)}/RR_{invasive, (p = 1+ vs. 0)}$
Brinton et al., 1983[c]	Case control	199 + 998	1.15 (0.92–1.46)	—	1.14 (0.66–1.96)
Weiss et al., 1996a	Population case control	228 + 1388	0.92 (0.77–1.11)	0.89 (0.76–1.03)	0.62 (0.33–1.15)
Longnecker et al., 1996[c,d]	Population case control	233 + 2057	1.01 (0.84–1.22)	0.90 (0.78–1.05)	—
Trentham-Dietz et al., 2000	Population case control	301 + 3789	1.05 (0.89–1.24)	0.95 (0.88–1.02)	—
Wohlfahrt et al., 2002	Cohort	872 + 15,418	1.06 (0.96–1.17)	1.03 (0.93–1.14)	1.12 (0.88–1.42)
Summary			1.04 (0.97–1.11)	0.96 (0.91–1.01)	1.05 (0.86–1.29)

[a]The largest study on reproductive risk factors for CIS lesion did not present comparable estimates for invasive cancer (Lambe et al., 1998). Information on the association between reproductive history and invasive cancer could, however, be found in Lambe et al. (1996b). Using information from both studies the ratio for age at first birth and multiparity was 0.91 and 1.08.
[b]The trend ratios are estimated as described in the statistical appendix.
[c]Includes also non-DCIS cases of carcinoma in situ.
[d]Results from pre- and postmenopausal women combined.
Abbreviations: DCIS, ductal carcinoma in situ; RR, risk ratio; CIS, carcinoma in situ.

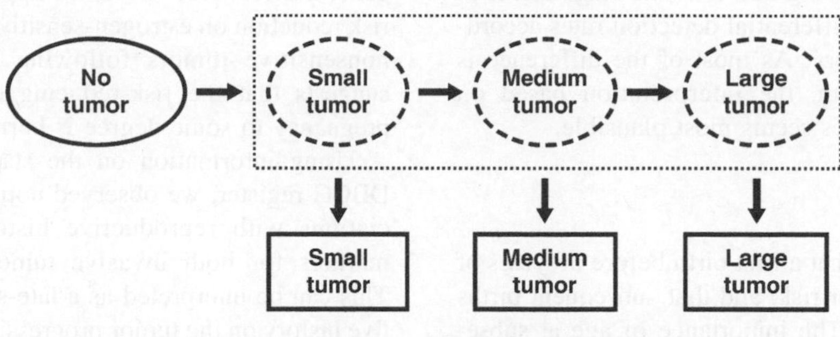

Figure 4 Simplified illustration of the transformation from having no tumor, an undetected tumor to a diagnosed tumor.

in nulliparous compared with parous women or in women with a late compared to early age at first childbirth. The breast tissue of a nulliparous woman is more firm and homogenous than the breast tissue of a parous woman, which might make detection of a tumor more difficult. However, it is equally conceivable that the nodularity present in a parous woman's breast would make it difficult to distinguish glandular tissue from tumor tissue. Thus, the extent and direction in which reproductive factors may influence detection of tumors is difficult to predict. Differential use of mammography according to reproductive history could also cause differences in time of detection. The vast majority of women in our study, however, were under age 50. In Denmark, mammography is offered only to women aged 50 years or older, and even today, only in few parts of the country. The association between reproductive history and tumor size could also be due to social differences, however, a study based on data from the DBCG register showed no association between tumor size and social class in Denmark (Norredam et al., 1998).

The two interpretations discussed in (Wohlfahrt et al., 1999b) can be further evaluated taking advantage of the later developed approach applied when investigating age at any birth (Wohlfahrt and Melbye, 2001). Table 9 shows the effect of each first to fourth birth by age-at and time-since birth according to tumor size.

This approach reveals that most of the stage differences are related to the effect of first birth although the result is not unequivocal. Thus, after first birth, and only first birth, the mothers have a clear increased risk of being diagnosed with a tumor less than 21 mm regardless of age-at and time-since birth. This indicates that the detection rate is lower in nulliparous women compared with parous women. Furthermore, the relative reduction in the incidence of very large tumors (>50 mm) in young compared with older mothers is especially expressed after first birth. Such a parity-specific difference in the effect of age at first birth can most easily be ascribed to a higher detection rate, especially in young mothers compared with nulliparous women, if the biological effect of a birth is thought to be independent of parity. Thus, taking these observations into account, an interpretation based on differences in detection rate between nulliparous and parous women appears the most plausible.

In conclusion, differential associations with reproductive history according to stage marker for both invasive and DCIS were observed in the Danish cohort. This can

Table 9 Effect[a,b] of First to Fourth Birth ≥10 Years After Birth According to Age at Birth on the Risk of Being Diagnosed with a Tumor with a Diameter of Less than 21 mm, 21 to 50 mm, and More than 50 mm

		Tumor size <21 mm RR (95% CI)	Tumor size 21–50 mm RR (95% CI)	Tumor size >50 mm RR (95% CI)
Age at first birth	<30	1.12 (1.01–1.25)	0.81 (0.71–0.91)	0.64 (0.49–0.84)
	≥30	1.23 (1.06–1.41)	0.96 (0.81–1.13)	0.94 (0.65–1.35)
Age at second birth	<30	0.89 (0.82–0.97)	0.89 (0.81–0.99)	0.78 (0.61–1.00)
	≥30	1.00 (0.91–1.10)	1.02 (0.90–1.15)	0.74 (0.54–1.02)
Age at third birth	<30	0.87 (0.79–0.95)	0.80 (0.71–0.90)	0.89 (0.66–1.19)
	≥30	0.88 (0.79–0.97)	1.01 (0.90–1.14)	1.06 (0.78–1.43)
Age at fourth birth	<30	0.64 (0.52–0.80)	0.90 (0.71–1.15)	0.98 (0.56–1.71)
	≥30	0.99 (0.84–1.17)	1.05 (0.85–1.29)	1.23 (0.76–2.00)

[a]The estimates are based on the DBCG data, the method described in Wohlfahrt and Melbye (2001) and tumor size definition in Wohlfahrt et al. (1999b).
[b]The reference group is women with one birth less.
Abbreviation: risk ratio.

either be interpreted as being due to a late-stage effect of reproductive history or differential detection rates according to reproductive history. As most of the difference is observed after first birth, the interpretation based on differential detection rates seems most plausible.

Conclusion

It is generally accepted that a first birth before 30 years of age reduces breast cancer risk, and that subsequent births further reduce the risk. The importance of age at subsequent births is less known. Using the Danish cohort, we found that the long-term risk reduction after birth depends on the age at birth in a similar way for first and subsequent births, i.e. any birth at early age has a similar long-term reducing effect. Furthermore, we observed a latency period of at least 10 years of the effect of each birth. In general, our findings suggest that the risk-reducing effect of any birth at young age represents an early-stage long-term effect with a short-term latency period.

A possible negative effect of induced abortion on breast cancer risk has been much debated. The validity of previous retrospective case-control studies on the subject has, however, been questioned due to the sensitive nature of the issue. Using the Danish cohort with register-based information on induced abortions, we showed that induced abortion is not associated with subsequent breast cancer risk.

Using the total information on gestational age for induced abortions, stillbirths, and livebirths in the Danish national registries, we found that breast cancer risk is not associated with gestational age in pregnancies with short duration (induced abortions), whereas women with a term birth had a lower risk compared with women with a preterm birth. Taken together this suggests that the risk reduction after a birth is due to factors occurring late in pregnancy, and combined with the finding of even higher relative risks in women with an extremely preterm birth, this is a novel support to Russo and Russo's hypothesis.

Whereas our studies of the gestational effect on risk of breast cancer provided support to the hypothesis by Russo and Russo that differentiation of the breast cells protects against breast cancer, there are clearly other factors that need be considered. If differentiation was the sole explanation, one would assume that the first child birth resulted in by far the greatest reduction in breast cancer risk on the assumption that most breast cells would have become differentiated. Our finding that any birth at young age contributes equally to the risk of breast cancer conflicts somewhat with that interpretation.

Based on clinical information on subtype at disease from the DBCG register we concluded that the risk-reducing effect following a birth is observed for most traditional subtypes of breast cancer and in that sense is a general effect. However, an apparently relatively larger risk reduction on estrogen-sensitive tumors compared with nonsensitive tumors following births at an early age suggests that the risk-reducing effect occurring late in pregnancy to some degree is hormonally mediated.

Using information on the stage of disease from the DBCG register, we observed noticeable differential associations with reproductive history according to stage markers for both invasive tumors and in situ lesions. This can be interpreted as a late-stage effect of reproductive history on the tumor progression. However, as most of the difference is observed after first birth, a plausible interpretation is that detection rates are different in women with and without children.

In conclusion, a plausible biological interpretation of the epidemiological data in the Danish cohort is that a pregnancy at an early age after a latency period has a general long-term reducing effect on breast cancer risk due to an early-stage prohibiting effect induced by hormonally mediated events late in pregnancy.

THE SHORT-TERM EFFECT

Endogenous hormones are important for cell growth and are likely to be involved not only in the initiation of breast cancer, but also in the progression of the disease. During pregnancy, endogen hormonal levels are drastically changed, and it is therefore natural to speculate that mothers, in addition to the long-term protective effect of childbirth, experience a short-term increased risk of breast cancer in the immediate years following birth. A simplified illustration of this idea is seen in Figure 5; shortly after birth the mother experiences a short-term increase in

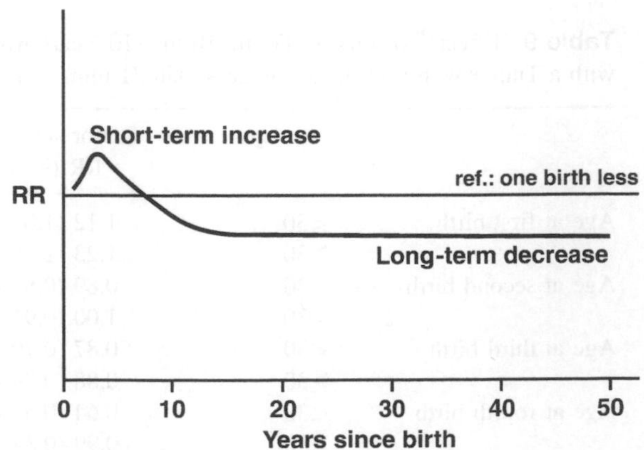

Figure 5 Simplified illustration of the short-term increase in risk and the long-term decrease in risk after a birth when comparing with women with one birth less.

breast cancer risk followed by the well-known long-term decrease in breast cancer risk.

The first signs of the short-term effect of a birth were observed as differential effects of reproductive history according to attained age. Several papers have reported that the protective effect of a childbirth only was seen in older women (Velentgas and Daling, 1994). The differential effect of parity, the "crossover" effect, led to the idea that a birth might have a dual effect, i.e. a short-term negative effect followed by a long-term protective effect (Janerich and Hoff, 1982). This was in line with the surprising finding of MacMahon and colleagues that mothers aged more than 35 years at first birth had a higher risk than nulliparous women (MacMahon et al., 1970) and was further supported by the elegant mathematical modeling by Malcome Pike (Pike et al., 1983) showing that the long-term protective effects alone were inadequate to fit the epidemiological data. These findings nourished the ground for a series of studies more or less directly investigating the risk of breast cancer according to time since birth. In 1988 and 1990, two hospital-based case-control studies observed a large increased risk shortly after birth. Some of this risk increase is probably due to selection bias, i.e. mothers with babies delay going into hospitals for less severe procedures, thereby inducing an overrepresentation of mothers with young children among breast cancer cases (Bruzzi et al., 1988; Williams et al., 1990). Two subsequent Scandinavian population-based studies found no evidence for an increased short-term effect (Adami et al., 1990; Vatten and Kvinnsland, 1992). In the mid 1990s three of six large United States and international studies found a small tendency toward an increased risk shortly after childbirth (Rosner et al., 1994; Hsieh et al., 1994; Cummings et al., 1994; Shapiro et al., 1994; Cummings et al., 1997; Thompson et al., 2002), and three large Scandinavian register-based case-control and cohort studies from 1994 and 1995 found significant but mostly small effects (Lambe et al., 1994; Albrektsen et al., 1995; Leon et al., 1995). The Swedish study (Lambe et al., 1994) was later updated (Liu et al., 2002). In the Danish cohort from 2001, a small but significant effect was likewise observed (Wohlfahrt et al., 2001).

The studies have been dominated by two statistical approaches. Firstly, an investigation of the risk in women after a birth compared with women in which everything else was equal but the birth. Secondly, studies on the effect of time since latest birth among multiparous women. Table 10 shows the studies using the second approach. The table presents the largest difference in risk between an early and late time period after birth. A generally higher risk in the early years after the latest birth compared with long time after latest birth is observed. However, this difference could simply be an expression of a delayed long-term protection. Figure 5 illustrates how the maximum measured difference is the risk difference between the top of the short-term increase and the long-term risk decrease. It has therefore been argued that a comparison should be performed directly between women with *n*-birth and women with one birth less (*n*-1 births) to directly investigate the short-term effect (Cummings et al., 1997). This comparison would in Figure 5 be the more reasonable comparison between the short-term increase and the reference line.

Table 11 presents the studies on the transient effect after first to fifth birth. The largest effects have emerged from case-control studies by Lambe and Hsieh (Senie et al., 1980; Lambe et al., 1994; Hsieh et al., 1994). Calculating the average risk increase in the first 10 years based on their results, an increase of more than 40% is observed. Later studies have not been able to confirm such a large effect. In the Danish cohort, a much more modest effect of 7% has been observed. An increase of the same magnitude has been observed after the second birth, whereas there is no clear evidence of an increase

Table 10 Studies on the Relative Risk of Breast Cancer the First Years After Latest Birth Compared with Many Years Since Latest Birth

Study	Design	Cases	Early and late time intervals	Max relative difference
Bruzzi et al., 1988	Hospital case control	573	0–2 vs. 10+	166%
Williams et al., 1990	Hospital case control	422	0–2 vs. 10+	192%
Adami et al., 1990	Population case control	422	1–4 vs. 5+	10%
Vatten and Kvinnsland, 1992	Cohort	340	0–5 vs. 11–15	20%
Shapiro S et al., 1994	Hospital case control	?	5–6 vs. 10+	60%
Cummings et al., 1994	Population case control	2,279	3–6 vs. 10+	21%
Leon et al., 1995	Population case control	3,439	0–2 vs. 10+	21%
Albrektsen et al., 1995	Cohort	4,787	3–4 vs. 10+[a]	63%
Wohlfahrt et al., 2001	Cohort	10,790	2–3 vs. 15+	26%

[a]The level in the late time interval was estimated from subintervals based on inverse variance–weighted estimation.

Table 11 Studies on the Relative Risk of Breast Cancer up to 11 Years After First to Fifth Birth Compared to Women with Zero to Four Births

Study[a]	Design	Cases	Time interval[b]	First birth	Second birth	Third birth	Fourth birth	Fifth birth
Lambe et al., 1994	Population case control	9,619	0–9 yr	42%	Small	–	–	–
Hsieh et al., 1994	Hospital case control	?	0–9 yr	64%	Small	–	–	–
Leon et al., 1995	Population case control	3,439	0–2 yr	–	11%	14%	−22%	4%
Albrektsen et al., 1996	Cohort	4,787	0–4 yr	–	15%	−3%	3%	−24%
Cummings et al., 1997	Population case control	8,104	0–11 yr	−22%	−Effect	–	–	–
McCredie et al., 1998	Population case control	890	0–9 yr	−14%	27%	43%	–	–
Wohlfahrt et al., 2001	Cohort	10,790	0–9 yr	7%	7%	−1%	−11%	–

[a]Thompson et al. (2002) apparently observed a transient increase after first and second birth but not following subsequent births. The study is not included as it was impossible to determine the definition of the short-term effect from the SER abstract. Pike et al. (1983) and Rosner et al. (1994) found a transient increase, but their models could not be included in this framework. The study by Lambe et al. is later updated (Liu et al., 2002).
[b]Time interval after birth. Estimates for subintervals are combined by inverse variance–weighted estimation. In Lambe et al. (1994), (Hsieh and Lan (1996, first result row in table III in the parallel method paper)), Hsieh et al. (1994, first result row in table 3), Cummings et al. (1997, table 4), and Wohlfahrt et al. (2001), the risk in the time interval after birth is compared with women with one birth less. In Albrektsen et al. (1996, table 1), Leon et al. (1995, table 5), and McCredie et al. (1998, table V), the extracted comparisons are with women with one birth less and more than five, two, and nine years since latest birth, respectively.

following subsequent births. In conclusion, there is evidence for a transient increase in breast cancer risk following a birth, but the size of the increase is relatively small compared with what was believed earlier.

The two statistical approaches can be viewed as two perspectives rather than as a statistical issue per se. However, correct statistical analysis of the transient change in risk has been discussed. Early studies using the "breast tissue age" approach modeled the short-term effect by including an instantaneous, one-time increase in risk after birth (Pike et al., 1983; Rosner et al., 1994). In the later years, many studies have been based on the concept of a model proposed by Hiseh and Lan (Hsieh and Lan, 1996). However, the use of continuous variables has limited its potentials to investigate the non-linear effects of time since delivery (Liu et al., 2002). In the Danish cohort, a categorical modeling of the transient increase following time-since-birth has been used. The approach was first used by a Norwegian study group (Albrektsen et al., 1995) and "circumvents" the generic linear dependency between age, age at birth, and time since birth in time-since-birth studies by imposing reasonable assumptions (primarily that the age effect is the same regardless of parity) (Albrektsen et al., 1999; Heuch et al., 1999). As of yet, this approach has to a surprisingly low extent been used in breast cancer research.

Hormonally Related Characteristics of Pregnancy

The dominating theory used to explain the transient increase in breast cancer risk is that the drastic change in hormonal levels during pregnancy induces rapid progression of occult tumors. An alternative approach to evaluate the short-term effect is therefore to correlate the short-term maternal breast cancer risk with characteristics of the pregnancy suggested to be related to the hormonal level during pregnancy.

Several studies have investigated the overall risk following birth according to characteristics of pregnancy, however, only few have focused on the short-term risk. Table 12 presents studies on breast cancer risk in the first five years after the latest/last birth according to hormonally related pregnancy characteristics. In one case-control study, self-reported treatment of nausea/vomiting was significantly associated with the short-term breast cancer risk (Enger et al., 1997), but in another case-control study self-reported experience of nausea was found to be unrelated to short-term breast cancer risk (Troisi et al., 1998). However, the pregnancy characteristics were in these studies self-reported which may cause bias, although such a bias would probably be small considering the short time interval between event and interview (Lumey et al., 1994; Sanderson et al., 1998; Tomeo et al., 1999). In addition, the pregnancy characteristics in these studies were not necessarily related to the latest birth, which may dilute associations. In the Danish cohort with register-based pregnancy information, we found a significantly larger short-term breast cancer increase following a multiple compared with a singleton birth (Wohlfahrt and Melbye, 1999). A few studies of mothers with multiple births have previously reported an increased risk of breast cancer in the first years following a multiple birth (Hsieh et al., 1993; La Vecchia et al., 1996; Lambe et al., 1996a). However, these studies have compared the incidence with singleton mothers irrespective of the time since birth in these mothers, and one can therefore not

Table 12 Studies on the Maternal Breast Cancer Risk Less Than Five Years Since Latest Birth According to Hormonally Related Pregnancy Characteristics

Study	Design	Source of information	Pregnancy characteristics	Cases <5 yr since latest birth	Relative risk <5 yr since latest birth[a]
Enger et al., 1997	Population case control	Self reported	Ever treatment of nausea/vomiting	35/134	103% (5–292%)
Troisi et al., 1998	Population case control	Self reported	Ever gestational diabetes	25/338	−12% (−52–60%)
			Ever toxemia	27/338	−3% (−45–70%)
			Ever nausea/vomiting[b]	180/338	−6% (−32–30%)
Hsieh et al., 1999	Population case control	Register based	Latest a preterm birth	15/245	−9% (−50–65%)
Wohlfahrt and Melbye, 1999	Cohort	Register based	1 kg higher birth weight of latest	663/663	20% (−4–50%)
			Latest a multiple birth	18/681	80% (10–280%)
			Latest a girl	332 /663	0% (−10–20%)

[a]In women with birth characteristics compared with women without.
[b]Experience of frequent nausea or vomiting.

determine how the short effect differs. In the Danish cohort there was also an indication of an association between high birth weight of offspring and short-term breast cancer increase. Although insignificant, the finding was further underlined by the fact that the association was only observed for the incidence of breast cancer with tumors larger than 2 cm. Birth weight has been found to be the anthropometrical marker of foetal growth that was strongest associated with maternal pregnancy estriol levels. However, the predictive value has been questioned (Kaijser et al., 2000; Peck et al., 2003). The association between high birth weight and maternal breast cancer risk could be attributed to the fact that these mothers are at risk of diabetes mellitus or high BMI, both groups known to have higher breast cancer risk (Talamini et al., 1997; Weiderpass et al., 1997; Weiss et al., 1999).

The significant associations above can be interpreted as support for the hypothesis that estrogen plays a significant role in the short-term effect of a birth: estrogens stimulate the proliferation of premalignant mammary cells and thereby promote breast cancer (Innes and Byers, 1999). Associations between hormonal level during pregnancy and birth characteristics, however, do not necessarily mean that the difference is large enough to create a notable difference in the breast cancer risk. Thus, studies on the direct correlation between hormonal level and breast cancer risk are obviously preferable. However, only a few studies have directly evaluated the association between hormonal level at birth and the subsequent breast cancer risk taking time since birth into account. The first study to evaluate the serum steroid hormone levels during pregnancy as a maternal risk factor included only 40 cases to evaluate the short-term effect (Peck et al., 2002). In a study based on the Danish cohort, no differences according to time since birth in the effect of AFP during pregnancy were observed (Melbye et al., 2000).

Another way to evaluate the short-term effect is to investigate at which gestational week it acts. In a Swedish study Hsieh et al. (1999) found that in uniparous women, the breast cancer risk in the first five years after birth was slightly smaller 0.91 (0.50–1.65) in women with a preterm birth compared to a term birth, but five to nine years after birth the risk was slightly higher 1.07 (0.67–1.72). These estimates are, however, not significantly different and can therefore only to a very limited degree be taken as support for the hypothesis that the high hormonal level in the final weeks of a term pregnancy is responsible for the negative short-term effect after a birth. However, the approach is indeed interesting and may prove especially fertile if one is able to differentiate further by gestational age.

In the above review, there is no mention of studies that do not try to separate the short-term and long-term effects associated with pregnancy characteristics or studies that did so by stratifying by age. However, studies that investigated characteristics of pregnancies that were not necessarily the latest pregnancy are included. In the Danish cohort only pregnancy characteristics of the latest birth were considered. An even better approach would be to estimate the pregnancy characteristic–specific short-term effect of each birth, or, if data are sparse, to estimate a common pregnancy characteristic–specific short-term effect for all births, assuming that the effect of the pregnancy characteristics is independent of parity (an assumption that can be evaluated by a statistical test). This approach was used in the Danish cohort in the investigation of whether the short-term effect differs according to family history (Wohlfahrt et al., 2002) and tumor invasiveness (Wohlfahrt et al., 2004). However, it is probably not essential in the investigation of the short-term effect because the latest birth will play a dominant role in the cumulative short-term effects of previous births, but it is important for long-term effects. An illustration of estimation of the long-term effect of each birth using the Danish cohort is given in (Wohlfahrt and Melbye, 2000). The interpretation of differences in the long-term effect by hormonally related pregnancy characteristics is probably different from the interpretation of differences in the short-term effect. It could for example be argued that differences would be opposite, i.e. a special hormonal level induces both a relatively higher short-term increased risk and a relatively higher long-term risk reduction through a more comprehensive cell maturation. Thus, stratification by time since birth seems essential in this context. It may be difficult to address this due to small numbers of cases; however, the condensed models mentioned above could be a useful approach (e.g. Wohlfahrt et al. (2002)).

Characteristics of the Mother

The short-term effect is thought to affect occult tumors. Therefore some interest has been directed toward the short-term effect in women with a higher risk of having occult tumors, i.e. high-risk women. The strongest risk factor for breast cancer is age, and the short-term risk has been observed to vary by age at birth. However, the results have been conflicting. In the Danish cohort, attained age did not appear to modify the short-term effect.

Also nulliparous women represent a high-risk group, with a higher risk of occult tumors due to a hypothesized lower degree of final differentiation of the breast cells. Most studies have observed a stronger effect after first and second birth. Also in the Danish cohort, a stronger transient increase was observed after first and second birth (Wohlfahrt et al., 2001).

Another group with a high risk of having occult tumors, at least in the reproductive years, consists of women with a family history of breast cancer due to their higher breast cancer risk in the young years. Two studies have focused on the short-term effect according to family history, both observing a larger short-term effect in women with family history than in women without. In the Nurses' health study including 2249 cases aged 30 to 55 years, a 50% larger transient increased effect was observed in women with a family history of breast cancer (Colditz et al., 1996). In the Danish cohort, including 2770 incident cases of breast cancer diagnosed in women below 40 years, the short-term increase in risk in the first five years after a birth was 30% (3–64%) larger in women with a family history of breast cancer than in women without. After the first five years there was no difference in the effect of a birth between women with and women without family history (Wohlfahrt et al., 2002).

Stage at Diagnosis

If a pregnancy changes the growth pattern of occult tumors, this might very well be reflected in tumor characteristics at the time of diagnosis. Yet another approach to investigate the existence and features of the transient increase is therefore to analyze the risk by time since birth according to tumor characteristics at diagnosis and especially stage at diagnosis. This was addressed in the Danish cohort, where it was found that not only do mothers experience a transient increased risk of breast cancer after childbirth, they also, in particular, experience a relatively high risk of late-stage disease (Wohlfahrt et al., 2001). Thus, the risk of being diagnosed with a tumor with a diameter larger than 5 cm was on average 53% higher the first 10 years after birth compared with later. The risk of being diagnosed with a tumor less than 2 cm was not significantly associated with time since latest birth. Figure 6 illustrates the clearly larger transient increase in the incidence of large tumors (>50 mm) compared with "non-large" tumors ($\leq$50 mm) after second and third birth. The transient increase after first birth is not shown, as it is too heavily confounded by a lower detection rate in nulliparous women. The observed enhanced risk of being diagnosed with a relatively larger tumor shortly after birth supports the idea that pregnancy-related factors transiently induce a high growth rate in cells that are already malignant.

Nonhormonal Explanations

The short-term effect has primarily been perceived by a hormonal explanation, but non-hormonal explanations should also be considered.

Especially the finding of a higher risk of late-stage diagnoses in the first years after a birth supports an alternative explanation that the short-term effect is due to delayed diagnosis because of difficulties in detecting the tumor during pregnancy. This idea is supported by the finding of an increased risk shortly after birth in other non-hormonal cancer types (Lambe and Ekbom, 1995). However, a delayed diagnosis/surgery due to pregnancy would not only result in larger tumors after delivery, but also in a correspondingly low breast cancer rate during pregnancy. In four studies, including the Danish cohort, an approximately 70% lower risk of breast cancer during pregnancy was observed (Haas, 1984; Albrektsen et al., 1995; Lambe and Ekbom, 1995; Wohlfahrt et al., 2001). Some of this lower rate might very well be explained by a "healthy women" effect.

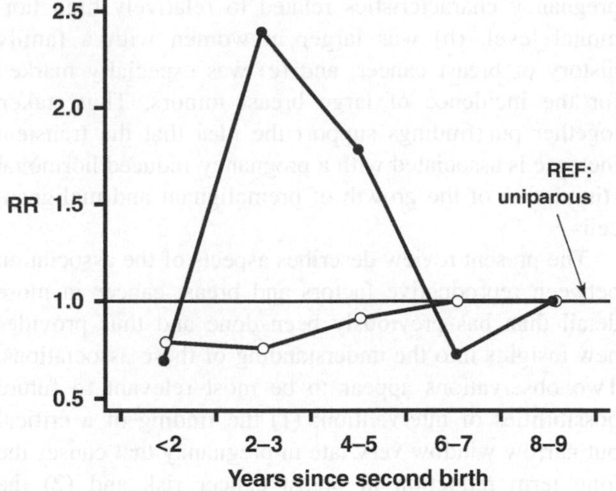

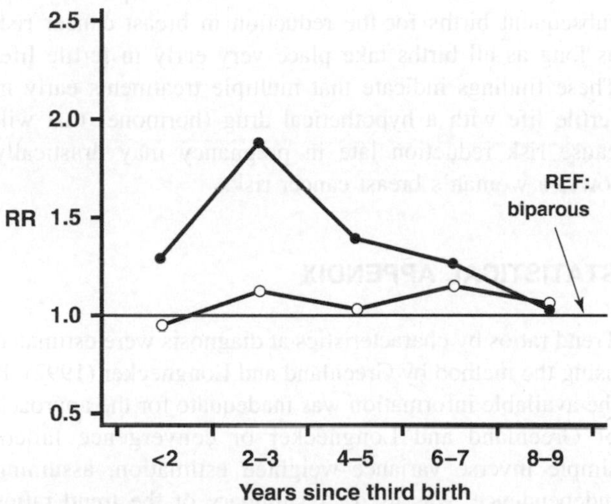

Figure 6 Effect of second birth (*top*) and third birth (*bottom*) by time since birth on the risk of being diagnosed with a tumor size less or equal to 50 cm (*circles*) and larger than 50 cm (*dots*). Reference group is the group of mothers with one birth less. *Source*: Wohlfahrt et al., 2001.

Nevertheless, calculations in the Danish cohort based on breast cancer rates before and after pregnancy did not support the idea that pregnancy-induced delay in diagnosis/surgery could explain the entire excess of cases in the years following pregnancy. Thus, the estimated number of cases that were "missing" during pregnancy was less than the observed excess of cases after birth. Pregnancy-induced diagnostic delay could at maximum account for an excess of cases equivalent to the observed increased breast cancer rate in the first four or five years after first and second delivery (Wohlfahrt et al., 2001). In other words, delayed diagnosis/surgery due to pregnancy does not appear to explain the entire excess of cases in the years following pregnancy.

Conclusion

In addition to the long-term reduction in breast cancer risk after birth, a birth is followed by a short-term increase in breast cancer risk. Data from the Danish cohort revealed that the transient increase is not as large as suggested by earlier studies, thus a nonhormonal explanation cannot be ruled out. However, we evaluated the possible cause using three different approaches. The transient increase (a) was larger following a birth with pregnancy characteristics related to relatively high hormonal levels, (b) was larger in women with family history of breast cancer, and (c) was especially marked for the incidence of large breast tumors. Thus, taken together, our findings support the idea that the transient increase is associated with a pregnancy-induced hormonal stimulation of the growth of premalignant and malignant cells.

In conclusion, a plausible biological interpretation of the epidemiological data in the Danish cohort is that a pregnancy has a short-term increased effect on a woman's breast cancer risk induced by the enhanced hormonal level during pregnancy.

SUMMARY

It is well known that a woman's reproductive history is strongly associated with her risk of breast cancer and generally accepted that a better understanding of this association holds a key to intervention. Thus, the overall aim of this review was to investigate in more detail the association between pregnancy and breast cancer risk. The focus was on the following questions: Is the importance of age at birth restricted to the first birth or do the ages of subsequent births also influence breast cancer risk? Besides a child birth, do other types of pregnancies affect breast cancer risk, and is the duration of the pregnancy of importance for the risk? Is the association between the different reproductive factors and breast cancer restricted to certain subtypes or certain stages of the malignancy? Is there, as suggested by others, a short-term increased risk of breast cancer after childbirth, prior to the well-known long-term protective effect?

It is generally accepted that a first birth before 30 years of age reduces breast cancer risk, and that subsequent births further reduce the risk. However, the long-term risk reduction after birth depends on the age at birth in a similar way for first and subsequent births, i.e. any birth at early age has a similar long-term reducing effect on the incidence of breast cancer. We furthermore observed a latency period of the effect of each birth of at least 10 years. In general, our findings suggest that the risk-reducing effect of any birth at young age represents an early-stage long-term effect with a 10-year latency period.

In contrast to the protective effect of childbirth, a negative effect of induced abortion on breast cancer risk has been suggested—an effect thought to be due to the relatively large amount of undifferentiated breast cells at the time of abortion. The validity of previous retrospective case-control studies on the subject has, however, been questioned due to a likely differential misclassification of the exposure caused by the sensitive nature of the issue. Using the Danish cohort with register-based information on induced abortions, we showed that induced abortion is not associated with subsequent breast cancer risk.

Furthermore, breast cancer risk is not associated with gestational age in pregnancies with short duration (induced abortions), whereas women with a term birth had a lower risk compared with women with an extremely preterm birth. Taken together this suggests that the risk reduction after a birth is due to factors occurring very late in pregnancy and the finding therefore lends novel support to Russo and Russo's hypothesis.

Although the studies of the gestational effect on risk of breast cancer provided support for the hypothesis by Russo and Russo that differentiation of the breast cells protects against breast cancer, there are clearly other factors that need be considered. If differentiation was the sole explanation, one would assume that the first childbirth resulted in by far the greatest reduction in breast cancer risk on the assumption that most breast cells would have become differentiated. The finding that any birth at young age induce the same reduction in the risk of breast cancer conflicts somewhat with this interpretation.

On the basis of clinical information on disease subtype, we concluded that the reduction in risk following a birth is observed for most subtypes of breast cancer and is as such a general effect. However, a relatively larger reduction in risk of estrogen-sensitive tumors compared with nonsensitive tumors following births at an early age suggests that the risk-reducing effect occurring late in pregnancy to some degree is hormonally mediated.

Noticeable differential associations with reproductive history exist according to stage markers for both invasive tumors and in situ lesions. This can be interpreted as a late-stage effect of reproductive history on the tumor progression. However, as most of the difference is observed following the first birth, a plausible interpretation is that detection rates are different in women compared with women without children.

In addition to the long-term reduction in risk of breast cancer following childbirth, a short-term increase in risk was observed. Data from the Danish cohort revealed that the transient increase is very modest and far from the figures reported earlier. Furthermore, a nonhormonal explanation cannot be ruled out. However, we evaluated the possible cause using three different approaches. The transient increase (a) was larger following a birth with pregnancy characteristics related to relatively high hormonal level, (b) was larger in women with a family history of breast cancer, and (c) was especially marked for the incidence of large breast tumors. Thus, taken together our findings support the idea that the transient increase is associated with a pregnancy-induced hormonal stimulation of the growth of premalignant and malignant cells.

The present review describes aspects of the association between reproductive factors and breast cancer in more detail than has previously been done and thus provides new insights into the understanding of these associations. Two observations appear to be most relevant to future possibilities of intervention: (1) the finding of a critical but narrow window very late in pregnancy that causes the long term reduction in breast cancer risk and (2) the finding that the first birth is no more important than subsequent births for the reduction in breast cancer risk as long as all births take place very early in fertile life. These findings indicate that multiple treatments early in fertile life with a hypothetical drug (hormone) that will cause risk reduction late in pregnancy may drastically lower a woman's breast cancer risk.

STATISTICAL APPENDIX

Trend ratios by characteristics at diagnosis were estimated using the method by Greenland and Longnecker (1992). If the available information was inadequate for the approach of Greenland and Longnecker or convergence failed, simple inverse variance–weighted estimation, assuming independence, was used. A summary of the trend ratios for presented studies in the review tables was estimated using inverse variance–weighted regression analyses of trend ratios. The presented estimates should not be interpreted as a complete meta-analysis, but rather as a condensed quantification of the results from selected papers.

REFERENCES

Adami HO, Bergstrom R, Lund E, Meirik O. Absence of association between reproductive variables and the risk of breast cancer in young women in Sweden and Norway. Br J Cancer 1990; 62:122–126.

Albrektsen G. Time-related effects of a pregnancy on the risk of female cancers. PhD thesis, University of Bergen, Norway. 1998.

Albrektsen G, Heuch I, Kvale G. The short-term and long-term effect of a pregnancy on breast cancer risk: a prospective study of 802,457 parous Norwegian women. Br J Cancer 1995; 72:480–484.

Albrektsen G, Heuch I, Kvale G. Further evidence of a dual effect of a completed pregnancy on breast cancer risk. Cancer Causes Control 1996; 7:487–488.

Albrektsen G, Heuch I, Kvale G. Joint effects on cancer risk of age at childbirth, time since birth and attained age: circumventing the problem of collinearity. Stat Med 1999; 18:1261–1277.

Albrektsen G, Heuch I, Tretli S, Kvale G. Breast cancer incidence before age 55 in relation to parity and age at first and last births: a prospective study of one million Norwegian women. Epidemiology 1994; 5:604–611.

Beral V, Bull D, Doll R, Peto R, Reeves G. Breast cancer and abortion: collaborative reanalysis of data from 53 epidemiological studies, including 83?000 women with breast cancer from 16 countries. Lancet 2004; 363(9414): 1007–1016.

Braaten T, Weiderpass E, Kumle M, Adami HO, Lund E. Education and risk of breast cancer in the Norwegian-Swedish women's lifestyle and health cohort study. Int J Cancer 2004; 110(4):579–583.

Brind J, Chinchilli VM, Severs WB, Summy-Long J. Induced abortion as an independent risk factor for breast cancer: a comprehensive review and meta-analysis. J Epidemiol Community Health 1996; 50:481–496.

Brinton LA, Hoover R, Fraumeni JF Jr. Epidemiology of minimal breast cancer. JAMA 1983; 249:483–487.

Britton JA, Gammon MD, Schoenberg JB, Stanford JL, Coates RJ, Swanson CA, Potischman N, Malone KE, Brogan DJ, Daling JR, Brinton LA. Risk of breast cancer classified by joint estrogen receptor and progesterone receptor status among women 20–44 years of age. Am J Epidemiol 2002; 156:507–516.

Bruzzi P, Negri E, La Vecchia C, Decarli A, Palli D, Parazzini F, Del Turco MR. Short term increase in risk of breast cancer after full term pregnancy. BMJ 1988; 297:1096–1098.

Chen CL, Weiss NS, Newcomb P, Barlow W, White E. Hormone replacement therapy in relation to breast cancer. JAMA 2002; 287:734–741.

Chie WC, Hsieh C, Newcomb PA, Longnecker MP, Mittendorf R, Greenberg ER, Clapp RW, Burke KP, Titus-Ernstoff L, Trentham-Dietz A, MacMahon B. Age at any full-term pregnancy and breast cancer risk. Am J Epidemiol 2000; 151:715–722.

Colditz GA, Rosner BA, Speizer FE. Risk factors for breast cancer according to family history of breast cancer. For the Nurses' Health Study Research Group. J Natl Cancer Inst 1996; 88:365–371.

Collaborative Group on Hormonal Factors in Breast Cancer. Alcohol, tobacco and breast cancer—collaborative reanalysis of individual data from 53 epidemiological studies, including 58,515 women with breast cancer and 95,067 women without the disease. Br J Cancer 2002a; 87: 1234–1245.

Collaborative Group on Hormonal Factors in Breast Cancer. Breast cancer and breastfeeding: collaborative reanalysis of individual data from 47 epidemiological studies in 30 countries, including 50302 women with breast cancer and 96973 women without the disease. Lancet 2002b; 360:187–195.

Cooper JA, Rohan TE, Cant EL, Horsfall DJ, Tilley WD. Risk factors for breast cancer by oestrogen receptor status: a population-based case-control study. Br J Cancer 1989; 59:119–125.

Cummings P, Stanford JL, Daling JR, Weiss NS, McKnight B. Risk of breast cancer in relation to the interval since last full term pregnancy. BMJ 1994; 308:1672–1674.

Cummings P, Weiss NS, McKnight B, Stanford JL. Estimating the risk of breast cancer in relation to the interval since last term pregnancy. Epidemiology 1997; 8:488–494.

Daling JR, Malone KE, Voigt LF, White E, Weiss NS. Risk of breast cancer among young women: relationship to induced abortion. J Natl Cancer Inst 1994; 86:1584–1592.

Dano H, Andersen O, Ewertz M, Petersen JH, Lynge E. Socioeconomic status and breast cancer in Denmark. Int J Epidemiol 2003; 32(2):218–224.

Decarli A, La Vecchia C, Negri E, Franceschi S. Age at any birth and breast cancer in Italy. Int J Cancer 1996; 67:187–189.

Ekbom A, Adami HO, Trichopoulos D, Lambe M, Hsieh CC, Ponten J. Epidemiologic correlates of breast cancer laterality (Sweden). Cancer Causes Control 1994; 5:510–516.

Enger SM, Ross RK, Henderson B, Bernstein L. Breastfeeding history, pregnancy experience and risk of breast cancer. Br J Cancer 1997; 76:118–123.

Ewertz M, Duffy SW. Risk of breast cancer in relation to reproductive factors in Denmark. Br J Cancer 1988; 58: 99–104.

Friedenreich CM. Review of anthropometric factors and breast cancer risk. Eur J Cancer Prev 2001; 10:15–32.

Greenland S, Longnecker MP. Methods for trend estimation from summarized dose-response data, with applications to meta-analysis. Am J Epidemiol 1992; 135:1301–1309.

Haas JF. Pregnancy in association with a newly diagnosed cancer: a population-based epidemiologic assessment. Int J Cancer 1984; 34:229–235.

Habel LA, Stanford JL. Hormone receptors and breast cancer. Epidemiol Rev 1993; 15:209–219.

Heuch I, Albrektsen G, Kvale G. Modeling effects of age at and time since delivery on subsequent risk of cancer. Epidemiology 1999; 10:739–746.

Hildreth NG, Kelsey JL, Eisenfeld AJ, LiVolsi VA, Holford TR, Fischer DB. Differences in breast cancer risk factors according to the estrogen receptor level of the tumor. J Natl Cancer Inst 1983; 70:1027–1031.

Hinkula M, Pukkala E, Kyyronen P, Kauppila A. Grand multiparity and the risk of breast cancer: population-based study in Finland. Cancer Causes Control 2001; 12:491–500.

Hislop TG, Coldman AJ, Elwood JM, Skippen DH, Kan L. Relationship between risk factors for breast cancer and hormonal status. Int J Epidemiol 1986; 15:469–476.

Hsieh C, Pavia M, Lambe M, Lan SJ, Colditz GA, Ekbom A, Adami HO, Trichopoulos D, Willett WC. Dual effect of parity on breast cancer risk. Eur J Cancer 1994; 30A: 969–973.

Hsieh CC, Chan HW, Lambe M, Ekbom A, Adami HO, Trichopoulos D. Does age at the last birth affect breast cancer risk? Eur J Cancer 1996; 32A:118–121.

Hsieh CC, Goldman M, Pavia M, Ekbom A, Petridou E, Adami HO, Trichopoulos D. Breast cancer risk in mothers of multiple births. Int J Cancer 1993; 54:81–84.

Hsieh CC, Lan SJ. Assessment of postpartum time-dependent disease risk in case-control studies: an application for examining age-specific effect estimates. Stat Med 1996; 15:1545–1556.

Hsieh CC, Wuu J, Lambe M, Trichopoulos D, Adami HO, Ekbom A. Delivery of premature newborns and maternal breast-cancer risk. Lancet 1999; 353:1239.

Huang WY, Newman B, Millikan RC, Schell MJ, Hulka BS, Moorman PG. Hormone-related factors and risk of breast cancer in relation to estrogen receptor and progesterone receptor status. Am J Epidemiol 2000; 151:703–714.

Innes KE, Byers TE. Preeclampsia and breast cancer risk. Epidemiology 1999; 10:722–732.

Janerich DT, Hoff MB. Evidence for a crossover in breast cancer risk factors. Am J Epidemiol 1982; 116:737–742.

Kaijser M, Granath F, Jacobsen G, Cnattingius S, Ekbom A. Maternal pregnancy estriol levels in relation to anamnestic and fetal anthropometric data. Epidemiology 2000; 11: 315–319.

Kalache A, Maguire A, Thompson SG. Age at last full-term pregnancy and risk of breast cancer. Lancet 1993; 341:33–36.

Kelsey JL, Gammon MD, John EM. Reproductive factors and breast cancer. Epidemiol Rev 1993; 15:36–47.

Kelsey JL, Horn-Ross PL. Breast cancer: magnitude of the problem and descriptive epidemiology. Epidemiol Rev 1993; 15:7–16.

Klip H, Burger CW, Kenemans P, van Leeuwen FE. Cancer risk associated with subfertility and ovulation induction: a review. Cancer Causes Control 2000; 11:319–344.

Kvale G, Heuch I. A prospective study of reproductive factors and breast cancer. II. Age at first and last birth. Am J Epidemiol 1987; 126:842–850.

La Vecchia C, Negri E, Braga C, Fanceschi S. Multiple births and breast cancer. Int J Cancer 1996; 68:553–554.

Lambe M, Ekbom A. Cancers coinciding with childbearing: delayed diagnosis during pregnancy? BMJ 1995; 311:1607–1608.

Lambe M, Hsieh C, Trichopoulos D, Ekbom A, Pavia M, Adami HO. Transient increase in the risk of breast cancer after giving birth. N Engl J Med 1994; 331:5–9.

Lambe M, Hsieh C, Tsaih S, Ekbom A, Adami HO, Trichopoulos D. Maternal risk of breast cancer following multiple births: a nationwide study in Sweden. Cancer Causes Control 1996a; 7:533–538.

Lambe M, Hsieh CC, Chan HW, Ekbom A, Trichopoulos D, Adami HO. Parity, age at first and last birth, and risk of breast cancer: a population-based study in Sweden. Breast Cancer Res Treat 1996b; 38:305–311.

Lambe M, Hsieh CC, Tsaih SW, Ekbom A, Trichopoulos D, Adami HO. Parity, age at first birth and the risk of carcinoma in situ of the breast. Int J Cancer 1998; 77:330–332.

Leon DA, Carpenter LM, Broeders MJ, Gunnarskog J, Murphy MF. Breast cancer in Swedish women before age 50: evidence of a dual effect of completed pregnancy. Cancer Causes Control 1995; 6:283–291.

Li CI, Malone KE, Porter PL, Weiss NS, Tang MT, Daling JR. Reproductive and anthropometric factors in relation to the risk of lobular and ductal breast carcinoma among women 65–79 years of age. Int J Cancer 2003; 107(4):647–651.

Li CI, Weiss NS, Stanford JL, Daling JR. Hormone replacement therapy in relation to risk of lobular and ductal breast carcinoma in middle-aged women. Cancer 2000; 88: 2570–2577.

Liu Q, Wuu J, Lambe M, Hsieh SF, Ekbom A, Hsieh CC. Transient increase in breast cancer risk after giving birth: postpartum period with the highest risk (Sweden). Cancer Causes Control 2002; 13(4):299–305.

LiVolsi VA, Kelsey JL, Fischer DB, Holford TR, Mostow ED, Goldenberg IS. Effect of age at first childbirth on risk of developing specific histologic subtype of breast cancer. Cancer 1982; 49:1937–1940.

Longnecker MP, Bernstein L, Paganini-Hill A, Enger SM, Ross RK. Risk factors for in situ breast cancer. Cancer Epidemiol Biomarkers Prev 1996; 5:961–965.

Lumey LH, Stein AD, Ravelli AC. Maternal recall of birth-weights of adult children: validation by hospital and well baby clinic records. Int J Epidemiol 1994; 23:1006–1012.

MacMahon B, Cole P, Brown J. Etiology of human breast cancer: a review. J Natl Cancer Inst 1973; 50:21–42.

MacMahon B, Cole P, Lin TM, Lowe CR, Mirra AP, Ravnihar B, Salber EJ, Valaoras VG, Yuasa S. Age at first birth and breast cancer risk. Bull World Health Organ 1970; 43:209–221.

McCredie M, Paul C, Skegg DC, Williams S. Reproductive factors and breast cancer in New Zealand. Int J Cancer 1998; 76:182–188.

McTiernan A, Thomas DB, Johnson LK, Roseman D. Risk factors for estrogen receptor-rich and estrogen receptor-poor breast cancers. J Natl Cancer Inst 1986; 77:849–854.

Melbye M, Wohlfahrt J, Andersen AM, Westergaard T, Andersen PK. Preterm delivery and risk of breast cancer. Br J Cancer 1999; 80:609–613.

Melbye M, Wohlfahrt J, Lei U, Norgaard-Pedersen B, Mouridsen HT, Lambe M, Michels KB. alpha-fetoprotein levels in maternal serum during pregnancy and maternal breast cancer incidence. J Natl Cancer Inst 2000; 92:1001–1005.

Melbye M, Wohlfahrt J, Olsen JH, Frisch M, Westergaard T, Helweg-Larsen K, Andersen PK. Induced abortion and risk of Breast cancer. N Engl J Med 1997; 336:81–85.

Miller WR. Hormonal factors and risk of breast cancer. Lancet 1993; 341:25–26.

Norredam M, Groenvold M, Petersen JH, Krasnik A. Effect of social class on tumour size at diagnosis and surgical treatment in Danish women with breast cancer. Soc Sci Med 1998; 47:1659–1663.

Oestreicher N, White E, Malone KE, Porter PL. Hormonal factors and breast tumor proliferation: do factors that affect cancer risk also affect tumor growth? Breast Cancer Res Treat 2004; 85(2):133–142.

Olsson H. Reproductive events, occurring in adolescence at the time of development of reproductive organs and at the time of tumour initiation, have a bearing on growth characteristics and reproductive hormone regulation in normal and tumour tissue investigated decades later—a hypothesis. Med Hypotheses 1989; 28:93–97.

Peck JD, Hulka BS, Poole C, Savitz DA, Baird D, Richardson BE. Steroid hormone levels during pregnancy and incidence of maternal breast cancer. Cancer Epidemiol Biomarkers Prev 2002; 11:361–368.

Peck JD, Hulka BS, Savitz DA, Baird D, Poole C, Richardson BE. Accuracy of fetal growth indicators as surrogate measures of steroid hormone levels during pregnancy. Am J Epidemiol 2003; 157:258–266.

Pike MC, Krailo MD, Henderson BE, Casagrande JT, Hoel DG. 'Hormonal' risk factors, 'breast tissue age' and the age-incidence of breast cancer. Nature 1983; 303: 767–770.

Polednak AP, Janerich DT. Characteristics of first pregnancy in relation to early breast cancer. A case-control study. J Reprod Med 1983; 28:314–318.

Robertson C, Primic-Zakelj M, Boyle P, Hsieh CC. Effect of parity and age at delivery on breast cancer risk in Slovenian women aged 25–54 years. Int J Cancer 1997; 73:1–9.

Rookus MA, van Leeuwen FE. Breast cancer risk after induced abortion, a Dutch case-control study (Abstract). Am J Epidemiol 1995; 141:554.

Rosner B, Colditz GA, Willett WC. Reproductive risk factors in a prospective study of breast cancer: the Nurses' Health Study. Am J Epidemiol 1994; 139:819–835.

Russo J, Russo IH. Toward a unified concept of mammary carcinogenesis. Prog Clin Biol Res 1997; 396:1–16.

Sanderson M, Williams MA, White E, Daling JR, Holt VL, Malone KE, Self SG, Moore DE. Validity and reliability of subject and mother reporting of perinatal factors. Am J Epidemiol 1998; 147:136–140.

Schieve LA, Cogswell ME, Scanlon KS, Perry G, Ferre C, Blackmore-Prince C, Yu SM, Rosenberg D. Prepregnancy body mass index and pregnancy weight gain: associations with preterm delivery. The NMIHS Collaborative Study Group. Obstet Gynecol 2000; 96:194–200.

Senie RT, Rosen PP, Lesser ML, Snyder RE, Schottenfeld D, Duthie K. Epidemiology of breast carcinoma II: factors related to the predominance of left-sided disease. Cancer 1980; 46:1705–1713.

Shapiro S, Rao RS, Palmer J, Rosenberg L. Pregnancy and breast cancer risk (Abstract). Am J Epidemiol 1994; 139(suppl): S69.

Slattery MM, Morrison JJ. Preterm delivery. Lancet 2002; 360:1489–1497.

Smith GD, Whitley E, Gissler M, Hemminki E. Birth dimensions of offspring, premature birth, and the mortality of mothers. Lancet 2000; 356:2066–2067.

Stalsberg H, Thomas DB, Noonan EA. Histologic types of breast carcinoma in relation to international variation and breast cancer risk factors. WHO Collaborative Study of Neoplasia and Steroid Contraceptives. Int J Cancer 1989; 44:399–409.

Stanford JL, Szklo M, Boring CC, Brinton LA, Diamond EA, Greenberg RS, Hoover RN. A case-control study of breast cancer stratified by estrogen receptor status. Am J Epidemiol 1987; 125:184–194.

Stanford JL, Szklo M, Brinton LA. Estrogen receptors and breast cancer. Epidemiol Rev 1986; 8:42–59.

Talamini R, Franceschi S, Favero A, Negri E, Parazzini F, La Vecchia C. Selected medical conditions and risk of breast cancer. Br J Cancer 1997; 75:1699–1703.

Thompson WD, Wu M, Janerich DT. Increase in risk of breast cancer following pregnancy (Abstract). Am J Epidemiol 2002; 141(suppl):S53.

Tomeo CA, Rich-Edwards JW, Michels KB, Berkey CS, Hunter DJ, Frazier AL, Willett WC, Buka SL. Reproducibility and validity of maternal recall of pregnancy-related events. Epidemiology 1999; 10:774–777.

Trentham-Dietz A, Newcomb PA, Storer BE, Remington PL. Risk factors for carcinoma in situ of the breast. Cancer Epidemiol Biomarkers Prev 2000; 9:697–703.

Trichopoulos D, Hsieh CC, MacMahon B, Lin TM, Lowe CR, Mirra AP, Ravnihar B, Salber EJ, Valaoras VG, Yuasa S. Age at any birth and breast cancer risk. Int J Cancer 1983; 31:701–704.

Troisi R, Weiss HA, Hoover RN, Potischman N, Swanson CA, Brogan DR, Coates RJ, Gammon MD, Malone KE, Daling JR, Brinton LA. Pregnancy characteristics and maternal risk of breast cancer. Epidemiology 1998; 9: 641–647.

Vatten LJ, Kvinnsland S. Pregnancy-related factors and risk of breast cancer in a prospective study of 29,981 Norwegian women. Eur J Cancer 1992; 28A:1148–1153.

Velentgas P, Daling JR. Risk factors for breast cancer in younger women. J Natl Cancer Inst Monogr 1994; 16:15–24.

Weiderpass E, Gridley G, Persson I, Nyren O, Ekbom A, Adami HO. Risk of endometrial and breast cancer in patients with diabetes mellitus. Int J Cancer 1997; 71:360–363.

Weiss HA, Brinton LA, Brogan D, Coates RJ, Gammon MD, Malone KE, Schoenberg JB, Swanson CA. Epidemiology of in situ and invasive breast cancer in women aged under 45. Br J Cancer 1996a; 73:1298–1305.

Weiss HA, Brinton LA, Potischman NA, Brogan D, Coates RJ, Gammon MD, Malone KE, Schoenberg JB. Breast cancer risk in young women and history of selected medical conditions. Int J Epidemiol 1999; 28:816–823.

Weiss HA, Devesa SS, Brinton LA. Laterality of breast cancer in the United States. Cancer Causes Control 1996b; 7: 539–543.

Williams EM, Jones L, Vessey MP, McPherson K. Short term increase in risk of breast cancer associated with full term pregnancy. BMJ 1990; 300:578–579.

Wohlfahrt J, Andersen PK, Melbye M. Multivariate competing risks. Stat Med 1999a; 18(9):1023–1030.

Wohlfahrt J, Andersen PK, Mouridsen HT, Adami HO, Melbye M. Reproductive history and stage of breast cancer. Am J Epidemiol 1999b; 150(12):1325–1330.

Wohlfahrt J, Andersen PK, Mouridsen HT, Melbye M. Risk of late-stage breast cancer after a childbirth. Am J Epidemiol 2001; 153(11):1079–1084.

Wohlfahrt J, Melbye M. Age at any birth is associated with breast cancer risk. Epidemiology 2001; 12(1):68–73.

Wohlfahrt J, Melbye M. Gender of offspring and long-term maternal breast cancer risk. Br J Cancer 2000; 82(5): 1070–1072.

Wohlfahrt J, Melbye M. Maternal breast cancer risk and birth characteristics of offspring by time since birth. Epidemiology 1999; 10(4):441–444.

Wohlfahrt J, Mouridsen HT, Andersen PK, Melbye M. Reproductive risk factors for breast cancer by receptor status, histology, laterality and location. Int J Cancer 1999c; 81:49–55.

Wohlfahrt J, Olsen JH, Melbye M. Breast cancer risk after childbirth in young women with family history (Denmark). Cancer Causes Control 2002; 13(2):169–174.

Wohlfahrt J, Rank F, Kroman N, Melbye M. A comparison of reproductive risk factors for CIS lesions and invasive breast cancer. Int J Cancer 2004; 108(5):750–753.

Yoo KY, Tajima K, Miura S, Takeuchi T, Hirose K, Risch H, Dubrow R. Breast cancer risk factors according to combined estrogen and progesterone receptor status: a case-control analysis. Am J Epidemiol 1997; 146:307–314.

4

The Cellular Origins of Breast Cancer Subtypes

ANDREW H. SIMS and ROBERT B. CLARKE

Breast Biology Group, Division of Cancer Studies, University of Manchester, Christie Hospital, Manchester, U.K.

ANTHONY HOWELL and SACHA J. HOWELL

CRUK Department of Medical Oncology, Division of Cancer Studies, University of Manchester, Christie Hospital, Manchester, U.K.

INTRODUCTION

Breast cancers arise from the epithelial cells of the breast. The histology of the normal breast epithelium reveals that it is composed of a relatively simple bilayer of inner luminal cells required for milk production and an outer layer of myoepithelial cells required for milk ejection (Daniel and Smith, 1999). This apparent simplicity hides a more complex cellular hierarchy, which is revealed during carcinogenesis, and several histological and molecular subtypes of breast cancer can be defined by the use of immunological, genetic, and gene expression analysis methods.

There is now unequivocal evidence in rodents that a single mammary cell can give rise to the whole of the breast structure, which indicates the presence of mammary stem cells (Shackleton et al., 2006). Stem cells give rise to all other epithelial cell types within the breast by proliferating and differentiating into luminal and myoepithelial cells. Breast carcinomas are highly heterogeneous, and tumorigenesis must involve particular epithelial targets. Stem cells are possibly the prime target because they are long lived. It is possible that they give rise to the variety of breast carcinomas because aberrant signaling affects the differentiation process. There is also evidence that some estrogen receptor alpha positive (ERα+) cells are progenitors on the differentiation pathway. An alternative hypothesis to this differentiation pathway is that ERα-positive tumor arises from these cells by acquiring the capacity to self-renew (Clarke et al., 2005).

The aim of this review is to summarize the various approaches to breast cancer classification and to suggest the origin of the breast cancer subtypes by considering current knowledge concerning the stem cell/differentiation model. Clinicians can already predict response to current therapies (e.g., endocrine therapy, trastuzumab) and determine prognosis according to tumor characteristics, but a greater understanding of the origins of all subtypes will undoubtedly lead to new approaches to treatment.

BREAST CANCER SUBTYPES

Classification of Breast Tumors

The reason for segregating breast tumors into subtypes is to determine whether this gives prognostic information concerning tumor behavior (e.g., the propensity to metastasize) or predicts responsiveness to various therapies. Methods of subtyping include standard histopathology, molecular pathology, genetic analysis, and gene expression profiling. By far the clearest delineation between tumors appears to be the distinction between luminal tumors and basal-like tumors. Luminal tumors generally express the ER with or without coexpression of the progesterone receptor (PR). Basal-like tumors are defined by expression of cytokeratins (CK) 5/14/17 and a lack of ER, PR, and ERBB2 expression. Here we will briefly outline the utility of these methods in a historical context for characterizing breast cancer subtypes (summarized in Fig. 1) and then relate the subtypes described to the differentiation pathway, i.e., from stem cells to differentiated cells that exist in normal breast epithelium.

Early Divergence of the Breast Cancer Subtypes

Recent studies looking at the possible developmental pathways from normal and premalignant lesions to in situ carcinoma and invasive malignancy have resulted in two major pathways leading to two broad types of breast carcinoma (Fig. 2). One pathway comprises well-differentiated ductal or lobular carcinoma in situ (DCIS, LCIS), which progresses to grade I invasive ductal or lobular carcinoma (IDC, ILC). The grade I IDC and ILC are of low nuclear grade, usually ERα/PR-positive and HER2-negative, genetically stable, and often have chromosome 16q loss. The other pathway to invasive cancer comprises poorly differentiated DCIS, which progresses to grade III IDC; these grade III tumors have high nuclear atypia, are more frequently ERα/PR-negative and HER2-positive, and are genetically unstable with a combination of recurrent genomic gains and losses (Simpson et al., 2005). This division is supported by Kronenwett et al. (2006) who reported that a measure of genomic instability called the stemline scatter index divided invasive breast tumors into two categories: genomically stable and unstable, and these categories are irrespective of alterations in DNA content of the tumor (i.e., diploid, tetraploid, and aneuploid). Transcriptomic analysis of matched DCIS and IDC has also shown conservation of gene expression (Schuetz et al., 2006).

METHODS OF BREAST TUMOR CLASSIFICATION

Histopathology

Careful examination of breast lobules indicates that most breast tumors arise at the junction between the terminal duct and lobule, in an area described by Wellings et al. (1975) as the terminal ductal lobular units. All precursor lesions including DCIS are thought to arise in enlarged lobules that have been termed atypical lobules (AL) by Wellings et al. (1975) and hyperplastic enlarged lobular units (HELUs) by Lee and colleagues (Lee et al., 2006). A sixfold increase in ER-positive and proliferating cells in HELUs compared with terminal duct lobular units was recently observed (Lee et al., 2006), which might imply that HELUs are the first potential precursor of luminal rather than basal breast cancer subtypes identified by histology. Histological type does not provide much prognostic or predictive information although some information might be given about sites of metastasis (e.g., lobular cancers tend to spread under epithelium in the GI and GU tracts) or subtype association with gene overexpression (e.g., medullary cancer association with *BRCA1* or *BRCA2* mutation). Histological grade, however, is important for prognosis and prediction of responsiveness to chemotherapy and endocrine therapy.

Molecular Pathology

Microscopy, immunochemical methods, and fluorescence in situ hybridization (FISH) are important clinical and research tools. In modern clinical practice, immunochemical quantitation of ER and PR expression levels along with HER2 (ERBB2) analysis by both immunohistochemistry (IHC) and FISH is indispensable for directing the use of endocrine and antigrowth factor therapies (e.g., trastuzumab and lapatinib). Multiple other cellular antigens in univariate and multivariate analyses have been identified by IHC that provide prognostic information although none has entered routine clinical use to date. Cell proliferation markers appear to be the most valuable of such markers (e.g., Ki67), although defining the ideal cut off values for high versus low proliferative rate by IHC has proved difficult (Colozza et al., 2005).

Genetic Profile

Several recent studies using comparative genomic hybridization (CGH) approaches have demonstrated genetic differences among breast tumor molecular subtypes (Bergamaschi et al., 2006; Roylance et al., 2006; Wennmalm et al., 2006). Loss of genomic material in chromosome 16q has been proposed as an early event in a low-grade, good-prognosis pathway of breast cancer progression. Roylance et al. (1999) used CGH to compare invasive ductal grade I tumors, which are predominantly ER-positive, with grade III breast carcinomas, which are predominantly ER-negative. The authors found that 65% of grade I tumors had lost the long arm of chromosome 16 compared with only 16% of grade III tumors. This pattern of chromosomal loss led the investigators to conclude that the majority of grade I tumors do not progress to grade III tumors (Fig. 2) because this would necessitate the recovery of lost genetic material (Wennmalm et al., 2006). A clear genetic distinction was observed between the luminal A or normal-like tumors and other breast cancer

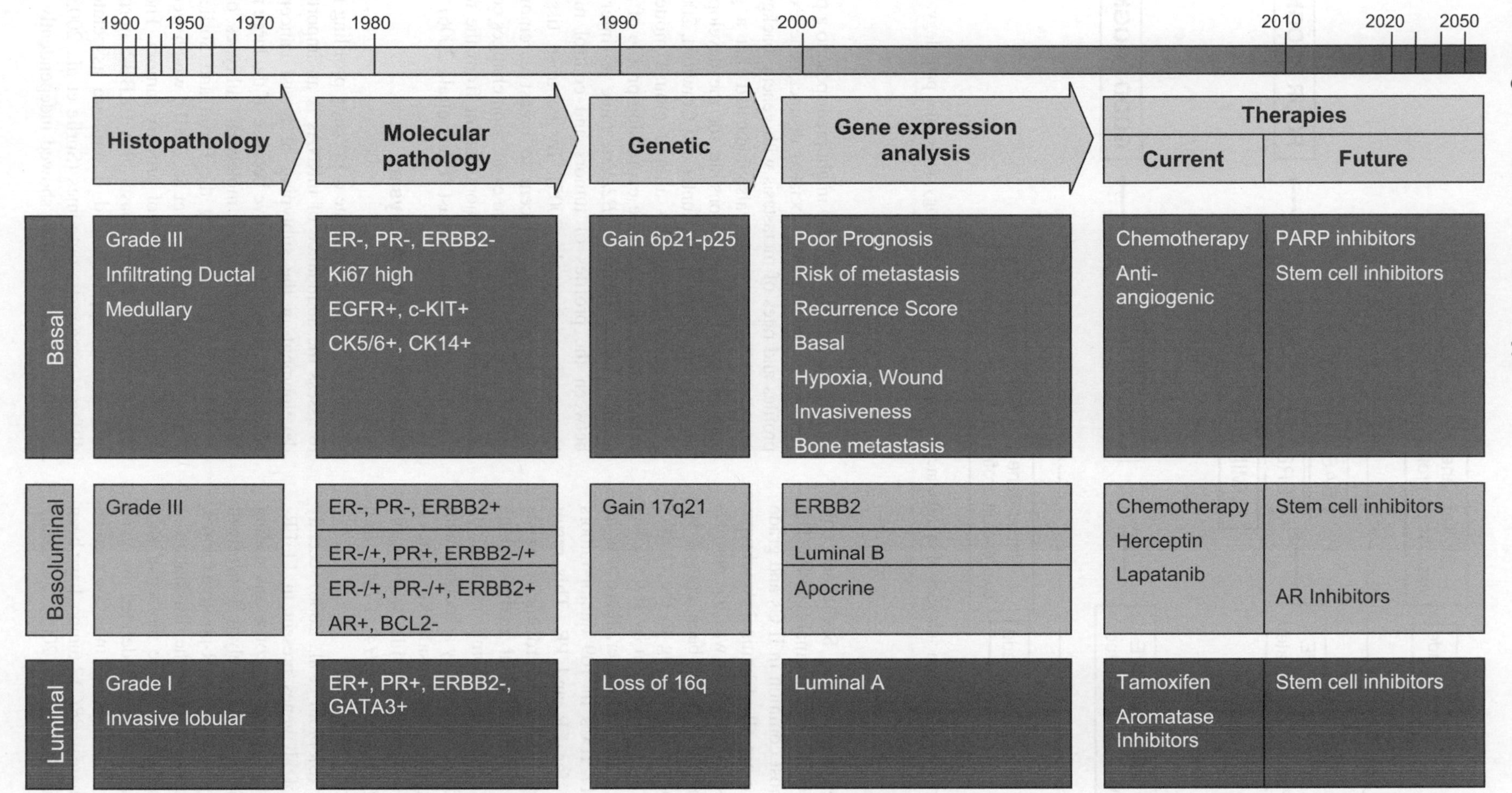

Figure 1 Comparison of the histopathology, molecular pathology, genetic, and gene expression methods used to delineate breast cancer tumor subtypes and suggested current and future therapies in a historical context. *Abbreviations*: CK, cytckeratin; ER, estrogen receptor; ERBB2 (HER2), erythroblastic leukemia viral oncogene homolog 2; PR, progesterone receptor; AR, androgen receptor.

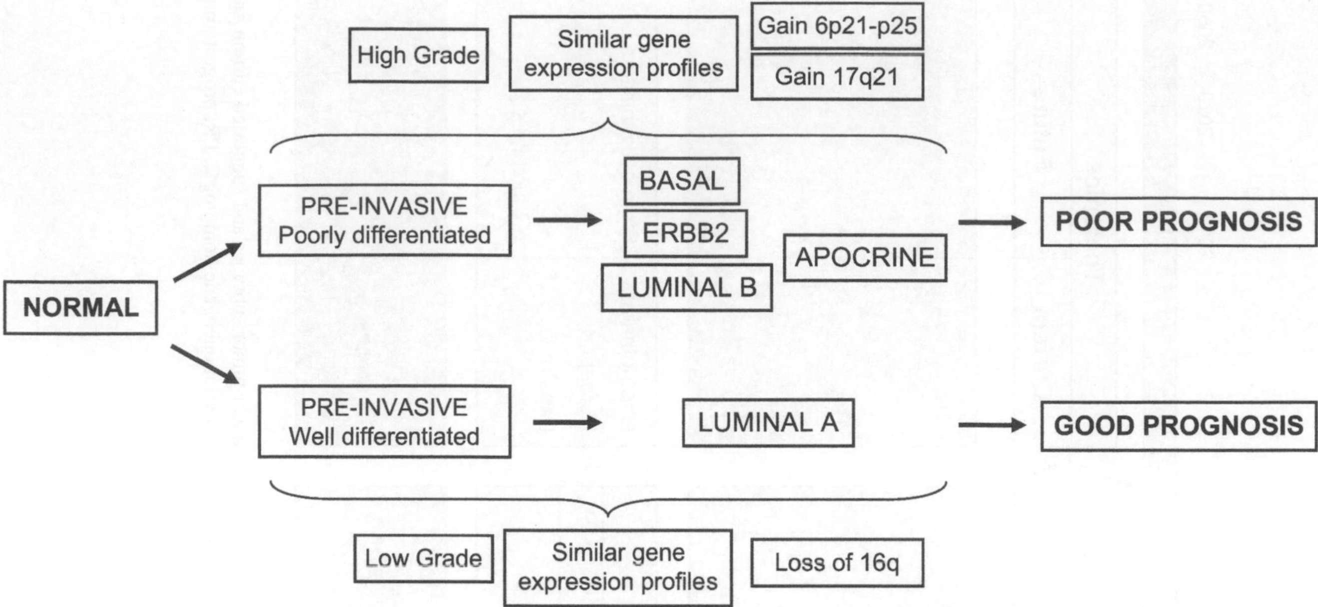

Figure 2 Early divergence between the main subtypes of breast cancer is supported by histopathology, molecular pathology, genetic, and gene expression analysis.

subtypes described by Perou et al. and Sorlie and colleagues (i.e., basal-like, ERBB2, and luminal type B). The 16q chromosome loss is most common in ILCs and grade 1 IDCs; however, ILCs are not all of luminal A subtype. The major cluster of ILCs in one study was the normal-like subtype, although this may have been caused by normal stromal cell contamination owing to the characteristic noncohesive pattern of infiltration by ILCs (Zhao et al., 2004). In a second study, however, there was no significant clustering of 17 ILCs in 109 ductal tumors including those negative for ER and PR. This result reveals that a broader intertumor heterogeneity exists than that suggested by histopathalogical analysis alone (Korkola et al., 2003). A gain of genomic material on chromosome six (6p21-p25) is particularly associated with ER-negative tumor subtypes and basal-like tumors, and several candidate oncogenes reside within this region such as *DEK*, *E2F3*, *NOTCH4*, *PIM1*, and *CCND3* (Bergamaschi et al., 2006).

Sjöblom and colleagues (Sjöblom et al., 2006) recently determined the sequence of all genes present in 11 ER-negative breast cancer cases using the consensus coding sequences database (CCDS). It seems likely that there will be genes that are specifically mutated in ER-positive tumors, and it will be interesting to see whether the distribution of the somatic mutations correlates with the molecular subtypes of breast cancer that have been defined by gene expression analysis. Tumors from *BRCA1* mutation carriers are often basal subtypes, whereas *BRCA2* tumors have been shown to be mainly luminal (Sorlie et al., 2003), indicating that the genetic background might predispose to a particular subtype. A study that associated distinct gene expression profiles and rates of metastasis with genetic background in 30 inbred mouse strains also indicated that a germline component might be responsible for the development of specific tumor subtypes (Hunter and Crawford, 2006).

Studies of genetically altered mouse models have demonstrated that the gene expression profile of adjacent normal tissue from *ErbB2/Neu* mice is intermediate between the profiles of tumors and control mammary tissues (Landis et al., 2005). By contrast, tissue with normal morphology adjacent to breast carcinomas did not contain significant gene expression changes compared with breast tissue taken more distant from the tumor or from the contralateral breast (Finak et al., 2006).

Gene Expression Analysis

The use of a variety of gene expression profiling methods to assess the abundance of mRNAs is an important new development in the subtyping of breast cancer and is potentially more informative because of the large numbers of genes analyzed. Five molecular subtypes of breast cancer were identified by the Perou and Sorlie groups (Perou et al., 2000; Sorlie et al., 2001), which were based on the "intrinsic" profile of primary tumors. These subtypes have been termed basal-like, ERBB2, normal-like, and luminal types A and B and are associated with different prognostic outcomes (Sorlie et al., 2003). More recently, the same groups showed independently that the molecular portraits are conserved across microarray platforms (Hu et al., 2006b; Sorlie et al., 2006). Other investigators have utilized gene expression profiling to identify tumor subtypes (Farmer et al., 2005; Richardson et al., 2006); however, not all of the subtypes identified by the Stanford group have been clearly identified in other molecular studies. In a study that identified a new gene expression subtype termed molecular aprocrine tumors, the majority of ERBB2-positive tumors were shown to be ER-negative and androgen receptor (AR)-positive and comprised a third major group alongside luminal and basal subtypes (Figs. 2 and 3) (Farmer et al., 2005). Using the largest combined dataset of breast tumors to date, the Perou group recently identified a possible "new" subtype characterized by the high expression of interferon-regulated genes (Hu et al., 2006b), and suggested that rare molecular subtypes of breast cancer might only be identified in very large population-based studies. There is also some doubt as to whether the normal-like subtype described by Perou's group and Sorlie's group actually represents cancerous tissue (Perou et al., 2000; Sorlie et al., 2001, 2003, 2006). Histopathological examination of tumor samples categorized as "normal-like" has revealed normal tissue contamination (Hu et al., 2006b). Despite variations between the microarray studies, it seems that distinct molecular mechanisms underlie the clinically relevant subtypes of breast cancer and that perturbations in these mechanisms can be reliably detected by different microarray platforms (Sims et al., 2006). It must be emphasized that the distinction between the subtypes in these transcriptomic studies is based on a large panel of genes rather than single markers. Nonetheless, the ER appears to be one of a number of genes where expression is almost exclusively limited to one of these major subtypes, making it one of the strongest discriminatory genes.

Gene expression analysis has been used to characterize histologically distinct subtypes of breast cancer at the molecular level. Bertucci et al. (2006) recently demonstrated that medullary breast cancer is a subtype of basal (i.e., ER-negative) breast cancers, and while inflammatory breast cancers can represent any of the main molecular subtypes identified, most are predominantly ER-negative (Nguyen et al., 2006). Gene expression analysis reveals that lobular and ductal cancers do not cluster separately, demonstrating that histology alone is an inaccurate way of subtyping breast cancer (Korkola et al., 2003; Zhao et al., 2004). Other approaches for subtyping breast cancer using gene expression analysis have focused on outcome; gene signatures were generated for poor prognosis (van 't Veer et al., 2002), recurrence score (Paik et al., 2004), and prediction of metastasis (Wang et al., 2005). Despite having few genes in common, these profiles show significant overlap in the outcome predicted for the same patients (Fan et al., 2006). The alternatives to these outcome-driven methods to stratify patients are those based on the actual characteristics of the tumors. These approaches have demonstrated the important role of cancer-associated fibroblasts in tumor progression (Chang et al., 2005) and that evasion of hypoxic conditions can identify particularly aggressive subtypes (Chi et al., 2006). The patients with these so-called "wound response" and "hypoxic" profiles also have a poor clinical outcome (Chang et al., 2005; Chi et al., 2006). It has been demonstrated that genes characterized by the "wound response" profile can be induced/repressed in MCF10A cells by transfection with the genes *CSN5* and *MYC*, suggesting that the signatures might be derived from small numbers of genetic events, which could be dependent on the cell of origin (Adler et al., 2006).

ORIGINS OF SUBTYPES AND THERAPEUTIC IMPLICATIONS

Normal Mammary Stem Cells

Adult breast epithelial stem cells are long lived, generally quiescent cells defined by their ability to self-renew and to produce progeny that can differentiate into functional cell types within the breast (Smalley and Ashworth, 2003; Reya and Clevers, 2005). This differentiation might occur either by symmetric or asymmetric cell division, giving rise to either new stem cells or an undifferentiated progenitor cell. The progenitors then undergo differentiation into luminal alveolar secretory and myoepithelial cells (Clarke et al., 2003; Dontu et al., 2003; Smalley and Ashworth, 2003; Smith and Boulanger, 2003). Although the stem cell is thought to be the target for carcinogenesis, it is possible that transit-amplifying progenitors are the targets and acquire the capacity to self-renew during the carcinogenesis process (Reya and Clevers, 2005). Seminal transplantation experiments in mice demonstrated that isolated segments from any portion of the mammary gland are capable of regenerating a complete mammary ductal and alveolar network (Deome et al., 1959; Daniel and Deome, 1965). More recently, this transplantable, reconstitutive capacity was shown in the progeny of a single retrovirally marked mammary epithelial cell (Kordon and Smith, 1998). Recently, parallel experiments in two laboratories have confirmed that an entire mouse mammary gland can be regenerated by transplanting single cells with defined cell surface markers into mammary fat pads cleared of epithelium (Shackleton et al., 2006; Stingl et al., 2006).

The position of the ER-positive cell within the hierarchy of stem cell to differentiated cell is important because estrogen is the major controller of the proliferating activity of the breast. In the mouse, the stem cell seems to be ER-negative (Asselin-Labat et al., 2007). In humans,

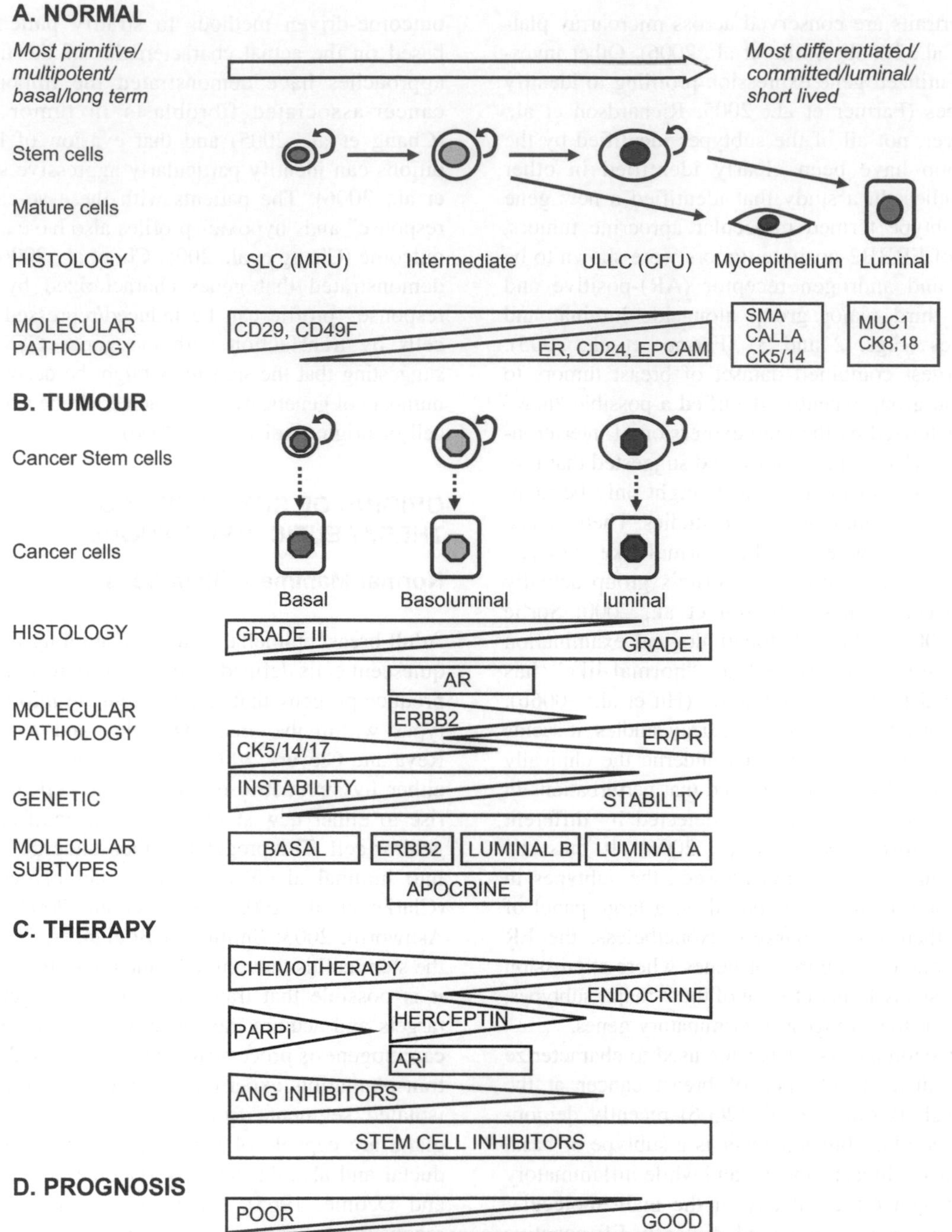

Figure 3 A model of stem cell hierarchy and how it may account for the origins of different subtypes of breast cancer via cancer stem cells. *Abbreviations*: ER, estrogen receptor; PR, progesterone receptor; SMA, = smooth muscle actin; ERBB2 (HER2), v-erb-b2 erythroblastic leukemia viral oncogene homolog 2; MRU, mammary repopulating unit; CFU, colony forming unit (Stingl et al., 2006); SLC, small light cell; ULLC, undifferentiated large light cell (Chepko and Smith, 1999). Cellular markers: CALLA, common acute lymphoblastic leukemia antigen; CK, cytokeratin; AR, androgen receptor; CD24, small cell lung carcinoma cluster 4 antigen; EPCAM, epithelial cell adhesion molecule; CD29, integrin β1; CD49f, integrin α chain α6; MUC1, mucin 1, cell surface associated; ANG, angiogenesis; PARPi, Poly (ADP-ribose) polymerase inhibitors; ARi, androgen receptor inhibitors.

ER-positive cells are long lived and have been found in the side population of precursor cells (Clarke et al., 2005). In the normal gland, ER-positive cells rarely divide and there is evidence to indicate that they control the cellular proliferation in response to estrogen (Wilson et al., 2006). These and other data have led to the proposed scheme in Figure 3A where the stem cell gives rise to ER-positive progenitors, which in turn control the development of differentiated breast luminal and myoepithelial cells by paracrine factors such as amphiregulin (Wilson et al., 2006). This scheme is supported by in vitro experiments, which show that a single breast epithelial cell negative for common differentiation markers can give rise to cells with luminal surface markers (e.g., EMA, MUC1), myoepithelial markers (e.g., KRT14 and SMA), and milk protein–expressing cells (Dontu et al., 2004; Stingl et al., 2006). The epithelial cells can also give rise to lobule-like structures in matrigel. Potential morphological correlates of the stem cell hierarchy are best seen by electron micrograph studies of the normal mouse mammary gland (Fig. 3A). Chepko and Smith (1999) described small light cells containing few cytoplasmic inclusions as putative stem cells, which gave rise to large undifferentiated light cells (candidates to be ER-positive) and a series of cells that were more differentiated.

Studies of ER expression in stem cells and normal breast epithelium suggest that differentiated lineages are derived from progenitors with different potentials at different times in development; the long-term ER-negative developmental stem cell is the most primitive and capable of reconstituting a cleared mammary fat pad as a single cell and the ER-positive short-term stem cell capable of producing colonies in vitro and patches of epithelium in the adult during tissue homeostasis. These stem cell types are most likely an in vivo continuum of phenotypes that give rise to the dividing ER-negative transit-amplifying cells that ultimately produce differentiated myo- and luminal epithelial cells in the adult tissue (Fig. 3A).

Breast Cancer Stem Cells

The presence of cancer stem cells (CSCs) can be inferred from studies where a single teratoma cell could produce a tumor and, more recently, from studies of leukemias in mice (Bonnet and Dick, 1997). Using different systems, a number of investigators have demonstrated that only a minority of cells in human cancers (i.e., CSCs) are capable of self-renewal and reconstitution of the original tumor (Reya and Clevers, 2005). The seminal work of Al-Hajj et al. (2003) indicates that a small subpopulation of breast cancer cells (ESA^{+},$CD44^{+}$,$CD24^{-/low}$) produce tumors in nonobese diabetic/severe combined immunodeficient mice (Al-Hajj et al., 2003), whereas very large numbers of other cancer cells were required to form tumors or did not form tumors. In addition, putative breast CSCs have been isolated from three breast cancer lesions and propagated in vitro and in vivo; stem-like cells have been identified in breast cancer cell lines (Locke et al., 2005; Ponti et al., 2005). These reports indicate the existence of stem-like cells in breast tumors and have important implications for tumor therapy. Most traditional cancer treatments target proliferating cells and while this might eliminate most of the tumor, relatively quiescent tumor stem cells could escape cancer treatment. It is important to understand the pathways that govern the self-renewal of normal stem cells because these same pathways might be active in CSCs. Inhibition of these signaling pathways has recently been proposed to be a novel therapeutic modality that could be used to target stem-like cells within the tumor (Behbod and Rosen, 2005; Liu et al., 2005; Kalirai and Clarke, 2006). Our group has recently described a novel culture technique for studying primary cells isolated from DCIS with stem-like properties. Inhibition of the EGFR or Notch signaling pathways reduced the self-renewal capacity of these DCIS mammospheres, thus targeting these pathways may have therapeutic value as adjuvant therapy for DCIS (Farnie et al., 2007).

The Origins of Breast Cancer Subtypes

The existence of a continuum of stem cells active at different points in development may provide an explanation for the existence of the breast cancer subtypes identified by the various histological, immunochemical, gene expression and genetic analysis approaches. On the basis of stem cell model of mammary carcinogenesis, one would predict that poorly differentiated, ER-negative breast tumors would arise from the most primitive stem cells, and the particular subset of mutations in these tumors must prevent differentiation into ER-positive cells. The basal-like breast cancer subtype expresses basal CK, the basal marker p63, and this subtype is highly EGFR-positive and ER-negative (Fig. 3B). The ERBB2 and luminal B subtypes have also been described as basoluminal (Laakso et al., 2006) or molecular apocrine (Farmer et al., 2005) and might be derived from a stem cell midway along the continuum. The luminal A subtype does not express the basal markers and is ER positive. The well-differentiated, ER-positive (luminal A) subtype would be predicted to arise from the transformation of ER-positive stem cells (Fig. 3B). Korsching et al. evaluated a panel of potential prognostic markers in 166 breast cancer cases using tissue microarray analysis. They were among the first to put forward a model describing the specific cellular origins of breast cancer subtypes based on differentiation into cytogenetic pathways (Korsching et al., 2002). Recent studies have indicated that *GATA3* expression may best classify this group of tumors and is responsible for maintaining differentiation of the luminal cell fate in the normal mammary gland development (Kouros-Mehr et al., 2006; Asselin-Labat et al., 2007).

The model of how different stem or progenitor cells give rise to the different subtypes of breast cancer is highly intuitive. It is difficult to identify, purify, and study the functional properties of normal stem cells, however, because of their scarcity. An even greater challenge is the characterization of CSCs that develop along a continuum and lead to different breast cancer subtypes. A very recent gene expression profiling study has compared tumorigenic CD44^{+}, CD24$^{-/low}$ cancer cells with normal breast epithelium to generate an "invasiveness" gene signature (Liu et al., 2007). This approach appears to identify the very worst-prognosis breast cancers, suggesting that the proportion or characteristics of CSCs in a tumor indicates its malignant potential. Breast cancer cells with CD44^{+}, CD24$^{-/low}$ subpopulation have previously been shown to express higher levels of proinvasive genes and are highly invasive. Only a subset of cell lines containing a CD44^{+}, CD24$^{-/low}$ subpopulation, however, was able to migrate to and proliferate in the lungs. The microenvironment is thought to have a strong influence on tumor progression, and patients who have breast tumors that express a "wound response" signature have been shown to have a poor clinical outcome (Chang et al., 2005). The prognostic power of the invasiveness gene signature was increased when combined with the wound response signature (Sheridan et al., 2006). Balic et al. demonstrated that most disseminated cancer cells detected in bone marrow of breast cancer patients have a putative breast cancer stem cell phenotype (i.e., CD44^{+},CD24$^{-/low}$), which suggests that these cells may display biological properties that facilitate their metastatic spread, enabling them to colonize distant sites (Balic et al., 2006).

Current and Future Therapies

Over the past two to three years, a paradigm shift in the way breast cancers are treated has begun. Until recently, the decision to use chemotherapy to treat a woman with early-stage breast cancer was based largely on the estimated population risk of recurrence derived from a number of histopathological features such as tumor size, grade, lymph node status, and expression of the biomarkers ER, PR, and ERBB2 based on IHC. Tools that more accurately calculate this risk, combined with the publication of treatment guidelines, have helped to guide clinicians and patients alike, but these advances have inevitably led to gross overtreatment for the majority of women concerned (Haybittle et al., 1982; Ravdin et al., 2001; Goldhirsch et al., 2005). Supervised gene expression analysis methods have been utilized in an attempt to improve the standard methods for prognostication (van 't Veer et al., 2002; Wang et al., 2005). Prospective validation of two such gene signatures is currently under way in very large multinational studies (MINDACT and TAILORx, which began recruitment in December 2006 and April 2006, respectively). The identification of prognostic groups differs fundamentally from the prediction of response to therapy, and a single retrospective study has demonstrated only one gene signature with predictive value (Paik et al., 2004). The unsupervised classification of breast cancers into biologically relevant subtypes could improve prediction of response to therapy, although this remains to be demonstrated. To date, such classification has not led to changes in therapeutic approach because therapy with agents targeting the ER and HER2 is based on detection of receptor protein expression rather than gene-based classification. A study by Rouzier et al. (2005) showed that molecular subtype was not independent of conventional clinicopathological predictors of response to neoadjuvant cytotoxic chemotherapy such as ER status and nuclear grade. However, complete pathological response rates were seen significantly more frequently in basal and erbB2+ subtypes (45% for both) compared with luminal (6%) and normal-like tumors (0%). None of the 61 genes associated with pathological complete response in the basal-like group were associated with pathological complete response in the ERBB2 subtype, suggesting that the molecular mechanisms of chemotherapy sensitivity, and presumably resistance, might vary between these two ER-negative subtypes (Rouzier et al., 2005).

The critical role of gene expression and genetic analysis of breast tumors lies in the identification of key pathways against which novel therapies can be targeted. If the CSC theory holds true then the "noise" from microarray analyses of heterogenous primary tumors might obscure the "signal" from the treatment-resistant CSC subpopulation responsible for relapse to therapy. Recent data indicate that breast cancer cells resistant to chemotherapy and radiotherapy are more clonogenic than treatment-sensitive populations. This resistance to therapy and clonogenicity may be conferred by pathways known to regulate normal mammary stem cell fate such as the Notch, Wnt/B-catenin, and Hedgehog pathways, making validation of these pathways as targets for breast cancer therapy an attractive option (Hu et al., 2006a; Liu et al., 2006; Woodward et al., 2007). The observations of Adler et al. that the overexpression of only the *CSN5* and *MYC* genes could recapitulate the wound response signature in nontransformed breast epithelial cells suggests that utilizing techniques to prospectively identify functional regulators of the large-scale transcriptional cancer signatures could reveal the principle targets for future therapies (Adler et al., 2006). Such studies might reveal different key genes in the different breast cancer subtypes and enhance our ability to target specific tumors with specific therapies rather than adopting the "one-size-fits-all" approach to treatment.

CONCLUSIONS

It is perhaps not surprising that genomic signatures appear to outperform preexisting clinical markers for classifying breast cancer when one considers the large numbers of additional factors that are taken into account, and that the measurement of these factors is continuous rather than categorical (Sims et al., 2006). The improved description and confirmation of breast cancer subtypes by gene expression analysis have been paralleled by advances in molecular and cellular biology describing normal breast epithelial stem cell types. We speculate that ER-positive and ER-negative subtypes of breast cancer (and possibly intermediate subtypes) can be explained by their origins in the different stem cells that operate at different points in mammary gland development.

There is increasing proof that an infrequent population of breast CSCs can recapitulate the entire tumor, and these CSCs are likely candidates for the origin of cancer recurrence. Information on signaling pathways that regulate normal and cancer stem cell self-renewal might lead to novel therapies. For example, knowledge of signaling pathways regulating stem cells could be used to induce differentiation of the CSC or promote their apoptosis. This knowledge could potentially be used in conjunction with conventional cancer treatments to eradicate proliferative cells and the quiescent CSCs, thus achieving improved cure rates for breast cancer.

ACKNOWLEDGMENTS

We are very grateful for funding from Breakthrough Breast Cancer, Breast Cancer Campaign, Cancer Research, U.K., and Christie's Appeal.

REFERENCES

Adler AS, Lin M, Horlings H, Nuyten DS, van de Vijver MJ, Chang HY. Genetic regulators of large-scale transcriptional signatures in cancer. Nat Genet 2006; 38:421–430.

Al-Hajj M, Wicha MS, Benito-Hernandez A, Morrison SJ, Clarke MF. Prospective identification of tumorigenic breast cancer cells. Proc Natl Acad Sci U S A 2003; 100: 3983–3988.

Asselin-Labat ML, Sutherland KD, Barker H, Thomas R, Shackleton M, Forrest NC, Hartley L, Robb L, Grosveld FG, van der Wees J, Lindeman GJ, Visvader JE. Gata-3 is an essential regulator of mammary-gland morphogenesis and luminal-cell differentiation. Nat Cell Biol 2007; 9:201–209.

Balic M, Lin H, Young L, Hawes D, Giuliano A, McNamara G, Datar RH, Cote RJ. Most early disseminated cancer cells detected in bone marrow of breast cancer patients have a putative breast cancer stem cell phenotype. Clin Cancer Res 2006; 12:5615–5621.

Behbod F, Rosen JM. Will cancer stem cells provide new therapeutic targets? Carcinogenesis 2005; 26:703–711.

Bergamaschi A, Kim YH, Wang P, Sorlie T, Hernandez-Boussard T, Lonning PE, Tibshirani R, Borresen-Dale AL, Pollack JR. Distinct patterns of DNA copy number alteration are associated with different clinicopathological features and gene-expression subtypes of breast cancer. Genes Chromosomes Cancer 2006; 45:1033–1040.

Bertucci F, Finetti P, Cervera N, Charafe-Jauffret E, Mamessier E, Adelaide J, Debono S, Houvenaeghel G, Maraninchi D, Viens P, Charpin C, Jacquemier J, Birnbaum D. Gene expression profiling shows medullary breast cancer is a subgroup of basal breast cancers. Cancer Res 2006; 66:4636–4644.

Bonnet D, Dick JE. Human acute myeloid leukemia is organized as a hierarchy that originates from a primitive hematopoietic cell. Nat Med 1997; 3:730–737.

Chang HY, Nuyten DS, Sneddon JB, Hastie T, Tibshirani R, Sorlie T, Dai H, He YD, Van't Veer LJ, Bartelink H, van de Rijn M, Brown PO, van de Vijver MJ. Robustness, scalability, and integration of a wound-response gene expression signature in predicting breast cancer survival. Proc Natl Acad Sci U S A 2005; 102:3531–3532.

Chepko G, Smith GH. Mammary epithelial stem cells: our current understanding. J Mammary Gland Biol Neoplasia 1999; 4:35–52.

Chi JT, Wang Z, Nuyten DS, Rodriguez EH, Schaner ME, Salim A, Wang Y, Kristensen GB, Helland A, Borresen-Dale AL, Giaccia A, Longaker MT, Hastie T, Yang GP, van de Vijver MJ, Brown PO. Gene expression programs in response to hypoxia: cell type specificity and prognostic significance in human cancers. PLoS Med 2006; 3:e47.

Clarke RB, Anderson E, Howell A, Potten CS. Regulation of human breast epithelial stem cells. Cell Prolif 2003; 36(suppl 1):45–58.

Clarke RB, Spence K, Anderson E, Howell A, Okano H, Potten CS. A putative human breast stem cell population is enriched for steroid receptor-positive cells. Dev Biol 2005; 277:443–456.

Colozza M, Azambuja E, Cardoso F, Sotiriou C, Larsimont D, Piccart MJ. Proliferative markers as prognostic and predictive tools in early breast cancer: where are we now? Ann Oncol 2005; 16:1723–1739.

Daniel CW, Deome KB. Growth of mouse mammary glands in vivo after monolayer culture. Science 1965; 149:634–636.

Daniel CW, Smith GH. The mammary gland: a model for development. J Mammary Gland Biol Neoplasia 1999; 4:3–8.

Deome KB, Faulkin LJ Jr., Bern HA, Blair PB. Development of mammary tumors from hyperplastic alveolar nodules transplanted into gland-free mammary fat pads of female C3H mice. Cancer Res 1959; 19:515–520.

Dontu G, Al-Hajj M, Abdallah WM, Clarke MF, Wicha MS. Stem cells in normal breast development and breast cancer. Cell Prolif 2003; 36(suppl 1):59–72.

Dontu G, El-Ashry D, Wicha MS. Breast cancer, stem/progenitor cells and the estrogen receptor. Trends Endocrinol Metab 2004; 15:193–197.

Fan C, Oh DS, Wessels L, Weigelt B, Nuyten DS, Nobel AB, van't Veer LJ, Perou CM. Concordance among gene-expression-based predictors for breast cancer. N Engl J Med 2006; 355:560–569.

Farmer P, Bonnefoi H, Becette V, Tubiana-Hulin M, Fumoleau P, Larsimont D, Macgrogan G, Bergh J, Cameron D, Goldstein D, Duss S, Nicoulaz AL, Brisken C, Fiche M, Delorenzi M, Iggo R. Identification of molecular apocrine breast tumours by microarray analysis. Oncogene 2005; 24:4660–4671.

Farnie G, Clarke RB, Spence K, Pinnock N, Brennan K, Anderson NG, Bundred NJ. Novel cell culture technique for primary ductal carcinoma in situ: role of Notch and EGF receptor signaling pathways. J Natl Cancer Inst 2007; 99:616–627.

Finak G, Sadekova S, Pepin F, Hallett M, Meterissian S, Halwani F, Khetani K, Souleimanova M, Zabolotny B, Omeroglu A, Park M. Gene expression signatures of morphologically normal breast tissue identify basal-like tumors. Breast Cancer Res 2006; 8:R58.

Goldhirsch A, Glick JH, Gelber RD, Coates AS, Thurlimann B, Senn HJ. Meeting highlights: international expert consensus on the primary therapy of early breast cancer 2005. Ann Oncol 2005; 16:1569–1583.

Haybittle JL, Blamey RW, Elston CW, Johnson J, Doyle PJ, Campbell FC, Nicholson RI, Griffiths K. A prognostic index in primary breast cancer. Br J Cancer 1982; 45: 361–366.

Hu C, Dievart A, Lupien M, Calvo E, Tremblay G, Jolicoeur P. Overexpression of activated murine Notch1 and Notch3 in transgenic mice blocks mammary gland development and induces mammary tumors. Am J Pathol 2006a; 168: 973–990.

Hu Z, Fan C, Oh DS, Marron JS, He X, Qaqish BF, Livasy C, Carey LA, Reynolds E, Dressler L, Nobel A, Parker J, Ewend MG, Sawyer LR, Wu J, Liu Y, Nanda R, Tretiakova M, Ruiz Orrico A, Dreher D, Palazzo JP, Perreard L, Nelson E, Mone M, Hansen H, Mullins M, Quackenbush JF, Ellis MJ, Olopade OI, Bernard PS, Perou CM. The molecular portraits of breast tumors are conserved across microarray platforms. BMC Genomics 2006b; 7:96.

Hunter KW, Crawford NP. Germ line polymorphism in metastatic progression. Cancer Res 2006; 66:1251–1254.

Kalirai H, Clarke RB. Human breast epithelial stem cells and their regulation. J Pathol 2006; 208:7–16.

Kordon EC, Smith GH. An entire functional mammary gland may comprise the progeny from a single cell. Development 1998; 125:1921–1930.

Korkola JE, DeVries S, Fridlyand J, Hwang ES, Estep AL, Chen YY, Chew KL, Dairkee SH, Jensen RM, Waldman FM. Differentiation of lobular versus ductal breast carcinomas by expression microarray analysis. Cancer Res 2003; 63:7167–7175.

Korsching E, Packeisen J, Agelopoulos K, Eisenacher M, Voss R, Isola J, van Diest PJ, Brandt B, Boecker W, Buerger H. Cytogenetic alterations and cytokeratin expression patterns in breast cancer: integrating a new model of breast differentiation into cytogenetic pathways of breast carcinogenesis. Lab Invest 2002; 82:1525–1533.

Kouros-Mehr H, Slorach EM, Sternlicht MD, Werb Z. GATA-3 maintains the differentiation of the luminal cell fate in the mammary gland. Cell 2006; 127:1041–1055.

Kronenwett U, Ploner A, Zetterberg A, Bergh J, Hall P, Auer G, Pawitan Y. Genomic instability and prognosis in breast carcinomas. Cancer Epidemiol Biomarkers Prev 2006; 15:1630–1635.

Laakso M, Tanner M, Nilsson J, Wiklund T, Erikstein B, Kellokumpu-Lehtinen P, Malmstrom P, Wilking N, Bergh J, Isola J. Basoluminal carcinoma: a new biologically and prognostically distinct entity between basal and luminal breast cancer. Clin Cancer Res 2006; 12:4185–4191.

Landis MD, Seachrist DD, Montanez-Wiscovich ME, Danielpour D, Keri RA. Gene expression profiling of cancer progression reveals intrinsic regulation of transforming growth factor-beta signaling in ErbB2/Neu-induced tumors from transgenic mice. Oncogene 2005; 24:5173–5190.

Lee S, Mohsin SK, Mao S, Hilsenbeck SG, Medina D, Allred DC. Hormones, receptors, and growth in hyperplastic enlarged lobular units: early potential precursors of breast cancer. Breast Cancer Res 2006; 8:R6.

Liu S, Dontu G, Mantle ID, Patel S, Ahn NS, Jackson KW, Suri P, Wicha MS. Hedgehog signaling and Bmi-1 regulate self-renewal of normal and malignant human mammary stem cells. Cancer Res 2006; 66:6063–6071.

Liu S, Dontu G, Wicha MS. Mammary stem cells, self-renewal pathways, and carcinogenesis. Breast Cancer Res 2005; 7:86–95.

Liu R, Wang X, Chen GY, Dalerba P, Gurney A, Hoey T, Sherlock G, Lewicki J, Shedden K, Clarke MF. The prognostic role of a gene signature from tumorigenic breast-cancer cells. N Engl J Med 2007; 356:217–226.

Locke M, Heywood M, Fawell S, Mackenzie IC. Retention of intrinsic stem cell hierarchies in carcinoma-derived cell lines. Cancer Res 2005; 65:8944–8950.

Nguyen DM, Sam K, Tsimelzon A, Li X, Wong H, Mohsin S, Clark GM, Hilsenbeck SG, Elledge RM, Allred DC, O'Connell P, Chang JC. Molecular heterogeneity of inflammatory breast cancer: a hyperproliferative phenotype. Clin Cancer Res 2006; 12:5047–5054.

Paik S, Shak S, Tang G, Kim C, Baker J, Cronin M, Baehner FL, Walker MG, Watson D, Park T, Hiller W, Fisher ER, Wickerham DL, Bryant J, Wolmark N. A multigene assay to predict recurrence of tamoxifen-treated, node-negative breast cancer. N Engl J Med 2004; 351:2817–2826.

Perou CM, Sorlie T, Eisen MB, van de Rijn M, Jeffrey SS, Rees CA, Pollack JR, Ross DT, Johnsen H, Akslen LA, Fluge O, Pergamenschikov A, Williams C, Zhu SX, Lonning PE, Borresen-Dale AL, Brown PO, Botstein D. Molecular portraits of human breast tumours. Nature 2000; 406:747–752.

Ponti D, Costa A, Zaffaroni N, Pratesi G, Petrangolini G, Coradini D, Pilotti S, Pierotti MA, Daidone MG. Isolation and in vitro propagation of tumorigenic breast cancer cells with stem/progenitor cell properties. Cancer Res 2005; 65:5506–5511.

Ravdin PM, Siminoff LA, Davis GJ, Mercer MB, Hewlett J, Gerson N, Parker HL. Computer program to assist in making decisions about adjuvant therapy for women with early breast cancer. J Clin Oncol 2001; 19:980–991.

Reya T, Clevers H. Wnt signalling in stem cells and cancer. Nature 2005; 434:843–850.

Richardson AL, Wang ZC, De Nicolo A, Lu X, Brown M, Miron A, Liao X, Iglehart JD, Livingston DM, Ganesan S. X chromosomal abnormalities in basal-like human breast cancer. Cancer Cell 2006; 9:121–132.

Rouzier R, Pusztai L, Delaloge S, Gonzalez-Angulo AM, Andre F, Hess KR, Buzdar AU, Garbay JR, Spielmann M, Mathieu MC, Symmans WF, Wagner P, Atallah D, Valero V, Berry DA, Hortobagyi GN. Nomograms to predict pathologic complete response and metastasis-free survival after preoperative chemotherapy for breast cancer. J Clin Oncol 2005; 23:8331–8339.

Roylance R, Gorman P, Harris W, Liebmann R, Barnes D, Hanby A, Sheer D. Comparative genomic hybridization of breast tumors stratified by histological grade reveals new insights into the biological progression of breast cancer. Cancer Res 1999; 59:1433–1436.

Roylance R, Gorman P, Papior T, Wan YL, Ives M, Watson JE, Collins C, Wortham N, Langford C, Fiegler H, Carter N, Gillett C, Sasieni P, Pinder S, Hanby A, Tomlinson I. A comprehensive study of chromosome 16q in invasive ductal and lobular breast carcinoma using array CGH. Oncogene 2006; 25:6544–6553.

Schuetz CS, Bonin M, Clare SE, Nieselt K, Sotlar K, Walter M, Fehm T, Solomayer E, Riess O, Wallwiener D, Kurek R, Neubauer HJ. Progression-specific genes identified by expression profiling of matched ductal carcinomas in situ and invasive breast tumors, combining laser capture microdissection and oligonucleotide microarray analysis. Cancer Res 2006; 66:5278–5286.

Shackleton M, Vaillant F, Simpson KJ, Stingl J, Smyth GK, Asselin-Labat ML, Wu L, Lindeman GJ, Visvader JE. Generation of a functional mammary gland from a single stem cell. Nature 2006; 439:84–88.

Sheridan C, Kishimoto H, Fuchs RK, Mehrotra S, Bhat-Nakshatri P, Turner CH, Goulet R, Jr., Badve S, Nakshatri H. CD44+/CD24- breast cancer cells exhibit enhanced invasive properties: an early step necessary for metastasis. Breast Cancer Res 2006; 8:R59.

Simpson PT, Reis-Filho JS, Gale T, Lakhani SR. Molecular evolution of breast cancer. J Pathol 2005; 205:248–254.

Sims AH, Ong KR, Clarke RB, Howell A. High-throughput genomic technology in research and clinical management of breast cancer. Exploiting the potential of gene expression profiling: is it ready for the clinic? Breast Cancer Res 2006; 8:214.

Sjöblom T, Jones S, Wood LD, Parsons DW, Lin J, Barber TD, Mandelker D, Leary RJ, Ptak J, Silliman N, Szabo S, Buckhaults P, Farrell C, Meeh P, Markowitz SD, Willis J, Dawson D, Willson JK, Gazdar AF, Hartigan J, Wu L, Liu C, Parmigiani G, Park BH, Bachman KE, Papadopoulos N, Vogelstein B, Kinzler KW, Velculescu VE. The consensus coding sequences of human breast and colorectal cancers. Science 2006; 314:268–274.

Smalley M, Ashworth A. Stem cells and breast cancer: a field in transit. Nat Rev Cancer 2003; 3:832–844.

Smith GH, Boulanger CA. Mammary epithelial stem cells: transplantation and self-renewal analysis. Cell Prolif 2003; 36(suppl 1):3–15.

Sorlie T, Perou CM, Tibshirani R, Aas T, Geisler S, Johnsen H, Hastie T, Eisen MB, van de Rijn M, Jeffrey SS, Thorsen T, Quist H, Matese JC, Brown PO, Botstein D, Eystein Lonning P, Borresen-Dale AL. Gene expression patterns of breast carcinomas distinguish tumor subclasses with clinical implications. Proc Natl Acad Sci U S A 2001; 98: 10869–10874.

Sorlie T, Tibshirani R, Parker J, Hastie T, Marron JS, Nobel A, Deng S, Johnsen H, Pesich R, Geisler S, Demeter J, Perou CM, Lonning PE, Brown PO, Borresen-Dale AL, Botstein D. Repeated observation of breast tumor subtypes in independent gene expression data sets. Proc Natl Acad Sci U S A 2003; 100:8418–8423.

Sorlie T, Wang Y, Xiao C, Johnsen H, Naume B, Samaha RR, Borresen-Dale AL. Distinct molecular mechanisms underlying clinically relevant subtypes of breast cancer: gene expression analyses across three different platforms. BMC Genomics 2006; 7:127.

Stingl J, Eirew P, Ricketson I, Shackleton M, Vaillant F, Choi D, Li HI, Eaves CJ. Purification and unique properties of mammary epithelial stem cells. Nature 2006; 439:993–997.

van 't Veer LJ, Dai H, van de Vijver MJ, He YD, Hart AA, Mao M, Peterse HL, van der Kooy K, Marton MJ, Witteveen AT, Schreiber GJ, Kerkhoven RM, Roberts C, Linsley PS, Bernards R, Friend SH. Gene expression profiling predicts clinical outcome of breast cancer. Nature 2002; 415: 530–536.

Wang Y, Klijn JG, Zhang Y, Sieuwerts AM, Look MP, Yang F, Talantov D, Timmermans M, Meijer-van Gelder ME, Yu J, Jatkoe T, Berns EM, Atkins D, Foekens JA. Gene-expression profiles to predict distant metastasis of lymph-node-negative primary breast cancer. Lancet 2005; 365:671–679.

Wellings SR, Jensen HM, Marcum RG. An atlas of subgross pathology of the human breast with special reference to possible precancerous lesions. J Natl Cancer Inst 1975; 55:231–273.

Wennmalm K, Calza S, Ploner A, Hall P, Bjohle J, Klaar S, Smeds J, Pawitan Y, Bergh J. Gene expression in 16q is associated with survival and differs between Sorlie breast cancer subtypes. Genes Chromosomes Cancer 2007; 46:87–97.

Wilson CL, Sims AH, Howell A, Miller CJ, Clarke RB. Effects of oestrogen on gene expression in epithelium and stroma of normal human breast tissue. Endocr Relat Cancer 2006; 13:617–628.

Woodward WA, Chen MS, Behbod F, Alfaro MP, Buchholz TA, Rosen JM. WNT/beta-catenin mediates radiation resistance of mouse mammary progenitor cells. Proc Natl Acad Sci U S A 2007; 104:618–623.

Zhao H, Langerod A, Ji Y, Nowels KW, Nesland JM, Tibshirani R, Bukholm IK, Karesen R, Botstein D, Borresen-Dale AL, Jeffrey SS. Different gene expression patterns in invasive lobular and ductal carcinomas of the breast. Mol Biol Cell 2004; 15:2523–2536.

5

The Importance of Estrogen Receptors in Breast Cancer

RACHEL SCHIFF, JENNIFER SELEVER, and SUZANNE A. W. FUQUA
Lester and Sue Smith Breast Center, Baylor College of Medicine, Houston, Texas, U.S.A.

INTRODUCTION

Breast cancer is a classic hormone-responsive malignancy. The association between estrogen and carcinoma of the breast was recognized over 100 years ago, in a report by Beatson showing that patients with inoperable breast tumors frequently responded to surgical oophorectomy (Beatson, 1896). Since then, a substantial body of experimental, clinical, and epidemiological evidence has indicated that steroid hormones, namely estrogens and progestins, play a role in the progression of breast cancer. In fact, the known risk factors for breast cancer largely reflect the extent of lifetime exposure of the breast to these two hormones (Thomas et al., 1997). The presence of an intracellular estrogen-binding protein, initially called estrophilin, in estrogen target organs of animals and also in human breast cancers was reported through the 1960s, after radiolabeled estrogens became available for research (Jensen and Jacobson, 1962). The importance of estrogen in the development and promotion of growth of normal breasts led to a massive research effort into the mechanisms whereby estrogen exerts its effects, and with the eventual elucidation (Toft and Gorski, 1966) and cloning of the first estrogen receptor (ER), now called ERα (Green et al., 1986a,b). Another level of intricacy to this research field was introduced with the discovery of a second ER, called ERβ.

The idea that therapeutic antagonists to estrogen action could also prevent breast cancer was first suggested by Lacassagne in 1936, long before either the target (ER) or antiestrogen drugs were identified. Following the identification of ERα, Jensen et al. (1971) took the concept of targeting ERα one step further by suggesting that the measurement of ERα levels in breast cancers could help to predict response to hormonal therapy. As the century turned, we can state that both the predictive value of ERα in breast cancer and the usefulness of targeting this receptor have clearly stood the test of time. Improved and newly developed methods for assessing receptor proteins have led to less expensive, simpler, and possibly more accurate and consistent measurements of ERα for clinical use. New insights into the biology of ER and its mechanism of action, resulting from an immense number of clinical and basic molecular studies, have already begun to lead to better therapies. As a result, the number of available compounds that interact with the receptor and selectively modulate its activity (called selective estrogen receptor modulators or SERMs) grows steadily each year in the clinical setting. This chapter will offer a current view of the dynamic research field of ER expression, function, and role in breast cancer etiology, progression, and treatment along with highlighting crucial open questions and significant future challenges.

ER-MEDIATED PROCESSES IN NORMAL AND CANCER BREAST CELLS

The development of the normal mammary gland, as well as the development and progression of breast cancer, is regulated by a number of steroid and polypeptide hormones and growth factors (Dickson and Lippman, 2000). Among these complex hormonal influences, estrogen is considered to play a major role in promoting the proliferation of both the normal and the neoplastic breast epithelium. Estrogen acts locally on mammary glands and, through autocrine and paracrine loops, stimulates DNA synthesis and promotes bud formation in the normal gland (Anderson et al., 1982; Dickson et al., 1986; Huseby et al., 1984; Russo and Russo, 1996; for a recent review see Russo et al., 2000). The use of antiestrogens targeting the ER, both in vitro and in vivo, in animal models and in the clinic, has revealed the broad spectrum of effects of this pathway on normal breast tissue and breast cancers included cell proliferation, cell survival, differentiation, and angiogenesis. Estrogens clearly have some nongenomic actions (Duval et al., 1983) (see section "ER cross talk with other signal transduction pathways and alternative signaling"); however, the majority of these cellular effects are thought to be mediated by their binding to the ERs, which leads to receptor activation as a transcription factor that then regulates the expression of a variety of specific target genes. Among these regulated genes, as has been shown in normal and cancerous cells, are genes encoding proteins that are involved in DNA synthesis, cell cycle control [Cyclin D1, c-myc (Altucci et al., 1996; Miller et al., 1996)], and cell survival [Bcl-2/BclX_L (Choi et al., 2001; Rosfjord and Dickson, 1999; Safe, 2001)]; several polypeptide growth factors, growth factor–binding proteins, and growth factor receptors [e.g., epidermal growth factor (EGF) and insulin-likc growth factor-1 (IGF-1) and their receptors (Clarke et al. 1991)]; other receptors [progesterone receptor (PR), laminin]; proteases [cathepsin D, plasminogen, collagenase (Fulco et al., 1998)]; angiogenic factors [vascular endothelial growth factor (Hyder et al., 2000)]; and many other proteins. This partial list can, at least in part, explain the pleiotropic effects of ER signaling in normal and pathological conditions of the mammary gland. For many of the aforementioned proteins, their pathological overexpression and functional relevance for breast cancer has received experimental support in vitro, in vivo, and/or in clinical studies.

The importance of the integrity of ERα in the normal mammary gland has been clearly demonstrated using ERα knockout (α-ERKO) mice (for a recent review see Couse and Korach, 1999 and references there). The mammary glands of these animals are poorly developed due to the loss of multiple stimuli that are downstream of ERα including several important mammary developmental regulators such as the PR. Notably, these studies indicate that stromal ERα is also essential to the mitogenic actions of estradiol in the mammary epithelium, thus suggesting an even more complex paracrine ER-mediated regulation in mammary glands that involves both epithelial-epithelial and epithelial-stromal interactions. The recognized involvement of the ER pathway in the regulation of pathological processes such as angiogenesis (Haynes et al., 2000a) and metastasis (Gorlich and Jandrig, 1996), in both endothelium and epithelium compartments, may also involve the stromal ER, and therefore should be considered among other therapeutic targets. However, the role of stromal ER in human normal and breast tumors is still, unfortunately, blurred. Transgenic mice constitutely overexpressing ERα have been generated (Frech et al., 2005). These mice develop abnormal ductal and lobular structures, and ductal carcinoma in situ, suggesting a role of altered ERα expression in the early stages of breast cancer development.

Only limited data are available on the expression and function of ERβ in normal breast and its potential role in breast carcinogenesis. In contrast to the dramatic underdevelopment observed in the α-ERKO, studies using β-ERKO mice suggest that ERβ has only a limited role in normal breast development and function, including late differentiation events and lactation (Couse and Korach, 1999; Krege et al., 1998). This KO phenotype agrees with the minor amounts of detectable ERβ mRNA in the adult mouse mammary gland, whereas ERα transcripts are easily detectable (Couse et al., 1997). However, ERβ appears to be important for the growth control of the urogenital tract epithelium (Couse et al. 2000; Couse and Korach, 1999), and it has been suggested that its expression affords a protective role against hyperproliferation and carcinogenesis in that tissue. But whether ERβ plays a significant role in breast neoplastic processes is still an open and controversial issue. Clearly additional animal models overexpressing ERβ, and other clinical studies, are needed to clarify this open question.

ER GENES AND MRNA TRANSCRIPTIONAL REGULATION

Until recently, estrogen action was thought to be mediated primarily through a single ER, now called ERα. However, a second ER, ERβ, was identified and cloned independently from rat, human, and mouse (Kuiper et al., 1996; Mosselman et al., 1996; Tremblay et al., 1997). The two receptor subtypes are not isoforms of each other but rather are distinct proteins encoded by separate genes located on different chromosomes. The human ERα and ERβ genes have been mapped to chromosomes 6 (Menasce et al., 1993) and 14 (Enmark et al., 1997), respectively.

ER Expression in Premalignant Disease and Breast Cancer

In normal mammary epithelial cells, the level of ERα fluctuates during the menstrual cycle in response to cyclical changes in estrogen, with only a small percentage of the luminal cell population expressing the receptor. The highest percentage of ERα-expressing cells is found in the undifferentiated lobule type 1 (Lob1 cell), with a progressive reduction of expression in the more differentiated lobules Lob2 and Lob3 (Russo et al., 1999). In addition, it has been recently shown that only some cells in premenopausal normal breast tissues have ER, and these are not the proliferating cells (Clarke et al., 1997; Russo et al., 2000). However, in precancerous and in breast cancer tissues, normal control of the ER gene expression is disrupted, such that ERα expression is significantly increased in premalignant (Shoker et al., 1999; Shoker et al., 2000) as well as malignant breast lesions (van Agthoven et al., 1994). Importantly, it has been shown in prospective studies that the percentage of ERα-positive cells within precancerous lesions correlates with the risk of developing cancer (Shoker et al., 1999). The percentage of ER-positive proliferating cells in these premalignant lesions is also significantly increased (Anderson et al., 1998). All these observations together strongly suggest that the development of breast cancer may be associated with misregulation of ER expression. On the other hand, some breast tumors initially present as ERα-negative, or progress to become ER-negative, and these tumors have poorer prognosis and more aggressive clinical behavior (McGuire, 1988). In these cases, it is the loss of ERα expression that implies further misregulation of the normal ER expression.

Transcriptional Regulation

The human ERα mRNA is transcribed from a complex gene that consists of eight exons. Its promoter lacks homology to known consensus initiator or basal promoter sequences, such as TATA- and CAAT-boxes (Grandien, 1996). The exact molecular mechanisms regulating ER expression in breast tumors are unclear, but studies suggest that they are partly at the level of transcription. The existence of multiple promoter regulatory regions, utilized in a cell- and tissue-specific mode (Donaghue et al. 1999; Grandien, 1996), has been described in both the 5′-upstream and untranslated sequences of the human ERα, though only a single open reading frame appears to exist. Some ER-positive cell lines and normal human mammary epithelium appear to use a more proximal promoter (called P1) located immediately upstream of the coding region (Weigel et al., 1995). In contrast, in some breast tumors, enhanced ERα levels correlate with elevated mRNA expression from a more distal promoter (called P0) (Hayashi et al., 1997; Tanimoto et al., 1999). The biological mechanisms responsible for promoter choice are not yet well understood, but it seems feasible that a specific promoter switch might accompany the ER upregulation event that occurs during breast cancer development and progression.

Several potential regulatory DNA elements within the ERα promoter and several transcription factors that bind these regions preferentially in ER-positive tumor cells have been identified. Among those are known members of the AP-1 (Tang et al., 1997), AP-2 (McPherson et al., 1997), SP-1 (deGraffenreid et al., 2002), and estrogen receptor promoter B–associated factor-1 (ERBF-1) (Tanimoto et al., 1999) transcription factor families. A third promoter of the ERα gene, located more than 21 kilobase (kb) upstream of the proximal promoter, has also been recently described, but its relative contribution to ERα gene transcription is still controversial (Donaghue et al., 1999).

In addition, it is also generally accepted that estrogens downregulate ER expression in breast cancer cells (Saceda et al., 1988). However, other recent findings have also suggested that ER may positively contribute in an indirect autoregulatory manner, via protein-protein interaction, to its own expression in some breast cancer cell lines (Castles et al., 1997). Interestingly, Donaghue et al. (1999) have shown that all three previously mentioned ERα promoters are modulated by estrogen in estrogen-responsive breast cancer cell lines, and that it is the unique repertoire of transcription factors present within a given cell that determines whether ERα gene expression is increased or decreased by estrogen. The regulatory mechanisms responsible for controlling ERβ gene expression, whose expression pattern in normal and malignant breast tissues is not yet known, have not yet been disclosed. The human ERβ promoter has been cloned, and this study suggests that ERβ expression, like ERα expression, may be regulated by estrogen (Li et al., 2000). Since the presence or absence of the ER plays a key role in the biology of breast cancer, the exact nature, complexity, and role of specific DNA regulatory sequences and transcription complexes in regulating ER expression, especially in clinical premalignant and cancerous tissues, must be better defined.

The absence of ER transcription in ER-negative tumors might also involve other regulatory sequences or specific mechanisms. One of these proposed mechanisms is DNA hypermethylation, an epigenetic process that has been suggested to serve as an alternative mechanism for the loss of key gene function in neoplastic cells (Baylin and Herman, 2000). Indeed, it has been demonstrated that methylation of CpG islands located within both the distal and the more proximal promoters of ERα is associated with ER-negativity in some human breast cancer cell lines and cancers (Iwase et al., 1999; Nass et al., 2000; Ottaviano et al., 1994), and moreover experimentally induced demethylation can reactivate ER gene expression in these cells (Ferguson et al., 1995). Recently, histone deacetylase (HDAC) inhibitors that are clinically relevant have been used to reactivate ERα in ER-negative cells and enhance tamoxifen sensitivity (Zhou et al., 2007a). Similarly, ERβ expression can be reactivated by DNA methyl transferase inhibitors (Skliris et al., 2003). These observations suggest that methylation is an important contributor for the control of ER expression and that methylation may also play a role in the progression to hormone independence, but this speculation still awaits experimental confirmation.

MOLECULAR MECHANISM OF ER ACTION AS A LIGAND-DEPENDENT TRANSCRIPTION FACTOR

With the discovery of ERβ, estrogen, like other steroid and nuclear hormones, is now known to signal through more than one form of receptor. ERs are members of a large superfamily of nuclear receptors (Jensen, 1991; Kumar and Thompson, 1999) that includes receptors for other steroid hormones, nonsteroid hormones such as thyroid hormones and retinoids, and a number of other members whose ligands have yet to be identified (known as orphan receptors). Upon binding of their respective ligands, these receptors function as transcription factors to modulate the transcription of target genes critical to such biological processes as development, reproduction, and homeostasis.

Estrogen diffuses into cells and binds to the ER protein. ER is predominantly a nuclear protein that exists in an inactive complex consisting of several chaperone proteins such as heat-shock protein 90 (hsp90) that appear to dissociate upon ligand binding, allowing a "transformation" of the receptor to an active state (Jensen, 1991). Ligand-bound ER then dimerizes and associates with specific consensus sites present in the promoters of target genes. Depending on the ligand bound to it, the ER also interacts with a number of coregulatory complexes and with elements of the basal transcriptional machinery that together coordinately modulate the transcription of estrogen target genes.

ERα Structure and Functional Domains

Human ERα protein consists of 595 amino acids and displays an approximate molecular weight of 66 kDa. It shares a common structural and functional organization with all of the nuclear receptors, being divided into six regions, termed A to F, which include at least five major functional domains (Fig. 1).

The amino-terminal A/B domain is the most variable, in both sequence and length, in the nuclear receptor superfamily. The A/B domain contains a hormone-independent transcription activation function (AF-1) that can stimulate transcription in the absence of hormone binding. AF-1 is also thought to be responsible for gene and cell specificity (Bocquel et al., 1989; Lees et al., 1989; Metzger et al., 1995; Tasset et al., 1990; Tora et al., 1989) and to be important for the agonist activity of mixed antiestrogens (McInerney and Katzenellenbogen, 1996), probably through phosphorylation of specific serine residues (Chen et al., 2000b; Weigel, 1996). It has therefore been proposed that the AF-1 domain may be involved in hormone-resistant breast cancer (Campbell et al., 2001; Weigel and Zhang, 1998).

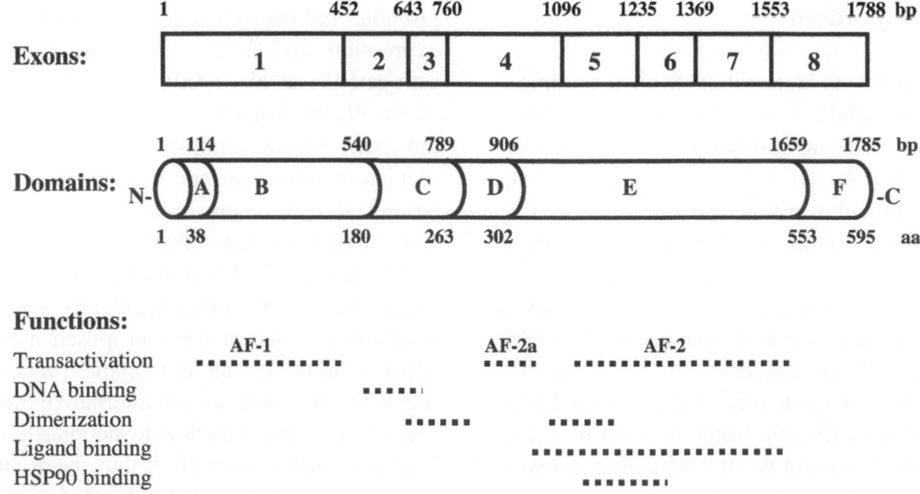

Figure 1 Schematic representation of ERα. At the top is the exon structure of ER mRNA and below are the structural domains (A–F) of the protein [base pair (bp) numbers above and amino acid (aa) numbers below the figures correspond to domain boundaries]. The functional domains of the receptor are indicated below the structural figures.

The C domain is highly conserved among the nuclear receptors and is the site that binds to DNA (DBD). This site contains nine cysteines in fixed positions that are arranged in two zinc fingers. Hormone binding induces conformational changes that allow the receptor to bind to hormone-responsive elements within target genes. For ER, these elements are inverted repeats of the sequence GGTCA separated by three variant bases, also known as estrogen response elements (EREs) (Klein-Hitpass et al., 1988; Martinez et al., 1987; Walker et al., 1984).

Region D is the hinge domain, which appears to function as a site of rotation, and may be an important binding site for accessory proteins (Jackson et al., 1997). Of particular interest is a putative phosphorylation site within this region that is found in all steroid receptors at essentially the same site (Knotts et al., 2001). A nuclear localization signal, responsible for the nuclear localization of ER, also resides in this region.

Region E is the ligand-binding domain (LBD). Structural studies of the ER LBD suggest that the "binding pocket" for the ligand is nearly twice the volume of its cognate estrogen ligand (Anstead et al., 1997; Pike et al., 2000). This difference might help explain the apparent high affinity of synthetic ER ligands that possess additional moieties to the receptor (Shiau et al., 1998). This phenomenon is not well expected for a "single-hormone" receptor such as ER and might suggest the existence of undiscovered endogenous ER modulators (Pike et al., 2000). Further crystallography studies with different ligands of the ERs have revealed that the structural and conformational changes induced by various ligands help contribute to their agonist versus antagonist effects (Brzozowski et al., 1997). A key event is the repositioning of helix 12 (H12) of the LBD in the presence of an agonist (such as estrogen) to seal the steroid in the hydrophobic pocket, allowing the ER complex to recruit coactivators to the transcriptional complex on the surface of helix 12. With antagonists like raloxifene, helix 12 realignment is prevented by bulky sidechain substituents that protrude from the ligand pocket and cause helix 12 to rotate away from an "agonist" position (Brzozowski et al., 1997; Pike et al., 2000). Moreover, using a novel assembly assay to examine structural changes in the LBD of the thyroid hormone receptor (TR), Pissios et al. (2000) have recently found that ligand binding, in addition to the induction of helix 12 repositioning, also have more global effects that dynamically alter and stabilize the structure of the entire LBD of the receptor.

Several reports have provided evidence for the phosphorylation of the ER at tyrosine 537 within the LBD region (Arnold et al., 1995b; Castoria et al., 1993). Tyrosine 537 phosphorylation was shown to be enhanced in response to hormone treatment (Auricchio et al., 1996; Migliaccio et al., 1986) and, in an in vitro study, by two Src family tyrosine kinases, p60c-Src and p56lck (Arnold et al., 1995a). Studies have also suggested that phosphorylation of this site is implicated in DNA binding and dimerization, and in the conformational changes of the ER (Arnold et al., 1995a; Arnold et al., 1995b) and its ability to activate transcription (Yudt et al., 1999).

Region E also contains another transactivation function, called AF-2, in addition to the AF-1 domain in the A/B region. AF-2 requires an agonist ligand for its activity and is also strongly influenced by the repertoire of coregulatory proteins within a given cell, as will be discussed in section "Nuclear receptor coactivator and corepressor proteins." A third activation domain, termed AF-2a (Norris et al., 1997; Pierrat et al., 1994) (Fig. 1), has been identified in the human ER within the amino-terminal part of the E domain. This particular region has either constitutive activity or a stimulatory effect on AF-1. Finally, just downstream of AF-2a domain is a negatively acting domain that is also involved in binding of the hsp 90 (Chambraud et al., 1990; Pierrat et al., 1994).

AF-1 exhibits some autonomous constitutive activity, but, in most cell types, both AF-1 and AF-2 are required to act in concert to promote full transcriptional activity on estrogen-responsive genes (Bocquel et al., 1989; Tzukerman et al., 1994). Nevertheless, depending on the particular promoter, ligand, or cell, AF-1 and AF-2 can function independently (Tzukerman et al., 1994). Furthermore, when AF-2 is not required for receptor activity, antiestrogens like tamoxifen exert their partial agonist activity through the activation of AF-1, contributing to the tissue selectivity found in the clinic for these molecules (McDonnell et al., 1995; Tzukerman et al., 1994).

ERβ

ERβ is somewhat shorter than ERα, with an approximate molecular weight of only 55 to 60 kDa, but is very similar in its overall structure to ERα (Ogawa et al., 1998) (Fig. 2). ERβ is reported to have 95% homology in the DBD and 53% homology in the LBD. The high degree of homology between the DBDs of the two receptors suggests that they both bind to EREs, and furthermore, the conservation in regions within the DBD required for dimerization suggests that the two receptors could heterodimerize. Indeed, the formation of mixed ER dimers has been shown both in vitro and in vivo (Ogawa et al., 1998), though a physiological role of the heterodimer is yet to be proven. In contrast, the A/B and the hinge domains are much less conserved. Furthermore, the AF-1 activity of ERβ is negligible or absent, a fact that helps explain, in part, the differences in transcriptional activation of specific estrogen-responsive genes between the two receptor subtypes (Cowley and Parker, 1999; Hyder et al., 1999). Furthermore, while mixed antiestrogens like tamoxifen and raloxifene show partial agonist/antagonist activity

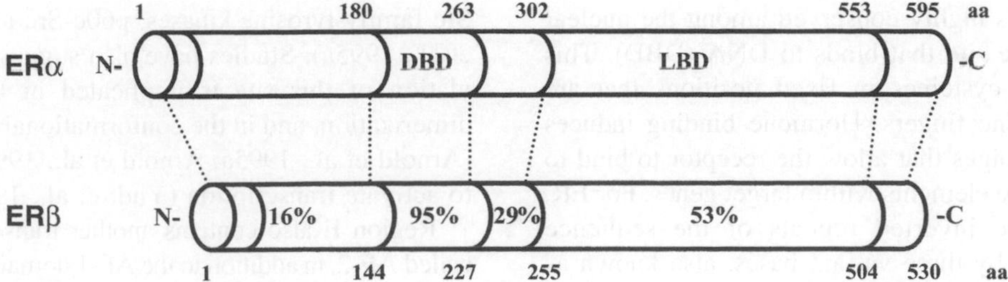

Figure 2 Comparison of the domain structures of ERα (*above*) and ERβ (*below*). The amino acid numbers of the domain boundaries, the structures, and the degree of homology between the receptor domains (in percentage) are shown. *Abbreviations*: DBD, DNA-binding domain; LBD, ligand-binding domain.

with ERα, these antiestrogens possess purely antagonistic effects though ERβ (Barkhem et al., 1998), again likely due to the absence of AF-1 activity. ERβ also appears to lack most of the carboxy-terminal F domain of ERα (Mosselman et al., 1996), an area known to have specific regulatory functions (Sladek et al., 1999) affecting the agonist/antagonist balance of certain antiestrogens. Since ERβ can signal to and activate AP-1 sites, even when bound to antiestrogens, ERβ expression might contribute to antiestrogen resistance, a prediction that is supported by a small clinical report (Speirs et al., 1999). Thus, one can predict that the balance of ERβ and ERα coexpression in breast tumors might prove to be an important biomarker for tumor progression (Hall and McDonnell, 1999; Speirs and Kerin, 2000).

The degree of homology of ERβ and ERα within the LBD, along with their different tissue distribution, also suggests that the two receptors may exert selective and different responses with distinct physiological roles, as was demonstrated in the knockout studies (Couse et al., 2000; Couse and Korach, 1999). Furthermore, while the binding affinity for estradiol is similar for ERα and ERβ, ERβ appears to have higher affinity for phytoestrogens, and certain ligands exhibit ERα or β-selective binding profiles (Katzenellenbogen et al., 2000; Kuiper et al., 1997). The three-dimensional structures of the ERβ LBD in the presence of the phytoestrogen genistein and the antagonist raloxifene were recently reported (Pike et al., 2000). The importance of the ligand-induced AF-2 helix 12 repositioning in the determination of the agonist/antagonist nature of the drug was again demonstrated, as was found previously in ERα studies. In the ERβ-genistein complex, helix 12 does not adopt the distinctive "agonist" position but, instead, lies in a suboptimal alignment that helps to explain genistein's partial agonist character in ERβ. ERα and ERβ ligand selectivity may become important in breast cancer patient management when a better understanding of ERβ role in breast cancer is achieved.

The ultimate way to address the potential significance of ERβ expression in breast cancer is to determine its role in clinical breast tumor progression. Results examining RNA expression of ERβ in clinical breast specimens, recently reviewed by Speirs and Kerin (2000), have been contradictory, perhaps due to the difficulty of accurately measuring RNA from heterogeneous tumor samples. In a study of 40 tumors, Dotzlaw and colleagues (1999) showed that ERβ expression was significantly lower in PR-positive tumors. This inverse relationship suggests that ERβ expression in some breast tumors may correlate with a poorer prognosis, since PR is a favorable prognostic marker and a predictor of response to tamoxifen therapy, and some subsequent studies appear to agree with this hypothesis. Another study, however, found that ERβ-positive cancers were also more frequently EGFR-positive than their negative counterparts (Knowlden et al., 2000), a feature normally associated with endocrine resistance and poorer prognosis. It has also been shown in an IHC study that ERβ is commonly coexpressed with ERα at the protein level (Jarvinen et al., 2000). Specific antibodies suitable for immunohistochemistry (IHC) of formalin-fixed, paraffin-embedded tissue have become available (Skliris et al., 2001). Using one such antibody, we reported that low levels of ERβ predict resistance to tamoxifen therapy in a study of 305 axillary node-positive patients with high levels preciting an improved disease-free and overall survival (Hopp et al., 2004). Additional clinical studies are needed to confirm this finding (Speirs et al., 2004).

Nuclear Receptor Coactivator and Corepressor Proteins

ER-mediated gene regulation, like that of other nuclear receptors, is influenced not only by the nature of the ligand bound to it but also by a group of accessory proteins. These host proteins, which are present in the nucleus at rate-limiting levels, are recruited to and interact with the DNA-bound ligand-receptor complex to either enhance (coactivators) or to suppress (corepressors) ER function [for recent reviews see Klinge, 2000; McKenna et al., 1999] through direct interactions with the RNA

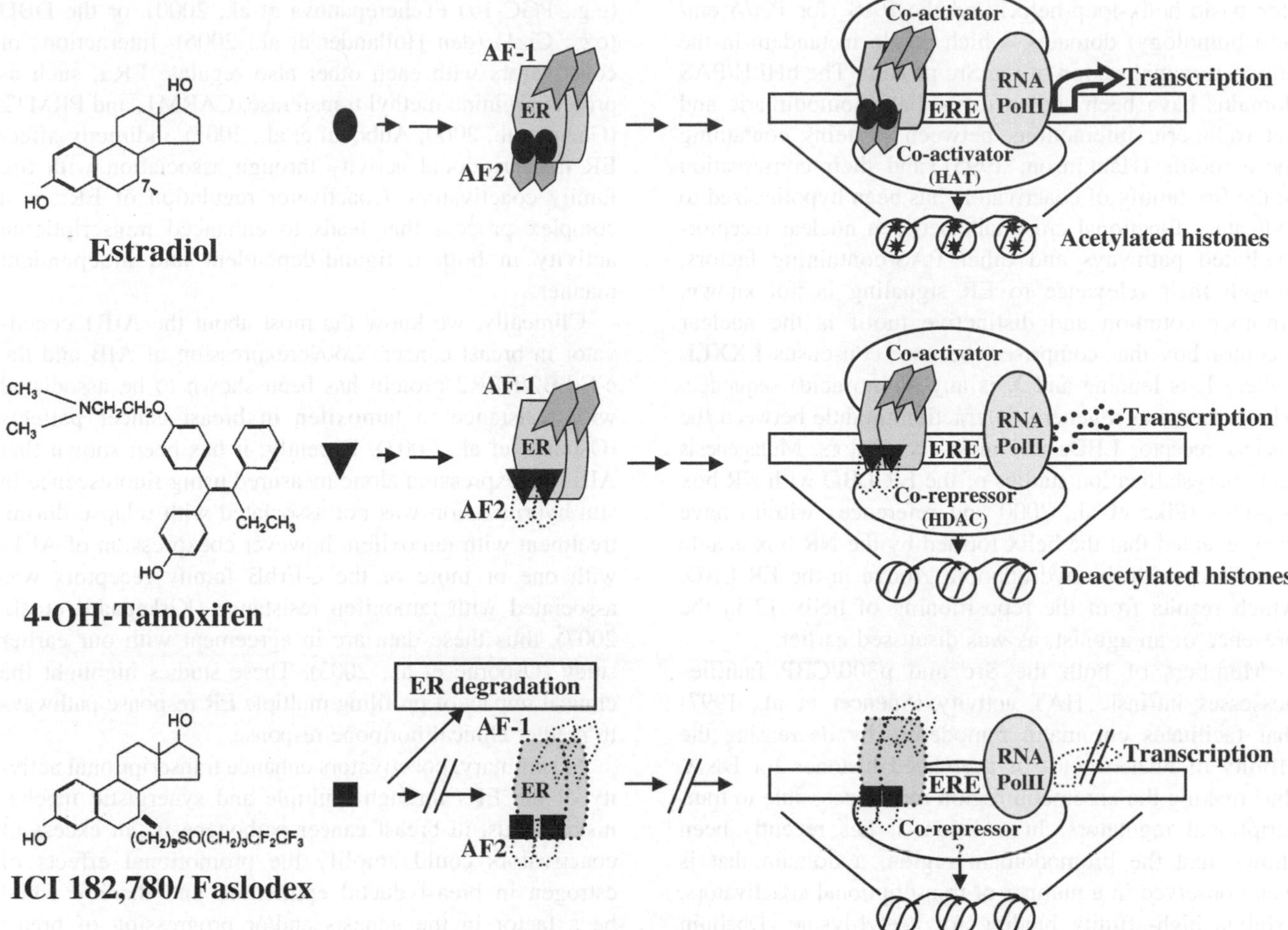

Figure 3 Model for the mechanism of action of estrogens and antiestrogens. The chemical structures of estrogen (estradiol), tamoxifen (4-OH-tamoxifen), and the pure antiestrogen ICI 182,780 (Faslodex) are shown on the right side. Estrogen (an oval shape) binds to the ER and induces conformational changes that result in dissociation of heat-shock protein 90 (hsp90), receptor dimerization, and nuclear localization. The ER homodimer then binds DNA sequences at palindromic estrogen response elements (EREs) within promoters of target genes. Due to receptor conformational changes, AF-1 and AF-2 domains juxtapose and associate both with transcriptional coactivators, which possess histone acetylase activity (HAT), and with elements of the basal transcriptional machinery. Subsequently, RNA polymerase II (RNA Pol II) is stimulated, and local chromatin (histones) is acetylated (stars), resulting in activation of transcription. Tamoxifen (a triangle shape), binding to the ER, also induces receptor dissociation from hsp, dimerization, nuclear localization, and binding to ERE DNA sequences. However, due to tamoxifen-induced receptor conformational changes, only AF-1 function is active and enhances agonistic mode of transcription. The ligand-dependent AF-2 domain, in contrast, interacts with components of the histone deacetylase (HDAC) corepressor complex. This results in chromatin deacetylation, repression of AF-2 transcriptional activity, and attenuation of transcription. ICI 182,780 (ICI) (a square shape) binds to the receptor and dissociates hsp90. However, receptor dimerization is impaired, a significant degradation is induced, and nuclear localization is disrupted. As a result, fewer of ICI-bound receptor complexes bind to ERE sequences. ICI also blocks both AF-1 and AF-2 functions, and therefore transcription of ER-regulated genes is inhibited.

polymerase II complex and also via histone acetyltransferase (HAT) activities (Fig. 3).

A variety of coactivators are already known to interact with ERα in a hormone-dependent manner to activate estrogen-driven transcription (Fig. 3). Among these is the p160 Src family of coactivators that includes Src-1 (also called NcoA-1), Src-2 (also called GRIP-1, TIF2, or NoA-2), and Src-3 (also called RAC-3, AIB1, PCIP, ACTR, or TRAM) (Anzick et al., 1997; Hong et al., 1996; Onate et al., 1995). Another class of accessory proteins, termed cointegrators, includes the CBP/p300 proteins and CBP/p300-associated factor (Chen and Li, 1998; Hanstein et al., 1996; Kamei et al., 1996; Torchia et al., 1997). These proteins form multiple contacts with the ER and each other, and act synergistically to enhance transcription.

The Src family of coactivators participates in transcriptional activation, and its members share a common domain structure. Two of these domains are the bHLH (for basic helix-loop-helix) and the PAS (for Per/Arent/Sim homology) domains, which reside in tandem in the amino-terminal region of the Src protein. The bHLH/PAS domains have been shown to mediate homodimeric and heterodimeric interactions between proteins containing these motifs (Hankinson, 1995), and their conservation in the Src family of coactivators has been hypothesized to indicate a functional cross talk between nuclear receptor-mediated pathways and other PAS-containing factors, though their relevance to ER signaling is not known. Another common and distinctive motif is the nuclear receptor box that comprises the core consensus LXXLL (where L is leucine and X is any amino acid) sequence, which serves as a general interaction module between the nuclear receptor LBDs and most coactivators. Mutagenesis and cocrystallization studies of the ER LBD with NR box peptides (Pike et al., 2000 and references within) have also revealed that the helix formed by the NR box is able to interact with the hydrophobic groove in the ER LBD, which results from the repositioning of helix 12 in the presence of an agonist, as was discussed earlier.

Members of both the Src and p300/CBP families possesses intrinsic HAT activity (Spencer et al., 1997) that facilitates chromatin remodeling by decreasing the affinity of nucleosomes of acetylated histones for DNA, thus making the chromatin region more accessible to transcriptional regulators. In addition, it has recently been shown that the bromodomain region, a domain that is well conserved in a number of transcriptional coactivators, exhibits high-affinity binding for acetyl-lysine (Dhalluin et al., 1999). This finding suggests that HAT activity may directly contribute to the formation of docking sites on the chromatin to which bromodomain-harboring factors may be recruited. One of such is the Brahma-related gene 1 (BRG-1) protein that belongs to the Swi/Snf family of transcriptional regulators that are involved in the ATP-dependent structural remodeling of chromatin. BRG-1 has been shown to be recruited to estrogen-responsive promoters and cooperates with factors involved in histone acetylation. Recently, it has been shown that BRG-1 deficiency in mice results in the development of mammary tumors (Bultman et al., 2008), directly implicating the Swi/Snf members in cancer. Also equally important is that both the nuclear receptors themselves (Wang et al., 2001; Cui et al., 2004, Cui et al., 2006) and their coactivators (Chen et al., 1999a) were recently found to be substrates for acetylation activity that can modulate their activity. This observation suggests that acetylation is engaged in an additional novel regulatory mechanism in hormone signaling.

In addition to ligand-dependent coactivators mentioned above, there are some coactivators that ligand-independently interact with the AF-1 domain (e.g., p68 RNA helicase) (Lonard and O'Malley, 2006), hinge domain (e.g., PGC-1α) (Tcherepanova et al., 2000), or the DBD (e.g., Ciz1) (den Hollander et al., 2006). Interactions of coactivators with each other also regulate ERα, such as protein arginine methyl transferase, CARM1, and PRMT2 (Chen et al., 2000; Auboeuf et al., 2007), indirectly affect ER transcriptional activity through association with Src family coactivators. Coactivator regulation of ERα is a complex process that leads to enhanced transcriptional activity in both a ligand-dependent and independent manner.

Clinically, we know the most about the AIB1 coactivator in breast cancer. Cooverexpression of AIB and the c-ErbB2/HER2 protein has been shown to be associated with resistance to tamoxifen in breast cancer patients (Osborne et al., 2003). Recently, it has been shown that AIB overexpression alone measured using fluorescence in situ hybridization was not associated with relapse during treatment with tamoxifen, however coexpression of AIB1 with one or more of the c-ErbB family receptors was associated with tamoxifen resistance (Kirkegaard et al., 2007), thus these data are in agreement with our earlier study (Osborne et al., 2003). These studies highlight the clinical impact of profiling multiple ER response pathways to predict clinical hormone response.

In summary, coactivators enhance transcriptional activity of the ERs through multiple and synergistic mechanisms. Thus, in breast cancer pathogenesis, an excess of coactivators could amplify the promotional effects of estrogen in breast ductal epithelium and thereby could be a factor in the genesis and/or progression of breast cancer (Kurebayashi et al., 2000). For instance, the coactivator Src-3 (AIB1) is often amplified or overexpressed in breast cancers (Anzick et al., 1997). In addition, Horwitz and coworkers have recently identified a novel coactivator termed L7/SPA (for Switch Protein for Antagonists) that is specifically bound to and enhances the transcriptional activities of steroid receptors, but only in the presence of mixed antagonists like tamoxifen and RU486 (Graham et al., 2000; Jackson et al., 1997). The clinical importance of this unique regulator in breast cancer etiology and endocrine resistance, however, has not been shown. The possible roles of other recently discovered coactivators, such as SRA (Lanz et al., 1999; Watanabe et al., 2001, Coleman et al., 2004), CIA (Sauve et al., 2001), and p68 RNA helicase (Endoh et al., 1999), which may work via different mechanisms, add to the complexity by which ER signaling is regulated and provides evidence that we have not yet entirely revealed all the subtleties of hormone action.

Like coactivators, the number of nuclear receptor corepressor proteins that may be important in ER pharmacology is steadily growing. These include the NcoR (Horlein et al., 1995), SMRT (Chen and Evans, 1995; Sande and Privalsky, 1996), REA (Delage-Mourroux et al., 2000; Montano et al., 1999), HET (Oesterreich et al., 2000), SHP (Seol et al., 1998), and BRCA-1 (Chen et al. 1999b). The corepressors NCoR and SMRT were initially characterized by their ability to bind and repress the unliganded TR and retinoid acid receptor (RAR). These factors, through direct interaction with mSin3 and HDACs, form a multisubunit repressor complex on promoters of target genes that facilitates chromatin condensation and subsequent inhibition of gene transcription. Upon the binding of their respective ligands, TR and RAR dissociate the repressor complex, which is then replaced by recruited coactivators to induce transcription. Steroid receptors, including ER, do not appear to interact with these corepressor complexes in the presence of agonist or in the absence of any ligand. However, in the presence of antiestrogens with mixed agonist/antagonist activity, these corepressor complexes can be recruited to ER, resulting in partial repression of transcription (Graham et al., 2000) (Fig. 3). In this context, a few key reports (Jackson et al., 1997; Smith et al., 1997) have shown that the relative expression and/or activity of coactivators and corepressors in a given cell can modulate the agonist/antagonist activity of drugs such as tamoxifen, providing one explanation for the different activities of these drugs in different tissues, and possibly also an explanation for acquired tamoxifen resistance in patients. The potential importance of corepressors in ER pharmacology has been suggested by us (Lavinsky et al., 1998) and others (Graham et al., 2000), in studies showing that the progression of human breast tumors from tamoxifen sensitivity to tamoxifen resistance is associated with a decrease in the expression level of the corepressor NcoR.

The corepressor REA was originally cloned from breast cancer cells (Montano et al., 1999). This protein is an ER-selective coregulator that is recruited to both hormone- and antihormone-occupied ER, and can decrease ER transcriptional activity. Haplodeficiency in the mice leads to faster mammary ductal elongation and increased lobuloaveolar development during pregnancy, suggesting that a reduction in REA function may cause overactivation of ER (Mussi et al., 2006). The orphan receptor SHP has also recently been shown to belong to this new category of negative coregulators for agonist-activated ER, though this regulator may work through different and yet not fully understood mechanisms compared with classical corepressors (Johansson et al., 2000, Suh et al., 2006). And finally, it has recently been discovered that BRCA-1, the first identified breast cancer susceptibility gene, is a specific repressor of estrogen-bound ERα, and that this repression is dose and AF-2 dependent (Chen et al., 1999b, Ma et al., 2005). These observations may implicate and link the function of BRCA-1, and perhaps other ER transcriptional corepressors, to the genesis and progression of breast cancer.

As with coactivators there are ligand-dependent and ligand-independent corepressors that interact with the AF-1 domain (HDAC4, RTA) (Leong et al., 2005), DBD, and hinge domains (MTA2) (Cui et al., 2006). Recently, we have shown that overexpression of MTA2 resulted in hormone-independent and antiestrogen-resistant cell growth (Cui et al., 2006). These findings, in combination with many additional corepressor studies, suggest that corepressors may be involved in the processes of antiestrogen function and the development of resistance as well. For further information on coregulators, the NURSA website (www.nursa.org) contains an extensive list of over 270 coregulators that can be searched (Auboeuf et al., 2007).

Realizing the importance of the coregulatory interacting molecules in SR signaling and their potential as therapeutic targets, McDonnell and colleagues (2000), utilizing the advanced technique of phage display in an elegant study, have now developed a series of high-affinity peptide antagonists that target the ER-coactivator interaction in a ligand and receptor subtype–specific manner. This novel approach, if successful in translation to the clinic (Gaillard et al., 2006), will provide a new class of pharmaceutical agents that could complement and improve the use of SERMs for the treatment of breast cancer and other ER-related diseases.

Posttranslational Modifications of ER

Posttranslational modifications of ERα, like other nuclear receptors, influence receptor conformation, ligand binding, DNA binding, and coactivator interactions (Likhite et al., 2006). DNA methylation is the addition of a methyl group on the 5′-carbon on the cytosine base by DNA methyltransferases (Wajed et al., 2001). Hypermethylation of the ERα promoter is associated with gene silencing by repressing transcription and can be associated with malignant transformation of cells, whereas hypomethylation of ERα is associated with gene activation indicating an inverse relationship between promoter methylation and transcriptional activity (Fan et al., 2006).

In addition to methylation, ERα is phosphorylated at multiple amino acid residues, ligand binding induces phosphorylation of serine (S) at amino acids 104, 106, and 118; MAP kinase pathway mediates the phosphorylation of S118 and S167; S236 is phosphorylated by protein kinase A (PKA) (Faus and Haendler, 2006); both PKA and p21-activated kinase 1 (PAK-1) signaling can mediate the modification of S305 (Cui et al., 2004). This illustrates that each pathway is possible of soliciting diverse responses from the receptor (Likhite et al., 2006). There is very little information on the specific phorphorylation sites in ERβ. The PKA-mediated phosphorylation of ERα at S305 allows the antagonist tamoxifen to act as an agonist of ERα, and PKA is known to be frequently overexpressed in breast tumors (Michalides et al., 2004). Interestingly, a somatic mutation of ERα at lysine 303, which introduces a substitution to arginine, enhances PKA phosphorylation of S305 (Cui et al., 2004).

Ubiquitination is another posttranslational modification of ERα that regulates its protein levels. Ubiquitination is the reversible covalent bonding of the highly conserved 76-amino acid ubiquitin to lysine residues on target proteins marking the protein for proteasome-mediated degradation. Ubiquitination is an important step in the transactivation of ERα (Ohta and Fukuda, 2004; Tateishi et al., 2004) and can be inhibited by proteasome inhibitor MG132 and lactocystin, indicating that the proteasome pathway is the major degradation pathway for ERα (Ascenzi et al., 2006; Tateishi et al., 2004).

One of the most recently discovered posttranslational modifications is sumoylation, which is biochemically analogous to ubiquitination, although sumoylation does not induce the degradation pathway (Sentis et al., 2005). SUMO-1, a small ubiquitin-like modifier, covalently and reversibly bonds to target proteins with the assistance of conjugating enzymes. It has been shown that SUMO-1 normally binds proteins at the SUMO-1-binding consensus site (hydrophobic amino acid-K-x-E). Recent experiments by Sentis et al. (2005) reveal that ligand-dependent sumoylation occurs on lysine residues within the hinge domain of ERα and that sumoylation regulates transcriptional activity of this nuclear receptor, although ERα does not contain the consensus motif (for a complete review see Selever and Fuqua, 2007).

ER CROSS TALK WITH OTHER SIGNAL TRANSDUCTION PATHWAYS AND ALTERNATIVE SIGNALING

Cross Talk with other Signal Transduction Pathways at the ER

Numerous studies have documented the effects of various growth factor signaling pathways, such as EGF and IGF-1, on the ER to upregulate its expression and/or activity (Nicholson et al., 1999b) (Fig. 4). Reagents or signaling molecules such as cAMP (Aronica and Katzenellenbogen, 1993), neurotransmitters (e.g., dopamine) (Smith et al., 1993), phosphatase inhibitors (Auricchio et al., 1995), and cyclin D1 (Neuman et al., 1997; Zwijsen et al., 1998) have also been shown to be involved in ER activation. Many of these pathways involve protein phosphorylation. Indeed, ER is known to be subject to phosphorylation at multiple sites (see section "ERα structure and functional domains"), and stimulation of a number of growth factor receptor and/or protein kinases leads to ligand-independent and/or a synergistic increase in transcriptional activation of ER in the presence of estrogen. Various kinases have been recently implicated as potential regulators of the ER; the list includes the kinases CyclinA-CDK2 (Rogatsky et al., 1999), the mitogen-activated protein kinases (MAPKs) p42/44 MAPK (Kato et al., 1995) and p38 (Lee et al., 2000), $pp90^{rsk1}$ (Joel et al., 1998a,b), and AKT (Campbell et al., 2001; Martin et al., 2000). Moreover, direct phosphorylation and potentiation of ER coactivators through these same kinase pathways have recently been demonstrated (Feng et al., 2001, Amazit et al., 2007, Zheng et al., 2005). For example, the transcriptional accessory activity of the important ER coactivator AIB1 is enhanced by MAPK phosphorylation (Font de Mora and Brown, 2000).

Additionally, evidence also suggests that in breast tumors, estrogens promote the autocrine and paracrine expression and/or activity of growth factor signaling pathway components including ligands (e.g., transforming growth factor α, IGF-II), receptors (EGF and IGF-I receptors), and key signal-transducing molecules (e.g., insulin receptor substrate-1), while also diminishing the expression of growth inhibitory factors (e.g., transforming growth factor β) and inhibiting expression of tyrosine phosphatases (Nicholson et al., 1999b and references within), thus leading to a net increase in growth factor mitogenic activity (Fig. 4). Taken together, these observations imply a positive feedback loop that augments essential signaling pathways of both the estrogen/ER and the growth factors/receptor systems. In this light, it has been suggested that advantageous aberrations within key growth factor signaling pathways in breast cancers may account for loss of estrogen dependence resulting in antiestrogen-resistant tumors (Nicholson et al., 1999b). The vital linkage of these two signaling pathways in breast tumors might predict synergistic and prolonged antitumor effects of antiestrogens combined with growth factor signal transduction inhibitors (Kunisue et al., 2000), a hypothesis that is now under active investigation. For example, Nicholson and colleagues (1999a) have shown that the treatment of breast cancer cells with a specific drug inhibitor of the EGF receptor tyrosine kinase can result in a very significant delay in the appearance of the endocrine-resistant phenotype. In preclinical models, inhibition of the c-Erb-B family members or the use of the pure antiestrogens delays and/or prevents the emergence of resistance in HER-2 overexpressing breast cancer cells (Arpino et al., 2007, Shou et al., 2004, Massarweh et al., 2006). If this strategy can be extended successfully to the clinical setting, it could profoundly affect the management of breast cancer patients.

Nonclassical Binding: ER Pathways Through AP-1

In addition to the classical response elements (EREs) that bind ER directly, ER can activate transcription through a number of other response elements, to which ER does not

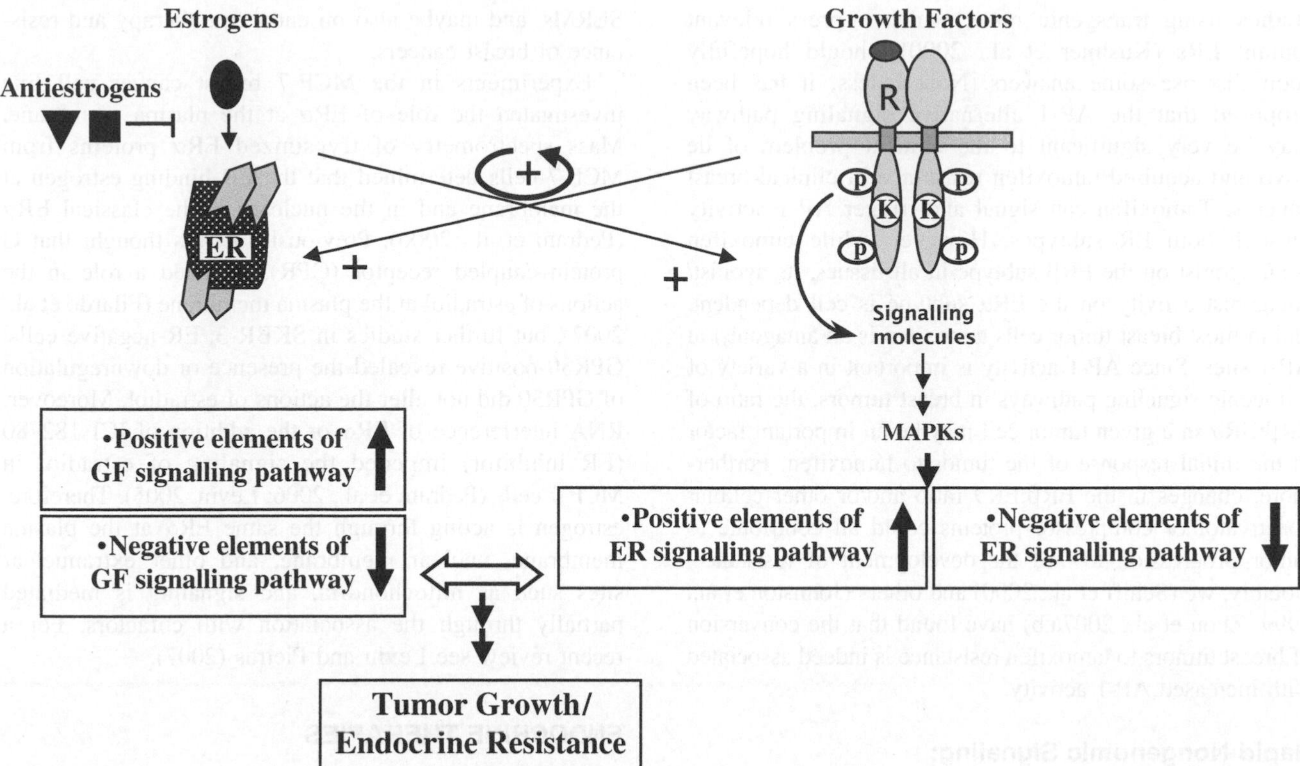

Figure 4 Model of steroid hormone and growth factor cross talk in endocrine response of breast cancer. ER signaling pathway (left side image) influences and stimulates growth factor pathways (right side image) through upregulation of positive elements (e.g., ligands, receptors, and signaling molecules) and downregulation of negative elements of growth factor signaling (e.g., inhibitory ligands and tyrosine phosphatases). In return, growth factor signaling pathways upregulate ER expression and/or activity, thus implying a positive feedback loop to augment essential signaling pathways of both estrogen and the growth factors. By contrast, antiestrogens [tamoxifen, (T) and ICI 182,780, (I)], countering estrogen action, generally downregulate growth factor signaling and controlled breast tumor cell growth. Advantageous anomalies within key growth factor signaling pathways in breast cancers may account for endocrine-resistant growth.

directly bind, but rather signals via protein-protein interactions. ER has been shown to interact and activate the quinone reductase gene through an electrophile response element (Montano and Katzenellenbogen, 1997), the cyclin D gene through a CRE-like element and an enhancer downstream of the coding region (Altucci et al., 1996, Eeckhoute et al., 2006)), and the collagenase and IGF-1 genes through AP-1 sites (Kushner et al., 2000; Umayahara et al., 1994). Most of these sites are known to be regulated by members of the AP-1 Jun/Fos transcription factor family, along with other factors. ER can also signal through sites that bind SP1 (Saville et al., 2000; Vyhlidal et al., 2000) and USF (Xing and Archer, 1998), or through other yet unidentified binding proteins.

The alternative pathway of ER action on AP-1 sites has been extensively studied (for a review see Kushner et al., 2000). These studies suggest at least two mechanisms by which ER can increase the activity of Jun/Fos complexes, and this depends on both the ER subtype present and the specific ligand used. One mechanism proposed is that estrogen- or tamoxifen-bound ERα complexes use their AF-1 and AF-2 domains to bind to the p160 Src component of the coactivator complex that has been prerecruited by Jun/Fos, triggering the coactivator pathway to a higher state of activity. In a proposed alternative mechanism, ERβ or truncated variants of ERα deficient in their AF-1 domain, when bound by specific SERMs, utilize their DBD region to titrate HDAC-corepressor complexes away from Jun/Fos complexes, thereby allowing unfettered activity of the coactivators on these AP-1 sites (Kushner et al., 2000). Not surprisingly, the ligand preference for AP-1 activation in this second AF-1-independent scenario is antiestrogens, with the pure antiestrogen ICI 182, 780 and raloxifene being most potent following by tamoxifen, while estrogens have almost no effect. In addition, it has been suggested that ERβ modulates ERα activity by altering the recruitment of AP-1 complexes to estrogen-responsive promoters (Matthews et al., 2006).

The importance of ER action at alternative response elements and particularly on AP-1 sites in the entire spectrum of ER action in vivo is yet unknown; ongoing studies using transgenic mice, which express relevant mutant ERs (Kushner et al., 2000), should hopefully soon disclose some answers. Nonetheless, it has been proposed that the AP-1 alternative signaling pathway may be very significant to the clinical problem of de novo and acquired tamoxifen resistance in clinical breast cancers. Tamoxifen can signal and trigger AP-1 activity through both ER subtypes. However, while tamoxifen is an agonist on the ERβ subtype in all tissues, its agonist/antagonist activity on the ERα subtype is cell dependent, and in most breast tumor cells tamoxifen is an antagonist at AP-1 sites. Since AP-1 activity is important in a variety of mitogenic signaling pathways in breast tumors, the ratio of ERβ:ERα in a given tumor cell may be an important factor in the initial response of the tumor to tamoxifen. Furthermore, changes in the ERβ:ERα ratio and/or other cellular coactivator or corepressor proteins could all contribute to tumor progression toward the development of resistance. Notably, we (Schiff et al., 2000) and others (Johnston et al., 1999, Zhou et al., 2007a,b) have found that the conversion of breast tumors to tamoxifen resistance is indeed associated with increased AP-1 activity.

Rapid Nongenomic Signaling: Membrane-Bound ER

Evidence for the existence of a plasma membrane ER was suggested more than 20 years ago (Pietras and Szego, 1977). Most of the studies in this field took place in the vascular system, where estrogen has important effects that are mediated at least in part by increased availability of the endothelium-derived signaling molecule nitric oxide (NO) (Farhat et al., 1996; Mendelsohn and Karas, 1999). More recently, a direct effect of estrogen on the vasculature has been identified. Research suggests that ER can mediate a rapid, nongenomic activation of endothelial NO synthase (eNOS) through a direct and estrogen-dependent interaction of membrane-bound ERα with the p85 regulatory subunit of phosphatidylinositol 3-kinase (PI3-K) that then leads to the activation of the PI3-K/Akt pathway (Haynes et al., 2000b). This novel pathway has only been shown for the ERα subtype. This pathway is fully inhibited by both ER and PI-3K pharmacological inhibitors such as the pure antagonist ICI 182,780 and wortmannin, respectively. Data also suggest that ERα appears to be localized to endothelial cell caveolae (Chambliss et al., 2000; Mendelsohn, 2000) and that the pathway is calcium dependent. Though there are yet many unclear molecular aspects of this novel pathway, the most important questions to be answered are, how broad is this new pathway beyond the vascular system and does it have any physiological role in the vasculature and other cell systems? Answers to these crucial inquiries may have an important impact on drug development of cardiovascular-targeted SERMs, and maybe also on endocrine therapy and resistance of breast cancers.

Experiments in the MCF-7 breast cancer cell line investigated the role of ERα at the plasma membrane. Mass spectrometry of trypsinized ERα proteins from MCF-7 cells determined that the ER-binding estrogen at the membrane and in the nuclease is the classical ERα (Pedram et al., 2006). Previously, it was thought that G protein–coupled receptor (GPR)30 played a role in the actions of estradiol at the plasma membrane (Filardo et al., 2002), but further studies in SKBR-3, ER-negative cells, GPR30-positive revealed the presence or downregulation of GPR30 did not alter the actions of estradiol. Moreover, RNA interference of ERα or the addition of ICI 182780 (ER inhibitor) impeded the signaling of estradiol in MCF-7 cells (Pedram et al., 2006; Levin, 2005). Therefore, estrogen is acting through the same ERα at the plasma membrane, nuclear membrane, and other extranuclear sites such as mitochondria, and signaling is mediated partially through the association with cofactors. For a recent review see Levin and Pietras (2007).

ENDOCRINE THERAPIES

Current endocrine therapies of breast cancer are based on three main known mechanisms of action, all of them targeting the ER signaling pathway: (1) antagonizing ER function by competitive binding (SERMs and pure antiestrogens); (2) downregulating ER (pure antiestrogens); and (3) reducing levels of estrogen [ovarian ablation, ovarian suppression by luteinizing hormone-releasing hormone (LHRH) agonists, and aromatase inhibitors (AIs)].

SERMs and Pure Antiestrogens

The significant discoveries in understanding the structure and function of ER, which help explain the agonist/antagonist activity of different ligands, have paved the way for the development of new classes of SERMs, drugs that act like estrogen in certain tissues (bone and cardiovascular tissues) but antagonize estrogen action in others (breast and uterus). Tamoxifen, the most commonly used drug for all breast cancers, is considered one of the first prototypic SERMs; however, it exhibits antagonist activity in the breast but undesired agonist activity in the uterus. The identification of tamoxifen as an SERM suggested that additional SERMs with unique and perhaps more desirable tissue selectivity could be developed. The development of raloxifene (Evista), which has similar properties on the breast (Wakeling et al., 1984), the bone, and lipid metabolism (Delmas et al., 1997; Johnston et al., 2000) but lacks significant uterotropic activity (Cohen et al., 2000; Gradishar et al., 2000), is a proof of this concept;

raloxifene is now an approved drug for the prevention and treatment of osteoporosis. It is also clear that SERMs with activities ranging from nearly full estrogenic to almost pure antiestrogenic activity can be developed for specific therapeutics ranging from the treatment and prevention of osteoporosis to the treatment and prevention of breast cancer. In addition, it is apparent that ERβ has unique biological functions and a potential role in breast cancer, as well as a distinct ligand-binding profile. Several laboratories and companies are searching for ER subtype-selective SERMs, and several candidates have been already reported (Katzenellenbogen et al., 2000).

SERMs can be conveniently divided into three major categories: the triphenylethylene derivatives like tamoxifen, other nonsteroidal compounds, and steroidal compounds that have complete antiestrogenic activity. Details of their behavioral spectrum as SERMs are beyond the focus of this chapter and can be found in recent reviews (Burger et al., 2000; Osborne et al., 2000, Gennari et al., 2007). Only a brief discussion will be undertaken here to address the importance of some key SERMs in breast cancer. Besides tamoxifen, several triphenylethylenes or other nonsteroidal compounds have been developed as antiestrogens for the treatment of breast patients. Some were not superior to tamoxifen in experimental models and did not make the passage to routine use in the clinic, while others, like droloxifene, have been tested and failed through different phases of clinical trial or are still currently under clinical evaluation. Clinical trials with the SERMs GW5638 (Rauschning and Pritchard, 1994), EM-652 (Tremblay et al., 1998a), and the more potent raloxifene analog LY353381 (Sato et al., 1998) are under way or planned.

Finally, the development of steroidal antiestrogens like ICI 182,780 (Faslodex), which demonstrate pure antiestrogen profiles on all genes and in all tissues studied to date (Howell et al., 2000), brings the promise of more potent first-line therapy for breast cancer patients than the other available SERMs, and may also override tamoxifen tumor resistance and recapture tumor growth inhibition responses. Faslodex is a very potent antiestrogen (Bowler et al., 1989). Its mechanism of action differs significantly from the "mixed" antiestrogens like tamoxifen. Faslodex blocks ER transactivation from both the AF-1 and AF-2 domains and also induces ER degradation (Wakeling, 1995) (Fig. 3). On the basis of our own results in a preclinical tamoxifen resistance xenograft model (Massarweh et al., 2006), as well as studies by others, Faslodex has been tested for use in women with resistance to tamoxifen. A phase II clinical trial has already found a high response rate with Faslodex in ER-positive tamoxifen-resistant patients (Howell et al., 1995), and a phase III clinical study suggests data supporting this earlier trial (Osborne, 2000). Clinical benefit of Faslodex was seen in postmenopausal women with advanced breast cancer or resistance to AIs (Perrey et al., 2007). These data suggest that although Faslodex may not be the most desirable SERM for breast cancer prevention in normal women because of its antagonist profile in the bone, it might useful for treating women with advanced disease.

Aromatase Inhibitors

AIs inhibit peripheral and tumor conversion of adrenal androgens to estrogens, resulting in lower estrogen levels in the circulation and in tumor tissues (Osborne, 1999a and references within). These inhibitors are effective in postmenopausal women, in whom estrogen levels are already low, probably due to the ability of breast tumor tissue to concentrate circulating estrogens to sustain substantial high levels of initial estrogens and to synthesize estrogens in situ (Osborne, 1999a). Alternatively, tumors may adapt and become "hypersensitive" to very low levels of estrogen, as has been suggested in experimental models (Masamura et al., 1995).

A number of potent and selective nonsteroidal AIs are now available and are rapidly becoming established as the second-line endocrine therapy in postmenopausal women with advanced disease who fail tamoxifen. Their full potential in the treatment of breast cancer is currently being investigated in a number of clinical trials. Of special interest is the finding (Ellis et al., 2001) that AIs achieved a higher response rate than tamoxifen in breast cancer patients expressing ERα, especially when they also express high levels of HER-2 [an EGF receptor family member that is known to increase tamoxifen resistance, probably via induction of tamoxifen's agonistic activity (Kurokawa et al., 2000)].

A shift in the standard of care for ER-positive breast cancer patients has occurred since the results of the Anastrozole or Tamoxifen Alone or in Combination (ATAC) trial and the International Breast International Group (BIG) 1-98 trial, which compared an AI to tamoxifen as first-line hormonal treatment. For years, adjuvant treatment of breast cancer patients with tamoxifen for five years was the most beneficial treatment improving relapse-free and overall survival. Recently, the AIs anastrozole, letrozole, and exemestane have been found to be a superior treatment option over tamoxifen in postmenopausal women (Wheler et al., 2006). The results of the ATAC trial suggest that treatment with anastrozole showed significant benefit in disease-free survival and time to tumor recurrence but showed no significant benefit for overall survival compared with tamoxifen alone or a combination of anastrozole and tamoxifen. Another benefit of anastrozole over tamoxifen is the reduction in side effects associated with treatment allowing more women a better quality of life while receiving treatment. In addition, the BIG 1-98 trial further verified that the adjuvant administration of AIs (letrozole) to postmenopausal women with early-stage breast cancer did reduce the time to recurrence and a reduction in distant metastasis. It has been suggested but is controversial whether tumors, which are ERα-positive, but PR-negative respond better to AIs (Fuqua et al., 2005, Cui et al., 2005). However, the recently reported results from BIG 1-98 suggest that the AI letrozole showed better clinical benefit than tamoxifen, regardless of the level of PR, when PR expression levels were uniformly reexamined by central review (Viale et al., 2007). Although AIs have proven effective, the most efficient treatment regimen and duration has yet to be determined (Buzdar et al., 2006). These results suggest the complementary potential of aromatase inhibition therapy with SERM therapy.

METHODS FOR THE MEASUREMENT OF ER IN BREAST CANCER

The assessment of ER status has been a useful prognostic indicator in breast carcinoma and can be used successfully to identify patients with a higher probability of response to hormone therapy (see section "ER in the clinical management of breast cancer patients") and therefore an improved prognosis.

Assay Methodology

A variety of assay methods have been used to measure ER values in clinical breast cancer specimens. The biochemical ligand-binding assay (LBA) was the first method that became the standard for ER detection and measurement. The prototype assay method and the most commonly used was the dextran-coated charcoal (DCC) radioactive LBA, followed by Scatchard analysis. This was carried out on cytosols from tumor tissue that had to be frozen instantaneously after removal from the patients and stored under special conditions. A key advantage of the DCC method is that it gives an objective numerical and reproducible quantitation of ER under conditions of good quality control (Hull et al., 1983). However, the assay requires a relatively large amount of tissue, which is made up of a heterogeneous mixture of tumor and normal components. In addition, endogenous ligands, if the patient is pregnant or is being treated with hormones or antihormones, may saturate the receptor sites and lead to low or false-negative results. The assay is also fairly sophisticated and involves the use of radioactive material, and thus usually compels centralization for accurate performance.

The development of specific antibodies to the receptor facilitates the development of new assay methods to overcome the difficulties allied with the LBA methodology. The antibody-based assays include enzyme immunoassays (EIA) for tumor cytosol and immunohistochemical assays (IHC). The IHC assay has many advantages (Harvey et al., 1999). The assay requires small tissue samples and can be done on fine needle aspirates and core needle biopsies, thus making it possible to monitor receptor status during therapy. Importantly, it works on routine fixed histological sections, so it allows retrospective analysis on archival material. The IHC assay can detect the presence of the receptor independent of its functionality or occupancy. In addition, the essence of the IHC method can ensure that the tissue sample contains tumor cells and can relate receptor content to morphology. These qualities are essential to increase the specificity and the accuracy of the ER assay because positive cells can be recognized even in tumors of low cellularity and false positive results due to ER in adjacent normal tissue can be avoided. And finally, the ability to employ in the IHC assays antibodies that can distinguish the new subtype ERβ will be important to study the role of this new receptor in the development and the progression of breast cancers and to assess its prognostic or predictive potential.

Due to the reasons outlined above and the relatively simplicity, low cost, and lack of requirements for specialized equipment, IHC using monoclonal antibodies is speedily and justly becoming the method of choice for measuring ER in the clinical setting. However, it should be emphasized that IHC analysis has a number of disadvantages. Results can vary substantially due to tissue fixation, procedural conditions, and type of antibody (Elledge et al., 1994) or antigen retrieval method (Jacobs et al., 1996) used. Depending on the epitope specificity, different antibodies may not detect a specific receptor isoform or variant. The subjective and semi-quantitative nature of IHC assessment, with limited standardization, quality control, and commonly accepted scoring and evaluation systems, complicates the easy use of IHC analysis of ER in the clinic.

Therefore, the switch to an IHC assay recalls the need for good quality assurance and for procedures that will allow at least semiquantitative reporting of results. As a result of recent major efforts assessing the quality and the scoring systems of many IHC techniques (Rhodes et al., 2000) and comparing the predictive value of ER status determined by IHC to that determined by LBA, a standard "working protocol" using a common scoring system is now emerging (Leake et al., 2000). Using this methodology, several laboratories find that results are highly reproducible. In reporting the results, scoring systems that include either a direct count of the proportion of positively stained tumor cells (Elledge et al., 2000) or a simple combination of proportion and intensity of positive-staining tumor cells (Leake et al., 2000; Rhodes et al., 2000) are found to work the best and to be highly reproducible.

Many comparative studies of DCC-LBA and IHC assay methods have been reported. In general, when good quality assurance procedures were used, a high correlation (80–90%) was found between the two methods (Allred et al., 1990; Molino et al., 1997). More importantly, for clinical use, assessing ER by IHC was proved to have an equivalent or even slightly better ability than the LBA method to predict response to adjuvant endocrine therapy. Thus, in the light of everything mentioned above, it is now clear that IHC analysis is likely to be the method used most often in the future.

Cutoff Point

A major concern with any of the ER assays, and particularly when it is used to predict response to endocrine therapy, is the cutoff point that distinguishes ER-"positive" from ER-"negative" tumors. Establishing a threshold range below which the probability of response is very low or negligible is important.

Early studies correlating assay results with clinical response to endocrine therapies indicated that tumors with even a small amount of detectable ER protein had a significantly higher response rate than those with undetectable ER levels (McGuire et al., 1975). For the DCC LBA, these levels were ~3 fmol/mg protein, which were at the limit of the assay's sensitivity. However, in the past, arbitrary cutoff points as high as 20 fmol/mg cytosol protein have been used by some laboratories, perhaps because tumors with higher ER levels were known to be most likely to benefit from hormonal therapy (Osborne et al., 1980). This most likely resulted in some patients being misclassified as ER-negative, and consequently being denied hormonal therapy from which they had a good chance of benefitting. Moreover, such misclassification could have led to the flawed impression that a substantial number of ER-negative patients benefit from hormonal therapy. It is therefore critical that stringently low cutoff points be adapted.

The optimal cutoff point for IHC assays is even more difficult to define. One of the problems is achieving a balance between sensitivity and specificity of the assay. There have been over 20 studies assessing the ability of ER by IHC to predict response to hormonal therapy. However, many of these studies were small, and in addition, were performed with antibodies most suitable for fresh-frozen tumor samples (Elledge et al., 2000), a procedure that is not very relevant at the present since practically all-ER IHC is now performed on formalin-fixed, paraffin-embedded samples. In addition, because of lack of validation and standardization regarding both technical and scoring aspects of these assays, the definition of positive and negative varied considerably. Therefore, the appropriate cutoff values for hormonal treatment using ER determination by IHC have yet to be determined. Importantly, however, recent reports using a validated prototype protocol and scoring system similar to that cited above, in large studies, are now suggesting a stringently low cut point. A score value >2, for example, specimens with >1% cells staining, was considered positive and was the optimal cutoff point for predicting improved outcome (Elledge et al., 2000; Harvey et al., 1999).

ER IN THE CLINICAL MANAGEMENT OF BREAST CANCER PATIENTS

ER as a Prognostic Factor

Prognostic factors are defined as "any measurements available at the time of diagnosis or surgery that are associated with disease-free or overall survival in the absence of systemic adjuvant therapy" (Clark, 2000), and may include both patient and tumor characteristics, such as age and menopausal status, tumor size and histological grade, lymph node status, and different biomarkers that are associated with biological processes. These factors are indicative of the intrinsic biological aggressiveness of a tumor and can be used to predict the natural history of the tumor.

Tumor ER status has been shown in many studies to correlate with a variety of patient and other tumor characteristics (Osborne, 1991) and to be age related. Using the biochemical LBA procedure with low cutoff, nearly 80% of tumors from postmenopausal patients are ER-positive, while only about 50% to 60% of tumors from premenopausal women express detectable ER levels. ER also positively correlates with several "good" prognostic markers such as lower S-phase (DNA-replicating) fraction, highly differentiated histology, and diploidy; whereas it negatively associates with tumors demonstrating mutation, loss, or amplification of breast cancer-related genes (Clark, 2000 and references within; Osborne, 1998). In addition, for unknown reasons, ER-positive tumors tend to involve soft tissue and bone, whereas ER-negative tumors more commonly metastasize to brain and liver. Importantly, ER status shows no consistent association with tumor size and axillary lymph node status. ER-negative tumors correlate with poor tumor differentiation, high proliferation rate, and other unfavorable characteristics. These correlations justified the studies of ER as a prognostic factor in patients with early breast disease.

Although there is not complete agreement in the literature, most studies found that patients with ER-positive tumors have longer disease-free time and overall survival compared with those with ER-negative tumors. However, later studies with longer follow-up suggested that disease-free survival curves tend to merge after the initial few years in which patients with ER-positive tumors enjoy lower relapse rate, so that with long follow-up the favorable prognostic significance of ER vanishes (Aamdal et al., 1984; Hahnel et al., 1979; Hilsenbeck et al., 1998). Because ER status does not correlate with axillary lymph node status and its prognostic significance probably diminishes over time, further studies are needed to clarify its significance as a marker of metastatic potential.

Gene expression profiling studies have classified breast cancer into five intrinsic subtypes with distinct ER status: luminal A and B (ERα-positive), normal-like, HER2-positive (predominantly ER-negative), and basal (ER-negative) with differing clinical outcomes (Perou et al., 2000). Current work is focused on elucidating other genes that are coexpressed with ER to use as novel prognostic variables and molecular targets for treatment. One such factor, recently identified is FOXA1 (Badve et al., 2007). FOXA1 has been shown to be a major factor in controlling proliferation and progression of the luminal A, ERα-positive subtype of tumors. These early studies are promising that subtypes of ERα-positive tumors can be identified with these new genomic profiling technologies.

ER as a Predictive Factor

A predictive factor is defined as "any measurement associated with response or lack of response to a particular therapy" (Clark, 2000); and ER status, as has been shown by numerous studies over the last 30 years, strongly predicts responses to hormonal therapy, and so is a strong predictive factor. In the advanced disease, it can be concluded that about 50% to 60% of all ER-positive patients will benefit from first-line hormonal therapy, whereas, at most, only 5% to 10% of ER-negative patients will benefit. The response rate is somewhat higher in patients with high ER concentrations, such as those with >100 fmol/mg protein by LBA. But it should be pointed out that, as mentioned before, it is the low cutoff that is most significant for clinical choices, since the major clinical use of the ER assay is not to define a group of patients with the highest probability of response to hormonal therapy, but rather a group of patients with little or no chance of response. ER status is also important in predicting benefit from second line and subsequent hormone manipulations; response rate for ER-positive patients is progressively lower but still significant (Buzdar et al., 1996; Dombernowsky et al., 1998), while hardly any ER-negative patients respond to second-line endocrine therapy.

In addition to the amount of ER, other tumor factors and biomarkers that reflect the functional integrity of the ER pathway are useful to further improve the ability to identify those patients who respond best. PR, which has its own clinical and biological significance in breast cancer, is positively regulated by ER and is therefore a candidate marker of an intact ER pathway; indeed, several clinical studies have confirmed the value of PR in predicting response to hormonal therapy in advanced breast cancer (Osborne, 1991; Ravdin et al., 1992).

At present, most breast cancer patients (>80%) appear with localized disease. Because these patients may already have subclinical or undetectable micrometastases, knowing their ER status in the primary tumor may predict the efficacy of adjuvant hormone therapy. Results of numerous studies in the adjuvant setting clearly demonstrate a significant benefit from five years of tamoxifen therapy, but only in patients with ER-positive tumors (Early Breast Cancer Trialists' Collaborative Group, 1992), and therefore today the major use of clinical ER measurement is in selection of adjuvant therapy.

ER in Prevention

Breast cancer affects more than 180,000 women yearly in the United States, and more than 40,000 women die each year of the disease (Landis et al., 1998). This malignancy is therefore a major health problem with an immediate need for strategies to prevent it, especially in women with high risk of the disease. The central role of estrogen and ER in breast cancer, as reviewed in this chapter, provided a rational for a chemoprevention strategy that was based on countering the action of the estrogen signaling pathway.

The antiestrogen tamoxifen was the first drug chosen to be tested in high-risk women because it was shown to reduce the incidence of contralateral breast cancer in the adjuvant setting. The recent NSABP P-1 breast cancer trial, with more than 13,000 healthy women at high risk for breast cancer randomized for treatment with tamoxifen or placebo for five years, found a striking 49% reduction in the incidence of invasive breast disease in these women (Fisher et al., 1998). Adverse effects included increases in endometrial cancers and thromboembolic vascular events, results that were expected in view of the estrogenic activity of this drug in certain non-breast tissues; however, the benefits appeared to outweigh these risks for women at high risk for breast cancer. Two other smaller European studies failed to confirm the U.S. study, perhaps due to differences in power, age, risk, compliance, and the use of estrogen-replacement therapy in the European studies (Osborne, 1999b).

Raloxifene, an approved drug for osteoporosis, is a second SERM with a potential as a chemoprevention agent for breast cancer. The Multiple Outcomes of Raloxifene Evaluation (MORE) trial, in which more than 7500 postmenopausal women with osteoporosis were randomized to receive raloxifene or placebo and followed up for a median of 40 months, found that raloxifene decreased the risk of invasive breast cancer in these women by 76% during three years of treatment (Cummings et al., 1999). As was seen with tamoxifen, raloxifene therapy in the MORE trial also increased the relative risk of thromboembolic disease, but, unlike tamoxifen, it did not increase the relative risk of endometrial cancer (Cummings et al., 1999), again an expected result due to the known antagonistic nature of raloxifene in the uterus.

A clinical trial designed to directly compare raloxifene and tamoxifen in the prevention of breast cancer was initiated in 1999 (Jordan, 1999). Results from this study, the study of tamoxifen and raloxifene (STAR), came out in 2006 and concluded that raloxifene was as effective as tamoxifen in reducing the risk of invasive breast cancer. But the downside to raloxifene is that it did not lower the risk of noninvasive breast cancer; however, raloxifene has reduced side effects including fewer cases of cataracts and thromboembolic events (Vogel et al., 2006). Overall the two drugs, tamoxifen and raloxifene, were comparable in their ability to prevent invasive breast cancer in at-risk patients with similar side effects. Therefore, raloxifene is another drug that clinicians can keep in their arsenal of treatments to fight breast cancer.

ER MUTATIONS AND VARIANTS IN CLINICAL BREAST CANCER

Mutations in the ER gene can profoundly affect the activity of the receptor protein. Accepting the central role of the ER in the development and progression of breast cancer, one could imagine that these mutations, if taking place in vivo, could contribute to breast cancer risk and evolution. Particularly, ER mutations have been suggested as a possible molecular mechanism to account for the de novo and acquired endocrine-resistant phenotype of tumors (Osborne and Fuqua, 1994; Tonetti and Jordan, 1997). However, deletions or insertions and missense mutations within the ER gene in primary breast cancer have been reported to be rare. In a study examining over 100 primary breast tumors, only 1% of the cancers revealed point mutations in the ERα gene (Roodi et al., 1995), though the frequency may be higher in metastatic lesions (Karnik et al., 1994). Several neutral polymorphisms were also found in this study in both ER-negative and ER-positive tumors, but there was no correlation of any of the polymorphic alleles with the ER phenotype or with other clinical parameters including tumor type, size, grade, or stage (Roodi et al., 1995).

In 2000, Fuqua et al. (2000) identified a common somatic mutation in the ERα gene in up to 30% of breast hyperplasias, a type of premalignant lesion that is probably a nonobligate precursor of invasive breast cancer. More recently, and with optimal primer extension sequencing detection methods, the A to G somatic mutation at ERα nucleotide 908 (A908G) was detected in 50% of invasive breast tumors (Herynk et al., 2007). The A908G nucleotide mutation replaces a lysine with an arginine residue at amino acid 303 (K303R) and at the border of the hinge and the hormone-binding domains of the receptor. The mutation shows greatly increased sensitivity to estrogen and enhanced binding to the Src-2 coactivator compared with wild-type ERα (Fuqua et al., 2000). It was determined that the K303R mutation is associated with poor outcome including node-positive tumors and larger tumor size. Likewise, the mutation is also correlated with unfavorable prognosis based on shorter time to recurrence, but this factor alone was not an independent predictor of outcome (Herynk et al., 2007). Furthermore, expression of this hypersensitive ERα mutant in breast cancer cells resulted in markedly increased proliferation at subphysiological levels of hormone. Therefore, K303R is a gain-of-function mutation that could have a significant biological role in early breast disease and awaits further studies for confirmation.

Another reported missense ER mutation is a tyrosine-to-asparagine substitution at the amino acid residue 537. This ER mutant possesses a potent, estradiol-independent transcriptional activity, compared with wild-type ER (Zhang et al., 1997). Similar mutations at the corresponding site in ERβ also result in a constitutive receptor (Tremblay et al., 1998b). On the basis of X-ray crystal structure, it has been suggested that the amino acid substitution introduced at position 537 facilitates the shift of helix 12 of the ER LBD into an active conformation and thus allows interaction with coactivators and transcription enhancement independent of the ligand (Weis et al., 1996).

A few years ago, Wolf and Jordan (1994) isolated a naturally occurring mutation that leads a tyrosine-to-aspartate substitution at amino acid 351 at the amino terminus of the LBD from a tamoxifen-resistant MCF-7 xenograft tumor. This mutant, which allows ERα to perceive tamoxifen and raloxifene as estrogens, appears to be the major form of ER expressed by this tumor. It has been recently suggested that the AF-2 activity of the mutant, in synergism with its AF-1 activity, is responsible for the mutant phenotype. A few other ERα missense mutations have been identified from primary and metastatic breast cancers (Hopp and Fuqua, 1998). Unfortunately, however, functional studies with most of these mutant receptors have not yet been reported, and their clinical significance has not yet been disclosed.

In contrast to the reportedly rare incidence of ER mutations, expression of ERα and ERβ mRNA splice variants in both normal and neoplastic tissue is common and abundant. Several variant forms, with single and multiple exons skipped, have been identified and are usually found along with the wild-type receptor (recently reviewed in (Hopp and Fuqua, 1998; Murphy et al., 1998). These exon-deleted mRNA isoforms encode ER-like proteins missing some of the functional domains of the wild-type receptor. However, whether these altered receptors are even expressed at the protein level in vivo and to what extent they can interfere with the wild-type ER signaling pathway are not yet known for the majority of these receptor species.

Some of the splice variants have been reported to be associated with various clinical parameters in breast tumors, and thus they have been suggested as potential prognostic markers in clinical samples. For example, ERα exon 4 deletion, which is missing the nuclear localization signal and part of the LBD, is preferentially detected in tumors with low histological grade or high PR levels, two "good" biological markers (Leygue et al., 1996). In contrast, variants deleted in exons 2 to 4 or exons 3 to 7 are associated with tumors of higher grade and high ER levels (Leygue et al., 1996). In addition, it has recently been shown that both the ratio of splice variants to wild-type ERα and the complexity of the variants (one-exon vs. multi-exon deletions) are increased in breast tumors compared with normal tissue (van Dijk et al., 2000). These observations suggest that specific ER variants may play a role in breast cancer development and progression.

Many studies designed to enable functional characterization of the different splice variants have been published. A recent report has shown that most individual variants display both similarities and differences compared with wild-type ERα and that selected splice variants (mainly exon 3 and exon 5 deletions) have the capacity to both positively and negatively regulate gene expression, depending on promoter context (Bollig and Miksicek, 2000). The exon 5 deletion variant is one of the best-studied ERα variants and the only ERα variant so far detected at the protein level in breast cancer cell lines and tumors (Desai et al., 1997). This variant is a truncated 40-kDa protein missing most of the LBD but retains AF-1 function (Fuqua and Wolf, 1995). The activity of the variant appears to be highly dependent on both the promoter context and the cellular environment. For instance, the variant is constitutively active and thus acts as a dominant positive receptor in ER-negative MDA-231 cell line (Fuqua et al., 1995) but, in another ER-negative cell line, HMT-35225S (Ohlsson et al., 1998), and in ER-positive MCF-7 cells (Desai et al., 1997), it behaves as a dominant-negative receptor. Interestingly, cells transfected with the exon 5 deletion variant were found to be resistant to tamoxifen in one study (Fuqua et al., 1995). Furthermore, the expression of this variant was also found to significantly increased in cancers from patients relapsing after tamoxifen treatment compared with the respective primary tumors (Gallacchi et al., 1998), but the variant's role in clinical tamoxifen resistance remains to be clarified.

For ERβ, multiple mRNA splice variants have also been described in several studies, and as with ERα, it has been suggested that changes in the relative expression of the ERβ mRNA variants occur during breast tumorigenesis and tumor progression (Leygue et al., 1999). Furthermore, we have recently shown, using Erβ-specific antibodies in Western blot analysis, that ERβ protein is expressed in breast cancer cell lines and tumors in various size isoforms, most likely corresponding to previously described splice variants (Fuqua et al., 1999). Clearly, more studies to determine the clinical relevance of any of the aforementioned ERα and ERβ mRNAs variants are needed (Davies et al., 2004), and those studies still await the development of specific reagents to permit quantification of protein expression of the specific isoforms.

SUMMARY AND CONCLUSIONS

Epidemiological, clinical, and experimental evidence suggest that estrogens are among the most important players contributing to the progression of breast cancer. Estrogens are now known to exert their cellular effects through the binding and activation of two specific nuclear receptors, ERα and ERβ. Since the original elucidation of ERα, there has been, over the past forty years, an explosion of information in the research field of steroid receptor action in general and of ERs in particular. These extensive biochemical and structural studies led to a significant progress in understanding ERs structure and cellular functions, which are now viewed to be influenced by the net effect of at least pentavalent ensemble components: the ER subtype, the ligand, the nature of specific elements within given target promoters, the coregulatory host proteins, and finally the host cellular signaling molecules that can modify and potentiate ER activity. These discoveries explain, at least in part, the agonist/antagonist activity of different ligands and pave the way for the ongoing progress in developing new classes of SERMs with the promise to offer optimal hormone replacement therapy along with better tools to treat or prevent the breast cancer disease.

On the contrary, in normal mammary development both the expression and function of the ERs are tightly regulated, in cancer, commonly, a perturbation in the ER signaling takes place. Two principal examples are the altered regulation of ER expression and the appearance of ER mutants and specific variants in both early hyperplastic and more progressed mammary lesions. ER status in breast cancer is most important for predicting which patients are most likely to benefit from endocrine therapy. The new method of IHC to detect ER is superior due to the advantages of use in paraffin-embedded tissue, and is more simple and sensitive than the old LBA method. This method should also help in further determination of the role of different ER mutants and variants and of the ERβ subtype in breast cancer. With better understanding of the ensemble of factors responsible for ERs action and response to endocrine therapy, simultaneous measurements of these key factors should further improve the predictive ability of receptor status in the future. Such preclinical and clinical studies are now in progress. Epidemiological, clinical, and experimental evidence suggests that estrogens are among the most important players contributing to the progression of breast cancer. Estrogens are now known to exert their cellular effects through the binding and activation of two specific nuclear receptors, ERα and ERβ. Whereas in normal mammary development both the expression and function of the ERs are tightly regulated, in cancer a perturbation in the ER signaling commonly takes place. Two principal examples are the altered regulation of ERα expression and the appearance of ERα mutants and specific variants in both early hyperplastic and more progressed mammary lesions.

Since the original elucidation of ERα over 30 years ago, there has been an explosion of information in the research field of steroid receptor action in general and of ERs in particular. These extensive biochemical and structural studies have led to significant progress in understanding ER's structure and cellular functions, which now appear to be influenced by at least five factors: the ER subtype, the ligand, the nature of specific elements within given target promoters, the coregulatory host proteins, and finally the host cellular signaling molecules that can modify and potentiate ER activity. These discoveries explain, at least in part, the agonist/antagonist activity of different ligands and pave the way for the current progress in developing new classes of SERMs, which promise to offer optimal hormone replacement therapy along with better tools to treat or prevent breast cancer.

ERα status in breast cancer is most important for predicting which patients are most likely to benefit from endocrine therapy. The newer method of IHC to detect ERα is superior due to the advantages of use in paraffin-embedded tissue, and is simpler and more sensitive than the old LBA method. This method should also help in further clarification of the role of different ERα mutants and variants and of the ERβ subtype in breast cancer. Most recently the Oncotype DX qRT/PCR assay, which incorporates ERα RNA measurements, has been reported to predict risk for distant recurrence (Paik et al., 2004). With better understanding of the ensemble of factors responsible for modulating ER's action and the response to endocrine therapy, simultaneous measurements of these key factors by efficient assays such as qRT/PCR and expression profiling should further improve the predictive ability of receptor status in the future. Such preclinical and clinical studies are now in progress.

REFERENCES

Aamdal S, Bormer O, Jorgensen O, Host H, Eliassen G, Kaalhus O, Pihl A. Estrogen receptors and long-term prognosis in breast cancer. Cancer 1984; 53:2525–2529.

Allred DC, Bustamante MA, Daniel CO, Gaskill HV, Cruz AB Jr. Immunocytochemical analysis of estrogen receptors in human breast carcinomas. Evaluation of 130 cases and review of the literature regarding concordance with biochemical assay and clinical relevance. Arch Surg 1990; 125:107–113.

Altucci L, Addeo R, Cicatiello L, Dauvois S, Parker MG, Truss M, Beato M, Sica V, Bresciani F, Weisz A. 17beta-Estradiol induces cyclin D1 gene transcription, p36D1-p34cdk4 complex activation and p105Rb phosphorylation during mitogenic stimulation of G(1)-arrested human breast cancer cells. Oncogene 1996; 12:2315–2324.

Amazit L, Pasini L, Szafran AT, Berno V, Wu RC, Marylin M, Jones ED, Mancini MG, Hinojos CA, O'Malley BW, Mancini MA. Regulation of Src-3 intercompartmental dynamics by estrogen receptor and phosphorylation. Mol Cell Biol 2007; 27:6913–6932.

Anderson E, Clarke RB, Howell A. Estrogen responsiveness and control of normal human breast proliferation. J Mammary Gland Biol Neoplasia 1998; 3:23–35.

Anderson TJ, Ferguson DJ, Raab GM. Cell turnover in the "resting" human breast: influence of parity, contraceptive pill, age and laterality. Br J Cancer 1982; 46:376–382.

Anstead GM, Carlson KE, Katzenellenbogen JA. The estradiol pharmacophore: ligand structure-estrogen receptor binding affinity relationships and a model for the receptor binding site. Steroids 1997; 62:268–303.

Anzick SL, Kononen J, Walker RL, Azorsa DO, Tanner MM, Guan XY, Sauter G, Kallioniemi OP, Trent JM, Meltzer PS. AIB1, a steroid receptor coactivator amplified in breast and ovarian cancer. Science 1997; 277:965–968.

Arnold SF, Obourn JD, Jaffe H, Notides AC. Phosphorylation of the human estrogen receptor on tyrosine 537 in vivo and by Src family tyrosine kinases in vitro. Mol Endocrinol 1995a; 9:24–33.

Arnold SF, Vorojeikina DP, Notides AC. Phosphorylation of tyrosine 537 on the human estrogen receptor is required for binding to an estrogen response element. J Biol Chem 1995b; 270:30205–30212.

Aronica SM, Katzenellenbogen BS. Stimulation of estrogen receptor-mediated transcription and alteration in the phosphorylation state of the rat uterine estrogen receptor by estrogen, cyclic adenosine monophosphate, and insulin-like growth factor-I. Mol Endocrinol 1993; 7:743–752.

Arpino G, Guiterrez C, Weiss H, Rimawi M, Massarweh S, Bharwani L, De Placido S, Osborne CK, Schiff R. Treatment of human epidermal growth growth receptor 2-overexpressing breast cancer xenografts with multiagent HER-targeted therapy. J Natl Cancer Inst 2007; 99:694–705.

Ascenzi P, Bocedi A, Marino M. Structure-function relationship of estrogen receptor alpha and beta: impact on human health. Mol Aspects Med 2006; 27(4):299–402.

Auboeuf D, Batsche E, Dutertre M, Muchardt C, O'Malley BW. Coregulators: transducing signal from transcription to alternative splicing. Trends Endocrinol Metab 2007; 18(3): 122–129.

Auricchio F, Di Domenico M, Migliaccio A, Castoria G, Bilancio A. The role of estradiol receptor in the proliferative activity of vanadate on MCF-7 cells. Cell Growth Differ 1995; 6:105–113.

Auricchio F, Migliaccio A, Castoria G, Di Domenico M, Bilancio A, Rotondi A. Protein tyrosine phosphorylation and estradiol action. Ann N Y Acad Sci 1996; 784:149–172.

Badve S, Turbin D, Thorat MA, Morimiya A, Nielsen TO, Perou CM, Dunn S, Huntsman DG, Nakshatri H. FOXA1 expression in breast cancer–correlation with luminal subtype A and survival. Clin Cancer Res 2007; 13:4415–4421.

Barkhem T, Carlsson B, Nilsson Y, Enmark E, Gustafsson J, Nilsson S. Differential response of estrogen receptor alpha and estrogen receptor beta to partial estrogen agonists/antagonists. Mol Pharmacol 1998; 54:105–112.

Baylin SB, Herman JG. DNA hypermethylation in tumorigenesis: epigenetics joins genetics. Trends Genet 2000; 16:168–174.

Beatson GT. On the treatment of inoperable cases of carcinogen of the mamma: suggestions for a new method of treatment with illustrative cases. Lancet 1896; 2:104–107, 162–167.

Bocquel MT, Kumar V, Stricker C, Chambon P, Gronemeyer H. The contribution of the N- and C-terminal regions of steroid receptors to activation of transcription is both receptor and cell-specific. Nucleic Acids Res 1989; 17:2581–2595.

Bollig A, Miksicek RJ. An estrogen receptor-alpha splicing variant mediates both positive and negative effects on gene transcription. Mol Endocrinol 2000; 14:634–649.

Bowler J, Lilley TJ, Pittam JD, Wakeling AE. Novel steroidal pure antiestrogens. Steroids 1989; 54:71–99.

Brzozowski AM, Pike AC, Dauter Z, Hubbard RE, Bonn T, Engstrom O, Ohman L, Greene GL, Gustafsson JA, Carlquist M. Molecular basis of agonism and antagonism in the oestrogen receptor. Nature 1997; 389:753–758.

Bultman SJ, Herschkowitz JI, Godfrey V, Gebuhr TC, Yaniv M, Perou CM, Magnuson T. Characterization of mammary tumors from Brg1 heterozygous mice. Oncogene 2008; 27:460–468.

Burger HG. Selective oestrogen receptor modulators. Horm Res 2000; 53:25–29.

Buzdar A, Chlebowski R, Cuzick J, Duffy S, Forbes J, Jonat W, Ravdin P. Defining the role of aromatase inhibitors in the adjuvant endocrine treatment of early breast cancer. Curr Med Res Opin 2006; 22(8):1575–1585.

Buzdar A, Jonat W, Howell A, Jones SE, Blomqvist C, Vogel CL, Eiermann W, Wolter JM, Azab M, Webster A, Plourde PV. Anastrozole, a potent and selective aromatase inhibitor, versus megestrol acetate in postmenopausal women with advanced breast cancer: results of overview analysis of two phase III trials. Arimidex Study Group. J Clin Oncol 1996; 14:2000–2011.

Campbell RA, Bhat-Nakshatri P, Patel NM, Constantinidou D, Ali S, Nakshatri H. Phosphatidylinositol 3-kinase/AKT-mediated activation of estrogen receptor alpha: a new model for anti-estrogen resistance. J Biol Chem 2001; 276:9817–9824.

Castles CG, Oesterreich S, Hansen R, Fuqua SA. Auto-regulation of the estrogen receptor promoter. J Steroid Biochem Mol Biol 1997; 62:155–163.

Castoria G, Migliaccio A, Green S, Di Domenico M, Chambon P, Auricchio F. Properties of a purified estradiol-dependent calf uterus tyrosine kinase. Biochemistry 1993; 32:1740–1750.

Chambliss KL, Yuhanna IS, Mineo C, Liu P, German Z, Sherman TS, Mendelsohn ME, Anderson RG, Shaul PW. Estrogen receptor alpha and endothelial nitric oxide synthase are organized into a functional signaling module in caveolae. Circ Res 2000; 87:E44–E52.

Chambraud B, Berry M, Redeuilh G, Chambon P, Baulieu EE. Several regions of human estrogen receptor are involved in the formation of receptor-heat shock protein 90 complexes. J Biol Chem 1990; 265:20686–20691.

Chen JD, Evans RM. A transcriptional co-repressor that interacts with nuclear hormone receptors. Nature 1995; 377:454–457.

Chen D, Huang SM, Stallcup MR. Synergistic, p160 coactivator-dependent enhancement of estrogen receptor function by CARM1 and p300. J Biol Chem 2000a; 275(52): 40810–40816.

Chen Y, Lee WH, Chew HK. Emerging roles of BRCA1 in transcriptional regulation and DNA repair. J Cell Physiol 1999b; 181:385–392.

Chen JD, Li H. Coactivation and corepression in transcriptional regulation by steroid/nuclear hormone receptors. Crit Rev Eukaryot Gene Expr 1998; 8:169–190.

Chen H, Lin RJ, Xie W, Wilpitz D, Evans RM. Regulation of hormone-induced histone hyperacetylation and gene activation via acetylation of an acetylase. Cell 1999a; 98:675–686.

Chen D, Riedl T, Washbrook E, Pace PE, Coombes RC, Egly JM, Ali S. Activation of estrogen receptor alpha by S118 phosphorylation involves a ligand-dependent interaction with TFIIH and participation of CDK7. Mol Cell 2000b; 6:127–137.

Choi KC, Kang SK, Tai CJ, Auersperg N, Leung PC. Estradiol up-regulates antiapoptotic bcl-2 messenger ribonucleic acid and protein in tumorigenic ovarian surface epithelium cells. Endocrinology 2001; 142:2351–2360.

Clark GM. Prognostic and predictive factors. In: Harris JR, ed. Diseases of the Breast. Philadelphia: Lippincott Williams & Wilkins, 2000:489–514.

Clarke R, Dickson RB, Lippman ME. The role of steroid hormones and growth factors in the control of normal and malignant breast. In: Parker M, ed. Nuclear Hormone Receptors. London: Academic Press, 1991.

Clarke RB, Howell A, Potten CS, Anderson E. Dissociation between steroid receptor expression and cell proliferation in the human breast. Cancer Res 1997; 57:4987–4991.

Cohen FJ, Watts S, Shah A, Akers R, Plouffe L Jr. Uterine effects of 3-year raloxifene therapy in postmenopausal women younger than age 60. Obstet Gynecol 2000; 95:104–110.

Coleman KM, Lam V, Jaber BM, Lanz RB, Smith CL. SRA coactivation of estrogen receptor alpha is phosphorylation-independent, and enhances 4-hydroxytamoxifen agonist activity. Biochem Biophys Res Commun 2004; 323:332–338.

Couse JF, Curtis Hewitt S, Korach KS. Receptor null mice reveal contrasting roles for estrogen receptor alpha and beta in reproductive tissues. J Steroid Biochem Mol Biol 2000; 74:287–296.

Couse JF, Korach KS. Estrogen receptor null mice: what have we learned and where will they lead us? Endocr Rev 1999; 20:358–417.

Couse JF, Lindzey J, Grandien K, Gustafsson JA, Korach KS. Tissue distribution and quantitative analysis of estrogen receptor-alpha (ERalpha) and estrogen receptor-beta (ERbeta) messenger ribonucleic acid in the wild-type and

ERalpha-knockout mouse. Endocrinology 1997; 138: 4613–4621.

Cowley SM, Parker MG. A comparison of transcriptional activation by ER alpha and ER beta. J Steroid Biochem Mol Biol 1999; 69:165–175.

Cui Y, Niu A, Pestell R, Kumar R, Curran EM, Liu Y, Fuqua SA. Metastasis-associated protein 2 is a repressor of estrogen receptor {alpha} whose overexpression leads to estrogen-independent growth of human breast cancer cells. Mol Endocrinol 2006; 20:2020–2035.

Cui X, Schiff R, Arpino G, Osborne CK, Lee AV. Biology of progesterone receptor loss in breast cancer and its implication for endocrine therapy. J Clin Oncol 2005; 23:7721–7735.

Cui Y, Zhang M, Pestell R, Curran EM, Welshons WV, Fuqua SA. Phosphorylation of estrogen receptor alpha blocks its acetylation and regulates estrogen sensitivity. Cancer Res 2004; 64(24):9199–9208.

Cummings SR, Eckert S, Krueger KA, Grady D, Powles TJ, Cauley JA, Norton L, Nickelsen T, Bjarnason NH, Morrow M, Lippman ME, Black D, Glusman JE, Costa A, Jordan VC. The effect of raloxifene on risk of breast cancer in postmenopausal women: results from the MORE randomized trial. Multiple Outcomes of Raloxifene Evaluation. JAMA 1999; 281:2189–2197.

Davies MP, O'Neill PA, Innes H, Sibson DR, Prime W, Holcombe C, Foster CS. Correlation of mRNA for oestrogen receptor beta splice variants ERbeta1, ERbeta2/ERbetacx and ERbeta5 with outcome in endocrine-treated breast cancer. J Mol Endocrinol 2004; 33:773–782.

de Graffenreid L, Hilsenbeck SG, Fuqua SAW. SP1 regulation of the estrogen receptor alpha gene promoter. J Steroid Biochem Mol Biol 2002; 82:7–18.

Delage-Mourroux R, Martini PG, Choi I, Kraichely DM, Hoeksema J, Katzenellenbogen BS. Analysis of estrogen receptor interaction with a repressor of estrogen receptor activity (REA) and the regulation of estrogen receptor transcriptional activity by REA. J Biol Chem 2000; 275: 35848–35856.

Delmas PD, Bjarnason NH, Mitlak BH, Ravoux AC, Shah AS, Huster WJ, Draper M, Christiansen C. Effects of raloxifene on bone mineral density, serum cholesterol concentrations, and uterine endometrium in postmenopausal women. N Engl J Med 1997; 337:1641–1647.

den Hollander P, Rayala SK, Coverley D, Kumar R. Ciz1, a Novel DNA-binding coactivator of the estrogen receptor alpha, confers hypersensitivity to estrogen action. Cancer Res 2006; 66(22):11021–11029.

Desai AJ, Luqmani YA, Walters JE, Coope RC, Dagg B, Gomm JJ, Pace PE, Rees CN, Thirunavukkarasu V, Shousha S, Groome NP, Coombes R, Ali S. Presence of exon 5-deleted oestrogen receptor in human breast cancer: functional analysis and clinical significance. Br J Cancer 1997; 75:1173–1184.

Dhalluin C, Carlson JE, Zeng L, He C, Aggarwal AK, Zhou MM. Structure and ligand of a histone acetyltransferase bromodomain. Nature 1999; 399:491–496.

Dickson RB, Huff KK, Spencer EM, Lippman ME. Induction of epidermal growth factor-related polypeptides by 17 beta-estradiol in MCF-7 human breast cancer cells. Endocrinology 1986; 118:138–142.

Dickson RB, Lippman ME. Autocrine and paracrine growth factors in the normal and neoplastic breast. In: Harris JR, ed. Diseases of the Breast. Philadelphia: Lippincott Williams & Wilkins, 2000:471–488.

Dombernowsky P, Smith I, Falkson G, Leonard R, Panasci L, Bellmunt J, Bezwoda W, Gardin G, Gudgeon A, Morgan M, Fornasiero A, Hoffmann W, Michel J, Hatschek T, Tjabbes T, Chaudri HA, Hornberger U, Trunet PF. Letrozole, a new oral aromatase inhibitor for advanced breast cancer: double-blind randomized trial showing a dose effect and improved efficacy and tolerability compared with megestrol acetate. J Clin Oncol 1998; 16:453–461.

Donaghue C, Westley BR, May FE. Selective promoter usage of the human estrogen receptor-alpha gene and its regulation by estrogen. Mol Endocrinol 1999; 13:1934–1950.

Dotzlaw H, Leygue E, Watson PH, Murphy LC. Estrogen receptor-beta messenger RNA expression in human breast tumor biopsies: relationship to steroid receptor status and regulation by progestins. Cancer Res 1999; 59:529–532.

Duval D, Durant S, Homo-Delarche F. Non-genomic effects of steroids. Interactions of steroid molecules with membrane structures and functions. Biochim Biophys Acta 1983; 737:409–442.

Early Breast Cancer Trialists' Collaborative Group. Systemic treatment of early breast cancer by hormonal, cytotoxic, or immune therapy: 133 randomized trials involving 31000 recurrences and 24000 deaths among 75000 women. Lancet 1992; 339:1–15, 71–85.

Eeckhoute J, Carroll JS, Geistlinger TR, Torres-Arzavus MI, Brown M. A cell-type specific transcriptional network required for estrogen regulation of cyclin D1 and cell cycle progression in breast cancer. Genes Dev 2006; 20: 2513–2516.

Elledge RM, Clark GM, Fuqua SA, Yu YY, Allred DC. p53 protein accumulation detected by five different antibodies: relationship to prognosis and heat shock protein 70 in breast cancer. Cancer Res 1994; 54:3752–3757.

Elledge RM, Green S, Pugh R, Allred DC, Clark GM, Hill J, Ravdin P, Martino S, Osborne CK. Estrogen receptor (ER) and progesterone receptor (PgR), by ligand-binding assay compared with ER, PgR and pS2, by immuno-histochemistry in predicting response to tamoxifen in metastatic breast cancer: a Southwest Oncology Group Study. Int J Cancer 2000; 89:111–117.

Ellis MJ, Coop A, Singh B, Mauriac L, Llombert-Cussac A, Jänicke F, Miller WR, Evans DB, Dugan M, Brady C, Quebe-Fehling E, Borgs M. Letrozole is more effective neoadjuvant endocrine therapy than tamoxifen for ErbB-1- and/or ErbB-2-positive, estrogen receptor-positive primary breast cancer: evidence from a phase III randomized trial. J Clin Oncol 2001; 19:3808–3816.

Endoh H, Maruyama K, Masuhiro Y, Kobayashi Y, Goto M, Tai H, Yanagisawa J, Metzger D, Hashimoto S, Kato S. Purification and identification of p68 RNA helicase acting as a transcriptional coactivator specific for the activation function 1 of human estrogen receptor alpha. Mol Cell Biol 1999; 19:5363–5372.

Enmark E, Pelto-Huikko M, Grandien K, Lagercrantz S, Lagercraxtz J, Fried G, Nordenskjöld M, Gustafsson J-Å, Human estrogen receptor β-gene structure, chromosomal localization, and expression pattern. J Clin Endocrinol 1997; 82:4258–4265.

Fan M, Yan PS, Hartman-Frey C, Chen L, Paik H, Oyer SL, Salisbury JD, Cheng AS, Li L, Abbosh PH, Huang TH, Nephew KP. Diverse gene expression and DNA methylation profiles correlate with differential adaptation of breast cancer cells to the antiestrogens tamoxifen and fulvestrant. Cancer Res 2006; 66(24):11954–11966.

Farhat MY, Lavigne MC, Ramwell PW. The vascular protective effects of estrogen. FASEB J 1996; 10:615–624.

Faus H, Haendler B. Post-translational modifications of steroid receptors. Biomed Pharmacother 2006; 60(9):520–528.

Feng W, Webb P, Nguyen P, Liu X, Li J, Karin M, Kushner PJ. Potentiation of estrogen receptor activation function 1 (AF-1) by Src/JNK through a serine 118-independent pathway. Mol Endocrinol 2001; 15:32–45.

Ferguson AT, Lapidus RG, Baylin SB, Davidson NE. Demethylation of the estrogen receptor gene in estrogen receptor-negative breast cancer cells can reactivate estrogen receptor gene expression. Cancer Res 1995; 55:2279–2283.

Filardo EJ, Quinn JA, Frackelton AR Jr., Bland KI. Estrogen action via the G protein-coupled receptor, GPR30: stimulation of adenylyl cyclase and cAMP-mediated attenuation of the epidermal growth factor receptor-to-MAPK signaling axis. Mol Endocrinol 2002; 16(1):70–84.

Fisher B, Costantino JP, Wickerham DL, Redmond CK, Kavanah M, Cronin WM, Vogel V, Robidoux A, Dimitrov N, Atkins J, Daly M, Wieand S, Tan-Chiu E, Ford L, Wolmark N. Tamoxifen for the prevention of breast cancer: report of the National Surgical Adjuvant Breast and Bowel Project P-1 Study. J Natl Cancer Inst 1998; 90:1371–1388.

Font de Mora J, Brown M. AIB1 is a conduit for kinase-mediated growth factor signaling to the estrogen receptor. Mol Cell Biol 2000; 20:5041–5047.

Frech MS, Halama ED, Tilli MT, Singh B, Gunther EJ, Chodosh LA, Flaws JA, Furth PA. Deregulated estrogen receptor α epxression in mammary epithelial cells of trangenic mice results in the development of ductal carcinoma in situ. Cancer Res 2005; 65:681–685.

Fulco RA, Petix M, Salimbeni V, Torre EA. Prognostic significance of the estrogen-regulated proteins, cathepsin-D and pS2, in breast cancer. Minerva Med 1998; 89:5–10.

Fuqua SAW, Cui Y, Lee AV, Osborne CK, Horwitz KR. Insights into the role of progesterone receptors in breast cancer. J Clin Oncol 2005; 23:931–932.

Fuqua SA, Schiff R, Parra I, Friedrichs WE, Su JL, McKee DD, Slentz-Kesler K, Moore LB, Willson TM, Moore JT. Expression of wild-type estrogen receptor beta and variant isoforms in human breast cancer. Cancer Res 1999; 59:5425–5428.

Fuqua SAW, Wiltschke C, Castles C, Wolf D, Allred DC. A role for estrogen-receptor variants in endocrine resistance. Endocr Relat Cancer 1995; 2:19–25.

Fuqua SA, Wiltschke C, Zhang QX, Borg A, Castles CG, Friedrichs WE, Hopp T, Hilsenbeck S, Mohsin S, O'Connell P, Allred DC. A hypersensitive estrogen receptor-alpha mutation in premalignant breast lesions. Cancer Res 2000; 60:4026–4029.

Fuqua SA, Wolf DM. Molecular aspects of estrogen receptor variants in breast cancer. Breast Cancer Res Treat 1995; 35:233–241.

Gaillard S, Grasfeder LL, Haeffele CL, Lobenhofer EK, Chu TM, Wolfinger R, Kazmin D, Koves TR, Muoio DM, Chang CY, McDonnell DP. Receptor-selective coactivators as tools to define the biology of specific receptor-coactivator pairs. Mol Cell 2006; 24:797–803.

Gallacchi P, Schoumacher F, Eppenberger-Castori S, Von Landenberg EM, Kueng W, Eppenberger U, Mueller H. Increased expression of estrogen-receptor exon-5-deletion variant in relapse tissues of human breast cancer. Int J Cancer 1998; 79:44–48.

Gennari L, Merlotti D, Valleggi F, Martini G, Nuti R. Medicinal chemistry and emerging strategies applied to the development of selective estrogen receptor modulators (SERMs). Curr Med Chem 2007; 14:1249–1261.

Gorlich M, Jandrig B. Estradiol receptors and metastasis in human breast cancer. Folia Biol (Praha) 1996; 42:3–10.

Gradishar W, Glusman J, Lu Y, Vogel C, Cohen FJ, Sledge GW, Jr. Effects of high dose raloxifene in selected patients with advanced breast carcinoma. Cancer 2000; 88:2047–2053.

Graham JD, Bain DL, Richer JK, Jackson TA, Tung L, Horwitz KB. Thoughts on tamoxifen resistant breast cancer. Are coregulators the answer or just a red herring? J Steroid Biochem Mol Biol 2000; 74:255–259.

Grandien K. Determination of transcription start sites in the human estrogen receptor gene and identification of a novel, tissue-specific, estrogen receptor-mRNA isoform. Mol Cell Endocrinol 1996; 116:207–212.

Green S, Walter P, Greene G, Krust A, Goffin C, Jensen E, Scrace G, Waterfield M, Chambon P. Cloning of the human oestrogen receptor cDNA. J Steroid Biochem 1986a; 24: 77–83.

Green S, Walter P, Kumar V, Krust A, Bornert J-M, Argos P, Chambon P. Human oestrogen receptor cDNA; sequence, expression and homology to v-erb-A. Nature 1986b; 320:134–139.

Hahnel R, Woodings T, Vivian AB. Prognostic value of estrogen receptors in primary breast cancer. Cancer 1979; 44: 671–675.

Hall JM, McDonnell DP. The estrogen receptor beta-isoform (ERbeta) of the human estrogen receptor modulates ERalpha transcriptional activity and is a key regulator of the cellular response to estrogens and antiestrogens. Endocrinology 1999; 140:5566–5578.

Hankinson O. The aryl hydrocarbon receptor complex. Annu Rev Pharmacol Toxicol 1995; 35:307–340.

Hanstein B, Eckner R, DiRenzo J, Halachmi S, Liu H, Searcy B, Kurokawa R, Brown M. p300 is a component of an estrogen receptor coactivator complex. Proc Natl Acad Sci U S A 1996; 93:11540–11545.

Harvey JM, Clark GM, Osborne CK, Allred DC. Estrogen receptor status by immunohistochemistry is superior to the ligand-binding assay for predicting response to adjuvant endocrine therapy in breast cancer. J Clin Oncol 1999; 17:1474–1481.

Hayashi S, Imai K, Suga K, Kurihara T, Higashi Y, Nakachi K. Two promoters in expression of estrogen receptor messenger RNA in human breast cancer. Carcinogenesis 1997; 18:459–464.

Haynes MP, Russell KS, Bender JR. Molecular mechanisms of estrogen actions on the vasculature. J Nucl Cardiol 2000a; 7:500–508.

Haynes MP, Sinha D, Russell KS, Collinge M, Fulton D, Morales-Ruiz M, Sessa WC, Bender JR. Membrane estrogen receptor engagement activates endothelial nitric oxide synthase via the PI3-kinase-Akt pathway in human endothelial cells. Circ Res 2000b; 87:677–682.

Herynk MH, Parra I, Cui Y, Beyer A, Wu MF, Hilsenbeck SG, Fuqua SA. Association between the estrogen receptor alpha A908G mutation and outcomes in invasive breast cancer. Clin Cancer Res 2007; 13:3235–3243.

Hilsenbeck SG, Ravdin PM, de Moor CA, Chamness GC, Osborne CK, Clark GM. Time-dependence of hazard ratios for prognostic factors in primary breast cancer. Breast Cancer Res Treat 1998; 52:227–237.

Hong H, Kohli K, Trivedi A, Johnson DL, Stallcup MR. GRIP1, a novel mouse protein that serves as a transcriptional coactivator in yeast for the hormone binding domains of steroid receptors. Proc Natl Acad Sci U S A 1996; 93: 4948–4952.

Hopp TA, Fuqua SA. Estrogen receptor variants. J Mammary Gland Biol Neoplasia 1998; 3:73–83.

Hopp TA, Weiss HL, Parra IS, Cui Y, Osborne CK, Fuqua SAW. Low levels of estrogen receptor β protein predicts resistance to tamoxifen therapy in breast cancer. Clin Cancer Res 2004; 10:7490–7499.

Horlein AJ, Naar AM, Heinzel T, Torchia J, Gloss B, Kurokawa R, Ryan A, Kamei Y, Soderstrom M, Glass CK, et al. Ligand-independent repression by the thyroid hormone receptor mediated by a nuclear receptor co-repressor. Nature 1995; 377:397–404.

Howell A, DeFriend D, Robertson J, Blamey R, Walton P. Response to a specific antioestrogen (ICI 182780) in tamoxifen-resistant breast cancer. Lancet 1995; 345:29–30.

Howell A, Osborne CK, Morris C, Wakeling AE. ICI 182,780 (Faslodex): development of a novel, "pure" antiestrogen. Cancer 2000; 89:817–825.

Hull DF, Clark GM, Osborne CK, Chamness GC, Knight WAI, McGuire WL. Multiple estrogen receptor assays in human breast cancer. Cancer Res 1983; 43:413–416.

Huseby RA, Maloney TM, McGrath CM. Evidence for a direct growth-stimulating effect of estradiol on human MCF-7 cells in vivo. Cancer Res 1984; 44:2654–2659.

Hyder SM, Chiappetta C, Stancel GM. Interaction of human estrogen receptors alpha and beta with the same naturally occurring estrogen response elements. Biochem Pharmacol 1999; 57:597–601.

Hyder SM, Huang JC, Nawaz Z, Boettger-Tong H, Makela S, Chiappetta C, Stancel GM. Regulation of vascular endothelial growth factor expression by estrogens and progestins. Environ Health Perspect 2000; 108:785–790.

Iwase H, Omoto Y, Iwata H, Toyama T, Hara Y, Ando Y, Ito Y, Fujii Y, Kobayashi S. DNA methylation analysis at distal and proximal promoter regions of the oestrogen receptor gene in breast cancers. Br J Cancer 1999; 80:1982–1986.

Jackson TA, Richer JK, Bain DL, Takimoto GS, Tung L, Horwitz KB. The partial agonist activity of antagonist-occupied steroid receptors is controlled by a novel hinge domain-binding coactivator L7/SPA and the corepressors N-CoR or SMRT. Mol Endocrinol 1997; 11:693–705.

Jacobs TW, Prioleau JE, Stillman IE, Schnitt SJ. Loss of tumor marker-immunostaining intensity on stored paraffin slides of breast cancer. J Natl Cancer Inst 1996; 88:1054–1059.

Jarvinen T, Pelto-Huikko M, Holli K, Isola J. Estrogen Receptor beta Is Coexpressed with ERalpha and PR and Associated with Nodal Status, Grade, and Proliferation Rate in Breast Cancer. Am J Pathol 2000; 156:29–35.

Jensen EV. Overview of the nuclear receptor family. In: Parker MG, ed. Nuclear hormone receptors: Molecular Mechanisms, Cellular Functions, Clinical Abnormalities. London: Academic Press, 1991:1–13.

Jensen EV, Block GE, Smith S, Kyser K, DeSombre ER. Estrogen receptors and breast cancer response to adrenalectomy. J Natl Cancer Inst Monogr 1971; 34:55–70.

Jensen EV, Jacobson HI. Basic guides to the mechanism of estrogen action. Recent Prog Horm Res 1962; 18: 387–414.

Joel PB, Smith J, Sturgill TW, Fisher TL, Blenis J, Lannigan DA. pp90rsk1 regulates estrogen receptor-mediated transcription through phosphorylation of Ser-167. Mol Cell Biol 1998a; 18:1978–1984.

Joel PB, Traish AM, Lannigan DA. Estradiol-induced phosphorylation of serine 118 in the estrogen receptor is independent of p42/p44 mitogen-activated protein kinase. J Biol Chem 1998b; 273:13317–13323.

Johansson L, Bavner A, Thomsen JS, Farnegardh M, Gustafsson JA, Treuter E. The orphan nuclear receptor SHP utilizes conserved LXXLL-related motifs for interactions with ligand-activated estrogen receptors. Mol Cell Biol 2000; 20:1124–1133.

Johnston CC Jr., Bjarnason NH, Cohen FJ, Shah A, Lindsay R, Mitlak BH, Huster W, Draper MW, Harper KD, Heath H, 3rd, Gennari C, Christiansen C, Arnaud CD, Delmas PD. Long-term effects of raloxifene on bone mineral density, bone turnover, and serum lipid levels in early postmenopausal women: three-year data from 2 double-blind, randomized, placebo-controlled trials. Arch Intern Med 2000; 160:3444–3450.

Johnston SR, Lu B, Scott GK, Kushner PJ, Smith IE, Dowsett M, Benz CC. Increased activator protein-1 DNA binding and c-Jun NH2-terminal kinase activity in human breast tumors with acquired tamoxifen resistance. Clin Cancer Res 1999; 5:251–256.

Jordan VC. Targeted Antiestrogens to Prevent Breast Cancer. Trends Endocrinol Metab 1999; 10:312–317.

Kamei Y, Xu L, Heinzel T, Torchia J, Kurokawa R, Gloss B, Lin SC, Heyman RA, Rose DW, Glass CK. Rosenfeld MGA CBP integrator complex mediates transcriptional activation and AP-1 inhibition by nuclear receptors. Cell 1996; 85:403–414.

Karnik PS, Kulkarni S, Liu XP, Budd GT, Bukowski RM. Estrogen receptor mutations in tamoxifen-resistant breast cancer. Cancer Res 1994; 54:349–353.

Kato S, Endoh H, Masuhiro Y, Kitamoto T, Uchiyama S, Sasaki H, Masushige S, Gotoh Y, Nishida E, Kawashima H, et al. Activation of the estrogen receptor through phosphorylation by mitogen-activated protein kinase. Science 1995; 270:1491–1494.

Katzenellenbogen BS, Choi I, Delage-Mourroux R, Ediger TR, Martini PG, Montano M, Sun J, Weis K, Katzenellenbogen JA. Molecular mechanisms of estrogen action: selective ligands and receptor pharmacology. J Steroid Biochem Mol Biol 2000; 74:279–285.

Kirkegaard T, McGlynn LM, Campbell FM, Muller S, Tovey SM, Dunne B, Nielsen KV, Cooke TG, Bartlett JM. Amplified in breast cancer 1 in human epidermal growth factor receptor-positive tumors of tamoxifen-treated breast cancer patients. Clin Cancer Res 2007; 13:1405–1411.

Klein-Hitpass L, Ryffel GU, Heitlinger E, Cato AC. A 13 bp palindrome is a functional estrogen responsive element and interacts specifically with estrogen receptor. Nucleic Acids Res 1988; 16:647–663.

Klinge CM. Estrogen receptor interaction with co-activators and co-repressors. Steroids 2000; 65:227–251.

Knotts TA, Orkiszewski RS, Cook RG, Edwards DP, Weigel NL. Identification of a phosphorylation site in the hinge region of the human progesterone receptor and additional amino-terminal phosphorylation sites. J Biol Chem 2001; 276:8475–8483.

Knowlden JM, Gee JM, Robertson JF, Ellis IO, Nicholson RI. A possible divergent role for the oestrogen receptor alpha and beta subtypes in clinical breast cancer. Int J Cancer 2000; 89:209–212.

Krege JH, Hodgin JB, Couse JF, Enmark E, Warner M, Mahler JF, Sar M, Korach KS, Gustafsson JA, Smithies O. Generation and reproductive phenotypes of mice lacking estrogen receptor beta. Proc Natl Acad Sci U S A 1998; 95:15677–15682.

Kuiper GG, Carlsson B, Grandien K, Enmark E, Haggblad J, Nilsson S, Gustafsson JA. Comparison of the ligand binding specificity and transcript tissue distribution of estrogen receptors alpha and beta. Endocrinology 1997; 138: 863–870.

Kuiper GG, Enmark E, Pelto-Huikko M, Nilsson S, Gustafsson JA. Cloning of a novel receptor expressed in rat prostate and ovary. Proc Natl Acad Sci U S A 1996; 93:5925–5930.

Kumar R, Thompson EB. The structure of the nuclear hormone receptors. Steroids 1999; 64:310–319.

Kunisue H, Kurebayashi J, Otsuki T, Tang CK, Kurosumi M, Yamamoto S, Tanaka K, Doihara H, Shimizu N, Sonoo H. Anti-HER2 antibody enhances the growth inhibitory effect of anti-oestrogen on breast cancer cells expressing both oestrogen receptors and HER2. Br J Cancer 2000; 82:46–51.

Kurebayashi J, Otsuki T, Kunisue H, Tanaka K, Yamamoto S, Sonoo H. Expression levels of estrogen receptor-alpha, estrogen receptor-beta, coactivators, and corepressors in breast cancer. Clin Cancer Res 2000; 6:512–518.

Kurokawa H, Lenferink AE, Simpson JF, Pisacane PI, Sliwkowski MX, Forbes JT, Arteaga CL. Inhibition of HER2/neu (erbB-2) and mitogen-activated protein kinases enhances tamoxifen action against HER2-overexpressing, tamoxifen-resistant breast cancer cells. Cancer Res 2000; 60:5887–5894.

Kushner PJ, Agard DA, Greene GL, Scanlan TS, Shiau AK, Uht RM, Webb P. Estrogen receptor pathways to AP-1. J Steroid Biochem Mol Biol 2000; 74:311–317.

Lacassagne A. Hormonal pathogenesis of adenocarcinoma of the breast. Am J Cancer 1936; 27:217–225.

Landis SH, Murray T, Bolden S, Wingo PA. Cancer statistics, 1998. CA Cancer J Clin 1998; 48:6–29.

Lanz RB, McKenna NJ, Onate SA, Albrecht U, Wong J, Tsai SY, Tsai MJ, O'Malley BW. A steroid receptor coactivator, SRA, functions as an RNA and is present in an Src-1 complex. Cell 1999; 97:17–27.

Lavinsky RM, Jepsen K, Heinzel T, Torchia J, Mullen TM, Schiff R, Del-Rio AL, Ricote M, Ngo S, Gemsch J, Hilsenbeck SG, Osborne CK, Glass CK, Rosenfeld MG, Rose DW. Diverse signaling pathways modulate nuclear receptor recruitment of N-CoR and SMRT complexes. Proc Natl Acad Sci U S A 1998; 95:2920–2925.

Leake R, Barnes D, Pinder S, Ellis I, Anderson L, Anderson T, Adamson R, Rhodes T, Miller K, Walker R. Immunohistochemical detection of steroid receptors in breast cancer: a working protocol. UK Receptor Group, UK NEQAS, The Scottish Breast Cancer Pathology Group, and The Receptor and Biomarker Study Group of the EORTC. J Clin Pathol 2000; 53:634–635.

Lee H, Jiang F, Wang Q, Nicosia SV, Yang J, Su B, Bai W. MEKK1 activation of human estrogen receptor alpha and stimulation of the agonistic activity of 4-hydroxytamoxifen in endometrial and ovarian cancer cells. Mol Endocrinol 2000; 14:1882–1896.

Lees JA, Fawell SE, Parker MG. Identification of two transactivation domains in the mouse oestrogen receptor. Nucleic Acids Res 1989; 17:5477–5488.

Leong H, Sloan JR, Nash PD, Greene GL. Recruitment of histone deacetylase 4 to the N-terminal region of estrogen receptor alpha. Mol Endocrinol 2005; 19(12):2930–2942.

Levin ER. Integration of the extranuclear and nuclear actions of estrogen. Mol Endocrinol 2005; 19(8):1951–1959.

Levin ER, Pietras RJ. Estrogen receptor outside the nucleus in breast cancer. Breast Cancer Res Treat 2007 Jun 26; [Epub ahead of print].

Leygue E, Dotzlaw H, Watson PH, Murphy LC. Expression of estrogen receptor beta1, beta2, and beta5 messenger RNAs in human breast tissue. Cancer Res 1999; 59:1175–1179.

Leygue E, Huang A, Murphy LC, Watson PH. Prevalence of estrogen receptor variant messenger RNAs in human breast cancer. Cancer Res 1996; 56:4324–4327.

Li LC, Yeh CC, Nojima D, Dahiya R. Cloning and characterization of human estrogen receptor beta promoter. Biochem Biophys Res Commun 2000; 275:682–689.

Likhite VS, Stossi F, Kim K, Katzenellenbogen BS. Katzenellenbogen JA Kinase-specific phosphorylation of the estrogen receptor changes receptor interactions with ligand, deoxyribonucleic acid, and coregulators associated with alterations in estrogen and tamoxifen activity. Mol Endocrinol 2006; 20(12):3120–3132.

Lonard DM, O'Malley BW. The expanding cosmos of nuclear receptor coactivators. Cell 2006; 125(3):411–414.

Ma YX, Tomita Y, Fan S, Wu K, Tong Y, Zhao Z, Song LN, Goldberg ID, Rosen EM. Structural determinants of the BRCA1:estrogen receptor interaction. Oncogene 2005; 24:1831–1846.

Martin MB, Franke TF, Stoica GE, Chambon P, Katzenellenbogen BS, Stoica BA, McLemore MS, Olivo SE, Stoica A. A role for Akt in mediating the estrogenic functions of epidermal growth factor and insulin-like growth factor I. Endocrinology 2000; 141:4503–4511.

Martinez E, Givel F, Wahli W. The estrogen-responsive element as an inducible enhancer: DNA sequence requirements and conversion to a glucocorticoid-responsive element. EMBO J 1987; 6:3719–3727.

Masamura S, Santner SJ, Heitjan DF, Santen RJ. Estrogen deprivation causes estradiol hypersensitivity in human breast cancer cells. J Clin Endocrinol Metab 1995; 80: 2918–2925.

Massarweh S, Osborne CK, Jiang S, Wakeling AE, Rimawi M, Mohsin SK, Hilsenbeck S, Schiff R. Mechanisms of tumor regression and resistance to estrogen deprivation and fulvestrant in a model of estrogen receptor-positive, HER-2/neu-positive breast cancer. Cancer Res 2006; 66: 8266–8273.

Matthews J, Wihlen B, Tujague M, Wan J, Strom A, Gustafsson JA. Estrogen receptor (ER) beta modulates ERalpha-mediated transcriptional activation by altering the recruitment of c-Fos and c-Jun to estrogen-responsive promoters. Mol Endocrinol 2006; 20:534–543.

McDonnell DP, Chang CY, Norris JD. Development of peptide antagonists that target estrogen receptor-cofactor interactions. J Steroid Biochem Mol Biol 2000; 74:327–335.

McDonnell DP, Clemm DL, Hermann T, Goldman ME, Pike JW. Analysis of estrogen receptor function in vitro reveals three distinct classes of antiestrogens. Mol Endocrinol 1995; 9:659–669.

McGuire WL. Estrogen receptor versus nuclear grade as prognostic factors in axillary node-negative breast cancer. J Clin Oncol 1988; 6:1071–1072.

McGuire WL, Carbone PP, Vollmer EP. Estrogen receptors in human breast cancer. New York: Raven Press, 1975.

McInerney EM, Katzenellenbogen BS. Different regions in activation function-1 of the human estrogen receptor required for antiestrogen- and estradiol-dependent transcription activation. J Biol Chem 1996; 271:24172–24178.

McKenna NJ, Lanz RB. O'Malley BW. Nuclear receptor coregulators: cellular and molecular biology. Endocr Rev 1999; 20:321–344.

McPherson LA, Baichwal VR, Weigel RJ. Identification of ERF-1 as a member of the AP2 transcription factor family. Proc Natl Acad Sci U S A 1997; 94:4342–4347.

Menasce LP, White GR, Harrison CJ, Boyle JM. Localization of the estrogen receptor locus (ESR) to chromosome 6q25.1 by FISH and a simple post-FISH banding technique. Genomics 1993; 17:263–265.

Mendelsohn ME. Nongenomic, ER-mediated activation of endothelial nitric oxide synthase: how does it work? What does it mean? Circ Res 2000; 87:956–960.

Mendelsohn ME, Karas RH. The protective effects of estrogen on the cardiovascular system. N Engl J Med 1999; 340:1801–1811.

Metzger D, Ali S, Bornert JM, Chambon P. Characterization of the amino-terminal transcriptional activation function of the human estrogen receptor in animal and yeast cells. J Biol Chem 1995; 270:9535–9542.

Michalides R, Griekspoor A, Balkenende A, Verwoerd D, Janssen L, Jalink K, Floore A, Velds A, van't Veer L, Neefjes J. Tamoxifen resistance by a conformational arrest of the estrogen receptor alpha after PKA activation in breast cancer. Cancer Cell 2004; 5(6):597–605.

Migliaccio A, Rotondi A, Auricchio F. Estradiol receptor: phosphorylation on tyrosine in uterus and interaction with anti-phosphotyrosine antibody. EMBO J 1986; 5:2867–2872.

Miller TL, Jin Y, Sun JM, Coutts AS, Murphy LC, Davie JR. Analysis of human breast cancer nuclear proteins binding to the promoter elements of the c-myc gene. J Cell Biochem 1996; 60:560–571.

Molino A, Micciolo R, Turazza M, Bonetti F, Piubello Q, Corgnati A, Sperotto L, Recaldin E, Spagnolli P, Manfrin E, Bonetti A, Nortilli R, Tomezzoli A, Pollini GP, Modena S, Cetto GL. Prognostic significance of estrogen receptors in 405 primary breast cancers: a comparison of immunohistochemical and biochemical methods. Breast Cancer Res Treat 1997; 45:241–249.

Montano MM, Ekena K, Delage-Mourroux R, Chang W, Martini P, Katzenellenbogen BS. An estrogen receptor-selective coregulator that potentiates the effectiveness of antiestrogens and represses the activity of estrogens. Proc Natl Acad Sci U S A 1999; 96:6947–6952.

Montano MM, Katzenellenbogen BS. The quinone reductase gene: a unique estrogen receptor-regulated gene that is activated by antiestrogens. Proc Natl Acad Sci U S A 1997; 94:2581–2586.

Mosselman S, Polman J, Kijkema R. Identification and characterization of a novel human estrogen receptor. FEBS Lett 1996; 392:49–53.

Murphy LC, Dotzlaw H, Leygue E, Coutts A, Watson P. The pathophysiological role of estrogen receptor variants in human breast cancer. J Steroid Biochem Mol Biol 1998; 65:175–180.

Mussi P, Liao L, Park SE, Ciana P, Maggi A, Katzenellenbogen BS, Xu J, O'Malley BW. Haploinsufficiency of the corepressor of estrogen receptor activity (REA) enhances estrogen receptor function in the mammary gland. Proc Natl Acad Sci U S A 2006; 103:16716–16721.

Nass SJ, Herman JG, Gabrielson E, Iversen PW, Parl FF, Davidson NE, Graff JR. Aberrant methylation of the estrogen receptor and E-cadherin 5′ CpG islands increases with malignant progression in human breast cancer. Cancer Res 2000; 60:4346–4348.

Neuman E, Ladha MH, Lin N, Upton TM, Miller SJ, DiRenzo J, Pestell RG, Hinds PW, Dowdy SF, Brown M, Ewen ME. Cyclin D1 stimulation of estrogen receptor transcriptional activity independent of cdk4. Mol Cell Biol 1997; 17: 5338–5347.

Nicholson RI, Gee JMW, Barrow D, Pamment JS, Knowlden JM, McClelland R. Endocrine resistance in breast cancer can involve a switch towards EGFR signaling pathways and a gain of sensitivity to an EGFR-selective tyrosine kinase inhibitor, ZD1839. In: AACR-NCI-EORTC International Conference on Molecular Targets and Cancer Therapeutics. Vol 5. Philadelphia: AACR; 1999a (supplement).

Nicholson RI, McClelland RA, Robertson JF. Gee JM Involvement of steroid hormone and growth factor cross-talk in endocrine response in breast cancer. Endocr Relat Cancer 1999b; 6:373–387.

Norris JD, Fan D, Kerner SA, McDonnell DP. Identification of a third autonomous activation domain within the human estrogen receptor. Mol Endocrinol 1997; 11:747–754.

Oesterreich S, Zhang Q, Hopp T, Fuqua SA, Michaelis M, Zhao HH, Davie JR, Osborne CK, Lee AV. Tamoxifen-bound estrogen receptor (ER) strongly interacts with the nuclear matrix protein HET/SAF-B, a novel inhibitor of ER-mediated transactivation. Mol Endocrinol 2000; 14:369–381.

Ogawa S, Inoue S, Watanabe T, Hiroi H, Orimo A, Hosoi T, Ouchi Y, Muramatsu M. The complete primary structure of human estrogen receptor β (hERβ) and its heterodimerization with ER α in vivo and in vitro. Biochem Biophys Res Commun 1998; 243:122–126.

Ohlsson H, Lykkesfeldt AE, Madsen MW, Briand P. The estrogen receptor variant lacking exon 5 has dominant negative activity in the human breast epithelial cell line HMT-3522S1. Cancer Res 1998; 58:4264–4268.

Ohta T, Fukuda M. Ubiquitin and breast cancer. Oncogene 2004; 23(11):2079–2088.

Onate SA, Tsai SY, Tsai MJ, O'Malley BW. Sequence and characterization of a coactivator for the steroid hormone receptor superfamily. Science 1995; 270:1354–1357.

Osborne CK. Receptors. In: Harris J, Hellman S, Henderson IC, Kinne W, eds. Breast Diseases. Philadelphia, PA: JB Lippincott Co, 1991:301–325.

Osborne CK. Steroid hormone receptors in breast cancer management. Breast Cancer Res Treat 1998; 51:227–238.

Osborne CK. Aromatase inhibitors in relation to other forms of endocrine therapy for breast cancer. Endocr Relat Cancer 1999a; 6:271–276.

Osborne CK. On behalf of the North American Faslodex Investigator Group: A double-blind randomized trail comparing the efficacy and tolerability of Faslodex™ (Fulvestrant) with Arimidex™ (Anastrozole) in post-menopausal women with advanced breast cancer. In: Lippman ME, ed. San Antonio Breast Cancer Symposium. Vol 64. San Antonio, TX: Kluwer Academic Publishers, 2000:27.

Osborne CK, Bardou V, Hopp TA, Chamness GC, Hilsenbeck SG, Fuqua SAW, Wong J, Allred DC, Clark GM, Schiff R. Role of the estrogen receptor coactivator AIB1 (Src-3) and HER-2/neu in tamoxifen resistance in breast cancer. J Natl Cancer Inst 2003; 85:352–361.

Osborne CK, Fuqua SA. Mechanisms of tamoxifen resistance. Breast Cancer Res Treat 1994; 32:49–55.

Osborne CK, Yochmowitz MG, Knight WA 3rd, McGuire WL. The value of estrogen and progesterone receptors in the treatment of breast cancer. Cancer 1980; 46:2884–2888.

Osborne CK, Zhao H, Fuqua SA. Selective estrogen receptor modulators: structure, function, and clinical use. J Clin Oncol 2000; 18:3172–3186.

Osborne MP. Breast cancer prevention by antiestrogens. Ann N Y Acad Sci 1999b; 889:146–151.

Ottaviano YL, Issa JP, Parl FF, Smith HS, Baylin SB, Davidson NE. Methylation of the estrogen receptor gene CpG island marks loss of estrogen receptor expression in human breast cancer cells. Cancer Res 1994; 54:2552–2555.

Paik S, Shak S, Tang G, Kim C, Baker J, Cronin M, Baehner FL, Walker MG, Watson D, Park T, et al. A multigene assay to predict recurrence of tamoxifen-treated, node-negative breast cancer. N Engl J Med 2004; 351:2817–2826.

Pedram A, Razandi M, Levin ER. Nature of functional estrogen receptors at the plasma membrane. Mol Endocrinol 2006; 20(9):1996–2009.

Perou CM Sorlie T, Eisen MB, et al. Molecular portraits of human breast tumors. Nature 2000; 406:747–752.

Perrey L, Paridaens R, Hawle H, Zaman K, Nole F, Wildiers H, Fiche M, Dietrich D, Clement P, Koberler D, Goldhirsch A, Thurlimann B. Clinical benefit of fulvestrant in postmenopausal women with advanced breast cancer and primary or acquired resistance to aromatase inhibitors: final results of phase II Swiss Group for Clinical Cancer Research Trial (SAKK 21/00). Ann Oncol 2007; 18:64–69.

Pierrat B, Heery DM, Chambon P, Losson R. A highly conserved region in the hormone-binding domain of the human estrogen receptor functions as an efficient transactivation domain in yeast. Gene 1994; 143:193–200.

Pietras RJ, Szego CM. Specific binding sites for oestrogen at the outer surfaces of isolated endometrial cells. Nature 1977; 265:69–72.

Pike AC, Brzozowski AM, Hubbard RE. A structural biologist's view of the oestrogen receptor. J Steroid Biochem Mol Biol 2000; 74:261–268.

Pissios P, Tzameli I, Kushner P, Moore DD. Dynamic stabilization of nuclear receptor ligand binding domains by hormone or corepressor binding. Mol Cell 2000; 6:245–253.

Rauschning W, Pritchard KI. Droloxifene, a new antiestrogen: its role in metastatic breast cancer. Breast Cancer Res Treat 1994; 31:83–94.

Ravdin PM, Green S, Dorr TM, McGuire WL, Fabian C, Pugh RP, Carter RD, Rivkin SE, Borst JR, Belt RJ, et al. Prognostic significance of progesterone receptor levels in estrogen receptor-positive patients with metastatic breast cancer treated with tamoxifen: results of a prospective Southwest Oncology Group study. J Clin Oncol 1992; 10:1284–1291.

Rhodes A, Jasani B, Barnes DM, Bobrow LG, Miller KD. Reliability of immunohistochemical demonstration of oestrogen receptors in routine practice: interlaboratory variance in the sensitivity of detection and evaluation of scoring systems. J Clin Pathol 2000; 53:125–130.

Rogatsky I, Trowbridge JM, Garabedian MJ. Potentiation of human estrogen receptor alpha transcriptional activation through phosphorylation of serines 104 and 106 by the cyclin A-CDK2 complex. J Biol Chem 1999; 274: 22296–22302.

Roodi N, Bailey LR, Kao WY, Verrier CS, Yee CJ, Dupont WD, Parl FF. Estrogen receptor gene analysis in estrogen receptor-positive and receptor-negative primary breast cancer. J Natl Cancer Inst 1995; 87:446–451.

Rosfjord EC, Dickson RB. Growth factors, apoptosis, and survival of mammary epithelial cells. J Mammary Gland Biol Neoplasia 1999; 4:229–237.

Russo J, Ao X, Grill C, Russo IH. Pattern of distribution of cells positive for estrogen receptor alpha and progesterone receptor in relation to proliferating cells in the mammary gland. Breast Cancer Res Treat 1999; 53:217–227.

Russo J, Hu YF, Yang X, Russo IH. Developmental, cellular, and molecular basis of human breast cancer. J Natl Cancer Inst Monogr 2000; 27:17–37.

Russo J, Russo IH. Estrogens and cell proliferation in the human breast. J Cardiovasc Pharmacol 1996; 28:19–23.

Saceda M, Lippman ME, Chambon P, Lindsey RL, Ponglikitmongkol M, Puente M, Martin MB. Regulation of the estrogen receptor in MCF-7 cells by estradiol. Mol Endocrinol 1988; 2:1157–1162.

Safe S. Transcriptional activation of genes by 17 beta-estradiol through estrogen receptor-Sp1 interactions. Vitam Horm 2001; 62:231–252.

Sande S, Privalsky ML. Identification of TRACs (T3 receptor-associating cofactors), a family of cofactors that associate with, and modulate the activity of, nuclear hormone receptors. Mol Endocrinol 1996; 10:813–825.

Sato M, Turner C, Wang T, Adrian M, Rowley E, Bryant H. LY353381: a novel raloxifene analog with improved SERM potency and efficacy *in vivo*. J Pharmacol Exp Ther 1998; 287:1–7.

Sauve F, McBroom LD, Gallant J, Moraitis AN, Labrie F, Giguere V. CIA, a novel estrogen receptor coactivator with a bifunctional nuclear receptor interacting determinant. Mol Cell Biol 2001; 21:343–353.

Saville B, Wormke M, Wang F, Nguyen T, Enmark E, Kuiper G, Gustafsson JA, Safe S. Ligand-, cell-, and estrogen receptor subtype (alpha/beta)-dependent activation at GC-rich (Sp1) promoter elements. J Biol Chem 2000; 275:5379–5387.

Schiff R, Reddy P, Ahotupa M, Coronado-Heinsohn E, Grim M, Hilsenbeck SG, Lawrence R, Deneke S, Herrera R, Chamness GC, Fuqua SA, Brown PH, Osborne CK. Oxidative stress and AP-1 activity in tamoxifen-resistant breast tumors *in vivo*. J Natl Cancer Inst 2000; 92: 1926–1934.

Selever J, Fuqua SAW. Sumoylation of estrogen receptor α: Are post-translational modifications coordinated? Breast Cancer Online 2007

Sentis S, Le Romancer M, Bianchin C, Rostan MC, Corbo L. Sumoylation of the estrogen receptor alpha hinge region regulates its transcriptional activity. Mol Endocrinol 2005; 19(11):2671–2684.

Seol W, Hanstein B, Brown M, Moore DD. Inhibition of estrogen receptor action by the orphan receptor SHP (short heterodimer partner). Mol Endocrinol 1998; 12:1551–1557.

Shiau AK, Barstad D, Loria PM, Cheng L, Kushner PJ, Agard DA, Greene GL. The structural basis of estrogen receptor/coactivator recognition and the antagonism of this interaction by tamoxifen. Cell 1998; 95:927–937.

Shoker BS, Jarvis C, Clarke RB, Anderson E, Hewlett J, Davies MP, Sibson DR, Sloane JP. Estrogen receptor-positive proliferating cells in the normal and precancerous breast. Am J Pathol 1999; 155:1811–1815.

Shoker BS, Jarvis C, Clarke RB, Anderson E, Munro C, Davies MP, Sibson DR, Sloane JP. Abnormal regulation of the oestrogen receptor in benign breast lesions. J Clin Pathol 2000; 53:778–783.

Shou J, Massarweh S, Osborne CK, Wakeling AE, Ali S, Weiss H, Schiff R. J Natl Cancer Inst 2004; 96:926–935.

Skliris GP, Carder PJ, Lansdown MR, Speirs V. Immunohistochemical detection of ERbeta in breast cancer: towards more detailed receptor profiling? Br J Cancer 2001; 84:1095–1098.

Skliris GP, Munot K, Bell SM, Carder PJ, Lane S, Horgan K, Lansdown MR, Parkes AT, Hanby AM, Markham AF. Reduced expression of oestrogen receptor beta in invasive breast cancer and its re-expression using DNA methyl transferase inhibitors in a cell line model. J Pathol 2003; 201:213–220.

Sladek FM, Ruse MD, Nepomuceno L, Huang SM, Stallcup MR. Modulation of transcriptional activation and coactivator interaction by a splicing variation in the F domain of nuclear receptor hepatocyte nuclear factor 4alpha1. Mol Cell Biol 1999; 19:6509–6522.

Smith CL, Conneely OM. O'Malley BW. Modulation of the ligand-independent activation of the human estrogen receptor by hormone and antihormone. Proc Natl Acad Sci U S A 1993; 90:6120–6124.

Smith CL, Nawaz Z, O'Malley BW. Coactivator and corepressor regulation of the agonist/antagonist activity of the mixed antiestrogen, 4-hydroxytamoxifen. Mol Endocrinol 1997; 11:657–666.

Speirs V, Carder PJ, Lane S, Dodwell D, Lansdown MR, Hanby AM. Oestrogen receptor beta: what it means for patients with breast cancer. Lancet Oncol 2004; 5:174–181.

Speirs V, Kerin MJ. Prognostic significance of oestrogen receptor beta in breast cancer. Br J Surg 2000; 87:405–409.

Speirs V, Malone C, Walton DS, Kerin MJ, Atkin SL. Increased expression of estrogen receptor beta mRNA in tamoxifen-resistant breast cancer patients. Cancer Res 1999; 59: 5421–5424.

Spencer TE, Jenster G, Burcin MM, Allis CD, Zhou J, Mizzen CA, McKenna NJ, Onate SA, Tsai SY, Tsai MJ, O'Malley BW. Steroid receptor coactivator-1 is a histone acetyltransferase. Nature 1997; 389:194–198.

Suh JH, Huang J, Park YY, Seong HA, Kim D, Shong M, Ha H, Lee IK, Wang L, Choi HS. Orphan nuclear recpetor small heterodimer partner inhibits transforming growth factor-beta signaling by repressing SMAD3 transactivation. J Biol Chem 2006; 281:39169–39178.

Tang Z, Treilleux I, Brown M. A transcriptional enhancer required for the differential expression of the human estrogen receptor in breast cancers. Mol Cell Biol 1997; 17:1274–1280.

Tanimoto K, Eguchi H, Yoshida T, Hajiro-Nakanishi K, Hayashi S. Regulation of estrogen receptor alpha gene mediated by promoter B responsible for its enhanced expression in human breast cancer. Nucleic Acids Res 1999; 27:903–909.

Tasset D, Tora L, Fromental C, Scheer E, Chambon P. Distinct classes of transcriptional activating domains function by different mechanisms. Cell 1990; 62:1177–1187.

Tateishi Y, Kawabe Y, Chiba T, Murata S, Ichikawa K, Murayama A, Tanaka K, Baba T, Kato S, Yanagisawa J. Ligand-dependent switching of ubiquitin-proteasome pathways for estrogen receptor. EMBO J 2004; 23(24): 4813–4823.

Tcherepanova I, Puigserver P, Norris JD, Spiegelman BM, McDonnell DP Modulation of estrogen receptor-alpha transcriptional activity by the coactivator PGC-1. J Biol Chem 2000; 275(21):16302–16308.

Thomas HV, Reeves GK, Key TJ. Endogenous estrogen and postmenopausal breast cancer: a quantitative review. Cancer Causes Control 1997; 8:922–928.

Toft D, Gorski J. A receptor molecule for estrogens: isolation from the rat uterus and preliminary characterization. Proc Natl Acad Sci U S A 1966; 55:1574–1581.

Tonetti DA, Jordan VC. The role of estrogen receptor mutations in tamoxifen-stimulated breast cancer. J Steroid Biochem Mol Biol 1997; 62:119–128.

Tora L, White J, Brou C, Tasset D, Webster N, Scheer E, Chambon P. The human estrogen receptor has two independent nonacidic transcriptional activation functions. Cell 1989; 59:477–487.

Torchia J, Rose DW, Inostroza J, Kamei Y, Westin S, Glass CK, Rosenfeld MG. The transcriptional co-activator p/CIP binds CBP and mediates nuclear-receptor function. Nature 1997; 387:677–684.

Tremblay GB, Tremblay A, Copeland NG, Gilbert DJ, Jenkins NA, Labrie F, Giguere V. Cloning, chromosomal localization, and functional analysis of the murine estrogen receptor beta. Mol Endocrinol 1997; 11:353–365.

Tremblay A, Tremblay G, Labrie C, Labrie F, Giguere V. EM-800, a novel antiestrogen, acts as a pure antagonist of the transcriptional function of estrogen receptors alpha and beta. Endocrinology 1998a; 139:111–118.

Tremblay GB, Tremblay A, Labrie F, Giguere V. Ligand-independent activation of the estrogen receptors alpha and beta by mutations of a conserved tyrosine can be abolished by antiestrogens. Cancer Res 1998b; 58:877–881.

Tzukerman MT, Esty A, Santiso-Mere D, Danielian P, Parker MG, Stein RB, Pike JW, McDonnell DP. Human estrogen receptor transactivational capacity is determined by both cellular and promoter context and mediated by two functionally distinct intramolecular regions. Mol Endocrinol 1994; 8:21–30.

Umayahara Y, Kawamori R, Watada H, Imano E, Iwama N, Morishima T, Yamasaki Y, Kajimoto Y, Kamada T. Estrogen regulation of the insulin-like growth factor I gene transcription involves an AP-1 enhancer. J Biol Chem 1994; 269:16433–16442.

van Agthoven T, Timmermans M, Foekens JA, Dorssers LC, Henzen-Logmans SC. Differential expression of estrogen, progesterone, and epidermal growth factor receptors in normal, benign, and malignant human breast tissues using dual staining immunohistochemistry. Am J Pathol 1994; 144:1238–1246.

van Dijk MA, Hart AA, van't Veer LJ. Differences in estrogen receptor alpha variant messenger RNAs between normal human breast tissue and primary breast carcinomas. Cancer Res 2000; 60:530–533.

Viale G, Regan MM, et al. Prognostic and predictive value of centrally reviewed expression of estrogen and progesterone receptors in a randomized trail comparing letrozole and tamoxifen adjuvant therapy for postmenopausal women with early breast cancer: Results from the BIG 1–98 collaborative groups. J Clin Oncol 2007; 25(25): 3846–3852.

Vogel VG, Costantino JP, Wickerham DL, Cronin WM, Cecchini RS, Atkins JN, Bevers TB, Fehrenbacher L, Pajon ER, Jr., Wade JL, 3rd, Robidoux A, Margolese RG, James J, Lippman SM, Runowicz CD, Ganz PA, Reis SE, McCaskill-Stevens W, Ford LG, Jordan VC, Wolmark N. Effects of tamoxifen vs raloxifene on the risk of developing invasive breast cancer and other disease outcomes: the NSABP Study of Tamoxifen and Raloxifene (STAR) P-2 trial. JAMA 2006; 295(23):2727–2741.

Vyhlidal C, Samudio I, Kladde MP, Safe S. Transcriptional activation of transforming growth factor alpha by estradiol: requirement for both a GC-rich site and an estrogen response element half-site. J Mol Endocrinol 2000; 24:329–338.

Wajed SA, Laird PW, DeMeester TR. DNA methylation: an alternative pathway to cancer. Ann Surg 2001; 234(1):10–20.

Wakeling AE. Use of pure antioestrogens to elucidate the mode of action of oestrogens. Biochem Pharmacol 1995; 49:1545–1549.

Wakeling AE, Valcaccia B, Newboult E, Green LR. Non-steroidal antioestrogens–receptor binding and biological response in rat uterus, rat mammary carcinoma and human breast cancer cells. J Steroid Biochem 1984; 20:111–120.

Walker P, Germond JE, Brown-Luedi M, Givel F, Wahli W. Sequence homologies in the region preceding the transcription initiation site of the liver estrogen-responsive vitellogenin and apo-VLDLII genes. Nucleic Acids Res 1984; 12:8611–8626.

Wang C, Fu M, Angeletti RH, Siconolfi-Baez L, Reutens AT, Albanese C, Lisanti MP, Katzenellenbogen BS, Kato S, Hopp T, Fuqua SA, Lopez GN, Kushner PJ, Pestell RG. Direct acetylation of the estrogen receptor alpha hinge region by p300 regulates transactivation and hormone sensitivity. J Biol Chem 2001; 276:18375–18383.

Watanabe M, Yanagisawa J, Kitagawa H, Takeyama K, Ogawa S, Arao Y, Suzawa M, Kobayashi Y, Yano T, Yoshikawa H, Masuhiro Y, Kato S. A subfamily of RNA-binding DEAD-box proteins acts as an estrogen receptor alpha coactivator through the N-terminal activation domain (AF-1) with an RNA coactivator, SRA. EMBO J 2001; 20:1341–1352.

Weigel NL. Steroid hormone receptors and their regulation by phosphorylation. Biochem J 1996; 319:657–667.

Weigel RJ, Crooks DL, Iglehart JD, deConinck EC. Quantitative analysis of the transcriptional start sites of estrogen receptor in breast carcinoma. Cell Growth Differ 1995; 6:707–711.

Weigel NL, Zhang Y. Ligand-independent activation of steroid hormone receptors. J Mol Med 1998; 76:469–479.

Weis KE, Ekena K, Thomas JA, Lazennec G, Katzenellenbogen BS. Constitutively active human estrogen receptors containing amino acid substitutions for tyrosine 537 in the receptor protein. Mol Endocrinol 1996; 10:1388–1398.

Wheler J, Johnson M, Seidman A. Adjuvant therapy with aromatase inhibitors for postmenopausal women with early breast cancer: evidence and ongoing controversy. Semin Oncol 2006; 33(6):672–680.

Wolf DM, Jordan VC. The estrogen receptor from a tamoxifen stimulated MCF-7 tumor variant contains a point mutation in the ligand binding domain. Breast Cancer Res Treat 1994; 31:129–138.

Xing W, Archer TK. Upstream stimulatory factors mediate estrogen receptor activation of the cathepsin D promoter. Mol Endocrinol 1998; 12:1310–1321.

Yudt MR, Vorojeikina D, Zhong L, Skafar DF, Sasson S, Gasiewicz TA, Notides AC. Function of estrogen receptor tyrosine 537 in hormone binding, DNA binding, and transactivation. Biochemistry 1999; 38:14146–14156.

Zhang QX, Borg A, Wolf DM, Oesterreich S, Fuqua SA. An estrogen receptor mutant with strong hormone-independent activity from a metastatic breast cancer. Cancer Res 1997; 57:1244–1249.

Zheng FF, Wu R-C, Smith CL, O'Malley BW. Rapid estrogen-induced phosphorylation of the Src-3 coactivator occurs in an extranuclear complex containing estrogen receptor. Mol Cell Biol 2005; 25:8273–8284.

Zhou Q, Atadja P, Davidson NE. Histone deacetylase inihibitor LBH589 reactivates estrogen receptor alpha (ER) gene expression without loss of DNA hypermethylation. Cancer Biol Ther 2007a; 1:64–69.

Zhou Y, Yau C, Gray YW, Chew K, Dairkee SH, Moore DH, Eppenberger U, Eppenberger-Castori S, Benz CC. Enhanced NF kappa V and AP-1 transcriptional acitvity associated with antiestrogen resistant breast cancer. BMC Cancer 2007b; 7:59.

Zwijsen RM, Buckle RS, Hijmans EM, Loomans CJ, Bernards R. Ligand-independent recruitment of steroid receptor coactivators to estrogen receptor by cyclin D1. Genes Dev 1998; 12:3488–3498.

6

Progesterone Receptor Isoforms and Human Breast Cancer

ANNE GOMPEL
Université Paris Descartes, Unité de Gynécologie Endocrinienne, APHP, Hôtel Dieu de Paris, and INSERM U673, Hôpital Saint Antoine, Paris, France

AURÉLIE COURTIN
INSERM U673, Hôpital Saint Antoine, Paris, France

INTRODUCTION

The biological and clinical effects of progesterone are mediated through progesterone receptor (PR). The implication of PR in breast cancer (BRCA) is known for a long time. In particular PR expression constitutes a marker of good prognosis, corresponding to differentiated tumors. It has been shown recently from laboratory and clinical studies that in estradiol receptor (ER)-positive tumors, downregulation of PR could be due to the consequences of excessive growth factor–receptor signaling and a feature characteristic of tamoxifen resistance (Osborne et al., 2005). The impact of progesterone on breast cancer history however remains controversial. Part of this discrepancy might be due to the difficulty in getting appropriate models to reproduce the breast cancer history in the human breast. Indeed, the physiology of the human breast is peculiar and there is no equivalent animal model. In addition, transformed breast cells are differently regulated from normal breast cells and progesterone and PR isoforms may have different impact in both cells. It is thus of importance to understand the role and function of PR in breast cancer.

PROGESTERONE RECEPTOR STRUCTURE

PR is a member of the superfamily of steroid receptors. It is composed of two isoforms PRA and PRB. A single gene on chromosome 11, using two distinct promoters, encodes the two isoforms (Fig. 1). PRB, a 114kDa protein, contains 933 amino acids and PRA, a 94 kDa protein, is shorter, lacking a 164 amino acid region on the N-terminal part also called the B-upstream segment (BUS). These receptors contain classical domains (Lessey et al., 1983). These domains correspond to the N-terminal region (A/B domain), DNA-binding zinc finger region (C domain), hinge region (D domain), and C-terminal ligand-binding region (E/F domain) (Fig. 1). Like for other type I steroid receptors, ligand interaction with the C-terminal ligand-binding domain (LBD) induces a major conformational change that promotes receptor dimerization and recognition via the DNA-binding domain (DBD) of specific hormone-responsive elements [here progesterone receptor element (PRE)] within promoter of target genes. In the majority of steroid receptors, there are two regions for the activation of transcription AF-1 and AF-2 (Meyer et al., 1990). The PRB isoform contains an additional region

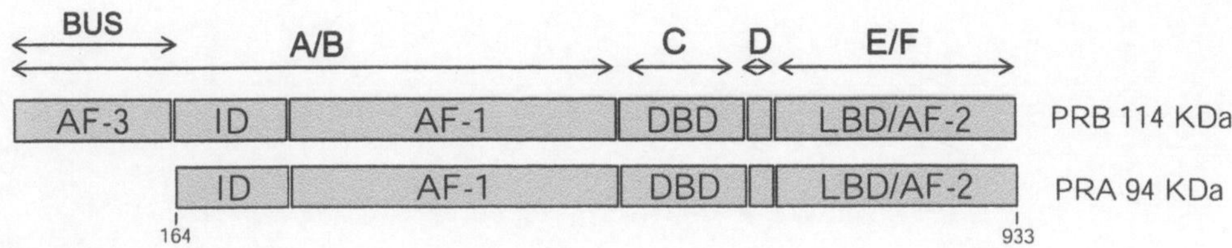

Figure 1 PRA and PRB isoforms structure. *Abbreviations*: DBD, DNA-binding domain; LBD, ligand-binding domain; ID, inhibitory domain; AF, transactivation domain; BUS, B-upstream segment.

with a third domain of activation of the transcription (AF-3) (Sartorius et al., 1994), whereas in PRA only the first two domains are present (Fig. 1). Close to the BUS domain exists a sequence thought to be inhibitory domain (ID) on the activation of transcription. Recent data show that BUS can act by stabilizing the conformational structure of PRB through an AF-3 synergism with AF-2 and AF-1 sites (Tung et al., 2006). Thus, the receptor complexes bound to DNA may be more active, if they contain at least two PREs. In addition, the mutation of AF-3 does not convert PRB into PRA and abolishes the PRB dependent transcription (Tung et al., 2006).

A third PR isoform has been described of 60 kD (PRC), truncated in the N-terminus and which does not contain the first zinc finger of the DNA-binding domain. It was reported to be able to enhance the transcriptional activity of PRA and PRB in breast cancer cells (T47-D cells) but has inhibitory action in uterine cells (Wei et al., 1996).

In absence of ligand, the protein is cytoplasmic and mainly nuclear and bound to chaperone molecule and a corepressor complex. Upon binding of agonist ligand, the LBD promotes the recruitment of coactivators, the release of corepressors, and an assembling of multiprotein complexes having either histone acetyltransferase (HAT) or non-HAT activity. Several coactivators are known to interact with PR, such as members of the p160/steroid receptor coactivator (SRC) family, cAMP response element-binding (CREB) activator, p300/CBP (Vicent et al., 2006). Recently HBO1 was described as a coactivator acting in synergy with the coupling of SRC-1 with AF3 of human progesterone receptor B (hPRB) and with AF2, through a hormone-dependent mechanism and strongly correlated to transcription (Georgiakaki et al., 2006). It is the first demonstration of a different effect of coactivator between PRB and PRA. This could contribute to explain the differential genes regulated by each isoform.

The two promoters, Promoter A (+464 to +1105) and Promoter B (−711 to +31), are responsible for the production of PRA and PRB, respectively with two different AUG sites for initiation of the transcription. The activities of these two promoters are increased by estrogen, but no consensus estradiol responsive elements (EREs) have been identified in either promoter A or promoter B (Kastner et al., 1990). Promoter A, however, contains an ERE half-site located upstream of two Sp1 sites (Petz et al., 2004). The presence of these adjacent binding sites suggests that the ER might be able to influence PR expression directly by binding to the ERE half-site, indirectly by interacting with proteins bound to the putative Sp1 sites, or a combination of additional Sp1 and AP1 sites in the PR promoter.

TRANSCRIPTION REGULATION BY PRA AND PRB

Ligand-Dependent Transcription

PR is a hormone-inducible transcription factor activated through a multistep mechanism. Before binding to DNA, it is necessary to displace a repressor complex, which sensibilizes the binding of PR to the nucleosome. The complexes are recruited by the sensitized chromatin. The accessibility of chromatin to PR necessitates a remodeling of chromatin by ATP-dependent proteins. It has been shown, at least in breast cancer cell lines that PR recruited by its ligand in the cytoplasm can cause a rapid ER kinase activation, which leads to phosphoacetylation of some histones and recruitment of the remodeling complex, coactivators and RNA polymerase II. Thus there might be a direct connection between the cytoplasmic fraction of PR, activation of the MAP kinase pathway and gene activation (Vicent et al., 2006). In addition, the same group has reported that PRB and ERα were associated via oncogene src in the cytoplasm, which could explain potentialization of PRB biological action by ER as described for the vascular endothelial growth factor (VEGF) promoter (Wu et al., 2004).

Ligand-Independent Transcription in Cancer: Aberrant Foci in Breast Cancer

Following ligand-binding activation of the receptors, PR isoforms dimerize as homo- or heterodimers, whereas in mouse tissues, PRA and PRB can be expressed in different cells (Gava et al., 2004). In normal human physiology, cells that express only one PR isoform are uncommon. Both PRA and PRB are coexpressed at equivalent levels in normal human epithelial breast cells (Graham and Clarke, 1997; Mote et al., 1999; Mote et al., 2002) and the coexpression and collocation of PRA and PRB in epithelial cells in normal tissues suggest that both PR isoforms are required to mediate the effects of progesterone in the human. The disruption of PRA/PRB in human appears to be a feature of tumor progression. In this condition, some abnormal control may occur from predominance of homodimers.

A recent study supports the view that abnormal transcription regulation occur in breast cancer cells (Arnett-Mansfield et al., 2007) when activated by the ligand, PRA/PRB, localized to foci in the nucleus. Disruption of chromatin by inhibition of histone deacetylase activity disrupted PR foci formation. PR foci were larger in cells treated with a histone deacetylase inhibitor, and there was reduced reliance on ligand for their formation. Conversely, blocking recruitment of coactivator SRC-1 to PR transcriptional complexes and subsequent inhibition of histone H4 acetylation abolished ligand-dependent PR foci, further linking foci to the formation of active PR-containing complexes on euchromatin (Arnett-Mansfield et al., 2007). Difference in size of foci between normal and cancer tissues is likely to be related to the known alterations in chromatin structure in cancers. It was shown that in breast cancer, foci were larger than in normal tissue and that the presence of PR in the foci does not need the presence of the ligand. In addition, at least in endometrial cancers, PRB was more localized to foci than PRA (Arnett-Mansfield et al., 2007). These observations suggest that PR dependent transcription can occur even without the presence of ligand in cancer cells, which might not be the case in normal cells, and that concerns mainly PRB.

Target Genes for PRA and PRB

Several studies have addressed the question of the PRA/PRB target genes (Graham et al., 2005; Jacobsen et al., 2005; Richer et al., 2002). In transient transfections PRB is generally a much stronger transcriptional activator than PRA. Contrary to what was initially thought, both isoforms have common and separate target genes. Different methodologies were used and do not provide identical results.

The group of K. Horwitz used T47-D PR-negative cells stably retransfected either by PRA or PRB. On these cells some genes appeared to be regulated by PRB ($n = 57$), PRA ($n = 12$) and both ($n = 10$) in the presence of ligand and respectively 4, 29, 18 in the absence of the ligand (Jacobsen et al., 2005). The independent ligand activation has been described in cancer cells and may be characteristic of transformed cells due to the deregulation or overexpression of some pathways.

In similar breast cancer cells (T47-D), but containing both isoforms (PR positive), which can be manipulated to induce a relative increase of PRA over PRB (Graham et al., 2005), when transcriptional regulation at 6 h of progestin treatment was measured, 77 progestin-regulated genes were identified, and there was a high level of concordance in regulation between cells with low and high PRA expression. In contrast, when transcriptional profiles were compared at 48 h of progestin treatment, more genes were progestin-regulated at this time overall, and many more genes were identified by as differentially regulated. In total, 601 genes were regulated twofold or more by 48 h of progestin treatment in cells with low PRA/PRB ratio, high PRA/PRB ratio, or both. However, there was small proportion (14%) of all progestin-regulated genes that were either switched on or off when PRA/PRB ratio was high at 48 h, or were regulated in the opposite direction in the two conditions. Fifty-four genes (66% of these genes) acquired responsiveness to progestins when the PRA/PRB ratio was high, 28 genes (34%) that were progestin regulated in cells with a low PRA/PRB ratio but which lost regulation when the PRA/PRB ratio was high. The genes, which acquired progestin responsiveness with time in condition with increased PRA/PRB ratio, were involved in cellular metabolism and regulation of cell shape and adhesion. This fits well with the previous observation in these cell lines that overexpression of PRA/PRB decreased cellular adhesion and modified cytoskeleton characteristics (McGowan et al., 2004) increasing stress fibers (see the following section) (Table 1).

ROLE OF PR ISOFORMS IN MAMMARY GLAND DEVELOPMENT AND FUNCTION

Knockout and Transgenic Mice

In order to examine the physiological significance of PR function in the murine mammary gland, a progesterone receptor knockout (PRKO) mouse model was generated in which PR isoforms were simultaneously abrogated through gene targeting approaches. Male and female embryos homozygous for the PR mutation developed normally to adulthood. However, the adult PRKO displayed significant defects in reproductive tissues (inability to ovulate, uterine hyperplasia and inflammation, severely limited mammary gland development and an inability to exhibit sexual behavior). PRKO mice failed to develop the pregnancy associated side-branching of the ductal epithelium with attendant lobular alveolar differentiation (Lydon et al., 1995). In addition the PRKO mice were resistant to the chemical carcinogens, DMBA (Ismail et al., 2003).

Ablation or overexpression of PRA or PRB in mice supports the view, that each isoform has distinct roles. In PRA-null mice that endogenously express only PRB, mammary gland development is apparently normal. The morphological changes in ductal side branching and

Table 1 Consequences of PRA or PRB Overexpression

	PRA overexpression	PRB overexpression
Basal proliferation	Similar to control (McGowan and Clarke, 1999)	Similar to control (Jacobsen et al., 2005)
Progestin antiproliferative effect	Greater in T47-D cells (McGowan and Clarke, 1999)	Greater in MDA-MB-231 (personal data)
Adhesion	Decreased (McGowan and Clarke, 1999)	No modification (Jacobsen et al., 2005)
Cell shape	Rounded (McGowan and Clarke, 1999)	
	Aggressive (more cell process) (Jacobsen et al., 2005)	
Migration	Lost of inhibitory effects of progestin (McGowan et al., 2004)	No modification (Jacobsen et al., 2005)
Tumors in nude mice		
Size	Smaller (Sartorius et al., 2003)	Larger (Sartorius et al., 2003)
Tamoxifen	Sensitive (Sartorius et al., 2003)	Resistance (Sartorius et al., 2003)
VEGF	No modification (Mote et al., 2004)	Increase expression (Wu et al., 2004)
Human breast cancer		
N+	Tamoxifen resistance (Hopp et al., 2004)	
BRCA carriers	Increased in normal tissues (Mote et al., 2004)	Loss of expression (Mote et al., 2004)

Abbreviations: PRA, progesterone receptor A; PRB, progesterone receptor B; VEGF, vascularendothelial growth factor; N+, node positive; BRCA, breast cancer.

lobular alveolar development in mammary gland were similar to those observed in wild type mice (Mulac-Jericevic et al., 2000). On the contrary, null mice lacking PRB, exhibit reduced mammary ductal side-branching and alveologenesis during pregnancy, demonstrating the importance of PRB rather than PRA in the mammary gland in mice (Mulac-Jericevic et al., 2003).

Furthermore, mammary glands of PRA transgenic mice exhibit excessive ductal growth, contain aberrant epithelial structures with ducts composed of multiple layers of epithelial cells, and a loss in basement membrane integrity and cell-cell adhesion (Shyamala et al., 2000); they carry morphological and biological features of transformed cells with a higher rate of proliferation and features characteristics of hyperplasia. By contrast, the mammary epithelial cells of PRB transgenics do not exhibit significant changes in the expression levels of the various defined molecular markers of cellular transformation, but have premature arrest in ductal growth without any alteration in the potential for lobulo-alveolar growth (Shyamala et al., 2000).

These models of transgenic mice are of great interest to understand the relative importance of each isoform in the mammary gland development and suggest that overexpression of PRA is linked with hyperplasia. However there are some differences in the physiology of the human mammary gland suggesting that these results cannot be entirely extrapolated to the human breast. In particular, the relative ratio of PRA/PRB is increased in the mammary gland of mice (Mote et al., 2006).

Normal Human Breast Tissue and Precancerous Lesion

PRA and PRB are coexisting in the same cells in the normal breast tissue and in an apparent equimolar amount (Mote et al., 1999, 2002). There are no or very small variation of the content of both isoforms during the menstrual cycle (Mote et al., 1999 and personal unpublished data). However the relative disruption of the isoforms expression seems to be a precocious event during tumorigenesis.

The group of C. Clarke has reported a disruption of the isoforms ratio in different conditions of precancerous breast tissues. In normal breast tissues as well as in benign breast disease with simple hyperplasia, the ratio A/B was conserved (Mote et al., 2002). In atypical lesions, however, there was a significant increase in predominant expression of PRA or PRB. In addition, in the normal breast and in hyperplasia without atypia, the relative expression of PRA and PRB in adjacent cells was homogenous. There was a significant increase in cell-to-cell heterogeneity of PR isoform expression in atypical hyperplasia and in the majority of breast cancers. Heterogeneous cell-to-cell expression of PR isoforms occurred prior to overall predominant expression of one isoform in premalignant breast lesions, demonstrating that loss of control of relative PRA/PRB expression is an early event in the development of breast cancer (Mote et al., 2002).

BREAST CANCER AND PROGESTERONE RECEPTOR

BRCA1 and PR expression

Abnormal Regulation of Estradiol and Progesterone Transduction Pathways in BRCA Tissues

BRCA1 mutation linked breast cancers are not expressing ER positivity in 70% of the cases and 30% in BRCA2 carriers. However, incidence of breast cancers in the carriers can be altered by reproductive factors and endocrine manipulations (Kotsopoulos et al., 2007). This raises the possibility that the initial stages of tumor formation in BRCA1 and BRCA2 mutation carriers are hormone dependent.

There are some strong evidences for direct and indirect interference between BRCA1 and ER expression and activity (Fan et al., 1999, 2001). The inhibition of ERα activity by Brca1 is due, in part, to a direct interaction between the BRCA1 and ERα proteins and, in part, to BRCA1-mediated downregulation of expression of p300, a transcriptional coactivator of ERα. BRCA1 mediates ligand-independent repression of ERα. activity. It was more recently shown that BRCA1 was also a repressor of PR activity and can interact with PR (Bramley et al., 2006). In breast cancer cell lines and naive cells transfected either by PRA or PRB or both, BRCA1 blocked the progesterone-stimulated activity of PRA alone, PRB alone, or a combination of PRA and PRB on various PR dependent genes (Ma et al., 2006). On the contrary, Brca1 silencing RNAs were unable to oppose PR transduction activity (Ma et al., 2006). Moreover, using a mouse model featuring a conditional mammary-targeted deletion of Brca1 the same authors confirmed the role played by BRCA1 in controlling the proliferative effects of progesterone and estradiol in the mammary gland (Ma et al., 2006). There was a significant increase in mammary gland volume in mice with intact ovaries with a conditional deletion of Brca1 as compared with wild-type control mice exposed to progesterone. In ovariectomized mice, the quantified mammary epithelial cell density was significantly increased in the Brca1 mutated mice in both the estrogen and estrogen plus progesterone treatment groups, as compared with the respective ovariectomized wild-type mouse treatment groups. More extensive dense alveolar-like growth was found in the estrogen plus progesterone treated Brca1 mutated female mice. This interaction between BRCA1 and PR could be involved during states of active proliferation and differentiation such as puberty and pregnancy, conditions associated with an increase in Brca1 expression (Marquis et al., 1995). In addition, since 30% to 40% of sporadic breast cancers are associated with a total or partial loss of expression of Brca1 the mechanism of modulation of ER and PR can be lost during tumorigenesis mechanism which could contribute to a different response of tumoral cells compared to normal cells to estradiol and progesterone (Staff et al., 2003).

Moreover in mice with Brca1/p53 deleted function, tumorigenesis was increased under progesterone and an antiprogestin was able to antagonize this effect (Poole et al., 2006) in contrast to a previous report showing that tamoxifen increased incidence of mammary tumors (Jones et al., 2005). This publication also confirmed the negative control of BRCA1 on PR expression at a posttranscriptional level (Poole et al., 2006).

Normal Breast Tissues from BRCA Patients Display PRA/PRB Ratio Disruption, Impaired Estradiol Transduction Pathways and Impaired PR Induction by Estradiol

There are also several reports from human breast tissues showing that Brca can interfere with the control of estradiol inducing PR transduction pathways.

ER and PR levels were reported as increased in the cancer peripheral breast tissue in patient carriers of Brca mutations (King et al., 2004).

The group of C. Clarke (Mote et al., 2004) using specific antibodies to each isoform, reported a predominant expression of PRA isoform (with a loss of PRB) in normal breast tissues prophylactically removed from patients bearing a germline mutation in one of the Brca genes. PR expression was also reduced whereas ERα expression was not different in Brca mutation carriers than in noncarriers, but there was a reduction in an ERE gene expression, namely PS2. The alterations in PS2 and PR expressions were similar in the Brca1 and Brca2 carriers, demonstrating that although these proteins are structurally and functionally distinct, there is overlap in their interaction with hormone-signaling pathways. This study provides evidence for altered hormone transduction pathways and suggests that heterozygosity for a germline mutation in Brca leads to changes in progesterone signaling in hormone-dependent tissues, which may be a factor in the increased risk of cancer in these women.

Similarly, a comparison of normal breast tissue samples from three groups of women (at high risk of breast cancer, with BRCA mutation or undergoing surgery for fibroadenoma) treated by estradiol after reimplantation in the nude mice showed that proliferation was equally stimulated by estradiol in the various samples (Bramley et al., 2006). However, there was a striking difference in the amount of estradiol-PR induction. Indeed the PR induction by estradiol was severely impaired in the samples from the Brca mutation carriers.

Thus it appears that in these conditions of impaired function of Brca, progesterone acquires different impact on the regulation of proliferation in breast tissues and this could explain the absence of protective effect of pregnancy on breast cancer risk in women carriers of Brca mutations (Bramley et al., 2006). This is an example of the modified effects of progesterone in transformed cells compared to normally regulated breast tissues.

If PR deregulation appears to be the feature of some breast cancer and can play a role in tumor progression it is still not very clear the role played by each isoform. Data coming from in vitro and in vivo studies remain contradictory in particular because the models and the methods used are not equivalent. Data obtained from in vitro studies have used clones expressing either PRA or PRB or clones containing both PRA and PRB but with a different amount. Since the control of genes expression may vary with the ratio in homo- and heterodimers, it may explain the difference in results generated from these models.

In Vitro Studies of Breast Cancer Cells

In models of engineered cells to express PRA/PRB in different amounts, various endpoints of breast cancer were studied.

The group of C. Clarke had studied the consequences of increasing the amount of PRA over PRB in T47-D cells containing an inducible PRA plasmid. Inducing PRA did not influence the proliferation rate, whether in basal conditions or after a treatment by progestin, except at long time where the cells became more sensitive to the inhibitory effect of progestins (Table 1) (McGowan and Clarkc, 1999). On the contrary, in T47-D original cells, progestin induced an increase in cell surface area and adherence, in cells overexpressing the PRA isoform, cells became rounded and there was decreased adherence of cells to culture flasks (Table 1) (McGowan and Clarke, 1999). The antiprogestin RU38486 decreased cell numbers similarly to progestin, but unlike progestin had no effect on cell surface. Various changes in the structure of the cytoskeleton and microfilament were described in these cells (Table 1) (McGowan et al., 2003). Changes in the microfilament system have been linked with cell transformation and tumorigenicity and stress fibers are commonly reduced in size and number and show altered organization after transformation (Pollack et al., 1975). The mechanisms underlying the changes in the cytoskeleton that occur in cancer are not fully understood; however, in light of the progestin effects on the cytoskeleton in cells overexpressing PRA, it is likely that cross talk between the cytoskeleton and endocrine signaling may be involved.

Using similar models, T47-D breast cancer cells demonstrated the ability to migrate into bone marrow fibroblasts and this was inhibited by progestin treatment (McGowan et al., 2004). The antiprogestin RU38486 abrogated the progestin effect on migration, demonstrating that it was PR-mediated. In cells expressing a predominance of PRA, the ability of progestin to inhibit breast cancer cell migration was lost. A number of integrins were progestin regulated in T47-D cells, but there was no difference in the progestin effect in cells with PRA predominance, nor were the levels of focal adhesion proteins altered in these cells (Table 1).

The group from K. Horwitz has used T47-D cells selected to be PR negative and then stably transfected them by an inducible PRA or PRB. The morphology of PRB cells was equivalent to the wild type. However, PRA cells exhibit greatly increased numbers of cellular processes and branching suggesting a more aggressive pattern (Jacobsen et al., 2005). No different profile of proliferation was seen in both cell lines but an increase in adhesiveness and cell migration in PRA clones (Table 1).

The same group demonstrated that PRB preferentially regulates VEGF expression in breast cancer cells, estradiol potentiates this induction, and antiestrogens function as agonists in PRB cells on VEGF expression (Table 1) (Wu et al., 2004). This suggests a more aggressive pattern (more angiogenesis) in tumors with PRB overexpression.

On models of estrogen-dependent breast tumor xenografts the same group showed that tumors expressing only PRA are half the size of tumors expressing only PRB, suggesting that PRA preferentially inhibit estrogen-dependent growth. The tamoxifen responsiveness is modulated by the PR isoforms but in this study, tumors expressing PRA are more sensitive to tamoxifen than tumors expressing PRB (Table 1) (Sartorius et al., 2003).

In ERα/PR-negative cells, MDA-MB-231 stably transfected by PRA or PRB, we observed that basal proliferation was identical in the several clones but that the antiproliferative effects of progestins were mainly observed in PRB clones (Courtin et al., submitted manuscript).

Thus, according to the model used it appears that either PRB or PRA may confer a more aggressive phenotype than cells with a conserved PRA/PRB ratio.

PR Isoforms Expression in Breast Cancer Tissues

PRA/PRB Disruption and Breast Cancer Prognosis

Approximately one-half of primary breast tumors are positive for both PR and ER, whereas less than 5% are negative for ER but still positive for PR. Several clinical studies have confirmed that elevated total PR levels correlate with an increased probability of response to tamoxifen, longer time to treatment failure, and longer overall survival (Osborne et al., 2005).

Using dual immunohistochemistry with specific antibodies against PRA and PRB (Fig. 2), compared to normal breast tissue, there was an increased PR level in proliferative disease without atypia but it was associated with maintenance of comparable levels of PRA and PRB. Nevertheless, a significant predominance of one isoform was noted in ductal carcinomas and invasive cancers. In half of cases examined, PRA predominated over PRB (Mote et al., 2002). These data are important because PR isoforms are functionally distinct and differentially inhibit ER-mediated transcription with PRA having stronger ER transrepressor properties than PRB (Abdel-Hafiz et al., 2002). Thus the PRA/PRB status of receptor-positive tumors may influence the outcome of endocrine therapies targeted at ER.

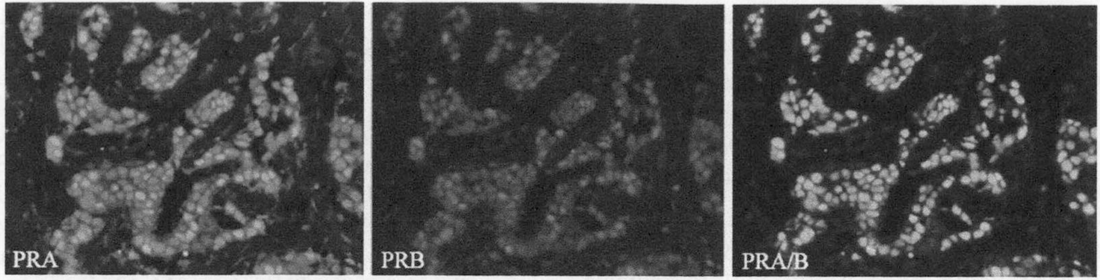

Figure 2 Dual fluorescence immunohistochemistry of PRA and PRB in breast cancer. PRA and PRB staining were obtained using hPRa7 or hPRa6 antibodies, respectively. Fluorescent microscope detected TXR (PRB) or FITC (PRA) fluorescence separately or simultaneously. *Source*: Dual fluorescence immunochemistry. Courtesy of P. Mote and C. Clarke. (Mote et al., 1999).

In another patient cohort study of exclusively node-positive patients, using western blot quantification of PRA and PRB tumor content, it was shown a predictive effect of PRA and PRB on disease-free survival in tamoxifen-treated patients. Specifically, tamoxifen-treated patients with higher PRA/PRB ratios had a significantly poorer disease-free survival than those with lower ratio. In this study, it has been reported that the high ratio was an effect of excess PRA rather than low PRB levels (Hopp et al., 2004). Thus it is suggested that loss of coordinate expression of PRA and PRB in favor of PRA might cause resistance to tamoxifen by direct repression of ER transcriptional activity or indirectly by PRA upregulation of genes known to be involved in tumor aggressiveness and poor prognosis. There was a nonsignificant association between PR isoform levels and HER-2 levels which is a predictor of tamoxifen resistance.

We have been involved in a study of a cohort of node-negative and node-positive breast cancer using the technique of dual immunohistochemistry (Fig. 2) (Mote et al., manuscript submitted). In this series, 53% of the tumors had a conserved PRA/PRB ratio, 29% were PRA > PRB and 18% PRB > PRA. PRA and PRB relative expression were linked to different grading and prognosis if sub-stratified as node-positive or node-negative patients.

From the sum of these data, no simple pattern is emerging. Additional work is needed to stratify the patients according to their PR isoforms status and the relationship with chemotherapy and endocrine therapy outcomes.

PR Polymorphism and PR Isoforms

Several polymorphisms have been identified in PR (De Vivo et al., 2002). But only two of them have known functional consequences. The +331G/A polymorphism was shown to increase PR gene transcription and favoring production of hPRB in an endometrial cancer cell line. Importantly, this phenotype was associated with endometrial cancer and breast cancer risks, in the Nurses Health study cohort (De Vivo et al., 2003).

The PROGINS variant is characterized by a 320 bp PV/HS-1 Alu insertion in intron G and two point mutations in exon 4 and 5. It decreases the antiproliferative activity and is less responsive to progestin compared with the most common PR because of reduced amounts of gene transcript and decreased protein activity (Romano et al., 2007).

Thus PR variants seem to be associated with breast cancer risk by modulating gene transcription efficiency.

PR Loss of Expression in Breast Cancer

The loss of expression of genes in cancer is often related to epigenetic modifications or mutation/deletion (De Vivo et al., 2003). PR promoter is frequently methylated. However, so far there is only scarce evidence for the role of methylation in the loss of expression in the relative isoforms (Xiong et al., 2005).

There is an inverse relationship between growth factors overexpression and hormone receptors, especially PR. Prolonged continuous exposure of MCF-7 breast cancer cells to an antiestrogen upregulates EGFR levels and downregulates PR expression as drug resistance develops (McClelland et al., 2001). Similarly, transfection of the HER2 oncogene into ER+ and PR+ breast cancer cells significantly reduces the expression of PR (Konecny et al., 2003). Exposure of cultured breast cancer cells to IGF-1, EGF, or heregulin markedly lowers PR levels while expression of other ER regulated genes such as PS2 is maintained (Cui et al., 2003). Finally, PI3K/Akt signaling working through an AP-1 negative regulatory site in the PR promoter has been implicated as the molecular mechanism by which GFs downregulate levels of PR (Cui et al., 2003; Lapidus et al., 1998). Thus, laboratory studies suggest that PR loss, like tamoxifen resistance, can be caused by excessive GF receptor signaling in the cells.

It is known for a long time that ER- and PR-positive tumors are more responsive to tamoxifen. Several clinical reports do suggest that high GF receptor content is associated with loss of PR (Balleine et al., 1999; Bamberger et al., 2000; Dowsett et al., 2001; Konecny et al., 2003). In addition, tamoxifen resistance is the hallmark of tumor with increased growth factors expression.

In conclusion, there are still lacking and contradictory information concerning the exact role of PR isoforms in breast cancer history and progression. However, disruption of their expression is the hallmark of less differentiated breast cancer and may be indicative of resistance to conventional treatment. Thus the analysis of their relative expression could be a useful tool to indicate adjuvant treatment in breast cancer patients.

REFERENCES

Abdel-Hafiz H, Takimoto GS, Tung L, Horwitz KB. The inhibitory function in human progesterone receptor N termini binds SUMO-1 protein to regulate autoinhibition and transrepression. J Biol Chem 2002; 277(37): 33950–33956.

Arnett-Mansfield RL, Graham JD, Hanson AR, Mote PA, Gompel A, Scurr LL, Gava N, de Fazio A, Clarke CL. Focal subnuclear distribution of progesterone receptor is ligand dependent and associated with transcriptional activity. Mol Endocrinol 2007; 21(1):14–29.

Balleine RL, Earl MJ, Greenberg ML, Clarke CL. Absence of progesterone receptor associated with secondary breast cancer in postmenopausal women. Br J Cancer 1999; 79(9–10):1564–1571.

Bamberger AM, Milde-Langosch K, Schulte HM, Loning T. Progesterone receptor isoforms, PR-B and PR-A, in breast cancer: correlations with clinicopathologic tumor parameters and expression of AP-1 factors. Horm Res 2000; 54(1):32–37.

Bramley M, Clarke RB, Howell A, Evans DG, Armer T, Baildam AD, Anderson E. Effects of oestrogens and anti-oestrogens on normal breast tissue from women bearing BRCA1 and BRCA2 mutations. Br J Cancer 2006; 94(7):1021–1028.

Cui X, Zhang P, Deng W, Oesterreich S, Lu Y, Mills GB, Lee AV. Insulin-like growth factor-I inhibits progesterone receptor expression in breast cancer cells via the phosphatidylinositol 3-kinase/Akt/mammalian target of rapamycin pathway: progesterone receptor as a potential indicator of growth factor activity in breast cancer. Mol Endocrinol 2003; 17(4):575–588.

De Vivo I, Hankinson SE, Colditz GA, Hunter DJ. A functional polymorphism in the progesterone receptor gene is associated with an increase in breast cancer risk. Cancer Res 2003; 63(17):5236–5238.

De Vivo I, Huggins GS, Hankinson SE, Lescault PJ, Boezen M, Colditz GA, Hunter DJ. A functional polymorphism in the promoter of the progesterone receptor gene associated with endometrial cancer risk. Proc Natl Acad Sci U S A 2002; 99(19):12263–12268.

Dowsett M, Bundred NJ, Decensi A, Sainsbury RC, Lu Y, Hills MJ, Cohen FJ, Veronesi P, O'Brien ME, Scott T, Muchmore DB. Effect of raloxifene on breast cancer cell Ki67 and apoptosis: a double-blind, placebo-controlled, randomized clinical trial in postmenopausal patients. Cancer Epidemiol Biomarkers Prev 2001; 10(9):961–966.

Fan S, Ma YX, Wang C, Yuan RQ, Meng Q, Wang JA, Erdos M, Goldberg ID, Webb P, Kushner PJ, Pestell RG, Rosen EM. Role of direct interaction in BRCA1 inhibition of estrogen receptor activity. Oncogene 2001; 20(1):77–87.

Fan S, Wang J, Yuan R, Ma Y, Meng Q, Erdos MR, Pestell RG, Yuan F, Auborn KJ, Goldberg ID, Rosen EM. BRCA1 inhibition of estrogen receptor signaling in transfected cells. Science 1999; 284(5418):1354–1356.

Gava N, Clarke CL, Byth K, Arnett-Mansfield RL, deFazio A. Expression of progesterone receptors A and B in the mouse ovary during the estrous cycle. Endocrinology 2004; 145(7):3487–3494.

Georgiakaki M, Chabbert-Buffet N, Dasen B, Meduri G, Wenk S, Rajhi L, Amazit L, Chauchereau A, Burger CW, Blok LJ, Milgrom E, Lombes M, Guiochon-Mantel A, Loosfelt H. Ligand-controlled interaction of histone acetyltransferase binding to ORC-1 (HBO1) with the N-terminal transactivating domain of progesterone receptor induces steroid receptor coactivator 1-dependent coactivation of transcription. Mol Endocrinol 2006; 20(9):2122–2140.

Graham JD, Clarke CL. Physiological action of progesterone in target tissues. Endocr Rev 1997; 18(4):502–519.

Graham JD, Yager ML, Hill HD, Byth K, O'Neill GM, Clarke CL. Altered progesterone receptor isoform expression remodels progestin responsiveness of breast cancer cells. Mol Endocrinol 2005; 19(11):2713–2735.

Hopp TA, Weiss HL, Hilsenbeck SG, Cui Y, Allred DC, Horwitz KB, Fuqua SA. Breast cancer patients with progesterone receptor PR-A-rich tumors have poorer disease-free survival rates. Clin Cancer Res 2004; 10(8):2751–2760.

Ismail PM, Amato P, Soyal SM, DeMayo FJ, Conneely OM, O'Malley BW, Lydon JP. Progesterone involvement in breast development and tumorigenesis—as revealed by progesterone receptor "knockout" and "knockin" mouse models. Steroids 2003; 68(10–13):779–787.

Jacobsen BM, Schittone SA, Richer JK, Horwitz KB. Progesterone-independent effects of human progesterone receptors (PRs) in estrogen receptor-positive breast cancer: PR isoform-specific gene regulation and tumor biology. Mol Endocrinol 2005; 19(3):574–587.

Jones LP, Li M, Halama ED, Ma Y, Lubet R, Grubbs CJ, Deng CX, Rosen EM, Furth PA. Promotion of mammary cancer development by tamoxifen in a mouse model of Brca1-mutation-related breast cancer. Oncogene 2005; 24(22):3554–3562.

Kastner P, Krust A, Turcotte B, Stropp U, Tora L, Gronemeyer H, Chambon P. Two distinct estrogen-regulated promoters generate transcripts encoding the two functionally different human progesterone receptor forms A and B. Embo J 1990; 9(5):1603–1614.

King TA, Gemignani ML, Li W, Giri DD, Panageas KS, Bogomolniy F, Arroyo C, Olvera N, Robson ME, Offit K, Borgen PI, Boyd J. Increased progesterone receptor expression in benign epithelium of BRCA1-related breast cancers. Cancer Res 2004; 64(15):5051–5053.

Konecny G, Pauletti G, Pegram M, Untch M, Dandekar S, Aguilar Z, Wilson C, Rong HM, Bauerfeind I, Felber M,

Wang HJ, Beryt M, Seshadri R, Hepp H, Slamon DJ. Quantitative association between HER-2/neu and steroid hormone receptors in hormone receptor-positive primary breast cancer. J Natl Cancer Inst 2003; 95(2):142–153.

Kotsopoulos J, Lubinski J, Lynch HT, Klijn J, Ghadirian P, Neuhausen SL, Kim-Sing C, Foulkes WD, Moller P, Isaacs C, Domchek S, Randall S, Offit K, Tung N, Ainsworth P, Gershoni-Baruch R, Eisen A, Daly M, Karlan B, Saal HM, Couch F, Pasini B, Wagner T, Friedman E, Rennert G, Eng C, Weitzel J, Sun P, Narod SA. Age at first birth and the risk of breast cancer in BRCA1 and BRCA2 mutation carriers. Breast Cancer Res Treat 2007; 105(2):221–228.

Lapidus RG, Nass SJ, Davidson NE. The loss of estrogen and progesterone receptor gene expression in human breast cancer. J Mammary Gland Biol Neoplasia 1998; 3(1):85–94.

Lessey BA, Alexander PS, Horwitz KB. The subunit structure of human breast cancer progesterone receptors: characterization by chromatography and photoaffinity labeling. Endocrinology 1983; 112(4):1267–1274.

Lydon JP, DeMayo FJ, Funk CR, Mani SK, Hughes AR, Montgomery CA Jr., Shyamala G, Conneely OM, O'Malley BW. Mice lacking progesterone receptor exhibit pleiotropic reproductive abnormalities. Genes Dev 1995; 9(18): 2266–2278.

Ma Y, Katiyar P, Jones LP, Fan S, Zhang Y, Furth PA, Rosen EM. The breast cancer susceptibility gene BRCA1 regulates progesterone receptor signaling in mammary epithelial cells. Mol Endocrinol 2006; 20(1):14–34.

Marquis ST, Rajan JV, Wynshaw-Boris A, Xu J, Yin GY, Abel KJ, Weber BL, Chodosh LA. The developmental pattern of Brca1 expression implies a role in differentiation of the breast and other tissues. Nat Genet 1995; 11(1):17–26.

McClelland RA, Barrow D, Madden TA, Dutkowski CM, Pamment J, Knowlden JM, Gee JM, Nicholson RI. Enhanced epidermal growth factor receptor signaling in MCF7 breast cancer cells after long-term culture in the presence of the pure antiestrogen ICI 182,780 (Faslodex). Endocrinology 2001; 142(7):2776–2788.

McGowan EM, Clarke CL. Effect of overexpression of progesterone receptor A on endogenous progestin-sensitive endpoints in breast cancer cells. Mol Endocrinol 1999; 13(10):1657–1671.

McGowan EM, Saad S, Bendall LJ, Bradstock KF, Clarke CL. Effect of progesterone receptor a predominance on breast cancer cell migration into bone marrow fibroblasts. Breast Cancer Res Treat 2004; 83(3):211–220.

McGowan EM, Weinberger RP, Graham JD, Hill HD, Hughes JA, O'Neill GM, Clarke CL. Cytoskeletal responsiveness to progestins is dependent on progesterone receptor A levels. J Mol Endocrinol 2003; 31(2):241–253.

Meyer ME, Pornon A, Ji JW, Bocquel MT, Chambon P, Gronemeyer H. Agonistic and antagonistic activities of RU486 on the functions of the human progesterone receptor. Embo J 1990; 9(12):3923–3932.

Mote PA, Arnett-Mansfield RL, Gava N, deFazio A, Mulac-Jericevic B, Conneely OM, Clarke CL. Overlapping and distinct expression of progesterone receptors A and B in mouse uterus and mammary gland during the estrous cycle. Endocrinology 2006; 147(12):5503–5512.

Mote PA, Balleine RL, McGowan EM, Clarke CL. Colocalization of progesterone receptors A and B by dual immunofluorescent histochemistry in human endometrium during the menstrual cycle. J Clin Endocrinol Metab 1999; 84(8):2963–2971.

Mote PA, Bartow S, Tran N, Clarke CL. Loss of co-ordinate expression of progesterone receptors A and B is an early event in breast carcinogenesis. Breast Cancer Res Treat 2002; 72(2):163–172.

Mote PA, Leary JA, Avery KA, Sandelin K, Chenevix-Trench G, Kirk JA, Clarke CL. Germ-line mutations in BRCA1 or BRCA2 in the normal breast are associated with altered expression of estrogen-responsive proteins and the predominance of progesterone receptor A. Genes Chromosomes Cancer 2004; 39(3):236–248.

Mulac-Jericevic B, Lydon JP, DeMayo FJ, Conneely OM. Defective mammary gland morphogenesis in mice lacking the progesterone receptor B isoform. Proc Natl Acad Sci U S A 2003; 100(17):9744–9749.

Mulac-Jericevic B, Mullinax RA, DeMayo FJ, Lydon JP, Conneely OM. Subgroup of reproductive functions of progesterone mediated by progesterone receptor-B isoform. Science 2000; 289(5485):1751–1754.

Osborne CK, Schiff R, Arpino G, Lee AS, Hilsenbeck VG. Endocrine responsiveness: understanding how progesterone receptor can be used to select endocrine therapy. Breast 2005; 14(6):458–465.

Petz LN, Ziegler YS, Schultz JR, Kim H, Kemper JK, Nardulli AM. Differential regulation of the human progesterone receptor gene through an estrogen response element half site and Sp1 sites. J Steroid Biochem Mol Biol 2004; 88(2):113–122.

Pollack R, Osborn M, Weber K. Patterns of organization of actin and myosin in normal and transformed cultured cells. Proc Natl Acad Sci U S A 1975; 72(3):994–998.

Poole AJ, Li Y, Kim Y, Lin SC, Lee WH, Lee EY. Prevention of Brca1-mediated mammary tumorigenesis in mice by a progesterone antagonist. Science 2006; 314(5804): 1467–1470.

Richer JK, Jacobsen BM, Manning NG, Abel MG, Wolf DM, Horwitz KB. Differential gene regulation by the two progesterone receptor isoforms in human breast cancer cells. J Biol Chem 2002; 277(7):5209–5218.

Romano A, Delvoux B, Fischer DC, Groothuis P. The PROGINS polymorphism of the human progesterone receptor diminishes the response to progesterone. J Mol Endocrinol 2007; 38(1–2):331–350.

Sartorius CA, Melville MY, Hovland AR, Tung L, Takimoto GS, Horwitz KB. A third transactivation function (AF3) of human progesterone receptors located in the unique N-terminal segment of the B-isoform. Mol Endocrinol 1994; 8(10):1347–1360.

Sartorius CA, Shen T, Horwitz KB. Progesterone receptors A and B differentially affect the growth of estrogen-dependent human breast tumor xenografts. Breast Cancer Res Treat 2003; 79(3):287–299.

Shyamala G, Yang X, Cardiff RD, Dale E. Impact of progesterone receptor on cell-fate decisions during mammary gland development. Proc Natl Acad Sci U S A 2000; 97(7):3044–3049.

Staff S, Isola J, Tanner M. Haplo-insufficiency of BRCA1 in sporadic breast cancer. Cancer Res 2003; 63(16): 4978–4983.

Tung L, Abdel-Hafiz H, Shen T, Harvell DM, Nitao LK, Richer JK, Sartorius CA, Takimoto GS, Horwitz KB. Progesterone receptors (PR)-B and -A regulate transcription by different mechanisms: AF-3 exerts regulatory control over coactivator binding to PR-B. Mol Endocrinol 2006; 20(11): 2656–2670.

Vicent GP, Ballare C, Zaurin R, Saragueta P, Beato M. Chromatin remodeling and control of cell proliferation by progestins via cross talk of progesterone receptor with the estrogen receptors and kinase signaling pathways. Ann N Y Acad Sci 2006; 1089:59–72.

Wei LL, Hawkins P, Baker C, Norris B, Sheridan PL, Quinn PG. An amino-terminal truncated progesterone receptor isoform, PRc, enhances progestin-induced transcriptional activity. Mol Endocrinol 1996; 10(11):1379–1387.

Wu J, Richer J, Horwitz KB, Hyder SM. Progestin-dependent induction of vascular endothelial growth factor in human breast cancer cells: preferential regulation by progesterone receptor B. Cancer Res 2004; 64(6):2238–2244.

Xiong Y, Dowdy SC, Gonzalez Bosquet J, Zhao Y, Eberhardt NL, Podratz KC, Jiang SW. Epigenetic-mediated upregulation of progesterone receptor B gene in endometrial cancer cell lines. Gynecol Oncol 2005; 99(1):135–141.

7

Compensatory Signaling Promoted by Antihormones and Anti–Growth Factor Therapies in Breast Cancer: A Starting Point for the Development of Resistance to Targeted Treatments

ROBERT I. NICHOLSON, I. R. HUTCHESON, H. E. JONES, K. TAYLOR, S. E. HISCOX, and J. M. W. GEE
Tenovus Centre for Cancer Research, Welsh School of Pharmacy, Cardiff University, Wales, U.K.

INTRODUCTION

Increasingly, anticancer drugs are being targeted to the signaling pathways that are believed to be responsible for the aberrant features of cancer cells. Unfortunately, although these drugs often improve the outcome for cancer sufferers, all too frequently resistance arises, and in some patients the benefits of drug treatment can be extremely short lived. In the Tenovus Centre for Cancer Research in Cardiff, our philosophy is that if we can identify the complex mechanisms involved in the development of drug resistance, then we can use this knowledge to devise more intelligent therapeutic strategies that could combat the cancer and significantly extend patient survival (Nicholson et al., 2007). Critically, recent experimental studies (primarily from our own group with regards to targeted treatments) have highlighted an important new phenomenon—"drug induction of compensatory signaling elements"—that acts to (*i*) limit initial response to anti-estrogen receptor (ER) (Gee et al., 2006) and anti–epidermal growth factor receptor (EGFR) (Hutcheson et al., 2006) therapies, (*ii*) permit drug resistance to develop (Nicholson et al., 2007) and (*iii*) facilitate invasive behavior and production of angiogenic factors (Gee et al., 2006). We believe that this phenomenon is likely to be shared by all current and future targeted therapies, where it may act to significantly reduce their effectiveness in patients. The current article describes our growing experience of drug-induced compensatory signaling in breast cancer and our initial attempts to target such signaling.

STUDIES REVEAL RESPONSES LIMITING ANTI-HORMONE ACTIONS

Many studies world wide have established that the intracellular signaling pathways associated with ER and insulin-like growth factor receptor (IGFR) action are highly interactive, as typified by models of hormone sensitive/endocrine responsive breast cancer (Yee and Lee, 2000; Hamelers and Steenbergh, 2003). As such, it has long been recognized that antihormonal drugs not only possess anti-estrogenic activity through their blockade of ER/estrogen response element (ERE) signaling, but also anti–growth factor actions through their ability to disrupt estrogen/IGFR signaling cross talk (Guvakova and Surmacz, 1997).

Indeed, it is most likely a combination of these antiestrogenic and anti–growth factor actions that is responsible for the growth inhibitory properties of antihormonal drugs. Intriguingly, however, it is now recognized that not all growth factors are used equally to drive hormone sensitive growth. Thus, estrogens suppress the expression of a number of other growth factor receptor signaling pathways, notably the tyrosine kinases EGFR and human epidermal growth factor receptor 2 (HER2). This suppression occurs at the transcriptional level in various ER-positive breast cancer models in vitro (Bates and Hurst, 1997; Newman et al., 2000; Yarden et al., 2001; Wilson and Chrysogelos, 2002; Gee et al., 2003), and is believed to involve events at negative regulatory elements within the first intron of the EGFR and HER2 genes (Newman et al., 2000; Wilson and Chrysogelos, 2002).

Importantly, there is pharmacological significance of this estrogen repression, since in turn antihormones can promote the expression of EGFR and HER2 and thereby considerably alter the cellular readout of growth factor receptors in some ER-positive cells (McClelland et al., 2001; Yarden et al., 2001; Gee et al., 2003). Our in vitro studies have firmly established that this drug-induced event can subsequently provide an efficient mechanism to drive antihormone-resistant growth. Although much is still to be learned about how antihormones induce such alternative growth factor pathways, it is now recognized as a key early event, where significantly altered EGFR/HER2 levels are already apparent by 10 days of response to tamoxifen or faslodex in MCF-7 human breast cancer cells (Gee et al., 2003). Such induction can be reversed by tamoxifen withdrawal (Gee et al., 2003) or as reported by Yarden et al. (2001) by prolonged reexposure to estrogens in ER-positive models. The increased growth factor receptor levels appear functional since they maintain modest levels of residual downstream activity through mitogen-activated protein kinase (MAPK) and protein kinase B (PKB/AKT). In turn, these kinases impact on ER activity, maintaining low levels of residual Serine118/Serine167 ER phosphorylation and detectable levels of the ER-regulated gene bcl-2 (Gee et al., 2003). This residual kinase, ER activity and thereby anti-apoptotic gene expression supports cell survival and low levels of proliferation and thus incomplete initial growth inhibitory effect in vitro. EGFR/HER2 expression, kinase activity and reactivation of ER incrementally increase during treatment, culminating in emergence of EGFR/HER2-promoted resistant growth (Knowlden et al., 2003; Britton et al., 2006). Such increases are also apparent in initially cloned cells, indicating that changes are adaptive in response to drug treatment, rather than due to outgrowth of particular cell populations apparent de novo (Fan et al., 2006). Excitingly, subversion of these events by use of the anti-EGFR agent gefitinib, alongside antihormone, reduces residual kinase and ER activity as well as maximally depleting bcl-2 expression, and thereby cotreatment is superior in promoting cell death and antiproliferative activity versus the single agents. This markedly improves the quality and duration of response to tamoxifen in culture and is able to significantly delay development of resistant growth (Gee et al., 2003; Nicholson et al., 2003, 2004a, 2005). Our studies (and others; Shou et al., 2004) have shown the efficacy of antihormone plus anti-EGFR agent is reproducible, and it extends to other ER-positive breast cancer models including those in vivo, and also to further antiestrogens such as faslodex (McClelland et al., 2001; Gee et al., 2003). Taken together, these data offer proof of principal that targeted therapies (in this instance ER blockade) can induce signaling which allows them to tolerate anticancer agents, maintaining a cohort of cells from which resistance can develop. Based on these various data, exploration of such combination treatment, and similarly inhibitory agents of HER2 or its dimerisation (as well as inhibitors of multiple erbB family members) alongside diverse antihormones, is currently under evaluation in breast cancer, with some promising emerging data (Argiris et al., 2004; Chu et al., 2005; Polychronis et al., 2005; Johnston et al., 2003; Johnston and Leary, 2006; Leary and Dowsett, 2006).

STUDIES REVEAL RESPONSES LIMITING ANTI-GROWTH FACTOR ACTIONS

Recognition of the use of alternative growth factor pathways as a potent means of promoting antihormone resistance in breast cancer cells has increasingly led us to employ selective inhibitors of growth factor signaling cascades to subvert established anti hormone resistant growth (Nicholson et al., 2007). Such studies with single agents, although in general terms successful in model systems (resulting in rapid antitumor effects), have once again revealed incomplete antiproliferative responses, a relatively poor induction of apoptosis, and the eventual emergence of anti–growth factor resistance (Jones et al., 2004). Significantly, our early signaling studies with such agents, as with antihormonal drugs, have revealed an incomplete block of proliferation and survival signaling pathways. Interestingly, we are again accumulating evidence that induction of signaling through alternative growth factor pathways begins early during the drug responsive phase (Hutcheson et al., 2006; Jones et al., 2006a,b,d; Knowlden et al., 2006). This drug-induced event appears, via maintaining residual activity of downstream kinases (and of ER where present), to limit initial growth inhibitory effect in cancer cells and ultimately to promote resistance. Indeed, so powerful are these drug-induced mechanisms that they may in some instances promote de novo resistance to the targeted therapy in cancer cells (Jones et al., 2006a,c).

EGFR Blockade Promotes Signaling Within Alternative Growth Factor Pathways

While we have observed that blockade of the significant levels of EGFR signaling in our ER-positive, acquired tamoxifen-resistant cell lines (e.g., TAMR and TAMR/T47D cells derived from MCF-7 and T47D cells respectively) is growth inhibitory (Knowlden et al., 2003; Jordan et al., 2004), it is equally associated with obvious inductive events at a signaling activity level and hence limited apoptotic impact and incomplete anti-tumor effect. Following seven day exposure to the anti-EGFR agent gefitinib, although EGFR and MAPK activity are substantially inhibited, levels of phosphorylated AKT are enhanced by drug treatment (Knowlden et al., 2006), an event that serves to maintain low levels of ER activity and residual TAMR growth. We believe, this drug-induced kinase activity is a consequence of EGFR blockade promoting type II receptor signaling (Knowlden et al., 2006) and alternative erbB receptor heterodimerisation (Hutcheson et al., 2007).

Type II Receptor Signaling

Classically, type II receptors [IGFR and the insulin receptor (InsR)] when activated by their ligands are believed to signal through insulin receptor substrate (IRS) adapter proteins, which are important docking sites for molecules such as Grb2 that promotes MAPK activity, and for phosphatidylinositol-3-kinase (PI3-kinase) that increases AKT activity (Sachdev and Yee, 2001). Such actions are driven by growth factor-induced phosphorylation of IRS1 on Tyrosine 896 and Tyrosine 612 residues respectively (White, 1997). Interestingly, however, we have recently discovered a novel cross-talk mechanism in cancer cells (Hutcheson et al., 2006; Knowlden et al., 2006) whereby EGFR can equally associate with IRS1, and indeed the phosphorylated NPXY motifs in activated type II receptors bound by IRS molecules are similarly found in the EGFR C-terminus (Songyang et al., 1995). Thus, IRS1 physically interacts with the increased levels of EGFR under basal conditions in TAMR cells, and it is EGFR that most efficiently induces IRS1 phosphorylation on Tyr896 and hence MAPK activity leading to enhanced cell proliferation (Hutcheson et al., 2006; Knowlden et al., 2006). In contrast to IGFs, EGF-like growth factors fail to induce Tyr612 phosphorylation of IRS1 and downstream AKT signaling. Moreover, TAMR cells treated with EGF and IGF in combination results in loss of IGFR/IRS1 association and Tyr612 IRS1 phosphorylation, while EGFR/IRS1 association and Tyr896 IRS1 phosphorylation are maintained. Thus, the EGFR in TAMR cells appears to recruit IRS1 away from IGF1R as part of its mechanism to engage MAPK mitogenic signaling. Significantly, we have noted that the dynamics of this EGFR/IGF1R/IRS1 cross-talk system are altered dramatically by EGFR blockade using gefitinib during early response [where such events are recapitulated by an EGFR small interfering RNA (siRNA) suggesting that the induced mechanism may be relevant to further anti-EGFR strategies]. As such, EGFR inhibition or depletion of EGFR level results in dissociation of IRS1 from EGFR, reducing Y896 IRS1 phosphorylation to deplete downstream MAPK activity and growth. In parallel, however, the drug significantly induces recruitment of IRS1 to IGFR and increases Y612 IRS1 phosphorylation and downstream activation of PI3-kinase/AKT (Hutcheson et al., 2006; Knowlden et al., 2006). We have shown that this promotion of the alternative IGFR pathway by drug in TAMR cells allows cells to survive anti-EGFR challenge in the short term. Moreover, our acquired gefitinib-resistant breast cancer cell line TAMR/TKIR, which utilizes the alternative receptor IGFR for autocrine mitogenic signaling (Jones et al., 2004a), also exhibits increased levels of Y612 IRS1 phosphorylation than its parental TAMR cells (Knowlden et al., 2006). Gefitinib-induced changes in IRS1, therefore, persist into the acquired resistant state, facilitating establishment of the IGFR/AKT pathway as the dominant growth mechanism. Indeed, while IRS1 has not been explored, for anti-EGFR agents (or indeed for herceptin) growth of the anti–growth factor resistant state has been linked to AKT hyperactivation, likely in part triggered by increased upstream IGFR signaling (in some instances further aggravated by the presence of drug). This has been revealed from model systems and is emerging from clinical material (Liu et al., 2001; Chakravarti et al., 2002; Jones et al., 2004a, 2006a; Desbois-Mouthon et al., 2006; Hutcheson et al., 2006; Nahta et al., 2006). Immunohistochemical assay development for Y896 and Y612 IRS1 phosphorylation is ongoing in our clinical breast cancer series where we have been able to show that IRS1 Y612 phosphorylation preferentially associates with the IGFR/AKT signaling pathway rather than EGFR-promoted mitogenic signaling in untreated clinical samples.

Although there is much to be learned about the molecular actions of IGFR signaling in anti-hormone resistant cells, parallel studies in other cancer types that overexpress EGFR have shown that type II receptors are also capable of cross talking with the EGFR to promote transactivation of key regulatory sites on this receptor under conditions of EGFR blockade. This again serves to limit anti-tumor response.

Thus, in A549 non–small cell lung carcinoma cells (NSCLC) that are partially responsive to EGFR selective tyrosine kinase inhibitors, drug treatment promotes a rapid phosphorylation of their substantial levels of IGFR, which in turn transactivates a specific site, Tyr1173, on EGFR to maintain residual downstream kinase activity (Jones et al., 2006a,d). Such signaling is subsequently maximized on emergence of acquired resistance, where IGFR comprises a key growth-promoting pathway. We have also obtained evidence that at its extremes, such type II receptor/EGFR interplay can lead to de novo insensitivity to EGFR blockade in cancer cells (Jones et al., 2006a,c). While deficient in mature IGFR, LoVo colorectal cancer cells have high intrinsic levels of activity of a further type II receptor, InsR-A, in a complex with HER2 (Jones et al., 2006c). However, InsR-A and HER2 activity are further elevated immediately on EGFR inhibition, and this promotes considerable transactivation of Tyr1173 EGFR and substantial levels of downstream AKT activity (Jones et al., 2006a,c). The impact of blockade of the EGFR pathway (and indeed also of anti-HER2 agents) is thereby completely overridden, resulting in de novo refractory growth (Jones et al., 2006c). It remains to be addressed whether such transactivation events occur in breast cancer. Interestingly, however, in the clinical breast cancer study 57, we observed that EGFR phosphorylation was invariably increased during early gefitinib treatment of the largely refractory ER-negative/EGFR-positive breast tumor cohort (Agrawal et al., 2005). This observation may again reflect its regulation in an EGFR kinase-independent manner by IGFR signaling which was readily detectable within such tumors (Gee et al., 2004a; Nicholson et al., 2004b; Jones et al., 2006a).

The considerable therapeutic promise of inhibiting such drug-induced type II receptor mechanisms is revealed by combined treatment with gefitinib plus selective IGFR tyrosine kinase inhibitors, notably ABDP [4-anilino-5-bromo-2-[4-(3-methylamino-1-propynyl) anilino]pyrimidine] or AG1024. Alongside effective inhibition of EGFR signaling, cotreatment with IGFR inhibitor blocked gefitinib-induction of IRS1, Y612, and AKT phosphorylation, and consequently a superior anti-tumor effect and delayed emergence of resistance was observed compared with the single agents in TAMR cells (Knowlden et al., 2006). Therapeutic inhibition of the PI3-kinase/AKT signaling downstream of the induced IGFR pathway similarly exerts an improved anti-tumor effect in combination with EGFR blockade in these cells (Hutcheson et al., 2007). These data complement the findings of Lu et al. (2004, 2005) and Camirand et al. (2005) who have noted an improved inhibitory effect on cancer cell growth by cotreating with the selective IGFR tyrosine kinase inhibitor AG1024 plus gefitinib, or using a recombinant bispecific antibody (Di-diabody). Moreover, we observed that cotreatment with ABDP plus gefitinib in A549 NSCLC was able to deplete IGFR-driven EGFR Tyr1173 phosphorylation and downstream kinase activity, and this strategy not only markedly improved anti-tumor activity in A549 cells (Jones et al., 2006a,d) but was also able to restore gefitinib sensitivity in LoVo cells (Jones et al., 2006c). In all instances, chronic exposure to cotreatment induced improved cell kill and thereby delayed resistance (Knowlden et al., 2006; Jones et al., 2006a,c,d).

Alternative ERBB Receptor Heterodimerisation

The phenomenon of receptor heterodimerisation is well established between the four erbB family members (EGFR, HER2, 3, 4), where the pattern of heterodimerisation plays a critical role in subsequent signaling events. For example, while dimers involving EGFR and HER2 efficiently promote cell proliferation through MAPK activation, dimers involving HER3 more efficiently promote survival signaling through PI3-kinase/AKT (Fedi et al., 1994; Prigent and Gullick, 1994). In this context, it is noteworthy that initial studies using specific anti-erbB strategies naturally focussed on the target erbB receptor and were less concerned with the effects of the drugs on subsequent heterodimerisation patterns across the family. Thus our early studies with gefitinib focussed on the ability of the drug to inhibit EGFR and its downstream signaling (Knowlden et al., 2003). Although this included blockade of the interaction of EGFR with other erbB family members, an evaluation of the interactions between HER2, HER3, and HER4 was not undertaken at that time. Subsequent studies have revealed that inhibition of EGFR activity in TAMR cells supports rapid formation and activation of HER2/HER3 heterodimers in the presence of HER3 ligands within the first week of treatment (Hutcheson et al., 2007). This shift toward an increased use of HER3, alongside drug-promoted IGFR signaling (Knowlden et al., 2006), increased AKT activity and residual cell survival during the drug responsive phase in TAMR cells. Similarly, preliminary studies indicate that the HER2 dimerisation inhibitor Omnitarg (pertuzumab) rapidly induces alternative EGFR/HER3 dimerisation under basal growth conditions. In this instance, the inductive event serves to maintain significant downstream MAPK activity. The important contribution for this mechanism in limiting maximal therapeutic response and its targeting potential is revealed by combining anti-EGFR and anti-HER2 treatments to impede EGFR/HER2, HER3/EGFR, and HER3/HER2-mediated signaling, or with anti-EGFR therapy plus a PI3-kinase/AKT inhibitor, LY294002, which in both instances improved anti-tumor effect (Hutcheson et al., 2007). Interestingly, gefitinib-promoted HER3/HER2 or Omnitarg-induced EGFR/HER3 heterodimer signaling is markedly exacerbated by exposure of cells to exogenous heregulin β1 (HRGβ1). Indeed, this growth factor can completely overcome anti-tumor effect of these single agents, in accordance with its potent promotion of growth and progression in breast cancer (Tsai et al., 2003). Such data are complemented by findings showing this ligand can override the effect of a further EGFR tyrosine kinase inhibitor, CGP59326, in the MKN7 gastric cancer model (Motoyama et al., 2002). While HRGβ1 is poorly expressed in our breast cancer models, it is commonly found in the epithelial and also stromal components of clinical breast cancers (Dunn et al., 2004; Hutcheson et al., 2007). Hence cell environment seems important if we are to consider the full consequences of drug-induced heterodimerisation. With regards to type II receptor inhibitors, we have obtained data from responsive LoVo colorectal cancer cells indicating blockade of InsR signaling with ABDP promoting an early reinstatement of EGFR/HER2 signaling that is subsequently fully recruited to promote acquired resistance (Jones et al., 2006a,d). In this instance, EGFR blockade plus ABDP cotreatment promoted substantial cell kill and subverted resistance to either agent, further illustrating the critical importance of drug-induced alternative receptor signaling.

Clearly our data (along with studies from other groups) are pointing toward a dynamic interplay between signaling pathways in cancer cells, which, when disturbed by targeted agents can lead to previously unpredicted signaling events that serve to limit the actions of such drugs. Importantly, our studies are also revealing that such rapid signaling responses appear to be compounded by additional drug-induced alterations in the patterns of gene expression, which not only have potential to affect cell survival or proliferation but also to promote features of disease progression.

MICROARRAY STUDIES REVEAL THE BREADTH OF DRUG-INDUCED GENES

Antihormones

As previously stated, it is established that gene expression can be repressed as well as promoted by estrogen/ER signaling in breast cancer cells, where in the former instance, antihormones can reinduce expression during the drug responsive phase (Inoue et al., 2002; Levenson et al., 2002; Cunliffe et al., 2003; Frasor et al., 2003, 2004; Hodges et al., 2003). Indeed, Frasor et al. (2003, 2004) suggested that transcriptional repression of genes actually comprises the bulk (70%) of the expression changes associated with estrogen challenge in ER-positive breast cancer models, and the microarray gene expression database recently assembled in the Tenovus Centre is in close agreement, with 63% suppression. In a number of these instances, the ontology of the estrogen-suppressed genes is antiproliferative or proapoptotic and therefore their increased levels undoubtedly form part of the growth inhibitory mechanism of antihormones. Thus our microarray studies (and those of Frasor et al., 2004) reveal induction of transforming growth factor beta (TGFβ) family members and cell cycle inhibitors during early anti-estrogen response (Shaw et al., 2005). However, we are increasingly recognizing using various microarray platforms applied to our model systems that antihormones also induce many genes whose ontology is not easily reconciled with growth inhibition. Indeed, their expression could contribute toward limiting maximal anti-tumor activity of these agents in ER-positive breast cancer cells (Gee et al. 2004b, 2006; Shaw et al., 2005).

While proof of principal for an adverse role for antihormone-induced genes has previously been provided by anti-estrogen induction of EGFR and HER2 (see Section II; Gee et al., 2003), there are clearly other genes that contribute in limiting therapeutic response since our own studies (Knowlden et al., 2003; Jones et al., 2004d) and those performed in xenograft models (Shou et al., 2004) indicate that EGFR targeting alongside anti-estrogens delays (rather than prevents) development of resistance. Among the genes emerging as antihormone induced on the microarrays, and subsequently verified at the mRNA and protein level, with potential to impact unfavorably on therapeutic response is CD44. This is reported to act as a facilitator of growth factor signaling via its ability to enhance ligand and receptor interactions, to act as coreceptor for erbB family members and to interact with protein kinase C (PKC) and Src (Ponta et al., 2003), and is obviously induced by tamoxifen (Harper et al., 2005). Further verified genes include the cochaperone Bcl-2-associated athanogene 1 (Bag1) and an adapter molecule, 14-3-3ζ (Gee et al., 2004b, 2006; Shaw et al., 2005), both induced by tamoxifen and faslodex. Bag1 can interact with the heat shock proteins HSC70/Hsp70 to enhance protein refolding, with bcl-2, ER, growth factor receptors, and Raf-1, as well as promoting proteasomal degradation of denatured proteins facilitating cell survival (Cutress et al., 2002; Townsend et al., 2005). 14-3-3ζ binds phospho-Ser/Thr-containing motifs, interplaying with PI3-kinase or AKT signaling and sequestering apoptotic proteins; it may contribute to InsR and EGFR signaling (Ogihara et al., 1997; Subramanian et al., 2001; Oksvold et al., 2004), and has recently been linked with clinical tamoxifen resistance (Frasor et al., 2006).

The transcription factor component nuclear factor kappa B1 (NFκB1; p105) was also induced at the mRNA and protein level both by antiestrogens (tamoxifen and faslodex and estrogen withdrawal), and subsequent studies have revealed parallel antihormone increases in NFκB1(p50) DNA binding and transcriptional activity of its target promoter (Gee et al., 2004b, 2006; Shaw et al., 2005). Bcl3 is reported to coactivate NFκB1(p50) homodimers and we noted that this gene was also elevated by antihormones in MCF-7 cells and indeed has been described as an estrogen repressed gene (Pratt et al., 2003). For all these induced genes, links have been reported with promotion of cell survival or proliferation [and in the case of NFκB and 14-3-3ζ with antihormone resistance (Gu et al., 2002; Pratt et al., 2003; Zhou et al., 2005; Frasor et al., 2006), and hence their induction may be important in the early evasion of anti-hormone-associated growth inhibition. We have substantiated the contribution for NFκB1 in limiting initial anti-tumor effect of antihormones by cotreating MCF-7 cells with faslodex plus the IκBα/IκBβ (IKK) inhibitor parthenolide (PA). This strategy depletes NFκB transcriptional activity (as measured by monitoring NFκB reporter luciferase activity) and in parallel substantially improves the growth inhibitory effect of faslodex (Gee et al., 2004b, 2006; Shaw et al., 2005). NFκB blockade is furthermore reported to be growth inhibitory and able to restore tamoxifen response in ER+ models overexpressing HER2 (MCF-7/HER2 or BT474 cells) (Zhou et al., 2005) and faslodex response in an established anti-estrogen resistant model (LCC9) (Riggins et al., 2005). Given these promising data cotargetting NFκB alongside antihormones, it is encouraging that NFκB signaling is already of clinical interest as a target in various cancers, for example, through use of the proteasomal inhibitor, Bortezomib, that prevents NFκB activation via inhibiting IkB degradation (Zhou et al., 2005).

Most recently, we have expanded our microarray studies to the powerful Affymetrix platform and have largely focussed our clustering and profiling on genes comprising the tyrosine kinase (TK) category of the "kinome" (as defined by the landmark paper from Manning et al., 2002), since these elements may prove particularly amenable to future therapeutic intervention (Vieth et al., 2005). Our studies have revealed induction of 15 TKs (in addition to EGFR) during anti-hormone treatment whose ontology suggests that they could promote compensatory signaling in the presence of such agents (Gee et al., 2006). For example, antiestrogens induce various Ephrin receptors that are of increasing interest in breast cancer (Fox and Kandpal, 2004). Furthermore, some genes, notably the Src-family member Lyn, are induced by all antihormones. Interestingly, Lyn is also reported to be glucose stress-activated, and to limit response to cytotoxic treatments in colon cancer (Bates et al., 2001) and also to imatinib in leukaemia (Kimura et al., 2005). Similar links have been reported for Bag1, 14-3-3ζ, and NFκB1 with cell survival in the presence of hypoxia, heat shock, and again in limiting radio- or chemo-response (Qi and Martinez, 2003; Townsend et al., 2005; Wu and Kral, 2005). Clearly, a number of anti-hormone-induced genes can be promoted by multiple therapies and may overlap with broader environmental stress survival mechanisms that can be recruited by cancer cells. Importantly, microarray technology is also beginning to reveal a number of further interesting features of anti-hormone-induced events.

Transient Versus Persistent Gene Changes

A comparison of the anti-hormone-induced gene expression database with our microarray data for anti-hormone resistant cells has revealed two major gene patterns (Gee et al., 2006). The first subset of genes represents those that are transiently induced during anti-hormone treatment, but which then decline in the resistant phenotype. The second induced subset persists through to the acquired resistant state. We are evaluating the biological relevance of these observations, but it is conceivable that the former may relate to generic mechanisms associated with the protection of cells that are growth arrested while the latter may be integral to the evolution and maintenance of drug resistant growth. Among the transiently-induced TKs on the Affymetrix arrays was Brk (PTK6) (Harvey and Crompton, 2004); a gene previously implicated in regulation of cell survival or proliferation in cancer and in limiting chemo-response. In contrast, the TKs, EGFR, and HER2 are retained through to anti-estrogen resistance where their signaling comprises an important mitogenic contribution (Benz et al., 1992; McClelland et al., 2001; Yarden et al., 2001; Knowlden et al., 2003). Indeed, in TAMR cells, we have shown the increased EGFR signaling promotes ER reactivation to trigger EGFR ligands such as amphiregulin, as well as ligands for the cross-talking IGFR pathway, that further facilitate the EGFR mitogenic signaling loop (Britton et al., 2006; Knowlden et al., 2006). Further induced genes retained at increased levels in resistance were Bagl and NFκB1, where there are particularly high levels of expression or activity in our MCF-7-derived models that have acquired resistance to severe estrogen deprivation (MCF-7X cells) or faslodex (FASRLT cells). Interestingly, constitutive NFκB activity has similarly been reported in further models of these acquired forms of resistance (Pratt et al., 2003; Riggins et al., 2005), as well as in ER-positive patients destined for relapse despite adjuvant tamoxifen treatment (Zhou et al., 2005). Finally, two members of the LIV-1 family of zinc transporters, SLC39A members 8 (BIGM103) and 7 (HKE4), were induced on the arrays during anti-hormone response and retained at elevated levels in resistance. Zinc is essential for cell growth and is a cofactor for more than 300 enzymes, representing over 50 different enzyme classes (Vallee and Auld, 1990). Its cellular levels are tightly regulated by various zinc transporter proteins, including the LIV-1 family (Taylor 2000; Taylor and Nicholson, 2003, 2004a, 2005), and we have previously shown that HKE4 acts to increase intracellular zinc level in several cell types (Taylor et al., 2004b). In parallel with the elevated HKE4 levels observed in our TAMR cells as verified at the PCR level, these cells also possess increased intracellular zinc (Taylor et al., 2007). Moreover, exposure of TAMR cells to exogenous zinc further enhances their EGFR/IGF1R signaling activity and growth (Taylor et al., 2007), while this in turn is significantly depleted by HKE4 siRNA (Taylor KM, unpublished). It is thus our hypothesis that increases in such transporters ensure zinc delivery is adequate to maximize efficiency of growth factor signaling and thereby allow emergence and maintenance of anti-hormone resistance in breast cancer cells.

Anti-Hormone Induced Genes Encourage Adverse Tumor Properties

Interestingly, while we believe many genes induced by antihormones may directly affect breast cancer cell growth under in vitro experimental conditions, it is likely that others only exert their cellular functions when in a more complex cell environment or genetic background. Examples of this not only relate to the provision of cell survival signaling, but also impinge on other key properties of cancer cells such as tumor spread and angiogenesis. In order for cancer cells to metastasize, they must invade the surrounding tissues, enter the circulatory system, survive in that environment, and eventually colonize other tissues, where interestingly some elements associated with these events appear to be antihormone induced. It has been reported that estrogens and ER confer a protective effect on invasiveness and motility (Platet et al., 2004), and in accordance with this ER-positive models such as MCF-7 cells exhibit an inherently low basal invasive behavior (Hiscox et al., 2006a,b, 2007). In turn, one would therefore expect that antihormones could reverse this process and indeed, although the effects are quite modest, we (and others; Platet et al., 2000, 2004) have recognized that anti-estrogen treatment can induce invasive behavior of anti-hormone responsive models in vitro (Gee et al., 2006; Hiscox et al., 2006c). Interestingly, our array studies have revealed that this treatment is paralleled by induction of several genes whose ontology implicates them in promotion of epithelial-mesenchymal transition (EMT), motility, and invasiveness. Of obvious interest is NFκB (Wu and Kral, 2005), and additionally RhoE and δ-catenin whose increased expression has been confirmed by PCR, immunocytochemistry, and Western blotting (Gee et al., 2004b, 2006; Shaw et al., 2005). RhoE is an antiproliferative Rnd family member, but also is reported to promote actin-cytoskeleton changes and cell rounding, and to augment cell migratory speed (Guasch et al., 1998). Overexpression of δ-catenin, an adhesive junction protein, can enhance growth factor–promoted cell scattering, increase cell spreading and formation of lamelipodia and filopodia (Lu et al., 1999). Similarly, many of the anti-hormone-induced TKs revealed by our Affymetrix studies [including Ephrin receptors (Fox and Kandpal, 2004), Lyn (Suzuki et al., 1998) and HER2] are implicated in cell migratory behavior. It is notable, however, that this significant induction of promigratory genes in anti-hormone responsive MCF-7 cells does not translate into substantial increases in invasiveness during the responsive phase. Intriguingly, our emerging data indicate that the full impact of anti-estrogen-induced genes may only be manifested under conditions of poor cell-cell contact. Thus, neutralising antibody (HECD-1) or siRNA depletion of E-cadherin-mediated intercellular adhesion (Gee et al., 2006; Hiscox et al., 2006c), that in itself affords only a small increase in invasiveness (twofold), dramatically enhances (up to 20-fold) the ability of antiestrogens to induce invasive behavior of MCF-7 cells, approaching levels observed in highly-aggressive ER-negative models such as MDAMB231 cells. Clearly, while antiestrogens confer only small increases in invasiveness under conditions of good cell-cell contact, this may be exacerbated where cell-cell contact is compromised. Our pharmacological studies indicate this event to be independent of EGFR, reinforcing the need to evaluate the anti-hormone induced-genes emerging from our array studies. Such observations could have major implications for anti-estrogen use in ER-positive tumors with inherently poor cell-cell contacts (potentially including tumors where E-cadherin expression is lost by genetic or epigenetic mechanisms (Droufakou et al., 2001) or its cellular mechanism for maintaining cell-cell contacts is dysfunctional (Rakha et al., 2005), where despite growth inhibition, anti-estrogen-induced aggressive behavior in any surviving cells may translate into aggressive disease spread to life-threatening sites and hence poorer prognosis.

Moreover, the in vivo milieu could further exacerbate the adverse impact of some anti-hormone-induced genes. For example, we have observed that increases in the TK c-Met arise as a consequence of chronic faslodex treatment, reaching its maximum level in the resultant faslodex acquired resistant model (FASRLT). Interestingly, while such cells fail to produce hepatocyte growth factor (HGF) or scatter factor (the ligand for Met), exposure to exogenous HGF (or coculturing FASRLT with fibroblasts that produce large quantities of this growth factor) is able to further increase their invasiveness (Hiscox et al., 2006b). Where HGF and Met are expressed in clinical breast cancer (Parr et al., 2004), their coexpression can associate with poor outcome (Lengyel et al., 2005). In addition to changes in genes implicated directly in invasive behavior, our microarray studies are also revealing that anti-hormone treatment is associated with altered expression profiles of some factors that are reported to be capable of promoting angiogenesis in vivo. These include modest changes on the Affymetrix arrays for a further TK Ephrin B4 receptor (Kumar et al., 2006) and also Angiopoietin-like 4 (Le Jan et al., 2003), with more substantial induction of the HIF1α-like factor EPAS1 (Leek et al., 2002; Giatromanolaki et al., 2006). It remains to be addressed what implications such drug-induced events might have in relation to local blood vessel formation and stabilization to permit residual cell survival and metastatic spread in vivo.

As a final example of the likely capacity of certain anti-hormone-induced genes to influence properties of breast cancer cells when in an appropriate context, several complement regulatory proteins (CRPs), including CD59, are significantly induced at the gene and protein level during acute response to tamoxifen or faslodex (Gee et al., 2004b, 2006; Shaw et al., 2005). CRPs are known to protect cells against immune-mediated cell death and are detectable in clinical breast cancer (Rushmere et al., 2004). Through collaborative studies, we have surmised that significant antihormone induction of CRPs could be functionally important in the in vivo context, defending tumor cells from immune surveillance during early treatment and thereby limiting overall cell kill in the presence of antiestrogens allowing disease spread. In support of this hypothesis, CD59 induction by these agents significantly increased resistance to complement-mediated lysis (Gee et al. 2004b, 2006; Shaw et al., 2005), while cell kill could be restored by cotreating with a CD59 neutralizing antibody alongside antiestrogens. Interestingly, induction of this gene also occurred during growth blockade of TAMR cells with gefitinib, implying this may comprise a fundamental drug-induced mechanism of cell survival recruited to evade the complement cascade.

Anti–Growth Factors

Excitingly, our microarray studies are also revealing that anti–growth factors can induce expression of signaling genes during the drug responsive phase that may, as with antihormones, limit maximal anti-tumor effect and contribute to the genesis of resistance. For example, the novel Ret coreceptor glial cell line–derived neurotrophic factor (GDNF) receptor alpha 3 (GFRα3; confirmed at the PCR and protein level) (Burmi et al., 2006) and several TKs (such as HER2 and Lyn) were significantly induced during the gefitinib responsive phase in TAMR cells (Hutcheson et al., 2006). In some instances, these induced elements have an adverse ontology, and are maintained at increased levels into the acquired resistant state. GFRα3 is a member of a family of 4 GFRα genes encoding plasma membrane-localized coreceptors of the TK Ret (Airaksinen and Saarma, 2002). On ligand binding, GFRα receptors are autophosphorylated and while they can signal independently, they commonly recruit and activate Ret to trigger downstream kinase signaling (Takahashi, 2001; Sariola and Saarma, 2003). Activation of Ret through Ret mutation or rearrangement is a key player in thyroid cancer (Asai et al., 2006), and GFRα signaling is reported to maintain survival of neuronal cells (Takahashi, 2001). However, other than the observation that Ret/PTC chimeric oncogene can promote mouse mammary tumorigenesis (Portella et al., 1996), such signaling has never previously been linked to human breast cancer. GFRα/Ret signaling has been implicated in promoting kinase survival signaling in other cell types, and we have shown that GFRα3 knockdown by siRNA can decrease proliferation and cell survival in TAMR cells (Burmi et al., 2006). Hence, its further induction by gefitinib may equally contribute toward maintaining residual viability and permitting emergence of resistance in the presence of this drug. In accordance with this concept, we have observed that exogenous GFRα3 ligand artemin is able to overcome the growth-inhibitory effects of gefitinib in TAMR cells in a dose-dependent manner (Burmi et al., 2006; Hutcheson et al., 2006). The microarray studies revealed that while there were several TKs induced uniquely by EGFR blockade, others overlapped with antihormone induction (again including Lyn and HER2) (Hutcheson et al., 2006).

A number of genes linked to cell motility and invasion (including Lyn and Met) have also been identified by the microarrays as gefitinib inducible (Hutcheson et al., 2006), again including GFRα3 where its signaling has recently been linked with pancreatic cancer invasiveness in vitro (Ceyhan et al., 2006). While it remains unknown if this induction translates out into a further increase in migratory capacity during early gefitinib response in our TAMR cells, invasion has certainly increased very substantially by the time of acquisition of resistance, as measured in our TAMR/TKIR cell line (Jones et al., 2004a). Equally, there is some literature evidence that tumor cell production of proangiogenic growth factors can be increased by EGFR blockade, stimulating blood vessel formation and thereby supporting resistant tumor growth. Thus, VEGF expression increased during long-term EGFR blockade and promoted resistance in a colon cancer model in vivo (Ciardiello et al., 2004; Bianco et al., 2005). Our microarray studies using gefitinib have revealed that EGFR blockade may promote further proangiogenic factors, notably ephrin B2 ligand (Heroult et al., 2006), platelet-derived growth factor-alpha (*PDGFα*) (Yu et al., 2003) and FGF2 (Bikfalvi et al., 1997), in drug responsive breast cancer cells.

CONCLUSIONS

In total, our novel data (complemented by previous reports largely using cytotoxic agents or radiotherapy) indicate that drug-induced signaling is critical in limiting initial anti-tumor response and in promoting therapeutic resistance and disease progression in the presence of targeted treatments, notably antihormones and anti–growth factors. Excitingly, we have been able to provide proof of principle data that combination strategies intelligently targeting drug-induced signaling alongside the primary therapy can promote a superior anti-proliferative effect and a previously unobtainable level of cell kill that dramatically hinders the development of resistance. As such, we believe that in the future, immense therapeutic benefit could emerge from focussed research in this area.

REFERENCES

Agrawal A, Gutteridge E, Gee JM, Nicholson RI, Robertson JF. Overview of tyrosine kinase inhibitors in clinical breast cancer. Endocr Relat Cancer 2005; 12(suppl 1):135–144.

Airaksinen MS, Saarma M. The GDNF family: signalling, biological functions and therapeutic value. Nat Rev Neurosci 2002; 3:383–394.

Argiris A, Wang CX, Whalen SG, DiGiovanna MP. Synergistic interactions between tamoxifen and trastuzumab (Herceptin). Clin Cancer Res 2004; 10:1409–1420.

Bates NP, Hurst HC. An intron 1 enhancer element mediates oestrogen-induced suppression of ERBB2 expression. Oncogene 1997; 15:473–481.

Bates RC, Edwards NS, Burns GF, Fisher DE. A CD44 survival pathway triggers chemoresistance via lyn kinase and PI3K/Akt in colon carcinoma cells. Cancer Res 2001; 61:5275–5283.

Benz CC, Scott GK, Sarup JC, Johnson RM, Tripathy D, Coronado E, Shepard HM, Osborne CK. Estrogen-dependent, tamoxifen-resistant tumorigenic growth of MCF-7 cells transfected with HER2/neu. Breast Cancer Res Treat 1992; 24:85–95.

Bianco R, Shin I, Ritter CA, Yakes FM, Basso A, Rosen N, Tsurutani J, Dennis PA, Mills GB, Arteaga CL. Loss of PTEN/MMAC1/TEP in EGF receptor-expressing tumor cells counteracts the antitumor action of EGFR tyrosine kinase inhibitors. Oncogene 2003; 22:2812–2822.

Bikfalvi A, Klein S, Pintucci G, Rifkin DB. Biological roles of fibroblast growth factor-2. Endocr Rev 1997; 18:26–45.

Britton DJ, Hutcheson IR, Knowlden JM, Barrow D, Giles M, McClelland RA, Gee JM, Nicholson RI. Bidirectional cross talk between ERα and EGFR signalling pathways regulates tamoxifen-resistant growth. Breast Cancer Res Treat 2006; 96:131–146.

Burmi RS, McClelland RA, Barrow D, Ellis IO, Robertson JFR, Nicholson RI, Gee JMW. Microarray studies reveal novel genes associated with endocrine resistance in breast cancer. Breast Cancer Res 2006; 8:S11.

Camirand A, Zakikhani M, Young F, Pollak M. Inhibition of insulin-like growth factor-1 receptor signaling enhances growth-inhibitory and proapoptotic effects of gefitinib (Iressa) in human breast cancer cells. Breast Cancer Res 2005; 7:R570–R579.

Ceyhan GO, Giese NA, Erkan M, Kerscher AG, Wente MN, Gisese T, Buchler MW, Friess H. The neurotrophic factor artemin promotes pancreatic cancer invasion. Ann Surg 2006; 244:274–281.

Chakravarti A, Loeffler JS, Dyson NJ. Insulin-like growth factor receptor I mediates resistance to anti-epidermal growth factor receptor therapy in primary human glioblastoma cells through continued activation of phosphoinositide 3-kinase signaling. Cancer Res 2002; 62:200–207.

Chu I, Blackwell K, Chen S, Slingerland J. The dual ErbB1/ErbB2 inhibitor, lapatinib (GW572016), cooperates with tamoxifen to inhibit both cell proliferation- and estrogen-dependent gene expression in antiestrogen-resistant breast cancer. Cancer Res 2005; 65:18–25.

Ciardiello F, Bianco R, Caputo R, Caputo R, Damiano V, Troiani T, Melisi D, De Vita F, De Placido S, Bianco AR, Tortora G. Antitumor activity of ZD6474, a vascular endothelial growth factor receptor tyrosine kinase inhibitor, in human cancer cells with acquired resistance to antiepidermal growth factor receptor therapy. Clin Cancer Res 2004; 10:784–793.

Cunliffe HE, Ringner M, Bilke S, Walker RL, Cheung JM, Chen Y, Meltzer PS. The gene expression response of breast cancer to growth regulators: patterns and correlation with tumour expression profiles. Cancer Res 2003; 63: 7158–7166.

Cutress RI, Townsend PA, Brimmell M, Bateman AC, Hague A, Packham G. BAG1 expression and function in human cancer. Br J Cancer 2002; 87:834–839.

Desbois-Mouthon C, Cacheux W, Blivet-Van Eggelpoel MJ, Barbu V, Fartoux L, Poupon R, Housset C, Rosmorduc O. Impact of IGF-1R/EGFR cross-talks on hepatoma cell sensitivity to gefitinib. Int J Cancer 2006; 119:2557–2566.

Droufakou S, Deshmane V, Roylance R, Hanby A, Tomlinson I, Hart IR. Multiple ways of silencing E-cardherin in lobular carcinoma of the breast. 2001; 92:404–408.

Dunn M, Sinha P, Campbell R, Blackburn E, Levinson N, Rampaul R, Bates T, Humphreys S, Gullick WJ. Co-expression of neuregulins 1, 2, 3 and 4 in human breast cancer. J Pathol 2004; 203:672–680.

Fan M, Yan PS, Hartman-Frey C, Chen L, Paik H, Oyer SL, Salisbury JD, Cheng AS, Li L, Abbosh PH, Huang TH, Nephew KP. Diverse gene expression and DNA methylation profiles correlate with differential adaptation of breast cancer cells to the antiestrogens tamoxifen and fulvestrant. Cancer Res 2006; 66:11954–11966.

Fedi P, Pierce JH, di Fiore PP, Kraus MH. Efficient coupling with phosphatidylinositol 3-kinase, but not phospholipase C gamma or GTPase-activating protein, distinguishes ErbB-3 signaling from that of other ErbB/EGFR family members. Mol Cell Biol 1994; 14:492–500.

Fox BP, Kandpal RP. Invasiveness of breast carcinoma cells and transcript profile: Eph receptors and ephrin ligands as molecular markers of potential diagnostic and prognostic application. Biochem Biophys Res Commun 2004; 318:882–892.

Frasor J, Chang EC, Komm B, Lin CY, Vega VB, Liu ET, Miller LD, Smeds J, Bergh J, Katzenellenbogen BS. Gene expression preferentially regulated by tamoxifen in breast cancer cells and correlations with clinical outcome. Cancer Res 2006; 66:7334–7340.

Frasor J, Danes JM, Komm B, Chang KC, Lyttle CR, Katzenellenbogen BS. Profiling of estrogen up- and down-regulated gene expression in human breast cancer cells: insights into gene networks and pathways underlying estrogenic control of proliferation and cell phenotype. Endocrinology 2003; 144:4562–4574.

Frasor J, Stossi F, Danes JM, Komm B, Lyttle CR, Katzenellenbogen BS. Selective estrogen receptor modulators: discrimination of agonistic versus antagonistic activities by gene expression profiling in breast cancer cells. Cancer Res 2004; 64:1522–1533.

Gee JMW, Gutteridge E, Robertson JF, Wakeling AE, Jones HE, Nicholson RI. Biological markers during early treatment of tamoxifen-resistant breast cancer with gefitinib ('Iressa'). Breast Cancer Res Treat 2004a; 88:S216.

Gee JM, Harper ME, Hutcheson IR, Madden TA, Barrow D, Knowlden JM, McClelland RA, Jordan N, Wakeling AE, Nicholson RI. The anti-epidermal growth factor receptor agent gefitinib (ZD1839/Iressa) improves anti-hormone response and prevents development of resistance in breast cancer *in vitro*. Endocrinology 2003; 144:5105–5117.

Gee J, Shaw V, Burmi R, McClelland R, Morgan H, Harper M, Hiscox S, Barrow D, Lewis P, Nicholson R. Array profiling of survival and resistance genes in anti-hormone-treated breast cancer cells. Int J Mol Med 2004b; 14:S81.

Gee JM, Shaw VE, Hiscox SE, McClelland RA, Rushmere NK, Nicholson RI. Deciphering anti-hormone-induced compensatory mechanisms in breast cancer and their therapeutic implications. Endocr Relat Cancer 2006; 13(suppl 1):S77–S88.

Giatromanolaki A, Sivridis E, Fiska A, Koukourakis MI. Hypoxia-inducible factor-2 alpha (HIF-2 alpha) induces angiogenesis in breast carcinomas. Appl Immunohistochem Mol Morphol 2006; 14:78–82.

Gu Z, Lee RY, Skaar TC, Bouker KB, Welch JN, Lu J, Liu A, Zhu Y, Davis N, Leonessa F, Brunner N, Wang Y, Clarke R. Association of interferon regulatory factor-1, nucleophosmin, nuclear factor-kappaB, and cyclic AMP response element binding with acquired resistance to Faslodex (ICI 182,780). Cancer Res 2002; 62:3428–3437.

Guasch RM, Scambler P, Jones GE, Ridley AJ. RhoE regulates actin cytoskeleton organization and cell migration. Mol Cell Biol 1998; 18:4761–4771.

Guvakova MA, Surmacz E. Tamoxifen interferes with the insulin-like growth factor I receptor signaling pathway in breast cancer cells. Cancer Res 1997; 57:2606–2610.

Hamelers IH, Steenbergh PH. Interactions between estrogen and insulin-like growth factor signaling pathways in human breast tumor cells. Endocr Relat Cancer 2003; 10:331–345.

Harper ME, Smith C, Nicholson RI. Upregulation of CD44s and variants in anti-hormone resistant breast cancer cells. Eur J Cancer 2005; 3(suppl):71 (abstract).

Harvey AJ, Crompton MR. The Brk protein tyrosine kinase as a therapeutic target in cancer: opportunities and challenges. Anticancer Drugs 2004; 15:107–111.

Heroult M, Schaffner F, Augustin HG. Eph receptor and ephrin ligand-mediated interactions during angiogenesis and tumor progression. Exp Cell Res 2006; 312:642–650.

Hiscox S, Jiang WG, Obermeier K, Taylor K, Morgan L, Burmi R, Barrow D, Nicholson RI. Tamoxifen resistance in MCF7 cells promotes EMT-like behaviour and involves modulation of beta-catenin phosphorylation. Int J Cancer 2006a; 118:290–301.

Hiscox S, Jordan NJ, Jiang W, Harper M, McClelland R, Smith C, Nicholson RI. Chronic exposure to fulvestrant promotes overexpression of the c-Met receptor in breast cancer cells: implications for tumour-stroma interactions. Endocr Relat Cancer 2006b; 13(4):1085–1099.

Hiscox SE, Jordan NJ, Morgan L, Green TP, Nicholson RI. Src kinase promotes adhesion independent activation of FAK and enhanced cell migration in tamoxifen resistant breast cancer cells. Clin Exper Metastasis 2007; 24:157–167.

Hodges LC, Cook JD, Lobenhofer EK, Li L, Bennett L, Bushel PR, Aldaz CM, Afshari CA, Walker CL. Tamoxifen functions as a molecular agonist inducing cell cycle-associated genes in breast cancer cells. Mol Cancer Res 2003; 1:300–311.

Hutcheson IR, Knowlden JM, Gee JMW, Harper ME, Barrow D, Nicholson RI. Inductive mechanisms limiting response to anti-epidermal growth factor receptor therapy. Endocr Relat Cancer 2006; 13(suppl 1):S89–S97.

Hutcheson IR, Knowlden JM, Hiscox SE, Barrow D, Gee JM, Robertson JF, Ellis IO, Nicholson RI. Heregulin β1 drives gefitinib-resistant growth and invasion in tamoxifen-resistant MCF-7 breast cancer cells. Breast Cancer Res 2007; 9:R50.

Inoue A, Yoshida N, Omoto Y, Oguchi S, Yamori T, Kiyama R, Hayashi S. Development of cDNA microarray for expression profiling of estrogen-responsive genes. J Mol Endocrinol 2002; 29:175–192.

Johnston SR, Leary A. Lapatinib: a novel EGFR/HER2 tyrosine kinase inhibitor for cancer. Drugs Today (Barc) 2006; 42:441–453.

Johnston SR, Head J, Pancholi S, Detre S, Martin LA, Smith IE, Dowsett M. Integration of signal transduction inhibitors with endocrine therapy: an approach to overcoming hormone resistance in breast cancer. Clin Cancer Res 2003; 9:524S–532S.

Jones HE, Gee JM, Barrow D, Tonge D, Holloway B, Nicholson RI. Inhibition of insulin receptor isoform-A signalling restores sensitivity to gefitinib in previously de novo resistant colon cancer cells. Br J Cancer 2006a; 95:172–180.

Jones HE, Gee JMW, Barrow D, Holloway B, Tonge D, Nicholson RI. Maintenance of EGFR phosphorylation by the IGF-1R in the presence of gefitinib in lung cancer cells: co-targeting the EGFR and IGF-1R maximises anti-tumour effects. Proc 4th Intl Symp Signal Transduction Modulators Cancer Therapy, 2006b:P210.

Jones HE, Gee JM, Hutcheson IR, Nicholson RI. Insulin-like growth factor-1 receptor and resistance in breast cancer. Expert Rev Endocrinol Metab 2006c; 1:33–46.

Jones HE, Gee JM, Hutcheson II, Knowlden JM, Barrow D, Nicholson RI. Growth factor receptor interplay and resistance in cancer. Endocr Relat Cancer 2006d; 13(suppl 1):S45–S51.

Jones HE, Goddard L, Gee JM, Hiscox S, Rubini M, Barrow D, Knowlden JM, Williams S, Wakeling AE, Nicholson RI.

Insulin-like growth factor-I receptor signalling and acquired resistance to gefitinib (ZD1839; Iressa) in human breast and prostate cancer cells. Endocr Relat Cancer 2004; 11:793–814.

Jordan NJ, Gee JM, Barrow D, Wakeling AE, Nicholson RI. Increased constitutive activity of PKB/AKT in tamoxifen resistant breast cancer MCF-7 cells. Breast Cancer Res Treat 2004; 87:167–180.

Kimura S, Naito H, Segawa H, Kuroda J, Yuasa T, Sato K, Yokota A, Kamitsuji Y, Kawata E, Ashihara E, Nakaya Y, Naruoka H, Wakayama T, Nasu K, Asaki T, Niwa T, Hirabayashi K, Maekawa T. NS-187, a potent and selective dual Bcr-Abl/Lyn tyrosine kinase inhibitor, is a novel agent for imatinib-resistant leukemia. Blood 2005; 106:3948–3954.

Knowlden JM, Hutcheson IR, Barrow D, Gee JMW, Wakeling AE, Nicholson RI. Insulin receptor substrate-1 involvement in epidermal growth factor receptor and insulin-like growth factor receptor signalling: implication for gefitinib ('IRESSA') response and resistance. Breast Cancer Res Treat 2007 Sep 28; [Epub ahead of print].

Knowlden JM, Hutcheson IR, Jones HE, Madden T, Gee JM, Harper ME, Barrow D, Wakeling AE, Nicholson RI. Elevated levels of epidermal growth factor receptor/c-erbB2 heterodimers mediate an autocrine growth regulatory pathway in tamoxifen-resistant MCF-7 cells. Endocrinology 2003; 144:1032–1044.

Le Jan S, Amy C, Cazes A, Monnot C, Lamande N, Favier J, Philippe J, Sibony M, Gasc JM, Corvol P, Germain S. Angiopoietin-like 4 is a proangiogenic factor produced during ischemia and in conventional renal cell carcinoma. Am J Pathol 2003; 162:1521–1528.

Leary A, Dowsett M. Combination therapy with aromatase inhibitors: the next era of breast cancer treatment? Br J Cancer 2006; 95:661–666.

Leek RD, Talks KL, Pezzella F, Turley H, Campo L, Brown NS, Bicknell R, Taylor M, Gatter KC, Harris AL. Relation of hypoxia-inducible factor-2 alpha (HIF-2 alpha) expression in tumor-infiltrative macrophages to tumor angiogenesis and the oxidative thymidine phosphorylase pathway in human breast cancer. Cancer Res 2002; 62:1326–1329.

Lengyel E, Prechtel D, Resau JH, Gauger K, Welk A, Lindemann K, Salanti G, Richter T, Knudsen B, Vande Woude GF, Harbeck N. c-Met overexpression in node-positive breast cancer identifies patients with poor clinical outcome independent of Her2/neu. Int J Cancer 2005; 113:678–682.

Levenson AS, Kliakhandler IL, Svoboda KM, Pease KM, Kaiser SA, Ward JE 3rd, Jordan VC. Molecular classification of selective oestrogen receptor modulators on the basis of gene expression profiles of breast cancer cells expressing oestrogen receptor alpha. Br J Cancer 2002; 87:449–456.

Liu B, Fang M, Lu Y, Mendelsohn J, Fan Z. Fibroblast growth factor and insulin-like growth factor differentially modulate the apoptosis and G1 arrest induced by anti-epidermal growth factor receptor monoclonal antibody. Oncogene 2001; 20:1913–1922.

Lu Q, Paredes M, Medina M, Zhou J, Cavallo R, Peifer M, Orecchio L, Kosik KS. Delta-catenin, an adhesive junction-associated protein which promotes cell scattering. J Cell Biol 1999; 144:519–532.

Lu D, Zhang H, Koo H, Tonra J, Balderes P, Prewett M, Corcoran E, Mangalampalli V, Bassi R, Anselma D, Patel D, Kang X, Ludwig DL, Hicklin DJ, Bohlen P, Witte L, Zhu Z. A fully human recombinant IgG-like bispecific antibody to both the epidermal growth factor receptor and the insulin-like growth factor receptor for enhanced anti-tumor activity. J Biol Chem 2005; 280:19665–9672.

Lu D, Zhang H, Ludwig D, Persaud A, Jimenez X, Burtrum D, Balderes P, Liu M, Bohlen P, Witte L, Zhu Z. Simultaneous blockade of both the epidermal growth factor receptor and the insulin-like growth factor receptor signaling pathways in cancer cells with a fully human recombinant bispecific antibody. J Biol Chem 2004; 279:2856–2865.

Manning G, Whyte DB, Martinez R, Hunter T, Sudarsanam S. The protein kinase complement of the human genome. Science 2002; 298:1912–1934.

McClelland RA, Barrow D, Madden TA, Dutkowski CM, Pamment J, Knowlden JM, Gee JM, Nicholson RI. Enhanced epidermal growth factor receptor signalling in MCF-7 breast cancer cells after long-term culture in the presence of the pure antiestrogen ICI 182,780 (Faslodex). Endocrinology 2001; 142:2776–2788.

Motoyama AB, Hynes NE, Lane HA. The efficacy of ErbB receptor-targeted anticancer therapeutics is influenced by the availability of epidermal growth factor-related peptides. Cancer Res 2002; 62:3151–3158.

Nahta R, Yu D, Hung MC, Hortobagyi GN, Esteva FJ. Mechanisms of disease: understanding resistance to HER2-targeted therapy in human breast cancer. Nat Clin Pract Oncol 2006; 3:269–280.

Newman SP, Bates NP, Vernimmen D, Parker MG, Hurst HC. Cofactor competition between the ligand-bound oestrogen receptor and an intron 1 enhancer leads to oestrogen repression of ERBB2 expression in breast cancer. Oncogene 2000; 19:490–497.

Nicholson RI, Hutcheson IR, Hiscox SE, Knowlden JM, Giles M, Barrow D, Gee JM. Growth factor signalling and resistance to selective oestrogen receptor modulators and pure anti-oestrogens: the use of anti-growth factor therapies to treat or delay endocrine resistance in breast cancer. Endocr Relat Cancer 2005; 12(suppl 1):29–36.

Nicholson RI, Hutcheson IR, Jones HE, Hiscox SE, Giles M, Taylor KM, Gee JM. Growth factor signalling in endocrine and anti-growth factor resistant breast cancer. Rev Endocr Metab Disord 2007; 8:241–253.

Nicholson RI, Hutcheson IR, Knowlden JM, Jones HE, Harper ME, Jordan N, Hiscox SE, Barrow D, Gee JM. Non-endocrine pathways and endocrine resistance: observations with antiestrogens and signal transduction inhibitors in combination. Clin Cancer Res 2004a; 10:346–354.

Nicholson RI, Jones HE, Gee JMW. EGFR inhibitors in breast cancer. Signal 2004b; 5:9–13.

Nicholson RI, Wakeling AE, Gee JM. Prospects for combining hormonal and anti-EGFR inhibition. Breast Cancer Online 2003; 6:2.

Ogihara T, Isobe T, Ichimura T, Taoka M, Funaki M, Sakoda H, Onishi Y, Inukai K, Anai M, Fukushima Y, Kikuchi M,

Yazaki Y, Oka Y, Asano T. 14-3-3 protein binds to insulin receptor substrate-1, one of the binding sites of which is in the phosphotyrosine binding domain. J Biol Chem 1997; 272:25267–5274.

Oksvold MP, Huitfeldt HS, Langdon WY. Identification of 14-3-3ζ as an EGF receptor interacting protein. FEBS Lett 2004; 569:207–210.

Parr C, Watkins G, Mansel RE, Jiang WG. The hepatocyte growth factor regulatory factors in human breast cancer. Clin Cancer Res 2004; 10:202–211.

Platet N, Cathiard AM, Gleizes M, Garcia M. Estrogens and their receptors in breast cancer progression: a dual role in cancer proliferation and invasion. Crit Rev Oncol Hematol 2004; 51:55–67.

Platet N, Cunat S, Chalbos D, Rochefort H, Garcia M. Unliganded and liganded estrogen receptors protect against cancer invasion via different mechanisms. Mol Endocrinology 2000; 14:999–1009.

Polychronis A, Sinnett HD, Hadjiminas D, Singhal H, Mansi JL, Shivapatham D, Shousha S, Jiang J, Peston D, Barrett N, Vigushin D, Morrison K, Beresford E, Ali S, Slade MJ, Coombes RC. Preoperative gefitinib versus gefitinib and anastrozole in postmenopausal patients with oestrogen-receptor positive and epidermal-growth-factor-receptor-positive primary breast cancer: a double-blind placebo-controlled phase II randomised trial. Lancet Oncol 2005; 6:383–391.

Ponta H, Sherman L, Herrlich PA. CD44: from adhesion molecules to signalling regulators. Nat Rev Mol Cell Biol 2003; 4:33–45.

Portella G, Salvatore D, Botti G, Cerrato A, Zhang L, Mineo A, Chiappetta G, Santelli G, Pozzi L, Vecchio G, Fusco A, Santoro M. Development of mammary and cutaneous gland tumors in transgenic mice carrying the RET/PTC1 oncogene. Oncogene 1996; 13:2021–2026.

Pratt MA, Bishop TE, White D, Yasvinski G, Menard M, Niu MY, Clarke R. Estrogen withdrawal-induced NF-kappaB activity and bcl-3 expression in breast cancer cells: roles in growth and hormone independence. Mol Cell Biol 2003; 23: 6887–6900.

Prigent SA, Gullick WJ. Identification of c-erbB-3 binding sites for phosphatidylinositol 3-kinase and SHC using an EGF receptor/c-erbB-3 chimera. EMBO J 1994; 13:2831–2841.

Qi W, Martinez JD. Reduction of 14-3-3 proteins correlates with increased sensitivity to killing of human lung cancer cells by ionizing radiation. Radiat Res 2003; 160:217–223.

Rakha EA, Abd El Rehim D, Pinder SE, Lewis SA, Ellis IO. E-cadherin expression in invasive non-lobular carcinoma of the breast and its prognostic significance. Histopathology 2005; 46:685–693.

Riggins RB, Zwart A, Nehra R, Clarke R. The nuclear factor kappa B inhibitor parthenolide restores ICI 182,780 (Faslodex; fulvestrant)-induced apoptosis in antiestrogen-resistant breast cancer cells. Mol Cancer Ther 2005; 4:33–41.

Rushmere NK, Knowlden JM, Gee JM, Harper ME, Robertson JF, Morgan BP, Nicholson RI. Analysis of the level of mRNA expression of the membrane regulators of complement, CD59, CD55 and CD46 in breast cancer. Int J Cancer 2004; 108:930–936.

Sachdev D, Yee D. The IGF system and breast cancer. Endocr Relat Cancer 2001; 8:197–209.

Sariola H, Saarma M. Novel functions and signalling pathways for GDNF. J Cell Sci 2003; 116:3855–3862.

Shaw VE, Gee JMW, McClelland RA, Morgan H, Rushmere N, Nicholson RI. Identification of anti-hormone induced genes as potential therapeutic targets in breast cancer. Proc Am Assoc Cancer Res 2005; 46:3706 (abstract).

Shou J, Massarweh S, Osborne CK, Wakeling AE, Ali S, Weiss H, Schiff R. Mechanisms of tamoxifen resistance: increased estrogen receptor-HER2/neu cross-talk in ER/HER2-positive breast cancer. J Natl Cancer Inst 2004; 96:926–935.

Songyang Z, Margolis B, Chaudhuri M, Shoelson SE, Cantley LC. The phosphotyrosine interaction domain of SHC recognizes tyrosine-phosphorylated NPXY motif. J Biol Chem 1995; 270:14863–14866.

Subramanian RR, Masters SC, Zhang H, Fu H. Functional conservation of 14-3-3 isoforms in inhibiting Bad-induced apoptosis. Exp Cell Res 2001; 271:142–151.

Suzuki T, Shoji S, Yamamoto K, Nada S, Okada M, Yamamoto T, Honda Z. Essential roles of Lyn in fibronectin-mediated filamentous actin assembly and cell motility in mast cells. J Immunol 1998; 161:3694–3701.

Takahashi M. The GDNF/RET signalling pathway and human diseases. Cytokine Growth Factor Rev 2001; 12: 361–373.

Taylor KM. LIV-1 breast cancer protein belongs to new family of histidine-rich membrane proteins with potential to control intracellular Zn2+ homeostasis. IUBMB Life 2000; 49: 249–253.

Taylor KM, Hiscox S, Nicholson RI. Zinc transporter LIV-1: a link between cellular development and cancer progression. Trends Endocrinol Metab 2004a; 15:461–463.

Taylor KM, Morgan HE, Johnson A, Nicholson RI. Structure-function analysis of HKE4, a member of the new LIV-1 subfamily of zinc transporters. Biochem J 2004b; 377:131–139.

Taylor KM, Morgan HE, Johnson A, Nicholson RI. Structure-function analysis of a novel member of the LIV-1 subfamily of zinc transporters, ZIP14. FEBS Lett 2005; 579:427–432.

Taylor KM, Nicholson RI. The LZT proteins; the LIV-1 subfamily of zinc transporters. Biochim Biophys Acta 2003; 1611:16–30.

Taylor KM, Morgan HE, Smart K, Zahari NM, Pumford S, Ellis IO, Robertson JF, Nicholson RI. The emerging role of the LIV-1 sub-family of zinc transporters in breast cancer. Mol Med 2007; 13:396–406.

Townsend PA, Stephanou A, Packham G, Latchman DS. BAG1: a multi-functional pro-survival molecule. Int J Biochem Cell Biol 2005; 37:251–259.

Tsai MS, Shamon-Taylor LA, Mehmi I, Tang CK, Lupu R. Blockage of heregulin expression inhibits tumorigenicity and metastasis of breast cancer. Oncogene 2003; 22: 761–768.

Vallee BL, Auld DS. Zinc coordination, function, and structure of zinc enzymes and other proteins. Biochemistry 1990; 29: 5647–5659.

Vieth M, Sutherland JJ, Robertson DH, Campbell RM. Kinomics: characterizing the therapeutically validated kinase space. Drug Discov Today 2005; 10:839–846.

White MF. The insulin signalling system and the IRS proteins Diabetologia 1997; 40:2–17.

Wilson MA, Chrysogelos SA. Identification and characterization of a negative regulatory element within the epidermal growth factor receptor gene first intron in hormone-dependent breast cancer cells. J Cell Biochem 2002; 85: 601–614.

Wu JT, Kral JG. The NF-kappaB/IkappaB signaling system: a molecular target in breast cancer therapy. J Surg Res 2005; 123:158–169.

Yarden RI, Wilson MA, Chrysogelos SA. Estrogen suppression of EGFR expression in breast cancer cells: a possible mechanism to modulate growth. J Cell Biochem 2001; 81:232–246.

Yee D, Lee AV. Crosstalk between the insulin-like growth factors and estrogens in breast cancer. J Mammary Gland Biol Neoplasia 2000; 5:107–115.

Yu J, Ustach C, Kim HR. Platelet-derived growth factor signaling and human cancer. J Biochem Mol Biol 2003; 36: 49–59.

Zhou Y, Eppenberger-Castori S, Eppenberger U, Benz CC. The NFkappaB pathway and endocrine-resistant breast cancer. Endocr Relat Cancer 2005; 12(suppl 1):S37–S46.

8

Apoptosis, Cell Death, and Breast Cancer

AYESHA N. SHAJAHAN and REBECCA B. RIGGINS
Department of Oncology, Lombardi Comprehensive Cancer Center, Georgetown University Medical Center, Washington D.C., U.S.A.

ROBERT CLARKE
Department of Oncology and Department of Physiology and Biophysics, Lombardi Comprehensive Cancer Center, Georgetown University Medical Center, Washington D.C., U.S.A.

INTRODUCTION

In 2007, approximately 178,480 new cases of invasive breast cancer were diagnosed and over 40,460 American women died of this disease (American Cancer Society, 2007). Lifetime risk of developing breast cancer is modified by several factors related to development (e.g., weight at birth, age at menarche), reproductive life (e.g., parity, lactation, age at menopause), lifestyle (e.g., obesity, alcohol consumption), and inheritance (e.g., mutant BRCA1) (Ahlgren et al., 2004; de Jong et al., 2002; Feigelson et al., 2004; Hulka and Stark, 1995). Despite the importance of family history, the altered expression/function of tumor suppressor genes such as BRCA1/2 and TP53 do not account for the high prevalence of sporadic or non-BRCA familial breast cancers. Among mutant BRCA1/2 carriers, the timing of breast cancer onset and progress can vary substantially, but the factors responsible for these variations are not fully understood (Nathanson et al., 2001). The precise molecular events responsible for affecting disease progression remain unknown in both sporadic and inherited breast cancers, but those that affect a breast cancer cell's choice to proliferate, differentiate, or die are likely to be key factors in this process.

Randomized trials and large meta-analyses clearly show that all breast cancer patients derive a statistically significant survival benefit from chemotherapy and endocrine therapy (EBCTCG, 1998; EBCTCG, 2002a; EBCTCG, 2002b; Fisher et al., 1996; Mansour et al., 1998), Tamoxifen (TAM; antiestrogen), Paclitaxel (taxane), and Adriamycin (anthracycline) being among the most effective single agents. The survival benefit gained from current systemic therapies largely reflects the abilities of cytotoxic and endocrine agents to modify cell survival such that cells are driven down an irreversible cell death pathway (Fischer and Schulze-Osthoff, 2005). Nonetheless, advanced breast cancer largely remains an incurable disease, and new treatment regimens and schedules have led to only incremental decreases in breast cancer–related mortality. A better understanding of the factors that regulate breast cancer cell survival or death is central to improving breast cancer outcomes in women.

MOLECULAR MECHANISM OF APOPTOSIS

Apoptosis, a type of programmed cell death (PCD), is an essential feature of normal mammary gland function. Failure to undergo apoptosis can lead to the development of cancer in breast epithelial cells (Green and Streuli, 2004). Cancer cells can evade apoptosis by modifying the signaling pathways that lead to apoptosis. Thus, significant effort is invested in the development of anticancer therapeutic agents that either selectively induce cell death in cancer cells or restore their apoptotic threshold (Meng et al., 2006).

The distinctive morphological and biochemical hallmarks of apoptosis include cell shrinkage, pyknosis (chromatin condensation), karyorhexis (nuclear fragmentation), membrane blebbing, and fragmentation of the cell into apoptotic bodies (Kerr et al., 1972). Phagocytic cells recognize and remove the apoptotic bodies, and thus avoid immune activation around the dying cell. Cell death by apoptosis requires the expenditure of ATP and the activation of proteases known as "caspases"(cysteine-dependent aspartate-specific proteases) (Wolf and Green, 1999). Caspases exist as latent zymogens that may be activated by autoactivation, transactivation, or proteolysis by other proteinases. In humans, over a dozen caspases have been identified (Hengartner, 2000); among these, caspases-3, -6, and -7 are called "executioner" caspases and they mediate their effect by the cleavage of specific cellular substrates. These executioner caspases are activated by the "initiator" caspases such as caspases-8, -9, and -10 (Denault and Salvesen, 2002; Riedl and Salvesen, 2007; Salvesen, 2002; Wolf and Green, 1999).

Overview of Extrinsic and Intrinsic Pathways

Many anticancer therapies activate caspases that cleave a number of different but selective substrates in the cytoplasm or nucleus, leading to many of the morphological features of an apoptotic cell death (Degterev et al., 2003). Caspase activation is initiated at the plasma membrane through death receptors either by an "extrinsic" pathway, or at the mitochondria by an "intrinsic" pathway (Fig. 1).

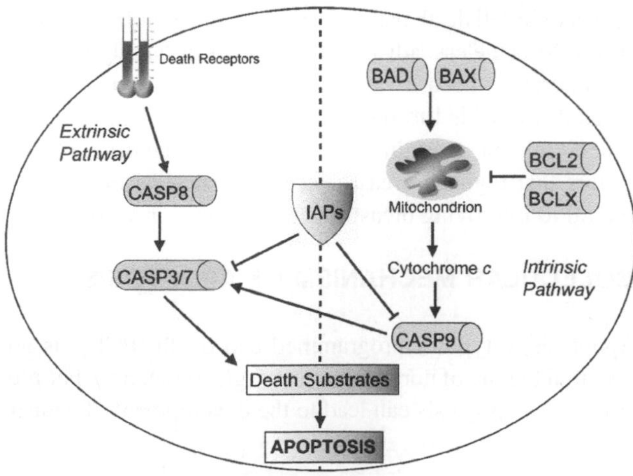

Figure 1 A simplified model of extrinsic and intrinsic signaling mechanisms involved in apoptotic cell death in the cell.

In normal tissue, apoptosis maintains homeostasis, and this process is tightly controlled at critical points of the signaling cascade (Green and Kroemer, 2004; Kroemer et al., 2007).

In the extrinsic or death receptor pathway, stimulation of death receptors of the tumor necrosis factor (TNF) receptor superfamily such as CD95 (APO-1/Fas) or TNF-related apoptosis-inducing ligand (TRAIL) receptors-1 and -2 result in the recruitment and oligomerization of the adapter molecule FADD (Fas-associating death domain-containing protein). The oligomerized FADD then localizes within the death-inducing signaling complex (Debatin and Krammer, 2004) followed by activation of initiator caspases-8, or -10 that contain death effector domains (Vandenabeele et al., 2006; Wolf and Green, 1999).

In the intrinsic or mitochondrial pathway, the executioner caspases are activated by caspase-9, which is activated by the adapter molecule apoptotic protease activating factor-1 (APAF-1) within a multiprotein complex called the "apoptosome." Activation of APAF-1 depends on both cytochrome *c* release from the intermembrane space of the mitochondria and ATP/dATP (Cain et al., 2002), leading to an increase in mitochondrial membrane potential (MMP) that is closely controlled by pro-(BAD, BAX) and antiapoptotic (BCL2) members of the BCL2 family of proteins (Decaudin et al., 1998; Green and Kroemer, 2004). A caspase-independent signal can also originate from within the mitochondria leading to irreversible loss of mitochondrial function; this can include the release of caspase-independent death effectors such as apoptosis-inducing factor (AIF) or endonuclease G (Cande et al., 2004; Kroemer and Martin, 2005; Li et al., 2001).

The intrinsic and extrinsic pathways converge at the executioner caspases. The executioner caspases selectively cleave their substrates in the primary sequence (always after an aspartate residue), and these target proteins can range from single polypeptide chain enzymes (poly ADP-ribose polymerse, PARP) to complex macromolecules (the lamin network) (Hengartner, 2000). PARP inactivation by caspase-specific cleavage, which forms an 89-kDa fragment, is a biochemical hallmark of apoptosis. Members of the heat shock protein (HSP) family, e.g., HSP70, can delay apoptosis by preventing the nuclear import of AIF (Ravagnan et al., 2001). The intrinsic drive for cancer cells to undergo apoptosis is held in check by inhibitor of apoptosis proteins (IAPs). Downstream of cytochrome *c* release, second mitochondrial activator of caspases/direct IAP binder with low pI (Smac/DIABLO) neutralize IAPs such as X-linked IAP (XIAP), survivin, and Apollon through their baculoviral inverted repeat (BIR) domains, and so indirectly promote caspase activation (Saelens et al., 2004; Vaux and Silke, 2003).

Alternative Death Pathways

Effectiveness of antineoplastic drugs can be assessed on the basis of their ability to induce apoptosis in tumor cells; however, it is now becoming evident that apoptosis may not be the only, or perhaps even the primary, mechanism of cell death in solid tumors (Brown and Attardi, 2005). Frequent failure to correlate apoptotic cell death with the effects of chemotherapeutic drugs on human tumors and cell lines (Brown and Attardi, 2005; Roninson et al., 2001) has prompted studies of other mechanisms of cell death.

Autophagy

Autophagy involves sequestration of cytosol and cytoplasmic organelles within double membranes called autophagosomes or autophagic vacuoles. The vesicular contents are broken down by pH-sensitive lysosomal hydrolases and the degradation products are recycled for use in macromolecular synthesis and/or bioenergetics (Kroemer and Jaattela, 2005). In general, autophagy is important in the developmental remodeling of cells, cellular adaptation to nutrient deprivation, and the elimination of damaged organelles (Edinger and Thompson, 2004; Edinger and Thompson, 2003; Klionsky and Emr, 2000). Paradoxically, autophagy can act both as a cell survival mechanism when extracellular nutrients or growth factors are limited and as an alternative cell death pathway to apoptosis (Jin, 2006) (Fig. 2). Removal of organelles such as mitochondria, which are apoptotic mediators, may protect the cell against apoptosis. Beclin-1/ATG6 (BECN1) is a key regulator of autophagy (Furuya et al., 2005), and monoallelic loss of the BECN1 locus is seen in over 40% of breast cancers (Liang et al., 1999). BCL2 antiapoptotic proteins can block autophagy by inhibiting BECN1 (Pattingre et al., 2005).

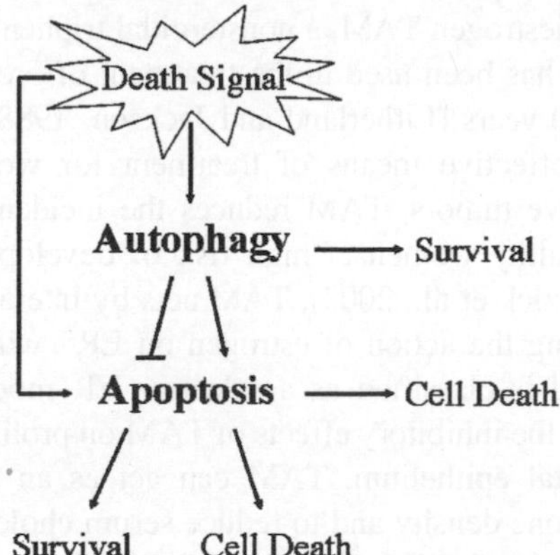

Figure 2 In response to a death signal, autophagy can prevent apoptosis to lead to survival or induce apoptosis to lead to cell death. The mechanism(s) that controls the balance between cell survival and cell death by autophagy, in response to a particular death signal, remains to be clarified.

Thus, antiapoptotic members of the BCL2 family may function as oncogenes not only by directly blocking apoptosis but also by blocking autophagy (Pattingre and Levine, 2006). Although the early events in autophagy are reversible, later events may share mechanism(s) with other death pathways. For example, cleavage of ATG5 by calpain (Yousefi et al., 2006) or upregulation of BID (Lamparska-Przybysz et al., 2006) can switch from autophagy to apoptosis.

Mitotic Catastrophe

Mitotic catastrophe is a type of cell death that occurs during or shortly after failed mitosis, which may occur following treatment with microtubule stabilizing or destabilizing agents or DNA damage (Mansilla et al., 2006; Roninson et al., 2001). The morphological alterations that occur during mitotic catastrophe are distinct from those that occur during apoptosis. These changes include multinucleation or the products of micronuclei because of faulty checkpoints, DNA structure checkpoints, or the spindle assembly checkpoint (also known as mitotic checkpoint) (Castedo et al., 2004; Roninson et al., 2001). The disruption of normal chromosome segregation of many chromosomes results in rapid cell death (Castedo et al., 2004). However, in the absence of cell death following mitotic catastrophe, the cell can divide asymmetrically, resulting in the generation of aneuploid daughter cells (Kops et al., 2005). Hence, mitotic catastrophe prevents irregular mitosis and, in turn, avoids aneuploidization that could lead to oncogenesis (Castedo et al., 2004; Kops et al., 2005).

Necrosis

A cell can undergo necrosis following physical damage or toxic insults when the intracellular level of ATP falls to a level incompatible with survival. The decision to undergo necrosis over apoptosis is dependent on the level of intracellular ATP, since apoptosis requires the presence of ATP, while necrosis results in ATP depletion (Nicotera et al., 1998). Morphologically, necrosis is identified by vacuolation of the cytoplasm, breakdown of the plasma membrane, and an induction of inflammation around the dying cell due to the release of cellular contents and proinflammatory molecules (Edinger and Thompson, 2004). The increase in cell volume (oncosis) during necrosis results in rupturing of the plasma membrane and the unorganized breakdown of swollen organelles (Kroemer et al., 2007). The ability of necrotic cells to promote local inflammation can support tumor growth (Vakkila and Lotze, 2004). While necrosis was previously thought to be a passive form of cell death, over the past several years the idea that cellular signaling pathways can specifically initiate necrosis has gained momentum (Proskuryakov et al., 2003).

Senescence

Cellular senescence was first identified as the state of permanent cell cycle arrest resulting from the replicative exhaustion of normal diploid cells in culture (Hayflick, 1965). Senescent cells appear static but are metabolically active, and appear large and flat with vacuoles and a large nucleus. In contrast to quiescent cells (reversible cell cycle arrest), senescent cells are unresponsive to mitogenic stimuli and are identified by cellular increase in β-galactosidase activity (Dimri et al., 1995). Thus, their inability to respond to serum or growth factors prevents immortalization and subsequent neoplastic transformation of the senescent cells. While apoptosis kills and eliminates potential cancer cells, cellular senescence irreversibly arrests cell growth (Campisi, 2001). Although the signaling mechanism for cellular senescence remains undetermined, DNA damage regulation by tumor suppressor genes such as TP53 and RB and epigenetic regulation of gene expression clearly play crucial roles (Campisi, 2001; Narita, 2007).

Telomeres are DNA-protein complexes that cap the end of linear eukaryotic chromosomes and range from 2 to 15 kb in humans (Martens et al., 1998). Telomeres prevent chromosomes from degradation, recombination, fusing with other chromosomes, and from being mistaken for DNA double-strand breaks. The de novo synthesis of telomeres is dependent on the enzyme telomerase, a reverse transcriptase (Cech, 2004). In most human cells, telomerase activity is gradually downregulated over time, resulting in successive telomere shortening that can ultimately limit their ability to proliferate; this is known as "cellular senescence," "mortality stage 1 (M1)," or "replicative senescence," since the maintenance of functional telomeres is crucial for continued proliferation. Inactivation of cell cycle checkpoint genes like TP53 can result in continued proliferation by bypassing the cell growth arrest in M1, eventually leading to critically short telomeres and massive cell death or "mortality stage 2 (M2)" or "crisis." Individual cells can evade M2 by maintaining their telomerase, resulting in immortal cancer cells that have been reported in 85% to 90% of human tumors (Kim et al., 1994). Thus, inhibition of telomerase activity may be a useful approach for mechanism-based anticancer therapy, reviewed in (Zimmermann and Martens, 2007).

ENDOCRINE THERAPIES

Endocrine therapy is often chosen as the first line of therapy in estrogen receptor α (ERα) and/or progesterone receptor (PR)-positive breast cancer patients because of its established efficacy and safety profile. However, endocrine resistance frequently arises. Two forms of endocrine resistance have been described: de novo resistance that is evident at the initial exposure to endocrine therapy or acquired resistance that arises over time after initiation of endocrine therapy. Absence of ERα expression is the most common de novo resistance mechanism, whereas a complete loss of ER expression is relatively uncommon in acquired resistance (Clarke et al., 2003; Moy and Goss, 2006). Improved knowledge of the mechanism of hormonal resistance, and the relationship between estrogen signaling and cell growth pathways, could provide the basis for combining signaling pathway inhibitors with endocrine therapies.

Antiestrogens, Aromatase Inhibitors, and Apoptosis

Endocrine therapy, administered as an antiestrogen (e.g., TAM or Faslodex) or an aromatase inhibitor (e.g., Letrozolc or Anastrazole), is the least toxic and most effective means to manage hormone-dependent breast cancers. Antiestrogens, and TAM in particular, have been the "gold standard" first-line endocrine therapy for over 20 years. Newer antiestrogens such as Faslodex are also showing significantly improved activity relative to TAM and some aromatase inhibitors (Howell et al., 1995; Howell et al., 2002). Third generation aromatase inhibitors have emerged as viable alternatives to antiestrogens for first-line endocrine therapy; overall response rates are generally greater for aromatase inhibitors (Ferretti et al., 2006). Aromatase inhibitors also have a different mechanism of action and toxicity profile to antiestrogens, but whether this toxicity profile favors aromatase inhibitors over antiestrogens is controversial (Ferretti et al., 2006). Aromatase inhibitors can only be given as single agents to postmenopausal women or to women who do not have functioning ovaries; antiestrogens can be given irrespective of a patient's menopausal status.

The antiestrogen TAM, a nonsteroidal triphenylethylene derivative, has been used in the treatment of breast cancer for over 30 years (Litherland and Jackson, 1988). Besides being an effective means of treatment for women with ERα-positive tumors, TAM reduces the incidence of disease in healthy women at high risk of developing breast cancer (Cuzick et al., 2003). TAM acts by interacting with and blocking the action of estrogen on ERα within breast tumors and is classified as a selective ER modulator. In addition to the inhibitory effects of TAM on proliferation of breast ductal epithelium, TAM can act as an agonist to maintain bone density and to reduce serum cholesterol and triglyceride levels (Osborne et al., 2000). Despite its beneficial activities, prolonged administration of TAM can increase the incidence of endometrial cancer in some postmenopausal women (Wilking et al., 1997). The partial agonist properties of TAM have prompted the use of Faslodex to substitute for TAM as first- or second-line endocrine treatment (Bundred and Howell, 2002; Howell, 2006). A steroidal analogue of 17β-estradiol, Faslodex (ICI 182,780; Fulvestrant) generally provides complete anatagonism without agonist effects, unlike TAM, which acts as a partial agonist. Faslodex prevents estrogen binding to ERα by inducing conformational changes and an eventual reduction of cellular ERα following polyubiquitination; Faslodex is classified as a selective downregulator of ER (SERD) (Osborne et al., 2004).

Antiestrogens primarily function through their ability to compete with estradiol (E2) for binding to ER and inducing growth arrest and cell death (Clarke et al., 2001). The consequences of occupying ER with an antiestrogen depend upon cellular context (i.e., expression of other proteins like ER coreguators), which ER is occupied (ERα, ERβ), and ligand structure (Clarke et al., 2001). The importance of ERα is established; that of ERβ is less clear (Speirs et al., 2004). Higher ERβ mRNA levels in resistant tumors have been reported (Arnold et al., 1995), but this cannot be causally linked to endocrine resistance because ERβ can also be associated with an aggressive phenotype (Dotzlaw et al., 1999; Speirs et al., 1999).

Aromatase inhibitors are often classed as type 1 (steroidal inactivator, e.g., Letrozole, Anastrozole), or type 2 (nonsteroidal inhibitor, e.g., exemestane). Third generation aromatase inhibitors are highly effective in blocking enzyme activity and exhibit notable specificity (Miller, 2004). These drugs act by blocking the ability of the P450 CYP19A1 gene product (aromatase) to convert androgen precursors to estrone or estradiol. Estradiol is the most potent estrogen and is found in high concentrations in breast tumors irrespective of menopausal status or the ER status of the tumor (Clarke et al., 2001; Clarke et al., 2003).

The extent of crossresistance among endocrine therapies is unclear. Since aromatase inhibitors can improve disease-free survival after two to three years of TAM as compared with a total of five years of TAM (Baum et al., 2003; Boccardo et al., 2001; Coombes et al., 2004; Jakesz et al., 2005; Thurlimann et al., 2005), it would seem that some TAM resistant tumors may retain sensitivity to an aromatase inhibitor. Second-and third-line responses to endocrine therapy have been widely documented, but lower response rates of shorter duration are usually observed with each successive line of treatment.

Both TAM and Faslodex can induce apoptosis in cells by inhibiting survival signaling mediated through ERα (Wang et al., 1995; Zhang et al., 1999; Diel et al., 1999). However, the precise mechanism for inducing apoptosis remains controversial. Administration of TAM results in activation of caspases-3, -8, -9 within 18 to 24 hours of drug treatment in rat mammary tumors (Mandlekar et al., 2000a). In addition, the effects of TAM can be mediated through an ERα-independent mechanism that results in an early activation of JNK1 followed by caspase activation (Mandlekar et al., 2000b). TAM can affect the level of proteins involved in cell growth including c-MYC (Kang et al., 1996), protein kinase C (Gelmann, 1996), and transforming growth factor β (TGFβ) (Perry et al., 1995) by ERα-independent mechanisms. However, since ER-negative tumors rarely respond to endocrine therapies (EBCTCG, 1998; EBCTCG, 2002a), these mechanisms are not likely to be responsible for significant apoptotic cell death in vivo.

About 25% of ER-positive/PR-positive tumors, 66% of ER-positive/PR-negative tumors and 55% of ER-negative/PR-positive tumors fail to respond to TAM (Clarke et al., 2003; Moy and Goss, 2006; Osborne and Schiff, 2003). Better predictors of endocrine responsiveness are clearly required. Many initially sensitive tumors become resistant (acquired resistance) (Clarke et al., 2001) and about one-third of all ER-positive breast tumors exhibit de novo endocrine resistance. The mechanisms of resistance to an antiestrogen remain unclear, reflecting a limited understanding of the signaling affecting cell proliferation, survival, and death and their hormonal regulation in breast cancer cells.

Of current interest is identification of the optimum choice and scheduling of antiestrogens and aromatase inhibitors. Evidence clearly shows improvements in overall response or disease-free survival for combined therapy (an aromatase inhibitor and an antiestrogen usually given sequentially) over single agent TAM (Baum et al., 2003; Boccardo et al., 2001; Coombes et al., 2004; Jakesz et al., 2005; Thurlimann et al., 2005). Recent data also imply that response rates are often greater to a first-line aromatase inhibitor than to TAM (Bonneterre et al., 2000; Mouridsen et al., 2001). However, the ability of aromatase inhibitors to induce a significant improvement in overall survival is uncertain. A recent meta-analysis failed to show an advantage for aromatase inhibitors with respect to overall survival, despite clear evidence favoring aromatase inhibitors in other end points (Ferretti et al., 2006). Thus, the optimum first-line endocrine therapy remains controversial for some women, as does the optimum choice and scheduling of combination endocrine therapy. Whichever way these controversies are eventually resolved, it is clear that both aromatase inhibitors and antiestrogens will remain as key modalities in the management of ER-positive breast cancers.

Understanding the signaling mechanism involved in antiestrogen-induced apoptosis is closely related to our knowledge of antiestrogen resistance. Through ongoing research in our laboratory, we have established interferon regulatory factor-1 (IRF-1) as a key node in a putative signaling network associated with responsiveness to endocrine therapy, where IRF-1 modifies ERα-mediated signaling to apoptosis (Bouker et al., 2004; Clarke et al., 2003; Gu et al., 2002). IRF-1 and a dominant negative IRF-1 (dnIRF-1) induce opposing effects on proliferation in vitro and tumorigenesis in vivo through regulation of caspase-3/7 and caspase-8 activities (Bouker et al., 2005). While TP53-dependent apoptosis occurs in the breast (Tu et al., 2005), T47D cells express mutant TP53 and our data show that TP53 is not required for the proapoptotic actions of IRF-1 (Bouker et al., 2004; Bouker et al., 2005). Expression of IRF-1 is reduced in neoplastic versus normal human breast (Doherty et al., 2001), and there is an inverse correlation between IRF-1 and tumor grade (Connett et al., 2005). In a study of mostly ERα-positive breast tumors, nuclear expression of IRF-1 is negatively correlated with NFκB expression, suggesting their expression pattern to be consistent with other genes implicated in our signaling network for endocrine resistance (Zhu et al., 2006).

Upregulation of NFκB is associated with E2-independence (Clarkson and Watson, 1999; Nakshatri et al., 1997) and antiestrogen resistance (Gu et al., 2002; Riggins et al., 2005). The NFκB p50/p65 heterodimer complex comprises two homologous proteins encoded by different genes; the p50 product of its p105 precursor (NFκB1) and NFκB p65 (RELA). While the predominant form in breast cancer cell lines is NFκB (p50/p65), another member of the family (p52) also is expressed in some breast cancers (Cogswell et al., 2000). Perhaps reflecting its regulation by both E2 and growth factors (Biswas et al., 2000; Nakshatri et al., 1997), which are also involved in endocrine resistance (Clarke et al., 2001; Dickson and Lippman, 1995), normal mammary gland development appears to be dependent on NFκB (Clarkson and Watson, 1999). NFκB is maintained in the cytosol in an inactive state, e.g., complexed with members of the *IκB* family that either inhibit nuclear transport or block NFκB's nuclear translocation signal (Tam and Sen, 2001). Generally, activation proceeds by phosphorylation of IκB by the IKK kinase complex, which results in the ubiquitination and degradation of IκB (Yaron et al., 1998). Elevated NFκB activity arises during neoplastic transformation in both the rat (Kim et al., 2000) and mouse mammary gland (Tonko-Geymayer and Doppler, 2002).

Antiestrogens, Aromatase Inhibitors, Autophagy, and the Unfolded Protein Response

While apoptosis is clearly implicated (Bouker et al., 2004; Gaddy et al., 2004; Kyprianou et al., 1991), some of the apoptosis end points in prior studies may not distinguish among earlier events that are more closely linked to signaling initiated through autophagy. Autophagy does occur in response to endocrine therapy (Bursch et al., 1996; Inbal et al., 2002). However, given very recent advances in the understanding of cell death mechanisms, it is not clear if signaling to both apoptosis and autophagy are involved in regulating cell survival, and/or if the initial signaling involves autophagy but later events include signaling to apoptosis.

One cell signaling process that may integrate autophagy and apoptosis in this context is the unfolded protein response (UPR), a key component of the endoplasmic reticulum stress response (Ron, 2002) and an adaptive signaling pathway that allows cells to survive the accumulation of unfolded proteins in the endoplasmic reticulum (Zhang and Kaufman, 2006). Initially a mechanism for allowing cells to recover normal endoplasmic reticulum function, prolonged UPR can induce cell death. UPR is activated by three molecular sensors: IRE1α, ATF6, and PERK (DuRose et al., 2006). Splicing of X-box binding protein 1 (XBP1) by IRE1α is obligatory for IRE1α- and ATF6-induced UPR (DuRose et al., 2006; Yoshida et al., 2001). XBP1 is a transcription factor; the unspliced form, XBP1(U), has a molecular weight (Mr) of approximately 33 kDa and acts as a dominant negative (Lee et al., 2003; Sriburi et al., 2004). The spliced, active form, XBP1(S), has a Mr of approximately 54 kDa. A very recent study shows that the UPR (initiated by XBP1 splicing) can induce autophagy (Ogata et al., 2006). Whether this is a prosurvival or prodeath form of autophagy is unknown, since UPR can induce both prodeath and prosurvival outcomes (Feldman et al., 2005). In MCF7 and T47D breast cancer cells, we have shown that overexpression of XBP1(S) prevents antiestrogen-induced cell cycle arrest and cell death via the mitochondrial apoptotic pathway. Therefore, XBP1 may be a useful molecular target for the development of novel predictive and therapeutic strategies in breast cancer (Gomez et al., 2007, in press). Figure 3

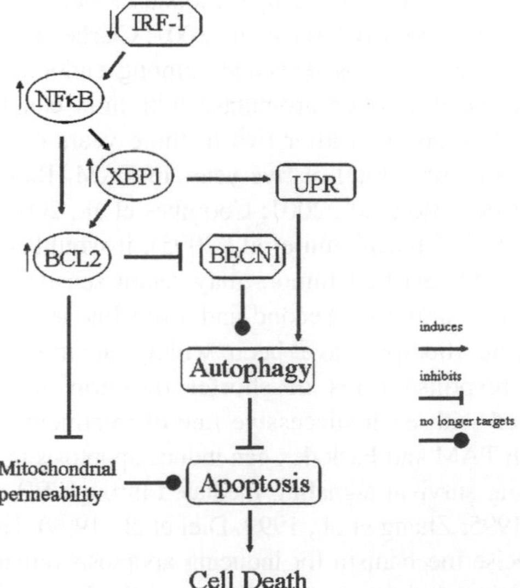

Figure 3 Some of the signaling mechanisms involved in endocrine resistance in breast cancer cells. *Abbreviations*: Interferon regulatory factor 1, IRF-1; nuclear factor kappa B, NFκB; X-box binding protein 1, XBP1; unfolded protein response, UPR; B-cell CLL/lymphoma 2, BCL2; beclin 1, BECN1.

shows some of the signaling mechanisms involved in endocrine resistance in breast cancer, based on the research done by others and our group.

CYTOTOXIC THERAPIES

Anthracyclines

Anthracyclines such as Doxorubicin are widely used in breast cancer treatment for the treatment of metastatic breast cancer. The mechanisms for the antineoplastic activities of doxorubucin are complex and include intercalation with DNA, direct cell membrane effects, initiation of DNA damage, apoptosis through inhibition of topoisomerase II, and the production of reactive oxygen species (Minotti et al., 2004). Despite its efficacy, Doxorubicin has several undesirable side effects, especially a cumulative cardiac toxicity (Singal and Iliskovic, 1998) (Table 1).

Doxorubicin-induced apoptosis occurs through a different signal transduction mechanism in nontransformed cells, such as endothelial cells and cardiomyocytes (H_2O_2-dependent), when compared with tumor cells that harbor a functional TP53 (Wang et al., 2004). Thus, targeted drug therapy could minimize cytotoxicity in normal cells and maximize cell death in cancer cells. The NF-κB/BCL2 pathway is a possible mechanism for tumor resistance to anthracyline-based chemotherapy. In breast tumor samples from patients treated with neoadjuvant Doxorubicin-based chemotherapy, nuclear localization of NF-κB is associated with expression of BCL2 and BAX. Moreover, the NF-κB/BCL2 pathway may be associated with a poor response to neoadjuvant Doxorubicin-based chemotherapy (Buchholz et al., 2005).

Alkylating Agents

Cyclophosphamide (CPA) is an alkylating agent that alkylates DNA, forming DNA-DNA cross-links that result in an inhibition of DNA synthesis and cell death. CPA is a prodrug that is metabolically activated in the liver by cytochrome P450 enzymes. Activated CPA metabolites, e.g., hydroxyl-CPA, are transported via the bloodstream to both tumor and healthy tissues, where DNA and protein damage can occur (Moore, 1991). Cisplatin (cis-diaminedichloroplatinum II), another alkylating agent, exerts its cytotoxic effects by reacting with DNA to

Table 1 Breast Cancer Therapeutics and Their Effect on Cell Death

Drug	Primary target	Selected cell death signaling
Endocrine agents		
Faslodex, Tamoxifen	Estrogen receptor α	Caspase activation, BCL2 downregulation, JNK activation caspase activation, BAK upregulation
Anastrazole, Letrozole	CYP19A1 aromatase	
Anthracyclines		
Doxorubicin, Epirubicin	DNA intercalation, topoisomerase II	BCL2 family regulation, NFκB inhibition, TP53 activation
Alkylating agents		
Cisplatin, Cyclophosphamide	DNA crosslinking	Caspase activation, TP53 activation, cytochrome c release
Antimetabolites		
5-fluorouracil, Capecitabine	Thymidylate synthase	TP53 activation, thymineless death
Microtubule inhibitors		
Docetaxel, Paclitaxel	Microtubule stabilization	Caspase activation, phosphorylation of BCL2 and BCLX, JNK activation, CD95/FAS expression
Vinorelbine, Vincristine	Microtubule dissolution	TP53 activation, posttranslational modification of BCL2 family members
Signal transduction inhibitors		
Gefitinib	EGFR kinase activity	Phosphorylation of BAD, downregulation of BCL2
Trastuzumab, CH401	HER2 extracellular domain	Inhibition of PI3K/AKT, phosphorylation of BAD, JNK activation
Dasatinib, AZD0530	c-Src kinase activity	Inhibition of PI3K/AKT, downregulation of BCLX
Genasense	BCL2	Downregulation of BCL2
ABT-737, others	BCL2 and BCLX	Prevention of BCL2 and BCLX interaction with proapoptotic BAX and BAK
Bortezomib	26S proteasome	Inhibition of PI3K/AKT, JNK activation, sensitization to TRAIL
Bevacizumab	VEGFR2	DNA fragmentation, inhibition of PI3K/AKT

yield a variety of adducts, the most common adduct being an intrastrand cross-link between adjacent guanines (Perez, 1998). Cisplatin can be administered as a first-line therapy for metastatic breast carcinoma (Sledge Jr., et al., 1988) or in combination with other chemotherapeutic drugs (Kourousis et al., 1998; Nagourney et al., 2000).

Besides targeting genomic DNA, Cisplatin can also bind to mitochondrial DNA, interact with phospholipids and phosphatidylserine in membranes, disrupt the cytoskeleton, and affect the polymerization of actin (Jamieson and Lippard, 1999). Thus, Cisplatin interaction with proteins is also a possible mechanism for Cisplatin-induced apoptosis (Perez, 1998). Cisplatin can activate caspases by stabilizing TP53 and releasing cytochrome *c* from mitochondria (Siddik, 2002). Cell death by both apoptosis and necrosis has been found in the same population of ovarian cancer cells treated with Cisplatin (Pestell et al., 2000). Studies in MCF7 breast cancer cell have shown that antisense BCL2 and Cisplatin combination therapy could potentially be useful in treating breast cancer overexpressing BCL2, perhaps by activating caspase-8 independent of TP53 status (Basma et al., 2005). High doses of Cisplatin (>312 μM) can damage molecules involved in cellular energy supply (such as ATP) or proteins involved in apoptosis (such as TP53, caspases, BCL2, and BAX), leading to necrotic cell death. Thus, dose of cisplatin or the context of the target cells could direct the mode of cell death either by a defective apoptotic program or by necrosis (Gonzalez et al., 2001). Mechanisms of resistance to Cisplatin include loss of damage recognition, overexpression of HER-2/neu, activation of the PI3K/AKT (also known as PI3K/PKB) pathway, loss of TP53 function, overexpression of BCL2, and interference in caspase activation (Siddik, 2002).

Antimetabolites

Antimetabolites, particularly the fluoropyrimidine 5-fluorouracil (5-FU), are widely used as chemotherapeutic agents in the treatment of breast cancer. Within the cell, 5-FU is metabolized to 5-fluoro-deoxyuridine monophosphate (FdUMP) that interacts with and inhibits thymidylate synthase (TS) and prevents the formation of thymidine 5′-monophosphate (dTMP), thus inhibiting DNA synthesis (Chu et al., 2003; Longley et al., 2003). Thymidine phosphorylase (TP) mediates the conversion of 5-FU into fluorouridine diphosphate (FUDP) by transfer of a ribose phosphate from phosphoribosylpyrophosphate (PRPP) performed by orotic acid phosphoribosyltransferase (OPRTase). FUDP can be phosophorylated to FUTP and incorporated into RNA-by-RNA polymerase. FdUMP is converted to fluorodeoxyuridine triphosphate (FdUTP) and is directly incorporated into DNA (Chu et al., 2003; Longley et al., 2003).

The cytotoxic effect of 5-FU can occur through a process called thymineless death (Houghton et al., 1997). At the level of DNA synthesis, FdUMP acts as a competitive inhibitor of TS that results in a dTTP/dUMP cellular pool imbalance with subsequent DNA damage (Hernandez-Vargas et al., 2006; Parker and Cheng, 1990). Breast cancer patients with high pretreatment levels of TS protein show increased response to 5-FU-based chemotherapy (Nishimura et al., 1999). In addition, inhibition of RNA metabolism (Longley et al., 2003) and interference with polyamine metabolism (Zhang et al., 2003) could also contribute to the antiproliferative effects of 5-FU. In response to 5-FU treatment of MCF7 breast cancer cells, increased expression of TP53 target genes that are involved in cell cycle and apoptosis including CDKN1A (CIP1, WAF1), TP53INP, CD95/FAS, and BBC3/PUMA, along with significant repression of *MYC* (Hernandez-Vargas et al., 2006). Low doses of 5-FU (IC_{50}, 10 μM) result in cell cycle arrest, while high doses (IC_{80}, 500 μM) result in apoptosis in breast cancer cells (Hernandez-Vargas et al., 2006). Thus, the TP53 status of tumors and tissue concentration of 5-FU could be important determinants of drug efficacy in breast cancer treatment. Capecitabine is an example of a rationally designed cytotoxic drug that generates 5-FU preferentially in tumor cells by exploiting their higher activity of the activating enzyme TP compared with healthy tissues. The use of such targeted therapies increases efficacy and minimizes toxicity. Capecitabine has good activity and a favorable safety profile when used for the treatment of metastatic breast cancer (Yarden et al., 2004).

Microtubule Inhibitors

Microtubules form an integral part of the cytoskeleton and consist of α- and β-tubulin heterodimers. Taxanes (e.g., Taxol/Paclitaxel, Taxotere/Docetaxel) and vinca alkaloids (e.g., Vincristine, Vinorelbine) target microtubules and are often used to treat breast cancer. However, these drugs have very distinct effects on microtubule stability. While taxanes promote tubulin polymerization and stabilization (Schiff et al., 1979), vinca alkaloids inhibit tubulin polymerization (Johnson et al., 1960). Cells can die through either apoptotic or nonapoptotic pathways, but the precise signaling pathways involved are not completely elucidated.

Paclitaxel induces aberrant mitotic spindle formation (Fuchs and Johnson, 1978) that results in G2-M cell cycle arrest followed by cell death. At concentrations lower than those required for microtubule disruption (2–4 nM), taxanes can inhibit cell growth, implying the existence of alternative mechanisms of action (Ganansia-Leymarie et al., 2003; Hernandez-Vargas et al., 2007). Several proapoptotic signaling mechanisms are implicated in response to antimicrotubule agents that appear independent of microtubule binding, such as phosphorylation of and binding to BCL2/$BCLX_L$ antiapoptotic proteins (Haldar et al., 1997), activation of jun N-terminal kinase (JNK) (Wang et al., 1998) and RAF1 kinase (Blagosklonny et al., 1996). Other apoptosis-related proteins including TP53, CDKN1A, and BAX, and caspases are involved in apoptotic cell death process induced by taxanes (Ganansia-Leymarie et al., 2003). Phosphorylation of caveolin-1, a regulator of proapoptotic proteins, increases Paclitaxel sensitivity in MCF7 breast cancer cells by facilitating BCL2 phosphorylation and regulating the induction of CDKN1A (Shajahan et al., 2007). The death receptor CD95/FAS, a mediator of apoptosis, is induced after taxane therapy (Hernandez-Vargas et al., 2007). Treatment of breast cancer cells with low levels of Docetaxel (2–4 nM) triggers necrosis, while a higher concentration of the drug (100 nM) induces apoptosis (Hernandez-Vargas et al., 2007). Moreover, cell death by autophagy has been described as a form of PCD following treatment with taxanes in breast cancer cells (Gorka et al., 2005). Thus, both apoptotic and nonapoptotic pathways are likely responsible for cell death in response to taxanes.

Vinorelbine is an antimitotic drug that impairs chromosomal segregation during mitosis by blocking cell cycle at G2/M phase. Like other mitotic poisons, vinorelbine can induce apoptosis in cancer cells but an understanding of the signaling mechanism(s) of cell death mediated by vinca alkaloids is incomplete. Disruption of microtubules by vinca alkaloids can cause induction of TP53 and regulation of a number of proteins involved in apoptosis including CDKN1A, RAS/RAF, and PKC/PKA (Wang et al., 1999). As is the case with taxanes, BCL2 phosphorylation/inactivation plays a role in apoptosis induction (Haldar et al., 1995), resulting in a decrease in BCL2 inhibition of the proapoptotic protein BAX (Wang et al., 1999).

TARGETED INHIBITORS OF SIGNALING TRANSDUCTION PATHWAYS

In addition to the conventional cytotoxic and endocrine therapies discussed above, novel signal transduction inhibitors are emerging as valuable tools for inducing breast cancer cell death in vitro and in vivo. The precise molecular targets of these agents are varied, ranging from cell surface receptors to components of the proteasomal degradation pathway (recently reviewed in (Bremer et al., 2006). The purpose of these agents is to induce death in malignant cells while leaving normal tissue relatively unaffected, a goal that is potentially achievable if the signaling pathways contributing to malignant transformation are known. Given that a comprehensive analysis of all such agents as they pertain to breast cancer therapy is beyond the scope of this review, we will instead focus on three broad classes of molecules and their targeted therapies that have shown promise in the clinic.

The epidermal growth factor receptor (EGFR) and its family member HER2 are important mediators of breast cancer cell proliferation and survival [reviewed in (Badache and Gonsalves, 2006)]. Overexpression of EGFR and HER2 are associated with poor prognosis. While HER2 is amplified in approximately one-third of breast cancers, it is rare for either EGFR or HER2 to exhibit activating mutations (Diehl et al., 2007). Other receptors, such as insulin-like growth factor 1 receptor (IGF-1R), TGFβ receptor, and vascular endothelial growth factor receptor (VEGFR; see below) are additional targets that are receiving increased attention for their potential in the treatment of breast cancer.

Downstream of growth factor receptors, many intracellular signaling molecules coordinate the aberrant pro-growth and prosurvival signals that lead to tumorigenesis. Other gene products are coupled to death receptors that transduce proapoptotic signals, while still others regulate cell proliferation and survival independent of growth factor receptors. The nonreceptor tyrosine kinase c-Src (Src) is overexpressed in approximately 70% of breast cancers, and the associated increase in its activity contributes significantly to tumor cell survival (recently reviewed in (Ishizawar and Parsons, 2004). The expression of intracellular signaling partners for TNF, FAS, TRAIL, and other cell surface death receptors may also be reduced, leaving cancer cells unable to respond to extrinsic apoptotic signals. More globally, deregulated expression of apoptotic gatekeepers like BCL2, or the ubiquitin-proteasome pathway, can disrupt the entire cell death program (Bremer et al., 2006).

In addition to the targeted therapies that directly disrupt cancer cell proliferation, others are designed to inhibit a tumor's ability to grow and spread by other means. Solid tumors such as breast cancer are particularly dependent on the formation of new blood vessels and capillary networks, both to supply fresh oxygen and nutrients and remove metabolic waste. The generation of new vascular tissue is known as angiogenesis; VEGF strongly induces angiogenesis by binding to the VEGFR2 expressed on endothelial cells. Many cancers, including those of the breast, overexpress VEGF, and agents that block angiogenesis via this signal transduction pathway have the capacity to induce apoptosis by starving the tumor [reviewed in (Schneider and Sledge, Jr., 2007).

Growth Factor Receptor Inhibitors

Preclinical studies of growth factor receptor inhibitors have revealed the potential of these agents to induce cell death by various means. The kinase inhibitor Gefitinib (ZD1839, Iressa) is an antagonist for EGFR but also has some activity toward HER2, and has been shown to induce apoptosis in breast cancer cell lines through the mitochondrial or intrinsic apoptotic pathway. These effects arise either by decreased phosphorylation of proapoptotic BAD [reviewed in (Motoyama and Hynes, 2003)], or by down regulation of prosurvival BCL2 (Okubo et al., 2004). Okubo et al. also show that Gefitinib enhances apoptosis induced by the steroidal antiestrogen Faslodex in ER-positive breast cancer cell lines. Others have reported that Gefitinib can restore antiestrogen sensitivity in MCF7/HER2 xenografts that have become resistant to either Faslodex or estrogen deprivation (Massarweh et al., 2006). EGFR inhibition also has the potential to enhance or restore sensitivity to other chemotherapeutic agents. MCF7/ADR breast cancer cells are resistant to multiple drugs because of overexpression of the transport pump gp170/*MDR1*, and they have also been shown to express high levels of EGFR and its ligand TGFα (Ciardiello et al., 2002). However, Gefitinib is able to restore Paclitaxel- and Docetaxel-mediated apoptosis in MCF7/ADR cells, despite persistent expression of the transporter. Gefitinib may also prove useful in the treatment of high-risk women with ductal carcinoma in situ (DCIS); ER-positive and ER-negative DCIS grown as subcutaneous xenografts in nude mice are both sensitive to growth inhibition and the induction of apoptosis by this drug (Chan et al., 2002).

Inhibition of HER2 using the targeted monoclonal antibody Trastuzumab can also induce apoptosis in breast cancer cells through blocking HER2-mediated phosphoinositol 3-kinase (PI3K) and AKT activity. HER2-induced PI3K/AKT activity would normally promote cell survival by phosphorylating and inhibiting the proapoptotic functions of BAD (Badache and Gonsalves, 2006; Meric-Bernstam and Hung, 2006; Zhou and Hung, 2003). In addition, a novel inhibitory antibody targeted toward HER2 (CH401) has been shown to not only inhibit PI3K/AKT activities but also to directly induce apoptosis through modulation of JNK and p38 in gastric cancer cells (Hinoda et al., 2004). Whether this antibody will show similar activity toward HER2 in breast cancer remains to be determined.

Other growth factor receptor inhibitors have shown promise in both in vitro and preclinical studies. IGF-IR regulates cell proliferation, survival, and migration in multiple cancer models, using intracellular signal transduction pathways similar to those utilized by EGFR and HER2 (e.g., PI3K/AKT and RAS/MAPK) [recently reviewed in (Sachdev and Yee, 2007)]. However, unlike these receptors, IGF-IR signaling events cannot be induced by overexpression of the receptor and are exclusively ligand dependent. Therefore, strategies for inhibition of this pathway focus on blocking expression and/or function of the IGF-I ligand and its receptor. Humanized, single-chain antibodies directed against IGF-IR can induce downregulation of receptor expression in MCF7 breast cancer cells in vitro and grown as xenografts (Maloney et al., 2003; Sachdev et al., 2003). Over-expression of signal-inhibitory IGF binding proteins is also reported to inhibit IGF-IR signaling and cell growth while inducing breast cancer cell death [reviewed in (Maloney et al., 2003; Sachdev and Yee, 2007)].

Finally, TGFβ signaling represents another promising target for specific inhibition in breast cancer. It is well established that the type 1 TGFβ receptor can activate PI3K survival pathways and promote mammary epithelial cell survival (Muraoka-Cook et al., 2006; Yi et al., 2005). In the context of overexpressed HER2, TGFβ1 potently stimulates cell migration (Ueda et al., 2004). In addition, Arteaga et al. have shown that inhibitory antibodies to TGFβ2 can prevent the growth of established MCF7/LCC2 TAM-resistant xenografts (Arteaga et al., 1999). A number of approaches have been explored for inhibiting the TGFβ pathway, including small-molecule inhibitors, antisense oligonucleotides, and monoclonal antibody therapy (recently reviewed in (Lahn et al., 2005). One of these compounds, LY-580276, has been shown to significantly inhibit tumor development in MX1 xenografts, a model of ER-negative/PR-negative breast cancer. More recently, the TGFβ receptor kinase inhibitor SB-431542 has been demonstrated to abrogate epithelial-to-mesenchymal transition and wound healing in mouse mammary epithelial cells and the ER-negative/PR-negative MDA-MB-231 breast cancer cell line (Halder et al., 2005). Cell proliferation, as measured by [^{3}H] thymidine incorporation, is also inhibited under these conditions. However the molecular mechanism of cell death induced by these agents is unknown, and it is also important to consider that in many cell types TGFβ signaling has growth-inhibitory rather than growth-promoting effects.

Intracellular Signaling Inhibitors and Activators

Growth factor and other cell surface receptors can use diverse intracellular signaling partners to control cell growth and apoptosis. Receptors on the surface of a tumor cell can make for a relatively easy target for molecular inhibition. However, if the normal function and regulation of the intracellular signaling network(s) upon which these receptors rely is also disrupted, inhibiting only the receptor will be often ineffective. For example, altered downstream signaling may explain, in part, why the in vivo efficacy of EGFR and HER2 inhibitors has been mixed (Johnston, 2006). The use of agents designed to target intracellular signaling partners such as c-Src, BCL2, components of the proteasome, and transcription factors such as signal transducer and activator of transcription (STAT), STAT3 and STAT5, is likely to improve our ability to selectively induce apoptosis in breast cancer, perhaps in combination with receptor-targeted therapies.

c-Src's overexpression in a large percentage of breast cancers makes it an attractive target for therapeutic intervention [reviewed in (Ishizawar and Parsons, 2004)]. It is well established that EGFR and c-Src kinase activities synergistically promote breast cancer cell growth and survival (Biscardi et al., 2000). c-Src activity can also be regulated by physical and functional interactions with other proteins that include p130Cas (Burnham et al., 2000), and this has recently been shown to play a critical role in antiestrogen resistance in breast cancer (Riggins et al., 2006), in part through attenuating TAM-induced apoptosis. Despite these findings, there are currently no c-Src-specific inhibitors in clinical use for the treatment of breast cancer. Dasatinib (BMS-354825) is a dual inhibitor of c-Src and the Abl kinase which has recently been approved for use in chronic myelogenous leukemia (CML), and this agent has also recently been shown to inhibit the growth of "triple negative" breast cancer cell lines that lack expression of ER, PR, and EGFR, a subset of tumors that is often difficult to treat (Finn et al., 2007). AZD0530 is another dual c-Src/Abl inhibitor that has been shown to inhibit breast cancer cell growth and motility in vitro (Hiscox et al., 2006). In models of lung cancer and CML, Dasatinib can reduce AKT activity and expression of the prosurvival protein BCLX (Nam et al., 2007), although it is not yet known whether this also occurs in breast cancer.

Growth factor receptors and c-Src share the STAT family of proteins, specifically STAT3 and STAT5, as targets. These transcription factors regulate apoptosis in normal mammary gland development (Clarkson et al., 2006) and therefore are important players in breast cancer. However, their lack of enzymatic and ligand binding activities makes them difficult to target. Multiple alternative approaches have been considered for the targeted inhibition of STAT3 and STAT5, including small hairpin RNA, peptide mimetics that prevent binding to signaling partners, and small molecules such as sulindac and cyclooxygenase inhibitors [reviewed in (Desrivieres et al., 2006)].

The prosurvival protein BCL2 and components of the ubiquitin-proteasome system represent two signaling pathways that are essential to the proper regulation of apoptosis. Like STAT3/5 these also lack enzymatic activity, making them more difficult to target in the treatment of breast and other cancers. However, inhibition of BCL2 by the antisense oligonucleotide Genasense (oblimersen sodium, G3139) has been successful in improving the sensitivity of breast cancer preclinical models to apoptosis induced by conventional chemotherapies [reviewed in (Nahta and Esteva, 2003)], even in models of multiple-drug-resistant breast cancer (Lopes de Menezes et al., 2003). Genasense has also been studied in phase I clinical trials in combination with standard chemotherapeutics in many types of cancer including breast (Marshall et al., 2004) and hormone-refractory prostate cancer (Kim et al., 2007; Tolcher et al., 2004). More recently, small molecule inhibitors of *BCL2* function have been developed that are designed to disrupt its interaction with (and inhibition of) proapoptotic family members BAK and BAX. HA14-1 and YC137 are early-generation BCL2 inhibitors that have been shown to induce apoptosis alone and in combination with other drugs in breast cancer cell lines (Real et al., 2004; Witters et al., 2007). A newer BCL2/BCLX inhibitor (ABT-737) that has recently been developed may also prove useful in the sensitization of breast cancer to apoptosis induced by chemotherapeutic drugs (Dai and Grant, 2007).

The ubiquitin-dependent proteasome degradative pathway plays a critical role in maintaining appropriate cellular function by regulating the stability of signaling proteins. The classical pathway relies on conjugation of multiple ubiquitin moieties to the target protein, which is then degraded by the 26S proteasome. In contrast, monoubiquitination appears to regulate endocytosis and/or trafficking within the nucleus [reviewed in (Ohta and Fukuda, 2004)]. Both of these processes are active in breast cancer, and many important mediators of breast cancer cell proliferation and apoptosis are targets of the ubiquitin-proteasome pathway, including EGFR and ER (Marx et al., 2007). Consequently, there is considerable interest in studying the ability of proteasome inhibitors for the treatment of breast cancer (Dees and Orlowski, 2006). Bortezomib (PS-341, Velcade) is a small-molecule peptide mimetic that inhibits the 20S core of the proteasome that has been approved for the treatment of multiple myeloma (Voorhees and Orlowski, 2006). In SKBR3, MDA-MB-453, MCF7 and MCF7/HER2 breast cancer cell lines, Bortezomib can enhance apoptosis induced by the HER2 inhibitor Trastuzumab (Cardoso et al., 2006) and downregulate AKT activity, while stimulating apoptotic JNK activity, in combination with the multikinase inhibitor sorafenib in MDA-MB-231 breast cancer cells (Yu et al., 2006). Brooks et al. have shown that Bortezomib can sensitize some breast cancer cell lines to apoptosis induced by TRAIL, but this does not occur in all breast cancer models (Brooks et al., 2005). In a phase I study of Bortezomib in 12 patients with metastatic breast cancer, the drug showed minimal toxicity but was not efficacious in either stabilizing disease or improving outcome (Yang et al., 2006). It is likely that this, and other signal transduction inhibitors, will need to be used in combination with other therapeutics to be a viable treatment option for breast cancer.

Antiangiogenic Agents

Specific inhibition of VEGFR2 is a common approach for targeting angiogenesis in solid tumors, including those of the breast. VEGFR2 is expressed in the vasculature, where proliferation during the process of angiogenesis can be stimulated in a paracrine manner by VEGF expressed by the tumor. Bevacizumab (Avastin) is a humanized monoclonal antibody directed against the VEGF ligand and the pursuit of similar angiogenesis inhibitors is an active focus of clinical breast cancer research [reviewed in (Schneider and Sledge Jr., 2007)]. Bevacizumab alone or in combination with Doxorubicin significantly inhibits VEGFR2 activation and angiogenic measures such as vascular permeability in women with inflammatory breast cancer (Wedam et al., 2006), and has been shown to significantly improve disease-free survival when combined with Paclitaxel in the treatment of metastatic breast cancer (Miller et al., 2005). Wedam et al. also showed that Bevacizumab induces apoptosis in vivo, as measured by terminal deoxynucleotidyl transferse-mediated dUTP nick-end labeling (TUNEL) staining (Wedam et al., 2006). In an in vitro model of lung tumorigenesis, Bevacizumab reduces AKT phosphorylation and activity (Inoue et al., 2007), although whether this occurs in the context of breast cancer is unknown.

SUMMARY AND CONCLUSIONS

We are now beginning to more clearly understand the molecular mechanisms of chemotherapy, endocrine therapy, and signal transduction inhibitor action and specifically how these compounds regulate tumor cell death. However, several key challenges remain. How we address these issues will directly affect our ability to be successful in the clinical management of breast cancer and in improving the outlook of women diagnosed with this disease.

One difficulty that is encountered is the heterogeneity among tumors and the multiple ways by which tumor cells can die in response to chemotherapeutic drugs. It is hoped that advancement of our knowledge of the molecular mechanisms of these drugs along with a greater understanding of tumorigenesis will enable more individualized treatment. In future, drug development and design must take into account the comprehensive cellular signaling mechanisms of inhibition of the target and the likely mechanisms by which resistance can develop to these drugs. In this regard, advances in biotechnology and bioinformatics will facilitate researchers and clinicians to assess high-throughput data gathered from DNA or proteomic arrays and tissue microarrays to enable molecular profiling of a patient's tumor. Thus, individual patients can be given a specific dose and type of chemotherapeutic drug that will increase efficacy and reduce unwanted toxicities.

A second challenge is redefining tumor cell death in the clinical setting. A reduction in tumor size is often considered evidence of a therapeutic agent's ability to induce cancer cell death. However, tumor shrinkage alone does not provide an understanding of the molecular mechanism(s) that control cell death in this context, and the signal transduction pathways that operate in vitro may not always be active in vivo. For many of the therapies discussed above, we do not yet understand whether the in vitro and in vivo cell death mechanisms of action are the same. This is particularly true for the newer, more specific signal transduction inhibitors. For example, when used in the neoadjuvant setting Trastuzumab can induce apoptosis in breast tumors, as measured by reduced AKT phosphorylation and increased cleavage of caspase-3 (Mohsin et al., 2005). In addition, Bevacizumab can induce DNA fragmentation in metastatic breast cancer (Wedam et al., 2006). However as more phase I/II clinical trials incorporate biomarker discovery into their design, we anticipate that these studies will generate important new data that clarify the in vivo apoptotic effects of these signal transduction inhibitors and other chemotherapeutic agents in breast cancer.

REFERENCES

Ahlgren M, Melbye M, Wohlfahrt J, Sorensen TI. Growth patterns and the risk of breast cancer in women. N Engl J Med 2004; 351:1619–1626.

American Cancer Society. Breast Cancer Facts & Figures 2007–2008. Atlanta: American Cancer Society, Inc.

Arnold SF, Obourn JD, Yudt MR, Carter, TH Notides, AC. In vivo and in vitro phosphorylation of the human estrogen receptor. J Steroid Biochem Mol Biol 1995; 52:159–171.

Arteaga CL, Koli KM, Dugger TC, Clarke R. Reversal of tamoxifen resistance of human breast carcinomas in vivo by neutralizing antibodies to transforming growth factor-beta. J Natl Cancer Inst 1999; 91:46–53.

Badache A, Gonsalves A. The ErbB2 signaling network as a target for breast cancer therapy. J Mammary Gland Biol Neoplasia 2006; 11:13–25.

Basma H, El-Refaey H, Sgagias MK, Cowan KH, Luo X, Cheng PW. BCL-2 antisense and cisplatin combination treatment of MCF-7 breast cancer cells with or without functional p53. J Biomed Sci 2005; 12:999–1011.

Baum M, Buzdar A, Cuzick J, Forbes J, Houghton J, Howell A, Sahmoud T. Anastrozole alone or in combination with tamoxifen versus tamoxifen alone for adjuvant treatment of postmenopausal women with early-stage breast cancer: results of the ATAC (Arimidex, Tamoxifen Alone or in Combination) trial efficacy and safety update analyses. Cancer 2003; 98:1802–1810.

Biscardi JS, Ishizawar RC, Silva CM, Parsons SJ. Tyrosine kinase signalling in breast cancer: epidermal growth factor receptor and c-Src interactions in breast cancer. Breast Cancer Res 2000; 2:203–210.

Biswas DK, Cruz AP, Gansberger E, Pardee AB. Epidermal growth factor-induced nuclear factor kappa B activation: A major pathway of cell-cycle progression in estrogen-receptor negative breast cancer cells. Proc Natl Acad Sci U S A 2000; 97:8542–8547.

Blagosklonny MV, Schulte T, Nguyen P, Trepel J, Neckers LM. Taxol-induced apoptosis and phosphorylation of

Bcl-2 protein involves c-Raf-1 and represents a novel c-Raf-1 signal transduction pathway. Cancer Res 1996; 56: 1851–1854.

Boccardo F, Rubagotti A, Amoroso D, Mesiti M, Romeo D, Caroti C, Farris A, Cruciani G, Villa E, Schieppati G, Mustacchi G. Sequential tamoxifen and aminoglutethimide versus tamoxifen alone in the adjuvant treatment of post-menopausal breast cancer patients: results of an Italian cooperative study. J Clin Oncol 2001; 19:4209–4215.

Bonneterre J, Buzdar A, Nabholtz JM, Robertson JF, Thurlimann B, von Euler M, Sahmoud T, Webster A, Steinberg M. Anastrozole is superior to tamoxifen as first-line therapy in hormone receptor positive advanced breast carcinoma. Cancer 2000; 92:2247–2258.

Bouker KB, Skaar TC, Fernandez DR, O'Brien KA, Riggins RB, Cao D, Clarke R. Interferon regulatory factor-1 mediates the proapoptotic but not cell cycle arrest effects of the steroidal antiestrogen ICI 182,780 (faslodex, fulvestrant). Cancer Res 2004; 64:4030–4039.

Bouker KB, Skaar TC, Riggins RB, Harburger DS, Fernandez DR, Zwart A, Wang A, Clarke R. Interferon regulatory factor-1 (IRF-1) exhibits tumor suppressor activities in breast cancer associated with caspase activation and induction of apoptosis. Carcinogenesis 2005; 26:1527–1535.

Bremer E, van Dam G, Kroesen BJ, de Leij L, Helfrich W. Targeted induction of apoptosis for cancer therapy: current progress and prospects. Trends Mol Med 2006; 12:382–393.

Brooks AD, Ramirez T, Toh U, Onksen J, Elliott PJ, Murphy WJ, Sayers TJ. The proteasome inhibitor bortezomib (Velcade) sensitizes some human tumor cells to Apo2L/TRAIL-mediated apoptosis. Ann N Y Acad Sci 2005; 1059: 160–167.

Brown JM, Attardi LD. The role of apoptosis in cancer development and treatment response. Nat Rev Cancer 2005; 5: 231–237.

Buchholz TA, Garg AK, Chakravarti N, Aggarwal BB, Esteva FJ, Kuerer HM, Singletary SE, Hortobagyi GN, Pusztai L, Cristofanilli M, Sahin AA. The nuclear transcription factor kappaB/bcl-2 pathway correlates with pathologic complete response to doxorubicin-based neoadjuvant chemotherapy in human breast cancer. Clin Cancer Res 2005; 11:8398–8402.

Bundred N, Howell A. Fulvestrant (Faslodex): current status in the therapy of breast cancer. Expert Rev Anticancer Ther 2002; 2:151–160.

Burnham MR, Bruce-Staskal PJ, Harte MT, Weidow CL, Ma A, Weed SA, Bouton AH. Regulation of c-SRC activity and function by the adapter protein CAS. Mol Cell Biol 2000; 20:5865–5878.

Bursch W, Ellinger A, Kienzl H, Torok L, Pandey S, Sikorska M, Walker R, Hermann RS. Active cell death induced by the anti-estrogens tamoxifen and ICI 164 384 in human mammary carcinoma cells (MCF-7) in culture: the role of autophagy. Carcinogenesis 1996; 17: 1595–1607.

Cain K, Bratton SB, Cohen GM. The Apaf-1 apoptosome: a large caspase-activating complex. Biochimie 2002; 84:203–214.

Campisi J. Cellular senescence as a tumor-suppressor mechanism. Trends Cell Biol 2001; 11:S27–S31.

Cande C, Vahsen N, Kouranti I, Schmitt E, Daugas E, Spahr C, Luban J, Kroemer RT, Giordanetto F, Garrido C, Penninger JM, Kroemer G. AIF and cyclophilin A cooperate in apoptosis-associated chromatinolysis. Oncogene 2004; 23:1514–1521.

Cardoso F, Durbecq V, Laes JF, Badran B, Lagneaux L, Bex F, Desmedt C, Willard-Gallo K, Ross JS, Burny A, Piccart M, Sotiriou C. Bortezomib (PS-341, Velcade) increases the efficacy of trastuzumab (Herceptin) in HER-2-positive breast cancer cells in a synergistic manner. Mol Cancer Ther 2006; 5:3042–3051.

Castedo M, Perfettini JL, Roumier T, Andreau K, Medema R, Kroemer G. Cell death by mitotic catastrophe: a molecular definition. Oncogene 2004; 23:2825–2837.

Cech TR. Beginning to understand the end of the chromosome. Cell 2004; 116:273–279.

Chan KC, Knox WF, Gee JM, Morris J, Nicholson RI, Potten CS, Bundred NJ. Effect of epidermal growth factor receptor tyrosine kinase inhibition on epithelial proliferation in normal and premalignant breast. Cancer Res 2002; 62:122–128.

Chu E, Callender MA, Farrell MP, Schmitz JC. Thymidylate synthase inhibitors as anticancer agents: from bench to bedside. Cancer Chemother Pharmacol 2003; 52(suppl 1): S80–S89.

Ciardiello F, Caputo R, Borriello G, Del BD, Biroccio A, Zupi G, Bianco AR, Tortora G. ZD1839 (IRESSA), an EGFR-selective tyrosine kinase inhibitor, enhances taxane activity in bcl-2 overexpressing, multidrug-resistant MCF-7 ADR human breast cancer cells. Int J Cancer 2002; 98:463–469.

Clarke R, Leonessa F, Welch JN, Skaar TC. Cellular and molecular pharmacology of antiestrogen action and resistance. Pharmacol Rev 2001; 53:25–71.

Clarke R, Liu MC, Bouker KB, Gu Z, Lee RY, Zhu Y, Skaar TC, Gomez B, O'Brien K, Wang Y, Hilakivi-Clarke LA. Antiestrogen resistance in breast cancer and the role of estrogen receptor signaling. Oncogene 2003; 22:7316–7339.

Clarkson RW, Boland MP, Kritikou EA, Lee JM, Freeman TC, Tiffen PG, Watson CJ. The genes induced by signal transducer and activators of transcription (STAT)3 and STAT5 in mammary epithelial cells define the roles of these STATs in mammary development. Mol Endocrinol 2006; 20: 675–685.

Clarkson RW, Watson JC. NF-kappaB and apoptosis in mammary epithelial cells. J Mammary Gland Biol Neoplasia 1999; 4:165–175.

Cogswell PC, Guttridge DC, Funkhouser WK, Baldwin AS Jr. Selective activation of NF-kappa B subunits in human breast cancer: potential roles for NF-kappa B2/p52 and for Bcl-3. Oncogene 2000; 19:1123–1131.

Connett JM, Badri L, Giordano TJ, Connett WC, Doherty GM. Interferon regulatory factor 1 (IRF-1) and IRF-2 expression in breast cancer tissue microarrays. J Interferon Cytokine Res 2005; 25:587–594.

Coombes RC, Hall E, Gibson LJ, Paridaens R, Jassem J, Delozier T, Jones SE, Alvarez I, Bertelli G, Ortmann O, Coates AS, Bajetta E, Dodwell D, Coleman RE, Fallowfield LJ, Mickiewicz E, Andersen J, Lonning PE, Cocconi G, Stewart A, Stuart N, Snowdon CF, Carpentieri M,

Massimini G, Bliss JM, d van V. A randomized trial of exemestane after two to three years of tamoxifen therapy in postmenopausal women with primary breast cancer. N Engl J Med 2004; 350:1081–1092.

Cuzick J, Powles T, Veronesi U, Forbes J, Edwards R, Ashley A, Boyle P. Overview of the main outcomes in breast-cancer prevention trials. Lancet 2003; 361:296–300.

Dai Y, Grant S. Targeting multiple arms of the apoptotic regulatory machinery. Cancer Res 2007; 67:2908–2911.

Debatin KM, Krammer PH. Death receptors in chemotherapy and cancer. Oncogene 2004; 23:2950–2966.

Decaudin D, Marzo I, Brenner C, Kroemer G. Mitochondria in chemotherapy-induced apoptosis: a prospective novel target of cancer therapy (review). Int J Oncol 1998; 12:141–152.

Dees EC, Orlowski RZ. Targeting the ubiquitin-proteasome pathway in breast cancer therapy. Future Oncol 2006; 2: 121–135.

Degterev A, Boyce M, Yuan J. A decade of caspases. Oncogene 2003; 22:8543–8567.

de Jong MM, Nolte IM, Te Meerman GJ, van der Graaf WT, Oosterwijk JC, Kleibeuker JH, Schaapveld M, de Vries EG. Genes other than BRCA1 and BRCA2 involved in breast cancer susceptibility. J Med Genet 2002; 39:225–242.

Denault JB, Salvesen GS. Caspases: keys in the ignition of cell death. Chem Rev 2002; 102:4489–4500.

Desrivieres S, Kunz C, Barash I, Vafaizadeh V, Borghouts C, Groner B. The biological functions of the versatile transcription factors STAT3 and STAT5 and new strategies for their targeted inhibition. J Mammary Gland Biol Neoplasia 2006; 11:75–87.

Dickson RB, Lippman ME. Growth factors in breast cancer. Endocr Rev 1995; 16:559–589.

Diehl KM, Keller ET, Woods-Ignastoski KM. Why should we still care about oncogenes? Mol Cancer Ther 2007; 6:418–427.

Diel P, Smolnikar K, Michna H. The pure antiestrogen ICI 182780 is more effective in the induction of apoptosis and down regulation of BCL-2 than tamoxifen in MCF-7 cells. Breast Cancer Res Treat 1999; 58:87–97.

Dimri GP, Lee X, Basile G, Acosta M, Scott G, Roskelley C, Medrano EE, Linskens M, Rubelj I, Pereira-Smith O, Peacocke M, Campisi J. A biomarker that identifies senescent human cells in culture and in aging skin in vivo. Proc Natl Acad Sci U S A 1995; 92:9363–9367.

Doherty GM, Boucher L, Sorenson K, Lowney J. Interferon regulatory factor expression in human breast cancer. Ann Surg 2001; 233:623–629.

Dotzlaw H, Leygue E, Watson PH, Murphy LC. Estrogen receptor-beta messenger RNA expression in human breast tumor biopsies: relationship to steroid receptor status and regulation by progestins. Cancer Res 1999; 59: 529–532.

DuRose JB, Tam AB, Niwa M. Intrinsic capacities of molecular sensors of the unfolded protein response to sense alternate forms of endoplasmic reticulum stress. Mol Biol Cell 2006; 17:3095–3107.

EBCTCG. Early Breast Cancer Trialists' Collaborative Group. Polychemotherapy for early breast cancer: an overview of randomised trials. Lancet 1998; 352:930–942.

EBCTCG. Early Breast Cancer Trialists' Collaborative Group. Multi-agent chemotherapy for early breast cancer. Cochrane Database Syst Rev 2002a CD000487.

EBCTCG. Early Breast Cancer Trialists' Collaborative Group. Radiotherapy for early breast cancer. Cochrane Database Syst Rev 2002b CD003647.

Edinger AL, Thompson CB. Death by design: apoptosis, necrosis and autophagy. Curr Opin Cell Biol 2004; 16:663–669.

Edinger AL, Thompson CB. Defective autophagy leads to cancer. Cancer Cell 2003; 4:422–424.

Feigelson HS, Jonas CR, Teras LR, Thun MJ, Calle EE. Weight gain, body mass index, hormone replacement therapy, and postmenopausal breast cancer in a large prospective study. Cancer Epidemiol Biomarkers Prev 2004; 13:220–224.

Feldman DE, Chauhan V, Koong AC. The unfolded protein response: a novel component of the hypoxic stress response in tumors. Mol Cancer Res 2005; 3:597–605.

Ferretti G, Bria E, Giannarelli D, Felici A, Papaldo P, Fabi A, Di CS, Ruggeri EM, Milella M, Ciccarese M, Cecere FL, Gelibter A, Nuzzo C, Cognetti F, Terzoli E, Carlini P. Second- and third-generation aromatase inhibitors as first-line endocrine therapy in postmenopausal metastatic breast cancer patients: a pooled analysis of the randomised trials. Br J Cancer 2006; 94:1789–1796.

Finn RS, Dering J, Ginther C, Wilson CA, Glaspy P, Tchekmedyian N, Slamon DJ. Dasatinib, an orally active small molecule inhibitor of both the src and abl kinases, selectively inhibits growth of basal-type/"triple-negative" breast cancer cell lines growing in vitro. Breast Cancer Res Treat 2007; 105(3):319–326. Epub 2007 Feb 1.

Fischer U, Schulze-Osthoff K. New approaches and therapeutics targeting apoptosis in disease. Pharmacol Rev 2005; 57: 187–215.

Fisher B, Dignam J, Mamounas EP, Costantino JP, Wickerham DL, Redmond C, Wolmark N, Dimitrov NV, Bowman DM, Glass AG, Atkins JN, Abramson N, Sutherland CM, Aron BS, Margolese RG. Sequential methotrexate and fluorouracil for the treatment of node-negative breast cancer patients with estrogen receptor-negative tumors: eight-year results from National Surgical Adjuvant Breast and Bowel Project (NSABP) B-13 and first report of findings from NSABP B-19 comparing methotrexate and fluorouracil with conventional cyclophosphamide, methotrexate, and fluorouracil. J Clin Oncol 1996; 14:1982–1992.

Fuchs DA, Johnson RK. Cytologic evidence that taxol, an antineoplastic agent from Taxus brevifolia, acts as a mitotic spindle poison. Cancer Treat Rep 1978; 62:1219–1222.

Furuya N, Yu J, Byfield M, Pattingre S, Levine B. The evolutionarily conserved domain of Beclin 1 is required for Vps34 binding, autophagy and tumor suppressor function. Autophagy 2005; 1:46–52.

Gaddy VT, Barrett JT, Delk JN, Kallab AM, Porter AG, Schoenlein PV. Mifepristone induces growth arrest, caspase activation, and apoptosis of estrogen receptor-expressing, antiestrogen-resistant breast cancer cells. Clin Cancer Res 2004; 10:5215–5225.

Ganansia-Leymarie V, Bischoff P, Bergerat JP, Holl V. Signal transduction pathways of taxanes-induced apoptosis. Curr Med Chem Anticancer Agents 2003; 3:291–306.

Gelmann EP. Tamoxifen induction of apoptosis in estrogen receptor-negative cancers: new tricks for an old dog? J Natl Cancer Inst 1996; 88:224–226.

Gomez BP, Riggins RB, Shajahan AN, Klimach U, Wang A, Crawford AC, Zhu Y, Zwart A, Wang M, Clarke R. Human X-Box binding protein-1 confers both estrogen independence and antiestrogen resistance in breast cancer cell lines. FASEB J 2007; 21:4013–4027.

Gonzalez VM, Fuertes MA, Alonso C, Perez JM. Is cisplatin-induced cell death always produced by apoptosis? Mol Pharmacol 2001; 59:657–663.

Gorka M, Daniewski WM, Gajkowska B, Lusakowska E, Godlewski MM, Motyl T. Autophagy is the dominant type of programmed cell death in breast cancer MCF-7 cells exposed to AGS 115 and EFDAC, new sesquiterpene analogs of paclitaxel. Anticancer Drugs 2005; 16:777–788.

Green DR, Kroemer G. The pathophysiology of mitochondrial cell death. Science 2004; 305:626–629.

Green KA, Streuli CH. Apoptosis regulation in the mammary gland. Cell Mol Life Sci 2004; 61:1867–1883.

Gu Z, Lee RY, Skaar TC, Bouker KB, Welch JN, Lu J, Liu A, Zhu Y, Davis N, Leonessa F, Brunner N, Wang Y, Clarke R. Association of interferon regulatory factor-1, nucleophosmin, nuclear factor-kappaB, and cyclic AMP response element binding with acquired resistance to Faslodex (ICI 182,780). Cancer Res 2002; 62:3428–3437.

Haldar S, Basu A, Croce CM. Bcl2 is the guardian of microtubule integrity. Cancer Res 1997; 57:229–233.

Haldar S, Jena N, Croce CM. Inactivation of Bcl-2 by phosphorylation. Proc Natl Acad Sci U S A 1995; 92:4507–4511.

Halder SK, Beauchamp RD, Datta PK. A specific inhibitor of TGF-beta receptor kinase, SB-431542, as a potent antitumor agent for human cancers. Neoplasia 2005; 7:509–521.

Hayflick L. The limited in vitro lifetime of human diploid cell strains. Exp Cell Res 1965; 37:614–636.

Hengartner MO. The biochemistry of apoptosis. Nature 2000; 407:770–776.

Hernandez-Vargas H, Ballestar E, Carmona-Saez P, von KC, Banon-Rodriguez I, Esteller M, Moreno-Bueno G, Palacios J. Transcriptional profiling of MCF7 breast cancer cells in response to 5-Fluorouracil: relationship with cell cycle changes and apoptosis, and identification of novel targets of p53. Int J Cancer 2006; 119:1164–1175.

Hernandez-Vargas H, Palacios J, Moreno-Bueno G. Telling cells how to die: docetaxel therapy in cancer cell lines. Cell Cycle 2007; 6:780–783.

Hinoda Y, Sasaki S, Ishida T, Imai K. Monoclonal antibodies as effective therapeutic agents for solid tumors. Cancer Sci 2004; 95:621–625.

Hiscox S, Morgan L, Green TP, Barrow D, Gee J, Nicholson RI. Elevated Src activity promotes cellular invasion and motility in tamoxifen resistant breast cancer cells. Breast Cancer Res Treat 2006; 97:263–274.

Houghton JA, Harwood FG, Tillman DM. Thymineless death in colon carcinoma cells is mediated via fas signaling. Proc Natl Acad Sci U S A 1997; 94:8144–8149.

Howell A. Fulvestrant ('Faslodex'): current and future role in breast cancer management. Crit Rev Oncol Hematol 2006; 57:265–273.

Howell A, DeFriend D, Robertson J, Blamey R, Walton P. Response to a specific antioestrogen (ICI 182780) in tamoxifen-resistant breast cancer. Lancet 1995; 345:29–30.

Howell A, Robertson JF, Quaresma AJ, Aschermannova A, Mauriac L, Kleeberg UR, Vergote I, Erikstein B, Webster A, Morris C. Fulvestrant, formerly ICI 182,780, is as effective as anastrozole in postmenopausal women with advanced breast cancer progressing after prior endocrine treatment. J Clin Oncol 2002; 20:3396–3403.

Hulka BS, Stark AT. Breast cancer: cause and prevention. Lancet 1995; 346:883–887.

Inbal B, Bialik S, Sabanay I, Shani G, Kimchi A. DAP kinase and DRP-1 mediate membrane blebbing and the formation of autophagic vesicles during programmed cell death. J Cell Biol 2002; 157:455–468.

Inoue S, Hartman A, Branch CD, Bucana CD, Bekele BN, Stephens LC, Chada S, Ramesh R. mda-7 In combination with bevacizumab treatment produces a synergistic and complete inhibitory effect on lung tumor xenograft. Mol Ther 2007; 15:287–294.

Ishizawar R, Parsons SJ. c-Src and cooperating partners in human cancer. Cancer Cell 2004; 6:209–214.

Jakesz R, Jonat W, Gnant M, Mittlboeck M, Greil R, Tausch C, Hilfrich J, Kwasny W, Menzel C, Samonigg H, Seifert M, Gademann G, Kaufmann M, Wolfgang J. Switching of postmenopausal women with endocrine-responsive early breast cancer to anastrozole after 2 years' adjuvant tamoxifen: combined results of ABCSG trial 8 and ARNO 95 trial. Lancet 2005; 366:455–462.

Jamieson ER, Lippard SJ. Structure, recognition, and processing of Cisplatin-DNA adducts. Chem Rev 1999; 99: 2467–2498.

Jin S. Autophagy, mitochondrial quality control, and oncogenesis. Autophagy 2006; 2:80–84.

Johnson IS, Wright HF, Svoboda GH, Vlantis J. Antitumor principles derived from Vinca rosea Linn. I. Vincaleukoblastine and leurosine. Cancer Res 1960; 20:1016–1022.

Johnston SR. Targeting downstream effectors of epidermal growth factor receptor/HER2 in breast cancer with either farnesyltransferase inhibitors or mTOR antagonists. Int J Gynecol Cancer 2006; 16(Suppl 2):543–548.

Kang Y, Cortina R, Perry RR. Role of c-myc in tamoxifen-induced apoptosis estrogen-independent breast cancer cells. J Natl Cancer Inst 1996; 88:279–284.

Kerr JF, Wyllie AH, Currie AR. Apoptosis: a basic biological phenomenon with wide-ranging implications in tissue kinetics. Br J Cancer 1972; 26:239–257.

Kim DW, Sovak MA, Zanieski G, Nonet G, Romieu-Mourez R, Lau AW, Hafer LJ, Yaswen P, Stampfer M, Rogers AE, Russo J, Sonenshein GE. Activation of NF-kappaB/Rel occurs early during neoplastic transformation of mammary cells. Carcinogenesis 2000; 21:871–879.

Kim NW, Piatyszek MA, Prowse KR, Harley CB, West MD, Ho PL, Coviello GM, Wright WE, Weinrich SL, Shay JW. Specific association of human telomerase activity with immortal cells and cancer. Science 1994; 266:2011–2015.

Kim R, Emi M, Matsuura K, Tanabe K. Antisense and non-antisense effects of antisense Bcl-2 on multiple roles of Bcl-2 as a chemosensitizer in cancer therapy. Cancer Gene Ther 2007; 14:1–11.

Klionsky DJ, Emr SD. Autophagy as a regulated pathway of cellular degradation. Science 2000; 290:1717–1721.

Kops GJ, Weaver BA, Cleveland DW. On the road to cancer: aneuploidy and the mitotic checkpoint. Nat Rev Cancer 2005; 5:773–785.

Kourousis C, Kakolyris S, Androulakis N, P. Heras, J. Vlachonicolis, L.Vamvakas, M. Vlata, Hatzidaki D, Samonis G, Georgoulias V. Salvage chemotherapy with paclitaxel, vinorelbine, and cisplatin (PVC) in anthracycline-resistant advanced breast cancer. Am J Clin Oncol 1998; 21: 226–232.

Kroemer G, Galluzzi L, Brenner C. Mitochondrial membrane permeabilization in cell death. Physiol Rev 2007; 87:99–163.

Kroemer G, Jaattela M. Lysosomes and autophagy in cell death control. Nat Rev Cancer 2005; 5:886–897.

Kroemer G, Martin SJ. Caspase-independent cell death. Nat Med 2005; 11:725–730.

Kyprianou N, English HF, Davidson NE, Isaacs JT. Programmed cell death during regression of the MCF-7 human breast cancer following estrogen ablation. Cancer Res 1991; 51:162–166.

Lahn M, Kloeker S, Berry BS. TGF-beta inhibitors for the treatment of cancer. Expert Opin Investig Drugs 2005; 14:629–643.

Lamparska-Przybysz M, Gajkowska B, Motyl T. BID-deficient breast cancer MCF-7 cells as a model for the study of autophagy in cancer therapy. Autophagy 2006; 2:47–48.

Lee AH, Iwakoshi NN, Anderson KC, Glimcher LH. Proteasome inhibitors disrupt the unfolded protein response in myeloma cells. Proc Natl Acad Sci U S A 2003; 100:9946–9951.

Li LY, Luo X, Wang X. Endonuclease G is an apoptotic DNase when released from mitochondria. Nature 2001; 412:95–99.

Liang XH, Jackson S, Seaman M, Brown K, Kempkes B, Hibshoosh H, Levine B. Induction of autophagy and inhibition of tumorigenesis by beclin 1. Nature 1999; 402: 672–676.

Litherland S, Jackson IM. Antioestrogens in the management of hormone-dependent cancer. Cancer Treat Rev 1988; 15:183–194.

Longley DB, Harkin DP, Johnston PG. 5-fluorouracil: mechanisms of action and clinical strategies. Nat Rev Cancer 2003; 3:330–338.

Lopes de Menezes DE, Hu Y, Mayer LD. Combined treatment of Bcl-2 antisense oligodeoxynucleotides (G3139), p-glycoprotein inhibitor (PSC833), and sterically stabilized liposomal doxorubicin suppresses growth of drug-resistant growth of drug-resistant breast cancer in severely combined immunodeficient mice. J Exp Ther Oncol 2003; 3:72–82.

Maloney EK, McLaughlin JL, Dagdigian NE, Garrett LM, Connors KM, Zhou XM, Blattler WA, Chittenden T, Singh R. An anti-insulin-like growth factor I receptor antibody that is a potent inhibitor of cancer cell proliferation. Cancer Res 2003; 63:5073–5083.

Mandlekar S, Hebbar V, Christov K, Kong AN. Pharmacodynamics of tamoxifen and its 4-hydroxy and N-desmethyl metabolites: activation of caspases and induction of apoptosis in rat mammary tumors and in human breast cancer cell lines. Cancer Res 2000a; 60:6601–6606.

Mandlekar S, Yu R, Tan TH, Kong AN. Activation of caspase-3 and c-Jun NH2-terminal kinase-1 signaling pathways in tamoxifen-induced apoptosis of human breast cancer cells. Cancer Res 2000b; 60:5995–6000.

Mansilla S, Bataller M, Portugal J. Mitotic catastrophe as a consequence of chemotherapy. Anticancer Agents Med Chem 2006; 6:589–602.

Mansour EG, Gray R, Shatila AH, Tormey DC, Cooper MR, Osborne CK, Falkson G. Survival advantage of adjuvant chemotherapy in high-risk node-negative breast cancer: ten-year analysis–an intergroup study. J Clin Oncol 1998; 16:3486–3492.

Marshall J, Chen H, Yang D, Figueira M, Bouker KB, Ling Y, Lippman M, Frankel SR, Hayes DF. A phase I trial of a Bcl-2 antisense (G3139) and weekly docetaxel in patients with advanced breast cancer and other solid tumors. Ann Oncol 2004; 15:1274–1283.

Martens UM, Zijlmans JM, Poon SS, Dragowska W, Yui J, Chavez EA, Ward RK, Lansdorp PM. Short telomeres on human chromosome 17p. Nat Genet 1998; 18:76–80.

Marx C, Yau C, Banwait S, Zhou Y, Scott GK, Hann B, Park JW, Benz CC. Proteasome-regulated ERBB2 and estrogen receptor pathways in breast cancer. Mol Pharmacol 2007; 71: 1525–1534.

Massarweh S, Osborne CK, Jiang S, Wakeling AE, Rimawi M, Mohsin SK, Hilsenbeck S, Schiff R. Mechanisms of tumor regression and resistance to estrogen deprivation and fulvestrant in a model of estrogen receptor-positive, HER-2/neu-positive breast cancer. Cancer Res 2006; 66:8266–8273.

Meng XW, Lee SH, Kaufmann SH. Apoptosis in the treatment of cancer: a promise kept? Curr Opin Cell Biol 2006; 18: 668–676.

Meric-Bernstam F, Hung MC. Advances in targeting human epidermal growth factor receptor-2 signaling for cancer therapy. Clin Cancer Res 2006; 12:6326–6330.

Miller KD, Chap LI, Holmes FA, Cobleigh MA, Marcom PK, Fehrenbacher L, Dickler M, Overmoyer BA, Reimann JD, Sing AP, Langmuir V, Rugo HS. Randomized phase III trial of capecitabine compared with bevacizumab plus capecitabine in patients with previously treated metastatic breast cancer. J Clin Oncol 2005; 23:792–799.

Miller WR. Biological rationale for endocrine therapy in breast cancer. Best Pract Res Clin Endocrinol Metab 2004; 18: 1–32.

Minotti G, Menna P, Salvatorelli E, Cairo G, Gianni L. Anthracyclines: molecular advances and pharmacologic developments in antitumor activity and cardiotoxicity. Pharmacol Rev 2004; 56:185–229.

Mohsin SK, Weiss HL, Gutierrez MC, Chamness GC, Schiff R, Digiovanna MP, Wang CX, Hilsenbeck SG, Osborne CK, Allred DC, Elledge R, Chang JC. Neoadjuvant trastuzumab induces apoptosis in primary breast cancers. J Clin Oncol 2005; 23:2460–2468.

Moore MJ. Clinical pharmacokinetics of cyclophosphamide. Clin Pharmacokinet 1991; 20:194–208.

Motoyama AB, Hynes NE. BAD: a good therapeutic target? Breast Cancer Res 2003; 5:27–30.

Mouridsen H, Gershanovich M, Sun Y, Perez-Carrion R, Boni C, Monnier A, Apffelstaedt J, Smith R, Sleeboom HP, Janicke F, Pluzanska A, Dank M, Becquart D, Bapsy PP, Salminen E, Snyder R, Lassus M, Verbeek JA, Staffler B,

Chaudri-Ross HA, Dugan M. Superior efficacy of letrozole versus tamoxifen as first-line therapy for postmenopausal women with advanced breast cancer: results of a phase III study of the International Letrozole Breast Cancer Group. J Clin Oncol 2001; 19:2596–2606.

Moy B, Goss PE. Estrogen receptor pathway: resistance to endocrine therapy and new therapeutic approaches. Clin Cancer Res 2006; 12:4790–4793.

Muraoka-Cook RS, Shin I, Yi JY, Easterly E, Barcellos-Hoff MH, Yingling JM, Zent R, Arteaga CL. Activated type I TGFbeta receptor kinase enhances the survival of mammary epithelial cells and accelerates tumor progression. Oncogene 2006; 25:3408–3423.

Nagourney RA, Link JS, Blitzer JB, Forsthoff C, Evans SS. Gemcitabine plus cisplatin repeating doublet therapy in previously treated, relapsed breast cancer patients. J Clin Oncol 2000; 18:2245–2249.

Nahta R, Esteva FJ. Bcl-2 antisense oligonucleotides: a potential novel strategy for the treatment of breast cancer. Semin Oncol 2003; 30:143–149.

Nakshatri H, Bhat-Nakshatri P, Martin DA, Goulet RJ Jr., Sledge GW Jr. Constitutive activation of NF-kappaB during progression of breast cancer to hormone-independent growth. Mol Cell Biol 1997; 17:3629–3639.

Nam S, Williams A, Vultur A, List A, Bhalla K, Smith D, Lee FY, Jove R. Dasatinib (BMS-354825) inhibits Stat5 signaling associated with apoptosis in chronic myelogenous leukemia cells. Mol Cancer Ther 2007; 6:1400–1405.

Narita M. Cellular senescence and chromatin organisation. Br J Cancer 2007; 96:686–691.

Nathanson KL, Wooster R, Weber BL. Breast cancer genetics: what we know and what we need. Nat Med 2001; 7: 552–556.

Nicotera P, Leist M, Ferrando-May E. Intracellular ATP, a switch in the decision between apoptosis and necrosis. Toxicol Lett 1998; 102–103:139–142.

Nishimura R, Nagao K, Miyayama H, Matsuda M, Baba K, Matsuoka Y, Yamashita H, Fukuda M, Higuchi A, Satoh A, Mizumoto T, Hamamoto R. Thymidylate synthase levels as a therapeutic and prognostic predictor in breast cancer. Anticancer Res 1999; 19:5621–5626.

Ogata M, Hino S, Saito A, Morikawa K, Kondo S, Kanemoto S, Murakami T, Taniguchi M, Tanii I, Yoshinaga K, Shiosaka S, Hammarback JA, Urano F, Imaizumi K. Autophagy is activated for cell survival after endoplasmic reticulum stress. Mol Cell Biol 2006; 26:9220–9231.

Ohta T, Fukuda M. Ubiquitin and breast cancer. Oncogene 2004; 23:2079–2088.

Okubo S, Kurebayashi J, Otsuki T, Yamamoto Y, Tanaka K, Sonoo H. Additive antitumour effect of the epidermal growth factor receptor tyrosine kinase inhibitor gefitinib (Iressa, ZD1839) and the antioestrogen fulvestrant (Faslodex, ICI 182,780) in breast cancer cells. Br J Cancer 2004; 90: 236–244.

Osborne CK, Schiff R. Growth factor receptor cross-talk with estrogen receptor as a mechanism for tamoxifen resistance in breast cancer. Breast 2003; 12:362–367.

Osborne CK, Wakeling A, Nicholson RI. Fulvestrant: an oestrogen receptor antagonist with a novel mechanism of action. Br J Cancer 2004; 90:S2–S6.

Osborne CK, Zhao H, Fuqua SA. Selective estrogen receptor modulators: structure, function, and clinical use. J Clin Oncol 2000; 18:3172–3186.

Parker WB, Cheng YC. Metabolism and mechanism of action of 5-fluorouracil. Pharmacol Ther 1990; 48:381–395.

Pattingre S, Levine B. Bcl-2 inhibition of autophagy: a new route to cancer? Cancer Res 2006; 66:2885–2888.

Pattingre S, Tassa A, Qu X, Garuti R, Liang XH, Mizushima N, Packer M, Schneider MD, Levine B. Bcl-2 antiapoptotic proteins inhibit Beclin 1-dependent autophagy. Cell 2005; 122:927–939.

Perez RP. Cellular and molecular determinants of cisplatin resistance. Eur J Cancer 1998; 34:1535–1542.

Perry RR, Kang Y, Greaves BR. Relationship between tamoxifen-induced transforming growth factor beta 1 expression, cytostasis and apoptosis in human breast cancer cells. Br J Cancer 1995; 72:1441–1446.

Pestell KE, Hobbs SM, Titley JC, Kelland LR, Walton, MI. Effect of p53 status on sensitivity to platinum complexes in a human ovarian cancer cell line. Mol Pharmacol 2000; 57:503–511.

Proskuryakov SY, Konoplyannikov AG, Gabai VL. Necrosis: a specific form of programmed cell death? Exp Cell Res 2003; 283:1–16.

Ravagnan L, Gurbuxani S, Susin SA, Maisse C, Daugas E, Zamzami N, Mak T, Jaattela M, Penninger JM, Garrido C, Kroemer G. Heat-shock protein 70 antagonizes apoptosis-inducing factor. Nat Cell Biol 2001; 3:839–843.

Real PJ, Cao Y, Wang R, Nikolovska-Coleska Z, Sanz-Ortiz J, Wang S, Fernandez-Luna, JL. Breast cancer cells can evade apoptosis-mediated selective killing by a novel small molecule inhibitor of Bcl-2. Cancer Res 2004; 64:7947–7953.

Riedl SJ, Salvesen GS. The apoptosome: signalling platform of cell death. Nat Rev Mol Cell Biol 2007; 8:405–413.

Riggins RB, Thomas KS, Ta HQ, Wen J, Davis RJ, Schuh NR, Donelan SS, Owen KA, Gibson MA, Shupnik MA, Silva CM, Parsons SJ, Clarke R, Bouton AH. Physical and functional interactions between Cas and c-Src induce tamoxifen resistance of breast cancer cells through pathways involving epidermal growth factor receptor and signal transducer and activator of transcription 5b. Cancer Res 2006; 66:7007–7015.

Riggins RB, Zwart A, Nehra R, Clarke R. The nuclear factor kappa B inhibitor parthenolide restores ICI 182,780 (Faslodex; fulvestrant)-induced apoptosis in antiestrogen-resistant breast cancer cells. Mol Cancer Ther 2005; 4:33–41.

Ron D. Translational control in the endoplasmic reticulum stress response. J Clin Invest 2002; 110:1383–1388.

Roninson IB, Broude EV, Chang BD. If not apoptosis, then what? Treatment-induced senescence and mitotic catastrophe in tumor cells. Drug Resist Updat 2001; 4:303–313.

Sachdev D, Li SL, Hartell JS, Fujita-Yamaguchi Y, Miller JS, Yee D. A chimeric humanized single-chain antibody against the type I insulin-like growth factor (IGF) receptor renders breast cancer cells refractory to the mitogenic effects of IGF-I. Cancer Res 2003; 63:627–635.

Sachdev D, Yee D. Disrupting insulin-like growth factor signaling as a potential cancer therapy. Mol Cancer Ther 2007; 6:1–12.

Saelens X, Festjens N, Vande WL, van GM, Van LG, Vandenabeele P. Toxic proteins released from mitochondria in cell death. Oncogene 2004; 23:2861–2874.

Salvesen GS. Caspases and apoptosis. Essays Biochem 2002; 38: 9–19.

Schiff PB, Fant J, Horwitz SB. Promotion of microtubule assembly in vitro by taxol. Nature 1979; 277:665–667.

Schneider BP, Sledge GW Jr. Drug insight: VEGF as a therapeutic target for breast cancer. Nat Clin Pract Oncol 2007; 4:181–189.

Shajahan AN, Wang A, Decker M, Minshall RD, Liu MC, Clarke R. Caveolin-1 tyrosine phosphorylation enhances paclitaxel-mediated cytotoxicity. J Biol Chem 2007; 282:5934–5943.

Siddik ZH. Biochemical and molecular mechanisms of cisplatin resistance. Cancer Treat Res 2002; 112:263–284.

Singal PK, Iliskovic N. Doxorubicin-induced cardiomyopathy. N Engl J Med 1998; 339:900–905.

Sledge GW Jr., Loehrer PJ Sr., Roth BJ, Einhorn LH. Cisplatin as first-line therapy for metastatic breast cancer. J Clin Oncol 1988; 6:1811–1814.

Speirs V, Carder PJ, Lane S, Dodwell D, Lansdown MR, Hanby AM. Oestrogen receptor beta: what it means for patients with breast cancer. Lancet Oncol 2004; 5:174–181.

Speirs V, Parkes AT, Kerin MJ, Walton DS, Carleton PJ, Fox JN, Atkin SL. Coexpression of estrogen receptor alpha and beta: poor prognostic factors in human breast cancer? Cancer Res 1999; 59:525–528.

Sriburi R, Jackowski S, Mori K, Brewer JW. XBP1: a link between the unfolded protein response, lipid biosynthesis, and biogenesis of the endoplasmic reticulum. J Cell Biol 2004; 167:35–41.

Tam WF, Sen R. IkappaB family members function by different mechanisms. J Biol Chem 2001; 276:7701–7704.

Thurlimann B, Keshaviah A, Coates AS, Mouridsen H, Mauriac L, Forbes JF, Paridaens R, Castiglione-Gertsch M, Gelber RD, Rabaglio M, Smith I, Wardley A, Price KN, Goldhirsch A. A comparison of letrozole and tamoxifen in postmenopausal women with early breast cancer. N Engl J Med 2005; 353:2747–2757.

Tolcher AW, Kuhn J, Schwartz G, Patnaik A, Hammond LA, Thompson I, Fingert H, Bushnell D, Malik S, Kreisberg J, Izbicka E, Smetzer L, Rowinsky EK. A Phase I pharmacokinetic and biological correlative study of oblimersen sodium (genasense, g3139), an antisense oligonucleotide to the bcl-2 mRNA, and of docetaxel in patients with hormone-refractory prostate cancer. Clin Cancer Res 2004; 10:5048–5057.

Tonko-Geymayer S, Doppler W. An essential link to mammary cancer? Nat Med 2002; 8:108–110.

Tu Y, Jerry DJ, Pazik B, Smith SS. Sensitivity to DNA damage is a common component of hormone-based strategies for protection of the mammary gland. Mol Cancer Res 2005; 3:435–442.

Ueda Y, Wang S, Dumont N, Yi JY, Koh Y, Arteaga CL. Overexpression of HER2 (erbB2) in human breast epithelial cells unmasks transforming growth factor beta-induced cell motility. J Biol Chem 2004; 279:24505–24513.

Vakkila J, Lotze MT. Inflammation and necrosis promote tumour growth. Nat Rev Immunol 2004; 4:641–648.

Vandenabeele P, Vanden BT, Festjens N. Caspase inhibitors promote alternative cell death pathways. Sci STKE 2006; 2006:pe44.

Vaux DL, Silke J. Mammalian mitochondrial IAP binding proteins. Biochem Biophys Res Commun 2003; 304: 499–504.

Voorhees PM, Orlowski RZ. The proteasome and proteasome inhibitors in cancer therapy. Annu Rev Pharmacol Toxicol 2006; 46:189–213.

Wang LG, Liu XM, Kreis W, Budman DR. The effect of antimicrotubule agents on signal transduction pathways of apoptosis: a review. Cancer Chemother Pharmacol 1999; 44:355–361.

Wang S, Konorev EA, Kotamraju S, Joseph J, Kalivendi S, Kalyanaraman B. Doxorubicin induces apoptosis in normal and tumor cells via distinctly different mechanisms. intermediacy of H(2)O(2)- and p53-dependent pathways. J Biol Chem 2004; 279:25535–25543.

Wang TH, Wang HS, Ichijo H, Giannakakou P, Foster JS, Fojo T, Wimalasena J. Microtubule-interfering agents activate c-Jun N-terminal kinase/stress-activated protein kinase through both Ras and apoptosis signal-regulating kinase pathways. J Biol Chem 1998; 273:4928–4936.

Wang TT, Phang JM. Effects of estrogen on apoptotic pathways in human breast cancer cell line MCF-7. Cancer Res 1995; 55:2487–2489.

Wedam SB, Low JA, Yang SX, Chow CK, Choyke P, Danforth D, Hewitt SM, Berman A, Steinberg SM, Liewehr DJ, Plehn J, Doshi A, Thomasson D, McCarthy N, Koeppen H, Sherman M, Zujewski J, Camphausen K, Chen H, Swain SM. Antiangiogenic and antitumor effects of bevacizumab in patients with inflammatory and locally advanced breast cancer. J Clin Oncol 2006; 24:769–777.

Wilking N, Isaksson E, von SE. Tamoxifen and secondary tumours. An update. Drug Saf 1997; 16:104–117.

Witters LM, Witkoski A, Planas-Silva MD, Berger M, Viallet J, Lipton A. Synergistic inhibition of breast cancer cell lines with a dual inhibitor of EGFR-HER-2/neu and a Bcl-2 inhibitor. Oncol Rep 2007; 17:465–469.

Wolf BB, Green DR. Suicidal tendencies: apoptotic cell death by caspase family proteinases. J Biol Chem 1999; 274: 20049–20052.

Yang CH, Gonzalez-Angulo AM, Reuben JM, Booser DJ, Pusztai L, Krishnamurthy S, Esseltine D, Stec J, Broglio KR, Islam R, Hortobagyi GN, Cristofanilli M. Bortezomib (VELCADE) in metastatic breast cancer: pharmacodynamics, biological effects, and prediction of clinical benefits. Ann Oncol 2006; 17:813–817.

Yarden Y, Baselga J, Miles D. Molecular approach to breast cancer treatment. Semin Oncol 2004; 31:6–13.

Yaron A, Hatzubai A, Davis M, Lavon I, Amit S, Manning AM, Andersen JS, Mann M, Mercurio F, Ben-Neriah Y. Identification of the receptor component of the IkappaBalpha-ubiquitin ligase. Nature 1998; 396:590–594.

Yi JY, Shin I, Arteaga CL. Type I transforming growth factor beta receptor binds to and activates phosphatidylinositol 3-kinase. J Biol Chem 2005; 280:10870–10876.

Yoshida H, Matsui T, Yamamoto A, Okada, T, Mori K. XBP1 mRNA is induced by ATF6 and spliced by IRE1 in response to ER stress to produce a highly active transcription factor. Cell 2001; 107:881–891.

Yousefi S, Perozzo R, Schmid I, Ziemiecki A, Schaffner T, Scapozza L, Brunner T, Simon HU. Calpain-mediated cleavage of Atg5 switches autophagy to apoptosis. Nat Cell Biol 2006; 8:1124–1132.

Yu C, Friday BB, Lai JP, Yang L, Sarkaria J, Kay NE, Carter CA, Roberts LR, Kaufmann SH, Adjei AA. Cytotoxic synergy between the multikinase inhibitor sorafenib and the proteasome inhibitor bortezomib in vitro: induction of apoptosis through Akt and c-Jun NH2-terminal kinase pathways. Mol Cancer Ther 2006; 5:2378–2387.

Zhang GJ, Kimijima I, Onda M, Kanno M, Sato H, Watanabe T, Tsuchiya A, Abe R, Takenoshita S. Tamoxifen-induced apoptosis in breast cancer cells relates to down-regulation of bcl-2, but not bax and bcl-X(L), without alteration of p53 protein levels. Clin Cancer Res 1999; 5:2971–2977.

Zhang K, Kaufman RJ. The unfolded protein response: a stress signaling pathway critical for health and disease. Neurology 2006; 66:S102–S109.

Zhang W, Ramdas L, Shen W, Song SW, Hu L, Hamilton SR. Apoptotic response to 5-fluorouracil treatment is mediated by reduced polyamines, non-autocrine Fas ligand and induced tumor necrosis factor receptor 2. Cancer Biol Ther 2003; 2:572–578.

Zhou BP, Hung MC. Dysregulation of cellular signaling by HER2/neu in breast cancer. Semin Oncol 2003; 30:38–48.

Zhu Y, Singh B, Hewitt S, Liu A, Gomez B, Wang A, Clarke R. Expression patterns among interferon regulatory factor-1, human X-box binding protein-1, nuclear factor kappa B, nucleophosmin, estrogen receptor-alpha and progesterone receptor proteins in breast cancer tissue microarrays. Int J Oncol 2006; 28:67–76.

Zimmermann S, Martens UM. Telomeres and telomerase as targets for cancer therapy. Cell Mol Life Sci 2007; 64:906–921.

9

Aromatase Inhibitors and Their Application to the Treatment of Breast Cancer

ANGELA M. H. BRODIE
University of Maryland School of Medicine, Baltimore, Maryland, U.S.A.

INTRODUCTION

Estrogens are known to be important in the growth of breast cancers in both pre- and postmenopausal women. However, estrogen receptor (ER) concentrations increase with the age of the patient. This results in a higher proportion of postmenopausal patients (approximately two-thirds) having hormone-sensitive cancers (McGuire, 1980). The incidence of breast cancer also increases with age. Thus, as the aging population is expanding, preventing and treating breast cancer become more important health concerns. Ovariectomy was the first treatment for breast cancer, but its efficacy is limited to premenopausal patients. After menopause, the ovary is no longer the major source of estrogens. However, estrogen production is increased in peripheral sites, such as adipose tissue (Hemsell et al., 1974), and contributes to the stimulation of breast cancers. Therefore, systemic treatment is required for postmenopausal patients. Two strategies that can be used to ameliorate the growth effects of estrogens on primary tumors and metastases are inhibition of estrogen action by compounds interacting with ERs (antiestrogens) and the inhibition of estrogen synthesis (aromatase inhibitors).

The efficacy of the antiestrogen tamoxifen in the treatment of breast cancer was first reported by Cole et al. in 1971 and has since become the most widely used endocrine therapy for breast cancer. The Early Breast Cancer Trialists' Collaborative Group (1992) established the efficacy of tamoxifen over chemotherapy as treatment of postmenopausal, hormone-responsive breast cancer. Tamoxifen increases long-term survival, reduces recurrences, and has few side effects (Jordan, 1995). Thus, tamoxifen treatment for ER-positive tumors has been an important therapeutic advance in breast cancer treatment. In the recent prevention trial, tamoxifen was found to reduce the risk of breast cancer by 42% (Fisher et al., 1998). While this reemphasizes the very important role of estrogen in breast cancer, some concerns remain about the long-term use of this antiestrogen. In addition to its function as an ER antagonist, tamoxifen also exhibits weak or partial agonist activities. The antiestrogenic activity of tamoxifen is limited to its effects on breast tumor cells, and tamoxifen may actually function as an estrogen agonist in other regions of the body, occasionally leading to secondary tumors of the endometrium and increasing the risk of strokes (Jordan, 1995). Several studies have reported a threefold increase in the incidence of endometrial carcinoma in tamoxifen-treated patients (Fornander et al., 1989, 1993). On the other hand, the beneficial effects of its estrogenic action in preventing osteoporosis could prove helpful in long-term disease management.

The agonist effects of tamoxifen were realized from its inception. Because of these concerns, we proposed selective inhibition of estrogen synthesis to reduce estrogen production as a different strategy. This approach would be unlikely to result in agonist effects and could therefore have more antitumor efficacy. Thus, selective aromatase inhibitors would be a safer and more effective approach than antiestrogens. We discovered the first of a number of compounds that are selective aromatase inhibitors (Schwarzel et al., 1973). Several of these agents reduced estrogen production concomitantly with marked regression of mammary tumors in animal models (Brodie et al., 1977, 1982). Subsequently, in clinical studies, one of these inhibitors, 4-hydroxyandrostenedione (4-OHA, formestane), was shown to be effective in reducing plasma estrogen levels and causing partial and complete regression of tumors in some patients with advanced breast cancer (Coombes et al., 1984; Goss et al., 1986; Bajetta et al., 2000). By reducing estrogen production, aromatase inhibitors can elicit further responses in some patients who have relapsed on antiestrogen therapy. Thus, aromatase inhibitors can extend the duration of response and quality of life for ER-positive breast cancer patients with advanced disease. Recent data on aromatase inhibitors in adjuvant and first-line treatment indicates that aromatase inhibitors are proving to be more effective than tamoxifen and are discussed in this review.

AROMATASE EXPRESSION

Aromatase plays an important role in reproduction in both males and females. Estrogens are synthesized in ovaries and testes and in large amounts by the placenta during pregnancy by the syncytiotrophoblasts in the outer layer of the chorionic villi (Inkster and Brodie, 1989; Fournet-Dulguerov et al., 1987). In men, aromatase is expressed in the Leydig cells of the adult male (Inkster and Brodie, 1995). The ovarian granulosa cells are the major source of estrogen synthesis in premenopausal women. Estrogen synthesis also occurs in the adipose tissue and muscle of both sexes. Adipose tissue is considered to be the main site of extragonadal estrogen synthesis contributing to circulating estrogen levels (Hemsell et al., 1974). However, breast tissue has been found to have several fold higher levels of estrogen than those in plasma (Thorsen et al., 1982; van Landeghem et al., 1985; Blankenstein et al., 1992). A number of reports, including our own, indicate that aromatase activity as well as aromatase mRNA is present in normal breast tissue and breast tumors (Perel et al., 1982; James et al., 1987; Killinger et al., 1987; Miller et al., 1982; Price et al., 1992; Koos et al., 1993; Lu et al., 1996). Approximately 60% of breast tumors express aromatase and have aromatase activity (Lipton et al., 1987). Aromatase in extragonadal sites is not regulated by follicle-stimulating hormone (FSH) but by glucocorticoids, cAMP, prostaglandin E2, and other factors. Thus, in postmenopausal breast cancer patients, estrogen synthesis is independent of feedback regulation between the pituitary gland and the ovary. The tissue-specific manner of aromatase regulation involves the use of alternative promoters (Simpson et al., 1993). The promoter utilized in the placenta is at least 40 kb upstream from the translational start site. In the gonads, a promoter proximal to the translational start site, promoter II, is used. Promoter II regulates the enzyme in breast cancer as a result of promoter switching (Simpson et al., 1993, 1981). Prostaglandin E_2, the product of the inducible form of cyclooxygenase-2 (COX-2), may be an important mediator of increased aromatase expression in breast cancer (Lu et al., 1996; Zhao et al., 1996; Brueggemeier et al., 1999).

AROMATASE AS TARGET FOR INHIBITION

Aromatase mediates the conversion of androgens, androstenedione, and testosterone to estrogens, estrone, and estradiol. This reaction is the last in the series of steps in steroid biosynthesis and is rate-limiting for estrogen synthesis. Therefore inhibition of aromatase will not interfere with any downstream steroid synthesis. In addition, the unique features of aromatization involving loss of the C-19 carbon and conversion of the steroidal A ring to an aromatic ring provide the opportunity to develop inhibitors selective for $P450_{arom}$, which do not interfere with other P450 enzymes such as 11β-hydroxylase. This enzyme mediates the synthesis of the adrenal steroid cortisol and is inhibited along with aromatase and other enzymes by general inhibitors of steroid biosynthesis, such as aminoglutethimide, used in breast cancer treatment initially to produce "medical adrenalectomies" but later used to inhibit aromatase in conjunction with cortisol replacement (Samojlik et al., 1977). For the above reasons, aromatase is an excellent target for selective inhibition and offers a rational approach to the treatment of breast cancer and other conditions in which estrogens play a role.

SELECTIVE AROMATASE INHIBITORS

Although the selective aromatase inhibitors were reported first in 1973 (Schwarzel et al., 1973), their use in the clinic began in the early 1980s (Coombes et al., 1984; Goss et al., 1986), following preclinical development (Brodie et al., 1976, 1977, 1980, 1982). Now, several inhibitors are available and are effective for the treatment of breast cancer, as discussed below. These inhibitors include steroidal compounds that are substrate analogs and are mechanism-based inhibitors (suicide inhibitors). They inactivate the enzyme and are irreversible. Formestane (lentaron, 4-OHA) and exemestane (aromasin) are part of this class of inhibitors. In addition, nonsteroidal compounds, imidazole and triazole derivatives, are also competitive inhibitors but act reversibly. While these compounds are intrinsically less specific for aromatase, several recent inhibitors with high specificity and potency have been developed, such as anastrozole (Arimidex) and letrozole (Femara). These two triazole inhibitors and exemestane are now approved by the FDA for breast cancer treatment in the United States. Fadrozole, an imadazole, is rather less specific for aromatase and is available in Japan. Vorazole, another triazole compound with similar activity to anastrozole and letrozole, has been discontinued.

High specificity and potency are important determinants in achieving drugs with few side effects. Both classes of inhibitors, steroidal enzyme inactivators and nonsteroidal triazole compounds, have proved to be well-tolerated agents in clinical studies.

Enzyme Inactivators

Formestane, 4-OHA, was among the first compounds discovered to be potent and specific inhibitors of aromatase (Brodie et al., 1976, 1977). In vitro, formestane interacts with human placental aromatase with an apparent K_I of 10.2 nM, causing a rapid, irreversible inactivation with a K_{inact} of 0.41×10^{-3}/sec (Brodie et al., 1981; Covey et al., 1982).

These types of compounds are thought to interact with the steroid-binding region of the enzyme and are converted by the normal catalytic mechanism to a product that binds either very tightly or irreversibly by covalent binding to the enzyme, causing its inactivation. Thus synthesis of estrogen is unable to occur until new enzyme is produced. As indicated above, a number of other steroidal derivatives of the substrate, androstenedione (Brodie et al., 1981; Covey et al., 1981; Metcalf et al., 1981; Brodie, 1993; Henderson et al., 1986), including exemestane, cause similar inactivation of aromatase. Because of this inactivation, it is unnecessary to have the drug present at all times to maintain inhibition of the enzyme, as is required with reversible inhibitors. Also, since the inhibitor interacts with the enzyme's catalytic mechanism, it is likely to be highly specific for the enzyme (Sjoerdsma, 1981). Both of these properties, high specificity and enzyme inactivation should have advantages for the patients, as any potential side effects of the drug are lessened. In vivo, formestane 50 mg/kg given subcutaneously twice daily almost completely inhibited ovarian estrogen synthesis and significantly reduced the growth of estrogen-dependent mammary tumors in rats (Brodie et al., 1977, 1982). Peripheral aromatization was also inhibited in male rhesus monkeys by formestane (Brodie and Longcope, 1980). These promising preclinical results (Brodie et al., 1977, 1982) and initial clinical studies (Coombes et al., 1984; Goss et al., 1986) provided the basis for further clinical trials of formestane. Formestane was the first selective aromatase inhibitor to become available and the first new treatment for breast cancer in 10 years at that time.

Nonsteroidal Aromatase Inhibitors

Nonsteroidal inhibitors possess a heteroatom such as a nitrogen-containing heterocyclic moiety. This interferes with steroidal hydroxylation by binding with the heme iron of cytochrome $P450_{arom}$. These compounds are reversible inhibitors of aromatase. Most nonsteroidal inhibitors are intrinsically less enzyme-specific and will inhibit, to varying degrees, other cytochrome P450-mediated hydroxylations in steroidogenesis. However, anastrozole and letrozole are two orally active achiral triazolyl compounds with excellent potency and pharmacokinetic properties and are highly selective for aromatase. Since many of the prospective nonsteroidal compounds that have been evaluated as inhibitors of aromatase are not potent inhibitors of the enzyme, it seems likely that the nature of the non-heterocyclic moiety is also important. This portion of the molecule may interact with aromatase via hydrogen and/or van der Waals bonding. The degree of compatibility or synergism between binding to the heme iron and interaction with the protein residue may also be crucial.

It is difficult to determine whether there is benefit from the inactivation mechanism of exemestane over competitive reversible inhibition by the current reversible nonsteroidal inhibitors, letrozole and anastrozole, since all three drugs reduce estrogen concentrations to the level of the assay sensitivity or below. The highly favorable pharmacokinetic profiles of the triazole compounds are likely to make important contributions to their efficacy. It is not yet established whether the two types of inhibitors could be used to advantage in sequential treatment when clinical resistance occurs with one class of inhibitors. There is some evidence that patients who were treated with nonsteroidal inhibitors and subsequently relapsed were found to respond to exemestane, as discussed below (Lönning et al., 1998; Thürlimann et al., 1997) and also to formestane (Murray and Pitt, 1995).

The extent of inhibition of peripheral aromatization and reduction in concentrations of circulating estrogens have been measured in patients treated with exemestane, letrozole, and anastrozole. All compounds were highly effective in reducing estrogen concentrations and required more sensitive assays than routinely used for measuring serum estrogen concentrations. Thus, solid-phase extraction and High Performance Liquid Chromatography (HPLC) purification preceded radioimmunoassay (Johannessen et al., 1997). The limits of detection were 2.6, 6.7, and 22 pmol/L for E_2, estrogen, and estrogen sulfate, respectively. Maximum suppression with exemestane was achieved with 25 mg/day. Although exemestane did inhibit estrogen levels ($p < 0.001$) in patients who had been treated previously with aminoglutethimide, no further reduction in concentration occurred after treatment with the nonsteroidal aromatase inhibitors (Johannessen et al., 1997; Lönning et al., 1990, 1996; Geisler et al., 1998a). Inhibition of peripheral aromatization measured by conversion of injected radiolabeled aromatase substrate (^{3}H androstenedione) was 97.9% for exemestane (Geisler et al., 1998a), 96% for anastrozole (Geisler et al., 1998b), and 98.9% for letrozole (Dowsett et al., 1995). In a crossover-design study (Geisler et al., 2002) inhibition of aromatization and estrogen levels by letrozole and anastrozole was compared. Twelve postmenopausal breast cancer patients were treated for six weeks with either 1 mg of anastrozole or 2.5 mg of letrozole, the recommended doses for these drugs. Aromatization was measured before and at the end of each treatment. Plasma estrone, estradiol, and estrone sulfate were also measured at each time in samples collected prior to injection of radiolabeled androstenedione. Patients were then crossed over to receive the other aromatase inhibitor for six weeks and measurements were performed as above. Aromatization was inhibited by 97.3% with anastrozole treatment. However, in all 12 patients treated with letrozole, no aromatization was detected. Estrone, estradiol and estrone sulfate levels were reduced by 81%, 84.9%, and 93.5% with anastrozole treatment and by 84.3%, 87.8%, and 98% with letrozole treatment, respectively. Thus, inhibition of estrone ($p = 0.019$) and estrone sulfate ($p = 0.0037$) was significantly greater with letrozole treatment. Estradiol concentrations were below the sensitivity of the assay for all patients during letrozole treatment and for 9 out of 12 patients treated with anastrozole. Because of the marked suppression of aromatization and estrogen levels by these two inhibitors, assay sensitivity and reliability were compromised. Only estrone sulfate levels were within assay limits and were concluded to provide the most accurate indication of estrogen suppression. Estrone sulfate levels were suppressed to 27.6 pmol/L (14–54.3) (93.5%) by anastrozole and to 8.9 pmol/L (4.9–16.10) (98%) by letrozole. It is presently not known whether these differences in inhibition of estrogen synthesis will result in differences in antitumor efficacy. However, this evidence together with results observed in the mouse tumor model discussed below suggests that breast tumors can respond to subtle changes in estrogen concentrations.

CLINICAL EFFICACY OF AROMATASE INHIBITORS

Second-Line Treatment for Advanced Breast Cancer

Although preclinical studies indicated 4-OHA to be highly potent and effective, clinical trials did not begin until the early 1980s. Initial studies were carried out in collaboration between Angela Brodie and colleagues at the University of Maryland and R. Charles Coombes and the team at the Royal Marsden Hospital in London. The first trial was in patients with advanced disease who had relapsed from hormone therapy, mainly tamoxifen. Nevertheless, significant responses were seen which provided the impetus needed for pharmaceutical interest to expand the trials. This subsequently led to the development of a number of new aromatase inhibitors. Ultimately, exemestane, anastrozole, and letrozole were the three compounds approved by the FDA for use in breast cancer in the United States.

Exemestane

Initial phase II studies were carried out in patients relapsing from tamoxifen and after second-line treatment with megestrol acetate and aminoglutethimide. The overall benefit was 25% to 30% (Jones et al., 1999; Poggesi et al., 1999). When exemestane was compared directly to megestrol acetate, no significant difference between overall response to treatment or overall benefit was seen in patients with advanced disease (Kaufmann et al., 2000). However, tolerability of exemestane was better than megase, which exhibits troublesome side effects such as excess weight gain (Crutz et al., 1990).

Anastrozole

In studies comparing this aromatase inhibitor with megestrol (40 mg four times daily), two doses of anastrozole 1 mg and 10 mg daily were administered to postmenopausal patients with advanced breast cancer (Buzdar et al., 1996; Jonat et al., 1996). There was no significant difference between the two doses in response or duration of response. Patients who had progressed after adjuvant treatment with tamoxifen as well as those who received tamoxifen for advanced breast cancer responded to anastrozole. Both 1- and 10-mg doses of anastrozole were well tolerated. The better tolerability of anastrozole was the main benefit over megestrol acetate.

Letrozole

Doses of 0.5 and 2.5 mg daily of letrozole were compared with megestrol. Letrozole was better tolerated and was statistically superior at the 2.5-mg dose compared to megestrol in overall response rate and time to treatment failure. In a non-blinded randomized trial of 555 patients previously treated with tamoxifen, the two doses (0.5 and 2.5 mg) of letrozole were compared with aminoglutethimide (250 with hydrocortisone or cortisone acetate replacement). After 33 months, the overall objective response rates and median duration of response were respectively 17.8% and 23.2 months for 2.5 mg of letrozole, 16.7% and 17.5 months for 0.5 mg of letrozole, and 11.2% and 12.3 months for 250 mg aminoglutethimide. Letrozole was significantly superior to aminoglutethimide for time to progression. Letrozole 2.5 mg/day was well tolerated, with minimal side effects, and is the recommended dose for the treatment of advanced breast cancer.

Aromatase inhibitors in First-Line Therapy Vs. Tamoxifen

Trials have now been carried out as first-line therapy with all three aromatase inhibitors in comparison with tamoxifen. The results are shown in Table 1.

All three FDA approved compounds inhibited peripheral aromatization between 97% and 99% (Jordan and Brodie, 2007). Double-blind studies demonstrated that anastrozole (1 mg daily) was slightly more effective than tamoxifen (20 mg daily) as first-line therapy in postmenopausal women with advanced breast cancer. Among those with ER+ tumors (Bonneterre et al., 2000, 2001; Nabholtz et al., 2000) the benefit was significant in terms of partial and complete responses including stable disease as well as time to progression. In a multicentered randomized double-blind study in advanced breast cancer, letrozole proved to be significantly better than tamoxifen in response rate, clinical benefit, time to progression, and time to treatment failure (Mouridsen et al., 2001). Exemestane was also significantly more effective than tamoxifen as first-line therapy in postmenopausal women with advanced breast cancer (Paridaens et al., 2000, 2003).

Aromatase Inhibitors in Adjuvant Therapy

Two adjuvant studies, the Arimidex, Tamoxifen, Alone or in Combination (ATAC) (anastrozole) and Breast International Group 1-98 (BIG1-98) (letrozole) trials comparing aromatase inhibitors as initial monotherapy, showed early disease-related benefit of treatment, although the ATAC trial with median follow-up of 68 months did not show an overall survival advantage. In the BIG1-98 trial, there were fewer deaths in the letrozole group than in the tamoxifen group but the difference was not statistically significant (Coates et al., 2007).

Currently, breast cancer patients receive tamoxifen for five years. Thus, most recurrences occur after tamoxifen is discontinued. The MA.17 trial evaluated whether extending adjuvant therapy with the aromatase inhibitor letrozole following tamoxifen would reduce recurrences in postmenopausal women (Goss et al., 2003). All patients completed five years of tamoxifen and were randomly assigned to a planned five years of letrozole ($n = 2593$) or placebo ($n = 2594$). Although overall survival was the same in both groups, in patients with positive lymph nodes, survival was significantly greater in the letrozole-treated group. Also, there was a reduction in contralateral breast cancer in patients treated with letrozole although the difference was not statistically significant, whereas disease-free and distant disease-free survival was significantly improved. Letrozole following tamoxifen was well tolerated although there were more hormonally related side effects than with placebo. However, the incidence of bone fractures and cardiovascular events were not different between placebo and letrozole groups.

A similar study has also been carried out with exemestane. In this trial, (Intergroup Exemestane Study) patients received two to three years of tamoxifen and then were randomly assigned to either continue tamoxifen treatment or to switch to exemestane for a total of five years of endocrine treatment. Patients switched to exemestane showed an improvement in disease-free survival and a modest improvement in overall survival. These findings support the idea that early improvement in disease-free survival would lead to greater overall survival. It was also observed that the benefit of the sequential use of tamoxifen and an aromatase inhibitor persist for some years after ending the aromatase inhibitor therapy (Coombes et al., 2007).

Table 1 Randomized Phase III Trials of Aromatase Inhibitors Versus Tamoxifen as First-Line Therapy in Metastatic Breast Cancer

Efficacy results, AI/tamoxifen	ORR (%)	Clinical benefit (%)	TTP (mo)
Anastrozole, $n = 1021$ (pooling)	29/27	57/52	8.5/7.0
Letrozole, $n = 907$ (1 trial)	30/20[a]	49/38[a]	9.4/6.0[a]
Exemestane, $n = 382$ (randomized phase II/III trial)	44/29[a]	72/66	10.9/6.7[a]

[a]Statistically significant; ORR, overall response; TTP, time to progression.
Source: From Refs. Bonneterre, Buzdar et al., 2001; Mouridsen et al., 2001; Paridaens, Dirix et al., 2003 and Pritchard 2005.

INTRATUMORAL AROMATASE MOUSE MODEL AS A GUIDE FOR FUTURE TRIALS

As indicated above, studies were carried out initially in patients with advanced disease who had received standard first-line therapy, usually tamoxifen, and then later relapsed before receiving an aromatase inhibitor as second-line treatment. The low response rates to aromatase inhibitors seen in these patients do not reflect the marked reduction in serum estrogen levels that occur during aromatase inhibitor treatment. This difference may be due to the insensitivity of some tumors to estrogens or to other forms of drug resistance that develops rather than to lack of efficacy of the inhibitors. Use of the inhibitors in first-line therapy or early stage disease is more likely to indicate the antitumor activity of the inhibitors. However, not all patients included in studies were known to be ER-positive. Therefore, in order to provide information that could predict the effects of these agents in the clinic and as a guide to the development of new protocols, we established an intratumoral aromatase model in nude mice to simulate the postmenopausal breast cancer patient (Yue et al., 1994, 1995). The model is useful for comparing aromatase inhibitors and antiestrogens since the tumors are ER-positive and express aromatase. For example, combining aromatase inhibitors and antiestrogens to inhibit both estrogen synthesis and estrogen action simultaneously could be explored, as this might be more effective than either type of agent alone. As the rodent has no significant production of estrogen from nonovarian tissue, we utilized estrogen-dependent human breast cancer cells (MCF-7) transfected with the human aromatase gene (MCF-7_{CA}) as an endogenous source of estrogen to stimulate tumor formation in ovariectomized nude mice (Yue et al., 1994, 1995). This intratumoral aromatase model was used to investigate the effects of the aromatase inhibitors letrozole and anastrozole and to compare them with tamoxifen and fulvestrant, the pure antiestrogen. We have also used these agents in various strategies in order to optimize treatment as a guide to future clinical trials (Long et al., 2004).

MCF-7 cells transfected with the human aromatase gene (MCF-7_{CA}) (3×10^7/mL cells in Matrigel) are inoculated into two sites in ovariectomized female BALB/c mice (aged 4–6 weeks). Animals are injected subcutaneously throughout the experiment with 0.1 mg/mouse/day of androstenedione, the substrate for aromatization to estrogens. Tumor growth is measured with calipers weekly and tumor volumes are calculated. When all tumors reach a measurable size ($\sim$500 mm^3), usually 28 to 35 days after tumor cell inoculations, animals are assigned to groups of four or five mice and treatment is begun. At autopsy, four to six hours after the last injected dose, tumors are removed, cleaned, and weighed.

These studies simulate first-line therapy and can directly compare antiestrogens with aromatase inhibitors. We found that while the antiestrogens tamoxifen and fulvestrant and the aromatase inhibitors letrozole and anastrozole were effective in reducing tumor growth, both aromatase inhibitors were more effective than tamoxifen (Lu et al., 1999; Brodie et al., 1999), as subsequently observed in the clinical trials described above.

Anastrozole (arimidex, 5 μg/day), in contrast with tamoxifen (3 μg/day), caused significant inhibition of tumor growth compared with the controls ($p < 0.05$) (Lu et al., 1999; Brodie et al., 1999). Letrozole (10 μg/day) was more potent than tamoxifen (60 μg/day) and fulvestrant (ICI 182,780) (5 mg/wk), although both fulvestrant and letrozole showed regression of established tumors. Letrozole (5 μg/day) was also able to cause marked regression of large tumors. Treatment with letrozole (5 μg/day) resulted in regression of tumor growth for up to approximately 15 weeks of continuous treatment. Thereafter, the tumors gradually resumed growth and almost reached their initial volume by 19 weeks of treatment.

As both antiestrogens and aromatase inhibitors are effective in treating breast cancer patients, combining these agents with different modes of action might result in greater antitumor efficacy than either alone. In these experiments, we used low doses of the compounds, which result in partial tumor suppression, to determine whether greater reduction in tumor growth could be achieved by combining the two types of agents. A dose of 5 μg/day of letrozole was compared to the same dose of anastrozole and 3 μg/day of tamoxifen. All compounds alone or in combination at these doses were effective in suppressing tumor growth in comparison to growth in the control mice. Weights of tumors removed at the end of treatment were significantly less for animals treated with the aromatase inhibitors, letrozole and anastrozole, than with tamoxifen ($p < 0.05$). However, treatment with either anastrozole or letrozole together with tamoxifen did not produce greater reductions in tumor growth, as measured by tumor weight, than either aromatase inhibitor treatment alone, but tumor weights were reduced more than with tamoxifen alone (Lu et al., 1999). Estrogen concentrations measured in tumor tissue of the letrozole-treated mice were markedly reduced from 460 pg/mg tissue to 20 pg/mg tissue. The combination of aromatase inhibitor and tamoxifen tended to be equivalent to or less effective than either aromatase inhibitor alone (Lu et al., 1999). Studies in patients treated with tamoxifen and letrozole suggest that the clearance rate of letrozole may be increased. This may also contribute to the combination being rather less effective than letrozole

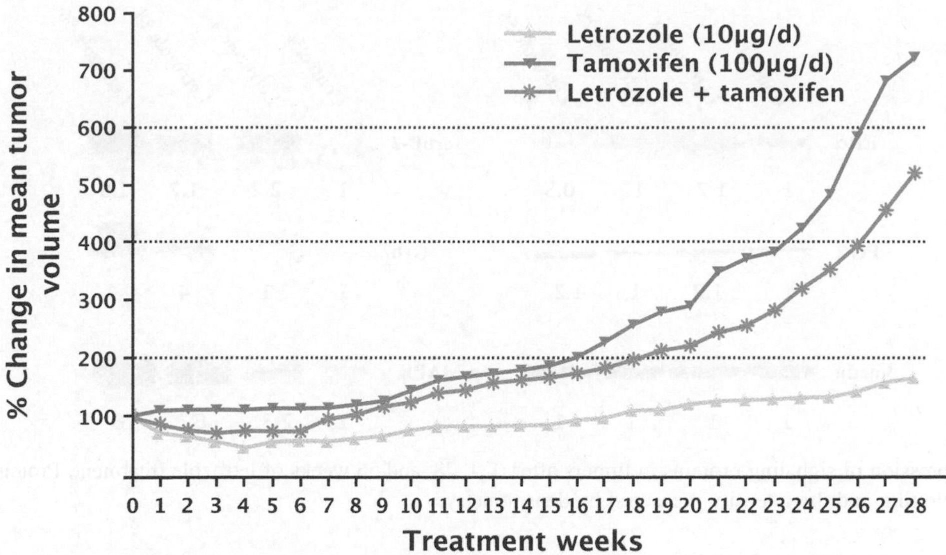

Figure 1 The effect of combining letrozole and tamoxifen compared to letrozole or tamoxifen alone. Mice with MCF-7$_{CA}$ tumors were treated with letrozole, tamoxifen, or the combination for 28 weeks.

alone. The same result was seen when other aromatase inhibitors, 4-OHA, and fadrozole were combined with tamoxifen. There was no additional benefit of the combination compared to these inhibitors alone (Yue et al., 1995). Similar results were obtained when ICI 182,780 was combined with tamoxifen (Lu et al., 1999). Taken together, these results suggest that combining aromatase inhibitors does not improve treatment. Tamoxifen may have a weak agonistic action on the tumors, which overrides the reduction in estrogen concentrations by the aromatase inhibitors and counteracts the effect of the pure antiestrogen. These results were subsequently mirrored in the ATAC trial. Tamoxifen was administered with or without anastrozole into breast cancer patients. However, the combination of tamoxifen and anastrozole was similar to the effect of tamoxifen and not as effective as anastrozole, consistent with the results from the xenograft model.

In the more recent studies, we have treated mice with tumors of MCF-7, cells with a higher dose of tamoxifen (100 µg/mouse/day) than previously used and 10-fold higher than the concentration of the aromatase inhibitor (letrozole 10 µg/mouse/day) (Long et al., 2004). Also, treatment was extended to determine the time to treatment failure. As shown in Figure 1, the combination of the nonsteroidal aromatase inhibitor letrozole with tamoxifen resulted in tumor suppression similar to treatment with tamoxifen alone, but was less effective than letrozole alone. A similar observation had been made with anastrozole in combination with tamoxifen indicating that treatment was not improved by either of the two nonsteroidal inhibitors combined with tamoxifen.

Following long-term tumor suppression during letrozole treatment, tumors eventually grew and were insensitive to the effects of letrozole or to second-line treatment with antiestrogens tamoxifen and fulvestrant. Understanding the mechanisms involved in loss of response to letrozole treatment could provide information that could be utilized to improve treatment for relapsing patients. The mechanisms associated with the cell's ability to proliferate despite treatment were studied in tumors from letrozole-treated mice collected at time points during treatment with letrozole (10 µg/mouse/day). First at week 4 when tumors regressed, then at week 28 when tumors were growing, and at week 56 during continued treatment with letrozole (Jelovac et al., 2005).

Analysis of tumor extracts revealed that ER levels were increased after the first four weeks of letrozole treatment when tumors were regressing. After 28 and 56 weeks of letrozole treatment, tumors were growing and ER expression had decreased by 50% compared with control tumors. Interestingly, phospho-ER (Ser167) was increased twofold in tumors collected at weeks 28 and 56, suggesting that ligand-independent activation of ER may be occurring in letrozole-insensitive tumors. Expression of tyrosine kinase receptor HER-2 and p-Shc protein was increased about

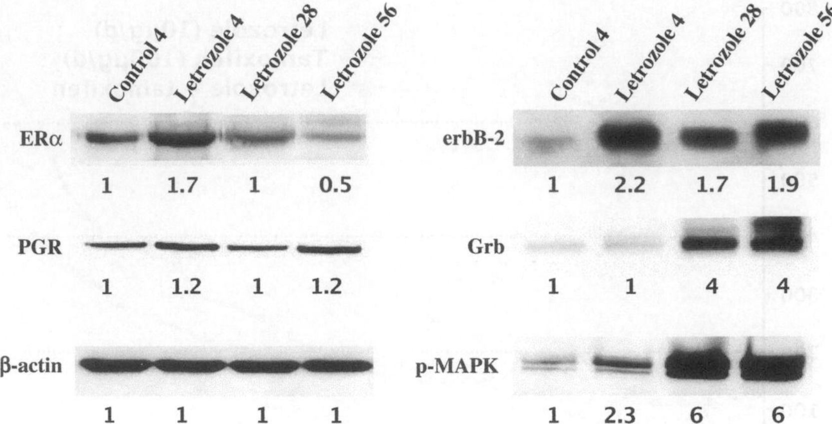

Figure 2 The expression of signaling proteins in tumors after 0, 4, 28, and 56 weeks of letrozole treatment. Proteins are detected by Western immuno-blotting and the intensity measured by densitometry.

twofold at weeks 4, 28, and 56 (Fig. 2). These findings suggest that the tumors may adapt to surviving without estrogens by activating hormone-independent pathways. However, expression of the adapter protein Grb-2 was increased in tumors by fourfold at weeks 28 and 56. Although phospho-MAPK was increased 2.3-fold in tumors that were responding to letrozole treatment at week 4, it was increased up to sixfold in tumors growing on letrozole at weeks 28 and 56 (Long et al., 2004) (Fig. 2).

Further studies were carried out on cells isolated from the Long-Term Letrozole Treated (LTLT) tumors collected at 56 weeks. Similar changes were found in signaling protein expression as in the tumors. Thus, ER expression in LTLT cells was decreased below the control level whereas HER-2, Grb-2, p-Shc, p-Raf, p-MAPK, pMER1/2, p-p90 RSK and p-elk were all upregulated two to sixfold (Jelovac et al., 2005). There was a dose-dependent inhibition of growth in LTLT cells in response to a series of doses of MEK1/2 inhibitor (UO126) or MAPK inhibitor (PD98059), whereas there was no effect on the parental MCF-7Ca cells. These findings indicate that the MAPK pathway has a functional role in enhancing LTLT cell proliferation. In addition, ER expression was restored to MCF-7Ca levels in LTLT cells treated with MEK inhibitor (PD98059). This finding suggests that hormone sensitivity could be regained by inhibiting the MAPK pathway.

The effect of inhibiting tyrosine kinase receptors in LTLT cells was explored with gefitinib (Iressa), an inhibitor of EGF receptor and also HER-2. There was a dose-dependent decrease in proliferation of LTLT cells treated with gefitinib, whereas the parental MCF-7_{CA} cells were unaffected. Gefitinib had a synergistic effect on proliferation when combined with the aromatase inhibitor, anastrozole, even though the LTLT cells were resistant to anastrozole alone and were only slightly inhibited by the same dose of gefitinib alone. The antibody herceptin which targets HER-2 was even more effective in causing a marked dose response inhibition of growth of LTLT cells and accompanied by reduced expression of p-HER-2 and p-MAPK. Furthermore, herceptin treatment completely restored ER levels and sensitivity to estradiol in LTLT cells. Herceptin combined with letrozole, had a synergistic effect and caused marked inhibition of LTLT cell growth. These studies indicate that blocking growth factor receptor signaling can restore sensitivity to hormones and aromatase inhibitor treatment. However, the addition of herceptin to letrozole treatment was very effective in causing regression of these tumors (Fig. 3) (Sabnis et al., 2006).

Although tumor growth grew unabated with letrozole, there was marked regression of tumors when herceptin was added to letrozole treatment. A number of clinical trials have now been initiated with tyrosine kinase inhibitors that will test the hypothesis that combining agents to inhibit estrogen signaling and signaling through other pathways will block cross talk and overcome resistance to therapy. As clinical trials in patients with advanced disease are challenging, valuable information will be gained from preclinical studies such as these that can guide the direction of the trials. Restoring sensitivity to aromatase inhibitors and hormone therapy could achieve important gains in treatment benefit and delay the need for chemotherapy.

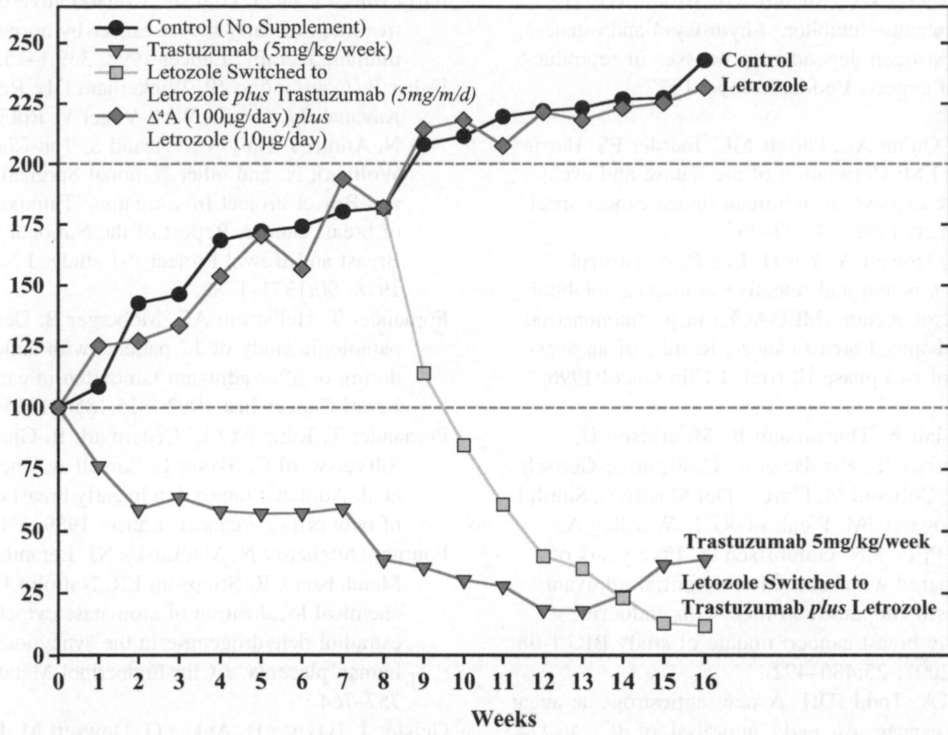

Figure 3 The effect of trastuzumab or trastuzumab plus letrozole on the growth of letrozole insensitive tumors (LTLT) in nude mice. Mice were treated with letrozole, trastuzumab, or vehicle for nine weeks, then trastuzumab injections were administered in addition to letrozole in one group. Treatment was continued in all other groups for 16 weeks.

CONCLUSION

In conclusion, aromatase inhibitors are proving to be more effective than tamoxifen with longer duration of benefit. Nevertheless, resistance may eventually develop. Investigations of the mechanism responsible indicate activation of tyrosine kinase receptor signaling. Evidence suggests that blocking these pathways could restore response to hormone therapy and delay the need for chemotherapy.

REFERENCES

Bajetta E, Zilembo N, Bichisao F, Pozzi P, Toffolati L. Steroidal aromatase inhibitors in elderly patients. Crit Rev Oncol Hematol 2000; 33:137–142.

Blankenstein MA, Maitimu-Smeele I, Donker GH, Daroszewski I, Milewicz A, Thijssen JHH. On the significance of *in situ* production of oestrogens in human breast cancer tissue. J Steroid Biochem Mol Biol 1992; 41:891–896.

Bonneterre J, Buzdar A, Nabholtz JM, Robertson JF, Thurlimann B, von Euler M, Sahmoud T, Webster A, Steinberg M. Arimidex Writing Committee; Investigators Committee Members. Anastrozole is superior to tamoxifen as first-line therapy in hormone receptor positive advanced breast carcinoma. Cancer 2001; 92:2247–2258.

Bonneterre J, Thürlimann B, Robertson JF, Krzakowski M, Mauriac L, Koralewski P, Vergote I, Webster A, Steinberg M, von Euler M. Anastrozole versus tamoxifen as first-line therapy for advanced breast cancer in 668 postmenopausal women-Results of the TARGET (Tamoxifen or Arimidex Randomized Group Efficacy and Tolerability) study. J Clin Oncol 2000; 18:3748–3757.

Brodie A. Aromatase, its inhibitors and their use in breast cancer treatment. Pharmacol Ther 1993; 60:501–515.

Brodie AMH, Garrett WM, Hendrickson JR, Marcotte PA, Robinson CH. Inactivation of activity in placental and ovarian rnicrosomes by 4-hydroxyandrostene-3, 17-dione and 4-acetoxyandrostene-3,1 7-dione. Steroids 1981; 38:693–702.

Brodie AMH, Garrett WM, Hendrickson JR, Tsai-Morris CH. Effects of 4-hydroxyandrostenedione and other compounds in the DMBA breast carcinoma model. Cancer Res 1982; 42: 3360s–3364s.

Brodie AMH, Longcope C. Inhibition of peripheral aromatization by aromatase inhibitors, 4-hy-droxy- and 4-acetoxy-androstene-3,17-dione. Endocrinology 1980; 106:19–21.

Brodie A, Lu Q, Liu Y, Long B. Aromatase inhibitors and their antitumor effects in model systems. Endocr Relat Cancer 1999; 6:205–210.

Brodie AMH, Schwarzel WC, Brodie HJ. Studies on the mechanism of estrogen biosynthesis in the rat ovary-.1 J Steroid Biochem 1976; 7:787–793.

Brodie AMH, Schwarzel WC, Shaikh AA, Brodie HJ. The effect of an aromatase inhibitor, 4-hydroxy-4-androstene-3, 17-dione, on estrogen dependent processes in reproduction and breast cancer. Endocrinology 1977; 100:1684–1694.

Brueggemeier RW, Quinn AL, Parrett ML, Joarder FS, Harris RE, Robertson FM: Correlation of aromatase and cyclo-oxygenase gene expression in human breast cancer specimens. Cancer Lett 1999; 140:27–35.

Buzdar A, Jonat W, Howell A, Yin H, Lee P. Anastrozole (ARIMIDEX), a potent and selective aromatase inhibitor versus megesterol acetate (MEGACE) in postmenopausal women with advanced breast cancer: Results of an overview analysis of two phase III trial. J Clin Oncol 1996; 14:2000–2011.

Coates AS, Keshaviah A, Thurlimann B, Mouridsen H, Mauriac L, Forbes JF, Paridaens R, Castiglione-Gertsch M, Gelber RD, Colleoni M, Lang I, Del Mastro L, Smith I, Chirgwin J, Nogaret JM, Pienkowski T, Wardley A, Jakobsen EH, Price KN, Goldhirsch A. Five years of letrozole compared with tamoxifen as initial adjuvant therapy for postmenopausal women with endocrine-responsive early breast cancer: update of study BIG 1-98. J Clin Oncol 2007; 25:486–492.

Cole MP, Jones CTA, Todd IDH. A new antiestrogenic agent in late breast cancer: An early appraisal of ICI 46,474. Br J Cancer 1971, 25:270–275.

Coombes RC, Goss P, Dowsett M, Gazet JC, Brodie A. 4-Hydroxyandrostenedione treatment of postmenopausal patients with advanced breast cancer. Lancet 1984; 2:1237–1239.

Coombes RC, Kilburn LS, Snowdon CF, Paridaens R, Coleman RE, Jones SE, Jassem J, Van de Velde CJH, Delozier T, Alvarez I, Del Mastro L, Ortmann O, Diedrich K, Coates AS, Bajetta E, Holmberg SB, Dodwell D, Mickiewicz E, Andersen J, Lonning PE, Cocconi G, Forbes J, Castiglione M, Stuart N, Stewart A, Fallowfield LJ, Bertelli G, Hall E, Bogle RG, Carpentieri M, Colajori E, Subar M, Ireland E, Bliss M, on behalf of the Intergroup Exemestane Study. Survival and safety of exemestane versus tamoxifen after 2-3 yeasrs' of tamoxifen treatment (Intergroup Exemestane Study): a randomized controlled trial. Lancet 2007; 369:559–570.

Covey DF, Hood WF. Aromatase enzyme catalysis is involved in the potent inhibition of estrogen biosynthesis caused by 4-acetoxy and 4-hydroxy-4-androstene-3,17-dione. Mol Pharmacol 1982; 21:173–180.

Covey DF, Hood WF, Parikh VD. 10β-Propynyl-substituted steroids: Mechanism-based enzyme-activated irreversible inhibitors of estrogen biosynthesis. J Biol Chem 1981; 256:1076.

Crutz JM, Muss HB, Brockschmidt JK, Evans GW. Weight changes in women with rnetastic breast cancer treated with megestcrol acetate: A comparison of standard versus high-dose therapy. Semin Oncol 1990; 17:63–67.

Dowsett M, Jones A, Johnston SR, Jacobs S, Trunet P, Smith IE. *In vivo* measurement of aromatase inhibition by letrozole (CGS 20267) postnienopausal patients with breast cancer. Clin Cancer Res 1995; 1:1511–1515.

Early Breast Cancer Trialists' Collaborative Group. Systemic treatment of early breast cancer by hormonal, cytotoxic, or immune therapy. Lancet 1992; 339:1–15.

Fisher B, Constantino JP, Wickerham DL, Redmond CK, Kavanah M, Cronin WM. Vogel V. Robidoux A, Dimitrov N, Atkins J. Daly M, Wieand S, Tan-Chiu E, Ford L, Wolmark N, and other National Surgical Adjuvant Breast and Bowel Project Investigators: Tamoxifen for prevention of breast cancer: Report of the National Surgical Adjuvant Breast and Bowel Project P-1 study. J Natl Cancer Inst 1998; 90:1371–1388.

Fornander T, Hellstrom AC, Moberger B. Descriptive clinicopathologic study of 17 patients with endometrial cancer during or after adjuvant tamoxifen in early breast cancer. J Natl Cancer Inst 1993; 815:1850–1855.

Fornander T, Rutqvist LE, Cedermark B, Glass U, Mattsson A, Silfverswärd C, Skoog L, Somell A, Theve T, Wilking N, et al. Adjuvant tamoxifen in early breast cancer: occurrence of new primary cancer. Lancet 1989; 1:117–120.

Fournet-Dulguerov N, MacLusky NJ, Leranth CZ, Todd R, Mendelson CR, Simpsom ER, Naftolin F. Immunohistochemical localization of aromatase cytochrome PF-450 and estradiol dehydrogenase in the syncytiotrophoblast of the human placenta. J Clin Endocrinol Metab 1987, 65(4): 757–764.

Geisler J, Haynes B, Anker G, Dowsett M, Lönning PE. Influence of letrozole and anastrozole on total body aromatization and plasma estrogen levels in postmenopausal breast cancer patients evaluated in a randomized, crossover-designed study. J Clin Oncol 2002; 104:27–34.

Geisler J, King N, Anker G, Ornati G, Di Salle E, Lønning PE, Dowsett M. *In vivo* inhibition of aromatization by exemestane, a novel irreversible aromatase inhibitor, in postmenopausal breast cancer patients. Clin Cancer Res 1998b; 4:2089–2093.

Geisler J, Lundgren S, Berntsen H, Greaves JL, Lønning PE. Influence of dexaminoglutethimide, an optical isomer of aminoglutethimide, on the disposition of estrone sulphate in postmenopausal breast cancer patients. Clin Endocrinol Metab 1998a; 83:2687–2693.

Goss PE, Powles TJ, Dowsett M, Hutchison G, Brodie AM, Gazet JC, Coombes RC. Treatment of advanced postmenopausal breast cancer with aromatase inhibitor, 4-hydroxyandrostenedione-Phase II report. Cancer Res 1986; 46:4823–4826.

Goss PE, Ingle JN, Martino S, Robert NJ, Muss HB, Piccart MJ, Castiglione M, Tu D, Shepherd LE, Pritchard KI, Livingston RB, Davidson NE, Norton L, Perez EA, Abrams JS, Therasse P, Palmer MJ, Pater JL. A randomized trial of letrozole in postmenopausal women after five years of tamoxifen therapy for early-stage breast cancer. N Engl J Med 2003; 349(19):1793–802.

Hemsell DL, Gordon J, Breuner PF, Siiteri PK. Plasma precursors of estrogen. II. Correlation of the extent of conversion of plasma androstenedione to estrone with age. J Clin Endocrinol Metab 1974; 38:476–479.

Henderson, Norbirath G, Kerb U. 1-Methyl-1,4-androstadiene-3, 17-dione (SH 489): Characterization of an irreversible inhibitor of estrogen biosynthesis. J Steroid Biochem 1986; 24:303–306.

Inkster SE, Brodie AMH. Immunocytochemical studies of aromatase in early and full-term human placental tissues: Comparison with biochemical assays. Biol Reprod 1989; 41:889–898.

Inkster SE, Brodie AMH. Human testicular aromatase: immunocytochemical and biochemical studies. J Clin Endocrinol Metab 1995; 80:1941–1947.

James VH, McNeill JM, Lai LC, Newton CJ, Ghilchik MW, Reed MJ. Aromatase activity in normal breast and breast tumor tissue: *In vivo* and *in vitro* studies. Steroids 1987; 50:269–279.

Jelovac D, Sabnis G, Long BJ, Goloubeva OG, Brodie AMH., Activation of MAPK in xenografts and cells during prolonged treatment with aromatase inhibitor letrozole. Cancer Res. 2005; 65:5380–5389.

Johannessen DC, Engan T, Di Salle E, Zurlo MG, Paolini J, Ornati G, Piscitelli G, Kvinnsland S, Lonning PE. Endocrine and clinical effects of exemenstane (PNU 155971), a novel steroidal aromatase inhibitor, in postmenopausal breast cancer patients: A phase I study. Clin Cancer Res 1997; 3:1101–1108.

Jonat W, Howell A, Blomqvist C, Eiermann W, Winblad G, Tyrrell C, et al. A randomized trial comparing two doses of the new selective aromatase inhibitor anastrozole (Arimidex) with meagasterol acetate in postmenopausal patients with advanced breast cancer. Eur J Cancer 1996; 32A:404–412.

Jones S, Vogel C, Arkhipov A, Fehrenbacher L, Eisenberg P, Cooper B, Honig S, Polli A, Whaley F, di Salle E, Tiffany J, Consonni A, Miller L. Multicenter, phase II trial of exemnestane as third-line hormonal therapy in postmenopausal women with metastatic breast cancer. J Chin Oncol 1999; 17:3418–3425.

Jordan VC. Tamoxifen: toxicities and drug resistance during the treatment and prevention of breast cancer. Annu Rev Pharmaeol Toxicol 1995; 35:195–211.

Kaufmann M, Bajetta E, Dirix LY, Fein LE, Jones SE, Zilembo N, Dugardyn J-L, Nasurdi C, Mennel RG, Cervek J, Fowst C, Polli A, di Salle E, Arkhipov A, Piscitelli G, Miller LL, Massimini G. Exemestane is superior to megestrol acetate after tamoxifen failure in postmenopausal women with advanced breast cancer: Results of a phase III randomized double-blind trial. J Clin Oncol 2000; 18:1399–1411.

Killinger DW, Perel E, Daniilescu D, et al. Aromatase activity in the breast and other peripheral tissues and its therapeutic regulation. Steroids 1987; 50:523–535.

Koos RD, Banks PK, Inkster SE, Yue W, Brodie AMH. Detection of aromatase and keratinocyte growth factor expression in breast tumors using reverse transcription-polymerase chain reaction. J Steroid Biochem Mol Biol 1993; 45:217–225.

Lipton A, Santner SJ, Santen RJ, Harvery HA, Feil PD, White-Hershey D, Bartholomew MJ, Antle CE. Aromatase activity in primary and metastatic human breast cancer. Cancer 1987; 59:779–782.

Long BJ, Jelovac D, Handratta V, Thiantanawat A, MacPherson N, Ragaz J, Goloubeva O, Brodie AM: Therapeutic Strategies Using the Aromatase Inhibitor Letrozole and Tamoxifen in a Breast Cancer Model. J Natl Cancer Inst 2004; 96:456–465.

Lönning PE. Pharmacology of new aromatase inhibitors. Breast 1996; 5:202–206.

Lönning PE. Pharmacological profiles of exemestane and formestane, steroidal aromatase inhibitors used for the treatment of postmenopausal breast cancer. Breast Cancer Res Treat 1998; 49:S45–S52.

Lönning PE, Dowsett M, Powles TJ. Postmenopausal estrogen synthesis and metabolism: Alterations caused by aromatase inhibitors used for treatment of breast cancer. J Steroid Biochem 1990; 35:355–366.

Lu Q, Liu Y, Long BJ, Grigoryev D, Gimbel M, Brodie A. The effect of combining aromatase inhibitors with antiestrogens on tumor growth in a nude mouse model for breast cancer. Breast Cancer Res Treat 1999; 57:183–192.

Lu Q, Nakamura J, Savinov A, Yue W, Weisz J, Dabbs DJ, Wolz G, Brodie AMH. Expression of aromatase protein and mRNA in tumor epithelial cells and evidence of functional significance of locally produced estrogen in human breast cancer. Endocrinology 1996; 137:3061–3068.

McGuire WL. An update on estrogen and progesterone receptors in prognosis for primary and advanced breast cancer. In: Iacobelli S, et al., eds. Hormones and Cancer. Vol 15. New York: Raven Press, 1980:337–344.

Metcalf BW, Wright CL, Burkhart JP, Johnston JO. Substrate-induced inactivation of aromatase by allenic and acetylenic steroids. Am Chem Soc 1981; 103:3221–3222.

Miller WR. Hawkins RA, Forrest APM. Significance of aromatase activity in human breast cancer. Cancer Res 1982; 42 (Suppl):3365s–3368s.

Mouridsen H, Gershanovich M, Sun Y, Pérez-Carrión R, Boni C, Monnier A, Apffelstaedt J, Smith R, Sleeboom HP, Jänicke F, Pluzanska A, Dank M, Becquart D, Bapsy PP, Salminen E, Snyder R, Lassus M, Verbeek JA, Staffler B, Chaudri-Ross HA, Dugan M. Superior efficacy of letrozole versus tamoxifen as first-line therapy for postmenopausal women with advanced breast cancer: results of a phase III study of the International Letrozole Breast Cancer Group. J Clin Oncol 2001;19:2596–2606.

Murray R, Pitt P. Aromatase inhibition with 4-OHA androstenedione after prior aromatase inhibition with aminoglutethimide in women with advanced breast cancer. Cancer Res Treat 1995; 35:249–253.

Nabholtz JM, Buzdar A, Pollak M, Harwin W, Burton G, Mangalik A, Steinberg M, Webster A, von Euler M. Anastrozole is superior to tamoxifen as first-line therapy for advanced breast cancer in postmenopausal women: results of a North American multicenter randomized trial. Arimidex Study Group. J Clin Oncol 2000; 18:3758–3767.

Paridaens R, Dirix LY, Beex L. et al. Exemestane (Aromasin) is active and well tolerated as first-line hormonal therapy (HT) of metastatic breast cancer (MBC) patients: Results of a randomized phase II trial (abstr 316). Proc Am Soc Clin Oncol 2000; 19:83a.

Paridaens R, Dirix L, Lohrisch C, Beex L, Nooij M, Cameron D, et al. Mature results of a randomized phase II multicenter study of exemestane versus tamoxifen as first-line hormone therapy for postmenopausal women with metastatic breast cancer. Ann Oncol 2003; 14:1391–1398.

Perel E, Blackstein ME, Killinger DW. Aromatase in human breast carcinoma. Cancer Res 1982; 42(Suppl):3369s–3372s.

Poggesi I, Jannuzzo MG, Di Salle E, et al. Effects of food and formulation on the pharmacokinetics (PK) and pharmacodynamics (PD) of a single oral dose of exemestane (Aromasin, EXE) (abstr 741). Proc Am Soc Clin Oncol 1999; 18:193a.

Price T, Aitken J, Head J, Mahendroo M, Means G, Simpson E. Determination of aromatase cytochrome P.450 messenger ribonucleic acid in human breast tissue by competitive polymerase chain reaction amplification. Clin Endocrinol Metab 1992; 174:1247–1252.

Pritchard KI. Aromatase inhibitors in adjuvant therapy of breast cancer: before, instead of, or beyond tamoxifen. J Clin Oncol 2005; 23:4850–4852.

Sabnis G, Macedo L, Schayowitz A, Goloubeva O, Brodie A. Herceptin restores sensitivity of letrozole resistant cells to hormone therapy. Proceedings of the VIII International Aromatase Conference, J Steroid Biochem Molec Biol, 2006.

Samojlik E, Santen RJ, Wells SA. Adrenal suppression with aminoglutethimide II. Differential effects of aminoglutethimide on plasma androstenedione and estrogen levels. J Clin Endocrinol Metab 1977; 45:480–487.

Schwarzel WC, Kruggel W, Brodie HJ. Studies on the mechanism of estrogen biosynthesis. VII. The development of inhibitors of the enzyme system in human placenta. Endocrinology 1973; 92:866–880.

Simpson ER, Ackerman GE, Smith ME, Mendelson CR. Estrogen formation in stromal cells of adipose tissue of women: Induction of glucocorticosteroids. Proc Natl Acad Sci U S A 1981; 78:5690–5694.

Simpson ER, Mahendroo MS, Means GD, Kilgore MW, Corbin CJ, Mendelson CR. Tissue-speci6c promoters regulate cytochrome P-450 expression. J Steroid Biochem Mol Biol 1993; 44:321–330.

Sjoerdsma A. Suicide inhibitors as potential drugs. Clin Pharmacol Ther 1981; 30:3–22.

Thorsen T, Tangen M, Stoa KF. Concentrations of endogeneous estradiol as related to estradiol receptor sites in breast tumor cytosol. Eur J Cancer Clin Oncol 1982; 18:333–337.

Thürlimann B, Paridaens R, Serin D, Bonneterre J, Roché H, Murray R, di Salle E, Lanzalone S, Zurlo MG, Piscitelli G. Third-line hormonal treatment with exemestane in postmenopausal patients with advanced breast cancer progressing on aminoglutethimide: A phase II multicentre multinational study. Eur J Cancer 1997; 33:1767–1773.

van Landeghem AAJ, Portman J, Nabauurs M. Endogeneous concentration and subcellular distribution of estrogens in normal and malignant human breast tissue. Cancer Res 1985; 45:2900–2906.

Yue W, Wang I, Savinov A, Brodie A. The effect of aromatase inhibitors on growth of mammary tumors in a nude mouse model. Cancer Res 1995; 55:3073–3077.

Yue W, Zhou D, Chen S, Brodie A. A new nude mouse model for postmenopausal breast cancer using MC-7 cells transfected with the human aromatase gene. Cancer Res 1994; 54:5092–5095.

Zhao Y, Agarwal VR, Mendelson CR, Simpson ER. Estrogen biosynthesis proximal to a breast tumor is stimulated by PGE2 via cyclic AMP, leading to activation of promoterII of the CYP19 (aromatase) gene. Endocrinology 1996; 137:5739–5742.

10

Aromatase Inhibition in Breast Cancer: Update of Clinical Applications

PAULA D. RYAN and PAUL E. GOSS

Massachusetts General Hospital Cancer Center and Harvard Medical School, Boston, Massachusetts, U.S.A.

INTRODUCTION

Endocrine manipulation is a highly effective strategy for the treatment of hormone receptor–positive breast carcinoma in both the adjuvant and metastatic settings. In recent decades, the selective estrogen receptor (ER) modulator tamoxifen has been the mainstay of adjuvant endocrine therapy for early stage hormone receptor–positive breast cancer in both pre- and postmenopausal women. In postmenopausal women, options for adjuvant hormonal therapy have recently expanded as the benefits of aromatase inhibitors (AIs) have been clearly and consistently demonstrated in large randomized clinical trials. In premenopausal women, the efficacy of tamoxifen and AIs in combination with ovarian function suppression (OFS) is currently being investigated.

AIs inhibit the enzyme complex, aromatase, responsible for the final step of estrogen synthesis. Unlike tamoxifen, AIs exert no partial estrogen agonist activity. AIs are classified as either steroidal (irreversible) inhibitors or nonsteroidal (reversible) inhibitors. The third-generation AIs in current clinical use include the steroidal AI, exemestane, and the nonsteroidal AIs, anastrozole and letrozole. Each of these has been shown to substantially suppress whole body aromatization by approximately 95% to 98% (Demers, 1994; Geisler et al., 1998; Geisler et al., 1996). AIs are effective antiestrogen therapy in postmenopausal women in whom estrogen synthesis depends solely on peripheral aromatization. However, the use of AIs as monotherapy is contraindicated in premenopausal women as there is a risk for reflex stimulation of gonadotropin secretion, ovarian stimulation with cyst formation, and increased estrogen levels. As such, to date, all clinical trials of adjuvant AI monotherapy have included postmenopausal women only. While changing the landscape of adjuvant hormonal therapy, new data have also highlighted the complexity of AI use. Results from ongoing trials and research strategies are awaited as attempts are made to optimize endocrine and in particular AI therapy.

AIs IN THE TREATMENT OF ADVANCED BREAST CANCER

Several studies demonstrated that AIs have superiority over megestrol acetate in patients with metastatic disease as either first-line therapy or second-line therapy after tamoxifen (Buzdar et al., 2001; Buzdar et al., 1997; Dombernowsky et al., 1998; Jonat et al., 1996; Kaufmann et al., 2000). In first-line treatment trials of metastatic disease with AIs compared with tamoxifen, each of the third-generation AIs has demonstrated improved clinical efficacy in postmenopausal women with advanced breast cancer (Bonneterre et al., 2000; Milla-Santos et al., 2003; Mouridsen et al., 2001; Nabholtz et al., 2000; Paridaens et al., 2003). On the basis of the collective results of these studies, AIs are the current treatment of choice for first-line metastatic breast cancer.

AIs IN THE ADJUVANT TREATMENT OF BREAST CANCER

Efficacy

In an attempt to improve outcomes with adjuvant endocrine therapy, recent clinical trials have probed the benefit of AIs. Over 30,000 women have been enrolled in large clinical trials of AI therapy in the adjuvant setting (Table 1). These trials have evaluated the use of AIs as up-front therapy, instead of tamoxifen, in combination with tamoxifen, in sequence after two to three years of tamoxifen therapy or as extended therapy after the completion of five years of tamoxifen therapy.

Up-front AI Therapy

Two large randomized trials have evaluated the use of up-front aromatase inhibition. The Anastrozole, Tamoxifen Alone or in Combination (ATAC) trial randomized 9366 postmenopausal women with ER-positive (ER+) or unknown invasive breast cancer to receive either five years of tamoxifen, five years of anastrozole, or five years of combination therapy with anastrozole and tamoxifen (Baum et al., 2002). The primary endpoints were disease-free survival (DFS) and safety/tolerability. The initial analysis published in 2002, presented at a median

Table 1 Results of Randomized Adjuvant Aromatase Inhibitor Trials

Study (reference)	Scheme	Eligibility criteria	Design, *N*	Median follow-up	Results[a]
ATAC (Howell et al., 2005)	ANZ × 5 yr vs. TAM × 5 yr vs. ANZ/TAM × 5 yr	Postmenopausal; ER-unknown and ER-negative also allowed	Double blind $N = 9366$	68 mo	DFS HR = 0.87, $p = 0.01$. Favors ANZ over TAM. Similar survival in combination arm (discontinued after first analysis)
BIG 1-98[b] (Coates et al., 2007)	LTZ × 5 yr vs. TAM × 5 yr vs. LTZ × 2 yr then TAM × 3 yr vs. TAM × 2 yr then LTZ × 3 yr	Postmenopausal; ER-positive	Double blind $N = 4922$	51 mo	DFS HR 0.82, $p = 0.007$. Favors LTZ over Tam. Analysis limited to patients on monotherapy arms. Crossover results not yet available
ITA (Boccardo et al., 2006)	TAM × 5 yr vs. TAM × 2–3 yr then ANZ × 3–2 yr	Postmenopausal; ER-positive, node-positive only; free of recurrence after 2–3 yr of TAM	Open label $N = 448$	64 mo	EFS HR = 0.57, $p = 0.005$. Favors TAM-ANZ over TAM.
ABCSG-8/ARNO-95 (Jakesz et al., 2005)	TAM × 5 yr vs TAM × 2 yr then ANZ × 3 yr	Postmenopausal; ER-positive	Open label $N = 3224$	28 mo	EFS HR = 0.60, $p = 0.0009$. Favors TAM-ANZ over TAM
IES (Coombes et al., 2004)	TAM × 5 yr vs TAM × 2–3 yr then EXE × 3–2 yr	Postmenopausal; ER-positive or unknown; free of recurrence after 2–3 yr of TAM	Double-blind $N = 4742$	30.6 mo	DFS HR = 0.68, $p = 0.00005$. Favors TAM-EXE over TAM
MA.17 (Goss et al., 2003)	Yr 6–10 LTZ × 5 yr vs. placebo × 5 yr	Postmenopausal; ER-positive, free of recurrence after 4.5–6 yr of TAM	Double-blind $N = 5187$	30 mo	DFS HR = 0.58, $p < 0.001$. Favors LTZ over placebo Improved OS in node-positive, HR = 0.61, $p = 0.04$

[a]Primary endpoint was disease-free survival for all studies except the ABCSG-8/ARNO-95 study where the primary endpoint was event-free survival.
[b]This analysis was limited to patients on the monotherapy arms on BIG 1-98.
Abbreviations: ANZ, anastrozole; TAM, tamoxifen; LTZ, letrozole; ATAC trial, Anastrozole, Tamoxifen Alone or in Combination trial; BIG 1-98, Breast International Group; IES, Intergroup Exemestane Study; MA.17, National Cancer Institute of Canada Clinical Trials Group MA.17 trial; ITA, Italian trial; ABCSG, Austrian Breast and Colorectal Cancer Study Group; ARNO, German Adjuvant Breast Cancer Group.

follow-up of 33 months, revealed superior DFS for the anastrozole arm compared with the tamoxifen arm (89.4% vs. 87.4%, respectively; $p = 0.013$) (Baum et al., 2002). The ATAC trial was updated at a median follow-up of 68 months, demonstrating that with only 8% of patients remaining on trial, DFS was significantly longer for anastrozole compared with tamoxifen, with a hazard ratio (HR) of 0.87 ($p = 0.01$) and an absolute difference of 3.7% between the two arms (Howell et al., 2005). The anastrozole arm experienced significantly fewer distant metastases and fewer incidences of contralateral breast cancers. To date, there has been no detectable difference in overall survival between the treatment groups (Baum et al., 2002; Baum et al., 2003; Howell et al., 2005). Of note, the combination arm of tamoxifen plus anastrozole in this trial showed equivalence or even a trend to worse outcome than tamoxifen monotherapy. Results from this arm was discontinued and not included in subsequent analyses.

Another large adjuvant trial, the Breast International Group (BIG) 1-98 randomized 8010 postmenopausal women with hormone receptor–positive breast cancer to one of the four treatment arms: five years of letrozole, five years of tamoxifen, two years of tamoxifen followed by three years of letrozole, or two years of letrozole followed by three years of tamoxifen. The first analysis published in 2005 compared the two groups assigned to receive initial letrozole with the two groups assigned to receive initial tamoxifen (Thurlimann et al., 2005). In the sequential treatment groups, events and follow-up were included only up to the time the therapy was switched. After a median follow-up of 25.8 months, letrozole resulted in a significantly lower risk of recurrence (HR, 0.81; 95% CI, 0.70–0.93; $p = 0.003$) with five-year DFS rate estimates of 84.0% for the letrozole group and 81.4% for the tamoxifen group, leading to an absolute difference of 2.6% between the two groups. Significantly, fewer recurrences at distant sites were noted in the letrozole group. Overall survival (OS) was not found to differ significantly between the tamoxifen and letrozole groups (Thurlimann et al., 2005). An analysis of BIG 1-98 that was limited to patients randomly assigned to the continuous therapy arms (2463 women receiving letrozole and 2459 women receiving tamoxifen) was recently published in 2007 (Coates et al., 2007). At a median follow-up of 51 months, there was an 18% reduction in the risk of an event (HR, 0.82; 95% CI, 0.71–0.95; $p = 0.007$). Anastrozole and letrozole are now both approved by the United States Food and Drug Administration as up-front therapy in postmenopausal women with early stage breast cancer (Table 2).

Sequential AI Therapy

Multiple trials have probed whether switching from tamoxifen to an AI is superior to tamoxifen alone. The Intergroup Exemestane Study (IES) randomized 4742 postmenopausal women with ER+ early breast cancer who were disease free following two to three years of tamoxifen either to continued tamoxifen or to exemestane to complete a total of five years of endocrine therapy (Coombes et al., 2004). With a median follow-up of 30.6 months, results indicated a decreased risk of breast cancer recurrence (HR, 0.68; 95% CI, 0.56–0.82; $p = 0.00005$), distant disease (HR, 0.66; 95% CI, 0.52–0.83; $p = 0.0004$), and contralateral breast cancer (HR, 0.44; 95% CI, 0.20–0.98; $p = 0.04$) for those women who received exemestane. No difference in OS was detected among treatment arms (Coombes et al., 2004). Updated analysis is pending.

A combined analysis at a median follow-up of 28 months of 3224 postmenopausal women participating in two smaller trials, the Austrian Breast and Colorectal Cancer Study Group (ABCSG)-8 and the German Adjuvant Breast Cancer Group (ARNO)-95 trial, also demonstrated improved event-free survival for two years of tamoxifen therapy followed by anastrozole for three years versus five years of tamoxifen alone (HR, 0.60; 95% CI, 0.44–0.81; $p = 0.0009$) (Jakesz et al., 2005). Similar results were noted in the Italian Tamoxifen Trial (ITA), which randomized 448 ER+, node-positive patients who had completed two to three years of adjuvant tamoxifen to either anastrozole or continued tamoxifen to complete a total of five years of therapy (Boccardo et al., 2005). Updated analysis at a median follow-up of 64 months' results demonstrated improved event-free survival (HR 0.57; 95% CI, 0.35–0.89; $p = 0.005$) for the anastrozole group (Boccardo et al., 2006). A meta-analysis of the ARNO-95, ABCSG-8, and ITA trials is awaited. The ongoing Tamoxifen and Exemestane Adjuvant Multicenter (TEAM) trial will provide additional data on the sequential use of AIs and tamoxifen.

Extended AI Therapy

After completion of five years of adjuvant hormonal therapy, women with ER+ breast cancer remain at risk of recurrence, and this risk appears to persist indefinitely [Early Breast Cancer Trialists Collaborative Group (EBCTCG, 2005)]. On the basis of this observation, the National Cancer Institute of Canada (NCIC) Clinical Trials Group MA.17 trial evaluated extending adjuvant endocrine therapy beyond five years of tamoxifen (Goss et al., 2003). Following the completion of five years of adjuvant tamoxifen therapy, 5187 postmenopausal women with hormone receptor–positive breast cancer were randomly assigned to letrozole or placebo for five years. After the initial prespecified interim efficacy analysis at a mean follow-up of 2.4 years, the decision was made to stop the trial and offer letrozole to those women

Table 2 Summary Table of Selected Predefined Adverse Events of Aromatase Inhibitors Vs. Tamoxifen as Up-front Adjuvant Therapy in ATAC and BIG 1-98

Study (reference)	Number of events *N* (%)	Number of events *N* (%)	*p* value
ATAC (Howell et al., 2005)	**Anastrozole** $N = 3092$	**Tamoxifen** $N = 3093$	
Hot flushes	1104 (35.7)	1264 (40.9)	0.02
Nausea and vomiting	393 (12.7)	384 (12.4)	0.7
Fatigue/tiredness	575 (18.6)	544 (17.6)	0.3
Mood disturbances	597 (19.3)	554 (17.9)	0.2
Arthralgia	1100 (35.6)	911 (29.4)	<0.0001
Vaginal bleeding	167 (5.4)	317 (10.2)	<0.0001
Vaginal discharge	109 (3.5)	408 (13.2)	<0.0001
Endometrial cancer	5 (0.2)	17 (0.8)	<0.0001
Bone fractures	340 (11.0)	237 (7.7)	<0.0001
Ischemic cardiovascular Disease	127 (4.1)	104 (3.4)	0.1
Ischemic cerebrovascular events	62 (2.0)	88 (2.8)	0.03
All venous thromboembolic events	87 (2.8)	140 (4.5)	0.0004
cataracts	182 (5.9)	213 (6.9)	0.1
BIG 1-98 (Coates et al., 2007)	**Letrozole** $N = 2448$	**Tamoxifen** $N = 2447$	
Vaginal bleeding	92 (3.8)	203 (8.3)	<0.001
Hot flashes	803 (32.8)	914 (37.4)	<0.001
Nausea	242 (9.9%)	231 (9.4%)	0.63
Vomiting	74 (3.0)	76 (3.1)	0.87
Night sweats	348 (14.2)	416 (17.0)	0.007
Fracture	211 (8.6)	141 (5.8)	<0.001
Arthralgia	489 (20.0)	331(13.5)	<0.001
Myalgia	174 (7.1)	150 (6.1)	0.19
Cerebrovascular accident or TIA	34 (1.4)	35 (1.4)	0.90
Thromboembolic event	50 (2.0)	94 (3.8)	<0.001
Cardiac event	134 (5.5)	122 (5.0)	0.48
Ischemic heart disease	54 (2.2)	41 (1.7)	0.21
Cardiac failure	24 (1.0)	14 (0.6)	0.14
Other cardiovascular event	19 (0.8)	6 (0.2)	0.014
Hypercholesterolemia	1238 (50.6)	601 (24.6)	<0.001

Abbreviations: ATAC, Anastrozole or Tamoxifen Alone or in Combination; BIG 1-98, Breast International Group; TIA, transient ischemic attack.

randomized to placebo. The interim analysis demonstrated the four-year DFS rate among women in the letrozole arm to be 93% compared with 87% in the placebo arm ($p < 0.001$) (Goss et al., 2003). A more complete and final analysis of the blinded study, at a median follow-up of 30 months, demonstrated that patients treated with letrozole experienced a significantly reduced HR for recurrences and contralateral breast cancer. While OS did not differ between treatment groups, a prespecified subset analysis of patients with node-positive disease, revealed a significant improvement in OS (HR, 0.61; 95% CI, 0.38–0.98; $p = 0.04$) (Goss et al., 2005b). Recent analyses were conducted to examine the relationships between duration of treatment in MA.17 trial and outcomes. All events up to the date of unblinding of the study were queried. A nonparametric kernel smoothing method was used to estimate the hazard rates for DFS, DDFS, and OS at 6, 12, 24, 36, and 48 months of follow-up, and the HRs of letrozole to placebo were determined. A Cox model with a time-dependent covariate was used to describe the trend in HRs over time. HRs for events in DFS and DDFS significantly decreased over time, with the trend favoring letrozole ($p \leq 0.0001$ and $p = 0.0013$, respectively). The trend for OS was not significant. For patients with node-positive status, the HRs for DFS, DDFS, and OS all decreased over time with tests for trend all showing significance ($p = 0.0004$, 0.0005, and 0.38, respectively) (Ingle et al., 2006).

Tolerability

The side effect profile of AI therapy must be carefully considered in clinical decision making regarding AI adjuvant therapy. When analyzing adverse events from the trials described above, it is important to note that toxicity of AI therapy has generally been assessed in comparison with tamoxifen. While MA.17 trial compared AI therapy to placebo, its toxicity results must be interpreted with some caution because all the women had recently completed five years of tamoxifen therapy, and presumably those who tolerated endocrine therapy least well did not complete tamoxifen and were therefore by definition excluded from randomization. Continued updated safety analyses from the AI adjuvant trials are also necessary to evaluate long-term toxicities.

General Tolerability/Quality of Life

AIs appear to be generally well tolerated. Not unexpectedly, the most common side effects are those related to estrogen deficiency and include hot flashes, vaginal complaints, myalgias, and arthralgias. In the MA.17 trial, these symptoms occurred significantly more frequently among women treated with letrozole than those treated with placebo (Goss et al., 2003). Other symptoms on study such as fatigue, sweating, constipation, headache, and dizziness occurred equally in both arms, suggesting no drug-related effect, while vaginal bleeding was significantly less frequent in the letrozole arm (Goss et al., 2003). The percentage of women discontinuing treatment because of adverse events was similar between the two arms. Published quality of life substudies of ATAC, MA.17, and IES all indicate that AI therapy has no adverse affect on overall self-reported quality of life (Fallowfield et al., 2004; Fallowfield et al., 2006; Whelan et al., 2005; Whelan and Pritchard, 2006). A recently published risk-benefit analysis of the ATAC trial concludes that anastrozole was better tolerated than tamoxifen with fewer serious adverse events (Buzdar et al., 2006).

Skeletal Effects

The most serious concern related to the profound estrogen suppression produced with AI therapy is the potential to decrease bone mineral density (BMD) and thereby to increase clinical fractures. While none of the three large trials incorporated a protocol-defined baseline fracture risk assessment or ongoing BMD monitoring (Winer et al., 2005), results from the overall study populations and bone metabolism substudies indicate that AIs do exert some adverse effects on bone health. In the ATAC trial, women taking anastrozole were significantly more likely to experience arthralgias (35.6% vs. 29.4%) and fractures (11.0% vs. 7.7%) (Howell et al., 2005). A bone substudy of 308 women enrolled in ATAC demonstrated that two years of anastrozole therapy resulted in median decreases in BMD of 4.1% and 3.9% at the lumbar spine and total hip, respectively. Moreover, one year of anastrozole therapy was associated with increases in markers of bone resorption and bone formation (Eastell et al., 2006).

Similarly, women treated with letrozole in the BIG 1-98 trial had a significantly increased rate of arthralgias (20.0% vs. 13.5%) and fractures (8.6% vs. 5.8%) (Coates et al., 2007). In the IES trial, women receiving exemestane experienced significantly higher rates of arthralgias (5.4% vs. 3.6%) and slight but nonsignificant increases in rates of osteoporosis and fractures (Coombes et al., 2004). Results from the IES bone substudy are awaited. The combined results of ABCSG-8 and ARNO-95 demonstrated significantly more fractures in patients receiving anastrozole than tamoxifen [odds ratio (OR), 2.14; 95% CI, 1.14–4.17; $p = 0.015$] (Jakesz et al., 2005). Results from the above trials, however, which compare AIs to tamoxifen, must be interpreted with caution as tamoxifen is known to have a beneficial effect on bone (Love et al., 1992; Powles et al., 1996).

In the MA.17 study, increased rates, which did not reach statistical significance, of new-onset osteoporosis and fractures occurred in the letrozole group compared with placebo (5.8% vs. 4.5% and 3.6% vs. 2.9%, respectively) (Goss et al., 2003). A recently published bone substudy of MA.17 evaluated bone turnover markers and BMD in a subset of 226 patients with a median follow-up of 1.6 years. At 24 months, patients receiving letrozole experienced significant decreases in total hip and lumbar spine BMD (−3.6% vs. −0.71% and −5.35% vs. −0.70%, respectively) (Perez et al., 2006). A significant decrease in BMD of the femoral neck (−2.72% vs. −1.48%) and a nonsignificant decrease in lumbar spine BMD were noted in a separate small trial assessing the effects of exemestane versus placebo on bone metabolism (Lonning et al., 2005).

Longer-term follow-up from the large clinical trials and further data from ongoing bone substudies are needed to better define the clinical implications of AI therapy on BMD and fracture risk. Current American Society of Clinical Oncology guidelines identify women receiving AI therapy to be at high risk for osteoporosis and recommend a baseline BMD study with interventions based on the result (Hillner et al., 2003). Two additional manuscripts published in 2006 also review the monitoring and management of bone in patients receiving AIs (Chien and Goss, 2006; Goss et al., 2005a).

Cardiovascular Effects

Most of the data, to date, suggest that AIs do not have adverse effects on lipid metabolism or cardiovascular disease. In the ATAC trial, no significant difference in ischemic cardiovascular disease was noted between treatment arms (Howell et al., 2005). Likewise, no significant difference in rates of myocardial infarctions was evident between treatment arms of either the ABCSG-8/ARNO-95 or IES trials (Coombes et al., 2004; Jakesz et al., 2005). In contrast, significantly more women in the letrozole group in the BIG 1-98 study experienced cardiovascular events other than ischemic heart disease and cardiac failure, with a trend for higher-grade cardiac events on letrozole compared with tamoxifen (Coates et al., 2007). Also, patients on letrozole experienced significantly more low-grade cholesterol elevation. Whether these cardiovascular effects reflect an adverse impact of letrozole or a cardioprotective effect of tamoxifen is unknown. In the MA.17 trial, no significant differences in cardiovascular events were noted between letrozole and placebo arms. A lipid substudy of the MA.17 trial demonstrated that five years of letrozole therapy did not alter serum cholesterol, high-density lipoproteins (HDL), low-density lipoproteins, or triglycerides (Wasan et al., 2005). Similarly, a small study examining lipid levels among 147 women randomized to either exemestane or placebo for two years demonstrated no significant change in lipid levels except for a modest reduction in HDL cholesterol and apolipoprotein AI in the exemestane group (Lonning et al., 2005).

Endometrial Cancer

Unlike tamoxifen, AIs have not been demonstrated to increase risk of endometrial cancer, stroke, or thromboembolic events. In the ATAC trial, treatment with an AI was associated with significantly lower incidence of endometrial carcinoma compared with tamoxifen (Howell et al., 2005). Similarly, the BIG 1-98, ABSCG-8/ARNO-95, and IES trials reported a nonsignificant trend toward fewer endometrial cancers in the AI arms compared with the tamoxifen arms (Coombes et al., 2004; Jakesz et al., 2005; Thurlimann et al., 2005).

Thromboembolic Events

Significantly lower incidences of thromboembolic events were noted in the AI arms of ATAC, BIG 1-98, and IES trials (Coates et al., 2007; Coombes et al., 2004; Howell et al., 2005; Thurlimann et al., 2005). The ABCSG-8/ARNO-95 trial demonstrated significantly fewer thromboses in patients treated with anastrozole and a trend toward fewer emboli (Jakesz et al., 2005). A statistically significantly lower incidence of ischemic cerebrovascular events was observed in the anastrozole arm of the ATAC trial. In MA.17 trial, there were similar numbers of thromboembolic events, stroke, or transient ischemic attacks between patients receiving letrozole and placebo (Goss et al., 2005).

Optimizing Adjuvant Endocrine Therapy

Current Recommendations

All trials, to date, have demonstrated a significant and consistent improvement in DFS among women who received an AI as part of their adjuvant therapy compared with women who received tamoxifen alone. Moreover, the MA.17 trial revealed an improvement in OS for node-positive patients receiving letrozole therapy after five years of tamoxifen. On the basis of these data, there is no doubt that the incorporation of AI therapy into adjuvant regimens for postmenopausal women with hormone responsive breast cancer is superior to tamoxifen alone. The American Society of Clinical Oncology Technology Assessment Panel, convened in 2005 to update guidelines to physicians and patients regarding the use of AIs in the adjuvant setting, concluded that "optimal adjuvant hormonal therapy for a postmenopausal woman with receptor-positive breast cancer should include an aromatase inhibitor either as initial therapy or after treatment with tamoxifen." The panel cautioned, "of course, women with breast cancer and their physicians must weigh the risks and benefits of all therapeutic options" (Winer et al., 2005).

Defining the Optimal Sequence, Duration, and Agent

To optimize AI therapy within adjuvant regimens several issues remain to be defined. These include among others: (1) the relative benefits of AIs as initial therapy, after two to three years of tamoxifen therapy, or after the completion of five years of tamoxifen; (2) the potential role for tamoxifen after AI therapy; (3) the optimal duration of AI therapy for those women who switch to an AI after two to three years of tamoxifen as well as for those who initiate AI therapy after five years of tamoxifen; and (4) whether there is a preferred agent among the currently prescribed AIs.

Several ongoing trials could provide insight and help guide clinical practice. Analysis of all four arms of BIG 1-98 trial, for example, should help clarify optimal sequencing strategies. The second rerandomization of MA.17 (MA.17R) trial will include women who received five years of letrozole and are then randomized to a further five years of AI therapy versus placebo. MA.17R has recently been amended to include women who have received five years of any prior AI alone or after two to three years of tamoxifen. The National Surgical Adjuvant Breast and Bowel Project (NSABP) B-42 study aims to compare five years of letrozole versus placebo in women who have completed five years of hormonal therapy either with tamoxifen and an AI or with an AI alone. These studies will better define optimal duration of AI therapy.

While all three AIs have demonstrated clinical efficacy in the adjuvant setting, certain differences are known to exist between them, and direct comparisons between agents have not yet been reported. Pharmacodynamic studies have demonstrated that both letrozole and exemestane are associated with greater suppression of aromatase than anastrozole (Geisler et al., 2002; Geisler et al., 1998; Geisler et al., 1996), and exemestane, because of its steroidal properties, is hypothesized to have a superior safety profile with regard to bone and lipid metabolism (Goss et al., 2004a; Goss et al., 2004b). Data are awaited from MA.27, a randomized phase III clinical trial comparing anastrozole with exemestane as initial adjuvant therapy, as well as from the Femara versus Anastrozole Clinical Evaluation (FACE) trial, which is comparing up-front adjuvant letrozole with anastrozole in postmenopausal women with node-positive breast cancer.

Identifying Predictive Biomarkers

Despite the great advances afforded by both tamoxifen and, more recently, by the AIs in the adjuvant setting, there are still subsets of women with hormone receptor–positive breast cancer who do not benefit from endocrine therapies. Improving patient selection through the identification of biomarkers that can predict response to endocrine therapies is under way.

One such strategy is to identify specific gene expression signatures of tumor cells. Oncotype DX, developed by Genomic Health, is a current commercially available assay (Paik et al., 2004) that uses an algorithm based on the expression of 21 genes to compute a recurrence score for a specific tumor sample. The recurrence score, which has been prospectively validated, quantifies the likelihood of distant recurrence in patients with node-negative, ER+ breast cancer treated with tamoxifen. Clinically, Oncotype DX is most useful in identifying patients with low-risk tumors that can be treated with tamoxifen alone without the addition of chemotherapy. Using microarray technology, the Massachusetts General Hospital two-gene -expression ratio, *HOXB13* versus *IL17BR,* and a 44-gene signature have been developed, which similarly claim to predict tamoxifen responsiveness in patients with ER+ breast cancer better than currently used clinicopathological criteria (Loi et al., 2006; Ma et al., 2006; Ma et al., 2004). The U.S. Food and Drug Administration approved MammaPrint^{TM}, developed by Agendia, in February 2007, which is a 70-gene prognostic signature that classifies patients into low risk or high risk of breast cancer recurrence within 5 to 10 years of their cancer diagnosis (van de Vijver et al., 2002).

Commonly tested tumor characteristics might also prove to be useful in differentiating tumors that are responsive to endocrine therapy. Emerging laboratory and clinical data suggest that among ER+ tumors, the progesterone receptor (PR) status may predict differential sensitivity to either AI or tamoxifen therapy (Cui et al., 2005). An exploratory retrospective subgroup analysis of the ATAC trial, for example, demonstrated that the benefit of anastrozole was substantially greater among women with ER+/PR– tumors than those with ER+/PR+ tumors (Dowsett et al., 2005). A similar, although nonsignificant trend of greater benefit of anastrozole in ER+/PR– patients was reported in the ABCSG-8/ARNO-95 trial (Jakesz et al., 2005). In BIG 1-98 trial, the benefits of letrozole over tamoxifen were the same in the ER+ tumors irrespective of PR status (Thurlimann et al., 2005). Outcomes according to tumor receptor status were measured in MA.17 trial using Cox's proportional hazards model, adjusting for nodal status and prior adjuvant chemotherapy (Goss et al., 2007, in press). The DFS HR for letrozole versus placebo in ER+/PR+ tumors ($N = 3809$) was 0.49 (95% CI, 0.36–0.67) versus 1.21 (95% CI, 0.63–2.34) in ER+/PR– tumors ($N = 636$). ER+/PR+ letrozole patients experienced significant benefit in distant DFS (DDFS; HR = 0.53, 95% CI, 0.35–0.80) and OS (HR = 0.58, 95% CI, 0.37–0.90). The authors caution against using these results for clinical decision making as this was a subset analysis and receptors were not measured centrally. Results from prospective randomized trials are needed before PR status can inform clinical decision making.

The human epidermal growth factor receptor (HER-2) might also have a predictive role. Preclinical models have suggested that tumors overexpressing HER-2 are resistant to tamoxifen, perhaps because of enhanced interactions between the ER and HER-2 signaling pathways (Osborne et al., 2003; Shou et al., 2004). Clinical evidence from small randomized trials comparing tamoxifen with AIs in the neoadjuvant setting suggest that tumors overexpressing HER-2 may be particularly responsive to AI therapy (Ellis et al., 2001; Zhu et al., 2004). As with PR status, though, HER-2 status should not yet guide clinical practice. In fact, the American Society of Clinical Oncology guidelines recommend that "HER-2 status not be considered when making choices about adjuvant hormonal therapy." The panel does note, however, "that some Panel members are more inclined to recommend initial therapy with an aromatase inhibitor in postmenopausal women with HER-2–positive tumors." (Winer et al., 2005).

Pharmacogenomic studies are identifying host characteristics that may provide information on endocrine responsiveness. It has recently been demonstrated, for example, that individuals with certain polymorphisms in the *CYP2D6* gene, an enzyme responsible for tamoxifen biotransformation, experience worse disease outcome and fewer adverse side effects with tamoxifen therapy (Goetz et al., 2005). Genetic polymorphisms have also recently been characterized in the aromatase gene (Ma et al., 2005) and may explain differences in response and toxicity among women receiving AI therapy.

Caution Regarding the Use of AIs in Perimenopausal women

Special attention should be addressed to perimenopausal women and those women who are premenopausal at diagnosis and who appear to have undergone menopause with chemotherapy. There is a lack of efficacy for AIs in these clinical situations; in fact, there is a potential for stimulation of the ovaries with reflex stimulation of gonadotropin secretion in premenopausal women. Although chemotherapy may result in amenorrhea, this does not necessarily equate with absence of ovarian function with premenopausal levels of estradiol found in some women with chemotherapy-induced amenorrhea. Letrozole at 2.5 mg/day given on days 3 to 7 following a menstrual cycle has been shown to be effective in inducing ovulation (Mitwally and Casper, 2001). The ATAC trial allowed entry of women who were amenorrheic for fewer than 12 months if amenorrhea resulted from chemotherapy and if follicle-stimulated hormone was in the postmenopausal range. This number of patients was very small and caution should be used in generalizing these results to all premenopausal patients with chemotherapy-induced amenorrhea. At present, there are no data supporting the use of an AI in combination with OFS, but several large ongoing randomized trials are addressing the value of AIs in premenopausal women. Suppression of Ovarian Function Trial (SOFT) has a target accrual of 3000 premenopausal women who either do not receive chemotherapy or who remain premenopausal after chemotherapy and who are randomly assigned to five years of treatment with tamoxifen, OFS plus tamoxifen, or OFS plus exemestane. Tamoxifen and Exemestane Trial (TEXT) has a target accrual of 1845 premenopausal women who are randomly assigned to five years of treatment with triptorelin plus tamoxifen or triptorelin plus exemestane. Premenopausal women in ABCSG-12 are randomly assigned to receive three years of either tamoxifen or anastrozole, in combination with goserelin.

AIs IN NEOADJUVANT TREATMENT OF BREAST CANCER

Each of the third-generation AIs has been evaluated in the neoadjuvant setting with the rationale to downstage hormone-responsive tumors before surgical resection in postmenopausal women (Dixon et al., 2000; Eiermann et al., 2001; Ellis et al., 2003; Miller and Dixon, 2002). All three are superior to tamoxifen with greater downstaging of tumor and disease control. The AIs are often employed as neoadjuvant therapy in elderly patients with comorbid disease to avoid the increased risk for complications with chemotherapy. There is an ongoing phase III randomized trial of neoadjuvant therapy (ACOSOG-Z1031) comprising exemestane versus letrozole versus anastrozole in postmenopausal women with ER+ stage II or stage III breast cancer. The results of this study will dictate which AI will then be used in a future study that will directly compare the efficacy of neoadjuvant AI therapy with neoadjuvant chemotherapy in postmenopausal women with early stage hormone responsive breast cancer.

THE POTENTIAL ROLE OF AIs IN THE TREATMENT OF DUCTAL CARCINOMA IN SITU AND IN CHEMOPREVENTION OF BREAST CANCER

The role of AIs in the treatment of ductal carcinoma in situ (DCIS) is currently being evaluated in the NSABP B 35 trial that randomizes women with DCIS to either anastrozole or tamoxifen after lumpectomy and radiation therapy.

Data from the large adjuvant AI trials provide a rationale for exploring the use of the AIs in the prevention setting. In patients receiving an AI, a consistent reduction in the rates of contralateral breast cancer was observed. In the ATAC trial there was a 53% reduction in the number of contralateral breast cancers in the anastrozole arm in hormone receptor–positive patients (95% CI, 27–71; $p = 0.001$) (Howell et al., 2005). Tamoxifen is known to reduce the incidence of contralateral tumors by 46% in women with predominantly ER+ tumors, suggesting that the overall reduction of hormone receptor–positive breast cancer associated with anastrozole may be about 70% to 80%. In the IES trial, women randomly assigned to two to three years of exemestane after two to three years of tamoxifen had a 56% reduction in contralateral breast cancer compared with those randomly assigned to continue tamoxifen (9 vs. 20 cases; $p = 0.04$) (Coombes et al., 2004). The ARNO-95/ABCSG-8 trial showed a 26% reduction in contralateral breast tumors (12 vs. 16; $p = 0.4$). In the MA.17 trial, women who were randomly assigned to five years of letrozole after five years of tamoxifen had a 46% reduction in new contralateral tumors compared with women randomly assigned to placebo (14 vs. 26 cases, respectively; $p \leq 0.01$).

Chemoprevention trials are now under way with AIs. MAP.3 is a phase III randomized prevention trial sponsored by NCIC Clinical Trials Group that compares exemestane to placebo in more than 4500 postmenopausal women at increased risk for breast cancer. The primary goal of this study is to determine if exemestane reduces the incidence of invasive breast cancer compared with placebo. Other key comparisons between the two treatment arms include the total incidence of invasive and noninvasive breast cancer, the incidence of receptor-negative breast cancer, lobular carcinoma in situ and atypical ductal hyperplasia events, the incidence of other malignancies, as well as the number of clinical fractures and clinical breast biopsies, cardiovascular events, and quality of life. The International Breast Cancer Intervention-II Trial (IBIS-II) began in February 2003 and is comparing anastrozole to placebo in postmenopausal women at increased risk for breast cancer. A second complimentary study to IBIS-II will compare anastrozole to tamoxifen for postmenopausal women with DCIS.

CONCLUSION

Recently, there has been remarkable progress in the treatment of hormone responsive postmenopausal breast cancer with AIs. Modest gains in progression-free survival with AI therapy in the metastatic setting versus tamoxifen have translated into substantial gains in the adjuvant setting. Recent large adjuvant clinical trials have proven that incorporation of AI therapy, either up front or in sequence after two to three years of tamoxifen, improves DFS. Likewise, extended adjuvant AI therapy after the completion of five years of tamoxifen improves DFS and also improves OS for women with node-positive disease. The third-generation AIs that are associated with myalgias, arthralgias, and with BMD reduction, tend to be otherwise fairly well tolerated with lower risks of endometrial carcinoma and thromboembolic events than tamoxifen. Data are awaited from ongoing trials to better define optimal sequence and duration of AI therapy, the optimal AI agent, and long-term safety profiles. AIs are also being studied in the neoadjuvant setting and ongoing trials will better define the efficacy of this approach in postmenopausal women. Attempts to further optimize endocrine adjuvant therapy by identifying predictive biomarkers of response as well as by developing strategies to overcome endocrine resistance are under way. For premenopausal women, the role of OFS in addition to either tamoxifen or AI therapy is being explored in ongoing clinical trials. The hope is that continued advances in endocrine therapy will translate into improved survival among all women with hormone receptor–positive breast cancer.

REFERENCES

Baum M, Budzar AU, Cuzick J, Forbes J, Houghton JH, Klijn JG, Sahmoud T. Anastrozole alone or in combination with tamoxifen versus tamoxifen alone for adjuvant treatment of postmenopausal women with early breast cancer: first results of the ATAC randomised trial. Lancet 2002; 359:2131–2139.

Baum M, Buzdar A, Cuzick J, Forbes J, Houghton J, Howell A, Sahmoud T. Anastrozole alone or in combination with tamoxifen versus tamoxifen alone for adjuvant treatment of postmenopausal women with early-stage breast cancer: results of the ATAC (Arimidex, Tamoxifen Alone or in Combination) trial efficacy and safety update analyses. Cancer 2003; 98:1802–1810.

Boccardo F, Rubagotti A, Guglielmini P, Fini A, Paladini G, Mesiti M, Rinaldini M, Scali S, Porpiglia M, Benedetto C, Restuccia N, Buzzi F, Franchi R, Massidda B, Distante V, Amadori D, Sismondi P. Switching to anastrozole versus continued tamoxifen treatment of early breast cancer. Updated results of the Italian tamoxifen anastrozole (ITA) trial. Ann Oncol 2006; 17(suppl 7):vii10–vii14.

Boccardo F, Rubagotti A, Puntoni M, Guglielmini P, Amoroso D, Fini A, Paladini G, Mesiti M, Romeo D, Rinaldini M, Scali S, Porpiglia M, Benedetto C, Restuccia N, Buzzi F, Franchi R, Massidda B, Distante V, Amadori D, Sismondi P. Switching to anastrozole versus continued tamoxifen treatment of early breast cancer: preliminary results of the Italian Tamoxifen Anastrozole Trial. J Clin Oncol 2005; 23:5138–5147.

Bonneterre J, Thurlimann B, Robertson JF, Krzakowski M, Mauriac L, Koralewski P, Vergote I, Webster A, Steinberg M, von Euler M. Anastrozole versus tamoxifen as first-line therapy for advanced breast cancer in 668 postmenopausal women: results of the Tamoxifen or Arimidex Randomized Group Efficacy and Tolerability study. J Clin Oncol 2000; 18:3748–3757.

Buzdar A, Douma J, Davidson N, Elledge R, Morgan M, Smith R, Porter L, Nabholtz J, Xiang X, Brady C. Phase III, multicenter, double-blind, randomized study of letrozole, an aromatase inhibitor, for advanced breast cancer versus megestrol acetate. J Clin Oncol 2001; 19:3357–3366.

Buzdar A, Howell A, Cuzick J, Wale C, Distler W, Hoctin-Boes G, Houghton J, Locker GY, Nabholtz JM. Comprehensive side-effect profile of anastrozole and tamoxifen as adjuvant treatment for early-stage breast cancer: long-term safety analysis of the ATAC trial. Lancet Oncol 2006; 7:633–643.

Buzdar AU, Jones SE, Vogel CL, Wolter J, Plourde P, Webster A. A phase III trial comparing anastrozole (1 and 10 milligrams), a potent and selective aromatase inhibitor, with megestrol acetate in postmenopausal women with advanced breast carcinoma. Arimidex Study Group. Cancer 1997; 79:730–739.

Chien AJ, Goss PE. Aromatase inhibitors and bone health in women with breast cancer. J Clin Oncol 2006; 24: 5305–5312.

Coates AS, Keshaviah A, Thurlimann B, Mouridsen H, Mauriac L, Forbes JF, Paridaens R, Castiglione-Gertsch M, Gelber RD, Colleoni M, Láng I, Del Mastro L, Smith I, Chirgwin J, Nogaret J-M, Pienkowski T, Wardley A, Jakobsen EH, Price KN, Goldhirsch A. Five years of letrozole compared with tamoxifen as initial adjuvant therapy for postmenopausal women with endocrine-responsive early breast cancer: update of study BIG 1-98. J Clin Oncol 2007; 25:486–492.

Coombes RC, Hall E, Gibson LJ, Paridaens R, Jassem J, Delozier T, Jones SE, Alvarez I, Bertelli G, Ortmann O, Coates AS, Bajetta E, Dodwell D, Coleman RE, Fallowfield LJ, Mickiewicz E, Andersen J, Lønning PE, Cocconi G, Stewart A, Stuart N, Snowdon CF, Carpentieri M, Massimini G, Bliss JM, van de Velde C. A randomized trial of exemestane after two to three years of tamoxifen therapy in postmenopausal women with primary breast cancer. N Engl J Med 2004; 350:1081–1092.

Cui X, Schiff R, Arpino G, Osborne CK, Lee AV. Biology of progesterone receptor loss in breast cancer and its implications for endocrine therapy. J Clin Oncol 2005; 23: 7721–7735.

Demers LM. Effects of Fadrozole (CGS 16949A) and Letrozole (CGS 20267) on the inhibition of aromatase activity in breast cancer patients. Breast Cancer Res Treat 1994; 30:95–102.

Dixon JM, Renshaw L, Bellamy C, Stuart M, Hoctin-Boes G, Miller WR. The effects of neoadjuvant anastrozole (Arimidex) on tumor volume in postmenopausal women with breast cancer: a randomized, double-blind, single-center study. Clin Cancer Res 2000; 6:2229–2235.

Dombernowsky P, Smith I, Falkson G, Leonard R, Panasci L, Bellmunt J, Bezwoda W, Gardin G, Gudgeon A, Morgan M, Fornasiero A, Hoffmann W, Michel J, Hatschek T, Tjabbes T, Chaudri HA, Hornberger U, Trunet PF. Letrozole, a new oral aromatase inhibitor for advanced breast cancer: double-blind randomized trial showing a dose effect and improved efficacy and tolerability compared with megestrol acetate. J Clin Oncol 1998; 16:453–461.

Dowsett M, Cuzick J, Wale C, Howell T, Houghton J, Baum M. Retrospective analysis of time to recurrence in the ATAC trial according to hormone receptor status: an hypothesis-generating study. J Clin Oncol 2005; 23:7512–7517.

Early Breast Cancer Trialists Collaborative Group (EBCTCG). Effects of chemotherapy and hormonal therapy for early breast cancer on recurrence and 15-year survival: an overview of the randomised trials. Lancet 2005; 365:1687–1717.

Eastell R, Hannon RA, Cuzick J, Dowsett M, Clack G, Adams JE. Effect of an aromatase inhibitor on bmd and bone turnover markers: 2-year results of the Anastrozole, Tamoxifen, alone or in Combination (ATAC) trial (18233230). J Bone Miner Res 2006; 21:1215–1223.

Eiermann W, Paepke S, Appfelstaedt J, Llombart-Cussac A, Eremin J, Vinholes J, Mauriac L, Ellis M, Lassus M, Chaudri-Ross HA, Dugan M, Borgs M, Semiglazov V. Preoperative treatment of postmenopausal breast cancer patients with letrozole: a randomized double-blind multicenter study. Ann Oncol 2001; 12:1527–1532.

Ellis MJ, Coop A, Singh B, Mauriac L, Llombert-Cussac A, Janicke F, Miller WR, Evans DB, Dugan M, Brady C, Que-Fehling E, Borgs M. Letrozole is more effective neoadjuvant endocrine therapy than tamoxifen for ErbB-1-and/or ErbB-2-positive, estrogen receptor-positive primary breast cancer: evidence from a phase III randomized trial. J Clin Oncol 2001; 19:3808–3816.

Ellis MJ, Coop A, Singh B, Tao Y, Llombart-Cussac A, Janicke F, Mauriac L, Quebe-Fehling E, Chaudri-Ross HA, Evans DB, Miller WR. Letrozole inhibits tumor proliferation more effectively than tamoxifen independent of HER1/2 expression status. Cancer Res 2003; 63:6523–6531.

Fallowfield LJ, Bliss JM, Porter LS, Price MH, Snowdon CF, Jones SE, Coombes RC, Hall E. Quality of life in the intergroup exemestane study: a randomized trial of exemestane versus continued tamoxifen after 2 to 3 years of tamoxifen in postmenopausal women with primary breast cancer. J Clin Oncol 2006; 24:910–917.

Fallowfield L, Cella D, Cuzick J, Francis S, Locker G, Howell A. Quality of life of postmenopausal women in the Arimidex, Tamoxifen, alone or in Combination (ATAC) Adjuvant Breast Cancer Trial. J Clin Oncol 2004; 22:4261–4271.

Geisler J, Haynes B, Anker G, Dowsett M, Lonning PE. Influence of letrozole and anastrozole on total body aromatization and plasma estrogen levels in postmenopausal breast cancer patients evaluated in a randomized, cross-over study. J Clin Oncol 2002; 20:751–757.

Geisler J, King N, Anker G, Ornati G, Di Salle E, Lonning PE, Dowsett M. In vivo inhibition of aromatization by exemestane, a novel irreversible aromatase inhibitor, in postmenopausal breast cancer patients. Clin Cancer Res 1998; 4:2089–2093.

Geisler J, King N, Dowsett M, Ottestad L, Lundgren S, Walton P, Kormeset PO, Lonning PE. Influence of anastrozole (Arimidex), a selective, non-steroidal aromatase inhibitor, on in vivo aromatisation and plasma oestrogen levels in postmenopausal women with breast cancer. Br J Cancer 1996; 74:1286–1291.

Goetz MP, Rae JM, Suman VJ, Safgren SL, Ames MM, Visscher DW, Reynolds C, Couch FJ, Lingle WL, Flockhart DA, Desta Z, Perez EA, Ingle JN. Pharmacogenetics of tamoxifen biotransformation is associated with clinical outcomes of efficacy and hot flashes. J Clin Oncol 2005; 23:9312–9318.

Goss PE, Chlebowski RT, LeBoff MS, Cosman F, Singer FR. Sledge GW Recommendations on bone health management for women with early stage breast cancer. Am J Oncol Rev 2005a; 5:34–43.

Goss PE, Ingle JN, Martino S, Robert NJ, Muss HB, Piccart MJ, Castiglione M, Tu D, Shepherd LE, Pritchard KI, Livingston RB, Davidson NE, Norton L, Perez EA, Abrams JS, Therasse P, Palmer MJ, Pater JL. A randomized trial of letrozole in postmenopausal women after five years of tamoxifen therapy for early-stage breast cancer. N Engl J Med 2003; 349:1793–1802.

Goss PE, Ingle JN, Martino S, Robert NJ, Muss HB, Piccart MJ, Castiglione M, Tu D, Shepherd LE, Pritchard KI, Livingston RB, Davidson NE, Norton L, Perez EA, Abrams JS, Cameron DA, Palmer MJ, Pater JL. Randomized trial of letrozole following tamoxifen as extended adjuvant therapy in receptor-positive breast cancer: updated findings from NCIC CTG MA.17. J Natl Cancer Inst 2005b; 97: 1262–1271.

Goss PE, Ingle JI, Martino S, Robert NJ, Muss HB, Piccart MJ, Castiglione M, Tu D, Shepherd L, Pritchard KI, Livingston RB, Davidson NE, Norton L, Perez EA, Abrams JS, Cameron DA, Palmer MJ, Pater JL. Efficacy of letrozole extended adjuvant therapy according to estrogen receptor and progesterone receptor status of the primary tumor from NCIC CTG MA.17. J Clin Oncol 2007; 25:2006–2011.

Goss PE, Qi S, Cheung AM, Hu H, Mendes M. Pritzker, K.P. Effects of the steroidal aromatase inhibitor exemestane and the nonsteroidal aromatase inhibitor letrozole on bone and lipid metabolism in ovariectomized rats. Clin Cancer Res 2004a; 10:5717–5723.

Goss PE, Qi S, Josse RG, Pritzker KP, Mendes M, Hu H, Waldman SD. Grynpas, M.D. The steroidal aromatase inhibitor exemestane prevents bone loss in ovariectomized rats. Bone 2004b; 34:384–392.

Hillner BE, Ingle JN, Chlebowski RT, Gralow J, Yee GC, Janjan NA, Cauley JA, Blumenstein BA, Albain KS, Lipton A, Brown S. American Society of Clinical Oncology 2003 update on the role of bisphosphonates and bone health issues in women with breast cancer. J Clin Oncol 2003; 21: 4042–4057.

Howell A, Cuzick J, Baum M, Buzdar A, Dowsett M, Forbes JF, Hoctin-Boes G, Houghton J, Locker GY, Tobias JS. Results of the ATAC (Arimidex, Tamoxifen, Alone or in Combination) trial after completion of 5 years' adjuvant treatment for breast cancer. Lancet 2005; 365:60–62.

Ingle JN, Tu D, Pater JL, Martino S, Robert NJ, Muss HB, Piccart MJ, Castiglione M, Shepherd LE, Pritchard KI, Livingston RB, Davidson NE, Norton L, Perez EA, Abrams JS, Cameron DA, Palmer MJ, Goss PE. Duration of letrozole treatment and outcomes in the placebo-controlled NCIC CTG MA.17 extended adjuvant therapy trial. Breast Cancer Res Treat 2006; 99:295–300.

Jakesz R, Jonat W, Gnant M, Mittlboeck M, Greil R, Tausch C, Hilfrich J, Kwasny W, Menzel C, Samonigg H, Seifert M, Gademann G, Kaufmann M. Switching of postmenopausal women with endocrine-responsive early breast cancer to anastrozole after 2 years' adjuvant tamoxifen: combined results of ABCSG trial 8 and ARNO 95 trial. Lancet 2005; 366:455–462.

Jonat W, Howell A, Blomqvist C, Eiermann W, Winblad G, Tyrrell C, Mauriac L, Roche H, Lundgren S, Hellmund R, Azab M. A randomised trial comparing two doses of the new selective aromatase inhibitor anastrozole (Arimidex) with megestrol acetate in postmenopausal patients with advanced breast cancer. Eur J Cancer 1996; 32A:404–412.

Kaufmann M, Bajetta E, Dirix LY, Fein LE, Jones SE, Zilembo N, Dugardyn JL, Nasurdi C, Mennel RG, Cervek J, Fowst C, Polli A, di Salle E, Arkhipov A, Piscitelli G, Miller LL, Massimini G. Exemestane is superior to megestrol acetate after tamoxifen failure in postmenopausal women with advanced breast cancer: results of a phase III randomized double-blind trial. The Exemestane Study Group. J Clin Oncol 2000; 18:1399–1411.

Loi S, Piccart M, Sotiriou C. The use of gene-expression profiling to better understand the clinical heterogeneity of estrogen receptor positive breast cancers and tamoxifen response. Crit Rev Oncol Hematol 2007; 61:187–194. (Epub 2006 Nov 7).

Lonning PE, Geisler J, Krag LE, Erikstein B, Bremnes Y, Hagen AI, Schlichting E, Lien EA, Ofjord ES, Paolini J, Polli A, Massimini G. Effects of exemestane administered for 2 years versus placebo on bone mineral density, bone biomarkers, and plasma lipids in patients with surgically resected early breast cancer. J Clin Oncol 2005; 23:5126–5137.

Love RR, Mazess RB, Barden HS, Epstein S, Newcomb PA, Jordan VC, Carbone PP, DeMets DL. Effects of tamoxifen on bone mineral density in postmenopausal women with breast cancer. N Engl J Med 1992; 326:852–856.

Ma CX, Adjei AA, Salavaggione OE, Coronel J, Pelleymounter L, Wang L, Eckloff BW, Schaid D, Wieben ED, Adjei AA, Weinshilboum RM. Human aromatase: gene resequencing and functional genomics. Cancer Res 2005; 65:11071–11082.

Ma XJ, Hilsenbeck SG, Wang W, Ding L, Sgroi DC, Bender RA, Osborne CK, Allred DC, Erlander MG. The HOXB13: IL17BR expression index is a prognostic factor in early-stage breast cancer. J Clin Oncol 2006; 24:4611–4619.

Ma XJ, Wang Z, Ryan PD, Isakoff SJ, Barmettler A, Fuller A, Muir B, Mohapatra G, Salunga R, Tuggle JT, Tran Y, Tran D, Tassin A, Amon P, Wang W, Wang W, Enright E, Stecker K, Estepa-Sabal E, Smith B, Younger J, Balis U, Michaelson J, Bhan A, Habin K, Baer TM, Brugge J, Haber DA, Erlander MG, Sgroi DC. A two-gene expression ratio predicts clinical outcome in breast cancer patients treated with tamoxifen. Cancer Cell 2004; 5:607–616.

Milla-Santos A, Milla L, Portella J, Rallo L, Pons M, Rodes E, Casanovas J, Puig-Gali M. Anastrozole versus tamoxifen as first-line therapy in postmenopausal patients with hormone-dependent advanced breast cancer: a prospective, randomized, phase III study. Am J Clin Oncol 2003; 26:317–322.

Miller WR, Dixon JM. Endocrine and clinical endpoints of exemestane as neoadjuvant therapy. Cancer Control 2002; 9:9–15.

Mitwally MF, Casper RF. Use of an aromatase inhibitor for induction of ovulation in patients with an inadequate response to clomiphene citrate. Fertil Steril 2001; 75: 305–309.

Mouridsen H, Gershanovich M, Sun Y, Perez-Carrion R, Boni C, Monnier A, Apffelstaedt J, Smith R, Sleeboom HP, Janicke F, Pluzanska A, Dank M, Becquart D, Bapsy PP, Salminen E, Snyder R, Lassus M, Verbeek JA, Staffler B, Chaudri-Ross HA, Dugan M. Superior efficacy of letrozole versus tamoxifen as first-line therapy for postmenopausal women with advanced breast cancer: results of a phase III study of the International Letrozole Breast Cancer Group. J Clin Oncol 2001; 19:2596–2606.

Nabholtz JM, Buzdar A, Pollak M, Harwin W, Burton G, Mangalik A, Steinberg M, Webster A, von Euler M. Anastrozole is superior to tamoxifen as first-line therapy for advanced breast cancer in postmenopausal women: results of a North American multicenter randomized trial. Arimidex Study Group. J Clin Oncol 2000; 18:3758–3767.

Osborne CK, Bardou V, Hopp TA, Chamness GC, Hilsenbeck SG, Fuqua SA, Wong J, Allred DC, Clark GM, Schiff R. Role of the estrogen receptor coactivator AIB1 (SRC-3) and HER-2/neu in tamoxifen resistance in breast cancer. J Natl Cancer Inst 2003; 95:353–361.

Paik S, Shak S, Tang G, Kim C, Baker J, Cronin M, Baehner FL, Walker MG, Watson D, Park T, Hiller W, Fisher ER, Wickerham DL, Bryant J, Wolmark N. A multigene assay to predict recurrence of tamoxifen-treated, node-negative breast cancer. N Engl J Med 2004; 351:2817–2826.

Paridaens R, Dirix L, Lohrisch C, Beex L, Nooij M, Cameron D, Biganzoli L, Cufer T, Duchateau L, Hamilton A, et al. Mature results of a randomized phase II multicenter study of exemestane versus tamoxifen as first-line hormone therapy for postmenopausal women with metastatic breast cancer. Ann Oncol 2003; 14:1391–1398.

Perez EA, Josse RG, Pritchard KI, Ingle JN, Martino S, Findlay BP, Shenkier TN, Tozer RG, Palmer MJ, Shepherd LE,

Liu S, Tu D, Goss PE. Effect of letrozole versus placebo on bone mineral density in women with primary breast cancer completing 5 or more years of adjuvant tamoxifen: a companion study to NCIC CTG MA.17. J Clin Oncol 2006; 24:3629–3635.

Powles TJ, Hickish T, Kanis JA, Tidy A, Ashley S. Effect of tamoxifen on bone mineral density measured by dual-energy x-ray absorptiometry in healthy premenopausal and postmenopausal women. J Clin Oncol 1996; 14:78–84.

Shou J, Massarweh S, Osborne CK, Wakeling AE, Ali S, Weiss H, Schiff R. Mechanisms of tamoxifen resistance: increased estrogen receptor-HER2/neu cross-talk in ER/HER2-positive breast cancer. J Natl Cancer Inst 2004; 96:926–935.

Thurlimann B, Keshaviah A, Coates AS, Mouridsen H, Mauriac L, Forbes JF, Paridaens R, Castiglione-Gertsch M, Gelber RD, Rabaglio M, Smith I, Wardly A, Price KN, Goldhirsh A. A comparison of letrozole and tamoxifen in postmenopausal women with early breast cancer. N Engl J Med 2005; 353:2747–2757.

van de Vijver MJ, He YD, van't Veer LJ, Dai H, Hart AA, Voskuil DW, Schreiber GJ, Peterse JL, Roberts C, Marton MJ, Parrish M, Atsma D, Witteveen A, Glas A, Delahaye L, van der Velde T, Bartelink H, Rodenhuis S, Rutgers ET, Friend SH, Bernards R. A gene-expression signature as a predictor of survival in breast cancer. N Engl J Med 2002; 347:1999–2009.

Wasan KM, Goss PE, Pritchard PH, Shepherd L, Palmer MJ, Liu S, Tu D, Ingle JN, Heath M, DeAngelis D, Perez EA. The influence of letrozole on serum lipid concentrations in postmenopausal women with primary breast cancer who have completed 5 years of adjuvant tamoxifen (NCIC CTG MA.17L). Ann Oncol 2005; 16:707–715.

Whelan TJ, Goss PE, Ingle JN, Pater JL, Tu D, Pritchard K, Liu S, Shepherd LE, Palmer M, Robert NJ, Martino S, Muss HB. Assessment of quality of life in MA.17: a randomized, placebo-controlled trial of letrozole after 5 years of tamoxifen in postmenopausal women. J Clin Oncol 2005; 23:6931–6940.

Whelan TJ, Pritchard KI. Managing patients on endocrine therapy: focus on quality-of-life issues. Clin Cancer Res 2006; 12:1056s–1060s.

Winer EP, Hudis C, Burstein HJ, Wolff AC, Pritchard KI, Ingle JN, Chlebowski RT, Gelber R, Edge SB, Gralow J, et al. American Society of Clinical Oncology technology assessment on the use of aromatase inhibitors as adjuvant therapy for postmenopausal women with hormone receptor-positive breast cancer: status report 2004. J Clin Oncol 2005; 23:619–629.

Zhu L, Chow LW, Loo WT, Guan XY, Toi M. Her2/neu expression predicts the response to antiaromatase neoadjuvant therapy in primary breast cancer: subgroup analysis from celecoxib antiaromatase neoadjuvant trial. Clin Cancer Res 2004; 10:4639–4644.

11

Testosterone, Other Androgens and Breast Cancer

JEAN-PIERRE RAYNAUD
Université Pierre et Marie Curie, Paris, France

MICHÈLE PUJOS-GAUTRAUD
Saint Emilion, France

JORGE R. PASQUALINI
Hormones and Cancer Research Unit, Institut de Puériculture et de Périnatalogie, Paris, France

INTRODUCTION

In the last years, androgens in women have become of particular interest because there is a lot of information demonstrating that these steroids play an important role in physiological and pathological conditions in pre- and postmenopausal women (Davis, 1999).

Androgens influence many functions or organs in women, such as hypothalamus-pituitary-ovary axis, mammary gland, bone, uterus, and cardiovascular system. However, the role of androgen treatment in women remains controversial. The proposed "female androgen insufficiency syndrome" describes a number of nonspecific symptoms as unexplained fatigue, decrease of well-being sensation, dysphoric mood and/or blunted motivation, and diminished sexual desire (Davison and Davis, 2003). An estimated 40% of women experience sexual dysfunction, highlighting the need for ongoing research in order to fully define the possible contribution of androgen insufficiency. Randomized controlled trials indicate that exogenous testosterone has a positive effect on sexual function, primarily desire, but also arousal, and orgasmic response in women after spontaneous or surgically induced menopause. Beneficial effects of testosterone treatment in postmenopausal women with lowered androgen levels have been well documented, and preliminary evidence suggests a role for treatment in premenopausal women with symptoms and lowered testosterone levels. (Shifren et al., 2000).

In the breast, androgens can exert their effect mainly in two ways: (1) as the breast tissues, normal or pathological, contain significant quantities of the androgen receptor (AR), the biological response can be carried out through this protein but also by binding to another receptor [e.g., estrogen receptor (ER), progesterone receptor (PR), or corticoid receptor (CR)] and (2) by the transformation into estrogens by the aromatase activity. Some observations support the concept that androgens may counteract the stimulatory effects of estrogens and progesterone in the mammary gland.

Mammography breast density and breast cell proliferation could be regarded as surrogate markers for the risk of breast cancer. The use of testosterone and other androgen levels as a prognostic factor in human breast cancer is widely debated. Early menarche, late menopause, and oral postmenopausal hormone replacement therapy (HRT) are all associated with increased risk of breast cancer, and these increased risks are generally interpreted as the result of a longer lifetime exposure to elevated sex steroids, particularly estrogens, which may inhibit apoptosis and stimulate proliferation of the mammary duct epithelium. Some authors suggest that testosterone may cause breast cancer and that testosterone and androstenedione may be more strongly associated with breast cancer than estradiol (Howard, 2005).

In this chapter, we review the biotransformation and the biological effects of testosterone and other androgens in normal and cancerous breast, the hormone concentration levels, and the breast cancer risk associated with androgens both in pre- and postmenopausal women, as well as in men. The risk of breast cancer will also be analyzed following androgen treatment.

BIOTRANSFORMATION

Biosynthesis of androgens takes place in the ovary, adrenals, and peripheral tissues as well as in the mammary gland. In the early steps of formation, two cytochrome P450 enzymes are involved: the P450 Sec, which catalyzes cholesterol side chain cleavage, and P450 C17, which catalyzes 17-hydroxylation and 17-20 bond cleavage (l7/20 lyase), which transforms pregnenolone into dehydroepiandrosterone (DHEA) and androstenediol, respectively. DHEA is extensively converted into DHEA-sulfate (DHEA-S), which is quantitatively the most important circulating steroid in women (Fig. 1). Androstenediol, DHEA, and DHEA-S are considered to be pro-androgens because they require conversion into testosterone, the biological active hormone testosterone. For the general interrelation of androgens and estrogens in the breast cancer tissue see Figure 2 in chapter 2.

Among living species, humans and other primates are the only ones having adrenals that secrete large amounts of the inactive precursor steroids (DHEA and especially DHEA-S), which are converted into potent androgens and/ or estrogens (Labrie, 2006).

In adult man, 50% of total androgens derive from the adrenal precursor steroids (Bélanger et al., 1986), and in women, the intracrine formation of estrogens in peripheral tissues is of the order of 75% before menopause and 100% after menopause. Between 20 and 50 years, circulating DHEA drops by more than 50%. Around 25% of testosterone derives from the ovaries, another 25% comes from the adrenals, and the remaining 50% derives mainly from peripheral tissues (Davis, 1999). Testosterone (T) by the action of 5α-reductases (type 1 and 2) is converted into 5α-dihydrotestosterone (DHT), a non-aromatizable androgen (Burger, 2002; Simpson, 2002). Testosterone is one of the most important aromatizable androgen, but as indicated in chapter 2 of this book, breast tissue (normal or cancerous) aromatase capacity is very limited and the most part of the transformation of androgens to estrogens (particularly in postmenopausal women) is peripheral.

The postmenopausal ovary is not a great androgen-producing gland (Couzinet et al., 2001), and the major

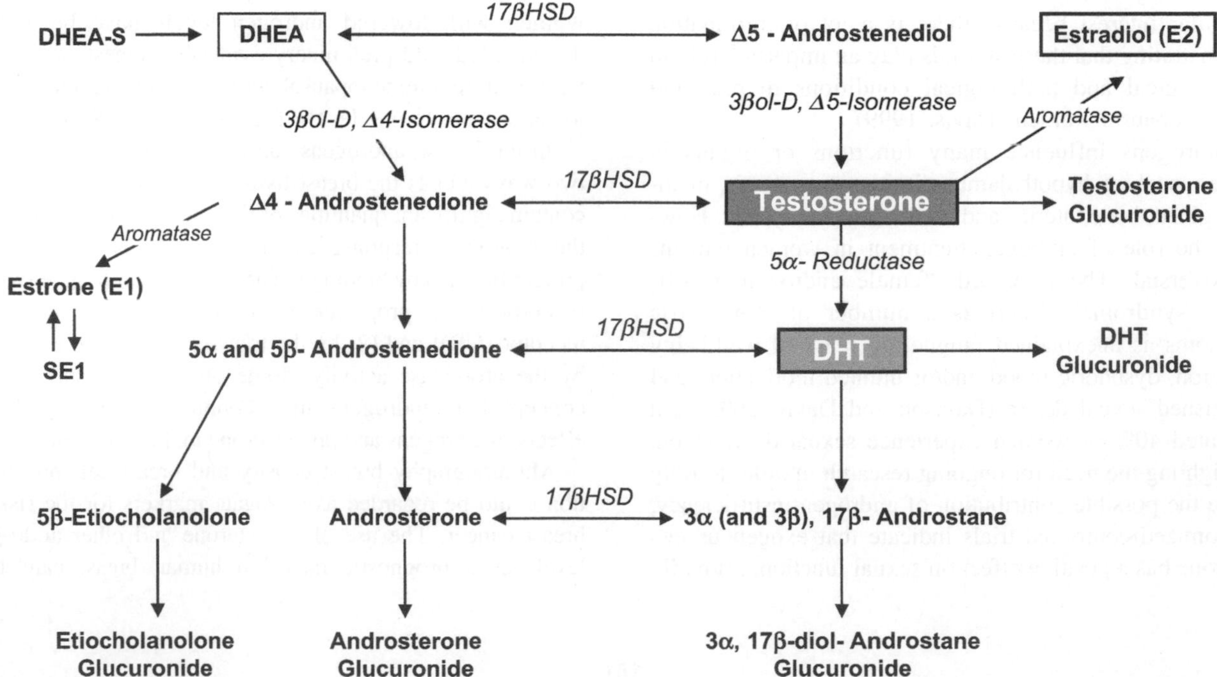

Figure 1 Biotransformation of androgens. *Abbreviations*: DHEA, dehydroepiandrosterone; DHEA-S, dehydroepiandrosterone-sulfate; DHT, 5α-dihydrotestosterone; 17β-HSD, 17β-hydroxysteroid dehydrogenase; 3βol-D, 3β-hydroxy dehydrogenase; Δ5 ⇒ Δ4 isomerase.

role of peripheral estrogen formation in postmenopausal women is clearly demonstrated by the high benefits of aromatase inhibitor treatment in breast cancer (Mouridsen et al., 2001; Goss et al., 2003) as well as by the decrease (76%) of breast cancer incidence in postmenopausal osteoporotic women who received the selective estrogen receptor modulator (SERM) raloxifene for three years (Cummings et al., 1999). Another important and biological active androgen is androstenediol, which has estrogenic properties; it can be formed and detected in normal breast and breast cancer (van Landeghem et al., 1985; Thijssen et al., 1991b, Boccuzzi and Bignardollo, 1996).

The classical concept of androgen and estrogen secretion in women assumed that all sex steroids had to be transported by the general circulation following secretion by the ovaries before reaching the target tissues. According to this classical concept, it was erroneously believed that the active steroids could be measured directly in the blood, thus providing a potential easily accessible measure of the general exposure to sex steroids. This concept does not apply to postmenopausal women where all estrogens and almost all androgens are made locally from DHEA in the peripheral tissues (Labrie et al., 1995), which possess the enzymes required to synthesize the physiologically active sex steroids (Labrie et al., 2006).

For general reviews on the formation and transformation of androgens in breast see Pasqualini (1993), Liao and Dickson (2002), and Labrie (2006).

BIOLOGICAL EFFECTS

The environment of sex hormones during pregnancy and neonatal life determines the pattern of the mammary gland in adult life, regardless of the genetic sex. Both, rats and mice of either sex, exposed to sex steroids in utero or during the neonatal period, exhibit permanent functional alterations in the endocrine and reproductive system (Bern et al., 1975; Mori et al., 1976; Yanai et al., 1981; Tomooka and Bern, 1982). Indeed, increased levels of circulating prolactin have been reported in neonatally androgenized female mice and rat (Christakos et al., 1976; Nagasawa et al., 1978), and prolactin exerts a considerable influence on chemically induced mammary carcinogenesis (Welsch and Nagasawa, 1977).

Both normal and cancerous breast tissues contain and produce several forms of androgens (Bonney et al., 1984; Thijssen and Blankenstein, 1989; Brignardello et al., 1995). A most important characteristic of the endocrine physiology of the mammary gland is that normal mammary gland, as well as early breast cancer, absolutely requires estrogens for proliferation and growth. Inhibitors of estrogen formation and action have shown very positive effects in the treatment of breast cancer (Labrie, 2006).

After the introduction of methyltrienolone (R1881) as a tag for AR (Bonne and Raynaud, 1977), the measurement of androgen binding sites in various conditions has been facilitated (Raynaud, 1977). AR is expressed in normal mammary epithelial and stroma cells (Wilson et al., 1996; Pelletier, 2000) and over 70% human breast are AR positive (Langer et al., 1990; Kuenen-Boumeester et al., 1996; Hackenberg and Schulz, 1996; Birrell et al., 1998; Brysacute, 2000), a value that is at least equivalent to those of ER (70–80%) and PR (50–70%) (Allegra et al., 1979; Miller et al., 1985). These facts provide the basis for a direct AR-mediated action of androgens in the normal and malignant breast tissues.

The AR gene contains a highly polymorphic CAG trinucleotide repeat, which encodes glutamines, in its first exon. The length of the CAG repeat is inversely associated with the degree of transcriptional activity of AR. Ovarian cancer patients who carried a short CAG repeat allele of AR were diagnosed on average of 7.2 years earlier than the patients who did not carry a short allele, indicating that a stronger AR activity might be associated with ovarian cancer development (Yong et al., 2000). In women who inherit a germline mutation in the BRCA1 gene, those who carry more CAG repeats in at least one AR allele have a higher risk of breast cancer development than those who carry less CAG repeats; shorter CAG repeat length in the AR gene is associated with more aggressive forms of breast cancer (Yu et al., 2000).

Several key enzymes responsible for metabolic conversions of various forms of androgens to estrogens are also present at significant amounts in normal breast and breast cancer tissues (Santen et al., 1986; Killinger et al., 1987; Thijssen et al., 1993; Pelletier et al., 2001), which provides the basis for the local biotransformation of androgens to estrogens, resulting in estrogen excess (Thijssen et al., 1991a; Newton et al., 1986; Mehta et al., 1987; Luu-The et al., 2001). The active androgens are inactivated to glucuronide (G) derivatives before their diffusion from the intracellular compartment into the circulation where they can be measured as Androsterone (ADT-G) and 3α-diol-G. It is now well established that uridine glucuronosyltransferases UGT 2 B7, UGT 2 B15, and UGT 2 B17 are the three enzymes responsible for the glucuronidation of all androgens and their metabolites in humans (Bélanger et al., 2003).

It has been proposed for many years that low levels of adrenal androgens may promote breast cancer and high levels may prevent it (Pasqualini, 1993). In the absence of estrogens, they stimulate growth of breast cancer cell via binding to ERα (this effect can be blocked by treatment with antiestrogens); in the presence of estrogens, they act as antiestrogens to inhibit estrogen stimulation of growth of breast cancer cells via binding to AR (this effect can be blocked by antiestrogens) (Boccuzzi et al., 1994; Boccuzzi and Brignardollo, 1996). In most premenopausal women who have relatively high circulating estrogens, androgens may exert mainly antiestrogenic effects via binding to AR, suppressing estrogen stimulation of the growth of mammary epithelial or cancer cells.

There is increasing evidence that androgens exert inhibitory effects on the proliferation of breast epithelial cells and play a protective role in the pathogenesis of breast cancer (Birrell et al., 1998; Labrie et al., 2003; Buchanan et al., 2005). Part of the mechanism of the inhibitory action of androgens on the stimulatory effect of estrogens could be the decrease of ERα caused by androgens in human breast cells in culture (Poulin et al., 1989) and in normal mammary gland epithelium (Dimitrakakis et al., 2003), and/or by the decreased expression of MYC, which is inversely correlated to that of the AR in breast cancer tissue (Bieche et al., 2001).

In vitro, androgens, especially those of adrenal origin, are able to bind to ERα, although the binding affinities are much lower compared to estrogens (Ojasoo and Raynaud, 1978; Kuiper et al., 1997; Ekena et al., 1998; Maggiolini et al., 1999; Katzenellenbogen et al., 2000). Downregulation of the expression of ERα and PR may be one of the mechanisms for androgens to achieve this effect (Rochefort, 1984; Labrie et al., 1990). Since progesterone has a dual influence on the mammary epithelia, including both growth stimulation and inhibition (Clarke and Sutherland, 1990), it remains possible that the reported dual functions of androgens may actually be a reflection of their progestational effects. Most androgens and progestins have various binding affinities to PR and AR, which mediate progestational and androgenic functions (Delettre et al., 1980). Kramer et al. (2006) have shown that medroxyprogesterone acetate (MPA) and chlormadinone acetate (CMA) induced proliferation of MCF10A cells. Progesterone, testosterone, norethisterone, levonorgestrel, dienogest, gestodene, and 3-ketodesogestrel had no significant effect, confirming that the choice of progestin for hormone therapy may be crucial for avoiding a potential risk of breast cancer.

MPA, a progestin used for oral contraception and HRT, has been implicated in increased breast cancer risk. Ghatge et al. (2005) have assessed the transcriptional effects of MPA as compared with those of progesterone and DHT in a new PR-negative (PR−), AR-positive human breast cancer cell line, designated Y-AR. Transcription assays using a synthetic promoter/reporter construct, as well as endogenous gene expression profiling comparing progesterone, MPA, and DHT, were performed in cells either lacking or containing PR and/or AR. In PR-positive (PR+) cells, MPA was found to be an effective progestin through both PR isoforms in transient transcription assays. Using Y-AR cells, an extensive gene regulatory overlap between DHT and MPA through AR was observed and none with progesterone. Thus, the increased breast cancer risk and/or the therapeutic efficacy of MPA in cancer treatment could be in part mediated by AR.

Ortmann et al. (2002) investigated the relationship between AR status and testosterone and DHT-dependent proliferation of the human breast carcinoma cell lines MCF-7, T47-D, MDA-MB 435S and BT-20. All four cell lines stained positively for AR. Western blot analysis revealed a strong expression of AR in MCF-7, in contrast to BT-20 cells. In the ER-negative (ER−) cell lines BT-20 and MDA-MB 435S, testosterone was a more potent inhibitor of cell proliferation than DHT, in contrast to the ER+ cell lines MCF-7 and T47-D in which a stronger inhibition of proliferation was achieved by DHT. A partial transformation of testosterone to estrogen in ER+ cells might explain a possible role of androgens in growth regulation of breast cancer.

In line with the observation of Ortmann et al. (2002), Sonne-Hansen et al. (2005) investigated cell proliferation, expression of estrogen-regulated proteins, and aromatase using the estrogen responsive human MCF-7 breast cancer cell line. Cells were cultured in a low estrogen milieu and treated with estrogens, aromatizable androgens, or non-aromatizable androgens. The MCF-7 cell line was observed to express sufficient aromatase enzyme activity in order to aromatize testosterone, providing significant cell growth stimulation. The testosterone-mediated growth effect was completely inhibited by the aromatase inhibitors letrozole and 4-hydroxy-androstenedione. Expression studies of estrogen-regulated proteins confirmed that testosterone was aromatized into estrogen in the MCF-7 cells. Thus, the results indicate that epithelial breast cancer cells possess the ability to aromatize circulating androgens into estrogens.

Gayosso et al. (2006) evaluated whether the antiproliferative effect induced by DHEA in MCF-7 cells is direct or indirect, through its conversion to estradiol or testosterone. Although DHEA had an antiproliferative effect at supraphysiological concentrations, when used at physiological concentrations it increased the proliferation of MCF-7 cells. 17β-Estradiol induced an increase in MCF-7 cell proliferation at physiological concentrations, whereas testosterone had a weak inhibitory effect at 100 μM. DHEA-induced antiproliferative and proliferative effects were not blocked by inhibitors of AR or ER, thus indicating that its effect is secondary to a direct interaction with a "putative" receptor rather than a conversion into steroid hormones. These results suggest that DHEA could be used at supraphysiologic concentrations in the treatment of breast cancer.

In summary, as pointed out by Liao and Dickson (2002), there are at least six possible mechanisms for androgen action:

1. Androgens serve as estrogens precursors and are converted to estrogens
2. Androgens exert estrogenic effects by directly binding to ERα; adrenal androgens have higher affinities for ERα than T and DHT
3. Androgens exert androgenic effect by binding to AR

4. Androgens may bind to PR and exert progestational effects
5. Androgens may stimulate the expression of prolactin and prolactin receptors
6. Androgens may act via AR-BRCA1 complex to inhibit the development of breast cancer; the length of the CAG repeat in the AR gene affects this mechanism

SEX HORMONE CONCENTRATIONS

Hormones assays of androgens in women require sensitive assays with the ability to detect low levels and a narrow range with precision. Circulating sex hormones are largely bound to sex hormone–binding globulin (SHBG). The relative binding of androgens to SHBG is, by decreasing order, DHT > testosterone > androstenediol > estradiol > estrone (Dunn et al., 1981). Only 1% to 2% of circulating testosterone is free (not bound to SHBG or albumin) (Haning et al., 1989). Debate exists on the importance of measurement of free or non-SHBG bound (calculated or assayed) versus total testosterone to assess testosterone availability (Giton et al., 2006).

There is an increasing trend to apply gas chromatography combined with mass spectrometry (GC-MS) or liquid chromatography tandem mass spectrometry (LC-MS/MS) assay methods to large-scale epidemiological studies for sex steroid serum levels measurement. These methods are unanimously considered as the gold standard for sex steroid measurements because of their accuracy, sensitivity, turnaround time, and ability to assess a more complete panel of steroid metabolites in the same run (Hsing et al., 2007). A high correlation between steroid levels measured by radioimmunoassay (RIA) and mass spectrometry (MS) has been shown, despite the significant differences in absolute measurements, probably due to the lack of specificity of RIA compared to GC or LCMS (Dorgan et al., 2002; Hsing et al., 2007).

It has been demonstrated that, in women, testosterone plasma levels are 10 times those of estradiol (Goebelsmann et al., 1974). Plasma total testosterone declines steeply with age in normal premenopausal women; at 40 years, the level is about half what it was at 21 years. Normal ranges of androgens for women of both reproductive and postreproductive age remain poorly defined. Since the great majority of circulating testosterone in normal women is derived from metabolic transformation of the adrenal androgens, DHEA and DHEA-S, and since their levels decline with age, the DHEA to T and DHEA-S to T ratios are invariant with age (Zumoff et al., 1981). In fact, the androgens, testosterone, and DHT, made in peripheral tissues from DHEA, exert their action locally in the same cells where synthesis takes place and are inactivated and transformed in the same cells into water-soluble glucuronide derivatives that diffuse quantitatively into the general circulation with only minimal release as active androgens.

In breast tumors of postmenopausal women, the estradiol concentration is 10- to 20-fold greater than in plasma (van Landeghem et al., 1985; Blankenstein et al., 1992; Pasqualini et al., 1996). Estrogenic activity in mammary tissue may thus be due to the local synthesis of estradiol from estrone and androgenic precursors (Thijssen et al., 1987). It will be of interest to know the level of androgenic activity in each specific tissue. But, such a direct measurement is not accessible in the human, except in exceptional circumstances such as samples obtained at surgery. The most practical and probably the most valid measure of androgenic activity in women seems to be that of androsterone glucuronide, the metabolite that accounts for 93% of the total androgen glucuronide derivatives, by a validated liquid chromatography tandem mass spectrometry technique, thus replacing measurement of serum testosterone (Labrie et al., 2006). Although the metabolic clearance rates of the three main androgen metabolites are likely to show differences between men and women, an estimate of the relative amount of total androgens in women and men calculated on the basis of the sum of these two metabolites suggests that total androgen production in women is more than 2/3 that found in men (Labrie et al., 1997).

ANDROGEN CONCENTRATION AND RISKS FACTORS

Most epidemiological studies use RIA to measure sex steroid hormones because they have acceptable turnaround times and are relatively inexpensive; however, precision and accuracy of certain RIAs, especially direct assay without extraction, are of concern in some studies (Fears et al., 2000; Rinaldi et al., 2001). GC or LC-MS have not been used in epidemiological studies to measure circulating levels of hormones, because historically these assays have required large volumes of serum and have been labor intensive and costly. Furthermore, for both logistic and financial reasons, only a single blood sample has been collected per study subject. Whether a single sample can reflect long-term hormone levels (generally the exposure of greatest etiologic interest) is therefore an important issue.

Although abundant biological data indicate that endogenous androgens play an important role in prostate cancer development, epidemiological data from human studies are inconclusive (Gann et al., 1996; Eaton et al., 1999; Hsing and Chokkalingam, 2006; Raynaud, 2006). Similarly, the association in case-control studies between serum androgen levels and breast cancer risk has led to contradictory data. Accordingly, subnormal levels of serum androgens

Table 1 Mean Plasma levels of Total Testosterone in Women with Breast Cancer and Control

Reference	Case/control	Values	Units	*p* value	Assay method/ sensitivity
Postmenopausal women					
Adly et al., 2006	179 159	0.7 (0.6–0.8) 0.7 (0.6–0.8)	nmol/L	0.92	RIA 0.07 nmol/L
Beatie et al., 2006	135 275	0.73 (0.42–0.98) 0.74 (0.50–0.90)	nmol/L	0.39	RIA 0.14 nmol/L
Berrino et al., 2005	31 Breast cancer survivors Relapses 79 Breast cancer survivors No Relapse	0.52 0.38	ng/mL	—	RIA 0.37 ng/mL
Cauley et al., 1999	97 244	0.73 (0–2.70) 0.62 (0–2.63)	nmol/L	0.005	RIA 0.03 nmol/L
Cummings et al., 2005	196 378	— —	pmol/L	—	RIA Lab 1, 0.9 ng/dL Lab 2, 3 ng/dL
Kaaks et al., 2005b	677 1309	1.27 (1.22–1.33) 1.15 (1.11–1.18)	nmol/L	<0.0001	RIA
Kahan et al., 2006	102 102	2.36 ± 0.11 1.82 ± 0.10	nmol/L	—	RIA variat coef Intra assay 7.0% Inter assay 12.6%
Missmer et al., 2004	312 628	22 (12–37) 19 (11–33)	ng/dL	<0.001	RIA 1 ng/dL
Schairer et al., 2005	179 152	0.7 (0.6–0.8) 0.7 (0.6–0.8)	nmol/L	0.39	RIA 0.07 nmol/L
Zeleniuch-Jacquotte et al., 2005	69 134	0.56 (0.19–1.54) 0.52 (0.18–1.30)	nmol/L	—	RIA variat coef Intra assay 8.7% Inter assay 15.8%
Premenopausal women					
Kaaks et al., 2005a	370 726	1.80 (1.71–1.88) 1.66 (1.60–1.72)	nmol/L	0.01	RIA

Abbreviation: RIA, radioimmunoassay.

have been reported in women with increased risk of breast cancer (Bulbrook et al., 1971; Brennan et al., 1973; Wang et al., 1975; Zumoff et al., 1981); the opposite finding has been also reported (Dorgan et al., 1996; Berrino et al., 1996; Secreto et al., 1984, 1991).

The inconsistencies in these epidemiological investigations are due, in part, to methodological limitations, including intra- and intersubject and interlaboratory variations. In many epidemiological studies, the coefficients of variation of steroid hormone RIA assays were larger than the intersubject variations, making it difficult to detect small (<15%) case-control differences (Lillie et al., 2003). The complexity and expense of hormone assays, coupled with the need to collect urine or blood samples from study subjects resulted in, until recently, relatively few epidemiological studies on these issues and small sample sizes for many of the earlier studies. These factors, in conjunction with error in the laboratory assays, likely contributed to an initial lack of consistent findings (Hankinson et al., 1998).

Many studies have documented higher testosterone levels in urine and blood of pre- and postmenopausal breast cancer patients, with or without a concurrent increase in circulating levels of estrogens, compared with the normal women at the same age (Grattarola, 1973; Adams, 1977; Secreto et al., 1983a,b,c, 1984, 1989, 1991; Dorgan et al., 1996, 1997a,b; Secreto and Zumoff, 1994; Stoll and Secreto, 1992; Zeleniuch-Jacquotte et al., 1997; Yu et al., 1999).

In the following section, the more recent studies are described and the results are summarized in Tables 1 to 3.

Premenopausal Women

Sturgeon et al. (2004) examined, in a case-control study, associations between serum levels of estradiol, SHBG, DHEA, testosterone, androstenedione and progesterone, and risk of premenopausal breast cancer. Cases of breast cancer under age 45 were identified in Seattle/Puget

Table 2 Plasmatic Androgens Levels in Pre- and Postmenopausal Women and Risk of Breast Cancer

Reference	Subjects distribution	Hormone level/(Subjects: cases/controls) Inferior	Superior	OR (CI 95%) Inferior	Superior	*p* Value
Postmenopausal women						
Testosterone						
Berrino et al., 2005	T1–T3	0.16–0.33 ng/mL	0.5–0.93 ng/mL	1	7.2 (2.4–21.4)	—
Zeleniuch-Jacquotte et al., 2005	T1–T3	(19/44)	(24/39)	1	1.63 (0.69–3.88)	0.26
Adly et al., 2006	Q1–Q4	≤0.45 nmol/L (32/39)	>1 nmol/L (33/36)	1	1.3 (0.6–2.6)	0.86
Cauley et al., 1999	Q1–Q4	<0.42 nmol/L (10/57)	≥0.97 nmol/L (32/60)	1	2.8 (1.2–6.5)	0.01
Kahan et al., 2006	Q1–Q4	<1.1 nmol/L (26/12)	>2.4 nmol/L (26/49)	1	4.1 (1.77–9.39)	0.001
Missmer et al., 2004	Q1–Q4	<15 ng/dL (66/164)	>26 ng/dL (97/171)	1	1.6 (1.0–2.4)	<0.001
Schairer et al., 2005	Q1–Q4	≤0.45 nmol/L (36/39)	>1 nmol/L (43/36)	1	1.4 (0.7–2.8)	0.34
Cummings et al., 2005	Q1–Q5	<381 pmol/L	>1.074 pmol/L	1	5.1 (2.5–10.3)	<0.001
Kaaks et al., 2005b	Q1–Q5	(107/259)	(171/255)	1	1.85 (1.33–2.57)	<0.001
Androstenedione						
Zeleniuch-Jacquotte et al., 2005	T1–T3	(19/47)	(19/48)	1	0.99 (0.44–2.24)	0.95
Adly et al., 2006	Q1–Q4	≤2.10 nmol/L (52/38)	>4.26 nmol/L (37/38)	1	1.2 (0.6–2.3)	0.31
Cauley et al., 1999	Q1–Q4	<0.84 nmol/L (14/60)	≥1.78 nmol/L (39/65)	1	2.4 (1.2–7.9)	0.017
Missmer et al., 2004	Q1–Q4	<43 ng/dL (64/159)	>78 ng/dL (91/151)	1	1.5 (1.0–2.3)	0.04
Schairer et al., 2005	Q1–Q4	≤2.10 nmol/L (39/38)	>4.26 nmol/L (44/38)	1	1.2 (0.6–2.5)	0.58
Kaaks et al., 2005b	Q1–Q5	(90/254)	(162/254)	1	1.94 (1.40–2.69)	<0.0001
DHEA						
Adly et al., 2006	Q1–Q4	≤6.30 nmol/L (52/38)	>15.50 nmol/L (36/38)	1	1.6 (0.8–3.2)	0.06
Missmer et al., 2004	Q1–Q4	<165 ng/dL (67/152)	>367 ng/dL (95/152)	1	1.4 (0.9–2.2)	0.02
Schairer et al., 2005	Q1–Q4	≤6.30 nmol/L (45/38)	>15.50 nmol/L (44/38)	1	1.2 (0.6–2.5)	0.65
DHEA-S						
Zeleniuch-Jacquotte et al., 2005	T1–T3	(23/42)	(23/43)	1	0.99 (0.45–2.20)	0.99
Cauley et al., 1999	Q1–Q4	<1 μmol/L (16/58)	≥2.71 μmol/L (33/61)	1	2.1 (1.0–4.4)	0.04
Missmer et al., 2004	Q1–Q4	<52 μg/dL (53/160)	>135 μg/dL (90/156)	1	1.7 (1.1–2.7)	0.003
Kaaks et al., 2005b	Q1–Q5	(101/254)	(162/254)	1	1.69 (1.23–2.33)	0.0002
Premenopausal women						
Testosterone						
Kaaks et al., 2005a	Q1–Q4	<1.13 nmol/L (70/176)	≥2.04 nmol/L (113/181)	1	1.73 (1.16–2.57)	0.01
Eliassen et al., 2006	Q1–Q4	Follicular phase 109/374		1	1.3 (0.8–2.4)	
Eliassen et al., 2006	Q1–Q4	Luteal phase 192/390		1	1.6 (0.9–2.8)	
Micheli et al., 2004	T1–T3	40/108		1	2.2 (0.6–7.6)	
Androstenedione						
Kaaks et al., 2005a	Q1–Q4	<3.32 nmol/L (83/180)	≥6.42 nmol/L (120/182)	1	1.56 (1.05–2.32)	0.01
DHEA-S						
Kaaks et al., 2005a	Q1–Q4	<2.25 μmol/L (77/181)	≥4.65 μmol/L (112/182)	1	1.48 (1.02–2.14)	0.1

Odds ratio, OR (95% CI) with tertile T1–T3, quartile Q1–Q4, or quintile Q1–Q5.

Sound, Washington, and control subjects were identified from the same area through random digit dialing methods. A total of 169 breast cancer cases were matched with 195 control subjects. The fully adjusted risk ratios and 95% CI for the highest versus lowest tertiles of estradiol, according to menstrual cycle phase, were 3.10 (0.8–12.7) for early follicular, 0.2–1.7 for late follicular, and 0.60 (0.3–1.4) for luteal phase. Risks for highest versus lowest quartiles

Table 3 Plasmatic SHBG Levels in Pre- and Postmenopausal Women and Risk of Breast Cancer

		SHBG level/subjects: cases/controls		OR (CI 95%)		
Reference	Subjects distribution	Inferior	Superior	Inferior	Superior	p Value
Postmenopausal women						
Berrino et al., 2005	T1–T3	—	>159.8 ng/mL	1	0.38 (0.14–1.00)	—
Zeleniuch-Jacquotte et al., 2005	T1–T3	(25/43)	(22/45)	1	0.81 (0.38–1.74)	0.9
Adly et al., 2006	Q1–Q4	≤76.73 nmol/L (62/38)	>135.85 nmol/L (37/38)	1	0.7 (0.4–1.3)	0.1
Beatie et al., 2006	Q1–Q4	<25 nmol/L	>49 nmol/L	1	1.15	0.86
Cauley et al., 1999	Q1–Q4	<29 nmol/L (22/58)	≥59 nmol/L (16/64)	1	0.7 (0.3–1.6)	>0.2
Kahan et al., 2006	Q1–Q4	<34.4 nmol/L	>67.9 nmol/L		No significance	—
Missmer et al., 2004	Q1–Q4	<34 nmol/L (88/150)	>67 nmol/L (75/157)	1	0.8 (0.6–1.3)	0.14
Schairer et al., 2005	Q1–Q4	<76.73 nmol/L (74/38)	>135.85 nmol/L (42/38)	1	0.7 (0.4–1.4)	0.05
Kaaks et al., 2005b	Q1–Q5	(155/260)	(103/260)	1	0.61 (0.44–0.84)	0.004
Premenopausal women						
Kaaks et al., 2005a	Q1–Q4	<31.1 nmol/L (92/180)	≥64.5 nmol/L (92/181)	1	0.95 (0.65–1.40)	0.72

ODDS ratios, OR (95% CI) with tertile T1–T3, quartile Q1–Q4, or quintile Q1–Q5.
Abbreviation: SHBG, sex hormone–binding globulin.

of SHBG and androgens were 0.81 (0.4–1.6) for SHBG, 2.42 (1.1–5.2) for DHEA, 1.12 (0.6–2.5) for testosterone, and 1.33 (0.6–2.8) for androstenedione. For luteal progesterone, the RR for the highest versus lowest tertile was 0.55 (0.2–1.4). Thus, there was not a convincing association between serum SHBG, estradiol, testosterone or androstenedione, and premenopausal breast cancer risk.

Micheli et al. (2004) have explored the relation of serum sex hormones to breast cancer in a prospective study in which 5963 postmenopausal women where recruited to the Hormones and Diet in the Etiology of Breast Tumors (ORDET) and had blood sampling 20 to 24 days after the start of their menstrual cycle. After 5.2 years of follow-up, 65 histologically confirmed breast cancer cases were identified and matched individually to four randomly selected controls. They found that in breast cancer cases, LH and FSH were lower than in controls and that free testosterone was significantly associated with breast cancer risk: RR [adjusted for age, body mass index (BMI), and ovarian cycle variables] of highest versus lowest tertile was 2.85 (1.11–7.33, p for trend = 0.030). Progesterone was inversely associated: RR = 0.40 (0.15–1.08, p for trend = 0.077). These findings support the hypothesis that ovarian hyperandrogenism associated with luteal insufficiency increases the risk of breast cancer in premenopausal women.

Kaaks et al. (2005a) observed, in a large multicenter cohort study within the European Prospective Investigation into Cancer and Nutrition (EPIC) of 370 premenopausal with a single prediagnostic serum samples who subsequently developed breast cancer and 726 matched cancer-free control subjects, that premenopausal women who had elevated serum levels of testosterone or androstenedione or low levels of progesterone had an increased risk of breast cancer. No clear relationship between breast cancer risk and premenopausal serum levels of estrone or estradiol was observed. The authors concluded that their results support the hypothesis that elevated blood concentrations of androgens are associated with an increased risk of breast cancer in premenopausal women.

Eliassen et al. (2006) found a correlation between circulating testosterone levels and breast cancer risk, particularly during the luteal phase of the cycle. Blood samples from 18,521 premenopausal women were collected during the early follicular and mid-luteal phases within the Nurses' Health Study. Breast cancer was diagnosed in 197 cases and matched with 394 control subjects. For women in the highest quartile of follicular phase, estradiol (total and free) levels had statistically significantly increased breast cancer risks. Luteal estradiol levels were not associated with breast cancer risk. Higher levels of testosterone (total and free) and androstenedione in both menstrual cycle phases were associated with modest, nonstatistically significant increases in overall breast cancer risk, but with stronger, statistically significant increases in risk of invasive and ER+/PR+ cancers.

Postmenopausal Women

Many studies were conducted in the past few years. It is very difficult to compare them on the ground of their diversity in patients' recruitment, in previous hormonal treatments, in the different hormones assayed, in the reliability of the assay method used, and in the cases themselves (breast cancer in situ or with metastases or recurrence).

Cauley et al. (1999) hypothesized that measurement of serum hormones could be used to identify women at high risk for developing breast cancer; they used a case-cohort approach to compare serum hormone concentrations in 97 incident case patients with breast cancer and 2444 randomly selected control. All women participated in the Study of Osteoporotic Fractures (United States), a prospective study of 9704 white, community-dwelling women over 65 years. Median concentrations of sex steroid hormones were higher in case patients than in controls; hormone concentrations were measured only once and a single measure is always imprecise to some degree. The association between serum hormone levels and breast cancer was stronger for bioavailable estradiol: Women in the highest quartile of estradiol concentration had a 3.6-fold greater risk for breast cancer than women in the lowest quartile of estradiol concentration (95% CI, 1.3–10). The risk was three times greater in women with the highest concentrations of testosterone. These associations were independent of age, BMI, and other conventional risk factors for breast cancer. The absolute concentrations of hormones, especially estradiol, were very low but are consistent with those previously reported in postmenopausal women (Hankinson et al., 1998). Nonetheless, a gradient of risk was observed across increasing concentrations suggesting that interventions such as a low-fat diet, weight reduction, or a vegetarian diet to reduce serum hormone concentrations may reduce risk for breast cancer. Thus, estradiol and testosterone could play important roles in the risk for breast cancer in older women.

Concentrations of these hormones may predict breast cancer risk and help clinicians to select the most appropriate treatment to decrease breast cancer risk.

Key et al. (2002) reanalyzed nine prospective studies of sex hormone levels in postmenopausal women, with a total of 663 breast cancer cases and 1765 healthy controls. The risk for breast cancer increased statistically significantly with increasing concentrations of all sex hormones examined: total estradiol, free estradiol, non-SHBG-bound estradiol (free plus albumin-bound estradiol), estrone, estrone sulfate, and testosterone. Therefrom, the authors concluded that the endogenous sex hormones levels are strongly associated with breast cancer risk in postmenopausal women.

Lamar et al. (2003) conducted a cross-sectional study among 133 postmenopausal women who gave blood to the serum bank (Columbia, Missouri, U.S.) and served as controls in a previous prospective nested case-control study of serum hormones and breast cancer risk. They evaluated associations of serum estrogen and androgen levels with age, anthropometrics, and reproductive history to assess whether these characteristics could potentially modify breast cancer risk through hormonal mechanisms. Serum levels of estradiol, bioavailable estradiol, estrone, estrone sulfate, and testosterone increased significantly with increasing BMI, whereas SHBG levels decreased. DHEA, DHEA-S, and androstenediol decreased significantly with increasing age. Although BMI and parity could potentially modify breast cancer risk through hormonal mechanisms, age-related increases in breast cancer incidence do not appear to be mediated through changes in serum levels of the hormones evaluated.

Missmer et al. (2004) have prospectively investigated the association between hormone levels and tumor receptor status or invasive versus in situ tumor status in a case-control nested within the Nurses' Health Study. Among eligible postmenopausal women, 322 cases of breast cancer [264 invasive, 41 in situ, 153 (ER+/PR+), and 39 (ER−/PR−) disease] were reported. For each case subject, two control subjects ($n = 643$) were matched. They found a statistically significant direct association between breast cancer risk and the level of both estrogens and androgens and any associations between this risk and the level of progesterone or SHBG. All hormones tended to be associated strongly with in situ disease. They concluded that circulating levels of sex steroid hormones might be most strongly associated with the risk of ER+/PR+ breast tumors.

Schairer et al. (2005) sought to determine whether serum concentrations of estrogens, androgens, and SHBG in postmenopausal women were related to the presence of mammary hyperplasia, an established breast cancer risk factor. A total of 179 subjects with breast hyperplasia were compared with 152 subjects with nonproliferative breast changes that are not associated with increased breast cancer risk. The odds ratios (ORs) associated with the three upper quartiles of estradiol in comparison with the lowest quartile were 2.2 (1.1–4.6), 2.5 (1.1–5.3), and 4.1 (2.0–8.5); p trend = 0.007. The corresponding ORs for bioavailable estradiol, estrone, and estrone sulfate were of similar magnitude. Serum concentrations of SHBG, testosterone, DHEA, androstenedione, and androstenediol were not associated with risk of hyperplasia. Serum concentrations of estrogens, but not of androgens or SHBG, were strongly and significantly associated with risk of breast hyperplasia in postmenopausal women, suggesting that estrogens are important in the pathologic process toward breast cancer.

Berrino et al. (2005) reported the results of the Diet and Androgens Trial-2 (DIANA-2, Italy), a dietary intervention study that required radical modifications of the usual diet over one year; blood samples were collected for hormone measurements as well as anthropometric measurements at the beginning and at one year. One-hundred and fifteen postmenopausal women were included after having been operated for breast cancer at least a year before, not undergoing chemotherapy and with no clinical evidence of disease recurrence, volunteered to participate. After 5.5 years of follow-up, 31 patients who recurred showed significantly greater serum values of testosterone, estradiol, glucose, and BMI than patients who did not, but only testosterone levels were strongly and significantly associated with recurrence or contra lateral cancer. 39 patients had testosterone levels above the median of 0.4 ng/mL both at baseline and after a year of dietary regimen, the recurrence rate was very high with 13 recurrences and 7 contralateral breast cancers. The 52 patients with testosterone levels <0.4 ng/mL both at baseline and after one year experienced three recurrence and three contralateral breast cancer only. This study indicated the potential effect of testosterone on breast cancer progression. If the predictive value of serum testosterone will be confirmed in larger studies, its measurement would become part of the standard diagnostic workup of breast cancer patients, and dietary or other medical intervention to reduce testosterone levels should be considered.

Zeleniuch-Jacquotte et al. (2005) conducted a case-control study nested within the cohort of the New York University Women's Health Study, a large prospective study documenting a positive association of circulating levels of estrogens and androgens with invasive breast cancer. The study included 69 cases of incident in situ carcinoma and 134 individually matched controls. No statistically significant trend of increasing risk with increasing level of any of the hormones was observed. ORs (95% CI) for the highest tertile relative to the lowest were 1.10 (0.51–2.39) for estradiol, 0.95 (0.41–2.19) for estrone, 1.63 (0.69–3.88) for testosterone, 0.99 (0.44–2.24) for androstenedione, 0.99 (0.45–2.20) for DHEA-S and 0.81 (0.38–1.74) for SHBG.

Kaaks et al. (2005b) published the results of a case-control study nested within the EPIC—a multicenter prospective study aimed at investigating the relationships between nutrition and other lifestyle factors, metabolism, genetic predisposition, and cancer risk. The study included 677 cases of breast cancer and 1309 matched control subjects, and thus was equal in size to all previously published cohort studies combined, but from an entirely European population in which standardized methods were used for collection of blood samples and questionnaire data, and for hormone assays. For all study centers combined, geometric mean levels of all sex steroids were significantly higher and SHBG levels significantly lower among cases compared with control subjects. The authors concluded that their large prospective cohort study confirmed earlier evidence that among postmenopausal women, breast cancer risk is directly related to circulating levels of both androgens and estrogens.

Cummings et al. (2005) assessed putative risk factors for breast cancer in a prospective cohort of 7678 women over 65 years from the Study of Osteoporotic Fractures (United States) with a follow up for breast cancer over 10.5 years, 196 cases of ER+ invasive breast cancer were included and 378 controls were randomly selected. Testosterone and estradiol levels were associated with an increased risk of ER+ invasive cancer. In models that included both testosterone and estradiol, only testosterone level remained significantly related to that risk. In models that included risk factors and hormone measurements, only testosterone level and advanced education remained significantly related to the risk of ER+ invasive breast cancer. The authors concluded that high serum testosterone and advanced education predicted ER+ breast cancer. If confirmed, high testosterone level may be more accurate than family history of breast cancer and other conventional risk factors for identifying older women who are most likely to benefit from chemoprevention with antiestrogens.

Beatie et al. (2006) using a case-cohort design studied 135 women with postmenopausal breast cancer and 275 postmenopausal women without breast cancer who were enrolled in the National Surgical Adjuvant Breast and Bowel Project Cancer Prevention Trial (P-1) and who had been treated with tamoxifen or placebo for 69 months. They found that median plasma levels of estradiol, testosterone, and SHBG were similar between the case and the cohort groups. The relative risk of breast cancer for women in the placebo group was not associated with sex hormone levels. Women with the highest levels of plasma estradiol or testosterone had a similar reduction in risk from treatment with tamoxifen, as did women with the lowest levels. Thus, among women who have a high risk of breast cancer, endogenous plasma levels of testosterone or estradiol are not useful for identifying women who will benefit most from treatment with tamoxifen.

Kahan et al. (2006) analyzed the risk of breast cancer with respect to circulating insulin-like growth factor (IGF)-1, IGF-binding protein (IGFBP)-3, sex steroid hormones, and SHBG, taking into consideration the characteristics of the tumors. Plasma hormone levels of 102 postmenopausal patients with breast cancer detected by mammography screening and 102 matched controls were analyzed in relation to the positivity of ER and PR. They found a significantly higher plasma concentration in the breast cancer cases than in the controls, a strong association between the risk of breast cancer and testosterone plasma level (there was no association with androstenedione), and a strong association between the risk of breast cancer and the IGF-1 concentration. When both plasma

IGF-1 and testosterone levels were in the highest quartile ranges, an OR = 26.4 was computed for breast cancer risk. The increased prevalence of ER+ breast cancers in patients with higher levels of IGF-1, IGFBP-3, or/and testosterone implicate these hormones in the etiology of hormone-dependent breast cancer.

Adrenal Androgen Concentration and Risk of Breast Cancer

In experimental studies, bioactive androgens (testosterone, DHT) or their precursors (e.g., DHEA or DHEA-S) have been found to either antagonize or enhance breast cell proliferation or mammary tumor growth (Liao and Dickson, 2002). The inverse associations of breast cancer risk with premenopausal DHEA levels and the apparent protective effects of androgens in some of the experimental studies have been cited to support the use of postmenopausal androgen replacement therapy for the prevention of osteoporosis, improved well-being, and/or sexual functioning and, possibly, breast cancer prevention (Basson, 1999; Shifren et al., 2000; Labrie et al., 2003).

The relationship between adrenal androgens and breast cancer is still confusing (Labrie et al., 1990; Pasqualini, 1993; Boccuzzi and Brignardollo, 1996). Epidemiological studies have generally observed a protective effect of DHEA on breast cancer, especially in Western women (Bulbrook et al., 1971; Wang et al., 1975; Zumoff et al., 1981). How serum DHEA levels have been associated with breast cancer in women, while women with breast cancer were found to have low urinary levels of ADT and etiocholanolone, two metabolites of DHEA (Cameron et al., 1970). A low urinary excretion of DHEA metabolites has been reported in women who subsequently develop breast cancer, in women with breast cancer, and in women with high risk of cancer recurrence after mastectomy. Subnormal plasma levels of DHEA and DHEA-S have also been reported in early, as well as advanced breast cancer patients, especially in premenopausal cancer patients (Lee et al., 1999). These data suggest that higher levels of adrenal androgens may be prophylactic for the development, progression, and reoccurrence of breast cancer.

Elevated plasma levels of DHEA have been found in women who subsequently developed postmenopausal breast cancer (Zeleniuch-Jacquotte et al., 1997; Dorgan et al., 1997b; Key et al., 2002; Manjer et al., 2003; Kaaks et al., 2005a,b). These data imply that similar to testosterone, elevated adrenal androgens may be associated with breast cancer development. One likely explanation for these direct associations is that elevated DHEA-S, androstenedione, and to some extent perhaps bioavailable testosterone may lead to increased mammary and adipose tissue synthesis of estrogens, which in turn may enhance tumor development. The direct association of breast cancer risk with serum DHEA-S and androstenedione concentrations indicates that elevated adrenal androgen synthesis is a risk factor for breast cancer.

Although theoretically DHEA (or DHEA-S) would have the advantage over other androgens that at physiological doses it is converted into more active androgens (testosterone, DHT) and/or estrogens only in those specific target tissues that possess the appropriate enzymes for such conversion, thus limiting the action of the sex steroids to those same tissues (Labrie et al., 2003), an association of DHEA-S levels with breast cancer risk strongly caution against the use of DHEA-S for postmenopausal hormone replacement (Kaaks et al., 2005b).

Recently, Adly et al. (2006) published the data of postmenopausal women about to undergo breast biopsy or mastectomy and who were not taking postmenopausal estrogens treatments or oral contraceptives at the time of the blood draw. In summary, they found that higher serum levels of estrogens, particularly estrone and estrone sulfate, were associated with increased risk of postmenopausal breast cancer independent of androgen levels. Associations with androgens were less consistent, with increasing levels of androstenediol and DHEA, but not testosterone or androstenedione.

The cumulative epidemiologic data to date leave the effects of androgens on breast cancer risk unresolved, suggesting both proliferative and antiproliferative effects of androgens on breast cancer cells.

TREATMENT

In the Female

Whether there is a role for the use of androgens in the management of postmenopausal women remains controversial (Burger, 2007). At present, a variety of testosterone-containing preparations are used in clinical practice or in investigational research protocols for the treatment of women sexual problems. All over the world, women are treated with different combinations of estrogen and progestin for hormonal contraception and to alleviate menopausal symptoms. Clinical and observational studies have reported an increased risk for breast cancer during postmenopausal combined oral estrogen/progestin treatment (Chlebowski et al., 2003; Beral, 2003). However, in many countries, testosterone treatment has gradually become a more accepted component of hormonal therapy in oophorectomized women, a prescription that, when the controversial issues will be resolved, could be extended to postmenopausal and even premenopausal women with symptoms of androgen deficiency (von Schoultz, 2007).

Findings from case-controlled studies of the relationship between endogenous testosterone levels and breast cancer risk do not necessarily translate to women treated with exogenous testosterone. If an association is found between endogenous circulating testosterone and breast cancer, it does not necessarily signify a causal relationship (Somboonporn and Davis, 2004a,b). Total testosterone, although the most common measure for clinical studies, does not yield specifically meaningful information about actual tissue androgen exposure. Labrie et al. (2003) demonstrated that the major proportion of androgenic effects in women is derived from an intracrine mode of action, which will not be detected by measurement of circulating testosterone or DHT.

Exogenous testosterone exerts either androgenic or indirect estrogenic actions, with the latter potentially increasing breast cancer risk. There is a justifiable concern that combined oral estrogen plus progestin therapy significantly increases the risk of breast cancer in postmenopausal women. The potential benefit or risk with regard to breast cancer of the administration of testosterone as part of hormone therapy should be taken into consideration (Somboonporn and Davis, 2004a,b). The results of in vivo and in vitro studies suggest that testosterone may serve as a natural endogenous protector of the breast and limit mitogenic and cancer-promoting effects of estrogen on mammary epithelium. Testosterone induced downregulation of mammary epithelial proliferation and ERα gene expression.

Dimitrakakis et al. (2003) evaluated the effect of physiological testosterone supplementation of estrogen replacement therapy in ovariectomized monkeys treated with estradiol, estradiol plus progesterone, estradiol plus testosterone or vehicle. They showed that addition of a physiological dose of testosterone to estradiol abolished estrogen-induced increases in mammary epithelial proliferation and found a significant reduction in mammary epithelial ERα and increased ERβ expression in estradiol plus testosterone group compared with estradiol alone. This effect of testosterone resulted in a reversal of the ERα/ERβ ratio, which was approximately 2.5 in the estradiol-treated group and approximately 0.7 in the estradiol-testosterone group. This suggests that the addition of testosterone might reduce the risk of breast cancer associated with estrogen-progestin therapy in postmenopausal women. Zhou et al. (2000) showed that estrogen therapy alone significantly increased mammary epithelial proliferation approximately sixfold and significantly increased the mammary epithelial level of ERα mRNA. When given concurrently, testosterone reduced estradiol-induced epithelial proliferation by approximately 40% and entirely abolished the estradiol-induced augmentation of ERα gene expression.

A transdermal testosterone patch designed for the use in women and releasing 300 μg of testosterone per day has been marketed in Europe and is evaluated in postmenopausal women (Mazer and Shifren, 2003). Hofling et al. (2007) published a six months prospective randomized double-blind placebo-controlled study. Postmenopausal women were given continuous combined estradiol 2 mg/norethisterone acetate 1 mg and were equally randomized to receive additional treatment with either the testosterone patch or a placebo patch. Breast cells were collected by fine needle aspiration biopsies at baseline and after six months. In the placebo group, there was a fivefold increase in total breast cell proliferation from baseline to six months. In contrast, during testosterone addition no significant increase in breast proliferation was recorded. These results indicate that testosterone addition to a common estrogen/progestin regimen may have a potential to modulate the stimulatory effects of hormones on the proliferation of breast cancer cells.

Brinton et al. (1986) undertook a case control study of postmenopausal estrogen use and breast cancer risk. A subgroup analysis in this study of 25 patients and 29 controls showed no significant increase in risk with oral methyltestosterone in combination with conjugated equine estrogen (RR, 1.05; 95% CI, 0.6–1.8). Ewertz (1986) studied the effects of IM injections containing estradiol-testosterone (2.5 mg estradiol plus 50 mg testosterone or 5.0 mg estradiol plus 100 mg testosterone) given at an interval of three to seven weeks in a subgroup analysis. This specific therapy was used for 56 of 1694 patients and 21 of 1705 controls. An RR of 2.3 (95% CI, 1.37–3.88) was reported. However, in these two studies the endpoint was not breast cancer risk and the sample sizes were very small.

After noting, in the setting of a specialized menopause clinical practice in South Australia, that women on testosterone in addition to usual hormone therapy rarely have abnormal mammograms compared with women on conventional hormone therapy, a systematic review of breast cancer incidence in this clinic population was undertaken. Dimitrakakis et al. (2004) hypothesized that the addition of testosterone to usual hormone therapy might protect women from breast cancer. In a retrospective, observational study, they followed 508 postmenopausal women receiving testosterone in addition to usual hormone therapy. Breast cancer status was ascertained by mammography at the initiation of testosterone treatment and biannually thereafter. The mean age at the start of follow-up was 56.4 years, and the mean duration of follow-up was 5.8 years. There were seven cases of invasive breast cancer in this population of testosterone users, for an incidence of 238 per 100,000 woman-years. The rate for estrogen/progestin and testosterone users was 293 per 100,000 woman-years, and was the same as for the general population in South Australia; substantially less than women receiving estrogen/progestin in the Schairer et al. (2000) study (628 per 100,000 woman-years), in the

Women's Health Initiative study (380 per 100,000 woman-years) or in the "Million Women" study (521 per 100,000 woman-years) (Beral, 2003). These observations suggest that the addition of testosterone to conventional hormone therapy for postmenopausal women does not increase and may indeed reduce the hormone therapy–associated breast cancer risk, thereby returning the incidence to the normal rates observed in the general, untreated population. A major weakness of the study is that the women were not randomly assigned to receive testosterone.

In contrast, Tamimi et al. (2006) published opposite results from a prospective cohort study conducted in 121,700 U.S. registered nurses between the ages of 30 to 50 years reporting every two years reproductive variables, medical history, postmenopausal hormone use. Over 99% of reported breast cancer was confirmed on review of the medical record. During the 24 years follow-up, 4610 breast cancer cases were identified; the percent of current estradiol plus testosterone users was very low (<2%) until year 2000. They found that compared to nonusers, estradiol only users had 15% greater risk of breast cancer and estradiol plus testosterone 77% (calculated in 852 cases and 29 cases, respectively) and concluded that although postmenopausal testosterone therapy may provide improvement with respect to sexual functioning, general well-being, and bone health, the increased risk of breast cancer may outweigh these benefits. It should be noted that the majority of women uses esterified estrogens and methyl testosterone (Estratest) as a postmenopausal treatment available in the United States since 1964 and that women reporting current use of therapy in 1998 were mostly past users of other types of hormones, including testosterone only (54.6%), estrogen only (28.8%), estradiol plus progesterone (19.1%), progesterone only (2.1%), and other types of hormone (7.5%). Only 2.4% of current estradiol plus testosterone users in 1998 were never users prior to initiating estradiol plus testosterone use. Thus, these results are not representative of the real situation in the world and use of testosterone by transdermal route instead of oral methyl testosterone, a 17β-alkylated steroid with a different metabolism and hormone specificity, can make a difference and modify the conclusion. It is not acceptable to draw conclusions from this prospective study as the authors did, paving the way of a conservative attitude from Scientific Societies (North American Menopause Society, 2005; Endocrine Society—Wierman et al., 2006).

Braunstein (2007) noted that most prospective studies have had duration of two years or less. Testosterone was administered in conjunction with estrogens or estrogens and progestins, which confound the interpretation of some of the studies. There does not appear to be an increase in cardiovascular risk factors. There are little data on endometrial safety, and most of the experimental data support a neutral or beneficial effect in regards to breast cancer and concluded that, except for hirsutism and acne, the therapeutic administration of testosterone in physiologic doses is safe for up to several years. Recently, Zang et al. (2007) published that the short-term treatment with testosterone of postmenopausal women does not stimulate endometrial proliferation. Testosterone appears to counteract endometrial estrogen-induced proliferation.

In the Male

Hypogonadism affects an estimated 2 to 4 million men in the United States, of which only 5% receive treatment (Rhoden and Morgentaler, 2004). In 2002, more than 1.75 million prescriptions were written for testosterone, which corresponds to a mean number of applications of 17.5 per patient per year. The incidence of male breast cancer is low. Rudan et al. (1995) gave a figure of 0.83/100,000 per year, meaning that one male breast cancer case per year should be expected among men being treated with testosterone. Sixty percent of male breast cancer patients have a history of a medical condition known to cause gynecomastia (Volpe et al., 1999) and men with Klinefelter's syndrome have a 50-fold increased lifetime risk of developing male breast cancer (Hulrborn et al., 1997). Male breast cancer was also described following estrogen therapy for prostate cancer.

Observations of male breast cancer are very scarce and anecdotal and studies inexistent in either testosterone levels or testosterone treatment and risk of breast cancer in the men. Krause (2005) reported a case of male breast cancer in a hypogonadal male who was supplemented with testosterone enanthate 200 mg every three weeks for 10 years. Pathologically, the tumor presented as an ER+ ductal carcinoma. This report poses questions, including whether the occurrence of the disease indicates an association with testosterone supplementation or whether this is merely a coincidence.

Medras et al. (2006) reported a study on 45 men with hypergonadotropic hypogonadism (aged 18–57 years) who received 250 mg of testosterone esters every 3 to 4 weeks for 5 to 26 years. Seventeen of them were treated for more than 10 years. Breast cancer was diagnosed in two subjects (11%), one after 11 years and another after 15 years of the therapy. A possible association between long-term androgen replacement therapy and a risk of breast cancer in men was suggested.

The suggestion that high testosterone levels contribute to the risk of male breast cancer similarly to the induction of female breast cancer by estrogens is questionable. No case-control study concerning testosterone supplementation in hypogonadism and the occurrence of male breast cancer is available to date.

CONCLUSIONS

As we have showed in this review, many studies have been conducted in the past few years. It appears to be very difficult to compare them on account of the diversity of their recruitments (cases only, case controlled, etc.), of the hormones chosen to be assayed (often only a single determination with no precision of the time of the day and of the time elapsed before detection of the cancer), of the sensitivity, variations, and specificity of the methods used, and at least, of the cases themselves (breast cancer in situ, with metastases, recurrences or contralateral recurrences).

For endogenous hormones, in premenopausal women, we found studies concluding that elevated blood concentrations of androgens are associated with elevated risk for all breast cancer (Micheli et al., 2004; Kaaks et al., 2005a,b), another one finds a significant increase in risk of invasive and ER+/PR+ cancer (Eliassen et al., 2006), and in contrast Sturgeon et al. (2004) concluded that there is no convincing association between serum levels of estrogens or androgens and premenopausal breast cancer risk. In postmenopausal women, some authors found that elevated levels of sex hormones may be predictors: estradiol and testosterone (Cauley et al., 1999), estrogens and androgens (Berrino et al., 2005; Kaaks et al., 2005a,b), testosterone (Cummings et al., 2005; Kahan et al., 2006; Hankinson, 2005–2006), all sex hormones (Key et al., 2002), and the risk elevated for only in situ and ER+/PR+ cancer (Missmer et al., 2004); conversely other investigators found a relation between elevated estrogens but not androgens (or SHBG) (Schairer et al., 2005) or no relation at all between hormones and breast cancer risk (Zeleniuch-Jacquotte et al., 2005; Lamar et al., 2003) and, in a more specialized study, Beatie et al. (2006) concluded that plasma dosing of estrogens or androgens is not useful to identify women who will benefit from treatment with tamoxifen.

For exogenous androgens, we have differences on the type of androgens, the route of administration (oral, parenteral, gels, or patches), and prospective studies allowing not to draw definite conclusions. As it is suggested (The WHI Study, 1998) that oral and particularly equine estrogens could induce a higher breast cancer risk and that methyl testosterone is deleterious for the liver, we need more studies with safer drugs as estrogens and testosterone gels or patches. Already, the few we have concluded that testosterone induces a downregulation of mammary epithelial proliferation and ERα gene expression. Even in postmenopausal women who are treated with estrogen and progestin, the addition of testosterone may have a modulating effect on the proliferation induced on breast cells.

The confusion is also increased by the scientific societies that do not give the same recommendations such as The Endocrine Society whose recommendations are "Against making a diagnosis of androgen deficiency in women at present" even when the North American Menopause Society recommends "transdermal patches or topical gels or creams to be preferred over oral products because of first-pass hepatics effects documented with oral formulations. Testosterone therapy should be administrated at the lowest dose for the shortest time that meets treatment goals".

Concerning the role of hormones in the incidence of breast cancer, there is one limitation in the fact that, in all studies, circulating serum hormone concentrations is only measured, but since the androgens made locally in peripheral tissues do not originate from circulating testosterone, only could reasonably expect that the measurement of serum levels of testosterone is of questionable biological and clinical significance (Labrie, 2006). We need a consensus for what hormone has to be dose and a harmonization of the different methods of assays.

Facing such contradictory observations and with no clinical randomized controlled studies available for a while, clinicians must follow the androgen treatment in the women as it is done for men who are treated with testosterone. The clinical investigations including physical examination, interview on different risk factors, mammography (most of the time, these women have one every year due to the estrogen treatment), and repeated assays to establish androgen deficiency are necessary before initiating the hormonal treatment. The objective of the hormonal treatment is to reach testosterone levels at the low normal concentration range (still to be defined) to treat the androgen deficiency symptoms. To achieve this goal, it is advisable to choose a safe way of administration as that of transdermal route either with a gel or a matricial patch.

REFERENCES

Adams JB. Steroid hormones and human breast cancer. An hypothesis. Cancer 1977; 40:325–333.

Adly L, Hill D, Sherman ME, Sturgeon SR, Fears T, Mies C, Ziegler RG, Hoover RN, Schairer C. Serum concentrations of estrogens, sex hormone-binding globulin, and androgens and risk of breast cancer in post-menopausal women. Int J Cancer 2006; 119:2402–2407.

Allegra JC, Lippman ME, Thompson EB, Simon R, Barlock A, Green L, Huff KK, Do HM, Aitken SC. Distribution, frequency and quantitative analysis of estrogen, progesterone, androgen and glucocorticoid receptors in human breast cancer. Cancer Res 1979; 39:1447–1454.

Basson SR. Androgens replacement for women. Can Fam Physician 1999; 45:2100–2107.

Beatie MS, Costantino JP, Cummings SR, Wickerham DL, Vogel VG, Dowsett M, Fomkerd EJ, Willett WC, Wolmark N, Hankinson SE. Endogenous sex hormones, breast cancer risk, and tamoxifen response: an ancillary study in the NSABP Breast Cancer Prevention Trial. J Natl Cancer Inst 2006; 98:110–115.

Bélanger A, Brochu M, Cliché J. Levels of plasma steroid glucuronides in intact and castrated men with prostatic cancer. J Clin Endocrinol Metab 1986; 62:812–815.

Bélanger A, Pelletier G, Labrie F, Barbier S, Chouinard. Inactivation of androgens by UDP-glucuronosyltranferase enzymes in humans. Trends Endocrinol Metab 2003; 14:473–479.

Beral V. Breast cancer and hormone replacement therapy in the Million Women Study. Lancet 2003; 362(9382):419–427.

Bern HA, Jones LA, Mori T, Young PN. Exposure of neonatal mice to steroids: long-term effects on the mammary gland and other reproductive structures. J Steroid Biochem 1975; 6:673–676.

Berrino F, Muti P, Micheli A, Bolelli G, Krogh V, Sciajino R, Pisani P, Panico S, Secreto G. Serum sex hormone levels after menopause and subsequent breast cancer. J Natl Cancer Inst 1996; 98:291–296.

Berrino F, Pasanini P, Bellati C, Venturelli E, Krogh V, Mastroianni A, Berselli E, Muti P, Secreto G. Serum testosterone levels and breast cancer recurrence. Int J Cancer 2005; 113:499–502.

Bieche I, Parfait B, Tozlu S, Lidereau R, Vidaud M. Quantitation of androgen receptor gene expression in sporadic breast tumours by real-time RT-PCR: evidence that MYC is an AR-regulated gene. Carcinogenesis 2001; 22:1521–1526.

Birrell SN, Hall RE, Tilley WD. Role of the androgen receptor in human breast cancer. J Mammary Gland Biol Neoplasia 1998; 3:95–103.

Blankenstein MA, Maitimu-Smeele I, Donker GH, Daroszewski J, Milewicz A. On the significance of in situ production of oestrogens in human breast cancer tissue. J Steroid Biochem Mol Biol 1992; 41:891–896.

Boccuzzi G, Brignardollo E. Adrenal androgen action in breast cancer. Ann N Y Acad Sci 1996; 784:349–361.

Boccuzzi G, Brignardello E, Di Monaco M, Gatto V, Leonardi L, Pizzini A, Gallo M. 5-En-androstene-3-β, 17-β-diol inhibits the growth of MCF-7 breast cancer cells when oestrogen receptors are blocked by oestradiol. Br J Cancer 1994; 70:1035–1039.

Bonne C, Raynaud JP. Androgen receptor assay with a specific ligand (^{3}H) methyltrienolone. In: Vermeulen A, Klopper A, Sciarra F, Jungblut P, Lerner L, eds. Research on Steroids. Vol 7. Amsterdam: Elsevier/North-Holland Biomedical Press, 1977:197–204.

Bonney RC, Scanlon MJ, Reed MJ, Jones DL, Beranek PA, James VH Adrenal androgen concentrations in breast tumors and in normal breast tissue. The relationship to oestradiol metabolism. J Steroid Biochem 1984; 20: 501–504.

Braunstein GD. Safety of testosterone treatment in postmenopausal women. Fertil Steril 2007; 88:1–17.

Brennan MJ, Wang DY, Hayward JL, Bulbrook RD, Deshpande N. Urinary and plasma androgens in begnin breast disease. Possible relation to breast cancer. Lancet 1973; 1: 1076–1079.

Brinton LA, Hoover R, Fraumeni JF Jr. Menopausal oestrogens and breast cancer risk: an expanded study case-control study. Br J cancer 1986; 54:825–832.

Brignardello E, Cassoni P, Migliardi M, Pizzini A, Di Monaco M, Boccuzzi G, Massobrio M. Dehydroepiandrosterone concentration in breast cancer tissue is related to its plasma gradient across the mammary gland. Breast Cancer Res 1995; 33:171–177.

Brysacute M. Androgens and androgen receptor: do they play a role in breast cancer? Med Sci Monit 2000; 6:433–438.

Buchanan G, Birrell SN, Peters AA, Bianco-Miotto T, Ramsay K, Cops EJ, Yang M, Harris JM, Simila HA, Moore NL, Bentel JM, Ricciardelli C, Horsfall DJ, Butler LM, Tilley WD. Decreased androgen receptor levels and receptor function in breast cancer contribute to the failure of response to medroxyprogesterone acetate. Cancer Res 2005; 65:8487–8496.

Bulbrook RD, Hayward DY, Spicer CC. Relation between urinary androgen and corticoid excretion and subsequent breast cancer. Lancet 1971; 2:395–398.

Burger HG. Androgen production in women. Fertil Steril 2002; 77(S4):3–5.

Burger HG. Should testosterone be added to estrogen-grogestin therapy for breast protection? Menopause 2007; 14(2): 159–162.

Cameron EHD, Griffiths K, Gleave EN, Stewart HJ, Forrest AMP, Campbell H. Benign and malignant breast disease in south Wales: a study of urinary steroids. Br Med J 1970; 4:768–771.

Cauley JA, Lucas FL, Kuller LH, Stone K, Browner W, Cummings SR. Elevated serum estradiol and testosterone concentrations are associated with a high risk for breast cancer. Ann Intern Med 1999; 130:270–277.

Chlebowski RT, Hendrix SL, Langer RD, Stefanick ML, Gass M, Lane D, Rodabough RJ, Gilligan MA, Cyr MG, Thomson CA, Khandekar J, Petrovitch H, McTiernan A, and WHI Investigators. Influence of estrogen plus progestin on breast cancer and mammography in healthy postmenopausal women: the Women's Initiative randomised controlled trial. JAMA 2003; 289:3243–3253.

Christakos S, Sinha D, Dao TL. Neonatal modification of endocrine functions and mammary carcinogenesis in the rat. Br J Cancer 1976; 34:58–63.

Clarke CL, Sutherland RL. Progestin regulation of cellular proliferation. Endocr Rev 1990; 11:266–301.

Couzinet B, Meduri G, Lecce MG, Young J, Brailly S, Loosfelt H, Milgrom E, Schaison G. The postmenopausal ovary is not a major androgen-producing gland. J Clin Endocrinol Metab 2001; 85:5060–5066.

Cummings SR, Eckert S, Krueger KA, Grady D, Powles TJ, Cauley JA, Norton L, Nickelsen T, Bjarnason NH, Morrow M, Lippman ME, Black D, Glusman E, Costa A, Jordan VC. The effect of Raloxifene on risk of breast cancer in postmenopausal women: results from the MORE randomized trial. Multiple outcomes of Raloxifene evaluation. J Am Med Assoc 1999; 281:2189–2197.

Cummings SR, Lee JS, Lui LY, Stone K, Ljung BM, Cauleys JA. Sex hormones, risk factors, and risk of estrogen receptor-positive breast cancer in older women: a long-term prospective study. Cancer Epidemiol Biomarkers Prev 2005; 14:1047–1051.

Davis SR. The therapeutic use of androgens in women. J Steroid Biochem Mol 1999; 69:177–184.

Davis SR. Androgen replacement in women: a commentary. J Clin Endocrinol Metab 1999; 84:1886–1891.

Davison SL, Davis SR. Androgens in women. J Steroid Biochem Mol Biol 2003; 85:363–366.

Delettre J, Mornon JP, Lepicard G, Ojasoo T, Raynaud JP. Steroid flexibility and receptor specificity. J Steroid Biochem 1980; 13:45–59.

Dimitrakakis C, Jones RA, Liu A, Bondy CA. Breast cancer incidence in postmenopausal women using testosterone in addition to usual hormone therapy. Menopause 2004; 11:531–535.

Dimitrakakis C, Zhou J, Wang J, Belanger A, Labrie F, Cheng C, Powell D, Bondy C. A physiologic role for testosterone in limiting estrogenic stimulation of the breast. Menopause 2003; 10:292–298.

Dorgan JF, Fears TR, McMahon RP, Aronson Friedman L, Patterson BH, Greenhut SF. Measurement of steroid sex hormones in serum: a comparison of radioimmunoassay and mass spectrometry. Steroids 2002; 67:151–158.

Dorgan JF, Longcope C, Stephenson HE Jr., Falk RT, Miller R, Franz C, Kahle L, Campbell WS, Tangrea JA, Schatzkin A. Relation of prediagnostic serum estrogen and androgen levels to breast cancer risk. Cancer Epidemiol Biomarkers Prev 1996; 5:533–539.

Dorgan JF, Longcope C, Stephenson HE, Falk RT, Miller R, Franz C, Kahle L, Campbell WS, Tangrea JA, Schatzkin A. Serum sex hormone levels are related to breast cancer risk in postmenopausal women. Environ Health Perspect 1997a; 105:583–585.

Dorgan JF, Stanczyk FZ, Longcope C, Stephenson HE, Chang L, Miller R, Franz C, Falk RT, Kahle L. Relationship of serum dehydroepiandrosterone (DHEA), DHEA sulfate, and 5-androstene-3 beta, 17 beta-diol to risk of breast cancer in postmenopausal women. Cancer Epidemiol Biomarkers Prev 1997b; 6:177–181.

Dunn IE, Nisula BC, Rodboard D. Transport of steroid hormones. Binding of 21 endogenous steroids to both testosterone-binding globulin and cortico-steroid-binding globulin in human plasma. J Clin Endocrinol Metab 1981; 53:58–68.

Eaton NE, Reeves GK, Appleby PN, Key TJ. Endogenous sex hormones and prostate cancer: a quantitative review of prospective studies. Br J Cancer 1999; 80:930–934.

Ekena K, Katzenellenbogen JA, Katzenellenbogen BS. Determinants of ligand binding specificity of estrogen receptor-alpha: estrogen versus androgen discrimination. J Biol Chem 1998; 273:693–699.

Eliassen AH, Missmer SA, Tworoger SS, Spjegelman D, Barbieri RL, Dowsett M, Hankinson SE. Endogenous steroid hormone concentrations and risk of breast cancer among premenopausal women. J Natl Cancer lnst 2006; 98: 1406–1415.

Ewertz M. Influence of non-contraceptive exogenous and endogenous sex hormones on breast cancer risk in Denmark. Int J Cancer 1986; 42:832–838.

Fears TR, Ziegler RG, Donaldson JL, Falk RT, Hoover RN, Stanczyk FZ, Vaught JB, Gail MH. Reproducibility studies and inter laboratory concordance for androgen assays in female plasma. Cancer Epidemiol Biomarkers Prev 2000; 9:403–412.

Gann PH, Hennekens CH, Ma J, Longcope C, Stampfer MJ. Prospective study of sex hormone levels and risk of prostate cancer. J Natl Cancer Inst 1996; 88:1118–1126.

Gayosso V, Montano LF, Lopez-Marure R. DHEA-induced antiproliferative effect in MCF-7 cells is androgen- and estrogen receptor-independent. Cancer J 2006; 12(2): 160–165.

Ghatge RP, Jacobsen BM, Schittone SA, Horwitz KB. The progestational and androgenic properties of medroxyprogesterone acetate: gene regulatory overlap with dihydrotestosterone in breast cancer cells. Breast Cancer Res 2005; 7:1036–1050.

Giton F, Fiet J, Guéchot J, Ibrahim F, Bronsard F, Chopin D, Raynaud JP. Serum bioavailable testosterone: assayed or claculated? Clin Chem 2006; 52:474–481.

Goebelsmann U, Arce JJ, Thorneycroft IH, Mishell DR Jr. Serum testosterone concentrations in women throughout the menstrual cycle and following HCG administration. Am J Obstet Gynecol 1974; 119:445–452.

Goss PE, Ingle JN, Martino S, Robert NJ, Muss HB, Picart MJ, Castiglione M, Tu D, Shepherd LE, Pritchard KI, Livingston RB, Davidson NE, Norton L, Perez EA, Abrams JS, Therasse P, Pamer MJ, Pater L A randomized trial of letrozole in postmenopausal women after five years of tamoxifene therapy for early-stage breast cancer. N Engl J Med 2003; 19:1793–1802.

Grattarola R. Androgens in breast cancer. Part I. Atypical endometrial hyperplasia and breast cancer in married premenopausal women. Am J Obstet Gynecol 1973; 116:423–428.

Hackenberg R, Schulz KD. Androgen receptor mediated growth control of breast cancer and endometrial cancer modulated by antiandrogen- and androgen-like steroids. J Steroid Biochem Mol Biol 1996; 56:113–117.

Haning RV Jr., Chabot M, Flood CA, Hackett R, Longcope C. Metabolic clearance rate (MCR) of dehydroepiandrosterone sulfate (DS) its metabolism to dehydroepiandrosterone, androstenedione, testosterone and dihydrotestosterone, and the effects of increased plasma DS concentration on DS MCR in normal women. J Clin Endocrinol Metab 1989; 9:1047–1052.

Hankinson SE. Endogenous hormones and risk of breast cancer in postmenopausal women. Breast Dis 2005–2006; 24:3–15.

Hankinson SE, Willett WC, Manson JE, Colditz GA, Hunter DJ, Spiegelman D, Barbieri RL, Speizer FE. Plasma sex steroid hormone levels and risk of breast cancer in postmenopausal women. J Natl Cancer Inst 1998; 90:1292–1299.

Hofling M, Hirschberg AL, Skoog L, Tani E, Hagerstrom T, von Schoultz B. Testosterone inhibits estrogen/progestogen-induced breast cell proliferation in post-menopausal women. Menopause 2007; 14:183–190.

Howard JM. Testosterone may cause breast cancer. Int J Cancer 2005; 115:497–498.

Hsing AW, Chokkalingam AP. Prostate cancer epidemiology. Front Biosci 2006; 11:1388–1413.

Hsing AW, Stanczyk FZ, Bélanger A, Schroeder P, Chang L, Falk RT, Fears TR. Reproducibility of serum sex steroid assays in men by RIA and mass spectrometry. Cancer Epidemiol Biomarkers Prev 2007; 16:1004–1008.

Hulrborn R, Hanson C, Kopf I, Verbiene I, Warnhammar E, Weimarck A. Prevalence of Klinefelter's syndrome in male breast cancer patients. Anticancer Res 1997; 17(6D): 4293–4297.

Kaaks R, Berrino F, Key T, Rinaldi S, et al. Serum sex steroids in premenopausal women and breast cancer risk within the European Prospective Investigation into Cancer and Nutrition (EPIC). J Natl Cancer Inst 2005a; 97:755–765.

Kaaks R, Rinaldi S, Key TJ, Berrino F, Peeters PH, Biessy C, Dossus L, Lukanova A, Bingham S, Khaw KT, Allen NE, Bueno-de-Mesquita HB, van Gils CH, Grobbee D, Boeing H, Lahmann PH, Nagel G, Chang-Claude J, Clavel-Chapelon F, Fournier A, Thiébaut A, González CA, Quirós JR, Tormo MJ, Ardanaz E, Amiano P, Krogh V, Palli D, Panico S, Tumino R, Vineis P, Trichopoulou A, Kalapothaki V, Trichopoulos D, Ferrari P, Norat T, Saracci R, Riboli E. Postmenopausal serum androgens, estrogens and breast cancer risk: the European prospective investigation into cancer and nutrition. Endocr Relat Cancer 2005b; 12:1071–1082.

Kahan Z, Gardi J, Nyari T, Földesi I, Hajnal-Papp R, Ormandi K, Lazar G, Thurzo L, Schally AV. Elevated levels of circulating insulin-like growth factor-I, IGF-binding globulin-3 and testosterone predict hormone-dependent breast cancer in postmenopausal women: a case-control study. Int J Oncol 2006; 29:193–200.

Katzenellenbogen BS, Montano MM, Ediger TR, Sun J, Ekena K, Lazennec G, Martini PG, McInerney EM, Delage-Mourroux R, Weis K, Katzenellenbogen JA. Estrogen receptors: selective ligands, partners, and distinctive pharmacology. Recent Prog Horm Res 2000; 55:163–193.

Key T, Appleby P, Barnes I, Reeves G. Endogenous Hormones and Breast Cancer Collaborative Group. Endogenous sex hormones and breast cancer in postmenopausal women: reanalysis of nine prospective studies. J Natl Cancer Inst 2002; 94:606–616.

Killinger DW, Perel E, Daniilescu, Kharlip L, Blankenstein MA. Aromatase activity in the breast and other peripheral tissues and its therapeutic regulation. Steroids 1987; 50:523–536.

Kramer EA, Seeger H, Kramer B, Wallwiener D, Mueck AO. The effect of progesterone, testosterone and synthetic progestogens on growth factor- and estradiol-treated human cancerous and benign breast cells. Eur J Obstet Gynecol Reprod Biol 2006; 129:77–83.

Krause W. Review of 54-year-old man with breast cancer after prolonged testosterone therapy. Clin Adv Hematol Oncol 2005; 3:714.

Kuenen-Boumeester V, Van der Kwast TH, Claassen CC, Claassen CC, Look MP, Liem GS, Klijn JG, Henzen-Logmans SC. The clinical significance of androgen receptors in breast cancer and their relation to histological and cell biological parameters. Eur J Cancer 1996; 32A:1560–1565.

Kuiper GG, Carlsson B, Grandien K, Enmark J, Haggblad J, Nilsson S, Gustafsson JA. Comparison of the ligand binding specificity and transcript tissue distribution of estrogen receptors alpha and beta. Endocrinology 1997; 138:863–870.

Labrie F. Dehydroepiandrotestosterone, androgens, and the mammary gland. Gynecol Endocrinol 2006; 22:118–130.

Labrie F, Bélanger A, Bélanger P, Bérubé R, Martel C, Cusan L, Gomez J, Candas B, Castiel I, Chaussade V, Deloche C, Leclaire J. Androgen glucuronides, instead of testosterone, as the new markers of androgenic activity in women. J Steroid Biochem Mol Biol 2006; 99:182–188.

Labrie F, Bélanger A, Cusan L, Candas B. Physiological changes in dehydroepiandrosterone are not reflected by serum levels of active androgens and estrogens but of their metabolites: intracrinology. J Clin Endocrinol Metab 1997; 82: 2403–2409.

Labrie F, Bélanger A, Simard J, Luu-The V, Labrie C. DHEA and peripheral androgen and estrogen formation: intracrinology. Ann N Y Acad Sci 1995; 774:16–28.

Labrie F, Luu-The V, Labrie C, Belanger A, Simard J, Lin S-X, Pelletier G. Endocrine and intracrine sources of androgens in women: inhibition of breast cancer and other roles of androgens and their precursor dehydroepiandrosterone. Endocr Rev 2003; 24:152–182.

Labrie F, Poulin R, Simard J, Zhao HF, Labrie C, Dauvois S, Dumont M, Hatton AC, Poirier D, Merand Y. Interactions between estrogens, androgens, progestins, and glucocorticoids in ZR-75-1 human breast cancer cells. Ann N Y Acad Sci 1990; 595:130–148.

Lamar CA, Dorgan JF, Longcope C, Stanczyk FZ, Falk RT, Stephenson HE Jr. Serum sex hormones and breast cancer risk factors in postmenopausal women. Cancer Epidemiol Biomarkers Prev 2003; 12:380–383.

Langer M, Kubista E, Schemper M, Spona J. Androgen receptors, serum androgen levels and survival of breast cancer patients. Arch Gynecol Obstet 1990; 247:203–209.

Liao DJ, Dickson RB. Roles of androgens in the development, growth, and carcinogenesis of the mammary gland. J Steroid Mol Biol 2002; 80:175–189.

Lee SH, Kim SO, Kwon SW, Chung BC. Androgen imbalance in premenopausal women with benign breast disease and breast cancer. Clin Biochem 1999; 32:375–380.

Lillie EO, Bernstein L, Ursin G. The role of androgens and polymorphisms in the androgen receptor in the epidemiology of breast cancer. Breast Cancer Res 2003; 5:164–173.

Luu-The V, Dufort I, Pelletier G, Labrie F. Type 5, 17-β-hydroxysteroid dehydrogenase: its role in the formation of androgens in women. Mol Cell Endocrinol 2001; 171:77–82.

Maggiolini M, Donze O, Jeannin E, Ando S, Picard D. Adrenal androgens stimulate the proliferation of breast cancer cells as direct activators of oestrogen receptor alpha. Cancer Res 1999; 59:4864–4869.

Manjer J, Johansson R, Berglund G, Janzon L, Kaaks R, Agren A, Lenner P. Postmenopausal breast cancer risk in relation to sex steroid hormones, prolactin and SHBG (Sweden). Cancer Causes Control 2003; 14:599–607.

Mazer NA, Shifren JL. Transdermal testosterone for women: a new physiological approach for androgen therapy. Obstet Gynecol Surv 2003; 58:489–500.

Medras M, Filus A, Jozkow P, Winowski J, Sicinska Werner T. Breast cancer and long-term hormonal treatment of male hypogonadism. Breast Cancer Res Treat 2006; 96:263–265.

Mehta RR, Valcourt L, Graves J, Green R. Subcellular concentrations of estrone, estradiol, androstenedione 17-β-hydroxysteroid dehydrogenase (17-β-OH-SDH) activity in malignant and non-malignant human breast tissues. Int J Cancer 1987; 40:305–308.

Micheli A, Muti P, Secreto G, Krogh V, Meneghini E, Venturelli E, Sieri S, Pala V, Berrino F. Endogenous sex hormones and subsequent breast cancer in premenopausal women. Int J Cancer 2004; 112:312–318.

Miller WR, Telford J, Dixon JM, Hawkins RA. Androgen receptor activity in human breast cancer and its relationship with estrogen and progesterone receptor activity. Eur J Cancer Clin Oncol 1985; 21:539–542.

Missmer SA, Eliassen AH, Barbieri RL, Hankinson SE. Endogenous estrogen, androgen, and progesterone concentrations and breast cancer risk among postmenopausal women. J Natl Cancer Inst 2004; 96:1856–1865.

Mori T, Bern HA, Mills KT, Young PN. Long-term effects of neonatal steroid exposure on mammary gland and tumorigenesis in mice. J Natl Cancer Inst 1976; 57:1057–1062.

Mouridsen H, Gershanovich M, Sun Y, Pérez-Carrión R, Boni C, Monnier A, Apffelstaedt J, Smith R, Sleeboom HP, Jänicke F, Pluzanska A, Dank M, Becquart D, Bapsy PP, Salminen E, Snyder R, Lassus M, Verbeek JA, Staffler B, Chaudri-Ross HA, Dugan M. Superior efficacy of letrozole versus tamoxifene as first-line therapy for postmenopausal women with advanced breast cancer: results of a phase III study of the International Letrozole Breast Cancer Group. J Clin Oncol 2001; 19:2596–2606.

Nagasawa H, Mori T, Yanai R, Bern HA, Mills KT. Long-term effects of neonatal hormonal treatments on plasma prolactin levels in female BALB/cfC3H and BALB/c mice. Cancer Res 1978; 38:942–945.

Newton CJ, Samuel DL, James VH. Aromatase activity concentrations of cortisol, progesterone and testosterone in breast and abdominal adipose tissue. J Steroid Biochem 1986; 24:1033–1039.

North American Menopause Society. The role of testosterone therapy in postmenopausal women: position statement of The North American Menopause Society. Menopause 2005; 12:496–511.

Ojasoo T, Raynaud JP. Unique steroid congeners for receptor studies. Cancer Res 1978; 38:4186–4198.

Ortmann I, Prifti S, Bohlmann MK, Rehberger-Schneider S, Strowitzki T, Rabe T. Testosterone and 5 alpha-dihydrotestosterone inhibit in vitro growth of human breast cancer cell lines. Gynecol Endocrinol 2002; 16:113–120.

Pasqualini JR. Role of androgens in breast cancer. J Steroid Biochem Mol Biol 1993; 45:167–172.

Pasqualini JR, Chetrite GS. The enzymatic systems in the formation and transformation of estrogen in normal and cancerous human breast. Control and potential clinical applications. In: Pasqualini JR, ed. Breast Cancer Prognosis, Treatment, and Prevention. 2nd ed. New York, London, Boca Raton, Singapore: Informa Healthcare, 2007:11–48.

Pasqualini JR, Chetrite G, Blacker C, Feinstein MC, Delalonde L, Talbi M, Maloche C. Concentrations of estrone, estradiol, and estrone sulfate and evaluation of sulfatase and aromatase activities in pre- and postmenopausal breast cancer patients. J Clin Endocrinol Metab 1996; 81: 1460–1464.

Pelletier G. Localization of androgen and estrogen receptors in rat and primate tissues. Histopathology 2000; 15: 1261–1270.

Pelletier G, Luu-The V, El Alfy M, Li S, Labrie F. Immunoelectron microscopic localization of 3-β-hydroxysteroid dehydrogenase in the human prostate and mammary gland. J Mol Endocrinol 2001; 26:11–19.

Poulin R, Simard J, Labrie C, Petitclerc L, Dumont M, Lagace L, Labrie F. Down regulation of estrogen receptor gene expression by androgens in the ZR-75-1 human breast cancer cell line. Endocrinology 1989; 125:392–399.

Raynaud JP. Receptors in breast cancer: an introduction. Ann N Y Acad Sci 1977; 286:87–89.

Raynaud JP. Prostate cancer risk in testosterone-treated men. J Steroid Biochem Mol Biol 2006; 102:261–266.

Rhoden EL, Morgentaler A. Risks of testosterone replacement therapy and recommendations for monitoring. N Engl J Med 2004; 350:482–492.

Rinaldi S, Déchaud H, Biessy C, Morin-Raverot V, Toniolo P, Zeleniuch-Jacquotte A, Akhmedkhanov A, Shore RE, Secreto G, Ciampi A, Riboli E, Kaaks R. Reliability and validity of commercially available, direct radioimmunoassay for measurements of blood androgens and estrogens in postmenopausal women. Cancer Epidemiol Biomarkers Prev 2001; 10:757–765.

Rochefort H. Biochemical basis of breast cancer treatment by androgens and progestins. Prog Clin Biol Res 1984; 142:79–95.

Rudan I, Rudan N, Strnad M. Differences between male and female breast cancer. I. Epidemiological features. Acta Med Croatica 1995; 49:117–120.

Santen RJ, Leszczynski D, Tilson-Mallet N, Feil PD, Wright C, Manni A, Santner JS. Enzymatic control of estrogen production in human breast cancer: relative significance of aromatase versus sulfatase pathways. Ann N Y Acad Sci 1986; 464:126–137.

Schairer C, Hill D, Sturgeon SR, Fears T, Mies C, Ziegler RG, Hoover RN, Sherman ME. Serum concentrations of estrogens, sex hormone binding globulin, and androgens and risk of breast hyperplasia in postmenopausal women. Cancer Epidemiol Biomarkers Prev 2005; 14:1660–1665.

Schairer C, Lubin J, Troisi R, Sturgeon S, Brinton L, Hoover R. Menopausal estrogen and estrogen-progestin replacement therapy and breast cancer risk. JAMA 2000; 283:485–491.

Secreto G, Recchione C, Cavalleri A, Miraglia M, Dati V. Circulating levels of testosterone, 17β-oestradiol, luteinising hormone and prolactin in postmenopausal breast cancer patients. Br J Cancer 1983a; 47:269–275.

Secreto G, Recchione C, Grignolio E, Cavalleri A. Increased urinary androgen excretion is a hormonal abnormality detectable before the clinical onset of breast cancer. Cancer Detect Prev 1983b; 6:435–438.

Secreto G, Recchione C, Miraglia M, Grignolio E, Cavalleri A. Increased urinary androgen levels in patients with carcinoma in situ of the breast with onset while taking oral contraceptives. Cancer Detect Prev 1983c; 6:439–442.

Secreto G, Toniolo P, Berrino F, C. Recchione, Di Pietro S, Fariselli G, De Carli A. Increased androgenic activity and breast cancer risk in premenopausal women. Cancer Res 1984; 44:5902–5905.

Secreto G, Toniolo P, Pasini P, Recchione C, Cavalleri A, Fariselli G, Totis A, Di Pietro S, Berrino F. Androgens and breast cancer in premenopausal women. Cancer Res 1989; 49:471–476.

Secreto G, Toniolo P, Berrino F, Recchione C, Cavalleri A, Pisani P, Totis A, Fariselli G, Di Pietro S. Serum and urinary androgens and risk of breast cancer in postmenopausal women. Cancer Res 1991; 51:2572–2576.

Secreto G, Zumoff B. Abnormal production of androgens in women with breast cancer. Anticancer Res 1994; 14:2113–2117.

Shifren JL, Braunstein GD, Simon JA, Casson PR, Buster JE, Redmond GP, Burki RE, Ginsburg ES, Rosen RC, Leiblum SR, Caramelli KE, Mazer NA. Transdermal testosterone treatment in women with impaired sexual function after oophorectomy. N Engl J Med 2000; 343:682–688.

Simpson ER. Aromatization of androgens in women: current concept and findings. Fertil Steril 2002; 77(S4):6–10.

Sonne-Hansen K, Lykkesfeldt AE. Endogenous aromatization of testosterone results in growth stimulation of the human MCF-7 breast cancer cell line. J Steroid Biochem Mol Biol 2005; 93:25–34.

Somboonporn W, Davis SR. Postmenopausal testosterone therapy and breast cancer risk. Maturitas 2004a; 49:267–275.

Somboonporn W, Davis SR. National Health and Medical Research Council. Testosterone effects on the breast: implications for testosterone therapy for women. Endocr Rev 2004b; 25:374–388.

Stoll BA, Secreto G. New hormone-related markers of high risk to breast cancer. Ann Oncol 1992; 3:435–438.

Sturgeon SR, Potischman N, Malone KE, Dorgan J, Daling J, Schaircr C, Brinton LA. Serum levels of sex hormones and breast cancer risk in premenopausal women: a case-control study (USA). Cancer Causes Control 2004; 15:45–53.

Tamimi RM, Hankinson SE, Chen WY, Rosner B, Colditz GA. Combined estrogen and testosterone use and risk of breast cancer in postmenopausal women. Arch Intern Med 2006; 166:1483–1489.

The Women's Health Initiative Study Group. Design of the Women's Health Initiative: clinical trial and observational study. Control Clin Trials 1998; 19:61–109.

Thijssen JH, Blankenstein MA, Miller WR, Milewicz A. Estrogens in tissues: uptake from the peripheral circulation or local production. Steroids 1987; 50:297–306.

Thijssen JH, Blankenstein MA. Endogenous oestrogens and androgens in normal and malignant endometrial and mammary tissues. Eur J Cancer Clin Oncol 1989; 25:1953–1959.

Thijssen JH, Blankenstein MA, Donker GH, Daroszewski J. Endogenous steroid hormones and local aromatase activity in the breast. J Steroid Biochem Mol Biol 1991a; 39:799–804.

Thijssen JH, Blankenstein MA, Donker GH, et al. Endogenous concentration and subcellular distribution of estrogens in normal and malignant human breast tissue. Cancer Res 1991b; 39:799–804.

Thijssen JH, Daroszewski J, Milewicz A, Blankenstein MA. Local aromatase activity in human breast tissues. J Steroid Biochem Mol 1993; 44:577–582.

Tomooka Y, Bern HA. Growth of mouse mammary gland after neonatal sex hormone treatment. J Natl Cancer Inst 1982; 69:1347–1352.

Van Landeghem AAJ, Poortman J, Nabuurs M, et al. Endogenous concentration and subcellular distribution of estrogens in normal and malignant human breast tissue. Cancer Res 1985; 45:2900–2906.

Volpe CM, Rafferra JD, Collure DW, Hoover EL, Doerr RJ. Unilateral male breast masses: cancer risk and their evaluation and mangement. Am J Surg 1999; 65:250–253.

von Schoultz B. Androgens and the breast. Maturitas 2007; 57:47–49.

Wang DY, Bulbrook RD, Hayward JL. Urinary and plasma androgens and their relation to familial risk of breast cancer. Eur J Cancer 1975; 11:873–877.

Welsch CW, Nagasawa H. Prolactin and murine mammary tumorigenesis: a review. Cancer Res 1977; 37:951–963.

Wierman ME, Basson R, Davis SR, Khosla S, Miller KK, Rosner W, Santoro N. Androgen therapy in women: an Endocrine Society clinical practice guideline. J Clin Endocrinol Metab 2006; 91:3697–3710.

Wilson CM, McPhaul MJ. A and B forms of the androgen receptor are expressed in a variety of human tissues. Moll Cell Endocrinol 1996; 120:51–57.

Yanai R, Nagasawa H, Mori T, Nakajima Yl. Long-term effects of neonatal exposure to 5-α-dihydrotestosterone on normal and neoplasic mammary development in mice. Endocrinol Jpn 1981; 28:231–234.

Yong EL, Lim J, Qi W, Ong V, Misfud A. Molecular basis of androgen receptor diseases. Ann Med 2000; 32:15–22.

Yu H, Bharaj B, Vassilikos EJ, Giai M, Diamandis EP. Shorter CAG repeat length in the androgen receptor gene is associated with more aggressive forms of breast cancer. Breast Cancer Res Treat 2000; 59:153–161.

Yu H, Diamandis EP, Hoffman B. Elevated estradiol and testosterone levels and risk for breast cancer. Ann Intern Med 1999; 131:715.

Zang H, Sahlin L, Masironi B, Eriksson E, Linden-Hirschberg A. Effects of testosterone treatment on endometrial proliferation in postmenopausal women. J Clin Endocrinol Metab 2007; 92:2169–2175.

Zeleniuch-Jacquotte A, Bruning PF, Bonfrer JM, Koening KL, Shore RE, Kim MY, Pasternack BS, Toniolo P. Relation of serum levels of testosterone and dehydroepiandrosterone sulfate to risk of breast cancer in postmenopausal women. Am J Epidemiol 1997; 145:1030–1038.

Zeleniuch-Jacquotte A, Gu Y, Shore RE, Koenig KL, Arslan AA, Kato I, Rinaldi S, Kaaks R, Toniolo P.

Postmenopausal levels of sex hormones and risk of breast carcinoma in situ: results of a prospective study. Int J Cancer 2005; 114:323–327.

Zeleniuch-Jacquotte A, Toniolo P, Levitz M, Shore RE, Koenig KL, Banerjee S, Strax P, Pasternack BS. Endogenous estrogens and risk of breast cancer by estrogen receptor status: a prospective study in postmenopausal women. Cancer Epidemiol Biomarkers Prev 1995; 4: 857–860.

Zhou J, Ng S, Adesanya-Famuiya O, Anderson K, Bondy CA. Testosterone inhibits estrogen-induced mammary epithelial proliferation and suppresses estrogen receptor expression. FASEB J 2000; 14:1725–1730.

Zumoff B, Levin J, Rosenfeld RS, Markham M, Strain GW, Fukushima DK. Abnormal 24-hr mean plasma concentrations of dehydroepiandrosterone and dehydroisoandrosterone sulfate in women with primary operable breast cancer. Cancer Res 1981; 41:3360–3363.

12

Combination of Breast Cancer Prevention with Tissue-Targeted Hormone Replacement Therapy

FERNAND LABRIE

Laboratory of Molecular Endocrinology and Oncology, Laval University Hospital Research Center (CRCHUL) and Laval University, Québec City, Québec, Canada

INTRODUCTION

Breast cancer is the most frequent (26%) and the second cause of cancer death (15%) in women (Jemal et al., 2007). In fact, it is estimated that in the United States alone, 178,480 women will be diagnosed with breast cancer in 2007 and that 40,460 women will die from the disease (Jemal et al., 2007). It is important to mention that during the 15 years between 1992 and 2007, the number of deaths from prostate cancer in the United States has decreased by 33% from 40,000 to 27,050, while the number of deaths from breast cancer has decreased by only 12% from 46,000 to 40,460.

The marked decrease in prostate cancer deaths can be attributed to early diagnosis and the high efficacy of early treatment, especially the use of androgen blockade at the localized stage of the disease (Labrie et al., 2002; Arnst, 2003; Cooperberg et al., 2003; Egawa et al., 2004; Mehring, 2004; Labrie et al., 2005a; Akaza et al., 2006). On the other hand, the much lower success achieved in breast cancer is likely related to the difficulty in diagnosing breast cancer at the true localized stage. In fact, when women treated by surgery for localized disease are followed for more than 10 years, cancer will reappear in approximately 50% of cases (EBCTCG, 1998), thus indicating that the cancer was already present as micrometastases in those women despite the clinical appearance of a localized disease. Since breast cancer has already metastasized in 50% to 60% of cases at the time of diagnosis and it is unlikely that improvements in the treatment of advanced disease will permit a cure in most cases in the foreseeable future, it is clear that an efficient and well-tolerated strategy for breast cancer prevention is urgently needed.

Moreover, with increased life expectancy, women now spend half their adult lifetime after menopause, thus indicating the need to find an alternative to traditional hormone replacement therapy (HRT), a source of concern mainly related to the risk of breast cancer. It is thus of major importance to develop a strategy that simultaneously takes into account the problems associated with menopause as well as breast cancer risk in order to better meet the needs of women's health and achieve a major decrease in deaths from breast cancer.

INHIBITION OF THE ESTROGENIC STIMULUS ON THE MAMMARY GLAND

Early menarche, late menopause, and use of estrogen replacement therapy (ERT) are all clearly associated with an increased risk of breast cancer (Beral et al., 2005). All these risk factors are linked to an increased exposure to estrogens, which stimulate the proliferation of the mammary duct epithelium and breast cancer (Pike et al., 1993; Key et al., 2001).

Among all the risk factors, estrogens are thus well recognized to play the predominant role in breast cancer development and growth (McGuire et al., 1975; Asselin and Labrie, 1978; Davidson and Lippman, 1989). Considerable attention has thus focused on the development of blockers of estrogen biosynthesis and action (Wakeling and Bowler, 1988; Dauvois et al., 1991; de Launoit et al., 1991a; Levesque et al., 1991; Gronemeyer et al., 1992; Labrie et al., 1992a, 1995c; Gauthier et al., 1997) for the treatment of breast cancer. In fact, a most important characteristic of the endocrine physiology of the mammary gland is that the normal mammary gland, as well as early breast cancer, absolutely requires estrogens for proliferation and growth.

Tamoxifen, Raloxifene, Fulvestrant, and Aromatase Inhibitors

In agreement with the important role of estrogens, inhibitors of estrogen formation and action have shown very positive results in breast cancer therapy, these benefits being accompanied by an exceptionally good tolerance compared with chemotherapy. Moreover, in addition to the well-recognized benefits of the antiestrogens tamoxifen, raloxifene (Fig. 1) and fulvestrant, these observations pertain to inhibitors of estrogen formation, namely the aromatase inhibitors anastrozole, letrozole, and exemestane (Bonneterre et al., 2000; Mouridsen et al., 2001; Goss et al., 2003), as well as to medical castration with gonadotropin-releasing hormone (GnRH) agonists (goserelin, leuprolide, decapeptyl, and buserelin). While being much better tolerated, these compounds used alone or in combination usually show results superior to chemotherapy, especially in early disease with a much better tolerance profile.

According to the latest Oxford analysis of the Early Breast Cancer Triallists' Collaborative Group (EBCTCG, 2005), five years of tamoxifen treatment in the adjuvant setting produced, after 15 years of follow-up, an 11.8 ± 1.3% absolute reduction in breast cancer mortality in women with estrogen receptor (ER)-positive tumors. In the National Surgical Adjuvant Breast and Bowel Project (NSABP) Breast Cancer Prevention Trial (P1), tamoxifen for 69 months reduced the risk of breast cancer diagnosis by 49% (Fisher et al., 1998), an effect which persisted at 43% at seven years of follow-up (Fisher et al., 2005).

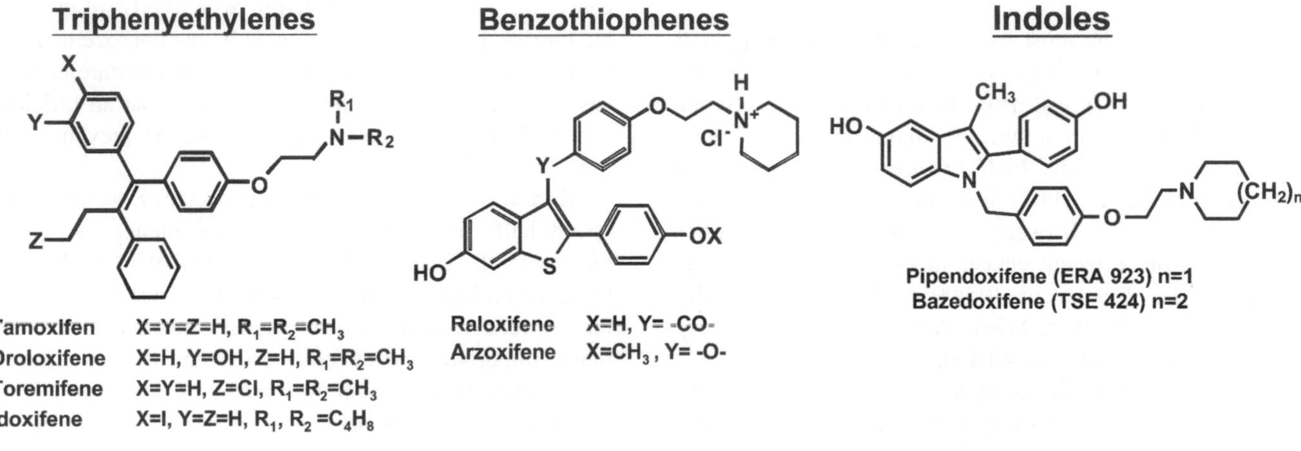

Figure 1 Structure of a series of SERMs.

Long-term treatment with tamoxifen, however, is well known to have side effects related to the partial estrogenic activity of this compound, especially the increased risk of endometrial cancer and thromboembolic events (Fisher et al., 1994; Jaiyesimi et al., 1995; EBCTCG, 1998; Wysowski et al., 2002; Braithwaite et al., 2003; Cuzick et al., 2003; EBCTCG, 2005). Accordinly, tamoxifen therapy for longer than five years does not seem to convey additional benefits and even seems to bring negative effects on breast cancer incidence (Fisher et al., 1996; Peto, 1996; Fisher et al., 2001). In addition, resistance to tamoxifen is a well-recognized phenomenon (Clarke et al., 2001). The limit of five years of tamoxifen administration and its estrogenic side effects indicate the need to search for improved selective estrogen receptor modulators (SERMs).

The observation that tamoxifen reduces the incidence of contralateral breast cancer (Cuzick and Baum, 1985) followed by the study of Powles et al., (Powles et al., 1989) has opened the way for the clinical trials that led to the approval of tamoxifen by the Federal Drug Administration in 1998 as the first agent to reduce the risk of breast cancer in high-risk women. The Breast Cancer Prevention Trial (P1) enrolled women at risk, which included age 60 or older, a history of lobular adenocarcinoma in situ, and age 35 to 59 years with a five-year predicted risk for breast cancer of 1.66%.

Despite approval by the U.S. Food and Drug Administration and endorsement by the American Society of Clinical Oncology, only 5% to 30% of high-risk women accept to take tamoxifen as a preventive agent (Vogel et al., 2002). Fear of the reported side effects of tamoxifen is a major drawback for healthy women, the two most serious side effects being, as mentioned above, endometrial cancer and thromboembolic events (Cuzick et al., 2002). In the study of tamoxifen and raloxifene (STAR Study), the results show nearly equal 50% benefits in preventing invasive breast cancer in postmenopausal women at high risk of breast cancer, although raloxifene was less efficient in preventing noninvasive disease (Wickerham and Fourchotte, 2006). Most importantly, half of the breast cancers are not prevented nor delayed by tamoxifen or raloxifene. The objective of new SERMs is thus to increase the benefit/risk ratio observed with tamoxifen or raloxifene. It is important to recognize that all SERMs are different and that the data obtained with tamoxifen, raloxifene, or any SERM cannot be extrapolated to other SERMs.

Aromatase inhibitors decrease the risk of breast cancer with a reduced risk of uterine cancer and blood clots (Baum et al., 2002; Goss et al., 2003; Coombes et al., 2004). Studies with anastrozole, letrozole, and exemestane have shown the benefits of switching from tamoxifen to an aromatase inhibitor (Goss et al., 2003; Coombes et al., 2004; Jakesz et al., 2005). It should be mentioned that despite the relatively short-term duration of the studies performed with aromatas inhibitors, an increased number of fractures have been found with all the aromatase inhibitors compared with tamoxifen (Baum et al., 2002; Coleman et al., 2004; Coombes et al., 2004; Jakesz et al., 2005; Lonning et al., 2005). Moreover, despite the advantages of switching to an aromatase inhibitor, the benefits obtained are still far from the prevention of recurrence in all patients, and resistance to aromatase inhibitors develops (Goss, 2002).

In this context of general estrogen deprivation caused by aromatase inhibitors, estrogen deficiency has been reported to have a negative effect on cognitive status, especially short- and long-term memory (Sherwin, 2003; Tralongo et al., 2005). Preliminary data have indicated a higher incidence of impaired word finding in women who were treated with the aromatase inhibitor exemestane compared with tamoxifen (Jones et al., 2003). Such data raise questions about the long-term effects of general estrogen deprivation on cognitive function, a problem that could be amplified under the long-term conditions of treatment needed for prevention.

Potential limitations of aromatase inhibitors, however, are related to the observation that these compounds do not block estradiol (E2) formation completely (Johannessen et al., 1997; Geisler et al., 2000). Moreover, aromatase inhibitors do not inhibit formation of the estrogenic androst-5-ene-3β, 17β-diol (5-diol) from dehydroepiandrosterone (DHEA) by 17β-hydroxysteroid dehydrogenase (17β-HSD) activity (Fig. 2). The estrogenic 5-diol is present in the blood of pre- and postmenopausal women at the levels of 0.49 ± 0.20 ng/mL and 0.27 ± 0.15 ng/mL, respectively (Labrie et al., 2006a). At these concentrations, 5-diol is known to stimulate the proliferation of human breast cancer cells (Poulin and Labrie, 1986) and other estrogen-sensitive tissues (Adams, 1985). As mentioned above, aromatase inhibitors thus leave 5-diol free to continue to stimulate breast cancer in the presence of an incomplete inhibition of E2 formation. The long-term effects of aromatase inhibitors, moreover, remain to be evaluated.

Fulvestrant, a steroidal pure antiestrogen, at the dose used, has been shown to be equivalent to tamoxifen as primary treatment of advanced breast cancer (Howell et al., 2004). On the other hand, fulvestrant has been shown to lead to a longer median time to progression compared with anastrazole in patients who had progressed with prior endocrine therapy (Howell et al., 2002; Osborne et al., 2002). Encouraging results have also been observed with fulvestrant in patients progressing under treatment with aromatase inhibitors (Johnston, 2005), a phenomenon possibly related to the upregulation of growth factor

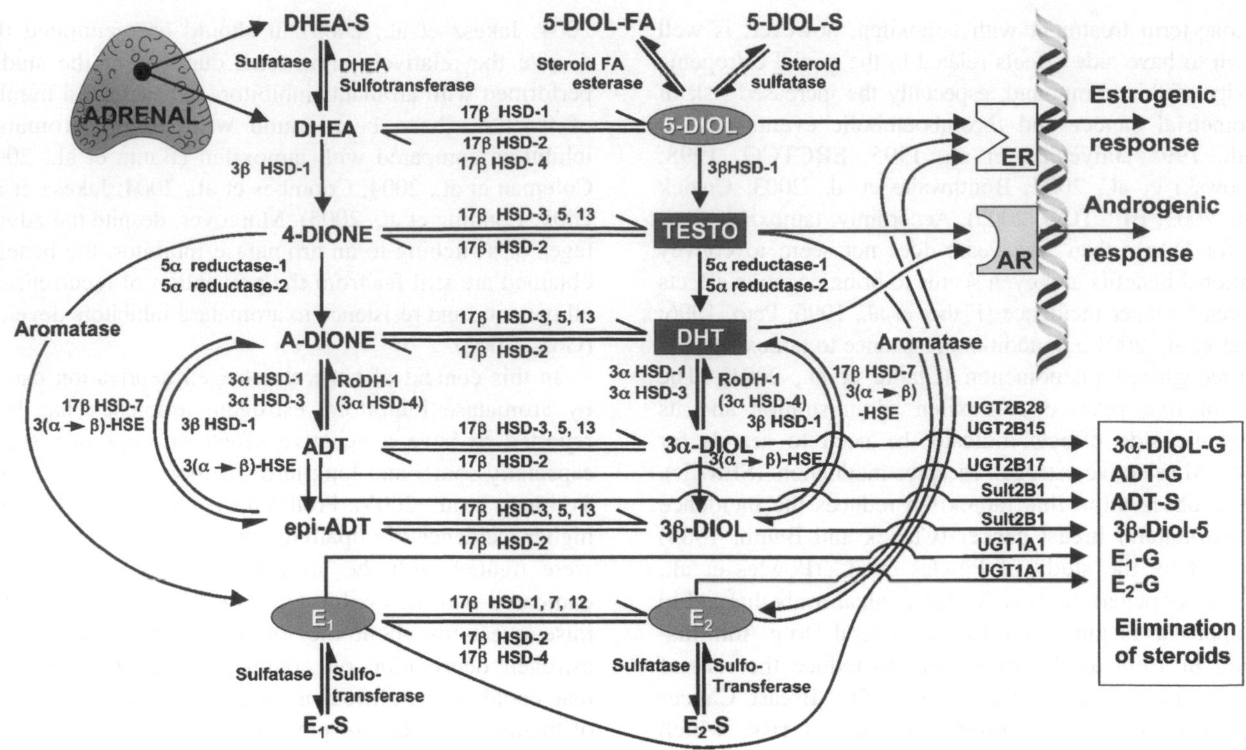

Figure 2 Human steroidogenic and steroid-inactivating enzymes in peripheral intracrine tissues.

signalling pathways under aromatase inhibitor treatment (Jelovac et al., 2005).

Despite the limitations mentioned above with the presently available drugs, it is well recognized that estrogens play the predominant role in the breast cancer development and growth and that blockade of estrogens has major beneficial effects. Therefore, estrogen deprivation should be part of the strategy of prevention. However, as mentioned above, it is unlikely that generalized estrogen deprivation, such as achieved with aromatase inhibitors or fulvestrant, will be acceptable for long-term use. It thus seems logical to suggest that SERMs, with their tissue-specific action, are the class of drugs upon which the best hope for an efficient and well-tolerated preventative therapy for breast cancer relies.

Novel SERMs

Characteristics of the Ideal SERM for Breast Cancer Prevention

One essential characteristic of the SERM chosen for prevention of breast cancer should be that it is a compound free of any estrogenic activity in the mammary gland and uterus while exerting estrogen-like activity in other tissues of importance for women's health. As well demonstrated in prostate cancer, the more efficient blockade of androgens achieved by combining medical (GnRH agonist) or surgical castration with a pure antiandrogen is more efficient than monotherapy, even at the advanced stage (Labrie et al., 1982, 1985; Crawford et al., 1989; Denis et al., 1993; Caubet et al., 1997; Prostate Cancer Triallists' Collaborative Group, 2000; Klotz, 2001; Labrie et al., 2002, 2005a). It is thus likely that the optimal long-term benefits of estrogen blockade in breast cancer will also be achieved with maximal estrogen blockade. For comparison, in localized prostate cancer, monotherapy with GnRH agonists alone achieves a one-third decrease in the death rate from prostate cancer (Peto and Dalesio, 2003), while at least 90% long-term control and probable cure of the disease is achieved when combining an GnRH agonist with a pure antiandrogen (Labrie et al., 2002).

That these observations made in men with localized prostate cancer could apply to breast cancer is supported by recent preclinical data showing that the combination of letrozole and fulvestrant is much more efficient than either compound used alone in inhibiting the growth of human MCF-7 (MCF-7 Ca) tumors in nude mice (Jelovac et al., 2005). In fact, with the combination therapy, tumor size was not only completely blocked, but it decreased 45% below baseline. It is noticeable that these important benefits of combined estrogen blockade observed on human breast tumor growth in nude mice were achieved in the presence of no additional inhibitory effect of the combination of the two drugs on uterine weight, thus indicating that the human breast tumor is more sensitive to low levels of estrogens remaining in the tissue after monotherapy with letrozole or fulvestrant than the normal uterus.

It should be mentioned that the experimental model used did not show an additive effect of anastrazole plus tamoxifen or letrozole plus tamoxifen (Lu et al., 1999; Long et al., 2004), a finding that was confirmed in breast cancer patients in the arimidex and tamoxifen alone versus their combination (Dowsett et al., 2001). Such data stress the importance of recognizing that all SERMs are different and that the data obtained with tamoxifen cannot be extrapolated to other SERMs or antiestrogens having less or no estrogenic activity in the mammary gland and uterus and vice versa.

The underlying principle is that in sex steroid-sensitive cancer, even low sex steroid levels permit continuous cancer cell division and growth with the risk of additional adverse gene mutations and adaptation of other growth pathways, especially the kinase pathways which more than compensate for the decreased estrogen levels and stimulate cancer cell growth independently from sex steroids. Such an adaptative phenomenon creates resistance to hormonal treatment (Schiff et al., 2005). The resistance to treatment observed with aromatase inhibitors in advanced breast cancer may in fact be related to the incomplete blockade of estrogens achieved with these compounds combined with the residual estrogenic stimulus of 5-diol.

SERMs Under Development

Arzoxifene

Among the SERMs under development, arzoxifene, an analog of raloxifene (Fig. 1) has shown a 10.3% response rate at the 20 and 50 mg doses in tamoxifen-resistant patients, while 26.1% and 8.0% response rates were seen at the same doses in tamoxifen-sensitive patients (Buzdar et al., 2003). On the other hand, in another phase II trial, a 30% response rate was observed with the 20 mg dose in previously untreated patients with a further 17% of patients showing stable disease (Baselga et al., 2003). A low 8% response rate was, however, seen with the 50 mg dose. The compound has moved to phase III where it is compared to tamoxifen (Johnston, 2005).

Acolbifene

Another SERM in development is acolbifene (Fig. 1). Possibly the most important property of acolbifene is that it has induced the disappearance or cure of 61% of human breast cancer tumors in nude mice (Fig. 3) (Roy et al., 2003). On the basis of the data obtained with tamoxifen, the effect of hormone therapy was so far believed to be limited to a tumorostatic action. In other words, following

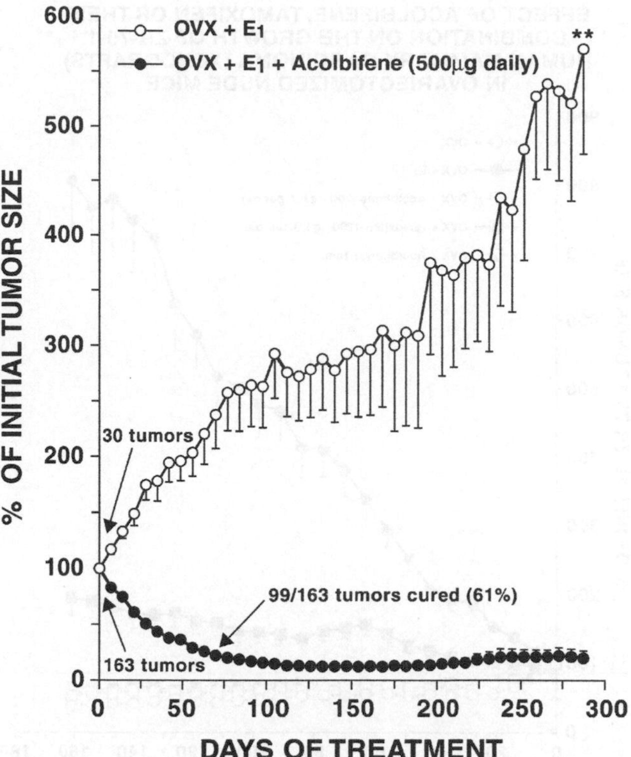

Figure 3 Effect of daily administration of EM-652 on the growth of human ZR-75-1 breast cancer xenografts in ovariectomized nude mice supplemented with estrone. Tumor size measured weekly is expressed as the percentage of initial tumor area. The average tumor size at the start of the study was 21.97 ± 1.52 mm^2 (range 4.71–40.42 mm^2). Individual tumor areas calculated on day 1 of the experiment were assigned a value of 100%. All subsequent tumor sizes were expressed as a percent of day 1 values (**$p < 0.01$). *Source*: From Roy et al. (2003).

the results originally obtained with tamoxifen (Gottardis et al., 1988), the effect of hormonal therapy has been traditionally believed to be limited to a slowing of tumor growth or a tumorostatic action. The tumorocidal action of acolbifene shown in Figure 3 is thus a new and most important paradigm of hormone therapy, which most likely results from a more complete blockade of the ER (Roy et al., 2003).

Acolbifene is the most potent of all available antiestrogens and SERMS to inhibit the stimulatory effect of estrogens on the proliferation of human breast cancer cells in vitro (Simard et al., 1997a; Labrie et al., 2001c, 2002). An example of the direct stimulatory effect of tamoxifen on the growth of human breast cancer can be seen in Figure 4. In fact, at 161 days, the daily oral administration of 200 μg of tamoxifen caused a fivefold stimulation of size of the ZR-75-1 human breast cancer xenografts compared with ovariectomy, while acolbifene, in

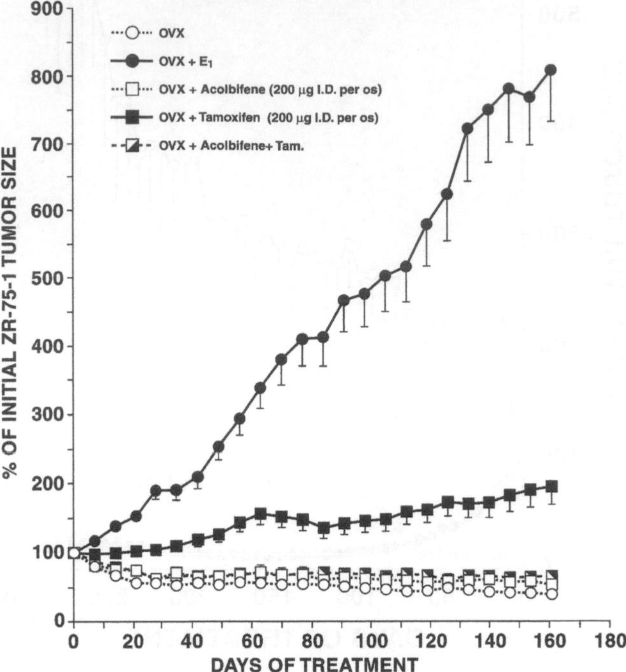

Figure 4 Effect of daily administration of acolbifene or tamoxifen alone or in combination for 161 days on the growth of human ZR-75-1 breast tumors (xenografts) in ovariectomized nude mice. The compounds were administered orally once daily at the dose of 200 µg per mouse. Mean tumor size of ovariectomized mice receiving the vehicle alone is shown for reference. Tumor size is expressed as percent of the pretreatment value (means ± S.E.M. of 18–30 tumors per group). *Source*: From Labrie et al. (2001a).

agreement with its pure antiestrogenic activity in the mammary gland, had absolutely no stimulatory effect. That the stimulatory effect of tamoxifen on tumor growth is an estrogenic effect is demonstrated in the same experiment by the observation of the complete reversal of the stimulatory effect of tamoxifen by simultaneous administration of the pure antiestrogen acolbifene. Many laboratories under in vitro as well as in vivo conditions have reported the stimulatory effect of tamoxifen or OH-tamoxifen on human breast cancer cell growth previously. Such an intrinsic estrogenic activity of tamoxifen is likely to limit its success in the treatment of breast cancer in women. It can also be mentioned that among seven tested antiestrogens, acolbifene is also the most potent inhibitor of the stimulatory effect of estrogens on the growth of human breast cancer tumors in nude mice (Gutman et al., 2002). In addition, while resistance to treatment is a major problem of cancer therapy, no resistance is observed with acolbifene in human breast cancer tumors in nude mice (Gutman et al., 2003).

It becomes important to make available a pure antiestrogen, which, due to its complete lack of estrogenic activity, should theoretically be more efficient than tamoxifen and raloxifene to treat breast cancer while simultaneously eliminating the excess risk of developing uterine carcinoma during its long-term use (Fisher et al., 1998; Bergman et al., 2000). We have thus compared the effect of EM-800 (precursor of acolbifene) or its active metabolite acolbifene with those of OH-tamoxifen, OH-toremifene, droloxifene, idoxifene, raloxifene, and its analog arzoxifene on estrogen-sensitive alkaline phosphatase (AP) activity in human endometrial carcinoma Ishikawa cells. AP activity is well known to be stimulated by estrogens, while the other steroids, namely androgens, progestins, mineralocorticoids, or glucocorticoids, have no effect on this parameter (Littlefield et al., 1990). Direct comparison of the estrogen-like activity of these mixed agonist/antagonist compounds can best be seen in Figure 5.

Incubation with the indicated concentrations of arzoxifene, raloxifene, OH-tamoxifen, OH-toremifene, droloxifene, or idoxifene increased AP activity by 3.1-, 2.1-, 4.3-, 4.8-, 4.0-, and 4.6-fold, respectively. The data obtained clearly demonstrate that the novel nonsteroidal antiestrogen acolbifene exerts pure antagonistic effects in human endometrial adenocarcinoma Ishikawa cells. In contrast to acolbifene, OH-tamoxifen, OH-toremifene, droloxifene, idoxifene, and raloxifene, as well as its analog arzoxifene, exert a stimulatory effect on this estrogen-sensitive parameter, an effect that can be competitively blocked by simultaneous exposure to the antiestrogen acolbifene. These data indicate that the stimulatory effect of these antiestrogens is mediated through activation of the ER (Simard ct al., 1997b). Similarly, in thc rat, acolbifcnc has no stimulatory effect on the endometrium, contrary to raloxifene, which exerts a significant stimulatory effect (Sato et al., 1998; Martel et al., 2000; Labrie et al., 2002). For the reasons mentioned above, namely pure antiestrogenic activity in the mammary gland and uterus, acolbifene is the only tissue-specific estrogen receptor modulator (TSERM), while all other SERMs show only partial tissue specificity or selectivity.

The phase II/III clinical program consisted of two studies (ERC-103 and C/197-042) evaluating the efficacy of acolbifene in the treatment of breast cancer in patients who had failed tamoxifen. In study ERC-103, forty-three postmenopausal women were enrolled: five patients (1 complete response, 4 partial responses) responded to therapy with acolbifene (Labrie et al., 2004a) for a response rate of 12%, while seven (16%) patients had stable disease for more than six months. These results are numerically comparable to the activity seen with the

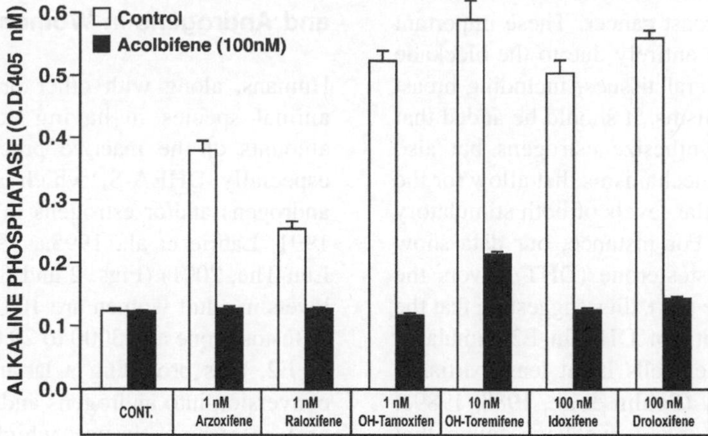

Figure 5 Blockade by EM-652 of the stimulatory effect of arzoxifene, raloxifene, OH-tamoxifen, OH-toremifene, idoxifene, and droloxifene on alkaline phosphatise activity in human Ishikawa carcinoma cells. Alkaline phosphatise activity was measured after a five-day exposure to the indicated concentrations of the specified compounds in the presence or absence of 100 nM acolbifene. The data are expressed as the means ± S.E.M. of four wells with the exception of the control groups where data are obtained from eight wells. *Source*: From Labrie et al. (2001a).

aromatase inhibitors anastrazole, letrozole, and exemestane in the same category of patients.

In the phase III study, the primary objective was to compare the progression-free survival between acolbifene and anastrozole in patients with advanced disease who had previously progressed with tamoxifen. An interim analysis based on a total of 110 events (progressions or death) was performed. Both the 20 mg and 40 mg doses of acolbifene were compared to anastrozole. Median progression free survival times were 3.19, 4.11, and 4.01 months for acolbifene 20 mg, acolbifene 40 mg, and anastrozole, respectively. On the basis of these results of the interim analysis indicating an activity of acolbifene similar to anastrazole in this category of patients with very advanced disease who had already failed hormone therapy, it was decided to focus on the development of acolbifene for breast cancer prevention. This approach would take advantage of the complete absence of estrogenic activity of acolbifene in the human mammary gland and uterus, thus permitting long-term treatment without any risk of estrogenic stimulatory effect in these two tissues. As mentioned earlier, prevention, but not treatment, offers the possibility of practically eliminating death from breast cancer.

An illustration of the unique properties of each SERM is the observation that different SERMs have a differential ability to block the expression of genes modulated by E2 (Frasor et al., 2004; Labrie et al., 2004b). These specific effects depend upon the variable interaction of the different coactivators and corepressors and other associated proteins with ER following the SERM-specific induced changes of 3D structure of ER (Brzozowski et al., 1997). Acolbifene induces changes in ER that block both AF-1 and AF-2 activation sites on ER (Labrie et al., 2001c), thus providing a potential explanation for the lack of development of resistance to treatment with acolbifenc in nude mice bearing human breast cancer ZR-75-1 xenografts (Gutman et al., 2002, 2003; Roy et al., 2003) as well as the 61% disappearance of human breast tumors in nude mice (Roy et al., 2003).

PHYSIOLOGY OF SEX STEROID FORMATION IN WOMEN

Intracrine Formation of Estrogens and Androgens in the Mammary Gland

Formation of Estrogens in the Mammary Gland

As mentioned above, transformation of the adrenal precursor steroids DHEA and dehydroepiandrosterone sulfate (DHEA-S) into androgens and/or estrogens in peripheral target tissues depends on the level of expression of the various steroidogenic and metabolizing enzymes in each cell of these tissues (Fig. 2). Knowledge in this area has recently made rapid progress with the elucidation of the structure of most of the tissue-specific genes that encode the steroidogenic enzymes responsible for the transformation of DHEA and DHEA-S into androgens and/or estrogens in peripheral intracrine tissues (Labrie, 1991; Labrie et al., 1992a, 1992b, 1995b; Luu-The et al., 1995b; Labrie et al., 2000, 2003b) (Fig. 2).

The now well demonstrated lack of correlation between serum testosterone and androgenic activity (Labrie et al., 2006a) is, by itself, sufficient to negate the value of the conclusions reached by these epidemiological studies. Ceasing at menopause, the major role of peripheral estrogen formation in postmenopausal women is clearly demonstrated, as mentioned above, by the major benefits of aromatase inhibitors in breast cancer. These important benefits on breast cancer are entirely due to the blockade of estrogens made in peripheral tissues, including breast cancer, by intracrine mechanisms. It should be added that mammary cells not only synthesize estrogens but also possess complex regulatory mechanisms that allow for the strict control of the intracellular levels of both stimulatory and inhibitory sex steroids. For instance, our data show that the androgen dihydrotestosterone (DHT) favors the degradation of E2 into estrone (E1), thus suggesting that the potent antiproliferative activity of DHT in E2-stimulated ZR-75-1 human breast cancer cells is, at least partially, exerted on 17β-HSD activity (Poulin et al., 1988, 1989c; Couture et al., 1993). Conversely, we have found that estrogens cause a marked increase in the production of the glucuronidated androgen metabolites androstane-3β, 17β-diol glucuronide (3α-diol-G), androstane-3β, 17β-diol-G (3β-diol-G), and androsterone glucuronide (ADT-G) in MCF-7 cells, thus decreasing the inhibitory androgenic activity (Roy et al., 1992). In fact, since glucuronidation is the predominant route of androgen inactivation, androgen-inactivating enzymes constitute an important site of regulation of breast cancer growth.

Formation of Androgens in the Mammary Gland

In the peripheral target tissues of both men and women, as well as in the ovary, the formation of testosterone from androstenedione is catalyzed by type 5 17β-HSD (Dufort et al., 1999) (Fig. 2). This enzyme is highly homologous with types 1 and 3, 3α-HSDs, as well as 20α-HSD and thus belongs to the aldo-keto reductase family.

Type 5 17β-HSD is not only expressed in the ovary but is also present in a large series of peripheral tissues including the mammary gland. The epithelium lining the acini and ducts of the mammary gland is composed of two layers, an inner epithelial layer and an outer discontinuous layer of myoepithelial cells. By immunocytochemistry, 3β-HSD is seen in the epithelial cells of acini and ducts as well as in stromal fibroblasts (Pelletier et al., 1999). Immunostaining is also observed in the walls of blood vessels, including the endothelial cells. On the other hand, the labeling is mainly cytoplasmic. No significant labeling was detected in the myoepithelial cells. On the other hand, immunostaining for type 5 17β-HSD gave results almost superimposable to those obtained for 3β-HSD, the cytoplasmic labeling being observed in both epithelial and stromal cells as well as in blood vessel walls (Pelletier et al., 1999). Studies performed at the electron microscopic level revealed that in sections stained for 3β-HSD or type 5 17β-HSD, labeling was not associated with any specific membrane-bound organelles in the different reactive cell types (Pelletier et al., 2001).

Double Source of Estrogens and Androgens in Women

Humans, along with other primates, are unique among animal species in having adrenals that secrete large amounts of the inactive precursor steroids DHEA and especially DHEA-S, which are converted into potent androgens and/or estrogens in peripheral tissues (Labrie, 1991; Labrie et al., 1995a, 1996c, 1997d, 2000, 2001b; Luu-The, 2001) (Figs. 2 and 6). In fact, plasma DHEA-S levels in adult women are 10,000 times higher than those of testosterone and 3000 to 20,000 times higher than those of E2, thus providing a large reservoir of substrate for conversion into androgens and/or estrogens in the peripheral intracrine tissues which possess the enzymatic machinery necessary to transform DHEA into active sex steroids.

The major importance of DHEA and DHEA-S in human sex steroid physiology is illustrated by the observation that approximately 50% of total androgens in adult men derive from the adrenal precursor steroids (Labrie et al., 1985; Bélanger et al., 1986; Labrie et al., 1993), while in women, our best estimate of the intracrine formation of estrogens in peripheral tissues is of the

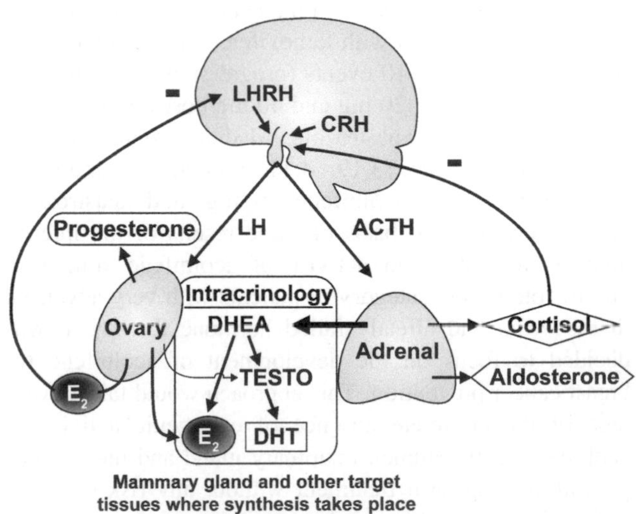

Figure 6 Schematic representation of ovarian and adrenal sources of sex steroids in premenopausal women. After menopause, the secretion of E2 by the ovaries ceases, and then 100% of estrogens and close to 100% of androgens are made locally in peripheral target intracrine tissues. The ovary secretes TESTO directly, while the adrenals secrete large amounts of DHEA that is converted into androgens (and/or estrogens) in peripheral tissues. *Abbreviations*: E2, estradiol; TESTO, testosterone; DHEA, dehydroepiandrosterone; ACTH, adrenocorticotropic hormone; CRH, corticotrophin-releasing hormone; DHT, dihydrotestosterone; LH, luteineizing hormone; LHRH, luteinising hormone-releasing hormone. *Source*: From Labrie et al. (2003b).

order of 50% before menopause and 100% after menopause. In fact, in women, the vast majority of androgens are made locally in target tissues throughout life (Labrie, 1991) (Fig. 2).

Valid Parameters of Androgenic Activity in Women

The traditional concept of androgen and estrogen secretion in women assumed that all sex steroids were transported by the general circulation following secretion by the ovaries before reaching the target tissues. According to this traditional concept, it was erroneously believed that the active sex steroids could be measured directly in the blood, thus providing a potentially easily accessible measure of the general exposure to sex steroids. In fact, this concept is valid only for animal species lower than primates where the gonads are the exclusive source of sex steroids. This concept does not apply to humans, especially potmenopausal women, where all estrogens and almost all androgens are made locally from DHEA in the peripheral tissues which possess the enzymes required to synthesize the physiologically active sex steroids from DHEA. Such local biosythesis and action of androgens in target tissues eliminates the exposure of other tissues to androgens and thus minimizes the risks of undesirable masculinising or other androgen-related side effects (Labrie et al., 1988; Bélanger et al., 1989). The same applies to estrogens, although a reliable parameter of total estrogen secretion (comparable to the glucuronides indentified for androgens) has yet to be determined. Although a fraction of androgens are aromatized to estrogens, the lack of sufficient information on the identity of the metabolites of estrogens does not permit one to make a sufficiently complete analysis of their metabolism at this time.

Serum Testosterone Is Not a Valid Parameter of Androgenic Activity in Women

All the clinical and most preclinical data clearly show that the administration of androgens inhibits proliferation of the normal mammary gland and breast cancer [reviewed in (Labrie et al., 2003b, 2006c)]. On the other hand, epidemiological data based on evaluation of the correlation between the risk of breast cancer and serum testosterone estimated by radioimmunoassays having a highly questionable accuracy (Taieb et al., 2003; Somboonporn and Davis, 2004; Kushnir et al., 2006; Wierman et al., 2006) have provided equivocal information, especially in postmenopausal women.

An explanation for these equivocal epidemiological conclusions based on serum testosterone levels has recently been provided by the demonstartion that serum testosterone, even when properly measured by mass spectrometry techniques, is not a valid marker of androgen activity in either pre- or postmenopausal women (Labrie et al., 2006a). Since the androgens made locally in peripheral tissues do not originate from circulating testosterone, one could reasonably have expected that measurement of the serum levels of testosterone is of questionable biological and clinical significance. In fact, the androgens testosterone and DHT made in peripheral tissues from DHEA exert their action locally in the same cells where synthesis takes place, with only minimal and highly variable release as active androgens in the circulation.

In women, serum testosterone essentially reflects the direct secretion of this steroid by the ovaries, while, as mentioned above, the majority of androgens are not of ovarian origin but are made locally in peripheral target tissues from the inactive precursor steroid DHEA (Labrie, 1991; Labrie et al., 2005b). Essentially, these androgens made locally act in the same cells where they have been synthesized and do not appear in significant amounts in the circulation (Fig. 7). The physiological mechanism of local androgen formation, action, inactivation, and elimination called intracrinology (Labrie et al., 1988, 1991) can, by itself, explain why no correlation has ever been unambiguously found in women between serum testosterone levels and any clinical situation known to be under androgen control.

Serum Androgen Glucuronides Are Presently the Only Valid Measure of Total Androgenic Activity

The active steroids made in peripheral target tissues are inactivated locally into the metabolites androsterone and 3α-diol that are further metabolized into the corresponding glucuronide derivatives (Bélanger et al., 2003; Labrie et al., 2006a). These metabolites can be measured with precision and accuracy in the circulation by mass spectrometry, thus providing the only valid estimate of androgenic activity in women (Labrie et al., 2006a).

While one would ideally like to know the level of androgenic activity in each specific tissue, such a direct measurement of the intratissue concentration of active androgens is not possible in the human except under exceptional circumstances such as in samples of tissue obtained at surgery (Poortman et al., 1983; Labrie et al., 1985; Bélanger et al., 1989). However, while not permitting the assessment of androgenic activity in specific tissues, measurement of the glucuronide derivatives of ADT-G and 3α-diol (3α-diol-G) by validated mass spectrometry techniques permits a precise measure of total androgenic activity in the whole organism (Fig. 7).

It is now well established that uridine glucurunosyl transferase (UGT) 2B7, UGT 2B15, and UGT 2B17 are the three enzymes responsible for the glucuronidation of

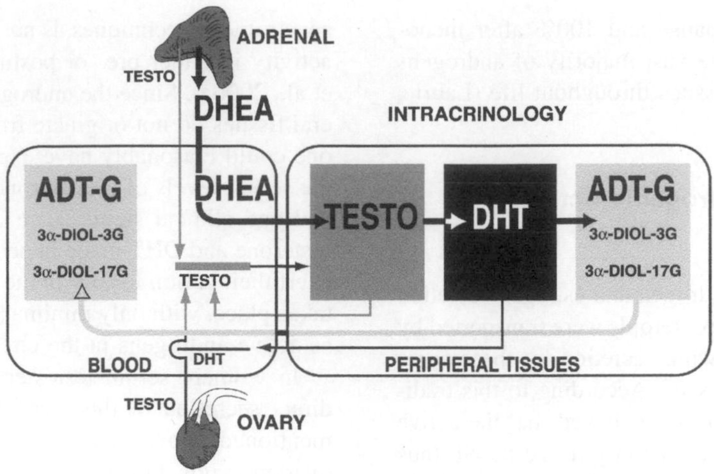

Figure 7 Schematic representation of the very important contribution of the precursor DHEA of adrenal origin to total androgenic activity in postmenopausal women with a parallel minor contribution of TESTO of two origins, i.e., the ovaries and adrenals. A very small proportion of the TESTO and DHT made intracellularly from DHEA by the steroidogenic enzymes of the intracrine pathways diffuse into the circulation where they can be measured. The height of the bars is proportional to the concentration estimated for each steroid. ADT-G, 3α-DIOL-3G, androstane-3α, 17β-diol 3-glucuronide, 3α-DIOL-17G, androstane-3α, 17β-diol 17 glucuronide. *Abbreviations*: TESTO, testosterone; DHT, dihydrotestosterone; DHEA, dehydroepiandrosterone; ADT-G, androsterone glucuronide.

all androgens and their metabolites in humans (Bélanger et al., 2003). This recent completion of the identification and characterization of all the human UDP-glucuronosyl transferases now makes possible the use of the glucuronide derivatives of androgens as markers of total androgenic activity in both women and men.

Lack of Correlation Between Serum Testosterone and Androgen Glucuronides

Since the glucuronide derivatives of androgens are the obligatory route of elimination of all androgens, these metabolites were measured by liquid chromatography tandem mass spectrometry under basal conditions in 377 healthy postmenopausal women aged 55 to 65 years as well as in 47 premenopausal women aged 30 to 35 years, while testosterone was assayed by gas chromatrography mass spectrometry (Labrie et al., 2006a).

As can be seen in Figure 8, no useful correlation is found between serum testosterone and ADT-G ($r = 0.37$), this metabolite accounting by itself for 93% of the obligatory metabolites of androgen elimination. An even lower correlation is observed between serum testosterone and the serum levels of the two other androgen glucuronides, namely 3α-diol-3G (androstane-3α, 17β-diol-3G) ($r = 0.27$) and 3α-diol-17G ($r = 0.22$) (Labrie et al., 2006a). A similar lack of correlation between testosterone and ADT-G ($r = 0.29$) is seen in normal cycling 30- to 35-year old women.

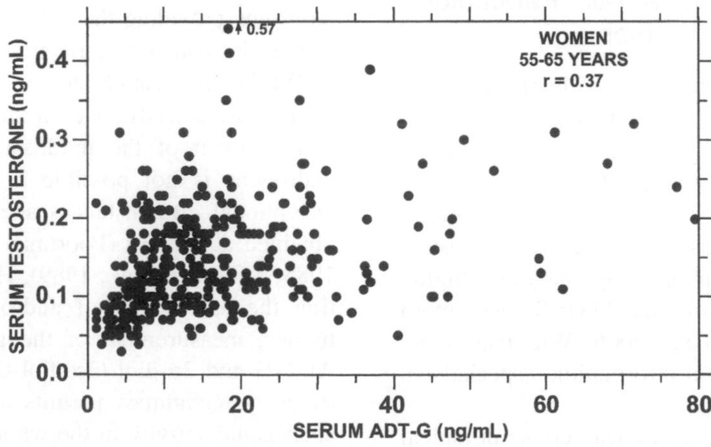

Figure 8 Lack of correlation between serum ADT-G and testosterone concentrations in three hundred seventy-seven (377) 55- to 65-year-old postmenopausal women. The Spearman correlation coefficient value of 0.37 is indicated. *Abbreviation*: ADT-G, androsterone glucuronide. *Source*: From Labrie et al. (2006a).

A somewhat better but still poor correlation is observed between serum testosterone and DHEA, the main source of androgens in women, with an *r*-value of 0.50 or between DHEA and ADT-G with an *r*-value of 0.65.

In fact, testosterone is, among all the steroids measured, the one showing the lowest correlation with the three glucuronide derivatives of androgens. Such data suggest that variable rates of secretion of testosterone by the ovary and/or adrenal could be responsible for the lack of correlation of ADT-G and 3α-diol-G with serum testosterone which is the sum of testosterone of ovarian and adrenal origins secreted directly into the blood plus the testosterone diffusing from the peripheral tissues following peripheral transformation of DHEA into androgens (Fig. 2). It is also possible that the peripheral tissue-made testosterone that diffuses at a low level into the circulation is highly variable, thus explaining, at least partially, the lack of correlation with serum androgen glucuronides. Better correlations are observed, however, between serum DHEA and its 17α-reduced metabolite 5-diol ($r = 0.83$), DHEA and androstenedione ($r = 0.79$), as well as between DHEA and its sulfated metabolite DHEA-S ($r = 0.77$) (Labrie et al., 2006a).

Our data thus show that the most practical and probably the most valid estimate (Labrie et al., 2006a) of androgenic activity in women is the serum concentration of ADT-G, the metabolite that accounts for 93% of the total androgen glucuronide derivatives, by a validated liquid chromatography tandem mass spectrometry technique, thus replacing measurement of serum testosterone.

Women Produce 50% As Much Androgens As Men

Using the serum concentrations of ADT-G, 3α-diol-G-3G, and 3α-diol-17G as estimates of total androgens, the sum of the average serum concentrations of these conjugated metabolites is 35.4 ng/mL in 69- to 80-year-old men (Vandenput et al., 2007) compared with 17.0 ng/mL in 55- to 65-year-old women (Labrie et al., 2006a). Although the metabolic clearance rates of the three main androgen metabolites are likely to show differences between men and women, an estimate of the relative amount of total androgens in women and men calculated on the basis of the sum of the serum concentrations of these three metabolites suggests that total androgen production in women is approximately 50% of that found in men (Labrie et al., 2006a; Vandenput et al., 2007).

Such data are based on the knowledge that the active androgens are inactivated to glucuronide derivatives before their diffusion from the intracellular compartment into the circulation where they can be measured as ADT-G and 3α-diol-G. Such data showing the presence of relatively high levels of androgens in women suggests that androgens play a major but so-far underestimated physiological role in women. Moreover, since the testicular secretion of androgens in men shows little decline with age while women rely almost exclusively on adrenal DHEA for their production of androgens, the 70% to 95% fall in serum DHEA after menopause leads to a major androgen deficiency in postmenopausal women, a situation which aggravates with increasing age.

Women Have Already Lost 60% of Total Androgens at Time of Menopause

The almost exclusive focus on the role of ovarian estrogens has removed attention from the dramatic 60% fall in circulating DHEA, which occurs between the ages of 20 to 30 and 40 to 50 years (Migeon et al., 1957; Vermeulen and Verdonck, 1976; Bélanger et al., 1994; Labrie et al., 1997b) (Fig. 9). That the 60% decrease in serum DHEA translates into a 60% loss in total androgens in women between the age of 30 to 35 years and 55 to 65 years of age is well illustrated in Fig. 10. The sum of the serum levels of ADT-G, 3α-diol-3G, and 3α-diol-17G thus decreases from 42.85 ng/mL to 17.04 ng/mL during this 25-year period (Labrie et al., 2006a) (Fig. 10). Since DHEA is transformed to both androgens and estrogens in peripheral tissues, such a fall in serum DHEA and DHEA-S explains why women at menopause, as mentioned above, are not only lacking estrogens but, starting in their 40s, have progressively been deprived of androgens.

Exogenous DHEA Is Mainly Transformed into Androgens in Women

As mentioned above, the active androgens and estrogens synthesized in peripheral target tissues exert their action in the cells of origin and very little extracellular diffusion of the active sex steroid occurs, thus resulting in very low levels of active sex steroids in the circulation after menopause for estrogens and throughout life for androgens (Labrie et al., 1997a). In fact, we have observed in postmenopausal women that the most striking effects of DHEA administration are seen on the circulating levels of the glucuronide derivatives of the metabolites of DHT, namely ADT-G and 3α-diol-G, these metabolites being produced locally in the peripheral intracrine tissues which possess the appropriate steroidogenic enzymes to synthesize testosterone and DHT from the adrenal precursors DHEA and DHEA-S.

INHIBITORY EFFECTS OF ANDROGENS IN THE NORMAL MAMMARY GLAND

There is strong evidence that androgens exert inhibitory effects on the proliferation of normal breast epithelial cells and play a protective role in the pathogenesis of breast

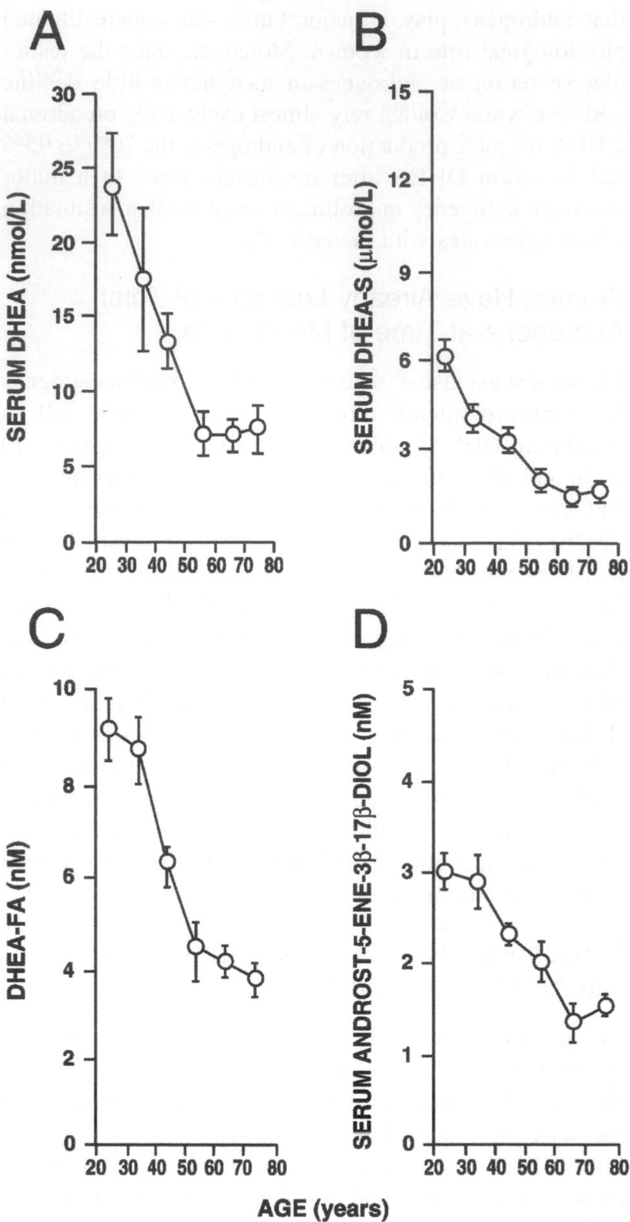

Figure 9 Effect of age (20–30 to 70–80 years) on serum concentration of (DHEA) (**A**), (DHEA-S) (**B**), (DHEA-FA) (**C**), and androst-e-ene-3β, 17β-diol (5-diol) (**D**) in women. *Abbreviations*: DHEA, dehydroepiandrosterone; DHEA-S, dehydroepiandrosterone sulfate; DHEA-FA, dehydroepiandrosterone fatty acid esters. *Source*: From Labrie et al. (1997).

cancer (Birrell et al., 1998; Labrie et al., 2003b; Labrie, 2006; Labrie et al., 2006c; Labrie, 2007).

Physiological Testosterone Levels Inhibit Mammary Gland Proliferation in the Monkey

The best estimate of the role of endogenous androgens on the proliferation of the epithelial cells of the mammary gland has been obtained in the Rhesus monkey model, the primate being the only species having a high secretion rate of DHEA by the adrenal glands (Leblanc et al., 2002, 2003, 2004). In an elegant series of experiments, after three menstrual cycles of blockade of the androgen receptor (AR) by the pure antiandrogen flutamide (FLU), the expression of the proliferation marker Ki67 was increased by twofold (Dimitrakakis et al., 2003). Such data indicate that androgens, under physiological conditions, counteract the proliferative effect of estrogens. Moreover, supplementation with low serum testosterone (0.4 ng/mL) completely blocked the 3.5-fold stimulation of epithelial cell proliferation in the mammary gland of the ovariectomized (OVX) monkeys (Fig. 11). This is a remarkable demonstration of the potent inhibitory effect of physiological levels of androgens on mammary epithelial cells.

Following the observation that testosterone inhibited the E2-stimulated proliferation of monkey epithelial mammary gland cells, Zhou et al., (Zhou et al., 2000) suggested that "combined estrogen-androgen hormone replacement might induce the risk of breast cancer associated with estrogen replacement." Such a complete reversal of the effect of E2 on mammary cell proliferation in the monkey by the low levels of testosterone found in normal women suggests that the low androgenic activity found in normal women after menopause, during contraceptive, HRT or ERT use. or following blockade of ovarian secretion could have a deleterious effect on breast cancer incidence and growth.

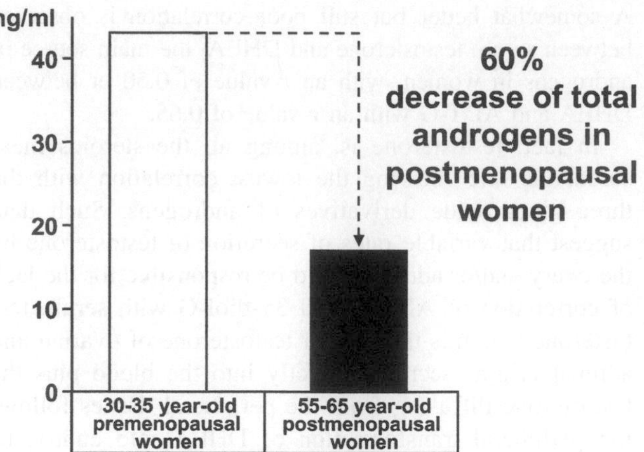

Figure 10 Sum of the serum levels of ADT-G, 3α-diol-3G, and 3α-diol 17G in 30- to 35-year-old normal premenopausal women ($n = 47$) and 55- to 65-year-old normal postmenopausal women ($n = 377$). The sum of the three metabolites of androgens decreases from 42.85 ng/mL in 30- to 35-year-old women to 17.04 ng/mL in postmenopausal women, thus showing a 60% loss of total androgens at time of menopause. *Source*: From Labrie et al. (2006a).

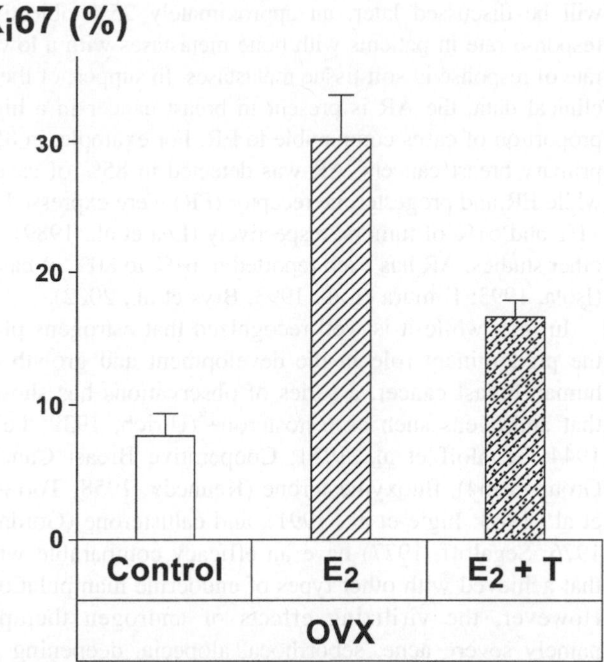

Figure 11 Effect of treatment of OVX monkeys with 17β-estradiol (E2; 2.5-mg pellet) alone or E2 plus testosterone (E2 + T; 35 μg/kg pellets) for three days on mammary gland epithelial cell proliferation estimated by Ki67 labeling. *Abbreviation*: OVX, ovariectomized. *Source*: From Dimitrakakis et al. (2003).

Part of the mechanism of the inhibitory action of androgens on the stimulatory effect of estrogens could be the decrease in ER-α levels caused by androgens as observed in normal mammary gland epithelium (Dimitrakakis et al., 2003) and in human breast cancer cells in culture (Poulin et al., 1989c). The inhibitory effect of androgens could also be related to decreased expression of MYC by androgens (Dimitrakakis et al., 2003) as supported by the observation that MYC expression is inversely correlated to that of AR in breast cancer tissue (Bieche et al., 2001). There has also been the suggestion that BRCA-1 could be an activator of AR, thus simultaneously providing an explanation for the high cancer risk in subjects having the BRCA-1 mutation (Park et al., 2000; Yeh et al., 2000). Moreover, AR mutation is associated with the growth of the breast in men (Grino et al., 1988), thus supporting the physiological role of androgens in inhibiting mammary epithelial cell proliferation.

That the addition of an androgen to HRT could have antiproliferative effects in the mammary gland and could thus reduce the risk of breast cancer is supported by the finding that the addition of methyltestosterone to a low dose oral contraceptive inhibited mammary gland epithelial proliferation in rats (Jayo et al., 2000).

Hyperandrogenism Inhibits Mammary Gland Proliferation in Women

Clinically, women with elevated androgen levels, whether endogenous or exogenous, experience breast atrophy, consistent with the notion that androgens, per se, are antiproliferative for the breast (Wierman et al., 2006). A strong argument against a potential positive correlation between androgens and breast cancer is provided by the polycystic ovarian syndrome (PCO), a situation characterized by androgen excess where the risk of breast cancer is decreased in the presence of hyperandrogenism (Wierman et al., 2006). In fact, an age-adjusted odds ratio for breast cancer in women with PCO of 0.52 (95% confidence interval 0.32–0.87) has been found (Gammon and Thompson, 1991).

As another example, female athletes as well as transsexuals taking androgens show an atrophy of the breast glandular tissue (Burgess and Shousha, 1993; Korkia and Stimson, 1997).

AR Mutations and Breast Cancer

Shorter alleles of the CAG repeat polymorphism in exon 1 of the AR gene, a condition known to be associated with high AR activity, has been associated with decreased risk of breast cancer in women having a history of breast cancer (Lobaccaro et al., 1993; Giguere et al., 2001; Haiman et al., 2002). Further follow-up of the Nurses' Health Study, however, did not confirm the initial data (Cox et al., 2006). In a panel of 95 advanced breast cancer cases, no association between the exon 1 CAG repeat in the AR gene and breast cancer risk was observed (Cox et al., 2006). Taken together, these data indicate the absence of a significant stimulatory effect of the AR on breast cancer inci dence (Cox et al., 2006) or even suggest an inhibitory effect (Lobaccaro et al., 1993; Giguere et al., 2001).

Testosterone Administration Inhibits Mammary Gland Proliferation in Women

In fact, the most direct and very convincing evidence for the inhibitory effect of androgens on epithelial mammary gland proliferation has recently been provided in women who received a testosterone patch for six months. At six months of treatment with continuous combined E2 2 mg/norethisterone acetate 1 mg, a fivefold increase in total breast cell proliferation was observed (Hofling et al., 2007; Von Schoultz, 2007). Notably, in the group who received a testosterone patch in addition to the E/NE HRT, the fivefold HRT-induced breast cell proliferation was completely inhibited. These data were followed by the following editorial comments: "There is considerable body of evidence that

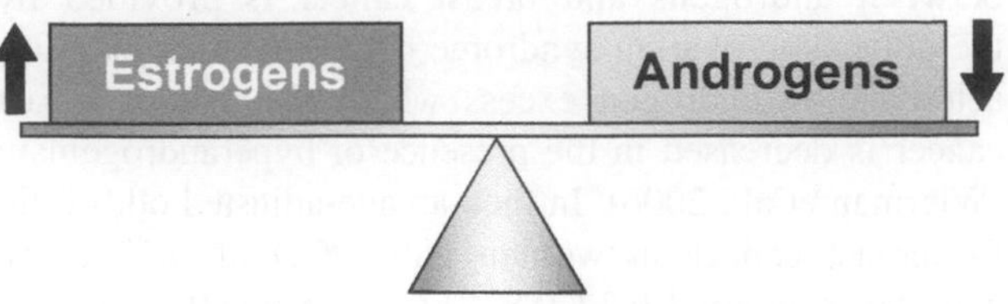

Mammary gland and
breast cancer proliferation results,
under physiological conditions,
from the balance between stimulation
by estrogens and inhibition by androgens
Estrogens
Androgens

Figure 12 Schematic representation of the balance between the stimulatory action of estrogens and the inhibitory effect of androgens on mammary gland and breast cancer proliferation. *Source*: From Labrie et al. (2006c).

both testosterone and its reduced derivative DHT exert inhibitory influences on the growth-promoting effects of E2 on the breast, though the evidence is not uniform" (Burger, 2007). As will be discussed later, this nonuniformity refers to epidemiological reports based on serum testosterone levels, which are not valid parameters of androgenic activity in women (Labrie et al., 2006a).

An inverse relationship has been found in women taking oral contraceptives between serum-free testosterone and breast cell proliferation (Isaksson et al., 2001). The long series of observations summarized above strongly suggest that the proliferation and growth of the mammary gland results from the balance between the stimulatory effect of estrogens and the inhibitory action of androgens (Fig. 12).

As support for the above-summarized data, in a retrospective, observational study of 508 postmenopausal women treated with testosterone implants in addition to traditional HRT, the incidence of breast cancer was markedly decreased (Dimitrakakis et al., 2004). The editorial accompanying this publication was entitled: "It might be wise to consider adding androgens to the estrogen and estrogen-progestin regimens in the appropriate patients (Gelfand, 2004).

INHIBITORY EFFECTS OF ANDROGENS AND DHEA IN BREAST CANCER

Clinical Evidence of the Beneficial Effects of Androgens in Breast Cancer

The best evidence that can be obtained to describe the activity of a compound is the observation of the effect obtained following the administration of this compound under rigorous experimental conditions. In the case of androgens, the administration of androgens has shown, as will be discussed later, an approximately 25% objective response rate in patients with bone metastases with a lower rate of response in soft tissue metastases. In support of these clinical data, the AR is present in breast cancer in a high proportion of cases comparable to ER. For example, in 852 primary breast cancers, AR was detected in 85% of cases, while ER and progesterone receptor (PR) were expressed in 71% and 61% of tumors, respectively (Lea et al., 1989). In other studies, AR has been reported in 61% to 80% of cases (Isola, 1993; Kimura et al., 1993; Brys et al., 2002).

In fact, while it is well recognized that estrogens play the predominant role in the development and growth of human breast cancer, a series of observations has shown that androgens such as testosterone (Ulrich, 1939; Fels, 1944; Segaloff et al., 1951; Cooperative Breast Cancer Group, 1964), fluoxymesterone (Kennedy, 1958; Tormey et al., 1983; Ingle et al., 1991), and calusterone (Gordan, 1976; Segaloff, 1977) have an efficacy comparable with that achieved with other types of endocrine manipulation. However, the virilizing effects of androgen therapy, namely severe acne, seborrhoea, alopecia, deepening of the voice, clitorimegalia, and intense libido in aged women greatly limited its use.

It should also be mentioned that androgens have been shown to induce an objective remission after failure of antiestrogen therapy and hypophysectomy. Such clinical observations indicate that the benefits obtained with androgen therapy in breast cancer cannot solely be due to the suppression of pituitary gonadotropin secretion but must result, at least in part, from a direct effect on tumor growth, a mechanism which is well supported by a series of experimental data described later. The virilizing secondary effects associated with treatment with testosterone and other androgens probably explain the limited interest devoted to androgens in breast cancer therapy, although androgens are still successfully used in the clinic.

The overwhelming clinical evidence for tumor regression observed in 20% to 50% of pre- and postmenopausal breast cancer patients treated with various androgens (Gordan, 1976) favors the view that naturally occurring androgens might constitute, as mentioned above, an as yet overlooked direct inhibitory control of mammary cancer cell growth. It is thus reasonable to suggest, as strongly supported by a series of preclinical data to be summarized later, that the balance between androgenic and estrogenic stimuli controls the proliferation of the normal mammary gland as well as breast tumors (Fig. 12).

EQUIVOCAL EPIDEMIOLOGICAL DATA BASED ON CORRELATION WITH SERUM TESTOSTERONE

Following the description of the effects of androgens summarized above on the normal mammary gland as well as in breast cancer in women, and the supporting data obtained in the monkey, it is important to remember that the administration of androgens has provided direct and unequivocal evidence of the inhibitory effect of androgens on the breast. However, since epidemiological data, despite the serious limitations already indicated above and described in more detail below, provide controversial evidence which can prevent women from receiving an efficient treatment for breast cancer, we will first summarize additional data demonstrating that the use of serum testosterone levels in women is not valid, thus very seriously questioning the scientific value of all the epidemiological studies based on correlation with serum testosterone in women.

The relatively recent understanding of the intracrine physiology in women provides an explanation for the equivocal and controversial data obtained from epidemiological studies that relied on the correlation between serum testosterone and breast cancer risk, especially in postmenopausal women. Before analyzing the epidemiological data reported using this approach, it is important to consider that in case-control studies using cancer cases and matched controls in postmenopausal women, a strong correlation is always found between serum E2 and all other steroids, including testosterone. Since it is well recognized that estrogens exert the predominant stimulatory role in breast cancer development and growth, it becomes very difficult or even impossible to assess the potential role of hormones other than E2 on breast cancer risk in epidemiological studies.

Lack of Value of Serum Testosterone as Indicator of Tissue Androgenic Activity in Women

Before referring to the value of serum testosterone as indicator of androgenic activity in the breast, it is important to remember, as mentioned above, that the majority of androgens in women are not of ovarian origin but are made in peripheral target tissues from the adrenal precursor DHEA. These androgens made by intracrine mechanisms act in the same cells where they have been synthesized before being inactivated, and being further transformed locally into glucuronide derivatives, which are released in the circulation where they can be measured accurately. Since the active androgens made locally are not released in the circulation in significant amounts, it is important to realize that the serum level of testosterone cannot be used to estimate androgenic activity in women (Figs. 2, 7, and 8) as well demonstrated recently (Labrie et al., 2006a).

As well recognized for more than 20 years, measurement of sex steroid concentrations in peripheral plasma does not reflect intracellular concentrations. In addition to the lack of reliability of serum testosterone for the reasons mentioned above, many of the women with breast cancer had a higher incidence of family history of breast cancer and obesity. It is also important to realize that the crucial event in androgen action is the binding of the hormone to its specific receptor, an event critically dependent on the concentration of intracellular steroids.

It is also appropriate to remember that a correlation observed in epidemiological studies with the serum level of sex steroids (or any other parameter) is not a proof of causal relationship. The observation of a correlation (assuming that the parameters are scientifically valid) can only serve as an indicator or as a suggestion to search for a potential direct causal relationship. It is also of particular importance to realize that in many epidemiological studies where a positive correlation has been reported between serum testosterone and breast cancer risk, there was an even greater correlation with serum estrogens, thus providing a more rational explanation for the correlation observed with breast cancer.

Lack of Reliability of the Immunoassays of Serum Testosterone in Women

In addition to the unavoidable physiological arguments clearly showing that serum testosterone has no value as estimate of androgenic activity in women (Fig. 8), all the epidemiological studies have used unreliable and insensitive radioimmunoassays to measure the low levels of testosterone present in women. In all these studies, true testosterone measured by mass spectrometry was, on average, 50% or less of the values measured by radioimmunoassay. Moreover, these studies did not take into account the marked diurnal variations of all serum steroids and the previous history of HRT.

At the low concentrations of testosterone in the plasma of women and with the serious limitations of the immunoassays used, the values obtained have little utility (Taieb et al., 2003; Kushnir et al., 2006). Knowledge of this serious problem has led to the development of a technology avoiding immunoassays, namely chromatography followed by sequential mass spectrometry (Van Uytfanghe et al., 2004; Kushnir et al., 2006; Labrie et al., 2006a).

Lack of Correlation Between Serum Sex Steroid Levels and Biological Activity

It has been well demonstrated that serum estrogen or androgen levels do not reflect tissue levels (Poortman et al., 1983; Labrie et al., 1985; Vermeulen et al., 1986a, 1986b; Thijssen et al., 1991; Pasqualini et al., 1996; Geisler et al., 2001; Geisler, 2003). In addition to the original suggestion of a variable uptake from the circulation, it is now understood that local biosynthesis of estrogens is mainly responsible for the high intratissue levels of estrogens in the breast tissue (Simpson, 2003). This is analogous to the situation in the human prostate where castration leads to a 95% decrease in serum testosterone, while intraprostatic DHT remains at 40% to 50% of the value found in intact men (Labrie et al., 1985; Bélanger et al., 1989).

Estrogens

As mentioned above, after menopause, all estrogens and almost all androgens are made locally in peripheral tissues (Labrie, 1991; Geisler, 2003; Simpson, 2003) by intracrine mechanisms. In fact, intratumoral levels of E2 in normal mammary gland and breast cancer show no or little difference between pre- and postmenopause (Edery et al., 1981; Poortman et al., 1983), while serum E2 decreases by 10-fold or more at menopause. In fact, breast tissue levels of E2 are 5- to 40-fold higher than plasma levels (Fishman et al., 1977; Poortman et al., 1983; Van Landedgem et al., 1985; Vermeulen et al., 1986a,b; Pasqualini et al., 1996; Geisler, 2003). Moreover, the tissue/plasma ratio of different estrogens varies; while estrone sulfate (E1S) is the major estrogen in blood followed by E1 and E2, the situation is different in postmenopausal breast tissue with E2 being predominant followed by E1 and E1S (Geisler, 2003).

The vast majority of studies show that tissue E2 concentrations are not correlated with circulating levels (Vermeulen et al., 1986; Pasqualini et al., 1996; Miller et al., 2002; Geisler, 2003; Simpson, 2003), while some have reported a correlation between serum and tumoral E2 levels (Recchione et al., 1995; Mady et al., 2000).

The variable serum/tissue radio of E2 between individuals for a single tissue is also found between tissues; following a 12 hour infusion of tritium-labeled E2 in postmenopausal women, the tissue/serum ratio was measured at 30, 20, and 10 in the endometrium, myometrium, and vagina, respectively (Poortman et al., 1983). In the mammary gland, the E2 gradient between the plasma and normal mammary gland or breast cancer tissue varied between 5 and 40 in different patients. Such data demonstrate the poor value of plasma E2 to assess estrogenic activity in breast tissue. Such high concentrations of intracellular E2 result from uptake from the circulation and, most importantly, from local biosynthesis (Labrie, 1991).

Androgens

The intratissular concentration of testosterone and DHT is the only biological significant parameter, and not the serum concentration of these steroids (Vermeulen et al., 1986). In this context, it is important to remember that the breast cancer tissue/plasma ratio of testosterone has been found to vary up to 100-fold with values ranging from 0.05 to 5 (Vermeulen et al., 1986), thus providing another strong argument showing that the circulating levels of testosterone cannot be used as a valid parameter of intracellular androgen action. While the breast cancer tissue/plasma ratio of E2 was measured at about 21 on average in breast cancer, the ratio of testosterone was at 1 (Vermeulen et al., 1986). In another study, the tissue (breast)/plasma ratio of E2 was approximately 3, while the tissue/plasma ratio of testosterone was approximately 0.5 (Szymczak et al., 1998). When looking at the total androgen pool, a complete lack of correlation has been found between serum testosterone and total androgens in both pre- and postmenopausal women (Labrie et al., 2006c).

DHEA A

A similar situation pertains to DHEA, namely a variable and high DHEA gradient between plasma and breast cancer tissue (Poortman et al., 1983; Vermeulen et al., 1986), while the breast cancer/plasma ratio of testosterone was measured at 1, a value of 8 was found for DHEA and a value of approximately 0.5 was measured for DHEA-S (Vermeulen et al., 1986). The high and variable intratumoral levels of DHEA can possibly be explained by the variable transformation of the particularly high plasma levels of DHEA-S in the μg/mL range into DHEA by sulfatase activity.

General Comments on Serum Steroid Levels

As well recognized for more than 20 years (Poortman et al., 1983), it is important to recognize that hormone concentrations in peripheral plasma do not reflect intracellular concentrations of the same hormones. Moreover, although mass spectrometry has been available for quite some time, it is somewhat unfortunate that immunoassays, mainly due to their low cost, remain the basis of steroid assays, thus removing the scientific value of the epidemiological studies based on plasma steroid values obtained by these assays. Finally, since the important event in hormone action is binding of the hormone with its specific receptor, the important parameter is not the concentration of the steroid in the circulation but its intracellular concentration available for receptor activation. In the case of androgens, it appears that measurement of ADT-G and 3α-diol-3G and 3α-diol-17G (Labrie et al., 2006c; Swanson et al., 2006; Labrie et al., 2007) provides an accurate estimate of total androgenic activity in an individual subject or patient. Such data, however, do not provide information about individual tissues.

Correlation of Breast Cancer Risk with Serum Estrogen Levels in Epidemiological Studies

Among the first 11 prospective studies published on serum or urinary estrogen levels and breast cancer risk in postmenopausal women, statistically significant results of a positive correlation were found in five studies (Toniolo et al.,

1995; Thomas et al., 1997; Hankinson et al., 1998; Cauley et al., 1999; Onland-Moret et al., 2003), while a positive but nonsignificant correlation was found in four others (Berrino et al., 1996; Dorgan et al., 1996; Key et al., 1996; Kabuto et al., 2000).

It is of interest that women in the Multiple Outcomes of raloxifene evaluation (MORE) study with serum E2 levels in the highest tertile (more than 10 pmol/L) had not only the greatest risk of breast cancer but also the greatest reduction in the relative risk (RR) of breast cancer with raloxifene (Cummings et al., 2002). On the other hand, women with E2 levels less than 5 pmol/L (limit of detectino) had very low risk of breast cancer and no further reduction in risk was seen following treatment with raloxifene.

Correlation of Breast Cancer Risk with Serum Testosterone and DHEA Levels in Epidemiological Studies

Since a strong correlation between the serum levels of E2 and all the other steroids is well known and E2 is recognized as the predominant stimulatory factor in breast cancer (Pike et al., 1993; EBCTCG, 1998; Cummings et al., 1999; Fisher et al., 2000), it is difficult or practically impossible to assess the potential role of hormones other than estrogens in breast cancer risk. This is an additional problem added to the lack of reliability of serum testosterone (Labrie et al., 2006a) and of the radioimmunoassay used to measure testosterone.

Early epidemiological data have indicated that high serum levels of DHEA in premenopausal women are associated with a lower risk of breast cancer (Bulbrook et al., 1971), although one positive correlation (Kaaks et al., 2005) and five negative or no association studies have been reported in premenopausal women (Helzlsouer et al., 1992; Wang et al., 2000; Micheli et al., 2004; Page et al., 2004; Sturgeon et al., 2004; Tworoger et al., 2006).

On the other hand, epidemiological data reported in postmenopausal women have provided equivocal evidence with no association or a tendency for decreased risk of breast cancer with higher serum testosterone or DHEA (Mady et al., 2000; Beattie et al., 2006) or an association of high serum DHEA with high risk of breast cancer (Dorgan et al., 1997; Key et al., 2002; Onland-Moret et al., 2003; Eliassen et al., 2006).

During the 17 years preceding 2002, nine research groups have published small size epidemiological cohort-based studies indicating an association of high risk of breast cancer with high levels of estrogens and other hormones. Since none of these individual studies was large enough to obtain sufficiently precise estimates of risks, an analysis of the pooled data was performed (Key et al., 2002). E2 data were available from all nine studies, while data for the other hormones were available in three to eight studies. Serum steroids were always measured by radioimmunoassay, a technique not appropriate, as mentioned earlier, especially for the low levels of testosterone found in women. In fact, while serum levels of testosterone have been measured at 0.14 ± 0.070 ng/mL (5th–95th centiles = 0.06–0.2 ng/mL) by mass spectrometry (Labrie et al., 2006a), the average serum testosterone values reported in these studies ranged between 0.22 and 0.35 ng/mL (average of means = 0.27), thus indicating that true testosterone accounted, on average, for only 48% of the values of serum testosterone reported (Key et al., 2002).

In any case, even when these serum concentrations of testosterone are measured by mass spectrometry, they are not representative of the androgenic activity, which can only be measured in the blood by the serum levels of ADT-G, 3α-diol-3G, and 3α-diol-17G (Labrie et al., 2006a) (Fig. 8). Despite the evidence that the epidemiological studies on breast cancer risk and their correlation with serum steroids are not valid for the multiple reasons mentioned above, we will briefly summarize the data reported.

When the pooled data from the nine available studies on endogenous sex hormone levels and breast cancer risk were examined in 2002 (663 cases and 1765 matched controls), none of the serum levels of any sex steroid hormones differed between cases and matched controls. However, for women who had been diagnosed with breast cancer, the RR was significantly increased between the lowest and highest quintiles for E2, E1, E1S, testosterone, DHEA, and DHEA-S, while it was decreased for SHBG (Key et al., 2002).

In the nested case-control study within the Nurses' Health Study II (Tworoger et al., 2006), serum DHEA and DHEA-S levels were similar between the 315 cases and 631 controls. No significant association was observed between serum DHEA and DHEA-S and breast cancer risk among all women. The only positive association found was between serum DHEA-S and ER+/PR+ breast cancer. Since there was no association between serum DHEA and DHEA-S levels for all cancers and, as mentioned above, the ER+/PR+ tumors were found in patients with somewhat higher serum DHEA and DHEA-S, such data could suggest an increased proportion of cancers having a better prognosis in women with high serum DHEA and DHEA-S, while the total number of cancers remains unchanged.

On the other hand, the trend for an inverse relationship between serum DHEA and DHEA-S in premenopausal women and cancer risk might argue in favor of less aggressive and slow growing tumors in young women during premenopause in the presence of higher serum DHEA and DHEA-S levels. The net result is the same number of total cases of breast cancer at all serum DHEA and DHEA-S levels during a woman's life, while high serum DHEA and DHEA-S levels would be accompanied by less aggressive (ER+/PR+) tumors. Moreover, a family history of breast cancer was 58% more frequent in the cases compared with controls, while the history of benign breast disease was 49% higher in the cases.

It is of particular interest to mention the data obtained in the NSABP Breast Cancer Prevention Trial (P1) where an analysis was performed to determine whether sex hormone levels were associated with breast cancer risk and with response to tamoxifen in that high-risk population (Beattie et al., 2006). In the NSABP-P1 study, there was no difference in the serum testosterone, E2, or SHBG levels in the 125 breast cancer cases and 280 controls (Beattie et al., 2006). The conclusion reached by the authors was that "these data do not support the use of endogenous sex hormone levels to identify women at high risk of breast cancer." On the other hand, there was a trend toward a lower risk of breast cancer with higher serum testosterone levels, the RRs being 1.0, 0.41, 0.58, and 0.51 with increasing quartiles of serum testosterone. Moreover, the serum concentration of E2 or testosterone was not associated with the response to tamoxifen.

In a small study, breast cancer was associated with low serum levels of testosterone (Mady et al., 2000), while in another one no difference was observed (Szymczak et al., 1998). In a nested case-control study within the Nurse's Health Study that included 418 breast cancer cases and 817 matched controls, a significant correlation was found with the highest and lowest risk patients but not those with intermediate risk for patients evaluated with the Gail predicted risk model. The risk for high E2, however, was 100% more elevated than for high testosterone.

In another nested case-control within the DOM cohort with 364 breast cancer cases and 382 controls, women with breast cancer more often reported a positive family history of breast cancer and were slightly heavier (Onland-Moret et al., 2003). In that study, no significant difference was noted in the urinary excretion levels of E2, testosterone, E1, 5α-androstane-3α, 17β-diol at enrolment (Onland-Moret et al., 2003). The trends for the highest versus the lowest quartiles were statistically significant for all steroids, the four steroids being correlated with each other, thus illustrating the same difficulty found in most studies, namely evaluation of the role of steroids other than E2, knowing that E2 is a well-recognized stimulus of breast cancer.

In another nested case-control study of 677 cases and 1309 matched controls within the EPIC cohort (Rinaldi et al., 2006), the indices of adiposity were higher, age of menarche was lower, and age at menopause was higher among breast cancer cases. Serum levels of E1, E2, androstenedione, testosterone, and DHEA-S were slightly higher (approximately 10%) in cases. It was found, however, that androgens had little effect on the strong association of breast cancer risk and obesity.

In the report of Tamimi et al. (Tamimi et al., 2006), also derived from data of the Nurses' Health Study, the users of estrogens plus testosterone therapy were more likely to have had benign breast disease and consumed more alcohol. Most importantly, since only 33 women were taking estrogens plus testosterone in 1988 and only 550 women responded positively in 1998, the exposure to testosterone in that study is extremely small, thus very seriously limiting the statistical power. In fact, in 2002, there were only 29 cases of breast cancer in patients who had used estrogen plus testosterone for some period of time. Compared to estrogen plus progestin users, the risk was similar at RRs of 1.77 (E + T) versus 1.58 (E + P). The small number of patients in the E + T group makes these results preliminary at best. Moreover, all users of E + T had used previous hormone therapies. Contrary to the above-mentioned data, in a study in postmenopausal women who received testosterone implants in addition to estrogen, the observed rates of breast cancer were not higher than the expected rates in never HRT users (Dimitrakakis et al., 2004).

Potential Explanations for the Equivocal Epidemiological Data

As discussed above, the controversial data obtained on the correlation between serum testosterone and breast cancer risk have three independent rigorous and clearly demonstrated scientific explanations, starting with the lack of correlation between serum and intratumoral levels of sex steroids (Vermeulen et al., 1986; Pasqualini et al., 1996; Miller et al., 2002; Geisler, 2003). The now well-demonstrated lack of correlation between serum testosterone and androgenic activity (Labrie et al., 2006a) is, by itself, sufficient to negate the value of the conclusions reached by these epidemiological studies. Another independent and very serious limitation of these studies relates to the use of insensitive and unreliable immunoassays that yielded values including, on average, 50% of compounds other than testosterone. Moreover, the failure to take into consideration the diurnal variation of testosterone when drawing blood (Somboonporn and Davis, 2004; Wierman et al., 2006) adds to the variability observed.

POTENT INHIBITORY EFFECT OF ANDROGENS IN HUMAN BREAST CANCER CELL LINES IN VITRO

Specificity of the Estrogen and Androgen Receptors Are Limited to Physiological Steroid Concentrations

ER and AR are highly specific for estrogens and androgens, respectively. However, at the supraphysiological or pharmacological concentrations of steroids sometimes used in vitro, some androgens can activate ER, while estrogens can activate AR. The observations reported in their summary without proper reference to the high concentrations used to obtain an effect can be highly misleading since many publications do not take into consideration the fact that the effects reported are limited to supraphysiological or pharmacological concentrations, which have no relevance to the physiological situation in women. Such characteristics of ER and AR, however, are not a risk to the specific stimulatory action of estrogens and to the specific inhibitory action of androgens in the mammary gland or breast cancer in women. For example, the affinities for ER of E2, DHT and testo have been determined at 0.055 nM, 105 nM, and 710 μM, respectively, in COS cells overexpressing ER-α (Ekena et al., 1998).

Physiological concentrations of androgens have been found to inhibit the growth of human breast cancer cell lines in nude mice (Engel et al., 1978; Poulin et al., 1988) as well as dimethylbenzyanthracene (DMBA)-induced mammary tumors in the rat (Dauvois et al., 1989; Gatto, Aragno et al., 1998). Another strong argument for the inhibitory role of AR is the constant neutralization of the effect of DHT by the pure androgen antagonist FLU, both in vivo and in vitro.

It is important to indicate that in all studies that used high pharmacological doses or concentrations of androgens or DHEA, the stimulatory effect was always blocked by estrogen antagonists, while the inhibitory effect was always blocked by androgen antagonists. Such data unequivocally demonstrate that the AR is always inhibitory, while ER activation always leads to stimulatory effects, even when each receptor is activated by pharmacological concentrations of compounds, which inappropriately interact with other receptors at such high and nonspecific concentrations.

Extremely Low Affinity of the Adrenal Sex Steroid Precursors for the Estrogen Receptor

Experiments were designed to study the competition by 5-diol, DHEA, and DHEA-S of the specific uptake of [^{3}H]-E2 by intact cells in monolayer culture. Figure 13 illustrates the characteristics of [^{3}H]-E2l specific uptake in intact ZR-75-1 cells. Linear Scatchard analysis (Scatchard, 1959) showed that, under the conditions used, E2 binds to 16.0 ± 2.8 fmol of specific binding sites per 10^6 cells (9600 ± 1700 sites per cell) at an apparent dissociation constant of 0.60 ± 0.09 nM.

In order to measure the relative affinity of the C19 steroids for the ER, cells were exposed to 5 nM [^{3}H]-E2 for 60 minutes in the presence of increasing concentrations of 5-diol, DHEA, or DHEA-S. As shown in Figure 13, only 5-diol has a marked ability to compete with E2 for high-affinity binding sites as assessed by the specific uptake of

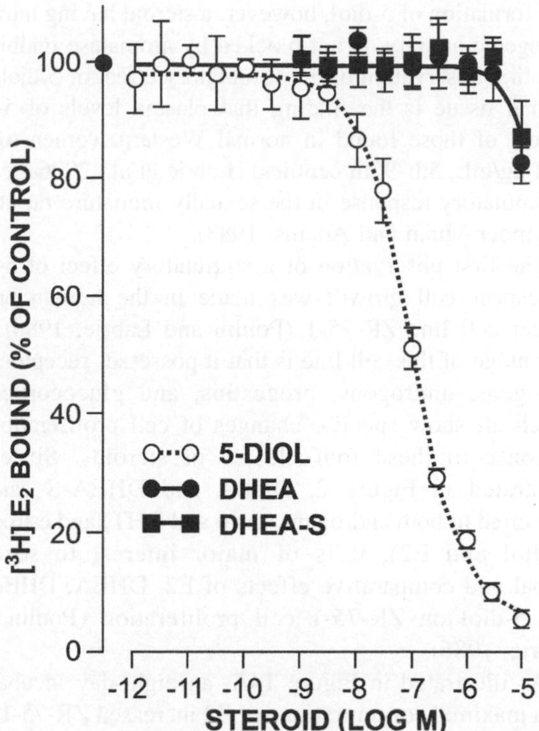

Figure 13 Specific uptake of [^{3}H]estradiol by ZR-75-1 cells incubated for 60 minutes at 37°C in the presence of C_{19}-Δ^5-steroids. Cells were plated and grown to confluency in RPMI 1640-5% DCC-treated FBS in the absence of steroids, as described in Poulin and Labrie (1986). The whole-cell specific uptake of radioligand was then measured in the presence of 5-diol (O), DHEA (●), or DHEA-S (■) at the indicated concentrations, in RPMI 1640 medium containing 5 nM [^{3}H]estradiol. Points, mean of triplicate determinations; bars, SE. For each treatment, the non-specific uptake of radioligand was determined by adding 500 nM diethylstilbestrol to parallel triplicate cultures. *Abbreviations*: DHEA, dehydroepiandrosterone; DHEA-S, dehydroepiandrosterone sulfate. *Source*: From Poulin and Labrie (1986).

the radioligand. The apparent dissociation constant (K_i) value for 5-diol, calculated according to Cheng and Prusoff (Cheng and Prusoff, 1973) was 11 nM. This value is in close agreement with those already obtained by other methods on breast cancer specimens as well as in MCF-7 cells (Kreitmann and Bayard, 1979).

Lack of Stimulatory Effect of DHEA or DHEA-S and Stimulatory Effect of 5-Diol, a Steroid Whose Formation Is Not Blocked by Aromatase Inhibitors

Several studies have shown that 5-diol could induce estrogenic effects in estrogen-sensitive tissues (Rochefort and Garcia, 1983; Adams, 1985; Poulin and Labrie, 1986).

The formation of 5-diol, however, a steroid having intrinsic estrogenic activity, is not blocked by aromatase inhibitors. The first observation of the stimulatory effect of 5-diol in a normal tissue is the finding that plasma levels of 5-diol typical of those found in normal Western women (0.25–0.84 ng/mL, 5th–95th centiles) (Labrie et al., 2006a) cause a stimulatory response in the sexually immature rat uterus (Seymour-Munn and Adams, 1983).

The first observation of a stimulatory effect of 5-diol on cancer cell growth was made in the human breast cancer cell line ZR-75-1 (Poulin and Labrie, 1986). An advantage of this cell line is that it possesses receptors for estrogens, androgens, progestins, and glucocorticoids which all show specific changes of cell proliferation in response to these four classes of steroids. Since, as illustrated in Figure 2, DHEA and DHEA-S can be converted to both androgens (testo and DHT) and estrogens (5-diol and E2), it is of major interest to see the global and comparative effects of E2, DHEA, DHEA-S, and 5-diol on ZR-75-1 cell proliferation (Poulin and Labrie, 1986).

As illustrated in Figure 14A, an eight-day incubation with maximal concentrations of E2 increased ZR-75-1 cell number by about 3.5-fold. The concentration of E2 required to induce half-maximal stimulation of cell proliferation was approximately 5 pM. It can be seen in Figure 14B that 5-diol has a strong mitogenic effect on ZR-75-1 cells; this steroid leading to a maximal increase in cell number 2.8-fold above control values, with a half-maximal effect being observed at approximately 2.5 nM. It should be mentioned that this concentration lies within the range of normal serum levels of 5-diol in women. On the other hand, DHEA had no effect on cell proliferation at physiological concentrations and had only a very weak stimulatory action on cell proliferation at pharmacological concentrations (Fig. 14C) and increased cell number up to about 75% above control at the maximal concentration used (10 μM). DHEA-S, on the other hand, showed no significant activity below 10 μM. It should be noticed that the first detectable action of DHEA was at 300 nM, a value at least 20 times higher than the plasma DHEA levels found in normal women (Labrie et al., 2006a).

The antiestrogen raloxifene (LY15678), a benzothiophene derivative having low agonistic activity in vivo (Clemens et al., 1983) was next used to assess the estrogenic nature of C_{19}-Δ^5-steroid action. It can be seen in Figure 14 that the antiestrogen alone exerted a 50% inhibition of cell growth, this inhibitory effect remaining maximal up to 0.3 nM E2 and 0.3 μM 5-diol. That the effect of LY156758 was not cytotoxic is indicated by the finding that 100 nM E2 could completely reverse the effect of the antiestrogen. The inhibitory effect of the antiestrogen was thus of a competitive nature for both E2 and 5-diol, the calculated (Cheng and Prusoff, 1973) K_d value of LY156758 action being 0.54 nM. Growth stimulation by high concentrations of DHEA was completely abolished by LY156758 at all steroid concentrations used, thus indicating the estrogenic nature of the stimulatory effect of all these steroids. It also shows that DHEA-derived androgens have no stimulatory effect on cell proliferation (Fig. 14). DHEA did not displace [^{3}H] E2 below the very high concentration of 3 μM. Such data indicate that the stimulation of ZR-75-1 cell proliferation seen at the concentrations of 300 nM DHEA and above is due to its transformation into 5-diol and/or E2.

Concerning DHEA-S, its maximal onefold stimulatory effect became significant at 10 μM (Fig. 14D), the effect being completely blocked by the antiestrogen LY156758. Using a high concentration of 22.8 μM DHEA-S in T47-D cells, a 0.35- to 1.0-fold increase in cell proliferation was observed, this effect being not significantly reversed by the antiestrogen fulvestrant (Calhoun et al., 2003). The large variation observed at various doses of fulvestrant indicates the questionable precision of the assay used, thus implying the low statistical power of that study. Moreover, the results obtained with fulvestrant were contradicted by the finding that tamoxifen, another estrogen antagonist, blocked the effect of DHEA-S, thus leading to the conclusion by the authors that it is an ER-mediated effect, possibly due to transformation into 5-diol. It should be mentioned, however, that the effects reported were small (43% stimulation) and highly variable (Toth-Fejel et al., 2004). In another study, DHEA-S was found to have no effect on MCF-7 cell proliferation up to 100 μM (Toth-Fejel et al., 2004). A small 80% "stimulation" of MCF-7 cell proliferation at low DHEA concentrations was not blocked by either FLU or fulvestrant, thus questioning the value of the data reported. At high concentrations, both DHEA and testosterone inhibited cell proliferation. It was also observed in the same report that DHEA-S inhibited cell growth in an ER-negative cell line.

While being the first study to show a stimulatory effect of 5-diol on human breast cancer cell proliferation, the study of Poulin and Labrie (1986) was also the first one to show a direct inhibitory effect of androgens on human breast cancer cell proliferation. Since 5-diol and DHEA can be converted into both androgens and E2, the preferential formation of androgens by DHEA (Labrie et al., 1997c), is the most reasonable explanation for an absence of stimulatory effect of DHEA on ZR-75-1 cell proliferation below 300 μM, a concentration 20 to 30 times above the plasma DHEA concentration found in normal women (Labrie et al., 2006a). Since 5-diol can also act as precursor of androgens, the inhibitory effect of 5-diol-derived androgens can explain why the maximal stimulatory effet of 5-diol is 2.8-fold compared with 3.5-fold for E2. Subsequently, the inhibitory effect of DHT on the E2-stimulated proliferation of human breast cancer ZR-75-1

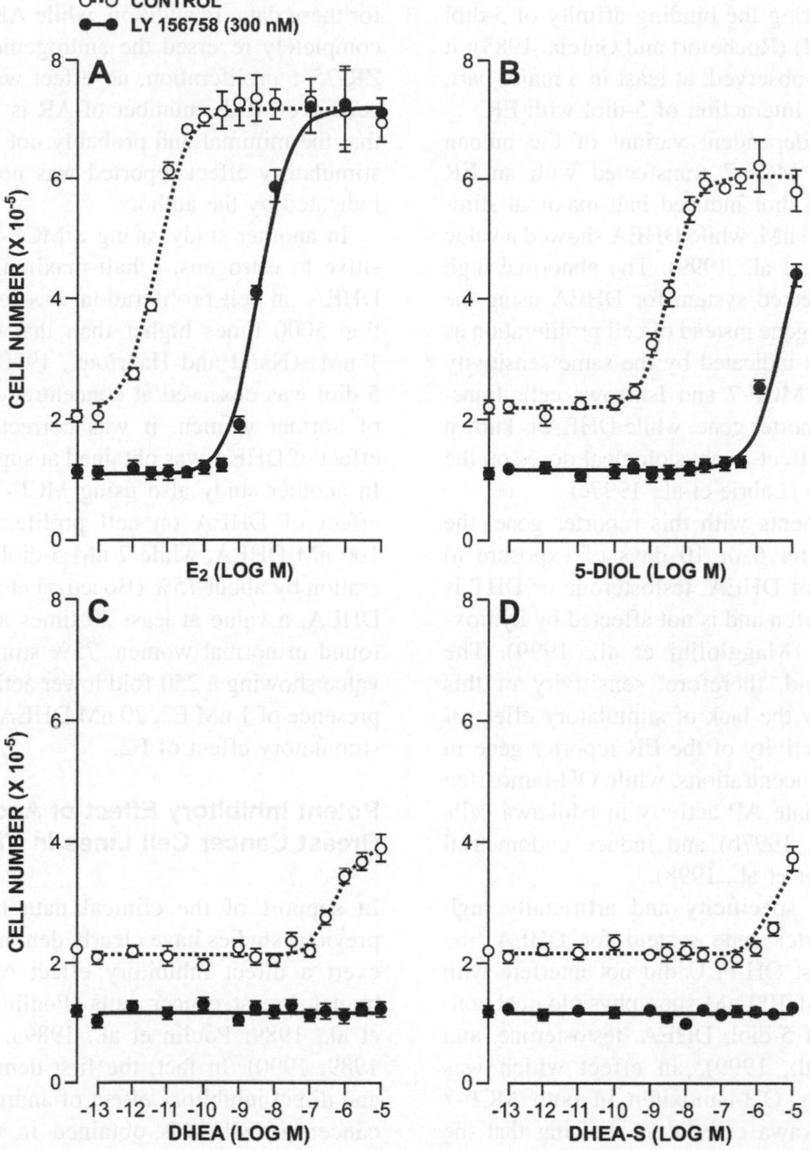

Figure 14 Effect of increasing concentrations of estradiol and C_{19}-Δ^5-steroids on the proliferation of ZR-71-1 cells in cluture and its inhibition by the antiestrogen LY156758. Cells were plated at an initial density of 2.0 × 104 cells/well in 24 well culture plates in RPMI 1640-5% DCC-treated FBS. After 48 hours, estradiol (A), Δ^5-diol (B), or DHEA (C) was added with fresh medium at the indicated concentrations in the presence (•) or absence (O) of 300 nM LY156758. Cell numbers were measured afer eight days in the presence of the steroids. Points, means of triplicate determinations from a representative experiement; bars, SE. *Abbreviation*: DHEA, dehydroepiandrosterone. *Source*: From Poulin and Labrie (1986).

(Poulin et al., 1988) and MCF-7 (Boccuzzi et al., 1992b) cells has been well demonstrated.

Such data also indicate the potential role of 5-diol on breast cancer growth in patients receiving aromatase inhibitors, which inhibit the formation of E2 but do not interfere with the formation of 5-diol (Fig. 2). It thus appears that even in postmenopausal women having no estrogenic contribution from the ovaries, aromatase inhibitors do not offer a complete blockade of estrogens.

In the human breast cancer cell line MCF-7, physiological concentrations of 5-diol have been found to stimulate the secretion of a 52K estrogen-sensitive glycoprotein (Adams et al., 1981). DHEA, however, required concentrations 100 to 200-fold higher than those found in the plasma of normal women to stimulate the secretion of the 52K protein. In these studies, attempts to find the presence of E2 potentially derived from 5-diol were negative (Adams et al., 1981; Seymour-Munn and

Adams, 1983). Considering the binding affinity of 5-diol for ER ($K_d = 4.5$–10 nM) (Rochefort and Garcia, 1983); it is likely that the effects observed, at least in a major part, resulted from the direct interaction of 5-diol with ER.

Using a hormone-independent variant of the human breast cancer cell line MCF-7 transfected with an ER reporter gene, E2 and 5-diol induced half-maximal stimulations at 0.2 nM and 10 nM, while DHEA showed a value of 100 nM (Maggiolini et al., 1999). The abnormal high sensitivity of this transfected system for DHEA using the activity of a ER reporter gene instead of cell proliferation as parameter of response is indicated by the same sensitivity of DHEA in wild type MCF-7 and Ishikawa cells transfected with the same resporter gene, while DHEA is known to have no stimulatory effect at physiological doses on the normal uterus in women (Labrie et al., 1997c).

As found in experiments with this reporter gene, the stimulation achieved after 6 or 10 days of exposure to pharmacological doses of DHEA, testosterone or DHT is abolished by OH-tamoxifen and is not affected by hydroxyflutamide (OH-FLU) (Maggiolini et al., 1999). The abnormal specificity and, therefore, sensitivity of this system is also shown by the lack of stimulatory effect of OH-tamoxifen on the activity of the ER reporter gene in Ishikawa cells at low concentrations, while OH-tamoxifen is well known to stimulate AP activity in Ishikawa cells in vitro (Simard et al., 1997b) and induce endometrial cancer in women (Fisher et al., 1998).

Despite the lack of specificity and artificially high sensitivity of this reporter gene system for DHEA, the pure androgen antagonist OH-FLU did not interfere with the stimulatory effects of 100 nM supraphysiological concentrations (100 nM) of 5-diol, DHEA, testosterone, and DHT (Maggiolini et al., 1999), an effect which was completely abolished by OH-tamoxifen in both MCF-7 and uterine cancer Ishikawa cells, thus showing that the abnormal action exerted at pharmacological concentrations of DHEA, 5-diol, testosterone, and DHT is mediated by ER and not by AR. In agreement with all the previous studies on the proliferation of MCF-7 cells, a pharmacological dose of DHEA and testosterone had to be used to observe these abnormal stimulatory effects in an artificial system lacking steroid specificity (Maggiolini et al., 1999).

A study using MCF-7 cells has reported a small 15% stimulatory effect of 1 nM DHT on cell proliferation when comparing with untreated control after 18 days of incubation (Birrell et al., 1995). Such a small effect after 18 days of treatment is unlikely to be significant. In the same report, the effect on ZR-75-1 cell proliferation started to appear after a delay of 8 days and reached only a 29% inhibitory effect at 18 days, while Figure 14 shows a 3.5-fold stimulation of ZR-75-1 cell proliferation after eight days (Poulin and Labrie, 1986). Particular incubation conditions can possibly offer an explanation for these data. In addition, while AR antisense nucleotides completely reversed the androgenic inhibitory effects on ZR-75-1 proliferation, no effect was observed in MCF-7 cells even if the number of AR is lower, thus suggesting that the minimal and probably not statistically significant stimulatory effect reported was not mediated by AR, as indicated by the authors.

In another study, using a MCF-7 cell line highly sensitive to estrogens, a half-maximal stimulatory effect of DHEA on cell proliferation was reported at a concentration 5000 times higher than that of 5-diol (0.5 μM vs. 1 nM) (Najid and Habrioux, 1990). While the effect of 5-diol was observed at concentrations found in the blood of normal women, it was correctly concluded that the effect of DHEA was obtained at supraphysiological levels. In another study also using MCF-7 cells, no stimulatory effect of DHEA on cell proliferation was seen up to 100 nM DHEA, while 2 nM 5-diol stimulated cell proliferation by about 75% (Boccuzzi et al., 1992b). At 500 nM DHEA, a value at least 20 times above the serum levels found in normal women, 75% stimulation was seen, this value showing a 250-fold lower activity than 5-diol. In the presence of 1 nM E2, 20 nM DHEA, however, reduced the stimulatory effect of E2.

Potent Inhibitory Effect of Androgens on Human Breast Cancer Cell Lines In Vitro

In support of the clinical data mentioned above, our previous studies have clearly demonstrated that androgens exert a direct inhibitory effect on the proliferation of human breast cancer cells (Poulin et al., 1988; Dumont et al., 1989; Poulin et al., 1989a, 1989c; Simard et al., 1989, 1990). In fact, the first demonstration of a potent and direct inhibitory effect of androgens on human breast cancer growth was obtained in the estrogen-sensitive human breast cancer cell line ZR-75-1 (Poulin and Labrie, 1986; Poulin et al., 1988). In that study, as shown in Figure 15, DHT not only completely blocked the stimulatory effect of E2 on cell proliferation but also reduced cell growth in the absence of estrogens. At low cell density (Fig. 12B), it can be seen that 10 nM DHT completely prevented breast cancer cell growth.

DHT has been shown to be formed from testosterone and 4-dione in human breast cancer tissue both in vitro in tissue pieces and in vivo (Thériault and Labrie, 1990). Such data indicate the presence of 5α-reductase in breast cancer tissue, an enzyme believed to be specific for androgen-dependent tissues. In ZR-75-1 cells, concentrations of DHT in the incubation medium similar to the plasma levels found in normal women (Abraham, 1974; Vermeulen and Verdonck, 1979; Rochefort and Garcia, 1983) and breast cancer patients (Mistry et al., 1986) (0.3–0.7 nM) are potent inhibitors of the mitogenic effect

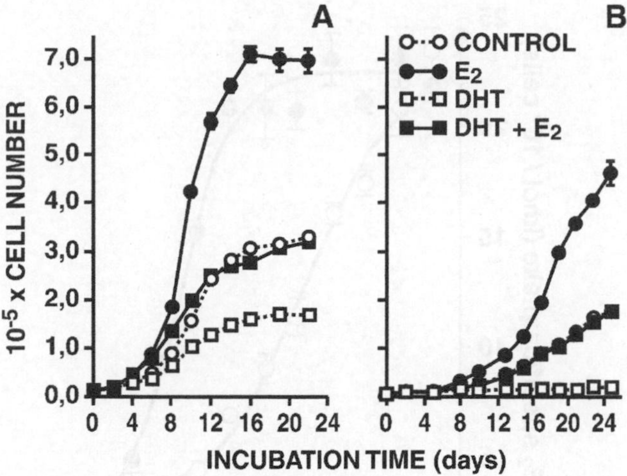

Figure 15 Time course of the effect of DHT and/or E2 on the proliferation of ZR-75-1 cells. (**A**) Cells were plated at 1×10^4 cells/2.0 cm^2 well and 48 hours later (zero time), 1 nM E2 (●), 10 nM DHT (□), or both steroids (■) were added and cell number determined at the indicated time intervals. Control cells received the ethanol vehicle only. (**B**) Same as in **A**. except that the initial density was 5.0×10^3 cells/2.0 cm^2 well. *Abbreviation*: DHT, dihydrotestosterone. *Source*: From Poulin et al. (1988).

of E2 and even inhibit growth in the absence of estrogens (Poulin et al., 1988). Furthermore, testosterone, at concentrations observed in adult women (1–3 nM) (Abraham, 1974; Vermeulen and Verdonck, 1979; Rochefort and Garcia, 1983; Mistry et al., 1986; Labrie et al., 2006a), is also a potent inhibitor of cell growth. 4-Dione also led to significant growth inhibition in ZR-75-1 cells, although the active concentrations (IC50, 15 nM) are in the upper range of the plasma concentrations (1–10 nM) found in women (Abraham, 1974; Vermeulen and Verdonck, 1979; Rochefort and Garcia, 1983; Mistry et al., 1986).

Several lines of evidence show that the potent growth-inhibitory effect of androgens observed in ZR-71-1 cells is mediated through their specific interaction with the AR. First, the potency of DHT and testosterone to induce antiproliferative effects (IC_{50}, ~0.10 and 0.50 nM, respectively) is in agreement with their relative binding affinity for androgen specific binding sites in intact ZR-75-1 cells as well as in other human breast cancer cells (Horwitz et al., 1978; MacIndoe and Etre, 1981). Such values compare well with the potency of DHT to specifically stimulate the secretion of the Zn-α2-glycoprotein (Chalbos et al., 1987) and the GCDFP-15 glycoprotein (Chalbos et al., 1987; Murphy et al., 1987) in T47-D human breast cancer cells. The ability of 4-dione to induce an antiproliferative effect (IC_{50} ~ 15 nM) most likely results from its metabolic transformation into testosterone and DHT (Griffiths et al., 1972; Perel and Killinger, 1983; Perel et al., 1985) than from its direct interaction with the AR (K_d ~ 200 nM). Secondly, the antiandrogen OH-FLU competitively reversed the effect of DHT and 4-dione with an apparent dissociation constant (K_i ~ 110 nM) consistent with its known affinity for the AR (Neri et al., 1979; Simard et al., 1986).

Because the benefits of combined treatment with an androgen and an antiestrogen have already been observed in women with breast cancer (Tormey et al., 1983; Ingle et al., 1991), and in agreement with the in vitro data mentioned above (Poulin et al., 1988; Dumont et al., 1989; Poulin et al., 1989a, 1989c; Simard et al., 1989), a more precise understanding of the mechanisms of action of androgens and antiestrogens in breast cancer cells becomes important. After a 12-d incubation of ZR-75-1 cells in the presence of 0.1 nM E2 in phenol red-free medium, cell number was increased 2.8-fold above control ($p < 0.01$) (Fig. 16A). The addition of 1 nM DHT, on the other hand, caused a 78% blockade ($p < 0.01$) of E2-induced ZR-75-1 cell growth, whereas the pure steroidal antiestrogen EM-139 (Levesque et al., 1991), on the other hand, not only completely reversed the effect of E2 but further inhibited cell number by 30% below control values ($p < 0.01$) (Fig. 16B). It can also be seen in Figure 16B

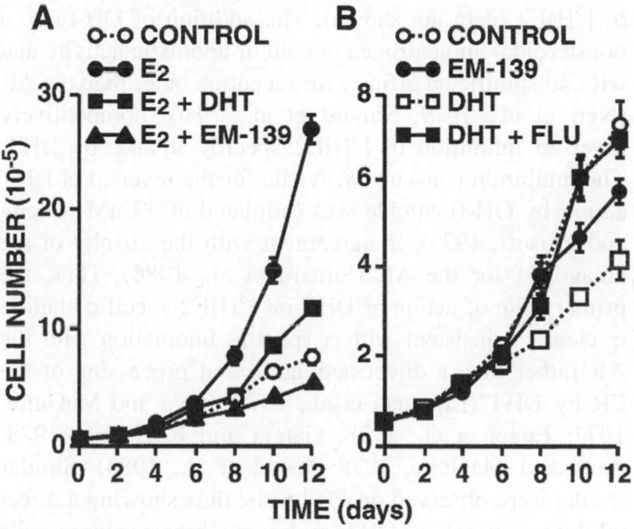

Figure 16 (**A**) Time course of the effect of 0.1 nM E2, 1 nM DHT + E2, 0.3 μM EM-139 + E2, or control medium on the proliferation of ZR-75-1 cells during a 12-day incubation period. (**B**) Time course of the effect of 1 nM DHT, 0.3 μM EM-139, DHT + EM-139, DHT + 0.3 μM OH-FLU, or control medium on the proliferation of ZR-75-1 cells. Three days after plating at an initial density of 5×10^5 cells/10 cm^2 per well, cells were incubated with the indicated concentrations of the compounds with medium changes every 48 hours for the indicated time periods. At the end of the indicated incubation periods, cell number was determined with a Coulter counter. Data are expressed as means ± SEM of quadriplicate wells. *Abbreviation*: DHT, dihydrotestosterone. *Source*: From deLaunoit et al. (1991).

that the inhibitory effect of DHT is completely prevented by the addition of the pure antiandrogen OH-FLU. Most interestingly, in another study, it was found that the growth-inhibitory effect of DHT is clearly additive to that induced by maximally effective concentrations of the antiestrogen LY156758, thus indicating an action mediated by a mechanism different from interaction with the ER (de Launoit et al., 1991a). Accordingly, the evidence obtained leaves little doubt that the antiproliferative effect of androgens does not result from competition for binding to the ER but rather is caused by a specific AR-mediated mechanism that is additive to blockade of the ER by an antiestrogen.

Considering the potential importance of androgens in breast cancer therapy, and to better understand the molecular mechanisms responsible for the antagonism between androgens and estrogens, we have investigated the effect of androgens on ER expression in the ZR-75-1 human carcinoma cell line. The specific uptake of [^{3}H]E2 in intact ZR-75-1 cell monolayers was decreased by as much as 88% after a 10-day preincubation with increasing concentrations of DHT (Fig. 17). A half-maximal effect of DHT on [^{3}H]E2 uptake was observed at 70 pM (Poulin et al., 1989a). Preincubation with dexamethasone and R5020 (100 nM each) had no effect on the specific uptake of [^{3}H]E2 (data not shown). The addition of OH-FLU, a nonsteroidal antiandrogen devoid of agonistic activity and with no significant affinity for receptors other than the AR (Neri et al., 1979; Simard et al., 1986) competitively reversed inhibition of [^{3}H]E2 specific uptake by DHT. The inhibition constant (K_i) value for the reversal of DHT action by OH-flutamide was estimated at 39 nM (Cheng and Prusoff, 1973), in agreement with the affinity of the antagonist for the AR (Simard et al., 1986). Thus, the primary site of action of DHT on [^{3}H]E2-specific binding is clearly consistent with a specific interaction with the AR rather than a direct activation and processing of the ER by DHT (Lippman et al., 1976; Zava and McGuire, 1977; Engel et al., 1978; Garcia and Rochefort, 1978; Zava and McGuire, 1978; Kasid et al., 1984). Similar results were observed on PR levels, thus showing a direct inhibitory effect of DHT in human breast cancer cells (Poulin et al., 1989a).

This study showed for the first time that androgens strongly suppress ER content in the human breast cancer cell line ZR-75-1, as measured by radioligand binding and anti-ER monoclonal antibodies. Similar inhibitory effects were observed on the levels of ER messenger RNA (mRNA) measured by ribonuclease protection assay (Poulin et al., 1989a). The androgenic effect was observed at subnanomolar concentrations of the nonaromatizable androgen DHT, regardless of the presence of estrogens, and was competitively reversed by the antiandrogen OH-flutamide. Such data on ER expression provide an explanation for at least part of the antiestrogenic effects of androgens on breast cancer cell growth and provide an explanation for the observations showing that the specific inhibitory effects of androgen therapy are additive to the standard treatment limited to blockade of estrogens by antiestrogens (de Launoit et al., 1991b). Another possible clue to the mechanism of action of DHT in breast cancer cells is provided by the observation that androgens and estrogens exert opposite effects on PR levels (MacIndoe and Etre, 1981).

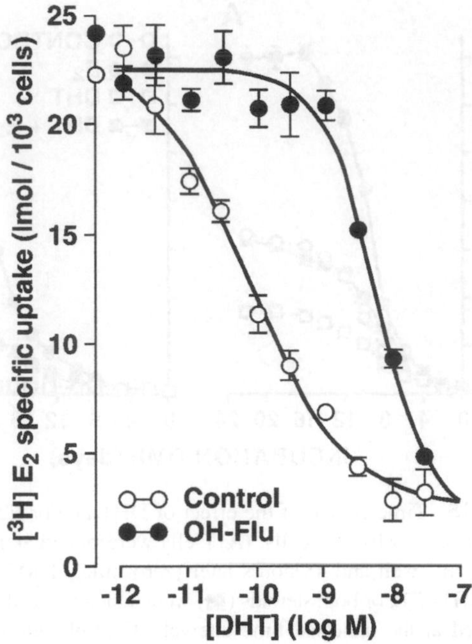

Figure 17 Effect of preincubation with increasing concentrations of DHT on [^{3}H] E2-specific binding in ZR-75-1 human breast cancer cells, a OH-lapatite exchange assay of specific [^{3}H] E2 specific binding of cytosol and nuclear (cytosol + nuclear = total) extracts obtained from AR-75-1 cells preincubated for 11 days with the indicated concentrations of DHT. B2 specific uptake of [^{3}H] E2 in intact ZR-75-1 cells preincubated for 10 days with the indicated concentrations of DHT alone (○, control) or in the presence of 3 μM antiandrogen OH-flutamide (●, OH-FLU). Values are given as means ± SE from triplicate determinations. *Abbreviation*: DHT, dihydrotestosterone. *Source*: From Poulin et al. (1989a).

The effect of androgens on ZR-75-1 cell proliferation, however, cannot be solely explained by the suppression of ER expression, since androgens still exert very potent inhibitory effects on growth in the absence of estrogens, even after prolonged periods of estrogen deprivation before exposure to androgens (Poulin et al., 1988; Simard et al., 1989). Moreover, the antiproliferative activity of androgens in estrogen-deprived ZR-75-1 cells is more pronounced and is additive to that exerted by antiestrogens (Poulin et al., 1988, 1989b).

Down-regulation of ER expression by androgens might be of crucial importance in their physiological mode of action, i.e., when estrogens are simultaneously present in normal as well as cancerous mammary gland tissue. In the specific case of human breast cancer, endogenous androgens may reduce the tumor cell sensitivity to estrogens by decreasing ER levels. Thus, in normal breast tissue, endogenous as well as locally produced androgens are likely to contribute to the regulation of the level of ER, thus modulating the sensitivity to estrogens. This inhibitory effect of androgens on intracellular ER concentrations may be expected to leave the relative effectiveness of the competitive blockade of estrogen action by antiestrogens unaffected or even imrpoved, while decreasing the efficiency of any residual estrogenic stimulation of cell growth.

In other studies, in the presence of estrogens, androgens have been found to inhibit breast cancer growth, this inhibitory effect being prevented by antiandrogens (Burak et al., 1997; Conde et al., 2004). While having no effect on MCF-7 cell line proliferation at physiological concentrations (0.1 to 10 nM), testosterone has been reported to inhibit at pharmacological concentrations (Gayosso et al., 2006). In ER-negative but AR-positive breast cancer cells, a high dose of DHEA-S inhibited cell proliferation; this inhibitory effect being blocked by the pure antiandrogen bicalutamide (Toth-Fejel et al., 2004). That the inhibitory effect of DHEA on breast cancer MCF-7 cell growth is due to interaction with AR is supported by the finding that the antiandrogen FLU reversed the inhibitory effect of DHEA on MCF-7 human breast cancer cell proliferation, while the antiestrogen tamoxifen had no effect (Boccuzzi et al., 1993).

A study in MCF-7 cells reported a small biphasic 80% stimulatory effect of DHEA on cell proliferation at 10 nM with no change between 100 and 10,000 nM (Gayosso et al., 2006). This reported small stimulatory effect at low DHEA concentrations has not been seen in the other studies mentioned above and was absent at higher concentrations. Moreover, in that study, E2 had only a 40% stimulatory effect at 1 nM, thus casting doubts on the purity of the compounds used and certainly the sensitivity of the cell line used and the precision of the assay. In fact, it can be asked if the two only stimulatory concentrations seen with DHEA could be due to the apparently high variability of the assays used? Such a possibility is strongly supported by the finding that neither FLU nor ICI 182780 (fulvestrant) affected the small and inconsistent effects observed on cell proliferation in that study.

While DHT exerts a potent inhibitory effect on breast cancer cell proliferation in ZR-75-1 human breast cancer cells (Poulin and Labrie, 1986; Poulin et al., 1988), DHT has not always been found to inhibit the growth of MCF-7 cells. The lack of inhibitory action of DHT in some MCF-7 cell lines can possibly be due to the presence of a high level of 3α-HSD activity in some cells, thus preventing DHT from exerting its inhibitory effect before its transformation into 3β-diol, a compound having intrinsic estrogenic activity (Labrie et al., unpublished data; Najid and Ratinaud, 1991).

Potent Inhibitory Effect of Androgens and DHEA in Human Breast Cancer Xenografts in Nude Mice and Breast Cancer Models in Rats and Mice

Lacassagne in 1936 first observed (Lacassagne, 1936) that treatment of mice with testosterone propionate delayed the occurrence of E1-stimulated mammary tumors. On the other hand, in DMBA-induced tumors, high doses of DHT (0.5–4.0 mg/day) for several weeks caused the regression of 60% of established tumors (Huggins et al., 1959). Similar effects have been observed with testosterone propionate (Costlow et al., 1976) and dromostanolone propionate (Quadri et al., 1974; Teller et al., 1978). Following our demonstration of the inhibitory effect of DHT and antiestrogens on ZR-75-1 cell proliferation in vitro (Poulin et al., 1988; Dumont et al., 1989; Poulin et al., 1989a, 1989c; Simard et al., 1989), we extended our study in vivo to OVX athymic mice using the same human breast cancer cells in order to more closely mimic the clinical situation in women. We thus examined the effect of DHT on tumor growth stimulated by "physiological" doses of E2 administered by silastic implants.

As illustrated in Figure 18, E2 caused a progressive increase in total tumor area from 100% (which corresponds to an average of 0.23 ± 0.08 cm^2) at start of the experiment to 226 ± 31% after 100 days of treatment. Treatment with DHT, on the other hand, not only completely reversed the stimulatory effect of E2 on tumor growth but it decreased total tumor area to 48 ± 10% of its original size. The androgen DHT is thus a potent inhibitor of the stimulatory effect of E2 on ZR-75-1 human breast carcinoma growth in in vivo athymic mice. Since OVX animals supplemented by exogenous estrogen were used in these studies, such data provide further support for a direct inhibitory action of androgens at the tumor cell level under in vivo conditions. In agreement with the in vitro data, Dauvois et al. (1989) and Dauvois (1991) have shown that constant release of the androgen DHT in OVX rats bearing DMBA-induced mammary carcinoma caused a marked inhibition of tumor growth induced by E2 (Fig. 19). That DHT acts through interaction with the AR in DMBA-induced mammary carcinoma is well supported by the finding that simultaneous treatment with the antiandrogen FLU completely prevented DHT action. Such data demonstrated, for the first time, that androgens are potent inhibitors of DMBA-induced mammary

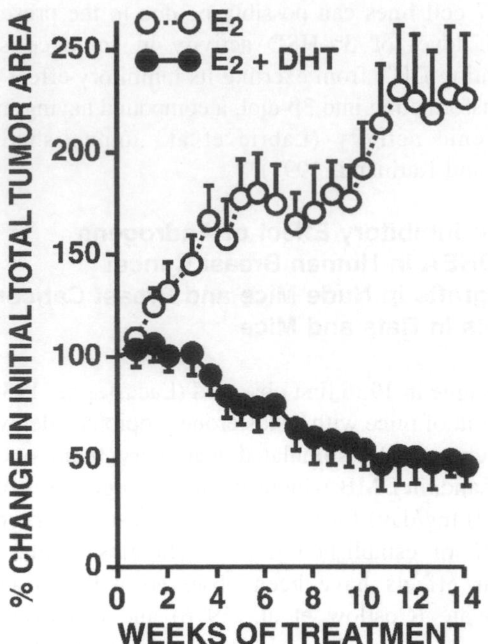

Figure 18 Effect of 100-day treatment of OVX athymic mice with silastic implants of 17β-estradiol (E2) (1/3000, E2/cholesterol, w/w) alone or in combination with silastic implants of DHT(1/5, DHT/cholesterol, w/w) on average total ZR-75-1 tumor area in nude mice. Results are expressed as percentage of pretreatment values (means ± SEM of 11 tumors in the E2 group and 9 tumors in the E2 group and 9 tumors in the E2 + DHT group). *Abbreviations*: OVX, ovariectomized; DHT, dihydrotestosterone. *Source*: From Dauvois et al. (1991).

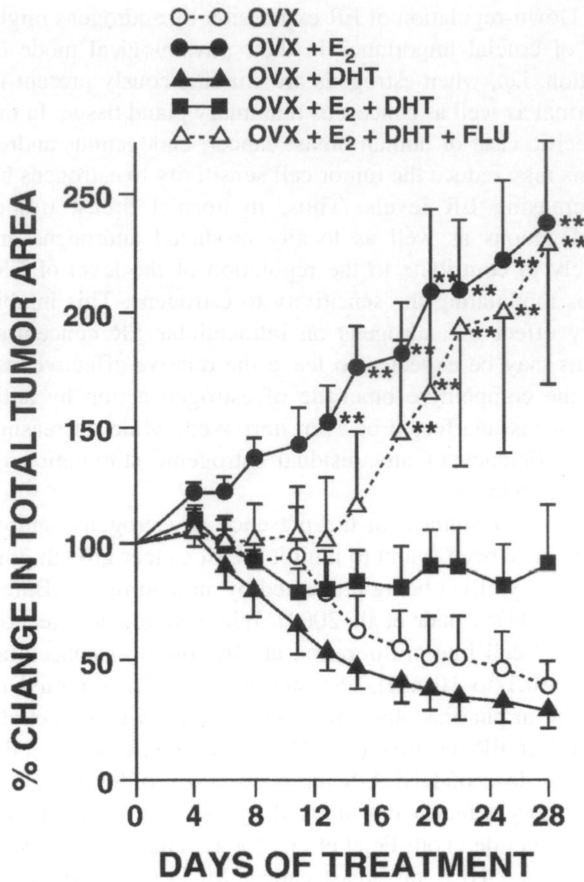

Figure 19 Effect of 28-day treatment of OVX rats with silastic implants of 17β-estradiol (E2), DHT, E2 + DHT, or E2 + DHT + twice daily injections of FLU, on average total DMBA-induced mammary tumor area in the rat. Results are expressed as percent of pretreatment values as means ± SEM of 22 to 26 tumors per group. $**p < 0.01$ OVX rats treated with the indicated steroid versus OVX animals at the same time interval. *Abbreviations*: OVX, ovariectomized; DHT, dihydrotestosterone; FLU, flutamide. *Source*: From Dauvois et al. (1989).

carcinoma growth by an action independent from inhibition of gonadotropin secretion and suggested an action exerted directly at the tumor level, thus further supporting in vitro data obtained with the human ZR-75-1 breast cancer cell line (Poulin et al., 1988, 1989a). The addition of DHEA to the diet has been shown to decrease the incidence of spontaneous mammary tumors in C3H mice (Schwartz, 1979). DHEA has also been found to inhibit mammary carcinogenesis in rats (Gordon et al., 1986; Schwartz et al., 1988; Ratko et al., 1991).

As illustrated in Figure 20, the size of the ZR-75-1 tumors increased by 9.4-fold over a 291-day period (9.5 months) in OVX nude mice supplemented with E1; in contrast, in control OVX mice that received the vehicle alone, tumor size decreased to 36.9% of the initial value during the course of the study (Couillard et al., 1998). On the other hand, treatment with increasing doses of percutaneous DHEA caused a progressive inhibition of E1-stimulated ZR-75-1 tumor growth. Inhibitions of 50.4%, 76.8%, and 80.0% were achieved at 9.5 months of treatment with the daily doses of DHEA of 0.3, 1.0, or 3.0 mg per animal, respectively (Fig. 20). In agreement with the decrease in total tumor load, treatment with DHEA led to a marked decrease in the average weight of the tumors remaining at the end of the experiment. To our knowledge, these data provide the first demonstration of the inhibitory effect of DHEA on the growth of human breast cancer xenografts in nude mice.

In the OVX mouse, exogenous DHEA represents the only source of sex steroids in peripheral tissues including the mammary gland. Moreover, by itself, DHEA does not possess any significant androgenic or estrogenic activity, its activity being dependent on its transformation into androgens and/or estrogens in peripheral target intracrine tissues (Labrie, 1991). Consequently, the inhibition of tumor growth seen after DHEA treatment in OVX animals results from its intracrine in situ conversion into androgens in the mammary gland (Labrie et al., 1988; Labrie,

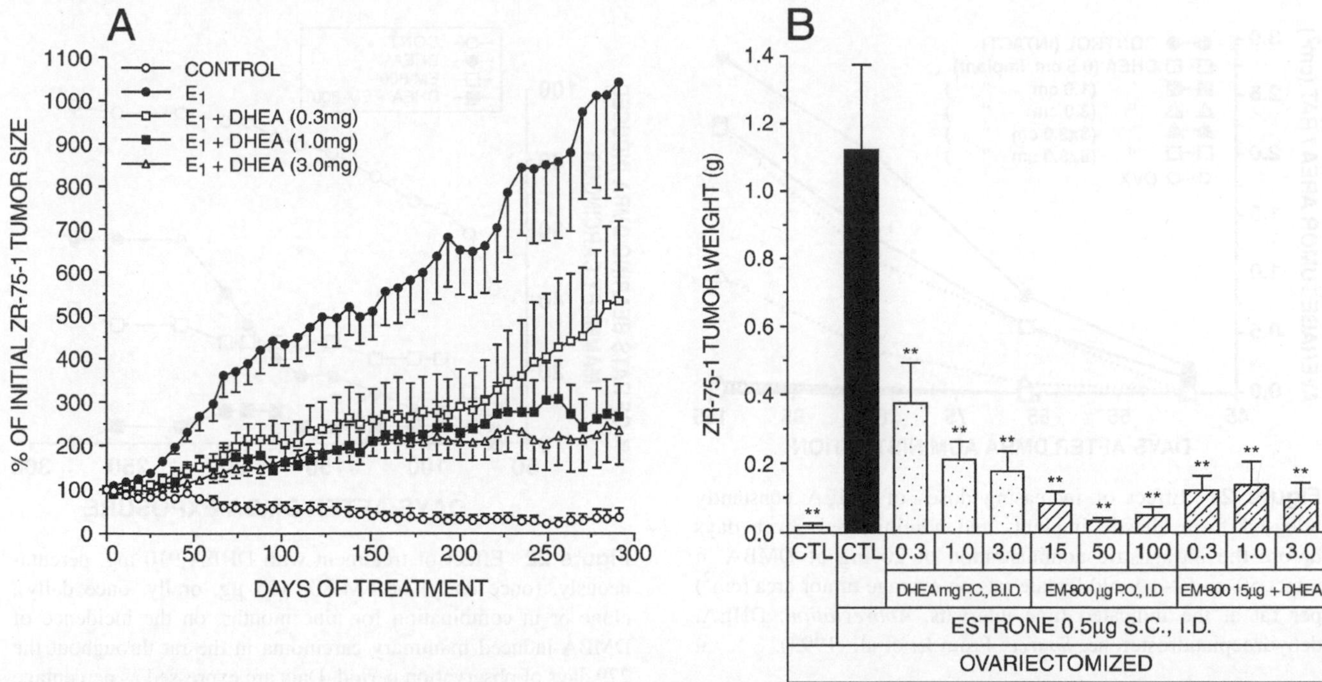

Figure 20 (A) Effect of increasing doses of DHEA (a total dose of 0.3, 1.0, or 23.0 mg) administered percutaneously in two doses daily on average ZR-75-1 tumor size in ovariectomized nude mice supplemented with 0.5 µg estrone (E1) daily. Ovariectomized mice receiving the vehicle alone were used as additional controls. The initial tumor size was taken as 100%. DHEA (0.3, 1.0, or 3.0 mg per animal per day) was administered percutaneously on the dorsal skin in a 0.02 mL solution of 50% ethanhol-50% propylene glycol. (**B**) Effect of treatment with increasing doses of DHEA (0.3, 1.0, or 3.0 mg) or EM-800 (15, 50, and 100 µg) in 0.2 mL of 4% ethanol-4% polyethylene glycol 600-1% gelatin-0.9% NaCl alone or in combination [EM-800 (acolbifene) at 15 µg and DHEA at 0.3, 1.0, or 3.0 mg] for 9.5 months on ZR-75-1 tumor weight in ovariectomized nude mice supplemented with E1. $^{**}p < 0.01$, treated versus control ovariectomized mice supplemented with E1. *Abbreviations*: CTL, control; PC, percutaneously; BID, twice daily; PO, by mouth; ID, once daily; SC, subcutaneously; DHEA, dehydroepiandrosterone.

1991, 1996b, 1996c; Labrie et al., 1995, 1997d). In fact, we have recently shown that DHEA exerts an almost exclusively androgenic effect in the rat mammary gland (Sourla et al., 1998b). Moreover, DHEA is well known to be converted into androgens, and treatment with DHEA is known to induce androgen-sensitive gene expression in the rat ventral prostate (Labrie et al., 1988, 1989, 2006b). Taken together, these data strongly suggest that DHEA exerts its inhibition of breast cancer development and growth through its conversion to androgens and activation of AR.

Prevention of Breast Tumor Development by DHEA

DHEA administration in mice and rats inhibits the development of experimental breast, colon, lung, colon, skin, and lymphatic tissue tumors (Schwartz et al., 1986; Levi et al., 2001). An example, in the skin tumorogenesis model in mice, DHEA inhibits tumor initiation as well as tumor promoter-induced epidermal hyperplasia and promotion of papillomas (Schwartz et al., 1986).

As described above, the human adrenals secrete large amounts of the precursor steroids DHEA and DHEA-S, both of which are converted into androgens in target intracrine tissues (Labrie et al., 1988, 1989; Labrie, 1991; Labrie et al., 1995, 1996a, 1996c, 1997d). In order to investigate the possibility that DHEA and its metabolites could have a preventive effect on the development of mammary carcinoma, we have studied the effect of increasing circulating levels of DHEA constantly released from silastic implants on the development of mammary carcinoma induced by DMBA in the rat. The DMBA-induced mammary carcinoma in the rat has been widely used as a model of hormone-sensitive breast cancer in women (Asselin et al., 1977; Asselin and Labrie, 1978; Dauvois et al., 1989).

Treatment with increasing doses of DHEA delivered constantly by Silastic implants of increasing length and number caused a progressive inhibition of tumor development (Li et al., 1993) (Fig. 21). It is of interest to see that tumor size in the group of animals treated with the highest dose (6 × 3.0-cm long implants) of DHEA was similar to that found in OVX animals, thus showing a

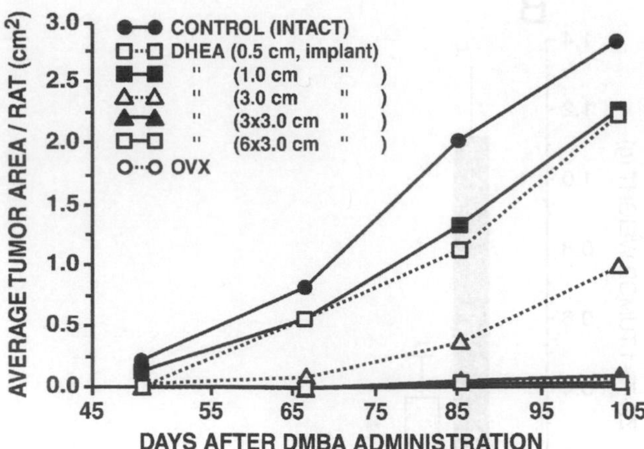

Figure 21 Effect of increasing doses of DHEA constantly released form silastic implants and administered seven days before the intragastric administration of 20 mg of DMBA in intact 50- to 52-day-old female rats on average tumor area (cm^2) per rat at the indicated time intervals. *Abbreviation*: DHEA, dehydroepiandrosterone. *Source*: From Li et al. (1993).

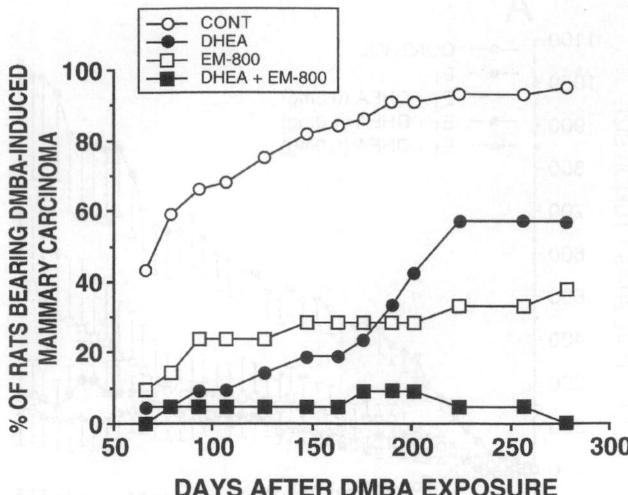

Figure 22 Effect of treatment with DHEA 910 mg, percutaneously, (once daily) or EM-800 (75 μg, orally, once daily), alone or in combination for nine months, on the incidence of DMBA-induced mammary carcinoma in the rat throughout the 279 days of observation period. Data are expressed as percentage of the total number of animals in each group. *Abbreviation*: DHEA, dehydroepiandrosterone. *Source*: From Luo et al. (1997d).

complete blockade of estrogen action by DHEA. Such data clearly demonstrate that circulating levels of the precursor adrenal steroid DHEA comparable to those observed in normal adult premenopausal women (Liu et al., 1990) exert a potent inhibitory effect on the development of mammary carcinoma induced by DMBA in the rat. It is of special interest to see that serum levels of DHEA of 7.09 ± 0.64 nM and 17.5 ± 1.1 nM led to a dramatic inhibition of tumor development to 22% and 11% of animals bearing mammary carcinoma compared with 68% in control intact animals. At the highest dose of DHEA used, which corresponds to serum DHEA values of 27.2 ± 2.2 nM, the incidence of tumors was reduced to only 3.8%. It should be mentioned that the serum DHEA levels in normal 20 to 30-year old women ranges between 8.3 and 17.3 nM (Liu et al., 1990).

It might be relevant to mention that treatment with DHEA markedly delayed the appearance of breast tumors in C3H mice that were genetically bred to develop breast cancer (Schwartz, 1979).

Prevention of Breast Tumorogenesis by DHEA Plus Acolbifene

Since antiestrogens (Jordan, 1976, 1978; Dauvois et al., 1991; Kawamura et al., 1991; Labrie et al., 1995c) as well as DHEA (Li et al., 1993) can independently inhibit the development of DMBA-induced mammary carcinoma, we have studied the potential benefits of combining the new antiestrogen EM-800 (precursor of acolbifene) with DHEA on the development of mammary carcinoma induced by DMBA in the rat. As illustrated in Figure 22, 95% of control animals developed palpable mammary tumors by 279 days after DMBA administration. Treatment with DHEA or acolbifene alone partially prevented the development of DMBA-induced mammary carcinoma, the incidence being thus reduced to 57% ($p < 0.01$) and 38% ($p < 0.01$), respectively. Interestingly, combination of the two compounds led to a significantly greater inhibitory effect than that achieved by each compound administered alone ($p < 0.01$ vs. DHEA or acolbifene alone). In fact, the only two tumors that developed in the group of animals treated with both compounds disappeared before the end of the experiment (Luo et al., 1997a).

Such data obtained in vivo support our previous findings that the inhibitory effects of androgens and antiestrogens on mammary carcinoma are exerted at least in part by different mechanisms and that the combination of an androgenic compound with a pure antiestrogen has improved efficacy compared with each compound used alone in the prevention and treatment of breast cancer in women. The antagonism between androgens and estrogens on breast cancer growth is illustrated schematically in Figures 23 and 24. DHEA, secondary to its predominant transformation into androgens in mammary gland tissue, exerts an inhibitory effect on mammary carcinoma development and growth, an effect that counteracts and can even completely neutralize the stimulatory effect of estrogens (Dimitrakakis et al., 2003; Hofling et al., 2007; Poulin, 1988).

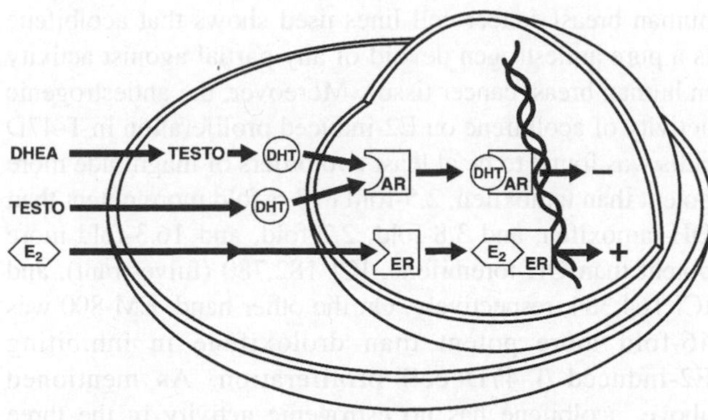

Figure 23 Antagonism between the inhibitory effects of androgens and DHEA and the stimulatory effects of estrogens on breast cancer proliferation. *Abbreviation*: DHEA, dehydroepiandrosterone.

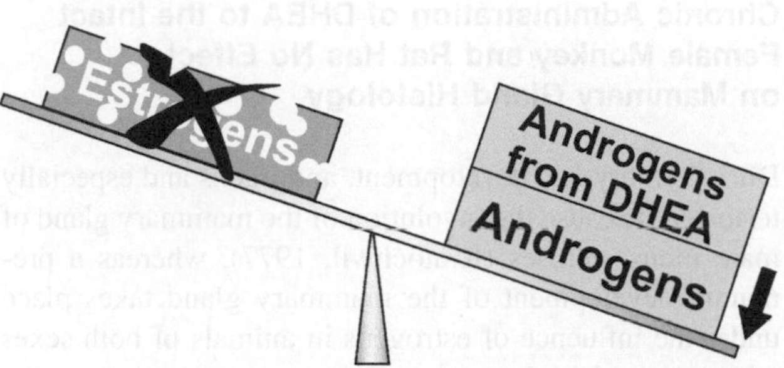

Figure 24 Mammary gland and breast cancer proliferation changes with the combination acolbifene plus DHEA. The estrogens are blocked by acolbifene, while additional androgens made form exogenous DHEA result in a marked inhibition of mammary gland and breast cancer proliferation. *Abbreviation*: DHEA, dehydroepiandrosterone.

A group of researchers have reported that DHEA is inhibitory on breast cancer growth in the presence of estrogens, while it can be stimulatory on experimental models where estrogens are absent (Secreto et al., 1991; Boccuzzi et al., 1992a). It should be mentioned, however, that an absence of estrogens does not exist in women where comparable levels of E2 are found in breast cancer tissue in pre- and postmenopausal women (Poortman et al., 1983). In fact, such a hypothetical situation of an absence of estrogens does not exist in normal women, even after menopause. Moreover, as well shown in Figure 14, very high and nonphysiological concentrations of DHEA are required to exert a stimulatory effect probably due to transformation into 5-diol and E2 at such high concentrations.

Although the above-mentioned data demonstrate the direct inhibitory effects of androgens and DHEA on breast cancer growth, it is likely that endogenous androgens and DHEA also play an important physiological role in the control of normal breast tissue growth and function and that the same antagonism between androgens and estrogens is operative in both the normal mammary gland and breast cancer (Figs. 12 and 25).

Combination Acolbifene plus DHEA in Nude Mice Bearing Human Breast Cancer Xenografts

As illustrated in Figure 20B, the sizes of the ZR-75-1 tumors increased by 9.4-fold over a 291-day period (9.5 months) in OVX nude mice treated with a daily 0.5-μg subcutaneously administered dose of E1; in agreement with the decrease in total tumor load, treatment with DHEA led to a marked decrease in the average weight of

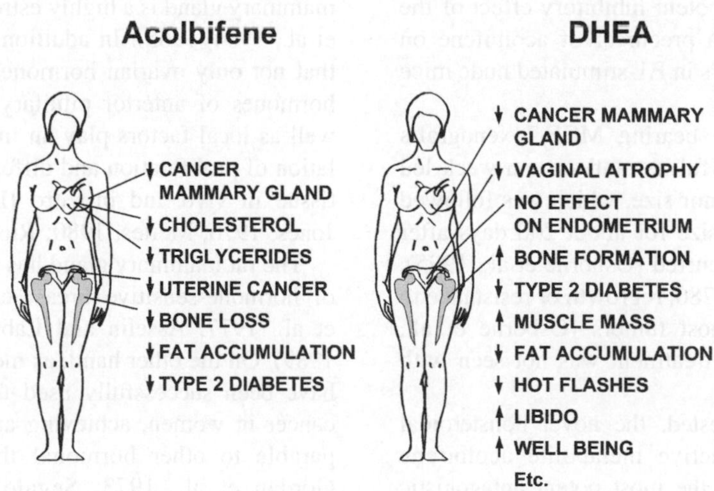

Figure 25 Schematic representation of the effects expected from the combination of a SERM and DHEA. The SERM should prevent breast and uterine cancer, while DHEA should replace the loss of sex steroids in postmenopausal women in the appropriate target tissues. Tissue-specific (TS-HRT) avoids exposure of the other tissues to sex steroids, thus eliminating the negative effects observed in the WHI and Million Women studies. *Abbreviation*: DHEA, dehydroepiandrosterone.

the tumors remaining at the end of the experiment. In fact, the average tumor weight decreased from 1.12 ± 0.26 g in control E1 supplemented, OVX nude mice to 0.37 ± 0.12 g ($p = 0.005$), 0.20 ± 0.06 g ($p = 0.001$), and 0.17 ± 0.06 g ($p = 0.0003$), respectively (Fig. 20A), when compared with the tumor size in control animals at 9.5 months. The tumor-size reductions achieved with the three EM-800 (precursor of acolbifene) doses were not significantly different between each other. As illustrated in Figure 20B, tumor weight at the end of the 9.5-month study was decreased from 1.12 ± 0.26 g in control E1 supplemented, OVX mice to 0.08 ± 0.03 g, 0.03± 0.01 g, and 0.04 ± 0.03 g in animals treated with they daily doses of 15, 50, or 100 μg of EM-800, respectively ($p < 0.0001$ at all doses of EM-800 vs. E1 supplemented, OVX).

As mentioned above, the antiestrogen EM-800 at a daily oral dose of 15 μg caused an 87.5% inhibition of E1-stimulated tumor growth measured at 9.5 months. The addition of DHEA at the three doses used had no statistically significant effect on the already marked inhibition of tumor size achieved with the 15-μg daily dose of EM-800 (Fig. 20B). Thus, the average tumor weight was dramatically reduced from 1.12 ± 0.26 g in control E1-supplemented mice to 0.08 ± 0.03 g ($p < 0.0001$), 0.11 ± 0.04 g ($p = 0.0002$), 0.13 ± 0.07 g ($p = 0.0004$), and 0.08 ± 0.05 g ($p < 0.0001$) in the animals that received the daily dose of 15 μg of Em-800 alone or in combination with 0.3, 1.0. or 3.0 mg of DHEA, respectively (no statistically significant difference was noted between the four groups) (Fig. 20B).

To our knowledge, these data provided the first demonstration of the inhibitory effect of DHEA on the growth of human breast cancer xenografts in nude mice. Moreover, this study shows that simultaneous treatment with DHEA (at daily doses ranging from 0.3 to 3.0 mg) has noninfluence on the highly potent inhibitory effect of the new antiestrogen EM-800, a precursor of acolbifene on the growth of ZR-75-1 tumors in E1-stimulated nude mice (Couillard et al., 1998).

Treatment of nude mice bearing MCF-7 xenografts with 10 mg of ICI 182,780 (fulvestrant) once a week led to a transient decrease in tumor size, which was followed by a stabilization of tumor size for about 200 days after which tumor progression occurred (Osborne et al., 1995). In mice treated with ICI 182,780, regrowth or resistance to ICI 182,780 occurred in most tumors (Osborne et al., 1995). Such a resistance to treatment was not seen with acolbifene (Roy et al., 2003).

Of all the compounds tested, the novel nonsteroidal prodrug EM-800 and its active metabolite acolbifene have been reported to exert the most potent antagonistic effects on E2-induced proliferation in T-47D, ZR-75-1, and MCF-7 human breast cancer cells in culture (Simard et al., 1997a). Furthermore, the absence of a stimulatory effect on basal cell proliferation in the three estrogen-sensitive human breast cancer cell lines used shows that acolbifene is a pure antiestrogen devoid of any partial agonist activity in human breast cancer tissue. Moreover, the antiestrogenic activity of acolbifene on E2-induced proliferation in T-47D cells was found to be at least two orders of magnitude more potent than tamoxifen, 2.5-fold to 3.6-fold more potent than OH-tamoxifen, and 3.8-fold, 2.7-fold, and 16.3-fold more potent than OH-toremifene, ICI 182,780 (fulvestrant), and ICI 164,384, respectively. On the other hand, EM-800 was 46-fold more potent than droloxifene in inhibiting E2-induced T-47D cell proliferation. As mentioned above, acolbifene has no estrogenic activity in the three breast cancer cell lines studied, while OH-tamoxifen, droloxifene, and toremifene cause a statistically significant stimulation of ZR-75-1 and or MCF-7 human breast cancer cell proliferation (Simard et al., 1997a).

Chronic Administration of DHEA to the Intact Female Monkey and Rat Has No Effect on Mammary Gland Histology

During embryonic development, androgens and especially testosterone cause the involution of the mammary gland of male mouse fetuses (Kratochwil, 1977), whereas a premature development of the mammary gland takes place under the influence of estrogens in animals of both sexes when injected in the pregnant mouse or directly into the embryo (Raynaud, 1971; Russo and Russo, 1989).

Although mammary gland histology and structure do not differ significantly in young male and female rats (Geriani, 1970), the first estrous cycle in female Sprague-Dawley rats results in a rapid growth and differentiation of the mammary gland, a change that can be prevented by ovariectomy (Cowie and Folley, 1961). In fact, the rat mammary gland is a highly estrogen-sensitive tissue (King et al., 1964, 1965). In addition, it has been demonstrated that not only ovarian hormones, but also mammotrophic hormones of anterior pituitary and of adrenal origin as well as local factors play an important role in the modulation of proliferation and differentiation of the mammary tissue in vivo and in vitro (Lyons, 1958; Forsyth and Jones, 1976; Meites, 1980; Russo and Russo, 1987).

The rat mammary gland has been widely used as model of hormone-sensitive breast cancer in women (Asselin et al., 1977; Asselin and Labrie, 1978; Dauvois et al., 1989). On the other hand, as mentioned earlier, androgens have been successfully used for the treatment of breast cancer in women, achieving an objective response comparable to other hormonal therapies (Kennedy, 1958; Gordan et al., 1973; Segaloff, 1977; Tormey et al., 1983). In addition, it has been shown that androgens such as dromostanolone propionate, testosterone, and DHEA, a precursor of androgens (Labrie et al., 1978; Labrie, 1991), exert a potent inhibitory effect on the development of DMBA-induced mammary carcinoma in the rat (Young et al., 1965; Quadri et al., 1974; Dauvois et al., 1989; Li et al., 1993). Despite the fact that a series of studies have shown the chemopreventive effect of DHEA on the development of rat mammary cancer, little is known about the effect of long-term administration of DHEA on mammary gland physiology and structure.

As mentioned earlier, the clinical evidence for tumor regression observed in 20% to 50% of breast cancer patients treated with various androgens suggests that naturally occurring androgens exert direct inhibitory control of mammary cancer cell growth. Moreover, as mentioned above, AR is expressed in 70% to 90% of breast cancers (Hall et al., 1995; Song et al., 2006), thus supporting the hypothesis of a direct inhibitory action of androgens on breast cancer. In animal models, DHEA has been shown to inhibit breast carcinogenesis. In fact, as mentioned above, treatment with increasing doses of DHEA induced a progressive inhibition of the development of DMBA-induced mammary carcinoma in the rat (Li et al., 1993). On the other hand, we have already reported that chronic treatment (12 months) of OVX rats with a pharmacological dose of DHEA stimulated alveolar and ductal growth as well as the secretory activity of the acinar cells (Sourla et al., 1998a). Since this stimulatory effect seen in OVX animals was completely inhibited by the concomitant administration of the pure antiandrogen FLU, it was concluded that it was related to the conversion of DHEA to androgens.

In order to clarify the potential influence of DHEA on the mammary gland in intact animals, we have studied the effect of chronic administration of DHEA to intact female monkeys and rats on mammary gland histopathology and circulating E2 and testosterone levels.

IN ANIMALS

Monkey

Serum Steroid Levels

The low dose of DHEA (2 mg/kg b.w./day), induced a 2.8-fold increase (from 4.9 ± 2.3 ng/mL to 13.6 ± 3.4 ng/mL at 359 days) of serum DHEA concentrations measured six hours after DHEA administration as compared with the serum levels measured before treatment. A much larger (18-fold) increase in serum DHEA-S levels (from 60.3 ± 19.6 ng/mL to 1099 ± 275 ng/mL) was measured following administration of DHEA at the low dose. At all the time intervals studied (1, 184, and 359 days), there was no significant change in serum testosterone or E2 levels.

At the highest dose of DHEA (10 mg/kg b.w./day) used, DHEA serum levels increased from 3.4 ± 1.0 ng/mL to 17.5 ± 4.0 ng/mL at 359 days (5.1-fold increase) when compared with the pretreatment levels. At this dose, serum DHEA-S concentrations were very high at all the time intervals studied, with values ranging from 44- to 47-fold above pretreatment values. Serum testosterone, on the other hand, was increased by 4.5-fold from 0.2 ± 0.08 ng/mL to 0.9 ± 0.2 ng/mL, while no significant change in E2 concentrations could be detected. It should be mentioned that the serum DHEA values obtained with the 10 mg/kg b.w./day are 8.9-fold higher than the values observed in 55- to 65-year-old postmenopausal women (1.97 ± 1.18 ng/mL) (Labrie et al., 2006a).

Histology of Mammary Glands

The monkey mammary gland consists of several lobules, each containing acini and a few ducts as well as adjacent stroma. The epithelial cells bordering the lumen ducts and acini are cuboidal to columnar and are separated from the basement membrane by a discontinuous layer of myoepithelial cells. Clear vacuoles and eosinophilic secretory materials can be occasionally seen in the epithelial cells (Fig. 26A). As shown in Figure 26B, long-term treatment (359 days) with either 2 mg or 10 mg DHEA/kg b.w.

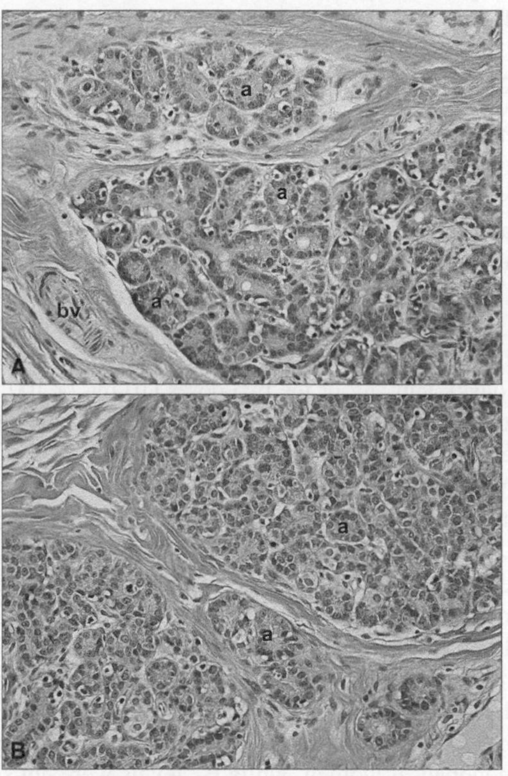

Figure 26 Representative micrographs illustrating mammary gland histology in control (**A**) and DHEA-treated (359 days) (**B**) the female monkey. The histological characteristics of acini (a) are not modified by the treatment. 400×. *Abbreviations*: DHEA, dehydroepiandrosterone; bv, blood vessel; a, acini. *Source*: From Pelletier et al. (2007).

administered daily orally did not modify the histology of the mammary gland.

Rat

Serum Steroid Levels

The effect of oral DHEA administration (10 and 100 mg/kg b.w./day) on circulating steroids was evaluated at the beginning (day 1) and end (day 175) of treatment. Neither DHEA nor DHEA-S could be detected in the plasma of control female rats. At the end of the study, the serum concentrations of both DHEA and DHEA-S were dose-related reaching 44.4 ± 9.8 ng/mL and 12507 ± 3500 ng/mL for DHEA and DHEA-S, respectively, following 175 days of daily treatment with the highest dose of DHEA. Such levels of DHEA are 22.5-fold above the serum DHEA levels observed in postmenopausal women. The same treatment increased serum testosterone concentrations to 1.85 ± 0.36 ng/mL at the highest DHEA dose (nondetectable in control rats). This increase in serum testosterone is 13.2-fold above the value of 0.14 ± 0.07 ng/mL found in 55- to 65-year-old normal postmenopausal women (Labrie et al., 2006a) No significant effect was observed on serum E2 levels.

Histology of Mammary Glands

In female rats, the mammary gland is mainly composed of ducts with very few acini. The ducts consist of one or two layers of epithelial cells, which are cuboidal or columnar. The acini are usually composed of one layer of cuboidal epithelial cells bordering the lumen. In both ducts and acini, myoepithelial cells are present forming a discontinuous layer. These epithelial structures are surrounded by stroma cells (Fig. 27A). Long-term oral treatment (175 days) with any of the two doses (10 mg or 100 mg/kg b.w./day) of DHEA did not induce any significant changes in the histology of the mammary gland (Fig. 27B).

The present data clearly demonstrate that chronic administration of DHEA at doses which increased serum DHEA levels 8.9-fold (monkeys) and 22.5-fold (rats) above the serum DHEA concentrations found in normal postmenopausal women has no effect on mammary gland histology. In the monkey, there was a significant increase in circulating levels of testosterone with the highest dose of DHEA (10 mg/kg b.w.) to 0.9 ± 0.2 ng/mL, a value 6.4-fold above the serum testosterone levels found in postmenopausal women, while E2 levels were not significantly modified. It has been reported that testosterone administration can prevent the stimulatory effect of E2 on mammary epithelial cell proliferation in the OVX monkey (Dimitrakakis et al., 2003; Labrie et al., 2006a). Moreover, in normal female monkeys, AR blockage induced an increase in mammary epithelial cell proliferation, thus

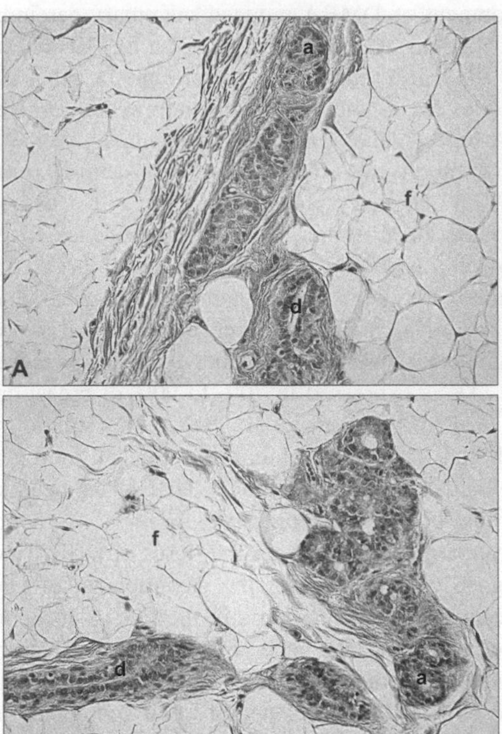

Figure 27 Representative micrographs illustrating mammary gland histology in control (**A**) and DHEA-treated (175 days) (**B**) in the female rat. No difference in the histological characteristics can be observed between the two groups. *Abbreviations*: DHEA, dehydroepiandrosterone; a, acini; d, duct; f, fat cells. 400×. *Source*: From Pelletier et al. (2007).

suggesting that endogenous androgens are involved in the negative regulation of mammary cell division (Dimitrakakis et al., 2003).

In the present experiment, we could not observe any changes in the histological characteristics of the acini and ducts in animals treated with the low or high dose of DHEA. It can be speculated that in normal monkeys treated with DHEA, the increase in circulating testosterone was not sufficient to interfere with the action of circulating and/or locally produced estrogens. Previous studies have shown that the oral or percutaneous administration of DHEA to postmenopausal women could increase serum testosterone without a significant influence on circulating E2 (Morales et al., 1994; Diamond et al., 1996; Baulieu et al., 2000; Nair et al., 2006).

In the female rat, the results obtained following DHEA administration are very similar to those obtained in the monkey. In control female rats, as expected, no circulating DHEA or DHEA-S could be detected. The exposure of DHEA and DHEA-S was dose-related following the oral administration of DHEA during 175 days. In fact, the serum levels of DHEA achieved with the highest dose of DHEA were 22.5-fold higher than the values found in 55- to 65-year-old postmenopausal women (Labrie et al., 2006a). Circulating testosterone which could not be detected in control rats was increased in treated animals with the highest levels being measured at 1.85 ± 0.3 ng/mL following the administration of 100 mg DHEA/kg b.w./day. Such a value is 13.2-fold above the serum testosterone concentration measured in postmenopausal women. As observed in monkeys, no statistically significant effect on serum E2 levels was observed.

In the rat mammary gland, the histological pattern was not modified in animals treated with 10 or 100 mg DHEA/kg b.w./day. We have already reported the effect of DHEA administered percutaneously during 12 months on the mammary gland in OVX rats (Sourla et al., 1998b). In that study, the very high dose used (30 mg twice daily percutaneously) stimulated acinar and ductal growth as well as the secretory activity of acinar cells. In that study, the addition of the pure antiandrogen FLU almost completely prevented the stimulatory effect of DHEA, thus indicating the almost exclusive androgenic component of the action of DHEA. The discrepancy between the results from that previous study and the present data demonstrating the absence of effect of DHEA in intact rats could be explained by the action of estrogens which might prevent the androgenic action of DHEA by mechanisms which remain to be clarified.

The present data show that in monkeys, a species having adrenals that produce high levels of DHEA as well as in rats where there is no circulating DHEA, the chronic administration of relatively higher doses of DHEA which increase serum DHEA levels 8.9- and 22.5-fold and serum testosterone levels 6.4- and 13.2-fold above the values found in normal postmenopausal women has no influence on mammary glands as evaluated by histopathological examination. Since the serum levels of DHEA obtained with the two doses of DHEA used are well above the serum concentrations found in young normal women and postmenopausal women who received DHEA percutaneously (Labrie et al., 2006a); this is a strong indication that long-term treatment of female patients with DHEA would not produce negative effects on the mammary gland and might even be beneficial for breast cancer prevention due to the increase in androgen biosynthesis from DHEA.

We have also used the OVX female Sprague-Dawley rat model to investigate the potential effect of DHEA and its active metabolites on the mammary gland histomorphology and structure in adult virgin female rats. We have also compared the effect of DHEA with that of E2, as well as the nonaromatizable androgen DHT, and we have also used the pure antiandrogen FLU and the pure antiestrogen EM-800 (precursor of acolbifene) to assess the specific androgenic and/or estrogenic actions of DHEA in the rat mammary gland.

The mammary gland of intact female rats aged approximately 14 months at the end of the experiment shows a mild to moderate lobular hyperplasia compared with young adults. The histological pattern is characterized by a large number and increased size of the lobular structures. The changes induced by the high dose of DHEA, in the OVX animals, namely histological changes characterized by a rather lobuloalveolar type of development of the mammary gland are analogous to those seen during pregnancy and lactation (Kelly et al., 1976; Russo and Russo, 1987).

The observed increase in parencymal surface area was mainly associated with an increase in the number of lobuloalveolar structures and to a lesser degree by an increase in the number of ducts present per square millimeter of total surface area of the mammary gland. Interestingly, the stimulation of lobuloalveolar growth of the mammary gland was almost completely abolished by the concomitant administration of the pure antiandrogen FLU, thus providing evidence for the predominant androgenic effect of DHEA, through its intracrine conversion to active sex steroids with androgenic activity.

It is also noteworthy that lobular development and lobular hyperplastic lesions, such as hyperplastic alveolar nodules, often accompanied by enhanced secretory activity (Russo et al., 1977) are not considered as preneoplastic lesions in the rat (Dao et al., 1975). Considering the predominant androgenic action of DHEA on normal mammary tissue as well as the well recognized and potent inhibitory action of DHEA on the development and growth of DMBA-induced mammary tumors, which is mainly considered an androgenic effect, we suggest that tissue DHEA metabolism plays an important role in the pathophysiology of the mammary gland and could be a useful preventive and therapeutic approach for breast cancer.

COMBINED TISSUE-SPECIFIC HRT AND BREAST CANCER PREVENTION

We feel that the increased understanding of androgen and estrogen formation and action in peripheral target tissues called intracrinology (Labrie, 1991; Labrie et al., 1992; Labrie et al., 1992, 1994, 1995b; Luu-The et al., 1995a; Labrie et al., 1996c, 1997a, 1997b, 1997c, 1997d, 2005b) as well as our recent observations indicating the predominant role of androgens over that of estrogens in the prevention of bone loss after ovariectomy in the rat (Martel et al., 1998), as well as the observation of a stimulatory action of DHEA on bone mineral density (BMD) in postmenopausal women (Labrie et al., 1997c) and the inhibitory action of adnrogens and DHEA on normal mammary gland and breast cancer in women have paved the way for a timely and potentially highly significant progress in the field of tissue-targeted sex steroid replacement therapy at menopause, especially after the issue raised by the use of estrogens and progestins (Women's Health Initiative, 2002; Beral et al., 2005).

The rapid fall in circulating E2 at menopause, coupled with the demonstrated beneficial effects of exogeneous estrogens on menopausal symptoms (Archer et al., 1999) and bone resorption (Christiansen et al., 1982; Lindsay et al., 2002; Women's Health Initiative, 2002), has focused most of the efforts of HRT on various forms of estrogens (ERT) as well as to combinations of estrogen and progestin (HRT). The traditional HRT, however, has recently been seriously questioned or even abandoned by many women and physicians following data indicating that the combination of Premarin and Provera (Prempro) increases the incidence of breast cancer with a potential negative impact on cardiovascular events (Women's Health Initiative, 2002). Similar concerns have also been raised in the Million Women Study (Beral et al., 2005).

As mentioned above, the almost exclusive focus on the role of ovarian estrogens has removed the attention from the dramatic 70% fall in circulating DHEA, which already occurs between the ages of 20 to 30 and 40 to 50 years (Migeon et al., 1957; Vermeulen and Verdonck, 1976; Vermeulen et al., 1982; Orentreich et al., 1984; Bélanger et al., 1994; Labrie et al., 1997a). Since DHEA is transformed to both androgens and estrogens in peripheral tissues, such a fall in serum DHEA and DHEA-S explains why all women at menopause are not only lacking estrogens but are also markedly deprived from androgens (Figs. 9, 10) (Labrie et al., 2006a). While men are protected from the age-related fall in serum DHEA by the continuous high rate of testosterone secretion by the testicles, the low amount of testosterone of direct ovarian and adrenal origins has a much lower protective role on the marked fall observed for serum DHEA and, therefore, the DHEA-derived androgens with age.

In order to avoid the problems illustrated by the WHI study, it appears logical to use a tissue-specific antiestrogenic/estrogenic compound (SERM) combined with a tissue-targeted androgenic/estrogenic replacement therapy at peri- and postmenopause (Fig. 27). This strategy appears as the best or possibly the only way able to maintain a physiological balance between androgens and estrogens in each cell of each tissue and simultaneously prevent breast cancer. Such an objective can only be met with DHEA, which permits the tissue-specific local formation of androgens and/or estrogens in each peripheral tissue (Labrie, 1991; Labrie et al., 2005b; Labrie, 2007).

As mentioned earlier, despite approval by the U.S. Food and Drug Administration and endorsement by the American Society of Clinical Oncology, only 5% to 30% of high-risk women accept to take tamoxifen as a preventive agent (Vogel et al., 2002). Fear of the reported side effects of tamoxifen is a major drawback for healthy women, the two most serious side effects being endometrial cancer and thromboembolic events (Cuzick et al., 2002). Moreover, half of the breast cancers are not prevented nor delayed by tamoxifen or rafloxifene. The objective of new SERMs is thus to increase the benefit/risk ratio observed with tamoxifen or raloxifene. It is important to recognize that all SERMs are different and that the data obtained with tamoxifen or raloxifene cannot be extrapolated to other SERMs and vice-versa.

Synergistic Effects of Acolbifene and DHEA on the Breast

With regard to the breast, DHEA is known to prevent the development (Luo et al., 1997d) and to inhibit the growth (Li et al., 1993) of DMBA-induced mammary tumors in the rat. DHEA, in addition, inhibits the growth of human breast cancer xenografts in nude mice (Couillard et al., 1998). Thus, contrary to estrogens and progestins, which exert stimulatory effects, DHEA at physiological doses is expected from a series of preclinical studies to inhibit both the development and the growth of breast cancer in women (Labrie et al., 2003b; Labrie, 2007).

In fact, androgens exert a direct antiproliferative activity on the growth of ZR-75-1 human breast cancer cells in vitro and such an inhibitory effect of androgens is additive to that of an antiestrogen (Poulin and Labrie, 1986; Poulin et al., 1988). Similar inhibitory effects have been observed in vivo on ZR-75-1 xenografts in nude mice (Dauvois et al., 1991). Androgens have also been shown to inhibit the growth of DMBA-induced mammary carcinoma in the rat, this inhibition being reversed by the simultaneous administration of the pure antiandrogen FLU (Dauvois et al., 1989). Most importantly, inhibitory effects comparable to those of other therapies have been observed in women with advanced breast cancer treated with androgenic compounds (Fels, 1944; Segaloff et al., 1951).

Since antiestrogens and sex steroid precursors exert inhibitory effects on breast cancer via different mechanisms, it is logical to believe that the combination of a SERM (acolbifene) and a sex steroid precursor (DHEA) could exert more potent inhibitory effects than each compound used alone on the development of breast cancer. As well illustrated in Figure 22, no DMBA-induced tumor was found at the end of an experiment in animals that had received both DHEA and a precursor of acolbifene.

Because of its highly potent and pure antiestrogenic activity, acolbifene should not only eliminate the risk of breast, uterine, and ovarian cancer associated with estrogen use (Lacey et al., 2002; Riman et al., 2002; Rodriguez et al., 2002; Women's Health Initiative, 2002; Beral et al.,

2005), but it should also reduce the spontaneous incidence of these cancers which are diagnosed in 13.3% (breast cancer), 2.7% (endometrial cancer), and 1.7% (ovarian cancer) of women during their lifetime.

Synergistic Effects on Bone

Since acolbifene and DHEA act by two different mechanisms following interaction with the estrogen and ARs, respectively, their combination appears well justified for the prevention and treatment of osteoporosis. In fact, in the rat, acolbifene is about 10 times more potent than raloxifene to protect against bone loss (Martel et al., 2000). On the other hand, we have found that DHEA exerts beneficial effects on bone in both the intact and OVX female rat (Luo et al., 1997a). Thus, in intact female rats, treatment with DHEA increases BMD of total skeleton, lumbar spine, and femur (Luo et al., 1997a).

In fact, our preclinical data clearly indicate that DHEA can provide the beneficial effects that are lacking with the use of a SERM alone. While a SERM has effects limited to inhibition of bone resorption, the addition of DHEA stimulates bone formation (an effect not found with a SERM, a bisphosphonate, an estrogen or calcitonin) and further reduces bone resorption above the effect achieved with acolbifene alone. Moreover, the antiresorptive therapies do not improve all the characteristics of the normal bone, especially the microarchitecture. While the effects of acolbifene on bone have been obtained at the preclinical level, treatment with DHEA has already been found to increase BMD in postmenopausal women (Labrie et al., 1997c). The observed stimulatory effect of DHEA in postmenopausal women on BMD and the increase in serum osteocalcin, a marker of bone formation, are of particular interest for the prevention and treatment of oestoporosis and indicate a unique activity of DHEA on bone physiology, namely a stimulatory effect on bone formation (Labrie et al., 1997c).

It is particularly important to indicate that the combination of DHEA and EM-800 (acolbifene) exerted unexpected beneficial effects on important biochemical parameters of bone metabolism (Table 1). In fact, DHEA alone did not affect the urinary OH-proline/ -creatinine ratio, a marker of bone resorption. Moreover, no effect of DHEA alone could be detected on daily urinary calcium or phosphorus excretion (Luo et al., 1997d). EM-800 (acolbifene), on the other hand, decreased the urinary OH-proline/ -creatinine ratio by 48% while, similarly to DHEA, no effect of EM-800 alone was seen on urinary calcium or phosphorus excretion. EM-800, alone, moreover, had no significant effect on serum AP activity, a marker of bone formation while DHEA increased the value of the parameter by about 75% (Luo et al., 1997d).

One of the unexpected effects of the combination of DHEA and EM-800 relates to the urinary OH-proline/ -creatinine ratio, a marker of bone resorption, which was reduced by 69% when both DHEA and EM-800 were combined; this value being statistically different ($p < 0.01$) from the 48% inhibition achieved by EM-800 alone, while DHEA alone did not show any effect (Table 1). Thus, the addition of DHEA to EM-800 increases by 50% of the inhibitory effect of EM-800 on bone reabsorption. Most importantly, another unexpected effect of the addition of DHEA to EM-800 was the approximately 84% decrease in urinary calcium (from 23.17 ± 1.55 to 3.71 ± 0.75 μmol/ 24 hr/100 g; $p < 0.01$) and the 55% decrease in urinary phosphorus (from 132.72 ± 6.08 to 59.06 ± 4.76 μmol/ 24 hr/100 g; $p < 0.01$), respectively (Luo et al., 1997d).

These results obtained in the rat clearly demonstrate that DHEA can provide the beneficial effects that are lacking with the use of a SERM alone, such as EM-800, raloxifene, etc. In fact, while a SERM has effects limited to inhibition of bone resorption, the addition of DHEA stimulates bone formation (an effect not found with a SERM or an estrogen) and further reduces bone resorption above the effect achieved with acolbifene alone.

Table 1 Effect of 12-Month Treatment with DHEA or EM-800 (Acolbifene) Alone or in Combination on Urinary Calcium and Phosphorus Excretion As Well As on Serum Alkaline Phosphatase

Group	Urine: Calcium (μmol/24 hr/100 g)	Urine: Phosphorus (μmol/24 hr/100 g)	Urine: HP/Cr (μmol/mmol)	Serum TALP (IU/L)
Control	23.17 ± 1.55	132.72 ± 6.08	13.04 ± 2.19	114.25 ± 14.04
DHEA (10 mg)	25.87 ± 3.54	151.41 ± 14.57	14.02 ± 1.59	198.38 ± 30.76[a]
EM-800 (75 μG)	17.44 ± 4.5	102.03 ± 25.13	6.81 ± 0.84[b]	114.11 ± 11.26
DHEA + EM-800	3.71 ± 0.75[b]	59.06± 4.76[b]	4.06 ± 0.28[b]	204.38 ± 14.20[b]

[a]$p < 0.01$;
[b]$p < 0.05$.
Abbreviations: DHEA, dehydroepiandrosterone; TALP, total alkaline phosphate.
Source: From Luo et al. (1997d).

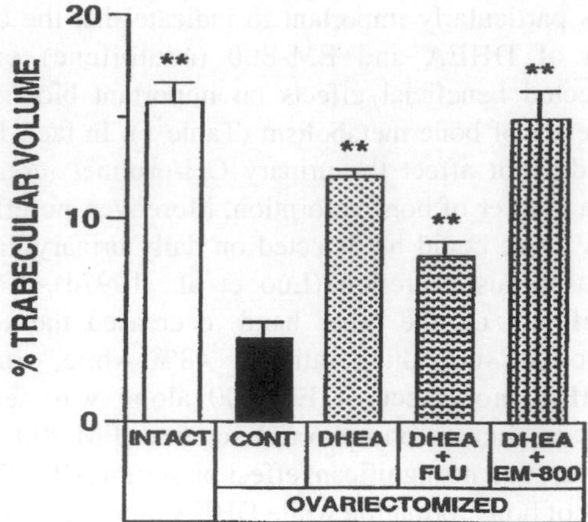

Figure 28 Effect of 12-month treatment with DHEA alone or in combination with flutamide or EM-800 (acolbifene) on trabecular bone volume in ovariectomized rats. Intact animals are added as additional controls. Data are presented as mean ± SEM $^{**}p < 0.01$ versus OVX control. *Abbreviations*: DHEA, dehydroepiandrosterone; OVX, ovariectomized. *Source*: From Luo et al. (1997).

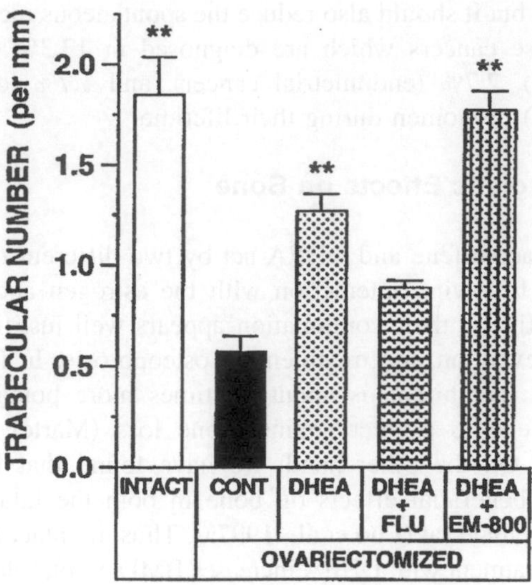

Figure 29 Effect of 12-month treatment with DHEA alone or in combination with flutamide or EM-800 (acolbifene) on trabecular number in ovariectomized rats. Intact animals are added as additional controls. Data are presented as mean ± SEM $^{**}p < 0.01$ versus OVX control. *Abbreviations*: DHEA, dehydroepiandrosterone; OVX, ovariectomized. *Source*: From Luo et al. (1997).

Importantly, the combination of EM-800 and DHEA in OVX rats treated for 12 months had beneficial effects on bone morphometry. Trabecular bone volume is particularly important for bone strength and to prevent bone fractures. Thus, in the above-mentioned study, trabecular bone volume of the tibia increased from 4.1 ± 0.7% in OVX rats to 11.9 ± 0.6% ($p < 0.01$) with DHEA alone, while the addition of EM-800 to DHEA further increased trabecular bone volume to 14.7 ± 1.4%, a value similar to that found in intact controls (Fig. 28).

From a value of 0.57 ± 0.08 per millimeter in OVX rats, treatment with DHEA resulted in a 137% increase in trabecular bone number compared with OVX controls. The stimulatory effect of DHEA thus reached 1.27 ± 0.1 per millimeter, while simultaneous treatment with EM-800 and DHEA resulted in an additional 28% increase in trabecular bone number ($p < 0.01$) compared with that achieved by DHEA alone (Fig. 29). Similarly, the addition of EM-800 to DHEA treatment resulted in an additional 15% ($p < 0.05$) decrease in trabecular bone separation, compared with the effect achieved with DHEA alone, thus leading to values not different from those seen in intact controls.

As complement to the numerical data presented in Figures 28 and 29, Figure 30 illustrates the increase in trabecular bone volume in the proximal tibia metaphysis induced by DHEA in OVX-treated animals (Fig. 30C) compared with OVX controls (Fig. 30B), as well as the partial inhibition of the stimulatory effect of DHEA after the addition of FLU to DHEA treatment (Fig. 30D). On the other hand, administration of DHEA in combination with EM-800 resulted in a complete prevention of the ovariectomy-induced osteopenia (Fig. 30E), the trabecular bone volume being comparable to that seen in intact controls (Fig. 30A).

The bone loss observed at menopause in women is believed to be related to an increase in the rate of bone resorption, which is not fully compensated by the secondary increase in bone formation. In fact, the parameters of both bone formation and bone resorption are increased in osteoporosis and both bone resorption and formation are inhibited by ERT. The inhibitory effect of estrogen replacement on bone formation is thus believed to result from a coupled mechanism between bone resorption and bone formation, such that the primary estrogen-induced reduction in bone resorption entrains a reduction in bone formation (Parfitt, 1984).

Cancellous bone strength and subsequent resistance to fracture do not only depend upon the total amount of cancellous bone but also on the trabecular microstructure, as determined by the number, size, and distribution of the trabeculae. The loss of ovarian function in postmenopausal women is accompanied by a significant decrease in total trabecular bone volume (Melsen et al., 1978; Vakamatsou et al., 1985), an effect mainly related to a decrease in the number and, to a lesser degree, in the width of trabeculae (Weinstein and Hutson, 1987).

In the above-summarized study, the androgenic stimulatory effect of DHEA was observed on almost all the bone histomorphometric parameters studied. DHEA thus resulted in a significant increase in trabecular bone

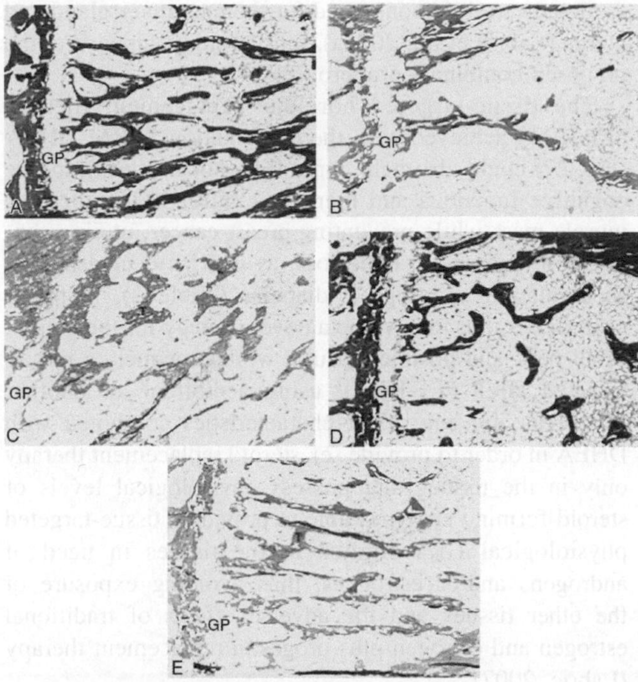

Figure 30 Proximal tibia metaphyses from intact control (**A**), ovariectomized control (**B**), and ovariectomized rats treated with DHEA alone (**C**) or in combination with flutamide (**D**) or EM-800 (acolbifene) (**E**). Note the reduced amount of trabecular bone (T) in ovariectomized control animals (**B**), and the significant increase in trabecular bone volume (T) induced after DHEA administration (**C**). The addition of flutamide to DHEA partially blocked the effect of DHEA on the trabecular bone volume (**D**), whereas the combination of DHEA and EM-800 provided complete protection against the ovariectomy-associated bone loss. Modified trichrome Masson-Goldner, magnification 80×. *Abbreviations*: DHEA, dehydroepiandrosterone; T, trabeculae; GP, growth plate. *Source*: From Luo et al. (1997).

volume as well as trabecular number, while it decreased the intertrabecular area.

In brief, the above-described data clearly demonstrate the beneficial effects of the combination of acolbifene and DHEA on the development of mammary carcinoma induced by DMBA as well as the protective effects of such a combination on bone mass, composition, and structure. Such data clearly suggest the additional beneficial effects of such a combination for the treatment and prevention of osteoporosis while improving the lipid profile and preventing breast and endometrial cancer.

Other Potential Beneficial Effects of the Combination Acolbifene DHEA

In addition to an increase in bone formation, DHEA has also been shown in postmenopausal women to stimulate vaginal maturation, and decrease skin dryness (Labrie et al., 1997c; Baulieu et al., 2000). DHEA has also been found to decrease fat mass, increase muscle mass, and decrease basal serum insulin and glucose (Diamond et al., 1996). It is also possible that SERMs could exert additional beneficial effects in postmenopausal women. It seems appropriate to mention some preclinical data obtained with acolbifene which could be very useful, if found in women. These data pertain to cholesterol and triglyceride lowering, reduced weight gain, and increased insulin sensitivity (Luo et al., 1997a; Picard et al., 2000; Lemieux et al., 2003, 2005). The inhibitory effect of acolbifene on serum cholesterol in the rat has been found to be due to an increase in the level of the LDL receptor in the liver (Lemieux et al., 2005). These effects of acolbifene on type 2 diabetes and fat accumulation would add to the already observed effects of DHEA in women (Diamond et al., 1996). Acolbifene has also been shown to increase NO synthesis in endothelial cells (Simoncini et al., 2002) (Fig. 27) (Table 2).

Table 2 Effect Already Observed or Expected in Women from DHEA, Acolbifene, and Their Combination

End organ-action	DHEA	Acolbifene	DHEA + acolbifene
Breast cancer	+$_{P}$	+C	+
Endometrial cancer	No effect, C	+$_{P}$	+
Bone mineral density	+$_{P}$+ C	+$_{P}$	+
Muscle mass and strength	+$_{P}$+ C	No effect	+
Cholesterol	No effect	+$_{P}$	+
Fat accumulation	+$_{P}$+ C	+$_{P}$	+
Type 2 diabetes	+$_{P}$+ C	+$_{P}$	+
Vaginal atrophy	+$_{P}$+ C	+^{P}	+
Hot flashes	+	TBD	TBD
Urine bleeding	+	+	+

Abbreviations: P, preclinical data; C, clinical data already observed; +, beneficial effect; TBD, to be determined.

CONCLUSION

Since, as mentioned above, breast cancer metastasizes early compared with prostate cancer (EBCTCG, 1998; Labrie et al., 2002, 2005a, 2007), prevention is essential in order to achieve a marked decrease in deaths from breast cancer. In fact, without an efficient, well-tolerated, and globally used prevention strategy, the majority of breast cancers will continue to be diagnosed at a true metastatic stage, despite being apparently clinically localized. For comparison purposes, in the field of prostate cancer, more than 99% of cancers can be diagnosed at the clinically localized stage with appropriate screening (Labrie et al., 1996b, 2002, 2005a). At that stage, cure is a possibility in most cases. Unfortunately, there is no marker for breast cancer equivalent to prostatic specific antigen for prostate cancer and, consequently, much too frequently (approximately 50% of cases), breast cancer has already spread at distant sites in the form of micrometastases at time of diagnosis, thus explaining the recurrence after apparently efficient local therapy by surgery and/or radiotherapy.

Knowing that estrogens play such a crucial role in breast cancer, the two most obvious choices for prevention of the disease are an aromatase inhibitor to block the formation of estrogens or a SERM to block the action of estrogens and, simultaneously, exert additional benefits of importance for women's health. Since the generalized estrogen ablation induced by aromatase inhibitors is unlikely to be acceptable for prevention of breast cancer due to the expected adverse effects in tissues other than the breast and uterus, it seems clear that major efforts should be devoted to the development of a SERM having a potent and pure antiestrogenic activity in the mammary gland and uterus while exerting beneficial effects in other systems of importance for women's health, especially the bones and metabolism. As mentioned above, all SERMs are different and detailed assays must be performed at the preclinical level to ensure the best chances of success of the new compounds chosen for use in the clinic. It should be remembered, however, that the clinical data provide the ultimate and only appropriate proof of efficacy and tolerance in a population with no apparent sign of cancer or disease.

While considering the need of a SERM to prevent breast and uterine cancer, it is clear that a SERM alone will not meet all the requirements of women after menopause. It thus appears important to develop an approach that takes into account the major decrease in sex steroids, including androgens, in postmenopausal women. With today's knowledge, DHEA, a tissue-targeted precursor of both androgens and estrogens (Labrie et al., 2005b) appears as an attractive if not the only available solution. In fact, estrogen formation from DHEA in peripheral tissues should not be an issue since the SERM can efficiently block the effect of estrogens in peripheral tissues as already well demonstrated for the mammary gland and uterus (Labrie et al., 2003a), thus strongly supporting the proposed combination approach.

The tissue-targeted hormone replacement therapy (TT-HRT) achieved with the combination SERM-DHEA (Fig. 27) could also help controlling hot flushes, improve cognitive functions and memory (Yaffe, 1998), increase muscle mass while preventing breast cancer, uterine cancer, ovarian cancer, bone loss, as well as decreasing fat accumulation and type 2 diabetes (Table 2). A major objective is thus to develop a novel strategy for the benefit of all peri- and postmenopausal women, namely a tissue-targeted HRT (TT-HRT), using acolbifene or another SERM having equivalent characteristics combined with DHEA in order to provide sex steroid replacement therapy only in the tissues that possess physiological levels of steroid-forming enzymes able to provide a tissue-targeted physiological HRT limited to the tissues in need of androgens and/or estrogens, thus avoiding exposure of the other tissues and the adverse effects of traditional estrogen and estrogen plus progestin replacement therapy (Labrie, 2007).

SUMMARY

Breast cancer is the most frequently diagnosed and the second cause of cancer death in women, thus making this cancer the most feared of all diseases in women. While the improvement in diagnosis and treatment of breast cancer has permitted a 12% decrease in deaths from this cancer during the last 15 years, much remains to be done, compared with the 33% decrease in deaths from prostate cancer during the same period. A possible explanation is that approximately 50% of breast cancers have already migrated as micrometastases at distant sites at time of diagnosis. Since cure of metastatic disease is an exception, it is essential to develop an efficient and well-tolerated strategy for breast cancer prevention, which would be acceptable for the general population of women. In this context, recent data have shown that estrogen plus progestin as well as estrogen alone used as replacement therapy increase the risk of breast cancer, thus indicating the need to find an alternative to traditional HRT if one wants to succeed in the fight against breast cancer.

The benefits of tamoxifen, raloxifene, fulvestrant, and aromatase inhibitors have clearly demonstrated the importance of blocking estrogens for breast cancer therapy. In terms of prevention, the adjuvant studies with tamoxifen and raloxifene have indicated that following five years of treatment, the incidence of breast cancer can be reduced by approximately 50%, thus leaving a large proportion of women at risk. Moreover, tamoxifen cannot be used for more than five years and it is unlikely that the more global estrogen blockade achieved with aromatase inhibitors will be acceptable for the long-term use required for prevention. The best hope for prevention of breast cancer appears to be a SERM having pure antiestrogenic activity in the breast and uterus.

While estrogens are well known to be the predominant stimulatory factor in the development and growth of the mammary gland and breast cancer, a long series of data indicate that androgens have an opposite inhibitory effect able to decrease or neutralize the action of estrogens. Accordingly, in women receiving testosterone in addition to estrogen, the stimulatory effect of estrogen on mammary gland proliferation was completely blocked. Moreover, clinical situations of hyperandrogenism such as the polycystic ovary syndrome and in athletes taking anabolic steroids, there is an inhibition of mammary gland development while the incidence of breast cancer is decreased by 50% in the polycystic ovary syndrome. In support of these data obtained in women, experiments performed in the monkey have clearly demonstrated that physiological doses of androgens completely inhibit mammary gland proliferation stimulated by estrogens.

In addition to the small quantity of androgens of ovarian origin, a major source of androgens in the mammary gland and other peripheral target tissues in women is provided by the adrenal precursor steroid DHEA, which can be converted at various levels into both androgens and/or estrogens in a tissue-specific manner according to local needs. The androgens made locally in peripheral tissues, including the breast, act in the same cells where their biosynthesis takes place by the mechanisms of intracrinology. Only a small and highly variable proportion of these androgens is released and is measurable in the circulation. These steroids are then inactivated and glucuronidated before being released into the circulation where they can be measured accurately by mass spectrometry. As a consequence, no correlation is found in women between the serum levels of testosterone and the sum of the serum concentration of the androgen metabolites, thus explaining why the epidemiological studies based on a correlation between serum testosterone and the risk of breast cancer are not valid. Moreover, as a second reason to invalidate the epidemiological studies, the radioimmunoassays used for measuring the low levels of testosterone found in the blood of women are not reliable. These conclusions are well supported by the measurements of androgens in the blood and in peripheral tissues where a complete lack of correlation is seen between the serum and tissue levels of androgens.

In clinical studies, androgens have been well demonstrated to inhibit breast cancer; as early as in 1939, testosterone and anabolic steroids have been used for the treatment of breast cancer in women with a success comparable to other hormonal therapies. However, the virilizing effects of androgens have limited the use of these compounds that have been replaced by the much better-tolerated tamoxifen. While the data obtained following administration of androgens are clear and straightforward, the epidemiological studies have shown equivocal results, which can be explained, as mentioned above, by the complete lack of reliability of serum testosterone as parameter of androgenic activity in women. Moreover, in all these studies, it should be noticed that a strong correlation is always found between serum E2, testosterone, and DHEA. Since E2 is the well-recognized and predominant stimulator of breast cancer, it becomes very difficult, or most likely impossible, to differentiate the effect of any steroid other than E2.

As strong support to the clinical studies showing that androgens and anabolic steroids have positive effects in women suffering from breast cancer, a long series of preclinical studies using human breast cancer cells in culture have demonstrated the direct and potent inhibitory effect of androgens on breast cancer cell proliferation, despite some reports, especially those using pharmaceutical concentrations of testosterone and DHEA, which have sometimes reported different results. The in vitro data are further strongly supported by a series of in vivo studies where androgens as well as DHEA have been found not only to prevent the development of carcinogen-induced mammary tumors in the rat and mouse but also to markedly inhibit the growth of established human tumors. Most interestingly, as found in in vitro studies, the combination of an androgen or DHEA with the novel SERM acolbifene have shown additive effects on the inhibition of the growth of human breast tumors in nude mice as well as on dimethylbenzenthracene-induced tumors in the rat.

Acolbifene is the most potent of all antiestrogens and it is the only compound having no intrinsic estrogenic stimulatory activity in the mammary gland and uterus. Most interestingly, this novel SERM has induced the disappearance of 60% of human breast cancer ZR-75-1 xenografts in nude mice, thus showing, for the first time, the tumorocidal action of antiestrogen therapy. On the basis of these data, acolbifene could reasonably be used for long periods of time without any risk of stimulation of the breast and uterus as found with tamoxifen.

Compared with traditional HRT, the advantage of DHEA, a tissue-specific precursor of androgens and estrogens, is that DHEA has no activity by itself. The precursor DHEA is transformed into androgens and/or estrogens in a tissue-specific manner according to the level of steroidogenic enzymes present in each tissue. Such a mechanism avoids exposing the other tissues to the active sex steroids, thus minimizing the risk of breast and uterine cancer found in the Women's Health Initiative and Million Women studies.

Since SERMs protect against bone loss and DHEA stimulates bone formation, it seems reasonable, as a novel approach of TT-HRT to use DHEA in combination with acolbifene or another SERM having similar properties. As an example of the benefits of such a combination, it has been shown in preclinical studies that the two compounds lead to synergistic effects on bone metabolism. Other expected beneficial effects of this combination are on muscle mass, vaginal atrophy, skin atrophy, fat accumulation, and type 2 diabetes.

Since, as mentioned above, breast cancer metastasizes early, prevention is essential if one wants to achieve a marked decrease in deaths from this disease. While the use of a SERM such as acolbifene having pure antiestrogenic activity in the breast and uterus is essential to prevent breast and uterine cancer, it is clear that such a compound used alone cannot meet all the requirements of women after menopause. It is thus important to combine with DHEA, a tissue-specific precursor of both androgens and estrogens and thus provide a tissue-targeted physiological HRT limited to the tissues in need of specific levels of each sex steroid, thus avoiding exposure of the other tissues and minimizing the adverse effects of traditional estrogen and estrogen plus progestin replacement therapy.

REFERENCES

Abraham GE. Ovarian and adrenal contribution to peripheral androgens during the menstrual cycle. J Clin Endocrinol Metab 1974; 39:340–346.

Adams JB. Control of secretion and the function of C19-D^5 steroids of the human adrenal gland. Mol Cell Endocrinol 1985; 41:1–17.

Adams J, Garcia M, Rochefort H. Estrogenic effects of physiological concentrations of 5-androstene-3-beta,17 beta-diol and its metabolism in MCF7 human breast cancer cells. Cancer Res 1981; 41:4720–4726.

Akaza H, Homma Y, Usami M, Hirao Y, Tsushima T, Okada K, Yokoyama M, Ohashi Y, Aso Y. Efficacy of primary hormone therapy for localized or locally advanced prostate cancer: results of a 10-year follow-up. BJU Int 2006; 98(3):573–579.

Archer DF, Furst K, Tipping D, Dain MP, Vandepol C. A randomized comparison of continuous combined transdermal delivery of estradiol-norethindrone acetate and estradiol alone for menopause. CombiPatch Study Group. Obstet Gynecol 1999; 94(4):498–503.

Arnst C. Why did prostate cancer death rates fall? Bus Week 2003; 3853:92.

Asselin J, Kelly PA, Caron MG, Labrie F. Control of hormone receptor levels and growth of 7,12-dimethylbenz(a)anthracene-induced mammary tumors by estrogens, progesterone and prolactin. Endocrinology 1977; 101:666–671.

Asselin J, Labrie F. Effects of estradiol and prolactin on steroid receptor levels in 7,12-dimethylbenz(a)anthracene-induced mammary tumors and uterus in the rat. J Steroid Biochem 1978; 9:1079–1082.

Baselga J, Llombart-Cussac A, Bellet M, Guillem-Porta V, Enas N, Krejcy K, Carrasco E, Kayitalire L, Kuta M, Lluch A, Vodvarka P, Kerbrat P, Namer M, Petruzelka L. Randomized, double-blind, multicenter trial comparing two doses of arzoxifene (LY353381) in hormone-sensitive advanced or metastatic breast cancer patients. Ann Oncol 2003; 14(9):1383–1390.

Baulieu EE, Thomas G, Legrain S, Lahlou N, Roger M, Debuire B, Faucounau V, Girard L, Hervy MP, Latour F, Leaud MC, Mokrane A, Pitti-Ferrandi H, Trivalle C, de Lacharriere O, Nouveau S, Rakoto-Arison B, Souberbielle JC, Raison J, Le Bouc Y, Raynaud A, Girerd X, Forette F. Dehydroepiandrosterone (DHEA), DHEA sulfate, and aging: contribution of the DHEAge Study to a sociobiomedical issue. Proc Natl Acad Sci U S A 2000; 97(8):4279–4284.

Baum M, Budzar AU, Cuzick J, Forbes J, Houghton JH, Klijn JG, Sahmoud T. Anastrozole alone or in combination with tamoxifen versus tamoxifen alone for adjuvant treatment of postmenopausal women with early breast cancer: first results of the ATAC randomised trial. Lancet 2002; 359(9324):2131–2139.

Beattie MS, Costantino JP, Cummings SR, Wickerham DL, Vogel VG, Dowsett M, Folkerd EJ, Willett WC, Wolmark N, Hankinson SE. Endogenous sex hormones, breast cancer risk, and tamoxifen response: an ancillary study in the NSABP Breast Cancer Prevention Trial (P-1). J Natl Cancer Inst 2006; 98(2):110–115.

Bélanger B, Bélanger A, Labrie F, Dupont A, Cusan L, Monfette G. Comparison of residual C-19 steroids in plasma and prostatic tissue of human, rat and guinea pig after castration: unique importance of extratesticular androgens in men. J Steroid Biochem 1989; 32:695–698.

Bélanger A, Brochu M, Cliche J. Levels of plasma steroid glucuronides in intact and castrated men with prostatic cancer. J Clin Endocrinol Metab 1986; 62:812–815.

Bélanger A, Candas B, Dupont A, Cusan L, Diamond P, Gomez JL, Labrie F. Changes in serum concentrations of conjugated and unconjugated steroids in 40- to 80-year-old men. J Clin Endocrinol Metab 1994; 79:1086–1090.

Bélanger A, Pelletier G, Labrie F, Barbier O, Chouinard S. Inactivation of androgens by UDP-glucuronosyltransferase enzymes in humans. Trends Endocrinol Metab 2003; 14:473–479.

Beral V, Bull D, Reeves G. Endometrial cancer and hormone-replacement therapy in the Million Women Study. Lancet 2005; 365(9470):1543–1551.

Bergman L, Beelen ML, Gallee MP, Hollema H, Benraadt J, van Leeuwen FE. Risk and prognosis of endometrial cancer after tamoxifen for breast cancer. Comprehensive Cancer Centres' ALERT Group. Assessment of liver and endometrial cancer risk following tamoxifen. Lancet 2000; 356(9233):881–887.

Berrino F, Muti P, Micheli A, Bolelli G, Krogh V, Sciajno R, Pisani P, Panico S, Secreto G. Serum sex hormone levels after menopause and subsequent breast cancer. J Natl Cancer Inst 1996; 88(5):291–296.

Bieche I, Parfait B, Tozlu S, Lidereau R, Vidaud M. Quantitation of androgen receptor gene expression in sporadic breast tumors by real-time RT-PCR: evidence that MYC is an AR-regulated gene. Carcinogenesis 2001; 22(9):1521–1526.

Birrell SN, Bentel JM, Hickey TE, Ricciardelli C, Weger MA, Horsfall DJ, Tilley WD. Androgens induce divergent proliferative responses in human breast cancer cell lines. J Steroid Biochem Mol Biol 1995; 52(5):459–467.

Birrell SN, Hall RE, Tilley WD. Role of the androgen receptor in human breast cancer. J Mammary Gland Biol Neoplasia 1998; 3(1):95–103.

Boccuzzi G, Aragno M, Brignardello E, Tamagno E, Conti G, Di Monaco M, Racca S, Danni O, Di Carlo F. Opposite effects of dehydroepiandrosterone on the growth of 7, 12-dimethylbenz(a)anthracene-induced rat mammary carcinomas. Anticancer Res 1992a; 12:1479–1484.

Boccuzzi G, Brignardello E, di Monaco M, Forte C, Leonardi L, Pizzini A. Influence of dehydroepiandrosterone and 5-en-androstene-3 beta, 17 beta-diol on the growth of MCF-7 human breast cancer cells induced by 17 beta-estradiol. Anticancer Res 1992b; 12(3):799–803.

Boccuzzi G, Di Monaco M, Brignardello E, Leonardi L, Gatto V, Pizzini A, Gallo M. Dehydroepiandrosterone antiestrogenic action through androgen receptor in MCF-7 human breast cancer cell line. Anticancer Res 1993; 13(6A):2267–2272.

Bonneterre J, Thurlimann B, Robertson JF, Krzakowski M, Mauriac L, Koralewski P, Vergote I, Webster A, Steinberg M, von Euler M. Anastrozole versus tamoxifen as first-line therapy for advanced breast cancer in 668 postmenopausal women: results of the Tamoxifen or Arimidex Randomized Group Efficacy and Tolerability study. J Clin Oncol 2000; 18(22):3748–3757.

Braithwaite RS, Chlebowski RT, Lau J, George S, Hess R, Col NF. Meta-analysis of vascular and neoplastic events associated with tamoxifen. J Gen Intern Med 2003; 18(11):937–947.

Brys M, Wojcik M, Romanowicz-Makowska H, Krajewska WM. Androgen receptor status in female breast cancer: RT-PCR and Western blot studies. J Cancer Res Clin Oncol 2002; 128(2):85–90.

Brzozowski AM, Pike AC, Dauter Z, Hubbard RE, Bonn T, Engstrom O, Ohman L, Greene GL, Gustafsson JA, Carlquist M. Molecular basis of agonism and antagonism in the oestrogen receptor. Nature 1997; 389(6652):753–758.

Bulbrook RD, Hayward JL, Spicer CC. Relation between urinary androgen and corticoid excretion and subsequent breast cancer. Lancet 1971; 2:395–398.

Burak WE, Quinn AL Jr., Farrar WB, Brueggemeier RW. Androgens influence estrogen-induced responses in human breast carcinoma cells through cytochrome P450 aromatase. Breast Cancer Res Treat 1997; 44(1):57–64.

Burger HG. Should testosterone be added to estrogen-progestin therapy for breast protection? Menopause 2007; 14(2): 159–162.

Burgess HE, Shousha S. An immunohistochemical study of the long-term effects of androgen administration on female-to-male transsexual breast: a comparison with normal female breast and male breast showing gynaecomastia. J Pathol 1993; 170(1):37–43.

Buzdar A, O'Shaughnessy JA, Booser DJ, Pippen JE, Jones SE Jr., Munster PN, Peterson P, Melemed AS, Winer E, Hudis C. Phase II, randomized, double-blind study of two dose levels of arzoxifene in patients with locally advanced or metastatic breast cancer. J Clin Oncol 2003; 21(6): 1007–1014.

Calhoun KE, Pommier RF, Muller P, Fletcher WS, Toth-Fejel S. Dehydroepiandrosterone sulfate causes proliferation of estrogen receptor-positive breast cancer cells despite treatment with fulvestrant. Arch Surg 2003; 138(8):879–883.

Caubet JF, Tosteson TD, Dong EW, Naylon EM, Whiting GW, Ernstoff MS, Ross SD. Maximum androgen blockade in advanced prostate cancer: a meta-analysis of published randomized controlled trials using nonsteroidal antiandrogens. Urology 1997; 49:71–78.

Cauley JA, Lucas FL, Kuller LH, Stone K, Browner W, Cummings SR. Elevated serum estradiol and testosterone concentrations are associated with a high risk for breast cancer. Study of Osteoporotic Fractures Research Group. Ann Intern Med 1999; 130(4 pt 1):270–277.

Chalbos D, Haagensen DE, Parish T, Rochefort H. Identification and androgen regulation of two proteins released by T47D human breast cancer cells. Cancer Res 1987; 47:2787–2792.

Cheng Y, Prusoff WH. Relationship between the inhibition constant (Ki) and the concentration of inhibitor which causes 50 per cent inhibition (I50) on an enzymatic reaction. Biochem Pharmacol 1973; 22:3099–3108.

Christiansen C, Christensen MS, Larsen NE, Transbol IB. Pathophysiological mechanisms of estrogen effect on bone metabolism. Dose-response relationships in early postmenopausal women. J Clin Endocrinol Metab 1982; 55:1124–1130.

Clarke R, Leonessa F, Welch JN, Skaar TC. Cellular and molecular pharmacology of antiestrogen action and resistance. Pharmacol Rev 2001; 53(1):25–71.

Clemens JA, Bennett DR, Black LJ, Jones CD. Effects of a new antiestrogen, keoxifene (LY156758), on growth of carcinogen-induced mammary tumors and on LH and prolactin levels. Life Sci 1983; 32(25):2869–2875.

Coleman RE, Banks LM, Hall E, Price D, Girgis S, Bliss JM, Coombes RC. Intergroup Exemestane Study: one year results of the bone sub-protocol. Breast Cancer Res Treat 2004; 88(1):S35.

Conde I, Alfaro JM, Fraile B, Ruiz A, Paniagua R, Arenas MI. DAX-1 expression in human breast cancer: comparison with estrogen receptors ER-alpha, ER-beta and androgen receptor status. Breast Cancer Res 2004; 6(3):R140–R148.

Coombes RC, Hall E, Gibson LJ, Paridaens R, Jassem J, Delozier T, Jones SE, Alvarez I, Bertelli G, Ortmann O, Coates AS, Bajetta E, Dodwell D, Coleman RE, Fallowfield LJ, Mickiewicz E, Andersen J, Lonning PE, Cocconi G, Stewart A, Stuart N, Snowdon CF, Carpentieri M, Massimini G, Bliss JM. A randomized trial of exemestane after two to three years of tamoxifen therapy in postmenopausal women with primary breast cancer. N Engl J Med 2004; 350(11):1081–1092.

Cooperative Breast Cancer Group. Testosterone propionate therapy of breast cancer. J Am Med Ass 1964; 188: 1069–1072.

Cooperberg MR, Grossfeld GD, Lubeck DP, Carroll PR. National practice patterns and time trends in androgen ablation for localized prostate cancer. J Natl Cancer Inst 2003; 95(13):981–999.

Costlow ME, Buschow RA, McGuire WL. Prolactin receptors and androgen-induced regression of 7,12-dimethylbenz(a) anthracene-induced mammary carcinoma. Cancer Res 1976; 36(9 pt 1):3324–3329.

Couillard S, Labrie C, Bélanger A, Candas B, Pouliot F, Labrie F. Effect of dehydroepiandrosterone and the antiestrogen EM-800 on the growth of human ZR-75-1 breast cancer xenografts. J Natl Cancer Inst 1998; 90:772–778.

Couture P, Thériault C, Simard J, Labrie F. Androgen receptor-mediated stimulation of 17b-hydroxysteroid dehydrogenase activity by dihydrotestosterone and medroxyprogesterone acetate in ZR-75-1 human breast cancer cells. Endocrinology 1993; 132:179–185.

Cowie AT, Folley SJ. The mammary gland and lactation. In: Young WC, ed. Sex and Internal Secretion. Baltimore: Williams and Wilkins, 1961:590–641.

Cox DG, Blanche H, Pearce CL, Calle EE, Colditz GA, Pike MC, Albancs D, Allcn NE, Amiano P, Berglund G, Boeing H, Buring J, Burtt N, Canzian F, Chanock S, Clavel-Chapelon F, Feigelson HS, Freedman M, Haiman CA, Hankinson SE, Henderson BE, Hoover R, Hunter DJ, Kaaks R, Kolonel L, Kraft P, Lemarchand L, Lund E, Palli D, Peeters PH, Riboli E, Stram DO, Thun M, Tjonneland A, Trichopoulos D, Yeager M. A comprehensive analysis of the androgen receptor gene and risk of breast cancer: results from the National Cancer Institute Breast and Prostate Cancer Cohort Consortium (BPC3). Breast Cancer Res 2006; 8(5):R54.

Crawford ED, Eisenberger MA, McLeod DG, Spaulding JT, Benson R, Dorr FA, Blumenstein BA, Davis MA, Goodman PJ. A controlled trial of leuprolide with and without flutamide in prostatic carcinoma. N Engl J Med 1989; 321(7):419–424.

Cummings SR, Duong T, Kenyon E, Cauley JA, Whitehead M, Krueger KA. Serum estradiol level and risk of breast cancer during treatment with raloxifene. JAMA 2002; 287(2): 216–220.

Cummings SR, Eckert S, Krueger KA, Grady D, Powles TJ, Cauley JA, Norton L, Nickelsen T, Bjarnason NH, Morrow M, Lippman ME, Black D, Glusman JE, Costa A, Jordan VC. The effect of raloxifene on risk of breast cancer in postmenopausal women: results from the MORE randomized trial. Multiple Outcomes of Raloxifene Evaluation. JAMA 1999; 281(23):2189–2197.

Cuzick J, Baum M. Tamoxifen and contralateral breast cancer. Lancet 1985; 2(8449):282.

Cuzick J, Forbes J, Edwards R, Baum M, Cawthorn S, Coates A, Hamed A, Howell A, Powles T. First results from the International Breast Cancer Intervention Study (IBIS-I): a randomised prevention trial. Lancet 2002; 360(9336): 817–824.

Cuzick J, Powles T, Veronesi U, Forbes J, Edwards R, Ashley S, Boyle P. Overview of the main outcomes in breast-cancer prevention trials. Lancet 2003; 361(9354):296–300.

Dao TL, Chistakos SS, Varela R. Biochemical characterization of carcinogen-induced mammary hyperplastic aveolar nodule and tumor in the rat. Cancer Res 1975; 35(5):1128–1134.

Dauvois S, Geng CS, Lévesque C, Mérand Y, Labrie F. Additive inhibitory effects of an androgen and the antiestrogen EM-170 on estradiol-stimulated growth of human ZR-75-1 breast tumors in athymic mice. Cancer Res 1991; 51:3131–3135.

Dauvois S, Li S, Martel C, Labrie F. Inhibitory effect of androgens on DMBA-induced mammary carcinoma in the rat. Breast Cancer Res Treat 1989; 14:299–306.

Davidson NE, Lippman ME. The role of estrogens in growth regulation of breast cancer. Crit Rev Oncog 1989; 1:89–111.

de Launoit Y, Dauvois S, Dufour M, Simard J, Labrie F. Inhibition of cell cycle kinetics and proliferation by the androgen 5 alpha-dihydrotestosterone and antiestrogen N,n-butyl-N-methyl-11-[16′ alpha-chloro-3′,17 beta-dihydroxy-estra-1′,3′,5′-(10′)triene-7′ alpha-yl] undecanamide in human breast cancer ZR-75-1 cells. Cancer Res 1991a; 51(11):2797–2802.

de Launoit Y, Veilleux R, Dufour M, Simard J, Labrie F. Characteristics of the biphasic action of androgens and of the potent antiproliferative effects of the new pure antiestrogen EM-139 on cell cycle kinetic parameters in LNCaP human prostatic cancer cells. Cancer Res 1991b; 51(19):5165–5170.

Denis L, Carnelro de Moura J, Bono A, Sylvester R, Whelan P, Newling D, Depauw M. Goserelin acetate and flutamide vs. bilateral orchiectomy: a phase III EORTC trial (30853). EORTC GU Group and EORTC Data Center. Urology 1993; 42:119–129.

Diamond P, Cusan L, Gomez JL, Bélanger A, Labrie F. Metabolic effects of 12-month percutaneous DHEA replacement therapy in postmenopausal women. J Endocrinol 1996; 150:S43–S50.

Dimitrakakis C, Jones RA, Liu A, Bondy CA. Breast cancer incidence in postmenopausal women using testosterone in addition to usual hormone therapy. Menopause 2004; 11(5):531–535.

Dimitrakakis C, Zhou J, Wang J, Belanger A, LaBrie F, Cheng C, Powell D, Bondy C. A physiologic role for testosterone in limiting estrogenic stimulation of the breast. Menopause 2003; 10(4):292–298.

Dorgan JF, Longcope C, Stephenson HE Jr., Falk RT, Miller R, Franz C, Kahle L, Campbell WS, Tangrea JA, Schatzkin A. Relation of prediagnostic serum estrogen and androgen levels to breast cancer risk. Cancer Epidemiol Biomarkers Prev 1996; 5(7):533–539.

Dorgan JF, Stanczyk FZ, Longcope C, Stephenson HE Jr., Chang L, Miller R, Franz C, Falk RT, Kahle L. Relationship of serum dehydroepiandrosterone (DHEA), DHEA sulfate, and 5-androstene-3 beta, 17 beta-diol to risk of breast cancer in postmenopausal women. Cancer Epidemiol Biomarkers Prev 1997; 6(3):177–181.

Dowsett M, Cuzick J, Howell A, Jackson I. Pharmacokinetics of anastrozole and tamoxifen alone, and in combination, during adjuvant endocrine therapy for early breast cancer in postmenopausal women: a sub-protocol of the 'Arimidex and tamoxifen alone or in combination' (ATAC) trial. Br J Cancer 2001; 85(3): 317–324.

Dufort I, Rheault P, Huang XF, Soucy P, Luu-The V. Characteristics of a highly labile human type 5 17beta-hydroxysteroid dehydrogenase. Endocrinology 1999; 140(2):568–574.

Dumont M, Dauvois S, Simard J, Garcia T, Schachter B, Labrie F. Antagonism between estrogens and androgens on GCDFP-15 gene expression in ZR-75-1 cells and correlation between GCDFP-15 and estrogen as well as progesterone receptor expression in human breast cancer. J Steroid Biochem 1989; 34:397–402.

EBCTCG. Tamoxifen for early breast cancer: an overview of the randomised trials. Early Breast Cancer Trialists' Collaborative Group. Lancet 1998; 351(9114):1451–1467.

EBCTCG. Effects of chemotherapy and hormonal therapy for early breast cancer on recurrence and 15-year survival: an overview of the randomised trials. Lancet 2005; 365(9472):1687–1717.

Edery M, Goussard J, Dehennin L, Scholler R, Reiffsteck J, Drosdowsky MA. Endogenous oestradiol-17beta concentration in breast tumours determined by mass fragmentography and by radioimmunoassay: relationship to receptor content. Eur J Cancer 1981; 17(1):115–120.

Egawa M, Misaki T, Imao T, Yokoyama O, Fuse H, Suzuki K, Namiki M. Retrospective study on stage B prostate cancer in the Hokuriku District, Japan. Int J Urol 2004; 11(5): 304–309.

Ekena K, Katzenellenbogen JA, Katzenellenbogen BS. Determinants of ligand specificity of estrogen receptor-alpha: estrogen versus androgen discrimination. J Biol Chem 1998; 273(2):693–699.

Eliassen AH, Missmer SA, Tworoger SS, Hankinson SE. Endogenous steroid hormone concentrations and risk of breast cancer: does the association vary by a woman's predicted breast cancer risk? J Clin Oncol 2006; 24 (12):1823–1830.

Engel LW, Young NA, Tralka TS, Lippman ME, O'Brien SJ, Joyce MJ. Establishment and characterization of three new continuous cell lines derived from human breast carcinomas. Cancer Res 1978; 38(10):3352–3364.

Fels E. Treatment of breast cancer with testosterone propionate. A preliminary report. J Clin Endocrinol 1944; 4:121–125.

Fisher B, Costantino JP, Lawrence Wickerham D, Redmond CK, Kavanah M, Cronin WM, Vogel V, Robidoux A, Dimitrov N, Atkins J, Daly M, Wieand S, Tan-Chiu E, Ford L, Wolmark N. Tamoxifen for prevention of breast cancer: report of the national surgical adjuvant breast and bowel project P-1 study. J Natl Cancer Inst 1998; 90:1371–1388.

Fisher B, Costantino C, Redmond ER, Fisher D, Wickerham L, Cronin WM, NSABP Contributors. Endometrial cancer in tamoxifen-treated breast cancer patients: findings from the National Surgical Adjuvant Breast and Bowel Project (NSABP) B-14. J Natl Cancer Inst 1994; 86:527–537.

Fisher B, Costantino JP, Wickerham DL, Cecchini RS, Cronin WM, Robidoux A, Bevers TB, Kavanah MT, Atkins JN, Margolese RG, Runowicz CD, James JM, Ford LG, Wolmark N. Tamoxifen for the prevention of breast cancer: current status of the National Surgical Adjuvant Breast and Bowel Project P-1 study. J Natl Cancer Inst 2005; 97(22):1652–1662.

Fisher B, Dignam J, Bryant J, DeCillis A, Wickerham DL, Wolmark N, Costantino J, Redmond C, Fisher ER, Bowman DM, Deschenes L, Dimitrov NV, Margolese RG, Robidoux A, Shibata H, Terz J, Paterson AHG, Feldman MI, Farrar W, Evans J, Lickley HL. Five versus more than five years of tamoxifen therapy for breast cancer patients with negative lymph nodes and estrogen-positive tumors. J Natl Cancer Inst 1996; 88:1529–1542.

Fisher B, Dignam J, Bryant J, Wolmark N. Five versus more than five years of tamoxifen for lymph node-negative breast cancer: updated findings from the National Surgical Adjuvant Breast and Bowel Project B-14 randomized trial. J Natl Cancer Inst 2001; 93(9):684–690.

Fisher B, Powles TJ, Pritchard KJ. Tamoxifen for the prevention of breast cancer. Eur J Cancer 2000; 36(2):142–150.

Fishman J, Nisselbaum JS, Menendez-Botet CJ, Schwartz MK. Estrone and estradiol content in human breast tumors: relationship to estradiol receptors. J Steroid Biochem 1977; 8(8):893–896.

Forsyth IA, Jones EA. Organ culture of mammary gland and placenta in the study of hormone action and placental secretion. In: Balls M, Monnickendam MA, eds. Organ Culture in Biomedical Research. England, UK: Cambridge University Press, 1976:201–221.

Frasor J, Stossi F, Danes JM, Komm B, Lyttle CR, Katzenellenbogen BS. Selective estrogen receptor modulators: discrimination of agonistic versus antagonistic activities by gene expression profiling in breast cancer cells. Cancer Res 2004; 64(4): 1522–1533.

Gammon MD, Thompson WD. Polycystic ovaries and the risk of breast cancer. Am J Epidemiol 1991; 134(8):818–824.

Garcia M, Rochefort H. Androgen effects mediated by estrogen receptor in 7,12-dimethylbenz(a)anthracene-induced rat mammary tumors. Cancer Res 1978; 38:3922–3929.

Gatto V, Aragno M, Gallo M, Tamagno E, Martini A, Di Monaco M, Brignardello E, Boccuzzi G. Dehydroepiandrosterone inhibits the growth of DMBA-induced rat mammary carcinoma via the androgen receptor. Oncol Rep 1998; 5(1):241–243.

Gauthier S, Caron B, Cloutier J, Dory YL, Favre A, Larouche D, Mailhot J, Ouellet C, Schwerdtfeger A, Leblanc G, Martel C, Simard J, Mérand Y, Bélanger A, Labrie C, Labrie F. (S)-(+)-4-[7-(2,2-dimethyl-1-oxopropoxy)-4-methyl-2-[4-[2-(1-piperidinyl)-ethoxy]phenyl]-2H-1-benzopyran-3-yl]-phenyl 2,2-dimethylpropanoate (EM-800): a highly potent, specific, and orally active nonsteroidal antiestrogen. J Med Chem 1997; 40:2117–2122.

Gayosso V, Montano LF, Lopez-Marure R. DHEA-induced antiproliferative effect in MCF-7 cells is androgen- and estrogen receptor-independent. Cancer J 2006; 12(2): 160–165.

Geisler J. Breast cancer tissue estrogens and their manipulation with aromatase inhibitors and inactivators. J Steroid Biochem Mol Biol 2003; 86(3–5):245–253.

Geisler J, Anker G, Dowsett M, Lonning PE. Letrozole supresses plasma estrogen levels in breast cancer patients more completely than anastrazole. Proc Am Assoc Clin Oncol 2000; 19:A102.

Geisler J, Detre S, Berntsen H, Ottestad L, Lindtjorn B, Dowsett M, Einstein Lonning P. Influence of neoadjuvant anastrozole (Arimidex) on intratumoral estrogen levels and proliferation markers in patients with locally advanced breast cancer. Clin Cancer Res 2001; 7(5):1230–1236.

Gelfand MM. It might be wise to consider adding androgen to the estrogen or estrogen-progestin regimens in the appropriate patients. Menopause 2004; 11(5):505–507.

Geriani RL. Fetal mammary gland differentiation in vitro in response to hormones I. Morphological findings. Dev Biol 1970; 21:506–529.

Giguere Y, Dewailly E, Brisson J, Ayotte P, Laflamme N, Demers A, Forest VI, Dodin S, Robert J, Rousseau F. Short polyglutamine tracts in the androgen receptor are protective against breast cancer in the general population. Cancer Res 2001; 61(15):5869–5874.

Gordan GS. Anabolic-androgenic steroids. In: Eichler O, Heffter A, Heubner W, eds. Handbook of Experimental Pharmacology. Berlin, New York: Springer-Verlag, 1976:499–513.

Gordan GS, Halden A, Horn Y, Fuery JJ, Parsons RJ, Walter RM. Calusterone (7b,17a-dimethyltestosterone) as primary and secondary therapy of advanced breast cancer. Oncology 1973; 28(2):138–146.

Gordon GB, Newitt JA, Shantz LM, Weng DE, Talalay P. Inhibition of the conversion of 3T3 fibroblast clones to adipocytes by dehydroepiandrosterone and related anticarcinogenic steroids. Cancer Res 1986; 46(7):3389–3395.

Goss P. Anti-aromatase agents in the treatment and prevention of breast cancer. Cancer Control 2002; 9(suppl 2):2–8.

Goss PE, Ingle JN, Martino S, Robert NJ, Muss HB, Piccart MJ, Castiglione M, Tu D, Shepherd LE, Pritchard KI, Livingston RB, Davidson NE, Norton L, Perez EA, Abrams JS, Therasse P, Palmer MJ, Pater JL. A randomized trial of letrozole in postmenopausal women after five years of tamoxifen therapy for early-stage breast cancer. N Engl J Med 2003; 19:1793–1802.

Gottardis MM, Robinson SP, Satyaswaroop PG, Jordan VC. Contrasting actions of tamoxifen on endometrial and breast tumor growth in the athymic mouse. Cancer Res 1988; 48:812–815.

Griffiths K, Jones D, Cameron EHD, Gleave EN, Forrest APM. Transformation of steroids by mammary cancer tissue. In: Dao TL, ed. Estrogen Target Tissues and Neoplasia. Chicago: University of Chicago Press, 1972:151–162.

Grino PB, Griffin JE, Cushard WG Jr., Wilson JD. A mutation of the androgen receptor associated with partial androgen resistance, familial gynecomastia, and fertility. J Clin Endocrinol Metab 1988; 66(4):754–761.

Gronemeyer H, Benhamou B, Berry M, Bocquel MT, Gofflo D, Garcia T, Lerouge T, Metzger D, Meyer ME, Tora L, Vergezac A, Chambon P. Mechanisms of antihormone action. J Steroid Biochem Mol Biol 1992; 41:217–221.

Gutman M, Couillard S, Labrie F, Candas B, Labrie C. Effect of treatment sequence with radiotherapy and the antiestrogen EM-800 on the growth of ZR-75-1 human mammary carcinoma in nude mice. Int J Cancer 2003; 103(2):268–276.

Gutman M, Couillard S, Roy J, Labrie F, Candas B, Labrie C. Comparison of the effects of EM-652 (SCH 57068), tamoxifen, toremifene, droloxifene, idoxifene, GW-5638 and raloxifene on the growth of human ZR-75-1 breast tumors in nude mice. Int J Cancer 2002; 99:273–278.

Haiman CA, Brown M, Hankinson SE, Spiegelman D, Colditz GA, Willett WC, Kantoff PW, Hunter DJ. The androgen receptor CAG repeat polymorphism and risk of breast cancer in the Nurses Health Study. Cancer Res 2002; 62(4): 1045–1049.

Hall M, Bates S, Peters G. Evidence for different modes of action of cyclin-dependent kinase inhibitors: p15 and p16 bind to kinases, p21 and p27 bind to cyclins. Oncogene 1995; 11:1581–1588.

Hankinson SE, Willett WC, Manson JE, Colditz GA, Hunter DJ, Spiegelman D, Barbieri RL, Speizer FE. Plasma sex steroid hormone levels and risk of breast cancer in postmenopausal women. J Natl Cancer Inst 1998; 90(17):1292–1299.

Helzlsouer KJ, Gordon GB, Alberg AJ, Bush TL, Comstock GW. Relationship of prediagnostic serum levels of dehydroepiandrosterone and dehydroepiandrosterone sulfate to the risk of developing premenopausal breast cancer. Cancer Res 1992; 52(1):1–4.

Hofling M, Hirschberg AL, Skoog L, Tani E, Hagerstrom T, von Schoultz B. Testosterone inhibits estrogen/progestogen-induced breast cell proliferation in postmenopausal women. Menopause 2007; 14(2):183–190.

Horwitz KB, Zava DT, Thilager AK, Jensen ET, McGuire WL. Steroid receptor analyses of nonhuman breast cancer cell lines. Cancer Res 1978; 38:2434–2439.

Howell A, Robertson JF, Abram P, Lichinitser MR, Elledge R, Bajetta E, Watanabe T, Morris C, Webster A, Dimery I, Osborne CK. Comparison of fulvestrant versus tamoxifen for the treatment of advanced breast cancer in postmenopausal women previously untreated with endocrine therapy: a multinational, double-blind, randomized trial. J Clin Oncol 2004; 22(9):1605–1613.

Howell A, Robertson J, Quaresma Albano J, Aschermannova A, Mauriac L, Kleeberg UR, Vergote I, Erikstein B, Webster A, Morris C. Fulvestrant, formerly ICI 182,780, is as effective as anastrozole in postmenopausal women with advanced breast cancer progression after prior endocrine treatment. J Clin Oncol 2002; 20(16):3396–3403.

Huggins C, Briziarelli G, Sutton HJ. Rapid induction of mammary carcinoma in the rat and the influence of hormone on the tumors. J Exp Med 1959; 109:25–42.

Ingle JN, Twito DI, Schaid DJ, Cullinan SA, Krook JE, Mailliard JA, Tschetter LK, Long HJ, Gerstner JG, Windschitl HE, Levitt R, Pfeifle DM. Combination hormonal therapy with tamoxifen plus fluoxymesterone versus tamoxifen alone in postmenopausal women with metastatic breast cancer. A phase II study. Cancer 1991; 67:886–891.

Isaksson E, von Schoultz E, Odlind V, Soderqvist G, Csemiczky G, Carlstrom K, Skoog L, von Schoultz B. Effects of oral contraceptives on breast epithelial proliferation. Breast Cancer Res Treat 2001; 65(2):163–169.

Isola JJ. Immunohistochemical demonstration of androgen receptor in breast cancer and its relationship to other prognostic factors. J Pathol 1993; 170(1):31–35.

Jaiyesimi IA, Buzdar AU, Decker DA, Hortobagyi GN. Use of tamoxifen for breast cancer: twenty-eight years later. J Clin Oncol 1995; 13(2):513–529.

Jakesz R, Jonat W, Gnant M, Mittlboeck M, Greil R, Tausch C, Hilfrich J, Kwasny W, Menzel C, Samonigg H, Seifert M, Gademann G, Kaufmann M, Wolfgang J. Switching of postmenopausal women with endocrine-responsive early breast cancer to anastrozole after 2 years' adjuvant tamoxifen: combined results of ABCSG trial 8 and ARNO 95 trial. Lancet 2005; 366(9484):455–462.

Jayo MJ, Register TC, Hughes CL, Blas-Machado U, Sulistiawati E, Borgerink H, Johnson CS. Effects of an oral contraceptive combination with or without androgen on mammary tissues: a study in rats. J Soc Gynecol Investig 2000; 7(4):257–265.

Jelovac D, Macedo L, Goloubeva OG, Handratta V, Brodie AM. Additive antitumor effect of aromatase inhibitor letrozole and antiestrogen fulvestrant in a postmenopausal breast cancer model. Cancer Res 2005; 65(12):5439–5444.

Jemal A, Siegel R, Ward E, Murray T, Xu J, Thun M. Cancer Statistics, 2007. CA Cancer J Clin 2007; 57:43–66.

Johannessen DC, Engan T, Di Salle E, Zurlo MG, Paolini J, Ornati G, Piscitelli G, Kvinnsland S, Lonning PE. Endocrine and clinical effects of exemestane (PNU 155971), a novel steroidal aromatase inhibitor, in postmenopausal breast cancer patients: a phase I study. Clin Cancer Res 1997; 3(7):1101–1108.

Johnston SR. 2005 Endocrinology and hormone therapy in breast cancer: selective oestrogen receptor modulators and down-regulators for breast cancer—have they lost their way? Breast Cancer Res 7(3):119–130.

Jones J, Vukelja S, Cantrell J. A planned comparison of menopausal symptoms during year 1 in patients receiving either examestane or tamoxifene in a double-blind adjuvant hormonal study. Breast Cancer Res Treat 2003; 82:S31.

Jordan VC. Effect of tamoxifen (ICI 46,474) on initiation and growth of DMBA-induced rat mammary carcinoma. Eur J Cancer 1976; 12:419–424.

Jordan VC. Use of the DMBA-induced rat mammary carcinoma system for the evaluation of tamoxifen as a potential adjuvant therapy. Rev Endocr Relat Cancer 1978; suppl 1:49–55.

Kaaks R, Berrino F, Key T, Rinaldi S, Dossus L, Biessy C, Secreto G, Amiano P, Bingham S, Boeing H, Bueno de Mesquita HB, Chang-Claude J, Clavel-Chapelon F, Fournier A, van Gils CH, Gonzalez CA, Gurrea AB, Critselis E, Khaw KT, Krogh V, Lahmann PH, Nagel G, Olsen A, Onland-Moret NC, Overvad K, Palli D, Panico S, Peeters P, Quiros JR, Roddam A, Thiebaut A, Tjonneland A, Chirlaque MD, Trichopoulou A, Trichopoulos D, Tumino R, Vineis P, Norat T, Ferrari P, Slimani N, Riboli E. Serum sex steroids in premenopausal women and breast cancer risk within the European Prospective Investigation into Cancer and Nutrition (EPIC). J Natl Cancer Inst 2005; 97(10): 755–765.

Kabuto M, Akiba S, Stevens RG, Neriishi K, Land CE. A prospective study of estradiol and breast cancer in Japanese women. Cancer Epidemiol Biomarkers Prev 2000; 9(6): 575–579.

Kasid A, Strobl JS, Huff K, Greene GL, Lippman ME. A novel nuclear form of estradiol receptor in MCF-7 human breast cancer cells. Science 1984; 225(4667):1162–1165.

Kawamura I, Mizota T, Kondo N, Shimomura K, Kohsaka M. Antitumor effects of droloxifene, a new antiestrogen drug, against 7,12-dimethylbenz(a)anthracene-induced mammary tumors in rats. Jpn J Pharmacol 1991; 57:215–224.

Kelly PA, Tsushima T, Shiu RP, Friesen HG. Lactogenic and growth hormone-like activities in pregnancy determined by radioreceptor assays. Endocrinology 1976; 99(3):765–774.

Kennedy BJ. Fluxymesterone therapy in treatment of advanced breast cancer. N Engl J Med 1958; 259:673–675.

Key T, Appleby P, Barnes I, Reeves G. Endogenous sex hormones and breast cancer in postmenopausal women: reanalysis of nine prospective studies. J Natl Cancer Inst 2002; 94(8):606–616.

Key TJ, Verkasalo PK, Banks E. Epidemiology of breast cancer. Lancet Oncol 2001; 2(3):133–140.

Key TJ, Wang DY, Brown JB, Hermon C, Allen DS, Moore JW, Bulbrook RD, Fentiman IS, Pike MC. A prospective study of urinary oestrogen excretion and breast cancer risk. Br J Cancer 1996; 73(12):1615–1619.

Kimura N, Mizokami A, Oonuma T, Sasano H, Nagura H. Immunocytochemical localization of androgen receptor with polyclonal antibody in paraffin-embedded human tissues. J Histochem Cytochem 1993; 41:671–678.

King RJB, Gordon J, Helfenstein JE. The metabolism of testosterone by tissue from normal and neoplastic rat breast. J Endocrinol 1964; 29:103–110.

King RJB, Panattoni M, Gordon J, Baker R. The metabolism of steroids by tissue from normal and neoplastic rat breast. J Endocrinol 1965; 33:127–132.

Klotz L. Combined androgen blockade in prostate cancer: meta-analyses and associated issues. BJU Int 2001; 87(9): 806–813.

Korkia P, Stimson GV. Indications of prevalence, practice and effects of anabolic steroid use in Great Britain. Int J Sports Med 1997; 18(7):557–562.

Kratochwil K. Development and loss of androgen responsiveness in the embryonic rudiment of the mouse mammary gland. Dev Biol 1977; 61(2):358–365.

Kreitmann B, Bayard F. Androgen interaction with the oestrogen receptor in human tissues. J Steroid Biochem 1979; 11:1589–1595.

Kushnir MM, Rockwood AL, Roberts WL, Pattison EG, Bunker AM, Fitzgerald RL, Meikle AW. Performance characteristics of a novel tandem mass spectrometry assay for serum testosterone. Clin Chem 2006; 52(1):120–128.

Labrie F. Intracrinology. Mol Cell Endocrinol 1991; 78: C113–C118.

Labrie F. Future perspectives of SERMs used alone and in combination with DHEA. Endocr Relat Cancer 2006; 13(2): 335–355.

Labrie F. Drug insight: breast cancer prevention and tissue-targeted hormone replacement therapy. Nat Clin Pract Endocrinol Metab 2007; 3(8):584–593.

Labrie F, Auclair C, Cusan L, Kelly PA, Pelletier G, Ferland L. Inhibitory effects of LHRH and its agonists on testicular gonadotropin receptors and spermatogenesis in the rat. Int J Androl Suppl 1978; 2:303–318.

Labrie F, Bélanger A, Bélanger P, Bérubé R, Martel C, Cusan L, Gomez JL, Candas B, Castiel I, Chaussade V, Deloche C,

Leclaire J. Androgen glucuronides, instead of testosterone, as the new markers of androgenic activity in women. J Ster Biochem Mol Biol 2006a; 99:182–188.

Labrie F, Bélanger A, Bélanger P, Bérubé R, Martel C, Cusan L, Gomez J, Candas B, Chaussade V, Castiel I, Deloche C, Leclaire J. Metabolism of DHEA in postmenopausal women following percutaneous administration. J Steroid Biochem Mol Biol 2007; 103(2):178–188.

Labrie F, Bélanger A, Candas B, Cusan L, Gomez JL, Labrie C, Luu-The V, Simard J. GnRH agonists in the treatment of prostate cancer. Endocrine Reviews 2005a; 26(3):361–379.

Labrie F, Belanger A, Cusan L, Candas B. Physiological changes in dehydroepiandrosterone are not reflected by serum levels of active androgens and estrogens but of their metabolites: intracrinology. J Clin Endocrinol Metab 1997a; 82(8):2403–2409.

Labrie F, Bélanger A, Cusan L, Gomez JL, Candas B. Marked decline in serum concentrations of adrenal C19 sex steroid precursors and conjugated androgen metabolites during aging. J Clin Endocrinol. Metab 1997b; 82:2396 2402.

Labrie F, Bélanger A, Dupont A, Luu-The V, Simard J, Labrie C. Science behind total androgen blockade: from gene to combination therapy. Clin Invest Med 1993; 16:475–492.

Labrie C, Bélanger A, Labrie F. Androgenic activity of dehydroepiandrosterone and androstenedione in the rat ventral prostate. Endocrinology 1988; 123:1412–1417.

Labrie F, Bélanger A, Simard J, Luu-The V, Labrie C. DHEA and peripheral androgen and estrogen formation: Intracrinology. Ann N Y Acad Sci 1995a; 774:16–28.

Labrie F, Candas B, Cusan L, Gomez JL, Diamond P, Suburu R, Lemay M. Diagnosis of advanced or noncurable prostate cancer can be practically eliminated by prostate-specific antigen. Urology 1996b; 47:212–217.

Labrie F, Candas B, Gomez JL, Cusan L. Can combined androgen blockade provide long-term control or possible cure of localized prostate cancer? Urology 2002; 60(1): 115–119.

Labrie F, Champagne P, Labrie C, Bélanger A, Roy J, Laverdière J, Deschênes L, Provencher L, Potvin M, Drolet Y, Pollak M, Panasci L, L'Espérance B, Dufresne J, Latreille J, Robert J, Samson B, Jolivet J, Yelle L, Cusan L, Diamond P, Candas B. Activity and safety of the orally active pure antiestrogen EM-800 (SCH 57050) in Tamoxifen-resistant breast cancer. J Clin Oncol 2004a; 22(5):864–871.

Labrie F, Diamond P, Cusan L, Gomez JL, Bélanger A. Effect of 12-month DHEA replacement therapy on bone, vagina, and endometrium in postmenopausal women. J Clin Endocrinol Metab 1997c; 82:3498–3505.

Labrie F, Dupont A, Bélanger A. Complete androgen blockade for the treatment of prostate cancer. In: de Vita VT, Hellman S, Rosenberg SA, eds. Important Advances in Oncology. Philadelphia: J.B. Lippincott, 1985: 193–217.

Labrie F, Dupont A, Bélanger A, Cusan L, Lacourcière Y, Monfette G, Laberge JG, Emond J, Fazekas AT, Raynaud JP, Husson JM. New hormonal therapy in prostatic carcinoma: combined treatment with an LHRH agonist and an antiandrogen. Clin Invest Med 1982; 5:267–275.

Labrie Y, Durocher F, Lachance Y, Turgeon C, Simard J, Labrie C, Labrie F. The human type II 17b-hydroxysteroid dehydrogenase gene encodes two alternatively-spliced messenger RNA species. DNA Cell Biol 1995b; 14:849–861.

Labrie F, El-Alfy M, Berger L, Labrie C, Martel C, Bélanger A, Candas B, Pelletier G. The combination of a novel SERM with an estrogen protects the mammary gland and uterus in a rodent model: the future of postmenopausal women's health? Endocrinology 2003a; 144(11):4700–4706.

Labrie C, Flamand M, Bélanger A, Labrie F. High bioavailability of DHEA administered percutaneously in the rat. J Endocrinol 1996a; 150:S107–S118.

Labrie F, Labrie C, Bélanger A, Simard J. Third and fourth generation SERMs. In: Manni A, Verderame M, eds. Selective Estrogen Receptor Modulators: Research and Clinical Applications. Totowa, NJ: Humana Press, 2002:167–187.

Labrie F, Labrie C, Bélanger A, Simard J, Giguère V, Tremblay A, Tremblay G. EM-652 (SCH 57068), a pure SERM having complete antiestrogenic activity in the mammary gland and endometrium. J Steroid Biochem Mol Biol 2001a; 79:213–225.

Labrie F, Labrie C, Simard J, Bélanger A. New generation selective estrogen receptor modulators (SERMS). Stéroïdes sexuels: Le point sur l'action des estrogènes et des progestatifs, Montpellier, France, 2004b.

Labrie F, Li S, Labrie C, Lévesque C, Mérand Y. Inhibitory effect of a steroidal antiestrogen (EM-170) on estrone-stimulated growth of 7,12 dimethylbenz(a)anthracene (DMBA)-induced mammary carcinoma in the rat. Breast Cancer Res Treat 1995c; 33:237–244.

Labrie F, Luu-The V, Bélanger A, Lin S-X, Simard J, Labrie C. Is DHEA a hormone? Starling Review. J Endocrinol 2005b; 187:169–196.

Labrie F, Luu-The V, Labrie C, Bélanger A, Simard J, Lin S-X, Pelletier G. Endocrine and intracrine sources of androgens in women: inhibition of breast cancer and other roles of androgens and their precursor dehydroepiandrosterone. Endocr Rev 2003b; 24(2):152–182.

Labrie F, Luu-The V, Labrie C, Simard J. DHEA and its transformation into androgens and estrogens in peripheral target tissues: intracrinology. Front Neuroendocrinol 2001b; 22(3):185–212.

Labrie F, Luu-The V, Lin SX, Labrie C, Simard J, Breton R, Bélanger A. The key role of 17b-HSDs in sex steroid biology. Steroids 1997d; 62:148–158.

Labrie F, Luu-The V, Lin SX, Simard J, Labrie C, El-Alfy M, Pelletier G, Bélanger A. Intracrinology: role of the family of 17b-hydroxysteroid dehydrogenases in human physiology and disease. J Mol Endocrinol 2000; 25(1):1–16.

Labrie F, Luu-The V, Martel C, Chernomoretz A, Calvo E, Morissette J, Labrie C. DHEA is an anabolic steroid like testosterone and THG. J Steroid Biochem Mol Biol 2006b; 100(103):52–58.

Labrie C, Martel C, Dufour JM, Lévesque C, Mérand Y, Labrie F. Novel compounds inhibit estrogen formation and action. Cancer Res 1992a; 52:610–615.

Labrie F, Poulin R, Simard J, Luu-The V, Labrie C, Bélanger A. Androgens, DHEA and breast cancer. In: Gelfand T, ed.

Androgens and Reproductive Aging. Oxsfordshire UK: Taylor and Francis, 2006c:113–135.

Labrie F, Simard J, Labrie C, Bélanger A. EM-652 (SCH 57068), a pure SERM in the mammary gland and endometrium. Références en Gynécologie Obstétrique 2001c; 8:331–336.

Labrie F, Simard J, Luu-The V, Bélanger A, Pelletier G. Structure, function and tissue-specific gene expression of 3b-hydroxysteroid dehydrogenase/5-ene-4-ene isomerase enzymes in classical and peripheral intracrine steroidogenic tissues. J Steroid Biochem Mol Biol 1992b; 43:805–826.

Labrie F, Simard J, Luu-The V, Bélanger A, Pelletier G, Morel Y, Mebarki F, Sanchez R, Durocher F, Turgeon C, Labrie Y, Rhéaume E, Labrie C, Lachance Y. The 3b-hydroxysteroid dehydrogenase/isomerase gene family: lessons from type II 3b-HSD congenital deficiency. In: Hansson V, Levy FO, Taskén K, eds. Signal Transduction in Testicular Cells. Ernst Schering Research Foundation Workshop. Berlin, Heidelberg, New York: Springer-Verlag, 1996c:185–218.

Labrie F, Simard J, Luu-The V, Pelletier G, Bélanger A, Lachance Y, Zhao HF, Labrie C, Breton N, de Launoit Y, Dumont M, Dupont E, Rhéaume E, Martel C, Couet J, Trudel C. Structure and tissue-specific expression of 3b-hydroxysteroid dehydrogenasc/5-cnc-4-ene isomerase genes in human and rat classical and peripheral steroidogenic tissues. J Steroid Biochem Mol Biol 1992c; 41:421–435.

Labrie F, Simard J, Luu-The V, Pelletier G, Belghmi K, Bélanger A. Structure, regulation and role of 3b-hydroxysteroid dehydrogenase, 17b-hydroxysteroid dehydrogenase and aromatase enzymes in formation of sex steroids in classical and peripheral intracrine tissues. In: Sheppard MC, Stewart PM, eds. Hormone, Enzymes and Receptors. London, UK: Baillière's Clinical Endocrinology and Metabolism, Baillière Tindall, 1994:451–474.

Labrie C, Simard J, Zhao HF, Bélanger A, Pelletier G, Labrie F. Stimulation of androgen-dependent gene expression by the adrenal precursors dehydroepiandrosterone and androstenedione in the rat ventral prostate. Endocrinology 1989; 124:2745–2754.

Labrie F, Sugimoto Y, Luu-The V, Simard J, Lachance Y, Bachvarov D, Leblanc G, Durocher F, Paquet N. Structure of human type II 5 alpha-reductase gene. Endocrinology 1992d; 131(3):1571–1573.

Lacassagne A. Hormonal Pathogenesis of Adenocarcinoma of the breast. Am J Cancer 1936; 27(2):217–228.

Lacey JV, Mink PJ, Lubin JH, Sherman ME, Troisi R, Hartge P, Schatzkin A, Schairer C. Menopausal hormone replacement therapy and risk of ovarian cancer. JAMA 2002; 288: 334–341.

Lea OA, Kvinnsland S, Thorsen T. Improved measurement of androgen receptors in human breast cancer. Cancer Res 1989; 49(24 pt 1):7162–7167.

Leblanc M, Bélanger MC, Julien P, Tchernof A, Labrie C, Bélanger A, Labrie F. Plasma lipoprotein profile in the male cynomolgus monkey under normal, hypogonadal and combined androgen blockade conditions. J Clin Endocrinol Metab 2004; 89:1849–1857.

Leblanc M, Labrie C, Bélanger A, Candas B, Labrie F. Pharmacokinetics of oral dehydroepiandrosterone (DHEA) in the ovariectomised cynomolgus monkey. J Steroid Biochem Mol Biol 2002; 81:159–164.

Leblanc M, Labrie C, Bélanger A, Candas B, Labrie F. Bioavailability and pharmacokinetics of dehydroepiandrosterone in the cynomolgus monkey. J Clin Endocrinol Metab 2003; 88(9):4293–4302.

Lemieux C, Gelinas Y, Lalonde J, Labrie F, Cianflone K, Deshaies Y. Hypolipidemic action of the SERM acolbifene is associated with decreased liver MTP and increased SR-BI and LDL receptors. J Lipid Res 2005; 46(6):1285–1294.

Lemieux C, Picard F, Labrie F, Richard D, Deshaies Y. The estrogen antagonist EM-652 and dehydroepiandrosterone prevent diet- and ovariectomy-induced obesity. Obes Res 2003; 11(3):477–490.

Levesque C, Merand Y, Dufour JM, Labrie C, Labrie F. Synthesis and biological activity of new halo-steroidal antiestrogens. J Med Chem 1991; 34(5):1624–1630.

Levi MS, Borne RF, Williamson JS. A review of cancer chemopreventive agents. Curr Med Chem 2001; 8(11): 1349–1362.

Li S, Yan X, Bélanger A, Labrie F. Prevention by dehydroepiandrosterone of the development of mammary carcinoma induced by 7,12-dimethylbenz(a)anthracene (DMBA) in the rat. Breast Cancer Res Treat 1993; 29:203–217.

Lindsay R, Gallagher JC, Kleerekoper M, Pickar JH. Effect of lower doses of conjugated equine estrogens with and without medroxyprogesterone acetate on bone in early postmenopausal women. JAMA 2002; 287(20):2668–2676.

Lippman ME, Bolan G, Huff K. The effect of androgens and antiandrogens on hormone-responsive human breast cancer in long-term tissue culture. Cancer Res 1976; 36:4610.

Littlefield BA, Gurpide E, Markiewicz L, McKinley B, Hochberg RB. A simple and sensitive microtiter plate estrogen bioassay based on stimulation of alkaline phosphatase in Ishikawa cells: estrogenic action of D^5 adrenal steroids. Endocrinology 1990; 127:2757–2762.

Liu CH, Laughlin GA, Fischer UG, Yen SS. Marked attenuation of ultradian and circadian rhythms of dehydroepiandrosterone in postmenopausal women: evidence for a reduced 17,20-desmolase enzymatic activity. J Clin Endocrinol Metab 1990; 71(4):900–906.

Lobaccaro JM, Lumbroso S, Belon C, Galtier-Dereure F, Bringer J, Lesimple T, Namer M, Cutuli BF, Pujol H, Sultan C. Androgen receptor gene mutation in male breast cancer. Hum Mol Genet 1993; 2:1799–1802.

Long BJ, Jelovac D, Handratta V, Thiantanawat A, MacPherson N, Ragaz J, Goloubeva OG, Brodie AM. Therapeutic strategies using the aromatase inhibitor letrozole and tamoxifen in a breast cancer model. J Natl Cancer Inst 2004; 96(6):456–465.

Lonning PE, Geisler J, Krag LE, Erikstein B, Bremnes Y, Hagen AI, Schlichting E, Lien EA, Ofjord ES, Paolini J, Polli A, Massimini G. Effects of exemestane administered for 2 years versus placebo on bone mineral density, bone biomarkers, and plasma lipids in patients with surgically resected early breast cancer. J Clin Oncol 2005; 23(22): 5126–5137.

Lu Q, Liu Y, Long BJ, Grigoryev D, Gimbel M, Brodie A. The effect of combining aromatase inhibitors with antiestrogens on tumor growth in a nude mouse model for breast cancer. Breast Cancer Res Treat 1999; 57(2):183–192.

Luo S, Labrie C, Bélanger A, Labrie F. Effect of dehydroepiandrosterone on bone mass, serum lipids, and dimethylbenz(a)anthracene-induced mammary carcinoma in the rat. Endocrinology 1997a; 138:3387–3394.

Luo S, Martel C, Gauthier S, Mérand Y, Bélanger A, Labrie C, Labrie F. Long term inhibitory effects of a novel antiestrogen on the growth of ZR-75-1 and MCF-7 human breast cancer tumors in nude mice. Int J Cancer 1997b; 73:735–739.

Luo S, Martel C, Sourla A, Gauthier S, Mérand Y, Bélanger A, Labrie C, Labrie F. Comparative effects of 28-day treatment with the new antiestrogen EM-800 and tamoxifen on estrogen-sensitive parameters in the intact mouse. Int J Cancer 1997c; 73:381–391.

Luo S, Sourla A, Labrie C, Bélanger A, Labrie F. Combined effects of dehydroepiandrosterone and EM-800 on bone mass, serum lipids, and the development of dimethylbenz(a) anthracene (DMBA)-induced mammary carcinoma in the rat. Endocrinology 1997d; 138:4435–4444.

Luu-The V. Analysis and characteristics of multiple types of human 17beta-hydroxysteroid dehydrogenase. J Steroid Biochem Mol Biol 2001; 76(1–5):143–151.

Luu-The V, Dufort I, Paquet N, Reimnitz G, Labrie F. Structural characterization and expression of the human dehydroepiandrosterone sulfotransferase gene. DNA Cell Biol 1995a; 14:511–518.

Luu-The V, Zhang Y, Poirier D, Labrie F. Characteristics of human types 1, 2 and 3 17b-hydroxysteroid dehydrogenase activities: oxidation-reduction and inhibition. J Steroid Biochem Mol Biol 1995b; 55:581–587.

Lyons WR. Hormonal synergism in mammary growth. Proc R Soc Biol 1958; 149:303–325.

MacIndoe JH, Etre LA. An antiestrogenic action of androgens in human breast cancer cells. J Clin Endocrinol Metab 1981; 53(4):836–842.

Mady EA, Ramadan EE, Ossman AA. Sex steroid hormones in serum and tissue of benign and malignant breast tumor patients. Dis Markers 2000; 16(3–4):151–157.

Maggiolini M, Donze O, Jeannin E, Ando S, Picard D. Adrenal androgens stimulate the proliferation of breast cancer cells as direct activators of estrogen receptor alpha. Cancer Res 1999; 59(19):4864–4869.

Martel C, Picard S, Richard V, Bélanger A, Labrie C, Labrie F. Prevention of bone loss by EM-800 and raloxifene in the ovariectomized rat. J Steroid Biochem Mol Biol 2000; 74(1–2):45–56.

Martel C, Sourla A, Pelletier G, Labrie C, Fournier M, Picard S, Li S, Stojanovic M, Labrie F. Predominant androgenic component in the stimulatory effect of dehydroepiandrosterone on bone mineral density in the rat. J Endocrinol 1998; 157:433–442.

McGuire WL, Carbone PP, Sears ME, Escher GC. Estrogen receptors in human breast cancer: an overview. In: McGuire WL, Carbone PP, Vollmer EP, eds. Estrogen Receptors in Human Breast Cancer. New York: Raven Press, 1975:1–7.

Mehring J. Do Drugs Make a Dent? Bus Week 2004; 3877:32.

Meites J. Relation of the neuroendocrine system to the development and growth of experimental mammary tumors. J Neural Transm 1980; 48(1):25–42.

Melsen F, Melsen B, Mosekilde L, Bergmann S. Histomorphometric analysis of normal bone from the iliac crest. Acta Pathol Microbiol Scand 1978 86:70–81.

Micheli A, Muti P, Secreto G, Krogh V, Meneghini E, Venturelli E, Sieri S, Pala V, Berrino F. Endogenous sex hormones and subsequent breast cancer in premenopausal women. Int J Cancer 2004; 112(2):312–318.

Migeon CJ, Keller AR, Lawrence B, Shepart TH II. Dehydroepiandrosterone and androsterone levels in human plasma. Effect of age and sex: day-to-day and diurnal variations. J Clin Endocrinol Metab 1957; 17:1051–1062.

Miller WR, Stuart M, Sahmoud T, Dixon JM. Anastrozole ('Arimidex') blocks oestrogen synthesis both peripherally and within the breast in postmenopausal women with large operable breast cancer. Br J Cancer 2002; 87(9):950–955.

Mistry P, Griffiths K, Maynard PV. Endogenous C19-steroids and estradiol levels in human primary breast tumor tissues and their correlation with androgen and estrogen receptors. J Steroid Biochem 1986; 24:1117–1125.

Morales AJ, Nolan JJ, Nelson JC, Yen SS. Effects of replacement dose of dehydroepiandrosterone in men and women of advancing age. J Clin Endocrinol Metab 1994; 78:1360–1367.

Mouridsen H, Gershanovich M, Sun Y, Perez-Carrion R, Boni C, Monnier A, Apffelstaedt J, Smith R, Sleeboom HP, Janicke F, Pluzanska A, Dank M, Becquart D, Bapsy PP, Salminen E, Snyder R, Lassus M, Verbeek JA, Staffler B, Chaudri-Ross HA, Dugan M. Superior efficacy of letrozole versus tamoxifen as first-line therapy for postmenopausal women with advanced breast cancer: results of a phase III study of the international letrozole breast cancer group. J Clin Oncol 2001; 19(10):2596–2606.

Murphy LC, Tsuyuki D, Myal Y, SHiu RPC. Isolation and sequencing of a cDNA clone for a prolactin-inducible protein (PIP). J Biol Chem 1987; 262:15236–15241.

Nair KS, Rizza RA, O'Brien P, Dhatariya K, Short KR, Nehra A, Vittone JL, Klee GG, Basu A, Basu R, Cobelli C, Toffolo G, Dalla Man C, Tindall DJ, Melton LJ III, Smith GE, Khosla S, Jensen MD. DHEA in elderly women and DHEA or testosterone in elderly men. N Engl J Med 2006; 355(16): 1647–1659.

Najid A, Habrioux G. Biological effects of adrenal androgens on MCF-7 and BT-20 human breast cancer cells. Oncology 1990; 47(3):269–274.

Najid A, Ratinaud MH. Comparative studies of steroidogenesis inhibitors (econazole, ketoconazole) on human breast cancer MCF-7 cell proliferation by growth experiments, thymidine incorporation and flow cytometric DNA analysis. Tumori 1991; 77(5):385–390.

Neri R, Peets E, Watnick A. Anti-androgenicity of flutamide and its metabolite Sch 16423. Biochem Soc Trans 1979; 7:565.

Onland-Moret NC, Kaaks R, van Noord PA, Rinaldi S, Key T, Grobbee DE, Peeters PH. Urinary endogenous sex hormone levels and the risk of postmenopausal breast cancer. Br J Cancer 2003; 88(9):1394–1399.

Orentreich N, Brind JL, Rizer RL, Vogelman JH. Age changes and sex differences in serum dehydroepiandrosterone sulfate concentrations throughout adulthood. J Clin Endocrinol Metab 1984; 59:551–555.

Osborne CK, Coronado Heinsohn EB, Hilsenbeck SG, McCue BL, Wakeling AE, McClelland RA, Manning DL, Nicholson RI. Comparison of the effects of a pure steroidal antiestrogen with those of tamoxifen in a model of human breast cancer. J Natl Cancer Inst; 1995. 87(10): 746–750.

Osborne CK, Pippen J, Jones SE, Parker LM, Ellis M, Come S, Gertler SZ, May JT, Burton G, Dimery A, Webster A, Morris R, Elledge R, Buzdar A. Double-blind, randomized trial comparing the efficacy and tolerability of Fulvestrant versus anastrozole in postmenopausal women with advanced breast cancer progressing on prior endocrine therapy: results of a North American Trial. J Clin Oncol 2002; 20(16):3386–3395.

Page JH, Colditz GA, Rifai N, Barbieri RL, Willett WC, Hankinson SE. Plasma adrenal androgens and risk of breast cancer in premenopausal women. Cancer Epidemiol Biomarkers Prev 2004; 13(6):1032–1036.

Parfitt AM. The cellular basis of bone remodeling: the quantum concept reexamined in light of recent advances in the cell biology of bone. Calcif Tissue Int 1984; 36(suppl 1): S37–S45.

Park JJ, Irvine RA, Buchanan G, Koh SS, Park JM, Tilley WD, Stallcup MR, Press MF, Coetzee GA. Breast cancer susceptibility gene 1 (BRCAI) is a coactivator of the androgen receptor. Cancer Res 2000; 60(21):5946–5949.

Pasqualini JR, Chetrite G, Blacker C, Feinstein MC, Delalonde L, Talbi M, Maloche C. Concentrations of estrone, estradiol, and estrone sulfate and evaluation of sulfatase and aromatase activities in pre- and postmenopausal breast cancer patients. J Clin Endocrinol Metab 1996; 81(4): 1460–1464.

Pelletier G, Labrie C, Martel C, Labrie F. Chronic administration of dehydroepiandrosterone (DHEA) to female monkey and rat has no effect on mammary gland histology. J Steroid Biochem Mol Biol 2007 (in press).

Pelletier G, Luu-The V, El-Alfy M, Li S, Labrie F. Immunoelectron microscopic localization of 3b-hydroxysteroid dehydrogenase and type 5 17b-hydroxysteroid dehydrogenase in the human prostate and mammary gland. J Mol Endocrinol 2001; 26(1):11–19.

Pelletier G, Luu-The V, Tetu B, Labrie F. Immunocytochemical localization of type 5 17b-hydroxysteroid dehydrogenase in human reproductive tissues. J Histochem Cytochem 1999; 47(6):731–737.

Perel E, Daniilescu D, Kharlip L, Blackstein ME, Killinger DW The relationship between growth and androstenedione metabolism in four cell lines of human breast carcinoma cells in culture. Mol Cell Endocrinol 1985; 41:197–203.

Perel E, Killinger DW. The metabolism of androstenedione and testosterone of C_{10}-metabolites in breast carcinoma, and benign prostatic hypertrophy tissue. J Steroid Biochem 1983; 19:1135–1139.

Peto R. Five years of tamoxifen–or more? J Natl Cancer Inst 1996; 88(24):1791–1793.

Peto R, Dalesio O. Breast and prostate cancer: 10-year survival gains in the hormonal adjuvant treatment trials. ECCO 12, Copenhagen. Eur J Cancer 2003 (abstr).

Picard F, Deshaies Y, Lalonde J, Samson P, Labrie C, Bélanger A, Labrie F, Richard D. Effects of the estrogen antagonist EM-652. HCl on energy balance and lipid metabolism in ovariectomized rats. Int J Obes Relat Metab Disord 2000; 24(7):830–840.

Pike MC, Spicer DV, Dahmoush L, Press MF. Estrogens, progestogens, normal breast cell proliferation, and breast cancer risk. Epidemiol Rev 1993; 15(1):17–35.

Poortman J, Thijssen JH, von Landeghem AA, Wiegerinck MA, Alsbach GP. Subcellular distribution of androgens and oestrogens in target tissue. J Steroid Biochem 1983; 19(1C): 939–945.

Poulin R, Baker D, Labrie F. Androgens inhibit basal and estrogen-induced cell proliferation in the ZR-75-1 human breast cancer cell line. Breast Cancer Res Treat 1988; 12:213–225.

Poulin R, Baker D, Poirier D, Labrie F. Androgen and glucocorticoid receptor-mediated inhibition of cell proliferation by medroxyprogesterone acetate in ZR-75-1 human breast cancer cells. Breast Cancer Res Treat 1989a; 13:161–172.

Poulin R, Labrie F. Stimulation of cell proliferation and estrogenic response by adrenal C19-D^5-steroids in the ZR-75-1 human breast cancer cell line." Cancer Res 1986; 46: 4933–4937.

Poulin R, Mérand Y, Poirier D, Lévesque C, Dufour JM, Labrie F. Antiestrogenic properties of keoxifene, trans-4-hydroxytamoxifen and ICI164384, a new steroidal antiestrogen, in ZR-75-1 human breast cancer cells. Breast Cancer Res Treat 1989b; 14:65–76.

Poulin R, Simard J, Labrie C, Petitclerc L, Dumont M, Lagacé L, Labrie F. Down-regulation of estrogen receptors by androgens in the ZR-75-1 human breast cancer cell line. Endocrinology 1989c; 125:392–399.

Powles TJ, Hardy JR, Ashley SE, Farrington GM, Cosgrove D, Davey JB, Dowsett M, McKinna JA, Nash AG, Sinnett HD. A pilot trial to evaluate the acute toxicity and feasibility of tamoxifen for prevention of breast cancer. Br J Cancer 1989; 60(1):126–31.

Prostate Cancer Trialists' Collaborative Group. Maximum androgen blockade in advanced prostate cancer: an overview of the randomised trials. Lancet 2000; 355:1491–1498.

Quadri SK, Kledzik GS, Meites J. Counteraction by prolactin of androgen-induced inhibition of mammary tumor growth in rats. J Natl Cancer Inst 1974; 52:875–878.

Ratko TA, Detrisac CJ, Mehta RG, Kelloff GJ, Moon RC. Inhibition of rat mammary gland chemical carcinogenesis by dietary dehydroepiandorsterone or a fluorinated analogue of dehydroepiandrosterone. Cancer Res 1991; 51(2):481–486.

Raynaud A. Fetal development of the mammary gland and hormonal effects on its morphogenesis. In: Falconer IR, ed. Lactation. University Park and London: Pennsylvania State University Press, 1971:1–29.

Recchione C, Ventrurelli E, Manzari A, Cavalleri A, Martinetti A, Secreto G. Testorterone, dihydrotestosterone and eostradiol levels in postmenopausal breast cancer tissue. J Steroid Biochem 1995; 52:541–546.

Riman T, Dickman PW, Nilsson S, Correia N, Nordlinder H, Magnusson CM, Weiderpass E, Persson IR. Hormone replacement therapy and the risk of invasive epithelial ovarian cancer in Swedish women J Natl Cancer Inst 2002; 94:497–504.

Rinaldi S, Key TJ, Peeters PH, Lahmann PH, Lukanova A, Dossus L, Biessy C, Vineis P, Sacerdote C, Berrino F, Panico S, Tumino R, Palli D, Nagel G, Linseisen J, Boeing H, Roddam A, Bingham S, Khaw KT, Chloptios J, Trichopoulou A, Trichopoulos D, Tehard B, Clavel-Chapelon F, Gonzalez CA, Larranaga N, Barricarte A, Quiros JR, Chirlaque MD, Martinez C, Monninkhof E, Grobbee DE, Bueno-de-Mesquita HB, Ferrari P, Slimani N, Riboli E, Kaaks R. Anthropometric measures, endogenous sex steroids and breast cancer risk in postmenopausal women: a study within the EPIC cohort. Int J Cancer 2006; 118(11):2832–2839.

Rochefort H, Garcia M. The estrogenic and antiestrogenic activities of androgens in female target tissues. Pharmacol Ther 1983; 23:193–216.

Rodriguez C, Patel AV, Calle EE, Jacob EJ, Thun MJ. Estrogen replacement therapy and ovarian cancer mortality in a large prospective study of US women. JAMA 2002; 285:1460–1465.

Roy J, Couillard S, Gutman M, Labrie F. A novel pure SERM achieves complete regression of the majority of human breast cancer tumors in nude mice. Breast Cancer Res Treat 2003; 81:223–229.

Roy R, Dauvois S, Labrie F, Bélanger A. Estrogen-stimulated glucuronidation of dihydrotestosterone in MCF-7 human breast cancer cells. J Steroid Biochem Mol Biol 1992; 41:579–582.

Russo J, Russo IH. Biological and molecular bases of mammary carcinogenesis. Lab Invest 1987; 57:112–137.

Russo J, Russo IH. Morphology and development of the mammary gland. In: Jones TC, Morh U, Hunt R, eds. Monographs on Pathology of Laboratory Animals: Integument and Mammary Glands. New York: Springer-Verlag, 1989:233–252.

Russo J, Saby J, William MI, Russo IH. Pathogenesis of mammary carcinomas induced in rats by 7,12-dimethylbenz (a)anthracene. J Natl Cancer Inst 1977; 59:435–445.

Sato M, Turner CH, Wang T, Adrian MD, Rowley E, Bryant HU. LY353381.HCl: a novel raloxifene analog with improved SERM potency and efficacy in vivo. J Pharmacol Exp Ther 1998; 287:1–7.

Scatchard G. The attraction of proteins for small molecules and ions. Ann N Y Acad Sci 1959; 51:660–672.

Schiff R, Massarweh SA, Shou J, Bharwani L, Arpino G, Rimawi M, Osborne CK. Advanced concepts in estrogen receptor biology and breast cancer endocrine resistance: implicated role of growth factor signaling and estrogen receptor coregulators. Cancer Chemother Pharmacol 2005; 56(suppl 1):10–20.

Schwartz AG. Inhibition of spontaneous breast cancer formation in female C3H (Avy/a) mice by long-term treatment with dehydroepiandrosterone. Cancer Res 1979; 39:1129–1132.

Schwartz AG, Pashko L, Whitcomb JM. Inhibition of tumor development by dehydroepiandrosterone and related steroids. Toxicol Pathol 1986; 14:357–362.

Schwartz AG, Whitcomb JM, Nyce JW, Lewbart ML, Pashko LL. Dehydroepiandrosterone and structural analogs: a new class of cancer chemopreventive agents. Adv Cancer Res 1988; 51:391–424.

Secreto G, Toniolo P, Berrino F, Recchione C, Cavalleri A, Pisani P, Toris A, Fariselli G, Di Pietro S. Serum and urinary androgens and risk of breast cancer in potmenopausal women. Cancer Res 1991; 51:2572–2576.

Segaloff A. The use of androgens in the treatment of neoplastic disease. Pharm Ther 1977; C2:33–37.

Segaloff A, Gordon D, Horwitt BN, Schlosser JV, Murison PJ. Hormonal therapy in cancer of the breast. 1. The effect of testosterone propionate therapy on clinical course and hormonal excretion. Cancer 1951; 4:319–323.

Seymour-Munn K, Adams J. Estrogenic effects of 5-androstene-3 beta, 17 beta-diol at physiological concentrations and its possible implication in the etiology of breast cancer. Endocrinology 1983; 112(2):486–491.

Sherwin BB. Estrogen and cognitive functioning in women. Endocr Rev 2003; 24(2):133–151.

Simard J, Dauvois S, Haagensen DE, Lévesque C, Mérand Y, Labrie F. Regulation of progesterone-binding breast cyst protein GCDFP-24 secretion by estrogens and androgens in human breast cancer cells: a new marker of steroid action in breast cancer. Endocrinology 1990; 126:3223–3231.

Simard J, Hatton AC, Labrie C, Dauvois S, Zhao HF, Haagensen DE, Labrie F. Inhibitory effects of estrogens on GCDFP-15 mRNA levels and secretion in ZR-75-1 human breast cancer cells. Mol Endocrinol 1989; 3:694–702.

Simard J, Labrie C, Bélanger A, Gauthier S, Singh SM, Mérand Y, Labrie F. Characterization of the effects of the novel non-steroidal antiestrogen EM-800 on basal and estrogen-induced proliferation of T-47D, ZR-75-1 and MCF-7 human breast cancer cells in vitro. Int J Cancer 1997a; 73:104–112.

Simard J, Luthy I, Guay J, Bélanger A, Labrie F. Characteristics of interaction of the antiandrogen Flutamide with the androgen receptor in various target tissues. Mol Cell Endocrinol 1986; 44:261–270.

Simard J, Sanchez R, Poirier D, Gauthier S, Singh SM, Mérand Y, Bélanger A, Labrie C, Labrie F. Blockade of the stimulatory effect of estrogens, OH-Tamoxifen, OH-Toremifene, Droloxifene and Raloxifene on alkaline phosphatase activity by the antiestrogen EM-800 in human endometrial adenocarcinoma Ishikawa cells. Cancer Res 1997b; 57:3494–3497.

Simoncini T, Fornari L, Mannella P, Varone G, Caruso A, Liao JK, Genazzani AR. Novel non-transcriptional mechanisms for estrogen receptor signaling in the cardiovascular system. Interaction of estrogen receptor alpha with phosphatidylinositol 3-OH kinase. Steroids 2002; 67(12):935–939.

Simpson ER. Sources of estrogen and their importance. J Steroid Biochem Mol Biol 2003; 86(3–5):225–230.

Somboonporn W, Davis SR. Testosterone effects on the breast: implications for testosterone therapy for women. Endocr Rev 2004; 25(3):374–388.

Song D, Liu G, Luu-The V, Zhao D, Wang L, Zhang H, Xueling G, Li S, Desy L, Labrie F, Pelletier G. Expression of aromatase and 17beta-hydroxysteroid dehydrogenase types 1, 7 and 12 in breast cancer. An immunocytochemical study. J Steroid Biochem Mol Biol 2006; 101(2–3):136–44.

Sourla A, Flamand M, Bélanger A, Labrie F. Effect of dehydroepiandrosterone on vaginal and uterine histomorphology in the rat. J Steroid Biochem Mol Biol 1998a; 66(3):137–149.

Sourla A, Martel C, Labrie C, Labrie F. Almost exclusive androgenic action of dehydroepiandrosterone in the rat mammary gland. Endocrinology 1998b; 139:753–764.

Sturgeon SR, Potischman N, Malone KE, Dorgan JF, Daling J, Schairer C, Brinton LA Serum levels of sex hormones and breast cancer risk in premenopausal women: a case-control study (USA). Cancer Causes Control 2004; 15(1):45–53.

Swanson C, Lorentzon M, Vandenput L, Labrie F, Rane A, Jakobsson J, Chouinard S, Belanger A, Ohlsson C. Sex steroid levels and cortical bone size in young men are associated with a uridine diphosphate glucuronosyltransferase 2B7 polymorphism (H268Y). J Clin Endocrinol Metab 2007; 92:3697–3704.

Szymczak J, Milewicz A, Thijssen JH, Blankenstein MA, Daroszewski J. Concentration of sex steroids in adipose tissue after menopause. Steroids 1998; 63(5–6):319–21.

Taieb J, Mathian B, Millot F, Patricot MC, Mathieu E, Queyrel N, Lacroix I, Somma-Delpero C, Boudou P. Testosterone measured by 10 immunoassays and by isotope-dilution gas chromatography-mass spectrometry in sera from 116 men, women, and children. Clin Chem 2003; 49(8):1381–1395.

Tamimi RM, Hankinson SE, Chen WY, Rosner B, Colditz GA. Combined estrogen and testosterone use and risk of breast cancer in postmenopausal women. Arch Intern Med 2006; 166(14):1483–1489.

Teller MN, Budinger JM, Zvilichovsky G, Watson AA, MdDonald JJ, Stohrer G, Brown GB. Oncogenicity of purine 3-oxide and unsubstituted purine in rats. Cancer Res 1978; 38:2229–2232.

Thériault C, Labrie F. Hormonal regulation of estradiol 17b-hydroxysteroid dehydrogenase activity in the ZR-75-1 human breast cancer cell line. Ann N Y Acad Sci 1990; 595:419–421.

Thijssen JH, Blankenstein MA, Donker GH, Daroszewski J. Endogenous steroid hormones and local aromatase activity in the breast. J Steroid Biochem Mol Biol 1991; 39 (5B):799–804.

Thomas HV, Key TJ, Allen DS, Moore JW, Dowsett M, Fentiman IS, Wang DY. A prospective study of endogenous serum hormone concentrations and breast cancer risk in post-menopausal women on the island of Guernsey. Br J Cancer 1997; 76(3):401–405.

Toniolo PG, Levitz M, Zeleniuch-Jacquotte A, Banerjee S, Koenig KL, Shore RE, Strax P, Pasternack BS. A prospective study of endogenous estrogens and breast cancer in postmenopausal women. J Natl Cancer Inst 1995; 87(3):190–197.

Tormey DC, Lippman ME, Edwards BK, Cassidy JG. Evaluation of tamoxifen doses with and without fluoxymesterone in advanced breast cancer. Ann Intern Med 1983; 98:139–144.

Toth-Fejel S, Cheek J, Calhoun K, Muller P, Pommier RF. Estrogen and androgen receptors as comediators of breast cancer cell proliferation: providing a new therapeutic tool. Arch Surg 2004; 139(1):50–54.

Tralongo P, Di Mari A, Ferrau F. Cognitive impairment, aromatase inhibitors, and age. J Clin Oncol 2005; 23(18):4243.

Tworoger SS, Missmer SA, Eliassen AH, Spiegelman D, Folkerd E, Dowsett M, Barbieri RL, Hankinson SE. The association of plasma DHEA and DHEA sulfate with breast cancer risk in predominantly premenopausal women. Cancer Epidemiol Biomarkers Prev 2006; 15(5):967–71.

Ulrich P. Testosterone (hormone mÀle) et son role possible dans le traitement de certains cancers du sein. Acta Unio Int Contra Cancrum 1939; 377–379.

Vakamatsou EH, Villanueva A, Stanciu J, Sudhaker RD, Parfitt AM. Calcif Tissue Int 1985, 37:594–597.

Van Landedgem AA, Poortman J, Nabuurs M, Thijssen JHH. Endogenous concentrations and subcellular distribution of estrogens in normal and malignant human breast cancer tissues. Cancer Res 1985; 45:2900–2906.

Van Uytfanghe K, Stockl D, Kaufman JM, Fiers T, Ross HA, De Leenheer AP, Thienpont LM. Evaluation of a candidate reference measurement procedure for serum free testosterone based on ultrafiltration and isotope dilution-gas chromatography-mass spectrometry. Clin Chem 2004; 50(11): 2101–2110.

Vandenput L, Labrie F, Mellstrom D, Swanson C, Knutsson T, Peeker R, Ljunggren O, Orwoll E, Eriksson AL, Damber JE, Ohlsson C. Serum levels of specific glucuronidated androgen metabolites predict BMD and prostate volume in elderly men. J Bone Miner Res 2007; 22(2):220–227.

Vermeulen A, Deslypere JP, Paridaens R. Steroid dynamics in the normal and carcinomatous mammary gland. J Steroid Biochem 1986a; 25(5B):799–802.

Vermeulen A, Deslypere JP, Paridaens R, Leclercq G, Roy F, Heuson JC. Aromatase, 17b-hydroxysteroid dehydrogenase and intratissular sex hormone concentrations in cancerous and normal glandular breast tissue in postmenopausal women. Eur J Cancer Clin Oncol 1986b; 22:515–525.

Vermeulen A, Deslypene JP, Schelfhout W, Verdonck L, Rubens R. Adrenocortical function in old age: response to acute adrenocorticotropin stimulation. J Clin Endocrinol Metab 1982; 54:187–191.

Vermeulen A, Verdonck L. Radioimmunoassays of 17b-hydroxy-5a-androstan-3-one, 4-androstene-3,17-dione, dehydroepiandrosterone, 17b-hydroxyprogesterone and progesterone and its application to human male plasma. J Steroid Biochem 1976; 7:1–10.

Vermeulen A, Verdonck L. Factors affecting sex hormone levels in postmenopausal women. J Steroid Biochem 1979; 11:899–904.

Vogel VG, Costantino JP, Wickerham DL, Cronin WM. Re: tamoxifen for prevention of breast cancer: report of the National Surgical Adjuvant Breast and Bowel Project P-1 Study. J Natl Cancer Inst 2002; 94(19):1504.

Von Schoultz B. Androgens and the breast. Maturitas doi:10.1016/j.maturitas.2007.02.012.

Wakeling AE, Bowler J. Biology and mode of action of pure antiestrogens. J Steroid Biochem 1988; 30:141–147.

Wang DY, Allen DS, De Stavola BL, Fentiman IS, Brussen J, Bulbrook RD, Thomas BS, Hayward JL, Reed MJ. Urinary androgens and breast cancer risk: results from a long-term prospective study based in Guernsey. Br J Cancer 2000; 82(9):1577–1584.

Weinstein RS, Hutson MS. Decreased trabecular width and increased trabecular spacing contribute to bone loss with aging. Bone 1987; 8:137–142.

Wickerham DL, Fourchotte V. An update on breast cancer prevention trials. Int J Gynecol Cancer 2006; 16 (suppl 2): 498–501.

Wierman ME, Basson R, Davis SR, Khosla S, Miller KK, Rosner W, Santoro N. Androgen therapy in women: an Endocrine Society Clinical Practice guideline. J Clin Endocrinol Metab 2006; 91(10):3697–710.

Women's Health Initiative. Risks and benefits of estrogen plus progestin in healthy postmenopausal women. JAMA 2002; 288:321–333.

Wysowski DK, Honig SF, Beitz J. Uterine sarcoma associated with tamoxifen use. N Engl J Med 2002; 346(23):1832–1833.

Yaffe K. Estrogen therapy in postmenopausal women: effects on cognitive function and dementia. JAMA 1998; 279: 688–695.

Yeh S, Hu YC, Rahman M, Lin HK, Hsu CL, Ting HJ, Kang HY, Chang C. Increase of androgen-induced cell death and androgen receptor transactivation by BRCA1 in prostate cancer cells. Proc Natl Acad Sci U S A 2000; 97(21):11256–11261.

Young SR, Baker A, Helfestein JE. The effects of androgens on induced mammary tumors in rats. Br J Cancer 1965; 19:155–159.

Zava DT, McGuire WL. Estrogen receptors in androgen-induced breast tumor regression. Cancer Res 1977; 37(6):1608–1610.

Zava DT, McGuire WL. Human breast cancer: androgen action mediated by estrogen receptor. Science 1978; 199(4330): 787–788.

Zhou J, Ng S, Adesanya-Famuiya O, Anderson K, Bondy CA. Testosterone inhibits estrogen-induced mammary epithelial proliferation and suppresses estrogen receptor expression. Faseb J 2000; 14(12):1725–1730.

13

Practical Progress in the Chemoprevention of Breast Cancer with Selective Estrogen Receptor Modulators

GREGOR M. BALABURSKI and V. CRAIG JORDAN

Fox Chase Cancer Center, Philadelphia, Pennsylvania, U.S.A.

INTRODUCTION

The known link between estrogen and breast cancer suggested an application for nonsteroidal antiestrogens as potential treatments for breast cancer. The majority of the compounds selected for evaluation were unsuccessful, but one compound ICI 46,474 an antiestrogenic, antifertility agent in the rat (Harper and Walpole, 1967) was noted to be as effective as high-dose estrogen or androgen therapy but with fewer side effects (Cole et al., 1971). The approval of tamoxifen (ICI 46,474) as an antiestrogen to treat breast cancer opened the door for a rigorous evaluation of the pharmacology of antiestrogens that ultimately led to the recognition of the concept of selective estrogen receptor modulation (SERM). The practical applications of the SERMs have facilitated the clinical goal of chemoprevention (Jordan, 2003) and the development of raloxifene, the first multifunctional medicine.

The first evidence to show that tamoxifen acts as a reversible antiestrogen in breast cancer was noted during in vitro studies utilizing MCF-7 cells (Lippman and Bolan, 1975). The conclusion that tamoxifen reversibly interfered with the trophic effects of estrogen was on the basis of three lines of evidence: (1) the inhibition of cell growth was reversible by addition of estradiol, (2) tamoxifen had no effect in cell lines unresponsive to estradiol, and (3) tamoxifen was capable of binding to the estrogen receptor (ER) (Jordan and Koerner, 1975; Lippman and Bolan, 1975). The antiestrogenic and antihormonal properties of tamoxifen were also demonstrated in vivo. Tamoxifen inhibited induction and growth of 7,12-dimethyl benz(a) anthracene (DMBA)-induced tumors in rats (Jordan, 1976; Jordan and Dowse, 1976; Jordon and Jaspan, 1976). In addition to research that demonstrated the antiestrogenic properties of tamoxifen, further studies illustrated the unusual pharmacology of the drug; it was antiestrogenic in some species but estrogenic in others. Tamoxifen is antiestrogenic in *Xenopus laevis* (Riegel et al., 1986) and the chick oviduct (Sutherland et al., 1977), estrogenic in dogs (Furr and Jordan, 1984) and yet both estrogenic and antiestrogenic in rats (Harper and Walpole, 1967; Jordan et al., 1977), mice (Harper and Walpole, 1966; Jordan et al., 1978) and humans (Furr and Jordan, 1984). The dichotomy of tamoxifen's actions was initially attributed to species-specific differences in metabolism. However, no differences in drug metabolites among various species were found (Jordan and Robinson, 1987). Thus, the new emerging concept to be developed was selective tissue targeting of the specific actions of the nonsteroidal antiestrogens.

THE RECOGNITION OF SERM

An understanding of the estrogen like pharmacology of tamoxifen in the mouse was crucial to developing the idea of tissue SERM. The implantation of MCF-7 breast cancer cells into athymic mice has been exploited as a model of estrogen-stimulated breast cancer growth (Osborne et al., 1985). Despite the fact that tamoxifen is estrogenic in the mouse and causes increases in uterine wet weight (Terenius, 1971), tamoxifen did not enhance the growth of MCF-7 cells in athymic mice (Jordan and Robinson, 1987). Therefore, the target tissue rather then the host is crucial for SERM.

The concept that tissues and not species were differentially stimulated or inhibited by tamoxifen was further clarified by the findings that ER-positive tumors from breast (MCF-7) and endometrial (EnCa101) origins behaved differently when implanted in the same athymic mouse despite the production of same drug metabolites (Gottardis et al., 1988). The estrogen stimulated growth of ER-positive breast tumor was inhibited by tamoxifen, while the endometrial tumor was stimulated by tamoxifen (Gottardis et al., 1988). These findings further established that metabolism does not play a role in the species-specific differences of tamoxifen action and that tamoxifen exhibits a tissue-specific pharmacology.

In parallel laboratory studies tamoxifen and raloxifene (originally known as LY 156,758 or keoxifene) (Clemens et al., 1983) prevented the development of estrogen-dependent N-nitrosomethylurea (NMU)-induced mammary carcinoma (Gottardis and Jordan, 1987) and maintained bone density in ovariectomized rats (Jordan et al., 1987). While both drugs exhibited similar effects in maintaining bone density (Jordan et al., 1987), raloxifene was less effective than tamoxifen in preventing tumor appearance at the same dose (Gottardis and Jordan, 1987). Tamoxifen, in contrast to raloxifene, increased the uterine wet weights of ovariectomized rats (Jordan et al., 1987). Most importantly, the fact that both antiestrogens delayed tumor formation and maintained bone density in the ovariectomized rat models indicated that these observations were a drug class effect.

Subsequent animal studies compared the effects of raloxifene treatment to those of ethynyl estradiol (Black et al., 1994). Raloxifene blocked decreases in bone mineral density (BMD) and had hypocholesteremic effects in rats that were almost identical to the effects of ethynyl estradiol and research previously reported for tamoxifen 15 years earlier (Harper and Walpole, 1967). There were no differences in triglyceride levels between the raloxifene-treated and ethynyl estradiol–treated animals as compared to ovariectomized controls. Most importantly, raloxifene did not exhibit any significant effects on the uterus. Uterine wet weights of raloxifene-treated animals were slightly higher than the ovariectomized controls, while the ethynyl estradiol–treated animals had substantially higher uterine wet weights than the ovariectomized controls. Additional uterine parameters considered were epithelial height, myometrial thickness, stromal expansion, and stromal eosinophilia. The raloxifene-treated animals exhibited no differences when compared to the ovariectomized controls in all parameters considered. The ethynyl estradiol–treated animals exhibited similar profiles to the intact controls and were statistically different from the ovariectomized controls.

The laboratory recognition of SERM was immediately translated to clinical advances, first to improve the safety of women treated by tamoxifen adjuvant therapy for node-positive and node-negative breast cancer, and subsequently, to introduce a new approach to the prevention of breast cancer by the development of drugs called SERMs. However, translational research does not follow a straight path and potentially good ideas with encouraging preliminary findings do not necessarily lead to improvements in health care. Billions of dollars have been invested in the development of the SERM concept, but clinical practice has not fulfilled the promise in its entirety. As a result, we have chosen to describe the twists and turns of the SERM story in some detail to illustrate how difficult and complicated it is to achieve success in therapeutics. The lesson learned is that the tantalizing clues that accumulate to indicate the advances in therapeutics are either possible or doomed once the evidence from prospective clinical trials are published.

TAMOXIFEN AND ENDOMETRIAL CANCER

The benefits of long-term tamoxifen therapy had to be carefully examined in light of the laboratory findings (Gottardis et al., 1988) that tamoxifen may be associated with increased incidence of endometrial cancer (Hardell, 1988; Jordan, 1988b; Fornander et al., 1989). Increases in endometrial cancer rates associated with tamoxifen therapy (Stewart and Knight, 1989; Neven et al., 1994) were not found in all studies, and the issue was further obscured by small sample sizes, lack of data collection, or usage of higher doses of tamoxifen (40 mg daily) (Fornander et al., 1989). The issue of dosage was resolved in the National Surgical Adjuvant Breast and Bowel Project (NSABP) B-14 trial that determined tamoxifen benefits and reduction in the incidence of breast cancer recurrence, contralateral breast cancer and mortality at the lower, 20-mg daily dose (Fisher et al., 1989). Furthermore, the B-14 trial contained a placebo arm that allowed for assessment of the rates of secondary cancers with emphasis on endometrial cancer. Subsequent analysis of secondary cancers, other then endometrial cancer, during the B-14 study indicated that there were no statistical differences in the rates of secondary cancers between the placebo- and tamoxifen-treated groups. Focus on the endometrial cancer rate of the patient population and subsequent analysis determined that the annual rate for the placebo group was 0.2 patients per 1000 and for the randomized tamoxifen-treated group, the annual rate was 1.6 patients per 1000. Overall analysis of all endometrial cancers observed in the study established that the vast majority of endometrial cancers occurred in postmenopausal women. Most importantly, the study found that when all categories of events were considered and combined, there was an overwhelming net benefit from tamoxifen treatment.

Meta-analysis of all randomized, placebo-controlled, adjuvant tamoxifen trials started before 1990 demonstrated significant tamoxifen benefits in breast cancer recurrence, contralateral breast cancer and mortality (EBCTCG, 1998). Of the 55 trials in the meta-analysis, 14 had a duration of less than one year, 32 trials had a two-year duration and 9 had a three- or more year duration (median 5 years). The analysis of recurrence as a first event and mortality indicated a highly statistically significant benefit with tamoxifen treatment. More importantly, breakdown of the trials by duration indicated that risk reduction may be dependent on the length of tamoxifen therapy and individuals who underwent longer duration of therapy received larger benefits. Additional breakdown of the study population based on ER status indicated a significant benefit to ER-positive individuals, which was most prominent in the five-year treatment trials. Tamoxifen did not benefit individuals with ER-negative tumors. The benefit of tamoxifen also applied to both node-negative and node-positive individuals and in both pre- and postmenopausal women, regardless of age. The meta-analysis also established that tamoxifen treatments increased the risk of endometrial cancer by approximately twofold, which translated in approximately fourfold increase in the risk of endometrial cancer during the duration of a five-year trial.

THE CLINICAL DEMONSTRATION OF SERM

Scientific principles for the effective applications of tamoxifen as a targeted adjuvant therapy (Jordan et al., 1979; Jordan and Allen, 1980) translated from the laboratory to clinical practice between the mid-1970s and the early 1990s. The targeting of long-term adjuvant tamoxifen therapy to patients with ER-positive breast cancers was shown to enhance survivorship (EBCTCG, 1998) and contribute to falling national death rates from breast cancer (EBCTCG, 2005). However, concerns were raised during the 1980s that the strategy of long-term tamoxifen treatment could result in toxicities related to the antiestrogenic effects of the drug. This debate initiated an interest in the clinical pharmacology of tamoxifen.

The effects of tamoxifen not related to breast cancer were first and specifically addressed in the Wisconsin Tamoxifen Study (Love et al., 1990). The study included postmenopausal women with breast cancer and histologically negative axillary lymph nodes, with a two-year follow-up. The primary focus of investigations was the effects of tamoxifen on plasma levels of lipids, lipoproteins, and coagulation proteins, changes in bone density, and symptomatic effects. Within three months of treatment the tamoxifen-treated group had statistically significant decreases in total cholesterol as compared with placebo, and more importantly, this decrease was persistent throughout all observed time points (Love et al., 1991b). The mean decrease in total cholesterol from baseline was approximately 12%. Initial results indicated decreases of high-density lipoprotein (HDL) levels in the tamoxifen group, which were statistically significant at the 12-month time point. The HDL cholesterol level reduction between the two groups was not observed at the 18- and 24- month time point. Triglyceride levels were modestly increased in the tamoxifen-treated group and continued to rise at 18 and 24 months. With the exception of the six-month time point, the increase in triglycerides was a statistically significant finding for all time points. The low-density lipoprotein (LDL) cholesterol levels decreased within the first three months of tamoxifen treatment and were significantly reduced for the 24-month period compared with placebo treatment (Love et al., 1990; Love et al., 1991b). Assessment of side effects associated with tamoxifen treatment indicated that tamoxifen was a well-tolerated agent, yet a significant number of patients developed chronic-moderate to chronic-severe vasomotor symptoms and/or mild gynecological symptoms (Love et al., 1991a). During the two-year study, the radius BMD in the tamoxifen-treated group decreased by 0.88% per year and the lumbar spine BMD increased 0.61% per year compared with baseline group (Love et al., 1992). In the placebo group, the BMD of the radius decreased by 1.29% per year and in the spine the BMD decreased by 1.00% per year, compared with baseline. Comparison of the tamoxifen-treated group to the placebo group indicated statistically significant differences for lumbar spine BMD but not for the radius BMD between the groups. It is important to note that the Wisconsin Tamoxifen Study included both pre- and postmenopausal women. Analysis of the BMDs based on menopausal status at the time of breast cancer diagnosis indicated that lumbar spine BMD increased 1.00% per year in the tamoxifen-treated group of women who were postmenopausal at time of diagnosis. There were no differences between the groups in osteocalcin levels, parathyroid hormone and 1,25-dihydroxyvitamin D. However, after 12 months there was a significant decrease in serum alkaline phosphatase levels in the tamoxifen-treated group compared with baseline and placebo groups.

The Wisconsin Tamoxifen Study indicated that toxicologically, tamoxifen is a well-tolerated agent with positive effects on BMD and potentially beneficial effects on overall lipid levels. Moreover, the study indicated that tamoxifen could potentially be used in breast cancer patients for stabilization of bone mass, particularly in women in whom estrogen and bisphosphonates are contraindicated.

The translation of laboratory observations that tamoxifen maintains bone density in ovariectomized rats (Jordan et al., 1987) into the clinic enhanced the possibility that the SERMs could become a novel drug group to aid postmenopausal women health.

CHEMOPREVENTION WITH TAMOXIFEN

Laboratory (Jordan et al., 1980; Jordan, 1981) and human epidemiological evidence (Miller and Bulbrook, 1980) supporting the hypothesis that estrogens are involved in breast cancer progression raised the possibility that endocrine intervention could prevent breast cancer development. Tamoxifen was the only candidate available to directly advance the strategy of decreasing breast cancer incidence in high-risk populations. However, a novel approach was also proposed to avoid many of the side effects noted with tamoxifen by developing the SERMs as multifunctional medicines. An indirect plan for breast cancer chemoprevention as a public health initiative was first described at the First International Chemoprevention Meeting in New York in 1987 as follows:

> The majority of breast cancers occur unexpectedly and from unknown origin. Great efforts are being focused on the identification of a population of high-risk women to test "chemopreventive" agents. But, are resources used less then optimally? An alternative would be to seize on the developing clues provided by an extensive clinical investigation of available antiestrogens. Could analogues be developed to treat osteoporosis or even retard the development of atherosclerosis? If this proved to be true, them majority of women in general would be treated for these conditions as soon as menopause occurred. Should the agent also retain antibreast tumor actions, then it might be expected to act as a chemosupressive on all developing breast cancers if these have an evolution from hormone-dependent disease to hormone-independent disease. A bold commitment to drug discovery and clinical pharmacology will potentially place us in a key position to prevent the development of breast cancer by the end of this century. (Jordan, 1988a)

This proposal was subsequently refined and presented at the American Association for Cancer Research (AACR) meeting in San Francisco in 1989. The proposal stated

> We have obtained valuable clinical information about this group of drugs that can be applied to other disease states. Research does not travel in straight lines and observations in one field are major discoveries in another. Important clues have been garnered about the effects of tamoxifen on bone and lipids, so apparently, derivatives could find targeted applications to retard osteoporosis or atherosclerosis. The ubiquitous application of novel compounds to prevent diseases associated with the progressive changes after menopause may, as a side effect, significantly retard the development of breast cancer. The target population would be postmenopausal women in general, thereby avoiding the requirement to select a high-risk group to prevent breast cancer (Lerner and Jordan, 1990).

Tamoxifen, a selective antiestrogen proven to delay the relapse and prolong survival (Adjuvant, 1987), was an ideal direct chemopreventive candidate because of the ease of administration and low acute toxicity, which in turn indicated good long-term compliance.

An overview of the characteristics of four major tamoxifen chemoprevention trials is shown in Table 1. Preliminary studies (Powles et al., 1989; Powles et al., 1994) established that patient's medication compliance was high and similar in both the tamoxifen and the placebo groups. Most commonly associated problems with tamoxifen treatment were hot flashes that occurred

Table 1 A Comparison of Patient Characteristics in the Tamoxifen Prevention Trials

Population characteristics	Royal Marsden	Italian	IBIS-I	NSABP P-1
Study size	2471	5408	7169	13388
Participants > 50 years old	62%	36%	49%	40%
Median follow-up	70 months	48 months	50 months	54.6 months
1° relative with breast cancer	55%	18%	48.1%	55%
> 1° relatives with breast cancer	17%	2.5%	61.7%	13%
Use of HRT	41%	8%	41%	0%
Breast cancer incidence per 1000 individuals				
Placebo	5.5	2.3	6.74	6.7
Tamoxifen	4.7	2.1	4.58	3.4

Abbreviations: IBIS, International Breast Cancer Intervention Study; NSAPB, National Surgical Adjuvant Breast and Bowel Project; HRT, hormone replacement therapy.

in 34% of the women in the tamoxifen group and in 20% of the women in the placebo group. The most significant differences in hot flashes, among the groups, were between the tamoxifen and the placebo groups of postmenopausal women. Menopausal women had similar incidences of hot flashes regardless of treatment.

Overall, tamoxifen was a well-tolerated agent with low acute toxicity. Even though hot flashes occurred more frequently in women on tamoxifen, the events were mild. Observed changes in lipid levels of tamoxifen-treated patients indicated the potentially positive effects of tamoxifen on overall cardiovascular health. Changes in clotting factors accompanied by decreases in the fibrinogen/antithrombin ratio indicated a potential decrease in risk of thrombosis.

It is very important to note that early studies such as the Royal Marsden study (Powles et al., 1998) and the Italian randomized trials (Veronesi et al., 1998), did not detect reduction of breast cancer risk associated with tamoxifen treatment. Both studies appeared to use large patient populations but the current consensus is that the populations were too small for practical purposes. The Royal Marsden study included 2462 pre- and postmenopausal women, while the Italian trials included 5408, pre- and postmenopausal, hysterectomized women at normal risk. The Italian trials (Veronesiet al., 1998) noted one crucial observation. Women who received hormone replacement therapy (HRT) and tamoxifen had significantly lower incidence of breast cancer compared with women in the placebo group who received HRT (Veronesi et al., 2003).

The International Breast Cancer Intervention Study (IBIS-I) (Cuzick et al., 2002) determined a 32% decrease in the rate of breast cancer between the tamoxifen- and the placebo- treated groups. The decrease was significant for both invasive and noninvasive cancers. Even though the tamoxifen-treated group had an approximately twofold excess of endometrial cancers as compared with the placebo-treated group, the finding was statistically insignificant. There were no differences in the rates of other cancers between the two groups. Moreover, the rate of venous thromboembolic events was 2.5 times higher in the tamoxifen group. A vast majority of these events (42%) occurred within three months of a major surgery or after prolonged immobility. Higher numbers of spontaneous thromboembolic events were also observed in the tamoxifen group as compared with the placebo group, but these findings were not statistically significant. In contrast to the Italian trials, the IBIS-I trial demonstrated no difference between the tamoxifen- and placebo-treated individuals receiving HRT.

The primary goal of the NSABP P-1 study (Fisher et al., 1998) was to determine whether five years of tamoxifen administration prevented invasive breast cancer in high-risk women. Secondary aims included determining incidence of myocardial infarctions (fatal and nonfatal) and the potential reduction of bone fractures. The NSABP P-1 trial found a highly statistically significant decrease in the number of invasive and noninvasive breast cancers in the tamoxifen-treated group compared with the placebo-treated group. The overall risk for invasive breast cancers in the tamoxifen-treated group was reduced by 49%. There was a 69% decrease in the annual rate of ER-positive cancers in the tamoxifen-treated group. The rates of ER-negative breast cancers remained similar in both the tamoxifen- and placebo-treated groups. The tamoxifen-treated patients had a 2.53 times greater risk of endometrial cancer than the placebo-treated individuals. No differences in the rates of other invasive carcinomas were observed between the tamoxifen and the placebo groups. In regard to the secondary end points there were no differences in the number and severity of ischemic events between the two groups. The protocol defined fractures of the hip and radius as primary fracture events. Fractures of the spine were added soon after initiation of the study. Fewer osteoporotic fracture events (hip, spine, and lower radius) occurred in women who received tamoxifen than in those who received placebo. There was an increase in the overall reduction in women over 50 years. The incidence of stroke was increased in the tamoxifen-treated group as was the incidence of thromboembolic events. There were no significant quality of life differences between the groups except for hot flashes and vaginal discharges.

It is important to note that the independent data monitoring committee of the NSABP P-1 trial, six months before the publication of the study, determined that the primary goal of the trial, the reduction of breast cancer incidence with tamoxifen treatment, was reached. Based on the overwhelming data that tamoxifen is an effective prophylactic breast cancer agent, the committee, based on ethical considerations, determined that the study be unblinded, thus allowing the placebo population of the trial consider tamoxifen treatment or enroll in a second prevention trial that compared tamoxifen to another SERM, raloxifene (Fisher, 1999).

Overview analysis (Cuzick et al., 2003) of the four major chemoprevention trials showed 46% reduction in the rates of breast cancer incidence. Moreover, even though statistically significant increases of endometrial cancer rates were not observed in the tamoxifen-treated group of all trials, a significant finding became apparent. Most of the endometrial cancer cases involved postmenopausal women. In addition to endometrial cancer, tamoxifen-treated individuals had elevated risk of death caused by pulmonary embolisms and significant increase of thromboembolic events.

The potential public health impact of the NSABP P-1 trial is difficult to ascertain. Initial analysis (Fisher, 1999) estimated that in a five year period approximately 500,000 invasive and 200,000 noninvasive breast cancers could be prevented among the approximately 29 million women in the United States eligible for tamoxifen chemoprevention. Yet, subsequent analysis (Rockhill et al., 2000) based on the findings of the NSABP P-1 trial and their application to the Nurses Health Study (Rockhill et al., 2001), deemed these estimates high. Analysis (Freedman et al., 2003) of nationally representative data from the year 2000 National Health Interview Survey (NHIS) tried to determine the benefits (reduction of invasive breast cancer and bone fractures) and risk of adverse events (increase in endometrial cancer and thromboembolic events) associated with tamoxifen treatment. The analysis concluded that 15.5% of women aged 35 to 79 in the Unites States would be eligible for tamoxifen chemoprevention, based on age and risk factors. However, the percentage of women eligible for chemoprevention varies with age. For example, 45% of white women over the age of 60 would be considered eligible for chemoprevention, but eligibility certainly does not translate into net chemoprevention benefit. Overall, from the 18.7% of white women eligible for chemoprevention, only 4.9% would receive a net benefit. Furthermore, even though the analysis indicates that the highest percentage of women eligible for chemoprevention is in the 60 to 79 years age group, the greatest percentage of white women who would benefit the most fall into the 40 to 49 and 50 to 59 years age groups.

The other issue to be considered with the availability of tamoxifen is efficacy based on compliance and cost. A recent study of tamoxifen compliance in the treatment setting found that over one-third of women stopped taking tamoxifen, a proven therapy that aids survival, after three to –five years (Barron et al., 2007). Additionally, cost of chemoprevention is an issue for health services. It is estimated that only very high-risk women (Gail score $\geq$3), those with a risk of few negative side effects, would benefit and only in an environment that provides cheap generic tamoxifen (Melnikow et al., 2006).

The risk-benefit analysis of any prophylactic agent must be carefully examined with a focus on the overall patient population. As a result, a new strategy (Jordan, 1988) was initiated that would improve on the net benefits achieved with tamoxifen.

CLINICAL EVALUATIONS OF RALOXIFENE TO PREVENT OSTEOPOROSIS

Overall, the story of the clinical development of raloxifene is the story of changing ideas about the relevance of models to predict population outcomes. The idea of a SERM is to address the prevention of three major diseases: osteoporosis, atherosclerosis, and breast cancer. The goal was to replace HRT for the treatment of osteoporosis with a SERM to reduce breast cancer risk. Unfortunately, the idea that a decrease in circulating cholesterol observed with HRT and raloxifene would translate into lives saved from coronary heart disease (CHD) proved to be wrong (Mosca et al., 2001; Rossouw et al., 2002; Anderson et al., 2004).

In pilot clinical trials, raloxifene was shown to lower serum cholesterol levels without increases in triglycerides or endometrial effects and decrease bone turnover, as determined by biochemical markers (Draper et al., 1996). These findings further supported the hypothesis that an antiestrogen may be used for treatment of breast cancer and can have beneficial effects on a number of other factors, including osteoporosis (Jordan, 1988). The effects of various doses of raloxifene on BMD (regional and total), bone turnover markers, serum lipids, and endometrial thickness were addressed in a two-year clinical trial (Delmas et al., 1997). The study population included 601 postmenopausal, 45 to 60 years old women with osteoporosis. The study groups received placebo, 30-, 60-, or 150-mg raloxifene daily supplemented with 400- to 600-mg elemental calcium. Serum lipids and bone turnover markers were measured every three months while spine and hip BMD, as well as endometrial thickness, were measured every six months. Within three months of raloxifene treatments, as compared with placebo, there was a decrease in the levels of the bone turnover markers within the levels of healthy postmenopausal women. Furthermore, raloxifene treatments increased the lumbar spine, femoral neck, total hip, and total body BMD. The population receiving the highest 150-mg daily raloxifene dose had the greatest increase in all categories with exception of total hip BMD (60-mg dose had the greatest increase). Raloxifene treatments decreased the levels of LDLs and total cholesterol in dose-dependent fashion without changes in the levels of HDLs and triglycerides. Raloxifene was relatively well tolerated and no differences in adverse events or proportion of women reporting hot flashes were observed between the placebo and raloxifene treatment groups. Most importantly no increases in endometrial thickness were observed in the raloxifene-treated population. The positive clinical profiles obtained during the study indicated that raloxifene might be useful in the prevention of osteoporosis and cardiovascular disease, without negative effects on the endometrium.

A subsequent clinical trial (Walsh et al., 1998) examined the lowest effective dose of raloxifene on intermediate cardiovascular end points and compared the effects to those of HRT. The primary end points considered were the levels of HDL and LDL cholesterol, triglycerides, and the clotting factor fibrinogen. The study population consisted of 390 healthy postmenopausal women aged 45 to 72. The treatments included placebo, 60 or 120-mg daily raloxifene and HRT (conjugated equine estrogen 0.625 mg daily and medroxyprogesterone acetate 2.5 mg daily). The duration of treatments was six months. Effects of treatment were apparent within the first three months and persisted during the duration of the study. LDL cholesterol levels, as compared with placebo, were decreased 12% with raloxifene treatments and 14% with HRT. HDL cholesterol levels were not affected by raloxifene treatments but increased 10% with HRT. Triglyceride levels were also unaffected by raloxifene treatments but increased 20% with HRT. In contrast, raloxifene treatments decreased the levels of fibrinogen while HRT did not affect the fibrinogen levels. The most common side effects reported were hot flashes, which were most common in the 120-mg raloxifene group. Overall, raloxifene had similar cardiovascular effects as HRT in healthy postmenopausal women. Most importantly, the decrease of LDL cholesterol further indicated to investigators at the time that raloxifene treatments may decrease the risk of coronary artery disease.

The Multiple Outcomes of Raloxifene Evaluation (MORE) trial (Ettinger et al., 1999) was initiated to determine the effects of raloxifene therapy on the risk of vertebral and nonvertebral fractures. The study population consisted of 7705 postmenopausal women, aged 31 to 80, with osteoporosis and the study population was subdivided into two subgroups. The first subgroup included women with femoral neck and lumbar spine BMD t score <2.5. The second subgroup included women with low BMD and one or more moderate to severe vertebral fractures and women who had at least two moderate fractures regardless of BMD. The treatments included placebo and 60- or 120-mg raloxifene, supplemented by 500-mg calcium and 400- to 600-IU calciferol. The primary end points considered were incidental vertebral fractures and BMD. The secondary end point consisted of any nonvertebral fractures. At the 36-month time point, overall and in each individual raloxifene treatment group, the raloxifene-treated individuals had fewer new vertebral fractures. Similar rates of nonvertebral fractures were observed for all study groups, with the exception of the statistically significant differences in ankle fractures between the pooled raloxifene groups and the placebo groups. Femoral neck and spine BMD were increased and bone turnover markers were decreased in the raloxifene-treated groups. No differences in endometrial cancer rates were observed between the raloxifene- and placebo-treated individuals. However, significant increases of thromboembolic events [including deep vein thrombosis (DVT) and pulmonary embolisms] were observed among the raloxifene-treated individuals. Therefore, raloxifene was considered to be a very well-tolerated agent.

Forty-eight-month follow-up (Delmas et al., 2002) indicated that raloxifene treatment significantly decreases the risk of vertebral fractures in both study subgroups without significant differences between the two raloxifene doses. However, there were no indications that raloxifene treatment decreased the risk of nonvertebral fractures. Similar to the 36-month time point, continuous raloxifene treatment significantly improved the lumbar spine and femoral neck BMDs. It is important to note that 36 months was the primary end point of the MORE trial. An additional year of follow-up was used primarily to determine the cumulative effects of raloxifene on vertebral fracture risks during a four-year time period.

More importantly, the MORE trial provided an appropriate arena for testing the breast cancer chemoprevention concept (Lerner and Jordan, 1990) so that an "antiestrogenic" medicine, in this case raloxifene, may not only treat a disease caused by overall physiological changes during menopause but also significantly reduce the development of breast cancer. Indeed, subsequent analysis (Cummings et al., 1999) of the MORE trial participants indicated that during the three year MORE trial the raloxifene-treated individuals had substantially lower rate of breast cancer. During the 40 months of median follow-up period, the rate of all breast cancers was 4.3 cancers per 1000 women years in the placebo and 1.5 cancers per 1000 women years.

The rates of invasive breast cancers were 3.6 cancers per 1000 women years in the placebo and 0.9 invasive breast cancers per 1000 women years in the raloxifene-pooled groups. It was determined that raloxifene decreased the risk of invasive ER-positive breast cancer by 90%, while the rate of invasive ER-negative breast cancer remained constant, albeit with a high-confidence interval. The positive effects of raloxifene on breast cancer were accompanied by negligible effects on the endometrium.

The Continuous Outcomes Relevant to Evista (CORE) (Ettinger et al., 1999) trial was an extension of the MORE trial. It examined the effects of four years of additional raloxifene treatment on a subset of the population from the MORE trial. Therefore, the study population consisted of postmenopausal women with osteoporosis. The primary end point of the CORE trial was incidence of invasive breast cancer, while the secondary end point considered was the incidence of ER-positive breast cancer. The treatments consisted of placebo and 60-mg daily raloxifene supplemented with 500-mg calcium and 400- to 600-IU Vitamin D. It is important to note that as the patient population had osteoporosis, the study population was allowed to take bone specific agents such as bisphosphonates, calcitonin, or fluoride.

During the four years of the CORE trial the raloxifene-treated individuals had 59% decreases in the incidence of invasive breast cancer. The incidence of invasive ER-positive breast cancer was decreased by 66% in the raloxifene-treated group. Most importantly, the incidence rate of invasive ER-negative breast cancer was not changed by raloxifene treatment. Overall, raloxifene decreased the rate of all breast cancers by 50%. Analysis of the combined data from the MORE and CORE trials indicated that after approximately eight years (range 4.8–8.5 years), raloxifene treatment reduced the incidence of invasive breast cancer by 66%. The incidence of invasive ER-positive breast cancers was decreased by 76% while the incidence of invasive ER-negative cancer remained the same. Overall, regardless of ER status, raloxifene treatments decreased the incidence of breast cancer by 58%. The incidence of adverse effects, vaginal bleeding, endometrial hyperplasia, and endometrial cancer were statistically insignificant between the placebo and raloxifene groups in the CORE trial and during the combined duration of the MORE and CORE trials.

The MORE or CORE study demonstrated the effectiveness of raloxifene to reduce fractures while reducing the risk of breast cancer. However, it must be stated that there were periods between the two trials when women were not treated with raloxifene. As a result, it is possible that if compliance to raloxifene had been maintained, the risk of breast cancer could be reduced more effectively.

STUDY OF TAMOXIFEN AND RALOXIFENE

The NSABP P-2 Study Of Tamoxifen And Raloxifene (STAR) trial was launched to compare the relative effects and safety of tamoxifen and raloxifene on the risk of developing invasive breast cancer in high-risk populations of women (Vogel et al., 2006). This study is an example of the distinct approach to chemoprevention in populations of postmenopausal women at high risk for breast cancer. Even though initially, and from a chronological aspect, the STAR trial appears to be a natural extension of the progress made in breast cancer chemoprevention with the MORE and CORE trials, in reality the STAR trial is an extension of the NSABP P-1 trial. The ethical considerations generated during the NSABP P-1 trial and the progress made during various adjuvant and chemopreventive tamoxifen trials laid the foundation for search of equivalent and/or superior breast cancer agents while minimizing undesired side effects.

The study, population of the STAR trial was 19,747 healthy postmenopausal women with increased five-year breast cancer risk. The treatments consisted of 20-mg daily tamoxifen and 60-mg daily raloxifene. The primary end point considered was invasive breast cancer. Secondary end points considered were diseases influenced by tamoxifen in previous breast cancer prevention trials and included endometrial cancer, in situ breast cancer, cardiovascular disease, stroke, pulmonary embolism, DVT, transient ischemic attack, osteoporotic fractures, cataracts, death, and quality of life (Vogel et al., 2006).

In regard to invasive breast cancer, both tamoxifen and raloxifene exhibited similar effects during the six-year follow-up (median follow-up 3.9 years). There were no significant differences in the rates of invasive breast cancer between the tamoxifen and raloxifene groups.

The incidence of invasive breast cancer for the tamoxifen group was 4.3 cases per 1000 women years and 4.41 cases per 1000 women years for the raloxifene group. Overall, there were fewer cases of in situ breast cancer in the tamoxifen group than in the raloxifene group, and this finding was statistically insignificant but approaching significance ($p = 0.052$). Tamoxifen and raloxifene also exhibited similar effects on uterine cancer. However, there was statistically insignificant trend of lower incidence of uterine cancer in the raloxifene group. Majority of uterine cancers occurred in women over 50 years. Even though the endometrial cancer rates were similar for both agents, the raloxifene group had 38% lower incidence rate then the tamoxifen group. The incidence of uterine hyperplasia (with and without atypia) was decreased by 84% in the raloxifene group. Importantly, the number of hysterectomies during follow-up in women not diagnosed with uterine cancer was significantly lower in the raloxifene group. No differences in the rates of other cancers were observed between the two groups. Lung cancers were more numerous in the raloxifene group but this finding was not statistically significant. Additionally, no differences in the incidence of ischemic heart disease, strokes, and fractures were observed between the two groups. Significant differences between the two groups were observed in regard to thromboembolic events, cataracts, and cataracts surgery. The raloxifene-treated group had a 30% decrease in thromboembolic events (pulmonary embolisms and DVT) and significantly less participants in the raloxifene group developed cataracts and had cataracts surgery.

The STAR trial indicates that raloxifene and tamoxifen are agents with similar breast cancer chemopreventive efficacy. Although the differences between the two treatment groups were not statistically significant in regard to invasive breast cancer, there were fewer instances of noninvasive breast cancer in the tamoxifen group, indicating that tamoxifen may be a more efficient agent in prevention of noninvasive breast carcinoma. However, even though both drugs exhibited similar chemopreventive efficacy, raloxifene exhibited a superior safety profile.

RALOXIFENE USE FOR THE HEART

Tamoxifen (Love et al., 1990) and raloxifene (Delmas et al., 1997; Ettinger et al., 1999; Delmas et al., 2002) therapy has been associated with positive changes in various cardiovascular markers. These observations raised the possibility that a potential side effect of SERM therapy may be an improved cardiovascular system. Combination of these findings with the observations that HRT may not significantly decrease the incidence of CHD in post menopausal women (Hulley et al., 1998; Rossouw et al., 2002; Anderson et al., 2004) led to the Raloxifene Use For The Heart (RUTH) trial (Barrett-Connor et al., 2006). The purpose of the RUTH trial was to determine the effects of raloxifene on cardiovascular events as compared to placebo. The trial included 10,101 postmenopausal women with established risk of CHD. The treatments included placebo and 60-mg daily raloxifene. When all combined coronary end points were considered there were no differences between the two groups. Additionally, no difference in the overall stroke incidence was observed. Nevertheless, the incidence of fatal stroke was 49% higher in the raloxifene group. Significant differences between the groups were observed in regard to venous thromboembolic events (44% higher in the raloxifene group), breast cancer (33% lower incidence of all breast cancers) and clinical vertebral fractures (35% lower incidence in the raloxifene group). Most importantly, the incidence of endometrial and other cancers did not differ between the groups. No differences in the numbers of adverse events were observed between the two groups, but a significantly larger number of women in the raloxifene group discontinued therapy because of adverse events.

Overall, extended raloxifene therapy (median 5.6 years) did not provide any significant cardiovascular benefits, but while significantly decreasing the rates of breast cancer and clinical vertebral fractures, it significantly increased the number of venous thromboembolic events. Concurrently, large clinical trials (Hulley et al., 1998; Rossouw et al., 2002; Anderson et al., 2004) of hormonally treated postmenopausal women have failed to demonstrate any benefits of estrogen therapy on cardiovascular health. These findings, though disappointing from a cardiovascular standpoint, further reinforce the need to further develop the SERM concept. Current trials support the idea that SERMs decrease the risk of breast cancer, and raloxifene (but not tamoxifen) does not increase the risk of endometrial cancer in postmenopausal women. Additionally, SERMs reduce the incidence of vertebral fractures in postmenopausal women, and raloxifene has a more favorable safety profile than tamoxifen in postmenopausal women. These clinical observations have now established a new drug group into medicine and it is appropriate to conclude with a discussion of their potential use in clinical practice.

CONCLUSION

Three issues are important to optimize the process of breast cancer chemoprevention: (1) identification of the target population, (2) selection of an appropriate agent, and (3) the burden of the cost of chemopreventive therapies on public health systems.

The Gail model (Gail et al., 1989) has been successfully used for identification of patient populations in the NSABP P-1 and STAR P-2 trials. However, in the Nurses Health Study (Rockhill et al., 2001), a study involving over 80,000 women, 44% of the observed breast carcinomas occurred in the high-risk group (Gail risk of $\geq$1.67) and 54% of the breast cancers occurred in population of women deemed not at risk for breast cancer as predicted by the Gail model. Therefore, it is important to develop models that could identify the desired target populations and distinguish various degrees of risks within the patient populations.

The link between ovarian hormones and breast cancer was noted over a century ago (Beatson, 1896) and the idea that creating a no-estrogen state may prevent breast cancer was suggested approximately 70 years ago (Lacassagne, 1936). Aromatase inhibitors that are currently used to treat breast cancer use this concept and current clinical trials have shown their superiority over tamoxifen in inhibiting contralateral breast cancer in postmenopausal women (Coombes et al., 2004; Goss et al., 2005; Howell et al., 2005; Thurlimann et al., 2005). However, what would be the cost, both to women and health care systems, if aromatase inhibitors were the agent of choice?

If one assumes a population similar to those described in the STAR trial (Vogel et al., 2006) and identifies a high-risk population of postmenopausal women based on the Gail model, then the incidence of breast cancer will be 8 per 1000 women annually. Chemopreventive application of aromatase inhibitors in the patient population may prevent three out of four breast cancers. Therefore, in order to prevent six breast cancers, an additional 992 women will need to be treated without other benefits and with potential for harmful side effects. Based on the National Health and Nutrition Examination Survey, up to 18% of women over the age of 50 in the United States suffer from osteoporosis and up to 50% suffer from osteopenia (Looker et al., 1997). Aromatase inhibitors will increase a woman's risk for osteoporosis and thus other alternative preventive strategies need to be considered.

The concept of chemoprevention with SERMs has been developed, tested in the laboratory, and refined over the past 20 years. The evidence-based laboratory concept (Jordan, 1988) has been successfully tested in the clinic and can now be used to extrapolate the results of the raloxifene clinical studies to estimate public health benefits. The MORE trial (Cummings et al., 1999) established the initial proof of the principle that a SERM could be successfully used to prevent osteoporotic fractures in a postmenopusal population while at the same time decreasing the breast cancer rate. The CORE trial (Martino et al., 2004) further documented a significant decrease in the breast cancer rates during long-term (up to 8 years) raloxifene treatments. However, it is interesting to point out that in contrast to the MORE and CORE trials that recorded 65% to 75% decrease in the breast cancer rates; there was only an estimated 50% decrease in the rates of breast cancer during the STAR trial. One reason for such a discrepancy may be the target population of the respective trials. Raloxifene may perform exceptionally well in low estrogen states such as those observed in osteoporotic women. This was the patient population in the MORE and the CORE trials. In contrast, the patient population of the STAR trial consisted of healthy postmenopausal women with possibly higher levels of circulating estrogen. Additional factors for such discrepancies may be low patient compliance combined with the raloxifene's poor bioavailability (Gottardis and Jordan, 1987; Snyder et al., 2000; Jordan, 2006). Raloxifene's poor bioavailability illustrates the need for long-lasting SERMs and indeed, new long-lasting alternatives such as arzoxifene (Sato et al., 1998; Suh et al., 2001), may become available in the near future. Arzoxifene is superior to raloxifene in prevention of rat mammary carcinogenesis (Suh et al., 2001) and clinical trials for the treatment and prevention of osteoporosis are nearing completion. Thus a SERM that reduces breast and endometrial cancers while increasing bone density will be a suitable intervention to prevent breast cancer in postmenopausal, high- and low-risk, women. The fact that SERMs are cheaper then aromatse inhibitor is also an advantage. But what of tamoxifen, the veteran SERM?

Tamoxifen is available in the United States as an effective chemopreventive agent in a high-risk postmenopausal population; however, there is significant increase in endometrial cancer. Evaluation of mortality outcomes (Melnikow et al., 2006) have projected that the use of tamoxifen in populations with Gail risk greater than or equal to 3 will have maximum benefit, but only in countries with affordable tamoxifen. Use of tamoxifen, particularly in managed health care systems, must be accompanied with comprehensive patient follow-up because of tamoxifen's significant side effects. Naturally, tamoxifen is a viable option in hysterectomized women. Nevertheless, tamoxifen is the only agent available to reduce the risk of breast cancer in premenopausal women. There are no elevations in endometrial cancer or blood clots in premenopausal women making tamoxifen a reasonable health choice. Compliance is also a major consideration for healthy women taking a medicine that decreases quality of life. In the case of tamoxifen, a large proportion of women report increase of hot flashes and menopausal symptoms. In recent years physicians have prescribed selective serotonin reuptake inhibitors (SSRIs) that significantly reduce hot flashes. However, the finding that tamoxifen must be converted to an active metabolite, i.e., endoxifen, for optimal activity and that some of the SSRIs block the CYP2D6 enzyme responsible for that conversion, is of concern (Jordan, 2007) (Fig. 1).

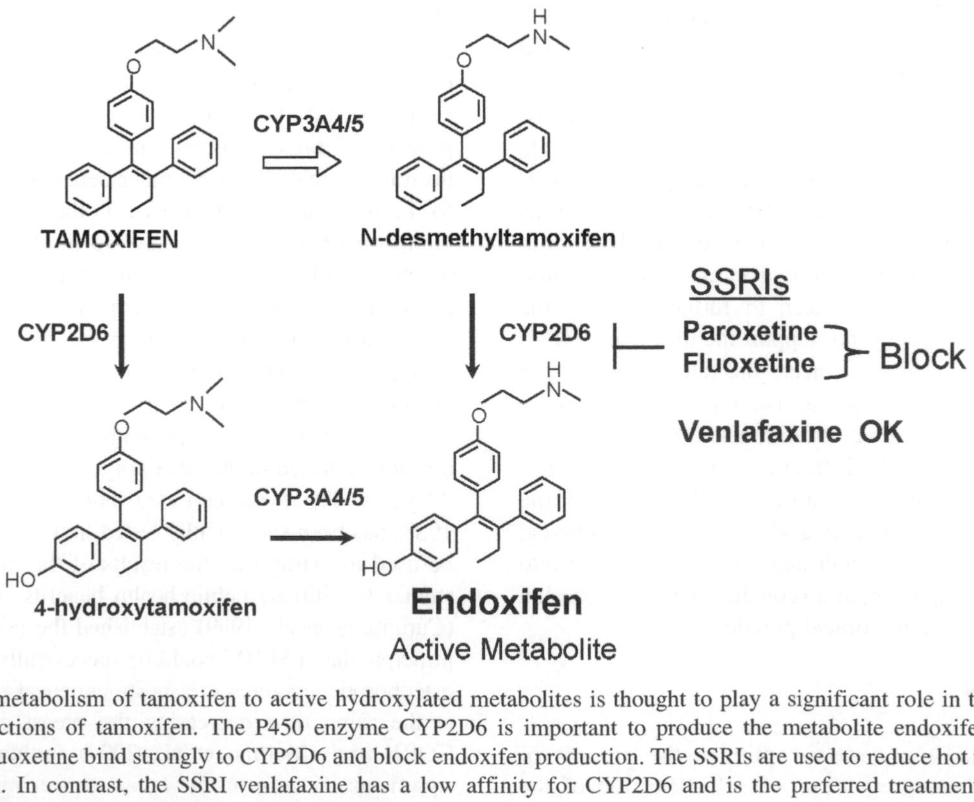

Figure 1 The metabolism of tamoxifen to active hydroxylated metabolites is thought to play a significant role in the antiestrogenic and anticancer actions of tamoxifen. The P450 enzyme CYP2D6 is important to produce the metabolite endoxifen but the SSRIs paroxetine and fluoxetine bind strongly to CYP2D6 and block endoxifen production. The SSRIs are used to reduce hot flashes in women taking tamoxifen. In contrast, the SSRI venlafaxine has a low affinity for CYP2D6 and is the preferred treatment for hot flashes. *Abbreviation*: SSRIs, selective serotonin reuptake inhibitors.

Also, there are individuals with nonfunctional alleles (CYP2D6 *4/*4) that have no enzymatic activity. It is therefore reasonable that if a woman is to complete five years of treatment for chemoprevention, she should determine whether she has an aberrant CYP2D6 enzyme and is not taking SSRI known to impair tamoxifen metabolism (Stearns et al., 2003; Goetz et al., 2005; Goetz et al., 2007).

In closing, it is now possible to recommend a practical strategy to patients to reduce the risks of breast cancer. Twenty years ago this was not possible. The SERM concept (Jordan, 1988a) has provided clues for further research development strategies for other members of the steroid receptors super family (Smith and O'Malley, 2004). Anabolic androgens that do not stimulate the prostate would be valuable medicines. Alternatively, glucocorticoids that can control inflammation without causing bone loss would be invaluable. A dedicated program of drug discovery and development is now possible to create targeted therapies previously thought to be impossible.

ACKNOWLEDGMENT

Supported by the Department of Defense Breast Program under award number BC050277 Center of Excellence (Views and opinions of, and endorsements by the author(s) do not reflect those of the U.S. Army or the Department of Defense), SPORE in Breast Cancer CA 89018, R01 GM067156, FCCC Core Grant NIH P30 CA006927, the Avon Foundation and the Weg Fund of Fox Chase Cancer Center.

REFERENCES

Adjuvant tamoxifen in the management of operable breast cancer: the Scottish Trial. Report from the Breast Cancer Trials Committee, Scottish Cancer Trials Office (MRC), Edinburgh. Lancet 1987; 2(8552):171–175.

Anderson GL, Limacher M, Assaf AR, Bassford T, Beresford SA, Black H, Bonds D, Brunner R, Brzyski R, Caan B, Chlebowski R, Curb D, Gass M, Hays J, Heiss G, Hendrix S, Howard BV, Hsia J, Hubbell A, Jackson R, Johnson KC, Judd H, Kotchen JM, Kuller L, LaCroix AZ, Lane D, Langer RD, Lasser N, Lewis CE, Manson J, Margolis K, Ockene J, O'Sullivan MJ, Phillips L, Prentice RL, Ritenbaugh C, Robbins J, Rossouw JE, Sarto G, Stefanick ML, Van Horn L, Wactawski-Wende J, Wallace R, Wassertheil-Smoller S. (2004). Effects of conjugated equine estrogen in postmenopausal women with hysterectomy: the Women's Health Initiative randomized controlled trial. JAMA (2004); 291(14):1701–1712.

Barrett-Connor E, Mosca L, Collins P, Geiger MJ, Grady D, Kornitzer M, McNabb MA, Wenger NK. Effects of raloxifene on cardiovascular events and breast cancer in postmenopausal women. N Engl J Med 2006; 355(2):125–37.

Barron TI, Connolly R, Bennett K, Feely J, Kennedy MJ. Early discontinuation of tamoxifen: a Lesson for oncologists. Cancer 2007; 110(11):2596.

Beatson GT. On the treatment of inoperable cases of the carcinoma of the mamma: suggestions for a new method of treatment with illustrative cases. Lancet 1896; ii; 104–107.

Black LJ, Sato M, Rowley ER, Magee DE, Bekele A, Williams DC, Cullinan GJ, Bendele R, Kauffman RF, Bensch WR, et al. Raloxifene (LY139481 HCI) prevents bone loss and reduces serum cholesterol without causing uterine hypertrophy in ovariectomized rats. J Clin Invest 1994; 93(1): 63–69.

Clemens JA, Bennett DR, Black LJ, Jones CD Effects of a new antiestrogen, keoxifene (LY156758), on growth of carcinogen-induced mammary tumors and on LH and prolactin levels. Life Sci 1983; 32(25):2869–2875.

Cole MP, Jones CT, Todd ID. A new anti-oestrogenic agent in late breast cancer. An early clinical appraisal of ICI46474. Br J Cancer 1971; 25(2):270–275.

Coombes RC, Hall E, Gibson LJ, Paridaens R, Jassem J, Delozier T, Jones SE, Alvarez I, Bertelli G, Ortmann O, Coates AS, Bajetta E, Dodwell D, Coleman RE, Fallowfield LJ, Mickiewicz E, Andersen J, Lonning PE, Cocconi G, Stewart A, Stuart N, Snowdon CF, Carpentieri M, Massimini G, Bliss JM, van de Velde C. A randomized trial of exemestane after two to three years of tamoxifen therapy in postmenopausal women with primary breast cancer. N Engl J Med 2004; 350(11):1081–1092.

Cummings SR, Eckert S, Krueger KA, Grady D, Powles TJ, Cauley JA, Norton L, Nickelsen T, Bjarnason NH, Morrow M, Lippman ME, Black D, Glusman JE, Costa A, Jordan VC. The effect of raloxifene on risk of breast cancer in postmenopausal women: results from the MORE randomized trial. Multiple Outcomes of Raloxifene Evaluation. JAMA 1999; 281(23):2189–2197.

Cuzick J, Forbes J, Edwards R, Baum M, Cawthorn S, Coates A, Hamed A, Howell A, Powles T. First results from the International Breast Cancer Intervention Study (IBIS-I): a randomised prevention trial. Lancet 2002; 360(9336): 817–824.

Cuzick J, Powles T, Veronesi U, Forbes J, Edwards R, Ashley S, Boyle P. Overview of the main outcomes in breast-cancer prevention trials. Lancet 2003; 361(9354):296–300.

Delmas PD, Bjarnason NH, Mitlak BH, Ravoux AC, Shah AS, Huster WJ, Draper M, Christiansen C. Effects of raloxifene on bone mineral density, serum cholesterol concentrations, and uterine endometrium in postmenopausal women. N Engl J Med 1997; 337(23):1641–1647.

Delmas PD, Ensrud KE, Adachi JD, Harper KD, Sarkar S, Gennari C, Reginster JY, Pols HA, Recker RR, Harris ST, Wu W, Genant HK, Black DM, Eastell R. Efficacy of raloxifene on vertebral fracture risk reduction in postmenopausal women with osteoporosis: four-year results from a randomized clinical trial. J Clin Endocrinol Metab 2002; 87(8):36093617.

Draper MW, Flowers DE, Huster WJ, Neild JA, Harper KD, Arnaud C. A controlled trial of raloxifene (LY139481) HCl: impact on bone turnover and serum lipid profile in healthy postmenopausal women. J Bone Miner Res 1996; 11 (6):835–842.

EBCTCG. Early Breast Cancer Trialists' Collaborative Group. Tamoxifen for early breast cancer: an overview of the randomised trials. Lancet 1998; 351(9114):1451–1467.

EBCTCG. Early Breast Cancer Trialists' Collaborative Group. Effects of chemotherapy and hormonal therapy for early breast cancer on recurrence and 15-year survival: an overview of the randomised trials. Lancet 2005; 365(9472):1687–1717.

Ettinger BD, Black M, Mitlak BH, Knickerbocker RK, Nickelsen T, Genant HK, Christiansen C, Delmas PD, Zanchetta JR, Stakkestad J, Gluer CC, Krueger K, Cohen FJ, Eckert S, Ensrud KE, Avioli LV, Lips P, Cummings SR. Reduction of vertebral fracture risk in postmenopausal women with osteoporosis treated with raloxifene: results from a 3-year randomized clinical trial. Multiple Outcomes of Raloxifene Evaluation (MORE) Investigators. JAMA 1999; 282(7): 637–645.

Fisher B. National Surgical Adjuvant Breast and Bowel Project breast cancer prevention trial: a reflective commentary. J Clin Oncol 1999; 17(5):1632–1639.

Fisher B, Costantino J, Redmond C, Poisson R, Bowman D, Couture J, Dimitrov NV, Wolmark N, Wickerham DL, Fisher ER, , and et al. A randomized clinical trial evaluating tamoxifen in the treatment of patients with node-negative breast cancer who have estrogen-receptor-positive tumors. N Engl J Med 1989; 320(8):479–484.

Fisher B, Costantino JP, Wickerham DL, Redmond CK, Kavanah M, Cronin WM, Vogel V, Robidoux A, Dimitrov N, Atkins J, Daly M, Wieand S, Tan-Chiu E, Ford L, Wolmark N. Tamoxifen for prevention of breast cancer: report of the National Surgical Adjuvant Breast and Bowel Project P-1 Study. J Natl Cancer Inst 1998; 90(18): 1371–1388.

Fornander T, Rutqvist LE, Cedermark B, Glas U, Mattsson A, Silfversward C, Skoog L, Somell A, Theve T, Wilking N, et al. Adjuvant tamoxifen in early breast cancer: occurrence of new primary cancers. Lancet 1989; 1(8630):117–120.

Freedman AN, Graubard BI, Rao SR, McCaskill-Stevens W, Ballard-Barbash R, Gail MH. Estimates of the number of US women who could benefit from tamoxifen for breast cancer chemoprevention. J Natl Cancer Inst 2003; 95(7):526–532.

Furr BJ, and Jordan VC. The pharmacology and clinical uses of tamoxifen. Pharmacol Ther 1984; 25(2):127–205.

Gail MH, Brinton LA, Byar DP, Corle DK, Green SB, Schairer C, Mulvihill JJ. Projecting individualized probabilities of developing breast cancer for white females who are being examined annually. J Natl Cancer Inst 1989; 81(24):1879–1886.

Goetz MP, Knox SK, Suman VJ, Rae JM, Safgren SL, Ames MM, Visscher DW, Reynolds C, Couch FJ, Lingle WL, Weinshilboum RM, Fritcher EG, Nibbe AM, Desta Z, Nguyen A, Flockhart DA, Perez EA, Ingle JN. The impact of cytochrome P450 2D6 metabolism in women receiving adjuvant tamoxifen. Breast Cancer Res Treat 2007; 101(1):113–121.

Goetz MP, Rae JM, Suman VJ, Safgren SL, Ames MM, Visscher DW, Reynolds C, Couch FJ, Lingle WL, Flockhart DA, Desta Z, Perez EA, Ingle JN. Pharmacogenetics of tamoxifen biotransformation is associated with clinical outcomes of efficacy and hot flashes. J Clin Oncol 2005; 23(36): 9312–9318.

Goss PE, Ingle JN, Martino S, Robert NJ, Muss HB, Piccart MJ, Castiglione M, Tu D, Shepherd, Pritchard KI, Livingston RB, Davidson NE, Norton L, Perez EA, Abrams JS, Cameron DA, Palmer MJ, Pater JL. Randomized trial of letrozole following tamoxifen as extended adjuvant therapy in receptor-positive breast cancer: updated findings from NCIC CTG MA.17. J Natl Cancer Inst 2005; 97(17): 1262–1271.

Gottardis MM, Jordan VC. Antitumor actions of keoxifene and tamoxifen in the N-nitrosomethylurea-induced rat mammary carcinoma model. Cancer Res 1987; 47(15): 4020–4024.

Gottardis MM, Robinson SP, Satyaswaroop PG, Jordan VC. Contrasting actions of tamoxifen on endometrial and breast tumor growth in the athymic mouse. Cancer Res 1988; 48(4):812–815.

Hardell L. Tamoxifen as risk factor for carcinoma of corpus uteri. Lancet 1988; 2(8610):563.

Harper MJ, Walpole AL. Contrasting endocrine activities of cis and trans isomers in a series of substituted triphenylethylenes. Nature 1966; 212(57):87.

Harper MJ, Walpole AL. A new derivative of triphenylethylene: effect on implantation and mode of action in rats. J Reprod Fertil 1967; 13(1):101–119.

Howell A, Cuzick J, Baum M, Buzdar A, Dowsett M, Forbes JF, Hoctin-Boes G, Houghton J, Locker GY, Tobias JS. Results of the ATAC (Arimidex, Tamoxifen, Alone or in Combination) trial after completion of 5 years' adjuvant treatment for breast cancer. Lancet 2005; 365(9453):60–62.

Hulley S, Grady D, Bush T, Furberg C, Herrington D, Riggs B, Vittinghoff E. Randomized trial of estrogen plus progestin for secondary prevention of coronary heart disease in postmenopausal women. Heart and Estrogen/progestin Replacement Study (HERS) Research Group. JAMA 1998; 280(7):605–613.

Jordan VC. Effect of tamoxifen (ICI 46,474) on initiation and growth of DMBA-induced rat mammary carcinomata. Eur J Cancer 1976; 12(6):419–424.

Jordan VC. Comparative antioestrogen action in experimental breast cancer. Adv Exp Med Biol 1981; 138:165–178.

Jordan VC. Chemosuppression of breast cancer with tamoxifen: laboratory evidence and future clinical investigations. Cancer Invest 1988a; 6(5):589–595.

Jordan VC. Tamoxifen and endometrial cancer. Lancet 1988b; 2(8618):1019.

Jordan VC. Tamoxifen: a most unlikely pioneering medicine. Nat Rev Drug Discov 2003; 2(3):205–213.

Jordan VC. Optimising endocrine approaches for the chemoprevention of breast cancer beyond the Study of Tamoxifen and Raloxifene (STAR) trial. Eur J Cancer 2006; 42(17): 2909–2913.

Jordan VC. Chemoprevention of breast cancer with selective oestrogen-receptor modulators. Nat Rev Cancer 2007; 7(1):46–53.

Jordan VC, Allen KE. Evaluation of the antitumour activity of the non-steroidal antioestrogen monohydroxytamoxifen in the DMBA-induced rat mammary carcinoma model. Eur J Cancer 1980; 16(2):239–251.

Jordan VC, Dix CJ, Allen KE. The effectivness of long term tamoxifen treatment in a laboratory model for adjuvant hormone therapy of breast cancer. In: Salmon SE, Jones SE, eds. Adjuvant Therapy of Cancer II. New York: Grunne & Stratton Inc.1979:19–26.

Jordan VC, Dix CJ, Rowsby L, Prestwich G. Studies on the mechanism of action of the nonsteroidal antioestrogen tamoxifen (I.C.I. 46,474) in the rat. Mol Cell Endocrinol 1977; 7(2):177–192.

Jordan VC, Dowse LJ. Tamoxifen as an anti-tumour agent: effect on oestrogen binding. J Endocrinol 1976; 68(02): 297–303.

Jordan VC, Jaspan T. Tamoxifen as an anti-tumour agent: oestrogen binding as a predictive test for tumour response. J Endocrinol 1976; 68(3):453–460.

Jordan VC, Koerner S. Inhibition of oestradiol binding to mouse uterine and vaginal oestrogen receptors by triphenylethylenes. J Endocrinol 1975; 64(1):193–194.

Jordan VC, Naylor KE, Dix CJ, Prestwich G. Anti-oestrogen action in experimental breast cancer. Recent Results Cancer Res 1980; 71:30–44.

Jordan VC, Phelps E, Lindgren JU. Effects of anti-estrogens on bone in castrated and intact female rats. Breast Cancer Res Treat 1987; 10(1):31–35.

Jordan VC, Robinson SP. Species-specific pharmacology of antiestrogens: role of metabolism. Fed Proc 1987; 46(5): 1870–1874.

Jordan VC, Rowsby L, Dix CJ, Prestwich G Dose-related effects of non-steroidal antioestrogens nad oestrogens on the measurement of cytoplasmic oestrogen receptors in the rat and mouse uterus. J Endocrinol 1978; 78(1):71–81.

Lacassagne A. Hormonal pathogenesis of adenocarcinoma of the breast. Am J Cancer 1936; 27:217–225.

Lerner LJ, Jordan VC. Development of antiestrogens and their use in breast cancer: eighth Cain memorial award lecture. Cancer Res 1990; 50(14):4177–4189.

Lippman ME, Bolan G. Oestrogen-responsive human breast cancer in long term tissue culture. Nature 1975; 256 (5518):592–593.

Looker AC, Orwoll ES, Johnston CC, Jr., Lindsay RL, Wahner HW, Dunn WL, Calvo MS, Harris TB, Heyse SP. Prevalence of low femoral bone density in older U.S. adults from NHANES III. J Bone Miner Res 1997; 12(11):1761–1768.

Love RR, Cameron L, Connell BL, Leventhal H. Symptoms associated with tamoxifen treatment in postmenopausal women. Arch Intern Med 1991a; 151(9):1842–1847.

Love RR, Mazess RB, Barden HS, Epstein S, Newcomb PA, Jordan VC, Carbone PP, DeMets DL. Effects of tamoxifen on bone mineral density in postmenopausal women with breast cancer. N Engl J Med 1992; 326(13):852–856.

Love RR, Newcomb PA, Wiebe DA, Surawicz TS, Jordan VC, Carbone PP, DeMets DL. Effects of tamoxifen therapy on lipid and lipoprotein levels in postmenopausal patients with node-negative breast cancer. J Natl Cancer Inst 1990; 82 (16):1327–1332.

Love RR, Wiebe DA, Newcomb PA, Cameron L, Leventhal H, Jordan VC, Feyzi J, DeMets DL. Effects of tamoxifen on cardiovascular risk factors in postmenopausal women. Ann Intern Med 1991b; 115(11):860–864.

Martino S, Cauley JA, Barrett-Connor E, Powles TJ, Mershon J, Disch D, Secrest RJ, Cummings SR. Continuing outcomes relevant to Evista: breast cancer incidence in postmenopausal osteoporotic women in a randomized trial of raloxifene. J Natl Cancer Inst 2004; 96(23): 1751–1761.

Melnikow J, Kuenneth C, Helms LJ, Barnato A, Kuppermann M, Birch S, Nuovo J. Chemoprevention: drug pricing and mortality: the case of tamoxifen. Cancer 2006; 107(5): 950–958.

Miller AB, Bulbrook RD. The epidemiology and etiology of breast cancer. N Engl J Med 1980; 303(21):1246–1248.

Mosca L, Barrett-Connor E, Wenger NK, Collins P, Grady D, Kornitzer M, Moscarelli E, Paul S, Wright TJ, Helterbrand JD, Anderson PW. Design and methods of the Raloxifene Use for The Heart (RUTH) study. Am J Cardiol 2001; 88(4):392–395.

Neven P, De Muylder X, Van Belle Y, Campo R, Vanderick G. Effects of tamoxifen on uterus. Lancet 1994; 344(8922): 623–624.

Osborne CK, Hobbs K, Clark GM. Effect of estrogens and antiestrogens on growth of human breast cancer cells in athymic nude mice. Cancer Res 1985; 45(2):584–590.

Powles T, Eeles R, Ashley S, Easton D, Chang J, Dowsett M, Tidy A, Viggers J, Davey J. Interim analysis of the incidence of breast cancer in the Royal Marsden Hospital tamoxifen randomised chemoprevention trial. Lancet 1998; 352(9122):98–101.

Powles TJ, Hardy JR, Ashley SE, Farrington GM, Cosgrove D, Davey JB, Dowsett M, McKinna JA, Nash AG, Sinnett HD, et al. A pilot trial to evaluate the acute toxicity and feasibility of tamoxifen for prevention of breast cancer. Br J Cancer 1989; 60(1):126–131.

Powles TJ, Jones AL, Ashley SE, O'Brien ME, Tidy VA, Treleavan J, Cosgrove D, Nash AG, Sacks N, Baum M, et al. The Royal Marsden Hospital pilot tamoxifen chemoprevention trial. Breast Cancer Res Treat 1994; 31(1):73–82.

Riegel AT, Jordan VC, Bain RR, Schoenberg DR. Effects of antiestrogens on the induction of vitellogenin and its mRNA in Xenopus laevis. J Steroid Biochem 1986; 24 (6):1141–1149.

Rockhill B, Colditz G, Kaye J. Re: tamoxifen prevention of breast cancer: an instance of the fingerpost. J Natl Cancer Inst 2000; 92(8):657A–657.

Rockhill B, Spiegelman D, Byrne C, Hunter DJ, Colditz GA. Validation of the Gail et al. model of breast cancer risk prediction and implications for chemoprevention. J Natl Cancer Inst 2001; 93(5):358–366.

Rossouw JE, Anderson GL, Prentice RL, LaCroix AZ, Kooperberg C, Stefanick ML, Jackson RD, Beresford SA, Howard BV, Johnson KC, Kotchen JM, Ockene J. Risks and benefits of estrogen plus progestin in healthy postmenopausal women: principal results From the Women's Health Initiative randomized controlled trial. JAMA 2002; 288(3):321–333.

Sato M, Turner CH, Wang T, Adrian MD, Rowley E, Bryant HU. LY353381.HCl: a novel raloxifene analog with improved SERM potency and efficacy in vivo. J Pharmacol Exp Ther 1998; 287(1):1–7.

Smith CL, O'Malley BW. Coregulator function: a key to understanding tissue specificity of selective receptor modulators. Endocr Rev 2004; 25(1):45–71.

Snyder KR, Sparano N, Malinowski JM. Raloxifene hydrochloride. Am J Health Syst Pharm 2000; 57(18):1669–1675 (quiz 1676–1678.

Stearns V, Johnson MD, Rae JM, Morocho A, Novielli A, Bhargava P, Hayes DF, Desta Z, Flockhart DA. Active tamoxifen metabolite plasma concentrations after coadministration of tamoxifen and the selective serotonin reuptake inhibitor paroxetine. J Natl Cancer Inst 2003; 95(23): 1758–1764.

Stewart HJ, Knight GM. Tamoxifen and the uterus and endometrium. Lancet 1989; 1(8634):375–376.

Suh N, Glasebrook AL, Palkowitz AD, Bryant HU, Burris LL, Starling JJ, Pearce HL, Williams C, Peer C, Wang Y, Sporn MB. Arzoxifene, a new selective estrogen receptor modulator for chemoprevention of experimental breast cancer. Cancer Res 2001; 61(23):8412–8415.

Sutherland R, Mester J, Baulieu EE Tamoxifen is a potent "pure" anti-oestrogen in chick oviduct. Nature 1977; 267(5610): 434–435.

Terenius L. Structure-activity relationships of anti-oestrogens with regard to interaction with 17-beta-oestradiol in the mouse uterus and vagina. Acta Endocrinol (Copenh) 1971; 66(3):431–447.

Thurlimann B, Keshaviah A, Coates, Mouridsen H, Mauriac L, Forbes JF, Paridaens R, Castiglione-Gertsch M, Gelber RD, Rabaglio M, Smith I, Wardley A, Price KN, Goldhirsch A. A comparison of letrozole and tamoxifen in postmenopausal women with early breast cancer. N Engl J Med 2005; 353(26):2747–2757.

Veronesi U, Maisonneuve P, Costa A, Sacchini V, Maltoni C, Robertson C, Rotmensz N, Boyle P. Prevention of breast cancer with tamoxifen: preliminary findings from the Italian randomised trial among hysterectomised women. Italian Tamoxifen Prevention Study. Lancet 1998; 352(9122): 93–97.

Veronesi U, Maisonneuve P, Rotmensz N, Costa A, Sacchini V, Travaglini, G. D'Aiuto, F. Lovison, G. Gucciardo, M. G. Muraca, M. A. Pizzichetta, S. Conforti, A. Decensi, C. Robertson and P. Boyle. Italian randomized trial among women with hysterectomy: tamoxifen and hormone-dependent breast cancer in high-risk women. J Natl Cancer Inst 2003; 95(2):160–165.

Vogel VG, Costantino JP, Wickerham DL, Cronin WM, Cecchini RS, Atkins JN, Bevers TB, Fehrenbacher L, Pajon ER Jr., Wade JL III, Robidoux A, Margolese RG, James J, Lippman SM, Runowicz CD, Ganz PA, Reis SE, McCaskill-Stevens W, Ford LG, Jordan VC, Wolmark N. Effects of tamoxifen vs raloxifene on the risk of developing invasive breast cancer and other disease outcomes: the NSABP Study of Tamoxifen and Raloxifene (STAR) P-2 trial. JAMA 2006; 295(23):2727–2741.

Walsh BW, Kuller LH, Wild RA, Paul S, Farmer M, Lawrence JB, Shah AS, Anderson PW. Effects of raloxifene on serum lipids and coagulation factors in healthy postmenopausal women. JAMA 1998; 279(18):1445–1451.

14

Oncostatic Effect of Analogs of LHRH on Breast Cancer

ANDREW V. SCHALLY

Miller School of Medicine, University of Miami, and Department of Veterans Affairs Medical Center, Miami, Florida, U.S.A.

JÖRG B. ENGEL

Frauenklinik der Julius Maximilians-Universität Würzburg, Germany

LUTEINIZING HORMONE-RELEASING HORMONE AND ITS ANALOGS

Introduction

In 1971, our laboratory was the first to accomplish the isolation, structural elucidation, and synthesis of porcine hypothalamic luteinizing hormone-releasing hormone-I (LH-RH-I) (1–6). It was then shown that the structure of hypothalamic LHRH I in all mammalian species examined, including human, is identical (7,8). Subsequently LHRH I was also identified in early bony fish, lungfish, and amphibians (7–11). At least 12 additional molecular forms of LHRH that differ structurally have been later identified in birds, reptiles, amphibians, fishes, other vertebrates, and protochordata and even coral (7–11). Another isoform of decapeptide LHRH, LHRH II, also known as chicken LHRH, since it was first isolated from chicken (12) has also been reported in mammalian brain, peripheral organs and some tumors such as breast carcinomas (13–16).

Because LHRH possessed major follicle-stimulating hormone (FSH)-releasing as well as LH-releasing activity, we established the concept that one hypothalamic hormone, designated LHRH/FSH-RH or simply gonadotropin-releasing hormone (Gn-RH) controls the secretion of both gonadotropins from the pituitary gland (4). Nevertheless, because the abbreviation Gn-RH for gonadotropin-releasing hormone can cause confusion, being too similar to GH-RH (growth hormone-releasing hormone) for which many agonistic and antagonistic analogs already exist, the use of the abbreviation LHRH is recommended (7,17,18). Besides the hypothalamus, LHRH I was also found in extrahypothalamic regions of the central nervous system, as well as in nonneuronal tissues, such as placenta, ovary, mammary gland, and lymphoid cells (15,19). The function of GnRH-I in extrapituitary tissues is unclear (15).

Development of Analogs of LHRH

In 1971, we postulated that the substitutions of one or more amino acids in the sequence of LHRH I should result in analogs with increased LH-releasing activity or antagonistic action (20). Since 1972, systematic work by various groups has been going on to synthesize agonistic and antagonistic analogs of LHRH I. In the past 30 years, more than 3000 analogs of LHRH I have been synthesized (7,21–29).

Agonists of LHRH and Their Effects

Replacement of amino acids in positions 6 and 10 can lead to superactive peptides and several LHRH analogs substituted in positions 6, 10, or both are 50 to 100 times more active than LHRH and also possess prolonged activity (7,24,26,27,30–32). Of these most important are: [D-Leu^6, Pro^9-NHET]LHRH (Leuprolide, Lupron), [D-Ser(Bu^t)^6,Pro^9-NHET]LHRH (Buserelin), [D-Trp^6]LHRH (Decapeptyl, Triptorelin), [D-Ser(Bu^t)^6,Aza-Gly^{10}]LHRH (Zoladex, goserelin) (7,24,26,27,30–32).

Receptors of LHRH on the Pituitary

The actions of LHRH I and its analogs on the pituitary are mediated by high-affinity 7 transmembrane receptors for LHRH I, found on the plasma membranes of the hypophyseal gonadotrophs (32–36). The initial step in the action of LHRH is the binding to its receptors (32,37). The binding of LHRH or its analogs causes an aggregation of LHRH receptors and formation of a complex, which is then internalized and degraded. The LHRH receptors are coupled to G proteins that act to stimulate phosphatase C, leading to the activation of protein kinase C and the relapse of LH and FSH (32,36–38). Normal LHRH secretion is pulsatile and physiological stimulation of secretion of LH and FSH requires an intermittent release of LHRH (39,40).

Mechanism of Action of LHRH and its Agonists

An acute injection of superactive agonists of LHRH induces a marked and sustained release of LH and FSH, but chronic administration produces inhibitory effects (7,22,24,27, 41–43). Thus continuous stimulation of the pituitary by repeated injections of superactive agonists of LHRH or monthly administration of depot preparations produces an inhibition of hypophyseal-gonadal axis through the process of "downregulation" of pituitary receptors for LHRH, desensitization of the pituitary gonadotrophs, and creation of a state of reversible medical castration with a suppression of circulating levels of LH and sex steroids (7,24,26,27,44,45). The inhibitory processes that can be produced by repeated administration or depot preparations of LHRH agonists have important clinical applications. Thus the therapy of sex hormone-dependent malignant neoplasms, such as prostate and breast cancer is based on the creation of a state of sex steroid deprivation. LHRH agonists and antagonists also exert direct inhibitory effects on breast, prostate, ovarian, and endometrial cancers mediated through specific LHRH receptors on the tumor cells (7,36,46–52). LHRH type II receptors have been detected in some mammals, but the presence of a functional LHRH II receptors in humans remains controversial (13,14,53). Most vertebrates have more than one LHRH receptor subtype concurrently with the expression of up to three LHRH ligands (54).

Antagonists of LHRH

Hundreds of LHRH antagonists have been also synthesized. In order to eliminate the undesirable effects caused by insertion of a D-arginine in position 6, analogs with neutral D-ureidoalkyl amino acids, such as D-Cit at position 6, were synthesized in our laboratory (7,21). Among these antagonists, AC-D-Nal(2)^1,D-Phe(4Cl)^2,D-Pal(3)^3, D-Cit^6,DAla^{10}]LHRH (SB-75, Cetrorelix) had the highest inhibitory activity and receptor binding affinity (7,21, 25,26). Other groups have also synthesized LHRH antagonists with diminished anaphylactoid activity. Among antagonists that were developed are antide [*N*-Ac-D-Nal (2)^1,D-Phe(4Cl)^2,DPal(3)^3,Lys(Nic)^5,D-Lys(Nic)^6,Lys (iPr)^8,D-Ala^{10}]LHRH (55) and Nal-Glu antagonist [Ac-D-Nal(2)^1,D-Phe(4Cl)^2,DPal(3)^3,Arg^5,D-Glu^6(AA),D-Ala^{10}] LHRH (56), Azaline B[Ac-D-Nal^1,DPhe(4Cl)^2,D-Pal^3, Aph^5(Atz),Aph^6(Atz),ILys^8,D-Ala^{10}]-LHRH (57), Ganirelix [*N*-Ac-D-Nal(2)^1,D-*p*-Cl-Phe^2,D-Pal(3)^3,DhArg(Et_2)^6, L-hArg(Et_2)^8,D-Ala^{10}]-LHRH (58) and Abarelix (PPI-149) [*N*-Ac-D-Nal(2)-D-(*p*-Cl)-Phe-D-Pal(3)-Ser- NM-Tyr-Asn-Leu-ILys-Pro-Gly-NH_2 (59).

LHRH antagonists have major uses in gynecology and oncology. LHRH antagonists produce a competitive blockade of LHRH receptors, preventing a stimulation by endogenous LHRH, and cause an immediate and dose-dependent inhibition of the release of gonadotropins and sex steroids (7,24–26) in contrast to the LHRH agonists, that require repeated administration. The use of antagonists reduce the time of the onset of therapeutic effects and prevents a clinical flare-up of disease caused by a transient LH and sex steroid release, which can occur in some cancer patients during initial agonist administration (7,24,26,60). While the principal mechanism of action of LHRH antagonists is based on a competitive receptor occupancy of LHRH receptors, chronic administration of high doses of LHRH antagonist, Cetrorelix, can also produces desensitization of gonadotrophs and downregulation of pituitary LHRH receptors (7,61). An orally active nonpeptide antagonist of the LHRH has recently been reported (62).

Sustained Delivery Systems for LHRH Analogs

Initially, agonists of LHRH were administered daily subcutaneously (s.c.) or intranasally (7,26). Subsequently, long-acting delivery systems for [D-Trp^6]LHRH (Decapeptyl) and other agonists in microcapsules of poly(DL-lactide-co-glycolide) (PLG) were developed which release a controlled dose of the peptide over a 30-day period (60). For administration, the microcapsules of Lupron or Decapeptyl are suspended in an injection vehicle and injected once every month intramuscularly. Cylindrical rods of Zoladex (Goserelin) are injected s.c (22,26). Improved depot preparations of LHRH agonists, which release the analogs for 60 to 90 days have been also developed recently. Depot formulations of LHRH antagonists Abarelix, Cetrorelix, Degarelex, and Teverelix have been reported.

Receptors for LHRH on Tumors

Besides their action on the pituitary (45,26) LHRH agonists and antagonists can also exert direct effects on tumor cells (7,28,63). The evidence for direct action of LHRH analogs on tumors is based on the detection of binding sites for LH-RH in various cancers, and the inhibitory effects of analogs on tumor cell lines in vitro (7,26,45,49). Thus specific membrane receptors for LHRH have been found in various human cancers (7,26,36,45,49). High-affinity binding sites for LHRH and the expression of mRNA for LHRH receptors were detected in human prostate cancer samples (52,64) and prostate cancer lines (51,52,65–67). We also detected high-affinity LHRH binding sites in more than 52% of human breast cancer samples (68). Other investigators reported the presence of LHRH receptors in various human mammary cancer cell lines (69–71). LHRH receptors on human cancers are similar to pituitary LH-RH receptors (72). In MCF-7 human breast cancer line, LHRH receptors are primarily intracellular and traffic to the cell surface (73). LHRH receptors were similarly found in 78% of human ovarian epithelial cancers specimens and human ovarian cancer lines (45,49,74–76). The presence of high-affinity membrane receptors for LHRH was also established in about 80% of human endometrial carcinomas (77) and in endometrial cancer lines (45,49,50). The expression of LHRH receptor gene in human breast, endometrial, ovarian tumors, and respective cancer cell lines was also demonstrated by reverse transcription polymerase chain reaction (RT-PCR) (45,74,78–80). These findings provided a motivation for the development of targeted cytotoxic LHRH analogs for therapy of malignancies in which specific receptors for LHRH are found (81–83). The presence of receptors for LHRH on tumors also explains the effect of LHRH analogs seen in vitro and occasional responses to LHRH agonists in post-menopausal women with breast cancer.

Signal Transduction Mechanisms of LHRH Receptors on Tumors

Tumoral LHRH receptors are reported to be linked to post receptor pathways distinct from pituitary LHRH receptors (49). Thus the signaling mechanism of LHRH receptors in human cancers is quite different from that in pituitary gonadotrophs (84). Initially Levy et al. (85) showed that in analogy to the known mechanism of LHRH action in the pituitary (38), LHRH analogues activate the phosphoinositide pathway in rat mammary tumor membranes. Later this group was able to demonstrate that high-affinity LHRH receptors in rat mammary tumors are modulated by guanine nucleotides (86). Imai et al. (87) found that LHRH receptors on ovarian carcinomas and uterine were coupled by Gi proteins to their effectors. Thus after binding of its ligand, the LHRH receptor in cancers couples to Gαi protein and activates a phosphotyrosine phosphatase (87–89). In turn phosphotyrosine phosphatase dephosphorylates the receptors for epidermal growth factor (EGF) (89). This abolishes mitogenic signaling induced by binding of EGF to its receptor and leads to an inhibition of mitogen activated protein kinase (MAPK), c-fos expression, and EGF-induced proliferation (88,90). In addition LHRH activates nuclear factor κB in human ovarian and endometrial cancer cells (91). This effect leads to an inhibition of apoptosis in tumor cells (90). The binding of LHRH analogs to their receptors in cancers also induces *c-jun* mRNA expression, *c-Jun* phosphorylation, and AP-1 activation (92). LHRH agonists induce Jun D-DNA binding in cancer cells, reduce DNA synthesis, and lead to accumulation of cells in the Gαi phase of the cell cycle (93). Emons, Grundker, and collaborators (49,88–93) made important contributions to the elucidation of the signal mechanisms of LHRH analogs in tumors and expertly reviewed this subject (84). A recent study by Imai (94) in ovarian cancer detected a Gi protein-mediated translocation of serine/threonine phosphatase 2A, a crucial enzyme in the control of apoptosis, to the plasma membrane after treatment with LHRH antagonist Cetrorelix. Thus, the cells were driven to apoptosis by the treatment, indicating that the observed effect was mediated through a Gi protein linked LHRH receptor (94). Another current report demonstrated that treatment with LHRH agonists and antagonists exerts an antimetastatic effect because of the inhibition of the activity of the plasminogen activator system, in addition to antiproliferative effects (95). In a collaborative effort with our group, Tang and coworkers (96) found that treatment of ovarian cancer cells with Cetrorelix-induced G1 cell cycle arrest coupled with downregulation of cyclin A-CDK2 complex levels, presumably due to an upregulation of the p21 and p53 protein levels. Although the existence of a LHRH II receptor has not been conclusively proven in mammals, some groups reported high-affinity binding sites for LHRH II on prostate, ovarian, and endometrial cancer cells (97,98). Thus, the antiproliferative effects after treatment with analogs of LHRH are caused by various mechanisms of action and may be mediated by more than one subtype receptor.

Direct Effects of LHRH Analogs on Tumors

A variety of findings on growth inhibition of cultured breast, prostate, ovarian, and endometrial cancers cells by LHRH analogs strongly support the concept of their direct effects (45,63). Thus the inhibition of human mammary, ovarian, endometrial, and prostatic cancer cell lines by LHRH agonists and LHRH antagonists, such as Cetrorelix, in vitro is well documented (69,70,79,99). Thus native LHRH and LHRH agonists were found to inhibit the proliferation of human breast, ovarian, and endometrial cancer cell lines (63). Interestingly in human ES-2 ovarian cancer cell line, stimulatory effects of the agonist D-Trp-6-LHRH were observed when a low concentration (10 ng/mL) was used and an antibody to LHRH inhibited cell proliferation (100). However in other studies using well-established human ovarian and endometrial cancer cell lines, stimulatory effects on proliferation were not observed even when low concentrations of LHRH analogs were used (101,102). Evidence for the production of an LHRH-like peptide and/or expression of mRNA for LHRH was obtained in human prostatic, mammary, endometrial, and ovarian cancer lines, suggesting that local LHRH may be involved in the growth of these tumors (7,28,49,79,103,104). The existence of regulatory LHRH loops in prostate, endometrial, and ovarian cancer consisting locally-produced LHRH-like peptides and specific LHRH receptors has also been postulated (46,49,87). Most reports in the literature suggest that in ovarian and endometrial cancers, LHRH and its receptor are part of a negative autocrine system (84,101,102). The ability of both LHRH agonists and antagonists to elicit inhibitory effects on tumor cells can be explained by the suppressive action of both types of analogs on LH and FSH secretion from the pituitary. Thus LHRH antagonist may operate in prostatic mammary, ovarian, and endometrial cancer cells by blocking the stimulatory effects of endogenous LHRH while LHRH agonist may be inducing a receptor downregulation and desensitization as in pituitary cells (71,28,105).

Targeted Cytotoxic Analogs of LHRH

An additional new class of antitumor compounds based on LHRH has been recently developed for targeted chemotherapy, which consists of LHRH agonists conjugated to chemotherapeutic agents (81–83,106,107). The hypothesis of a "magic bullet" that could specifically eradicate cancers was conceived in 1898 by Paul Ehrlich, but remained unexplored for many years (81). On the basis of the presence of LHRH receptors in breast, endometrial, ovarian, and prostatic cancers, our laboratory started more than 10 years ago the synthesis and evaluation of targeted antitumor compounds by linking cytotoxic compounds to LHRH analogs (81–83,106–108). Later we demonstrated that LHRH are also expressed by renal cell carcinoma (109), non Hodgkin's lymphomas (110) and even melanomas (111).

After exploring antineoplastic radicals and chemical linkages, we decided to conjugate [D-Lys6]LHRH through the ε-amino group of its D-Lys moiety and a glutaric acid spacer to the 14-OH group of doxorubicin (DOX), the most widely used anticancer agent to form cytotoxic LHRH analog AN-152 (106). Subsequently we synthesized an even more potent cytotoxic analog (AN-207) by linking 2-pyrrolino- DOX (AN-201), a daunosamine-modified derivative of DOX, which is 200 to 500 times more active in vitro than DOX to the same [D-Lys6]LHRH carrier (106). We have demonstrated that these cytotoxic LHRH analogs AN-152 and AN-207 powerfully inhibit growth of various experimental tumors. This therapeutic approach based on cytotoxic LHRH analogs is being tested clinically in women with breast, ovarian, and endometrial cancers.

BREAST CANCER

Endocrine Approaches to Treatment of Breast Cancer

Breast cancer is the most common malignancy in women over 40 years and the second leading cause of cancer related deaths among women in the United States and Western Europe (112). The mortality from breast cancer in women in the industrialized western world is second only to lung cancer (112). Breast cancer accounts for about one-third of all female cancers, and more than 800,000 new cases of breast cancer are reported worldwide each year (112). The annual mortality due to this malignancy is about 45,000 in the United States alone (113). The development of new treatment modalities is necessary.

The importance of endocrine therapy in breast cancer has been known for more than a century. In 1896, Beatson reported that ovarian ablation by bilateral oophorectomy can provide a treatment for premenopausal women with advanced metastatic breast cancer (114). However, only about 30% to 40% of unselected premenopausal patients with breast cancer showed objective tumor regression following ovarian ablation (115–117). Subsequently the development of analyses for steroid hormone receptors in breast cancers allowed a prediction of the likelihood of a favorable response to oophorectomy which was rated as 50% to 60% for women with estrogen receptor (ER)-positive tumors and a 70% to 75% for patients whose breast tumors contained both ER and progesterone receptors (PR) (118). Although 20% or more patients may not respond to oophorectomy, trial overview analyses have confirmed durable survival benefits of ovarian ablation in early breast cancer (119). Other early endocrine therapies used in the decades 1940 to 1960 included adjuvant treatment with oestrogens, ablative hypophysectomy and adrenalectomy, adjuvant treatment with glucocorticoids, androgens, and radiation of the ovaries (120–124).

Antioestrogen tamoxifen provided a welcome contemporary alternative to ovarian ablation by surgery or radiation in premenopausal patients with metastatic breast cancer (125). Clinical trials showed that the treatment with tamoxifen was as effective as ovarian ablation (115–117, 124), although the rise in serum estradiol levels induced by tamoxifen in premenopausal patients remained a concern (115). The optimal duration of adjuvant tamoxifen therapy appears to be five years (126). Overview analysis of a large number of clinical trials confirmed the efficacy of tamoxifen in ER-positive breast cancer (126). Tamoxifen is also effective for prevention of breast cancer (126).

In the late 1960s and early 1970s, the first generation aromatase inhibitor, aminoglutethimide was introduced in therapy of breast cancer in an endeavor to produce a medical adrenalectomy (124,127–129). Later modern aromatase inhibitors were developed which inhibit estrogen biosynthesis by blocking the conversion of androgens to estrogen in the adrenal gland (129,130).

After the discovery of the phenomena of induction of medical castration and sex steroid deprivation by LHRH agonists, it was found that the regression of rat mammary tumors could be induced by the administration of an LHRH analog (131–135). Successful treatment of premenopausal patients with metastatic breast cancer first reported by Klijn and DeJong (136) stimulated the initiation of a series of clinical trails. The purpose of this article is to review the existing experimental findings and various approaches to the therapy of breast cancer on the basis of agonists and antagonists of LHRH and targeted cytotoxic analogs of LHRH.

In Vivo Studies with LHRH Analogs in Animal Models of Mammary Tumors

Various groups have demonstrated a regression in the growth of 7,12-dimethylbenz(a)anthracene (DBMA)-induced estrogen-dependent mammary carcinoma in rats after administration of superactive LHRH agonists D-Leu-6-LHRH-ethylamide and Goserelin (Zoladex) (131–135). We have used D-Trp-6-LHRH (Triptorelin) in rat and mouse models of endocrine-dependent mammary tumors (137). Tumor weights in BDF-1 mice bearing the MXT adenocarcinoma were significantly decreased after administration of D-Trp-6-LHRH (Triptorelin) for 21 days. Treatment with D-Trp-6-LHRH (Triptorelin) lowered the plasma progesterone, but not the ovariectomy levels. In Wistar-Furth rats bearing the MT/W9A estrogen-dependent mammary adenocarcinoma, treatment with D-Trp-6-LHRH for 28 days significantly decreased tumor weights by more than 50% and tumor volume by 67% (137). Administration of D-Trp-6-LHRH (Triptorelin) significantly decreased progesterone levels by 74% and estradiol by 42%. After 28 days, tumor weights were decreased by more than 90% and in some rats the tumors had disappeared. The regression of mammary tumors in rats and mice after chronic administration of agonistic analogs of LHRH suggested that they could be tried for treatment of breast carcinoma in premenopausal women.

Two early but powerful antagonistic analogs LHRH were also tested by us in rat and mouse models of mammary tumors (137). Administration of Ac-D-*p*-CL-Phe-1,2,Phe-3,D-Ala-10-LHRH for three weeks significantly reduced the weight and volume of estrogen-dependent MXT mammary tumors in BDF1 mice. Ovarian weights and plasma levels of progesterone were also diminished after treatment with this antagonist.

N-Ac-D-p-CL-Phe-1,2,D-Trp-3-D-Arg-6,D-Ala-10-LHRH administered for four weeks to Wistar-Furth rats reduced the weight and volume of MT/W9A mammary tumor by 58% and 42%, respectively (137). LH, estrogen, and progesterone levels were also greatly reduced in rats treated with the antagonist. Suppression of tumor growth by antagonists was most likely linked with the inhibition of the levels of sex steroids, but some direct action of the antagonist on mammary tumors could not be excluded.

Subsequently we showed in BDF-1 mice bearing MXT estrogen-dependent tumors that 25 μg/day of modern antagonist Cetrorelix induced a greater reduction in tumor LHRH receptor levels and a more efficacious inhibition of tumor growth after three weeks than the same dose of [D-Trp^6]LHRH (Triptorelin) (138). Histologically, the regressive changes in the treated tumors were characteristic of apoptosis (programmed cell death). Both analogs also downregulated EGF receptors (138). In rats bearing DMBA-induced mammary carcinomas, administration of Cetrorelix also caused tumor regression and reduced uterine and ovarian weights, suggesting a suppression of pituitary LHRH receptors (139). In nude mice bearing estrogen sensitive MCF-7-MIII human breast cancers, both Cetrorelix at 30 μg/day and [D-Trp^6]LHRH (Triptorelin) at 25 μg/day completely arrested tumor growth over a period of six weeks and downregulated LHRH receptors on tumors (140).

Agonists and antagonists of LHRH could also suppress the growth of estrogen-independent breast cancers. Thus

BDF-1 mice bearing MXT (3.2) estrogen-independent mouse mammary carcinoma were treated for three weeks with microcapsules of LHRH agonist D-Trp-6-LHRH (Triptorelin) or the antagonist Cetrorelix (141). The lack of estrogen dependence of the tumor was proved by bilateral surgical ovariectomy, which had no effect. In two experiments, treatment with 25 μg/day doses of either analog resulted in a significant inhibition of tumor growth as shown by a 40% to 53% inhibition of tumor volumes (141), 38% to 43% decrease in tumor weights, and histological signs of tumor regression. The binding capacity of LHRH receptors was decreased by treatment with the analogs. A significant reduction in EGF-binding capacity was also observed following therapy with the two LHRH analogs (141).

Direct Effects of LHRH Analogs on Breast Cancer Cells

LHRH and LHRH Receptors in Breast Tumors

This concept of direct effects of LHRH analogs on breast cancer cells is supported by extensive experimental data (7,28,45,49,63,101,142,143). LHRH immunoreactivity has been detected in human milk at levels five to sixfold higher than in plasma, in samples of human breast cancer (144), as well as in human breast cancer cell lines (145). Normal and malignant human breast tissue express two forms of the neuropeptides LHRH, LHRH I, and LHRH II. These peptides are overexpressed in cancerous compared with normal tissues obtained from the same patients (15). The genes for LHRH and its receptor are also expressed in human breast with fibrocystic disease (146). The expression of LHRH gene in human breast cancer cell lines MDA-MB-23 I and ZR-75-1 was also demonstrated by nuclease protection assay, oligonucleotide primer extension studies, and RT-PCR (79). A peak of immunoreactive LHRH which coeluted with synthetic mammalian LHRH in two different high-performance liquid chromatography systems was similarly detected by antisera in cell extracts (79). These findings suggest the possibility of an autocrine role for LHRH in the regulation of breast carcinomas. Specific LHRH binding sites with low-affinity and high-capacity type were detected on human breast cancer cell lines and biopsy specimens of human breast cancer (69,70,145). Using the LHRH agonist $[^{125}I]$, [D-Trp6]LHRH as radioligand, we detected two classes of binding sites for LHRH analogues in human breast cancers, one with low affinity ($K_a = 2.8\ \mu M^{-1}$) and the other with high affinity ($K_a = 6\ \mu M^{-1}$) (68). These binding sites in human breast cancers had characteristics comparable to those of rat pituitary LHRH receptors and also bound potent LHRH antagonists with high affinity (147). About 52% of 500 breast cancer biopsies were classified as positive for LHRH receptors (68).

In Vitro Effects Of LHRH Analogs on Breast Cancer Lines

It is well established that LHRH agonists and antagonists can exert direct antiproliferative effects on human breast cancer lines in vitro (7,45,63,69,70,99). Direct antiproliferative effects of LHRH agonists and antagonists on a variety of human breast cancer cells have been shown by several groups (69,70,99,143). It was also demonstrated that LHRH antagonists of Cetrorelix class can inhibit growth of human breast cancers in vitro by direct action on tumor cells mediated by LHRH receptor (86,99).

Sharoni et al. (99) examined the inhibitory effects of LHRH antagonists (SB-29) [Ac-D-Nal(2)1,D-Phe(pCl)2,D-Trp3,D-Hci6,D-Ala10]-LHRH and (SB-30) [Ac-D-Nal(2) 1,D-Phe(pCl)2,D-Trp3,D-Cit6,D-Ala10]LHRH on the proliferation of estrogen-independent MDA-MB-231 human mammary tumor cells in culture based on $[^3H]$Thymidine incorporation into DNA and cell number. The antagonists induced up to 40% inhibition of $[^3H]$thymidine incorporation in MDA-MB-231 cells. This inhibition was dose-dependent in the 0.3 to 30 μM range and could be demonstrated after two days of incubation in the presence of the peptides. The agonist des-Gly10-[D-Ser(tBu)6] LHRH ethylamide (buserelin) had no effect on the tumor cells. The antagonists SB-29 and SB-30 also suppressed cell growth, as measured by cell number. These results support the concept that LHRH antagonists can directly inhibit the growth of human mammary tumors (99).

Segal-Abramson et al. (148) studied the binding of LHRH analogues to the human breast cancer cell line MCF-7 and the effect of these analogues on the cell proliferation to elucidate their direct action on estrogen-dependent mammary tumors. The growth rate of MCF-7 cells was increased by 200% in the presence of 1 nM estradiol. The basal growth was only slightly inhibited by Cetrorelix, but the estrogen-stimulated growth was completely nullified by this LHRH antagonist. In contrast, the LHRH agonist Buserelin stimulated cell growth in estrogen-deficient medium, but it was ineffective in the presence of estrogen. Cetrorelix inhibited the stimulation of growth by buserelin. High-affinity LHRH binding sites with a K_d of 1.4 ± 1.0 nM and with low-affinity sites ($K_d = 1.3 \pm 1.0\ \mu M$) were demonstrated in MCF-7 cells. These results suggest that antagonists directly inhibit mammary tumor growth (148). It was also reported that in estrogen-dependent MCF-7 breast cancer cells, Triptorelin (Decapeptyl) inhibited esterone sulfate-sulfatase activity and this effect is significantly augmented in the presence of heparin activity (149).

In collaboration we also evaluated the role of the insulin-like growth factors (IGFs) on the growth of MCF-7 mammary tumor cells and the effects of LHRH analogs on IGF action (150). When the mitogenic effects of IGF-I and IGF-II were compared, IGF-I was found to be three times more potent than IGF-II. MCF-7 cells secreted IGF-II, but not IGF-I. Estradiol (10^{-9} M/L) stimulated IGF-II release. The LHRH antagonist Cetrorelix inhibited basal growth as well as estrogen-induced and IGF-stimulated growth and blocked the release of IGF-II from MCF-7 cells. It was concluded that LHRH antagonist Cetrorelix can suppress the growth of breast tumors by blocking the autocrine secretion of IGF-II and by directly inhibiting the growth stimulatory effect of IGFs (150). LHRH analogs were also reported to decrease the invasiveness of human breast cancer cells in vitro (151). Thus LHRH analogs appear to reduce the metastatic potential of breast cancers (151).

Thus a large body of evidence supports the view that analogs of LHRH can act directly on human breast cancer and other cancers (7,26,28,45,63). It is well established that the proliferation of human breast cancer cells in vitro can be directly inhibited by LHRH agonists and antagonists. However it is not clear if this direct action of LHRH analogues on breast cancer is of clinical significance in the therapy of breast cancer. Considering that the concentrations of LHRH analogues required to induce antiproliferative effects in vitro are high (10^{-7} to 10^{-5} M), plasma concentrations of LHRH agonists achieved with depot preparations may not be adequate to produce therapeutic benefits, but since LHRH antagonists are used clinically in larger doses, they might exert some direct inhibitory effects.

Effects of Cytotoxic Analogs of LHRH on Breast Cancer

Cytotoxic analogs of LHRH bind with high affinity to human and murine breast cancers (78). In initial studies on breast cancer, we tested tumor inhibitory action of targeted cytotoxic LHRH analogs AN-152 and AN-207 in mice bearing estrogen-independent MXT mouse mammary cancers (152). Both AN-207 and AN-152 given intraperitoneally produced about 90% inhibition of tumor growth, but equimolar amounts of the cytotoxic radicals AN-201 and doxorubicin were toxic (152). Specific high-affinity LHRH receptors were present on MXT tumor samples of control untreated mice, but no binding sites for LHRH could be found on tumor membranes 15 to 17 days after the treatment with cytotoxic LHRH analogs (152). In the next study, we administered cytotoxic analogs intravenously as a single injection. AN-207 was effective in inhibiting growth of MXT breast cancers in doses 80 to 100 times smaller than AN-152 (153). Subsequent regimens of treatment for cytotoxic analogs were based on only one or two intravenous injections (154). Thus, in another investigation, one injection of AN-207 caused a complete regression of MX-1 hormone-independent doxorubicin-resistant human breast cancers in nude mice, which remained tumor free for at least 60 days after treatment (154). Significant levels of LHRH receptors and their mRNA were found in control tumors, but the receptor concentration could not be analyzed on treated tumors because of their complete regression (154).

When nude mice bearing MDA-MB-231 hormone-independent breast cancer were injected intravenously with a single dose of 250 nmol/kg cytotoxic LHRH analog AN-207, the growth of MDA-MB-231 tumors was inhibited for three weeks (155). Three weeks after treatment, the presence of mRNA for LHRH receptors was demonstrated by RT-PCR in all groups and radioreceptor assays demonstrated high-affinity binding sites for LHRH on tumor cell membranes of control animals, but not in tumors treated with AN-207 (155). Sixty days after the administration of AN-207, high-affinity LHRH binding sites were found again in MDA-MB-231 tumors (155).

Similar results were obtained in MDA-MB-435 human estrogen-independent mammary carcinomas implanted orthotopically in the mammary fat pad of nude mice (156). A single dose of 250 nmol/kg or two injections of AN-207 at 150 nmol/kg both resulted in about a 70% inhibition of tumor growth compared with controls. However, after treatment with radical AN-201 at the same doses, the tumor growth was not inhibited. In addition, six of eight control animals and three of eight mice given a single dose of AN-201 developed lymphatic metastases, but none of the animals treated with AN-207 showed metastatic lesions (156). This high efficacy of AN-207 could be partially blocked by pretreatment of nude mice with a large dose of agonist [D-Trp^6]LHRH one hour before the administration of AN-207. The level of mRNA for LHRH receptors showed a 26% decrease 33 days after treatment with AN-207, but by day 48 these levels returned to the control values. Our results show that high-affinity receptors for LHRH reappear on tumors. This observation provides a rationale for using repeated treatment with cytotoxic LHRH analogs (156).

Since AN-152 is in clinical trials, we evaluated its effects on the estrogen-independent, DOX-resistant human mammary carcinoma line MX-1, xenografted into nude mice (157). Nude mice bearing MX-1 tumors were given five IV injections of AN-152 or DOX at doses equivalent to 3 mg/kg of DOX. Tumor growth was followed and changes in the expression of LHRH receptors on tumors were evaluated. The effect of AN-152 on the expression of human epidermal growth factor receptor (HER)-2 was also investigated. Treatment with AN-152 significantly decreased the tumor volume compared with the control tumors and significantly extended tumor-doubling time. Therapy with AN-152, but not with DOX, resulted in a significant decrease of LHRH receptor levels on MX-1 tumors. The expression of mRNAs for HER-2, HER-3, and the levels of HER-2 and HER-3 proteins were also significantly reduced by AN-152. This favorable response in MX-1 tumors indicates that targeting can reverse the resistance to Doxorubicin. Cytotoxic LHRH analog AN-152 could be considered for targeted chemotherapy of DOX-resistant breast cancers expressing LHRH receptors (157).

In a collaborative study, we linked AN-152, the cytotoxic analog of LHRH containing doxorubicin, to a two-photon fluorophore (C625) to study its cellular pathway in tumors (158). Using two-photon laser-scanning microscopy, the AN-152 fluorophore conjugate could be observed directly as it interacted with LHRH receptors on MCF-7 breast cancer cell lines. The receptor-mediated entry of AN-152 into the cell cytoplasm and subsequently into the nucleus was clearly demonstrated (158).

Side Effects of Cytotoxic LHRH Analogs

In view of planned clinical use of targeted cytotoxic analogs of LHRH we investigated their effects on the pituitary, although the possible damage inflicted by cytotoxic analogs to pituitary cells secreting LH, FSH, thyroid stimulating hormone (TSH), ACTH, and GH might be acceptable to the cancer patient because hypophysectomy has been used for the treatment of some cancers including breast cancer (81).

Since gonadotroph cells of the anterior pituitary contain high levels of receptors for LHRH, therapy with cytotoxic analogs will result in the accumulation of DOX or AN-201 in this gland. To determine whether targeted cytotoxic therapy would cause a permanent damage to the pituitary, we tested the effects of AN-207 and its radical AN-201 in rats. It was found that AN-207 caused a selective damage to the gonadotroph cells one week after an IV injection, but the pituitary function completely recovered one week later (159). Similarly, only a transient decrease of the mRNA expression for LHRH receptors in rat pituitary was observed after the injection of AN-207 (160). Cytotoxic LHRH analog AN-207 decreased significantly the level of LHRH receptor mRNA in the pituitaries of ovariectomized rats five hours after administration, but one week after the treatment, the expression of LHRH receptor gene was similar to the controls. Because receptors for LHRH are not expressed in significant levels in most normal tissues, other side effects related to targeting of AN-207 or AN-152 are not expected after treatment with AN-207 or AN-152. The absence of toxicity of AN-207 to the pituitary cells, which are slowly proliferating, may be explained by the properties of the cytotoxic radical, AN-201, which is a strong DNA-intercalating agent that kills rapidly proliferating cell types such as cancer cells and cells of the bone marrow. Our findings indicate that cytotoxic LHRH analogs such as AN-152 and AN-207 have a selective transient effect on LH cells, but not on other cells, whereas cytotoxic radicals Doxorubicin and AN-201 nonselectively damages the LH, GH, and TSH cells (159). A possible damage to pituitary cells such as corticotrophs and thyrotrophs, could also be alleviated by replacement therapy (81). The dose-limiting toxicity of AN-152 and AN-207 will probably be myelotoxicity, caused by Doxorubicin and AN-201 respectively that are released by carboxylesterase enzymes from the peptide conjugates in the circulation (82,83). Because the activity of the carboxylesterase enzymes is low in humans, we can expect few adverse side effects in patients (82,83). These results suggest that targeted cytotoxic LHRH analogs such as AN-152 and AN-207 could be considered for treatment of LHRH receptor-positive advanced or metastatic breast cancers in women.

CLINICAL EFFECTS OF AGONISTIC ANALOGS OF LHRH

Introduction

Experimental studies suggested that agonists of LHRH should be considered for a new hormonal therapy for breast cancer in women. In clinical trials carried out since early 1980s, inhibitory effects of LHRH agonists on mammary tumors including regression of tumor mass and disappearance of metastases in premenopausal and some postmenopausal women with breast cancer treated with [D-Trp^6]LHRH, (Triptorelin), Buserelin, Zoladex (Goserelin), or Leuprolide have been clearly demonstrated (115,136,161–166). The efficacy of treatment with LHRH agonists of premenopausal patients with breast cancer is now accepted after various phase II and III trials.

Premenopausal Breast Cancer

Klijn and DeJong (136) were the first to report that two of four premenopausal women with metastatic breast cancer improved after seven weeks of treatment with buserelin. The successful treatment of premenopausal breast cancer patients with an agonist of LHRH by Klijn and De Jong (136) stimulated the initiation of a series of clinical trials. In these trials it was shown that the LHRH agonists buserelin, goserelin, triptorelin, and leuprorelin effectively suppressed plasma oestrogens to castrate levels (161–166). In clinical trials in France, Mathé et al. treated 23 patients with advanced breast carcinoma with microcapsules of Triptorelin (163). All patients showed a decrease in levels of LH. Five of 8 pre-menopausal patients were ER-positive and three of them responded.

Williams et al. (166) treated 53 premenopausal patients with advanced breast cancer with Goserelin (Zoladex). Tumor remissions after Zoladex therapy were observed in 31% of patients, the responses occurring primarily in women with ER-positive tumors. In a large trial in 134 premenopausal women with breast cancer, Kaufman et al. (161) utilized depot implant of Goserelin (Zoladex) and demonstrated 53% objective tumor responses. The response rates of about 40% and median duration of response of 10 to 15 months, as well as survival, corresponded to those achieved by oophorectomy and other endocrine therapies (161). Patients with ER-positive tumors showed higher objective responses (about 50%) than patients with ER negative tumors (7–33%) (115,116,161). Interestingly, Kaufman et al. (161) obtained a good response rate of 33% in patients whose tumors had a low ER content. Side effects were generally mild and mainly related to the estrogen deprivation and consisted of hot flashes and decreased libido (116,161). An irritation at the site of injection recorded in some patients was because of subcutaneous injections of then nonmicrocapsulated analogues. After the introduction of long-acting, sustained-release formulations of LHRH agonists, this irritation is avoided (161,116). Flare-up in disease, after initial treatment with LHRH agonist (recorded in about 15% of prostate cancer patients) and due to the transient rise in sex steroid levels, is very rare in patients with breast cancer (161,116). Only one patient with early disease reported an increase in bone pain after starting treatment with LHRH agonists.

Santen et al. (115) summarized various studies with LHRH agonists and computed a 41% objective response rate in unselective premenopausal patients and 51% in women with ER-positive tumors. These studies indicated that LHRH agonists are efficacious for the treatment of premenopausal women with estrogen-dependent, ER-positive breast cancer (26).

LHRH agonists can also be used for the treatment of fibrocystic disease of the breast in premenopausal women (167). When 66 patients with fibrocystic mastopathy, associated in most cases with a uterine fibroma or a fibromatous uterus, were treated for three to six months with microcapsules of [D-Trp^6]LHRH (Triptorelin) (167), a complete response was observed in nearly 50% of patients and a partial response in other patients. It was concluded that chronic mastopathy in premenopausal women can be successfully treated by LHRH analogs (167).

The Combination of LHRH Agonists with Tamoxifen, Chemotherapy or Aromatase Inhibitors

Various recent trials demonstrated beneficial effects of LHRH analogues in combination with tamoxifen in early breast cancer (168,169). In four clinical trials randomizing a total of 506 premenopausal women with advanced breast cancer, the combination of LHRH plus tamoxifen was superior to LHRH agonist alone (169).

It was also shown that combined estrogen blockade with an LHRH agonist and tamoxifen is superior to either treatment modality alone (168,169). In the trial of Klijn et al., combined treatment with buserelin and tamoxifen was more effective and resulted in longer overall survival than treatment with either drug alone (168). The five-year survival increased from 15% to 18% for single drugs to 34% for combination (168). Similar results were obtained with zoladex plus tamoxifen (170,171). Recently, two large multicenter studies reported that in premenopausal women with ER-positive breast cancer, adjuvant treatment with goserelin or goserelin plus tamoxifen is equally effective and burdened with fewer side effects than chemotherapy with six cycles of cyclophosphamide, methotrexate, and flourouracil (CMF) (172,173). Overall the results suggested that the goserelin-tamoxifen combination is significantly more effective than CMF chemotherapy in the adjuvant treatment of premenopausal patients with stage I and II breast cancer (173). The International Breast Cancer Study Group also compared in a group of 1063 premenopausal patients, three treatment regimens usual standard: (*i*) chemotherapy with CMF (cyclophosphamide, methotrexate, and 5-fluorouracil) (*ii*) CMF chemotherapy followed by ovarian suppression with goserelin, and (*iii*) goserelin alone (174). Overall, there were no statistically significant differences in five year disease-free survival (DFS) among the regimens. However patients with ER-negative tumors who received CMF or CMF followed by goserelin had better outcomes (84% to 88%, respectively) than patients in goserelin group (73% DFS). Patients with ER-positive tumors had very similar outcomes (81% DFS) irrespective of treatment regimen (174). Another randomized trial demonstrated that seven-year disease free and overall survival following endocrine therapy with triptorelin and tamoxifen for three years is not different from that after six cycles of chemotherapy with 5-flourouracil, epirubicin, and cyclophosphamide (FEC), in one to three node positive and hormone-receptor positive early breast cancer patients (175). A current study proposed endocrine treatment with a LHRH analog in combination with chemotherapy as primary treatment for premenopausal ER-positive T2-T4 breast cancer patients. Thus, the clinical response rate was 75% and in 58% of the patients breast conserving surgery could be performed after the treatment (176).

Goserelin (Zoladex) is reported to be the most extensively studied LHRH agonist for the treatment of breast cancer and data from a large clinical trial program indicate that alone or in combination with tamoxifen, goserelin is at least as effective as chemotherapy with CMF in patients with estrogen-dependent early disease (177). Goserelin has also been shown to be beneficial when used in addition to standard adjuvant therapy such as surgery, radiotherapy or chemotherapy (177).

However, to date it is not clear, whether adding a LHRH analog to adjuvant chemotherapy improves treatment results in premenopausal patients with estrogen and progesterone receptor-positive early breast cancer. Several studies demonstrated that adding treatment with goserelin to chemotherapeutic regimens might show some additional benefit by decreasing the risk of recurrence and DFS. However, the overall survival was not significantly improved (178,179). Accordingly, two recent randomized studies did not show any additional survival benefit of LHRH analogs (180,181). However, one of these studies reported a significant decrease in the risk of recurrence in patients younger than 40 years (181), and one metanalysis of four randomized trials found a significantly improved event-free and overall survival after 5.5 years follow-up in patients treated with chemotherapy and two years of goserelin (182). Further studies are required to define patient subgroups who may benefit from additional ovarian suppression.

Aromatase inhibitors and LHRH agonists seem to provide another feasible combination treatment (183,184). In premenopausal patients this combination suppresses estrogen levels below values obtained with LHRH agonist alone (129). It is still not clearly established, if the combination of an aromatase inhibitor to an LHRH agonist will lead to a further improvement in the adjuvant treatment of premenopausal ER-positive breast cancer. In one trial, 21 premenopausal women with advanced breast cancer were randomized to receive the LHRH agonist triptorelin alone or in combination with the aromatase inhibitor, formestane (185). Estradiol levels decreased by an average of 86.9% in the group treated with triptorelin alone and by 97.3% in the combination group. Three of the patients treated with triptorelin alone experienced tumor regression compared with four patients in the combination group (185). In another trial, 13 premenopausal women with metastatic breast cancer and three women with locally advanced primary breast cancer were treated with a combination of LHRH agonist, goserelin and a selective aromatase inhibitor anastrozole (184). All patients had previously been treated with goserelin and tamoxifen. Replacement of tamoxifen by anastrozole on tumor progression resulted in a further 76% fall in estradiol levels at three months. It was concluded that the combined use of goserelin and anastrozole as second-line endocrine therapy produces a significant clinical response in premenopausal women with advanced breast cancer (184).

Protection of the ovaries by LHRH analogs when given in combination with adjuvant chemotherapy (CMF and FEC) in premenopausal patients with early breast cancer was investigated in two recent studies. After treatment with CMF, all patients younger and 56% of the patients older than 40 years resumed normal menses (186). After therapy with FEC, normal menses occurred in 72% of the patients (187).

Side Effects of Agonists in Premenopausal Women

Side effects of treatment with LHRH agonists in premenopausal women are the typical symptoms which occur with the onset of menopause, i.e., amenorrhea, hot flashes, vaginal dryness, and mood swings. However, these symptoms are fully reversible after cessation of therapy. Decreased bone density is the most important side effect of long-term treatment with LHRH agonists, therefore treatment duration in early breast cancer was limited to two to three years.

In a randomized clinical trial, the premenopausal patients with breast cancer were randomly assigned to goserelin, goserelin plus tamoxifen, tamoxifen alone, or no endocrine therapy, and those with node-positive disease received chemotherapy with CMF (188). Goserelin and tamoxifen resulted in menopausal symptoms, which were reversible. However, women treated with CMF experienced physical symptoms throughout the whole study period and their quality of life was more affected (188).

Postmenopausal Breast Cancer

Several studies evaluated the effects of treatment with LHRH agonists in postmenopausal patients with metastatic breast cancer (163,164). Response rates varied between 0% and 20% with an overall response rate of about 8%. In the trial by Mathé (163), 3 of 15 postmenopausal patients responded to Triptorelin; two of them were ER-positive. Some anecdotal cases of successful treatment with triptorelin of metastatic breast cancer in postmenopausal women have been described (189). Radiological clearance of breast metastasis in a 70 year old woman with breast cancer after treatment with Triptorelin has also been reported (190). The results recorded in postmenopausal patients suggest that agonists have some direct antitumoral action. In premenopausal women with breast cancer, the beneficial effects of LHRH agonists are based on suppression of ovarian estrogen production by medical castration, but this mechanism cannot explain the responses observed in postmenopausal patients. Therefore, it is likely that LHRH analogues acted directly on the cancer cells.

Sensitive radioimmunoassays showed that in postmenopausal patients, levels of serum estradiol could be significantly higher than in ovariectomized women (116).

After therapy with LHRH agonists, serum estradiol levels are further suppressed by 15% to 20% to the values of ovariectomized women (191,192). Considering that androgens can be converted to estrogens, this fall in the estrogen levels in postmenopausal women after treatment with LHRH agonist may be the consequence of the decrease in androgen production by the ovaries caused by the inhibition of LH and FSH secretion (191,192).

However, most of the beneficial effects of LHRH agonists in the postmenopausal patients can be explained by direct inhibitory effects on tumors. This view is also supported by experimental data reviewed above.

A Case for the Use of LHRH Antagonists in Breast Cancer

On the basis of various experimental findings, LHRH antagonists should be superior to LHRH agonists in treatment of breast cancer (7,26,28), especially in the case of estrogen-independent tumors, but no clinical results exist till now. Cetrorelix has clear and significant direct effects on estrogen-independent breast cancers as various animal studies show, and it should be considered clinically for this indication (26,193). Thus Cetrorelix could compete with chemotherapy, which is considered the treatment of choice for ER-negative tumors and other drugs such as monoclonal antibody Herceptin (Trastuzumab), which is used in combination with Paclitaxel or Docetaxel in women who overexpress HER-2 protein (194). This genetic alteration is present only in 20% to 30% of women with breast cancer. Herceptin also has cardiac side effects. Cetrorelix could also compete with other drugs such as VEGF receptor antibody (Bevacizumab) or tyrosine kinase inhibitors (Lapatinib) and Gefitinib (Iressa), which are not yet used routinely in breast cancer (195). Direct effects of the LHRH agonists on breast cancer are smaller than those of the antagonists. LHRH agonists are used only in premenopausal women for estrogen-dependent breast cancers where they act by estrogen deprivation (161,168,169). In ER-negative breast cancers, LHRH agonists are therapeutically inferior to chemotherapy. LHRH antagonists such as Cetrorelix, so far have not been used clinically in women with breast cancers but deserve to be considered for trials.

FUTURE THERAPIES FOR BREAST CANCERS

Combinations of Antitumor Peptides

A detailed description of the effects of various proteins and peptides on the mammary gland is beyond the scope of this chapter. However, it must be stated that in addition to IGF-I and II, EGF and HER-2 ligand, α-TGF and other growth factors a number of proteins and peptides could act as promoters of breast cancer (26,28,150,194,196–198). Thus, Bombesin/gastrin releasing peptide may be involved in the growth and function of human breast cancers (26,28,197). Growth hormone (GH) plays a role in the differentiation of ductal epithelia and prolactin and is necessary for lobular epithelial cell proliferation and secretory function (198). Both GH and prolactin can be synthesized in the mammary gland tissue. Autocrine production of human growth hormone (hGH) was reported to generate an invasive phenotype in mammary carcinoma cells (199). Therapy with GH antagonists such as Pegvisomant or antagonists of Growth hormone-releasing hormone (GHRH) could nullify the autocrine effects of human GH on breast cancer (26,28,198–201).

GHRH peptide and its mRNA are also present in human breast cancers and GHRH could act as a growth factor. Antagonistic analogs of bombesin/GRP and of GHRH powerfully inhibit the growth of murine breast cancer and human breast cancers, xenografted into nude mice (200,201).

Receptors for vasoactive intestinal peptide (VIP) are also found in breast cancer (202). The growth of MDA-MB-231 cells breast cancer can be inhibited by a VIP-receptor antagonist (202).

Receptors for somatostatin, which is a growth inhibitor, are present in 33% of human breast cancers (68). Attempts have been made to use octapeptide somatostatin analogs for the therapy of human cancers (28). However the combination of analog somatostatin with tamoxifen did not have a greater therapeutic efficacy than tamoxifen alone in women with metastatic breast cancer (203).

The best suppression of experimental human breast cancers in vivo was obtained by using a combination of LHRH agonists or LHRH antagonist, Cetrorelix, with bombesin antagonists RC-3095 or RC-3940-II, which inhibit bombesin receptors and EGF receptors including HER-2 (197,204). The combination of Cetrorelix with GHRH antagonists should be also evaluated experimentally (26,200,201).

Cytotoxic Analogs of LHRH

It is possible that more than 50% of patients with LHRH receptor positive breast cancers might be successfully treated with cytotoxic LHRH analogues (81–83,107, 152,153).

Experimental studies show that cytotoxic analogs of LHRH, AN-152, and AN-207 containing radicals doxorubicin and 2-pyrrolinodoxorubicin respectively, can be targeted to mammary cancers expressing LHRH receptors producing a strong inhibition of the growth of these tumors (154–157). Clinical trials with AN-152 are in progress.

Safety pharmacology and toxicity studies in mice, rats, and dogs demonstrated a significantly reduced cardiotoxic potential of AN-152 compared with doxorubicin including no QT prolongation, myocarditis, or fibrosis in the various models (205,206). A Phase I clinical study assessed dose limiting toxicities, maximum tolerated dose (MTD), and pharmacokinetics of AN-152 given once every three weeks in patients with gynecological and breast cancers (205,206). Patients with tumors proven immunohistochemically to be LHRH-R positive were eligible if prior therapy did not exceed 70% of the recommended maximum lifetime dose for doxorubicin. Doses of AN-152 were doubled starting at 10 mg/m^2 until side effects occurred. Seventeen patients entered the study and received AN-152 by intravenous infusion over two hours at dosages of 10, 20, 40, 80, and 160 mg/m^2 and 267 mg/m^2. Infusion of AN-152 was well tolerated at all dosages, without supportive treatment. The cytotoxic LHRH analog AN-152 was stable in human plasma, a prerequisite for LHRH receptor-mediated uptake by tumor tissue. Pharmacokinetic analyses showed dose-dependent plasma levels of AN-152 and only minor release of doxorubicin (205,206). The infusion of AN-152 was well tolerated in female patients. No dose limiting toxicities were seen up to 160 mg/m^2 which is equimolar to a doxorubicin dose of 46 mg/m^2. Short lasting leukopenia/neutropenia of CTCAE Grade 4 was dose limiting in two patients at 267 mg/m^2.

Leukocytopenia was thus identified as a rapidly reversible dose-limiting toxicity of AN-152. A dose of 267 mg/m^2 of AN-152, given once every three weeks, was recommended for Phase II trial. Evidence of therapeutic activity was demonstrated, as disease stabilization and remission at 160 and 267 mg/m^2 dose levels of AN-152.

The continued development of targeted cytotoxic LHRH analogs may improve the present management of mammary cancers.

REFERENCES

1. Baba Y, Matsuo H, Schally AV. Structure of the porcine LH- and FSH-releasing hormone. II. Confirmation of the proposed structure by conventional sequential analysis. Biochem Biophys Res Commun 1971; 44:459–463.
2. Matsuo H, Arimura A, Nair RM, Schally AV. Synthesis of the porcine LH and FSH-releasing hormone by the solid-phase method. Biochem Biophys Res Commun 1971; 45: 822–827.
3. Matsuo H, Baba Y, Nair RM, Arimura A, Schally AV. Structure of the porcine LH- and FSH-releasing hormone. I. The proposed amino acid sequence. Biochem Biophys Res Commun 1971; 43:1334–1339.
4. Schally AV, Arimura A, Kastin AJ, Matsuo H, Baba Y, Redding TW, Nair RM, Debeljuk L, White WF. Gonadotropin-releasing hormone: one polypeptide regulates secretion of luteinizing and follicle-stimulating hormones. Science 1971; 173:1036–1038.
5. Schally AV, Kastin AJ, Arimura A. Hypothalamic FSH and LH regulating hormone, structure, physiology, and clinical studies. Fertil Steril 1971; 22:703–721.
6. Schally AV, Nair RM, Redding TW, Arimura A. Isolation of the LH- and FSH-releasing hormone from porcine hypothalami. J Biol Chem 1971; 246:7230–7236.
7. Schally AV. Luteinizing hormone releasing-hormone analogues: their impact on the control of tumorigenesis. Peptides 1999; 20:1247–1262.
8. Powell JFF, Fischer WH, Park M, Craig AG, Rivier JE, White SA, Francis RC, Fernald RD, Licht P, Warby C, Sherwood NM. Primary structure of solitary form of gonadotropin-releasing hormone (GnRH) in cichlid pituitary: three forms of GnRH in brain of cichlid and pumpkinseed fish. Regul Pept 1995; 57:43–53.
9. Sherwood NM, Adams BA. Gonadotropin-releasing hormone in fish: evolution, expression and regulation of the GnRH gene. In: Melamed P, Sherwood NM, eds. 5 Hormones and Their Receptors in Fish Reproduction. Singapore: World Scientific Publishing Co. 2005:1–39.
10. Joss JM, King JA, Millar RP. Identification of the molecular forms of and steroid hormone response to gonadotropin-releasing hormone in the Australian lungfish, *Neoceratodus forsteri*. Gen Comp Endocrinol 1994; 96:392–400.
11. King JA, Millar RP, Vallarino M, Pierantoni R. Localization and characterization of gonadotropin-releasing hormones in the brain, gonads, and plasma of a dipnoi (lungfish, *Protopterus annectens*). Regul Pept 1995; 57:163–174.
12. Miyamoto K, Hasegawa Y, Nomura M, Igarashi M, Kangawa K, Matsuo H. Identification of the second gonadotropin-releasing hormone in chicken hypothalamus: evidence that gonadotropin secretion is probably controlled by two distinct gonadotropin-releasing hormones in avian species. Proc Natl Acad USA. 1984; 81:3874–3878.
13. Millar R. GnRH II and type II GnRH receptors. Trends Endocrinol Metab 2003; 14:35–43.
14. Enamoto M Endo D, Kawashima S, Park MK. Human type II receptor mediates effects of GnRH on cell proliferation. Zoolog Sci 2004; 21:763–770.
15. Chen A, Kaganovsky E, Rahimipour S, Ben-Aroya N, Okon E, Koch Y. Two forms of gonadotropin-releasing hormone (GnRH) are expressed in human breast tissue and overexpressed in breast cancer: a putative mechanism for the antiproliferative effect of GnRH by down-regulation of acidic ribosomal phosphoproteins P1 and P21. Cancer Res 2002; 62:1036–1044.
16. Pawson AJ, Maudsley SR, Lopes J, Katz AA, Sun YM, Davidson JS, Millar RP. Multiple determinants for rapid agonist-induced internalization of a nonmammalian gonadotropin-releasing hormone receptor: a putative palmitoylation site and threonine doublet within the carboxyl-terminal tail are critical. Endocrinology 2003; 144:3860–3871.
17. Schally AV, McCann SM. The privileges of a Nobel Laureate. Fertil Steril 1995; 64:452–453.
18. Schally AV, Kastin AJ, Arimura A. FSH-releasing hormone and LH-releasing hormone. Vitam Horm 1972; 30:83–164.
19. Palmon A, Ben-Aroya N, Tel-Or S, Burstein, Y., Fridkin, M., and Koch, Y. The gene for the neuropeptide gonadotropin-releasing hormone is expressed in the mammary gland

of lactating rats. Proc Natl Acad Sci USA 1994; 91: 5748–5751.

20. Schally AV, Kastin AJ. Stimulation and inhibition of fertility through hypothalamic agents. Drug Ther 1971; 1:29–32.
21. Bajusz S, Csernus VJ, Janaky T, Bokser L, Fekete M, Schally AV. New antagonists of LHRH II. Inhibition and potentiation of LHRH by closely related analogs. Int J Peptide Prot Res 1988; 32:425–435.
22. Dutta AN. Luteinizing hormone-releasing hormone (LHRH) agonists. Drugs Future 1988; 13:43–57.
23. Dutta AN. Luteinizing hormone-releasing hormone (LHRH) antagonists. Drugs Future 1988; 13:761–787.
24. Karten MJ, Rivier JE. Gonadotropin-releasing hormone analog design. Structure-function studies toward the development of agonists and antagonists: rationale and perspective. Endocr Rev 1986; 7:44–66.
25. Reissmann T, Engel J, Kutscher B, Bernd M, Hilgard P, Peukert M, Szeleny I, Reichert S, Gonzalez-Barcena D, Nieschlag E, Comaru-Schally AM, Schally AV. Cetrorelix. Drugs Future. 1994, 19, 228-237.
26. Schally AV, Comaru-Schally AM. Hypothalamic and other peptide hormones In: Kufe DW, Pollock RE, Weichselbaum RR, et al. eds. Cancer Medicine 7th ed. Hamilton, Ontario: B.C. Dekker Publishers, 2006:802–816.
27. Vickery BH. Comparison of the potential for therapeutic utilities with gonadotrophin-releasing hormone agonists and antagonists. Endocr Rev. 1986; 7:115–124.
28. Schally AV, Comaru-Schally AM, Nagy A, Kovacs M, Szepeshazi K, Plonowski A, Varga JL, Halmos G. Hypothalamic hormones and cancer. Front Neuroendocrinol 2001; 22:248–291.
29. Schally AV, Kastin AJ, Coy DH. Edward T. Tyler Prize Oration-LH-releasing hormone and its analogs: recent basic and clinical investigations. Int J Fertil 1976; 21:1–30.
30. Coy DH, Vilchez-Martinez JA, Coy EJ, Schally AV. Analogs of luteinizing hormone-releasing hormone with increased biological activity produced by D-amino acid substitutions in position 6. J Med Chem 1976, 19; 423–425.
31. Fujino M, Fukuda T, Shinagawa S, Kobayashi S, Yamazaki I, Nakayama R, Seely JH, White WF, Rippel RH. Synthetic analogs of luteinizing hormone-releasing hormone (LHRH) substituted in positions 6 and 10. Biochem Biophys Res Commun 1974; 57:1248–1256.
32. Conn PM, Crawley WF. Gonadotropin-releasing hormone and its analogues. N Engl J Med 1991; 324:93–103.
33. Conn PM, Rogers DC, Stewart JM, Niedel J, Sheffield T. Conversion of a gonadotropin-releasing hormone antagonist to an agonist. Nature 1982; 296:653–655.
34. Clayton RN, Channabasavaiah K, Stewart JM, Catt KJ. Hypothalamic regulation of pituitary gonadotropin-releasing hormone receptors: effects of hypothalamic lesions and a gonadotropin-releasing hormone antagonist. Endocrinology 1982; 110:1108–1115.
35. Loumaye E, Wynn PC, Coy D, Catt KJ. Receptor-binding properties of gonadotropin-releasing hormone derivatives. J Biol Chem 1984; 259:12663–12671.
36. Stojilkovic S, Catt KJ. Expression and signal transduction pathways of gonadotropin releasing hormone receptors. Rec Prog Horm Res 1995; 30:161–205.
37. Hawes BE, Conn PM. Assessment of the role of G proteins and inositol phosphate production in the action of gonadotropin-releasing hormone. Clin Chem 1993; 39:325–332.
38. Naor Z. Signal transduction mechanism of Ca^{2+} mobilizing hormones: the case of gonadotropin releasing hormone. Endocr Rev 1990; 11:326–353.
39. Belchetz PE, Plant TM, Nakai Y, Keogh EJ, Knobil E. Hypophysial responses to continuous and intermittent delivery of hypothalamic gonadotropin-releasing hormone. Science 1978; 202:631–633.
40. Knobil E. The neuroendocrine control of the menstrual cycle. Recent Prog Horm Res 1980; 36:53–88.
41. Corbin A, Beattie CW, Tracy J, Jones R, Foell TJ, Yardley J, Rees RWA. The anti-reproductive pharmacology of LH-RH and the antagonistic analogs. Int J Fertil 1978; 23(2):81–92.
42. Johnson B, Gendrich RL, White WF. Delay of puberty and inhibition of reproductive processes in the rat by a gonadotropin-releasing hormone agonist analog. Fertil Steri 1976; 27:853–860.
43. Sandow J, von Rechenberg W, Jerzabek G, Stoll W. Pituitary gonadotropins inhibition by a highly active analog of luteinizing hormone-releasing hormone. Fertil Steril 1976; 30:205–209.
44. Conn PM, Crawley WF. Gonadotropin-releasing hormone and its analogs. N Engl J Med 1991; 324:93–103.
45. Emons G, Schally AV. The use of luteinizing hormone releasing hormone agonists and antagonists in gynecological cancers. Human Reprod 1994; 9:1364–1379 (review).
46. Dondi D, Limonta P, Moretti RM, Marrelli Montagnani M, Garattini E, Motta M. Antiproliferative effects of luteinizing hormone-releasing hormone (LHRH) agonists on human androgen-independent prostate cancer cell line DU 145: evidence for an autocrine-inhibitory LHRH loop. Cancer Res 1994; 54:4091–4095.
47. Emons G, Muller V, Ortmann O, Schulz KD. Effects of LHRH analogs on mitogenic signal transduction in cancer cells. J Steroid Biochem Mol Biol 1998; 65:199–206.
48. Emons G, Ortmann O, Becker M, Irmer G, Springer B, Laun R, Holzel F, Schulz K-D, Schally AV. High affinity binding and direct antiproliferative effects of LH-RH analogs in human ovarian cancer cell lines. Cancer Res 1993; 53:5439–5446.
49. Emons G, Ortmann O, Schulz K-D, Schally AV. Growth-inhibitory actions of analogs of luteinizing hormone releasing hormone on tumor cells. Trends Endocrinol Metab 1997; 8:355–362.
50. Emons G, Schröder B, Ortmann O, Westphalen S, Schulz K-D, Schally AV. High affinity binding and direct antiproliferative effects of luteinizing hormone-releasing hormone analogs in human endometrial cancer cell lines. J Clin Endocrinol Metab 1993; 77:1458–1464.
51. Limonta P, Dondi D, Moretti RM, Maggi R, Motta M. Antiproliferative effects of luteinizing hormone-releasing hormone agonists on the human prostatic cancer cell line LNCaP. J Clin Endocrinol Metab 1992; 75:207–212.
52. Qayum A, Gullick W, Clayton RC, Sikora K, Waxman J. The effect of gonadotrophin releasing hormone analogs in prostate cancer are mediated through specific tumour receptors. Br J Cancer 1990; 62:96–99.

53. Maudsley S, Davidson L, Pawson AJ, Chan R, de Maturana RL, Millar RP. Gonadotropin-releasing hormone (GnRH) antagonists promote proapoptotic signaling in peripheral reproductive tumor cells by activating a Galphai-coupling state of the type I GnRH receptor. Cancer Res. 2004, 64, 7533–7544.
54. Tello JA, Rivier JE, Sherwood NM. Tunicate gonadotropin-releasing hormone (GnRH) peptides selectively activate *Ciona intestinalis* GnRH receptors and the green monkey type II GnRH receptor. Endocrinology 2005; 146:4061–4073.
55. Ljungqvist A, Feng DM, Hook W, Shen ZX, Bowers C, Folkers K. Antide and related antagonists of luteinizing hormone release with long action and oral activity. Proc Natl Acad Sci USA 1988; 85:8236–8240.
56. Rivier JE, Porter J, Rivier CL, Perrin M, Corrigan A, Hook WA, Siraganian RP, Vale WW. New effective gonadotropin releasing hormone antagonists with minimal potency for histamine release in vitro. J Med Chem 1986; 29:1846–1851.
57. Jiang G, Miller C, Koerber SC, Porter J, Craig AG, Bhattacharjee S, Kraft P, Burris TP, Campen CA, Rivier CL, Rivier JE. Betidamino acid scan of the GnRH antagonist Acyline. J Med Chem 1997; 40:3739–3748.
58. Nelson LR, Fujimoto VY, Jaffe RB, Monroe SE. Suppression of follicular phase pituitary-gonadal function by a potent new gonadotropin-releasing hormone antagonist with reduced histamine-releasing properties (ganirelix). Fertil Steril 1995; 63:963–9.
59. Molineaux CJ, Sluss PM, Bree MP, Gefter ML, Sullivan LM, Garnick MB. Suppression of plasma gonadotropins by Abarelix: a potent new LHRH antagonist. Mol Urol 1998; 2:265–268.
60. Redding TW, Schally AV, Tice TR, Meyers WE. Long-acting delivery systems for peptide: inhibition of rat prostate tumours by controlled release of (D-Trp6)- luteinizing hormone-releasing hormone from injectable microcapsules. Proc Natl Acad Sci USA 1984; 81:5845–5848.
61. Pinski J, Lamharzi N, Halmos G, Groot K, Jungwirth A, Vadillo-Buenfil M, Kakar SS, Schally AV. Chronic administration of luteinizing hormone-releasing hormone (LHRH) antagonist Cetrorelix decreases gonadotroph responsiveness and pituitary LHRH receptor messenger ribonucleic acid levels in rats. Endocrinology 1996; 137:3430–3436.
62. Struthers RS, Chen T, Campbell B, Jimenez R, Pan H, Yen SS, Bozigian HP. Suppression of serum luteinizing hormone in postmenopausal women by an orally administered nonpeptide antagonist of the gonadotropin-releasing hormone receptor (NBI-42902). J Clin Endocrinol Metab 2006; 91:3903–3907.
63. Schally AV, Halmos G, Rekasi Z, Arencibia JM. The actions of LH-RH agonists, antagonists and cytotoxic analogs on the LH-RH receptors on the pituitary and tumors. In: Devroey P. ed. Infertility and Reproductive Medicine Clinics of North America: GnRH Analogs. Philadelphia: Saunders, 2001:17–44.
64. Halmos G, Arenciba JM, Schally AV, Davis R, Bostwick DG. High incidence of receptors for luteinizing hormone-releasing hormone (LHRH) and LHRH receptor gene expression in human prostate cancers. J Urol 2000; 163:623–629.
65. Lamharzi N, Halmos G, Jungwirth A, Schally AV. Decrease in the level and mRNA expression of LH-RH and EGF receptors after treatment with LH-RH antagonist Cetrorelix in DU-145 prostate tumor xenografts in nude mice. Int J Oncol 1998; 13:429–435.
66. Koppán M, Nagy A, Schally AV, Plonowski A, Halmos G, Arencibia JM, Groot K. Targeted cytotoxic analog of luteinizing hormone-releasing hormone AN-207 inhibits the growth of PC-82 human prostate cancer in nude mice. Prostate 1999; 38:151–158.
67. Limonta P, Dondi D, Moretti RM, Fermo D, Garattini E, Motta M. Expression of luteinizing hormone-releasing hormone mRNA in the human prostatic cancer cell line LNCaP. J Clin Endocrinol Metab 1993; 76:797–800.
68. Fekete M, Wittliff JL, Schally AV. Characteristics and distribution of receptors for [D-Trp^6]-luteinizing hormone-releasing hormone, somatostatin, epidermal growth factor and sex steroids in 500 biopsy samples of human breast cancer. J Clin Lab Anal 1989; 3:137–147.
69. Eidne KA, Flanagan CA, Harris NS, Millar RP. Gonadotropin-releasing hormone (GnRH)-binding sites in human breast cancer cell lines and inhibitory effects of GnRH antagonists. J Clin Endocrinol Metab 1987; 64:425–432.
70. Miller WR, Scott WN, Morris R, Fraser HM, Sharpe RM. Growth of human breast cancer cells inhibited by a luteinizing hormone-releasing hormone agonist. Nature 1985; 313:231–233.
71. Yano T, Korkut E, Pinski J, Szepeshazi K, Milovanovic S, Groot K, Clarke R, Comaru-Schally AM, Schally AV. Inhibition of growth of MCF-7 MIII human breast carcinoma in nude mice by treatment with agonists or antagonists of LH-RH. Breast Cancer Res Treat 1992; 21:35–45.
72. Kakar SS. Molecular structure of the human gonadotropin-releasing hormone receptor gene. Eur J Endocrinol 1997; 137:183–192.
73. Sedgley KR, Finch AR, Caunt CJ, McArdle CA. Intracellular gonadotropin-releasing hormone receptors in breast cancer and gonadotrope lineage cells. J Endocrinol 2006; 191:625–636.
74. Irmer G, Burger C, Muller R, Ortmann O, Peter U, Kakar SS, Neill JD, Schulz KD, Emons G. Expression of the messenger ribonucleic acids for luteinizing hormone-releasing hormone and its receptor in human ovarian epithelial carcinoma. Cancer Res 1995; 55:817–822.
75. Miyazaki M, Nagy A, Schally AV, Lamharzi N, Halmos G, Szepeshazi K, Groot K, Armatis P. Growth inhibition of human ovarian cancers by cytotoxic analogues of luteinizing hormone-releasing hormone. J Natl Cancer Inst 1997; 89:1803–1809.
76. Srkalovic G, Schally AV, Wittliff JL, Day TG Jr, Jenison EL. Presence and characteristics of receptors for [D-Trp^6]-luteinizing hormone-releasing hormone and epidermal growth factor in human ovarian cancer. Int J Oncol 1998; 12:489–498.
77. Srkalovic G, Wittliff JL, Schally AV. Detection and partial characterization of receptors for [D-Trp^6]-LH-RH and EGF in human endometrial carcinoma. Cancer Res 1990; 50:1841–1846.

78. Halmos G, Nagy A, Lamharzi N, Schally AV. Cytotoxic analogs of luteinizing hormone-releasing hormone bind with high-affinity to human breast cancers. Cancer Lett 1999; 36:129–136.
79. Harris N, Dutlow C, Eidne K, Dong KW, Roberts J, Millar R. Gonadotropin-releasing hormone gene expression in MDA-MB-231 and ZR-75-1 breast carcinoma cell lines. Cancer Res 1991; 51:2577–2581.
80. Kakar SS, Grizzle WE, Neil JD. The nucleotide sequences of human GnRH receptors in breast and ovarian tumors are identical with that found in pituitary. Mol Cell Endocrinol 1994; 106:145–149.
81. Schally AV, Nagy A. Chemotherapy targeted to hormone receptors on tumors. Cancer chemotherapy based on targeting of cytotoxic peptide conjugates to their receptors on tumors. Eur J Endocrinol 1999; 141:1–14.
82. Schally AV, Nagy A. New approaches to treatment of various cancers based on cytotoxic analogs of LHRH, somatostatin and bombesin. Life Sci 2003; 72:2305–2320.
83. Schally AV, Nagy A. Chemotherapy targeted to cancers through tumoral hormone receptors. Trends Endocrinol Metab 2004; 15:300–310.
84. Emons G, Grundker C, Gunthert AR, Westphalen S, Kavanagh J, Verschraegen C. GnRH antagonists in the treatment of gynecological and breast cancers. Endocr Relat Cancer 2003; 10:291–299.
85. Levy J., Segal T, Wiznitzer A, lnsler V, Sharoni Y. Molecular mechanisms of GnRH action on mammary tumors and uterine leiomyomata. In: Vickery BH, Lunenfeld B. eds. GnRH Analogues in Cancer and Human Reproduction, Vol. 1, Basic Aspeas. Kluwer: Dordrecht, 1989:127–135.
86. Segal-Abramson T, Giat J, Levy J, Sharoni Y. Guanine nucleotide modulations of high affinity gonadotropin-releasing hormone receptors in rat mammary tumors. Mol Cell Endocrinol 1992; 85:109–116.
87. Imai A, Takagi H, Horibe S, Fuseya T, Tamaya T. Coupling of gonadotropin-releasing hormone receptor to Gi protein in human reproductive tract tumors. J Clin Endocrinol Metab 1996; 81:3249–3253.
88. Emons G, Muller V, Ortmann O, Grossmann G, Trautner U, von Stuckrad B, Schulz KD & Schally AV. Luteinizing hormone-releasing hormone agonist triptorelin antagonizes signal transduction and mitogenic activity of epidermal growth factor in human ovarian and endometrial cancer cell lines. Int J Oncol 1996; 9:1129–1137.
89. Grundker C, Volker P, Gunthert AR, Emons G. Antiproliferative signaling of LHRH in human endometrial and ovarian cancer cells through G-protein αi-mediated activation of phosphotyrosine phosphatase. Endocrinology 2001; 142:2369–2380.
90. Grundker C, Volker P, Schulz KD, Emons G. Luteinizing hormone-releasing hormone (LHRH) agonist Triptorelin and antagonist Cetrorelix inhibit EGF-induced c-fos expression in human gynecological cancers. Gynecol Oncol 2000; 78:194–202.
91. Grundker C, Schulz K, Gunthert AR, Emons G. Luteinizing hormone-releasing hormone induces nuclear factor kappaB-activation and inhibits apoptosis in ovarian cancer cells. J Clin Endocrinol Metab 2000; 85:3815–3820.
92. Grundker C, Schlotawa L, Viereck V, Emons G. Protein kinase C (PKC)-independent stimulation of activator protein-1 (AP-1) and c-Jun N-terminal kinase (JNK) activity in human endometrial cancer cells by luteinizing hormone-releasing hormone (LHRH) agonist Triptorelin. Eur J Endocrinol 2001; 145:651–658.
93. Gunthert AR, Grundker C, Hollmann K, Emons G. Luteinizing hormone-releasing hormone induces JunD-DNA binding and extends cell cycle in human ovarian cancer cells. Biochem Biophys Res Comm 2002; 294:11–15.
94. Imai A, Sugiyama M, Furui T, Tamaya T. Gi protein-mediated translocation of serine/threonine phosphatase to the plasma membrane and apoptosis of ovarian cancer cell in response to gonadotropin-releasing hormone antagonist Cetrorelix. J Obstet Gynaecol 2006; 26:37–41.
95. Dondi D, Festuccia C, Piccolella M, Bologna M, Motta M. GnRH agonists and antagonists decrease the metastatic progression of human prostate cancer cell lines by inhibiting the plasminogen activator system. Oncol Rep 2006; 15:393–400.
96. Tang X, Yano T, Osuga Y, Matsumi H, Yano N, Xu J, Wada O, Koga K, Kugu K,Tsutsumi O, Schally AV, Taketani Y. Cellular mechanisms of growth inhibition of human epithelial ovarian cancer cell line by LH-releasing hormone antagonist Cetrorelix. J Clin Endocrinol Metab 2002; 87:3721–3727.
97. Grundker C, Schlotawa L, Viereck V, Eicke N, Horst A, Kairies B, Emons G. Antiproliferative effects of the GnRH antagonist cetrorelix and of GnRH-II on human endometrial and ovarian cancer cells are not mediated through the GnRH type I receptor. Eur J Endocrinol 2004; 151:141–149.
98. Maiti K, Oh DY, Moon JS, Acharjee S, Li JH, Bai DG, Park HS, Lee K, Lee YC, Jung NC, Kim K, Vaudry H, Kwon HB, Seong JY. Differential effects of gonadotropin-releasing hormone (GnRH)-I and GnRH-II on prostate cancer cell signaling and death. J Clin Endocrinol Metab 2005; 90:4287–4298.
99. Sharoni Y, Bosin E, Miinster A, Levy J, Schally AV. Inhibition of growth of human mammary tumor cells by potent antagonists of luteinizing hormone-releasing hormone. Proc Natl Acad Sci USA 1989; 86:1648–1651.
100. Arencibia JM, Schally AV. Luteinizing hormone-releasing hormone as an autocrine growth factor in ES-2 ovarian cancer cell line. Int J Oncol 2000; 16:1009–1013.
101. Emons G, Weiss S, Ortmann O, Grundker C, Schulz KD. LHRH might act as a negative autocrine regulator of proliferation of human ovarian cancer. Eur J Endocrinol 2000; 142:665–670.
102. Volker P, Grundker C, Schmidt O, Schulz KD, Emons G. Expression of receptors for luteinizing hormone-releasing hormone in human ovarian and endometrial cancers: frequency, autoregulation, and correlation with direct antiproliferative activity of luteinizing hormone-releasing hormone analogs. Am J Obstet Gynecol 2002; 186:171–179.
103. Irmer G, Bürger C, Ortmann O, Schulz KD, Emons G. Expression of luteinizing hormone-releasing hormone and its mRNA in human endometrial cancer cell lines. J Clin Endocrinol Metab 1994; 79:916–919.
104. Limonta P, Dondi D, Moretti RM, Fermo D, Garattini E, Motta M. Expression of luteinizing hormone-releasing

hormone mRNA in the human prostatic cancer cell line LNCaP. J Clin Endocrinol Metab 1993; 76:797–800.
105. Harris NJ, Wilcox JN, Dutlow CM, Flanagan CA, Prescott RA, Roberts JL, Eidne KA, Millar RP. A putative autocrine role for GnRH in mammary carcinoma cell lines. In: F. Bresciani, RJB King, ME Lippman, eds. Progress in Cancer Research and Therapy. Vol 35: Hormones and Cancer. New York: Raven Press, 1988:174–178.
106. Nagy A, Schally AV, Armatis P, Szepeshazi K, Halmos G, Kovacs M, Zarandi M, Groot K, Miyazaki M, Jungwirth A, Horvath J. Cytotoxic analogs of luteinizing hormone-releasing hormone containing doxorubicin or 2-pyrrolinodoxorubicin, a derivative 500- 1000 times more potent. Proc Natl Acad Sci USA 1996; 93:7269–7273.
107. Nagy A, Schally AV. Targeting of cytotoxic luteinizing hormone-releasing hormone analogs to breast, ovarian, endometrial, and prostate cancers. Biol Reprod 2005; 73:851–859.
108. Bajusz S, Janaky T, Csernus VJ, Bokser L, Fekete M, Srkalovic G, Redding TW, Schally AV. Highly potent analogs of luteinizing hormone-releasing hormone containing D-phenylalanine nitrogen mustard in position 6. Proc Natl Acad Sci USA 1989; 86:6318–6322.
109. Keller G, Schally AV, Gaiser T, Nagy A, Baker B, Halmos G, Engel JB. Receptors for luteinizing hormone releasing hormone expressed on human renal cell carcinomas can be used for targeted chemotherapy with cytotoxic luteinizing hormone releasing hormone analogues. Clin Cancer Res 2005; 11:5549–5557.
110. Keller G, Schally AV, Gaiser T, Nagy A, Baker B, Halmos G, Engel JB. Receptors for luteinizing hormone releasing hormone (LHRH) expressed in human non-Hodgkin's lymphomas can be targeted for therapy with the cytotoxic LHRH analogue AN-207. Eur J Cancer 2005; 41:2196–2202.
111. Keller G, Schally AV, Gaiser T, Nagy A, Baker B, Westphal G, Halmos G, Engel JB. Human malignant melanomas express receptors for luteinizing hormone releasing hormone allowing targeted therapy with cytotoxic luteinizing hormone releasing hormone analogue. Cancer Res 2005; 65:5857–5863.
112. Hortobagyi GN. The curability of breast cancer present and future Eur J Cancer 2003; 1:24–34.
113. Jemal A, Murray T, Samuels A, Ghafoor A, Ward E, Thun MJ. Cancer statistics, 2003. CA Cancer J Clin. 2003; 53:5–26.
114. Beatson GT. On the treatment of inoperable cases of carcinoma of the mamma. Suggestions for a new method of treatment with illustrative cases. Lancet 1896; 2:104–107.
115. Santen RJ, Manni A, Harvey H, Redmond C. Endocrine 'treatment of breast cancer in women. Endocr Rev 1990; 11:221–265.
116. Klijn JG. LH-RH agonists in the treatment of metastatic breast cancer: ten years' experience. Recent Results Cancer Res 1992; 124:76–90.
117. Hoffken K. LH-RH agonists in the treatment of premenopausal patients with advanced breast cancer. Recent Results Cancer Res 1992; 124:91–104.
118. Desombre ER, Holt JA, Herbst AL. Steroid receptors in breast, uterine, and ovarian malignancy. In Gold JJ, Josimovich JB. eds. Gynecologic Endocrinology. New York: Plenum Pub. Corp, 1987:511–528.
119. Clarke M, Collins R, Davies C, Goodwin J, Gray R. Ovarian ablation in early breast cancer: overview of the randomized trials. Lancet 1996; 348(9036):1189–1196.
120. Haddow A, Watkinson JM, Paterson E. Influence of synthetic oestrogens upon advanced malignant disease. Br Med J 1944; 2:393–398.
121. Luft R, Olivecrona H, Sjogren B. Hypophysectomy in man. Nordic Medicine 1952; 14:351–354.
122. Dao TL, Huggins C. Bilateral adrenalectomy in the treatment of cancer of the breast. Arch Surg 1955; 71:645–657.
123. Nosaquo ND. Androgens and estrogens in the treatment of disseminated mammary carcinoma. J Am Med Assoc1960; 172:135–147.
124. Lønning PE. Role of endocrine therapy in breast cancer-where are we going? Best Pract Res Clin Endocrinol Metabol 2004; 18:vii–ix.
125. Cole MP, Jones CT, Todd ID. A new anti-oestrogenic agent in late breast cancer. An early clinical appraisal of ICI46474. Br J Cancer 1971; 25:270–275.
126. Wickerham L. Tamoxifen–an update on current data and where it can now be used. Breast Cancer Res Treat 2002; 75(suppl):S7–S12.
127. Cash R, Brough AJ, Cohen MN, Satoh PS. Aminoglutethimide (Elipten-Ciba) is an inhibitor of adrenal steroidogenesis: mechanism of action and therapeutic trial. J Clin Endocrinol Metab 1967; 27:1239–1248.
128. Santen RJ, Lipton A, Kendall J. Successful medical adrenalectomy with aminoglutethimide. J Am Med Assoc 1974; 230:1661–1665.
129. Miller WR. Biological rationale for endocrine therapy in breast cancer. Best Pract Res Clin Endocrinol Metab 2004; 18:1–32.
130. Buzdar AU. New generation aromatase inhibitors—from the advanced to the adjuvant setting. Breast Cancer Res Treat 2002; 75(suppl 1):S13–7 (discussion S33–5) (review).
131. DeSombre ER, Johnson ES, White WF. Regression of rat mammary tumors effected by a gonadoliberin analog. Cancer Res 1976; 36:3830–3833.
132. Johnson ES, Seely JH, White WF. Endocrine-dependent rat mammary tumor regression: use of a gonadotropin releasing hormone analog. Science 1976; 194:329–330.
133. Rose DP, Pruitt B. Modification of the effect of a gonadoliberin analog of 7, 12-dimethylbenz(a)anthracene-induced rat mammary tumors by hormone replacement. Cancer Res 1979; 39:3968–3970.
134. Nicholson RI, Maynard PV. Anti-tumor activity of ICI 118630, a new potent luteinizing hormone-releasing hormone agonist. Brit J Cancer 1979; 39:268–273.
135. Danguy A, Legros N, Heuson-Stiennon JA, Pasteels JL, Atassi G, Heuson JC. Effects of a gonadotropinreleasing hormone (GnRH) analogue (A-438 18) on 7, 12dimethylbenz (a)anthracene-induced rat mammary tumors. Histological and endocrine studies. Eur J Canc 1977; 13:1089–1094.
136. Klijn JGM, De Jong FH. Treatment with a luteinizing hormone-releasing hormone analogue (Buserelin) in premenopausal patients with metastatic breast cancer. Lancet 1982; i:1213–1216.

137. Redding TW, Schally AV. Inhibition of mammary tumor growth in rats and mice by administration of agonistic and antagonistic analogs of luteinizing hormone releasing hormone. Proc Natl Acad Sci USA 1983; 80:1078–1082.
138. Szende B, Srkalovic G, Groot K, Lapis K, Schally AV. Growth inhibition of mouse MXT mammary tumor by the luteinizing hormone-releasing hormone antagonist SB-75. J Natl Cancer Inst 1990; 82:513–517.
139. Reissmann T, Engel J, Kutscher B, Bernd M, Hilgard P, Peukert M, Szeleny I, Reichert S, Gonzalez–Barcena D, Nieschlag E, Comaru– Schally AM, Schally AV. Cetrorelix. Drugs Future 1994; 19, 228–237.
140. Yano T, Korkut E, Pinski J, Szepeshazi K, Milovanovic S, Groot K, Clarke R, Comaru-Schally AM, Schally AV. Inhibition of growth of MCF-7 MIII human breast carcinoma in nude mice by treatment with agonists or antagonists of LH-RH. Breast Cancer Res Treat 1992; 21:35–45.
141. Szepeshazi K, Milovanovic S, Lapis K, Groot K, Schally AV. Growth inhibition of estrogen independent MXT mouse mammary carcinomas in mice treated with an agonist or antagonist of LH-RH, an analog of somatostatin, or a combination. Breast Cancer Res Treat 1992; 21:181–192.
142. Klijn JGM, Foekens JA. Extrapituitary actions. In: Vickery BH, Lunenfeld B eds. GnRH Analogues in Cancer and Human Reproduction, Vol I Basic Aspects. Kluwer: Dordrecht, 1989:71–84.
143. Foekens JA, Klijn JGM. Direct anti-tumor effects of LH-RH analogs. Recent Results Cancer Res 1992; 124:7–17.
144. Seppala M, Wahlstrom T. Identification of luteinizing hormone-releasing factor and alpha subunit of glycoprotein hormones in ductal carcinoma of the mammary gland. Int J Cancer 1980; 26:231–233.
145. Butzow R., Huthaniemi I, Clayton R, Wahlstrom T, Andersson LC and Seppala M. Cultured mammary carcinoma cells contain gonadotropin releasing hormone-like immunoreactivity, GnRH binding sites and chorionic gonadotropin. Int J Cancer 1987; 39:498–501.
146. Kottler ML, Starzec A, Carre MC, Lagarde JP, Martin A, Counis R. The genes for gonadotropin-releasing hormone and its receptor are expressed in human breast with fibrocystic disease and cancer. Int J Cancer 1997; 71:595–599.
147. Fekete M, Bajusz S, Groot K, Csernus VJ, Schally AV. Comparison of different agonists and antagonists of luteinizing hormone-releasing hormone for receptor-binding ability to rat pituitary and human breast cancer membranes. Endocrinology 1989; 124:946–955.
148. Segal-Abramson T, Kitroser H, Levy J, Schally AV, Sharoni Y. Direct effects of luteinizing hormone-releasing hormone agonists and antagonists on MCF-7 mammary cancer cells. Proc Natl Acad Sci USA 1992; 89:2236–2239.
149. Chetrite G, Blumberg-Tick J, Pasqualini JR. Effect of Decapeptyl (a GnRH analogue) and of transforming growth factor-alpha (TGF-alpha), in the presence of heparin, on the sulfatase activity of human breast cancer cells. J Steroid Biochem Mol Biol 1995; 52:451–457.
150. Hershkovitz E, Marbach M, Bosin E, Levy J, Roberts CT Jr, LeRoith D, Schally AV, Sharoni Y. Luteinizing hormone-releasing hormone antagonists interfere with autocrine and paracrine growth stimulation of MCF-7 mammary cancer cells by insulin-like growth factor. J Clin Endocrinol Metab 1993; 77:963–968.
151. von Alten J, Fister S, Schulz H, Viereck V, Frosch KH, Emons G, Grundker C. GnRH analogs reduce invasiveness of human breast cancer cells. Breast Cancer Res Treat 2006; 100:13–21.
152. Szepeshazi K, Schally AV, Nagy A, Halmos G, Groot K. Targeted cytotoxic luteinizing hormone releasing hormone (LH-RH) analogs inhibit growth of estrogen-independent MXT mouse mammary cancer in vivo by decreasing cell proliferation and inducing apoptosis. Anticancer Drugs 1997; 8:974–987.
153. Szepeshazi K, Schally AV, Nagy A. Effective treatment of advanced estrogen-independent MXT mouse mammary cancers with targeted cytotoxic LH-RH analogs. Breast Cancer Res Treat 1999; 56:267–276.
154. Kahan Z, Nagy A, Schally AV, Halmos G, Arencibia JM, Groot K. Complete regression of MX-1 human breast cancer xenografts after targeted chemotherapy with a cytotoxic analog of luteinizing hormone-releasing hormone, AN-207. Cancer 1999; 85:2608–2615.
155. Kahan Z, Nagy A, Schally AV, Halmos G, Arencibia JM, Groot K. Administration of a targeted cytotoxic analog of luteinizing hormone-releasing hormone inhibits growth of estrogen-independent MDA-MB-231 human breast cancers in nude mice. Breast Cancer Res Treat 2000; 59:255–262.
156. Chatzistamou L, Schally AV, Nagy A, Armatis P, Szepeshazi K, Halmos G. Effective treatment of metastatic MDA-MD-435 human estrogen independent breast carcinomas with a targeted cytotoxic analog of luteinizing hormone-releasing hormone, AN-207. Clin Cancer Res 2000; 6:4158–4165.
157. Bajo AM, Schally AV, Halmos G, Nagy A. Targeted doxorubicin-containing luteinizing hormone-releasing hormone analogue AN-152 inhibits the growth of doxorubicin-resistant MX-1 human breast cancers. Clin Cancer Res 2003; 9:3742–3748.
158. Wang X, Krebs LJ, Al-Nuri M. A chemically labeled cytotoxic agent: Two-photon fluorophore for optical tracking of cellular pathway in chemotherapy. Proc Natl Acad Sci USA 1999; 96:11081–11084.
159. Kovacs M, Schally AV, Nagy A, Koppan M, Groot K. Recovery of pituitary function after treatment with a targeted cytotoxic analog of luteinizing hormone-releasing hormone. Proc Natl Acad Sci 1997; 94:1420–1425.
160. Kovacs M, Schally AV, Csernus B, Busto R, Rekasi Z, Nagy A. Targeted cytotoxic analogue of luteinizing hormone-releasing hormone (LH-RH) only transiently decreases the gene expression of pituitary receptors for LH-RH. J Neuroendocrinology 2002; 14:5–13.
161. Kaufmann M, Jonat W, Kleeburg U, Eirmann W, Janicke F, Hilfrich J, Kreienberg R, Albrecht M, Weitzel HK, Schmid H, Strunz P, Schachner–Wunschmann E, Bastert G, Maass H. The German Zoladex trial group: goserelin, a depot gonadotropin releasing hormone agonist in the treatment of premenopausal patients with metastatic breast cancer. J Clin Oncol 1989; 7:1113–1119.

162. Manni A, Santen R, Harvey H, Lipton A, Max D. Treatment of breast cancer with gonadotropin-releasing hormone. Endocr Rev 1986; 7:89–94.
163. Mathé G, Keiling R, Prevot G, Vo Van ML, Gastiaburu J, Vannetzel JM, Despax R, Jasmin C, Levi F, Musset M, Machover D, Ribaud R, Misset JL. LHRH agonist: breast and prostate cancer. In: Klijn JGM, Paridaens R, Foekens JA, eds. Hormonal Manipulation of Cancer: Peptides, Growth Factors, and New (Anti) Steroidal Agents. New York: Raven Press, 1987:315–319.
164. Plowman PN, Nicholson RI, Walker KJ. Remission of postmenopausal breast cancer during treatment with the luteinizing hormone releasing hormone agonist ICI 118630. Br J Cancer 1986; 54:903–909.
165. Walker KJ, Turkes A, Williams MR, Blamey RW, Nicholson RI. Preliminary endocrinological evaluation of a sustained-release formulation of the LH-releasing hormone agonist D-Ser(But)6 Azgly 10 LHRH in premenopausal women with advanced breast cancer. J Endocrinol 1986; 111:349–53.
166. Williams MR, Walker KJ, Turkes A, Blamey RW, Nicholson RI. The use of an LHRH agonist (ICI 118630, Zoladex) in advanced premenopausal breast cancer. Br J Cancer 1986; 53:629–636.
167. Monsonego J, Destable MD, de Saint Florent G, Amouroux J, Kouyoumdjian JC, Haour F, Breau JL, Israel L, Comaru–Schally AM, Schally AV. Fibrocystic disease of the breast in premenopausal women: Histohormonal correlation and response to LHRH analog treatment. Am J Obstet Gynecol 1991; 164:1181–1189.
168. Klijn JG, Beex LV, Mauriac L, van Zijl JA, Veyret C, Wildiers J, Jassem J, Piccart M, Burghouts J, Becquart D, Seynaeve C, Mignolet F, Duchateau L. Combined treatment with buserelin and tamoxifen in premenopausal metastatic breast cancer: a randomized study. J Natl Cancer Inst 2000; 92:903–911.
169. Klijn JG, Blamey RW, Boccardo F, Tominaga T, Duchateau L, Sylvester R. Combined Hormone Agents Trialists' Group and the European Organization for Research and Treatment of Cancer. Combined tamoxifen and luteinizing hormone-releasing hormone (LHRH) agonist versus LHRH agonist alone in premenopausal advanced breast cancer: a meta-analysis of four randomized trials. J Clin Oncol 2001; 19:343–353.
170. Nicholson RI, Walker KJ, McClelland RA, Dixon A, Robertson JF, Blamey RW. Zoladex plus tamoxifen versus Zoladex alone in pre- and peri-menopausal metastatic breast cancer. J Steroid Biochem Mol Biol 1990; 37:989–995.
171. Jonat W, Kaufmann M, Blamey RW, Howell A, Collins JP, Coates A, Eiermann W, Janicke F, Njordenskold B, Forbes JF. A randomised study to compare the effect of the luteinising hormone releasing hormone (LHRH) analogue goserelin with or without tamoxifen in pre- and perimenopausal patients with advanced breast cancer. Eur J Cancer 1995; 31:137–142.
172. Jonat W, Kaufmann M, Sauerbrei W, Blamey R, Cuzick J, Namer M, Fogelman I, de Haes JC, de Matteis A, Stewart A, Eiermann W, Szakolczai I, Palmer M, Schumacher M, Geberth M, Lisboa B, and Zoladex Early Breast Cancer Research Association Study. Goserelin versus cyclophosphamide, methotrexate, and fluorouracil as adjuvant therapy in premenopausal patients with node-positive breast cancer: the Zoladex Early Breast Cancer Research Association Study. J Clin Oncol 2002; 20:4628–4635.
173. Jakesz R, Hausmaninger H, Kubista E, Gnant M, Menzel C, Bauernhofer T, Seifert M, Haider K, Mlineritsch B, Steindorfer P, Kwasny W, Fridrik M, Steger G, Wette V, Samonigg H, and Austrian Breast and Colorectal Cancer Study Group Trial 5. Randomized adjuvant trial of tamoxifen and goserelin versus cyclophosphamide, methotrexate, and fluorouracil: evidence for the superiority of treatment with endocrine blockade in premenopausal patients with hormone-responsive breast cancer—Austrian Breast and Colorectal Cancer Study Group Trial 5. J Clin Oncol 2002; 20:4621–4627.
174. Castiglione-Gertsch M, O'Neill A, Price KN, Goldhirsch A, Coates AS, Colleoni M, Nasi ML, Bonetti M, Gelber RD, and International Breast Cancer Study Group. Adjuvant chemotherapy followed by goserelin versus either modality alone for premenopausal lymph node-negative breast cancer: a randomized trial. J Natl Cancer Inst 2003; 95:1833–1846.
175. Roche H, Kerbrat P, Bonneterre J, Fargeot P, Fumoleau P, Monnier A, Clavere P, Goudier MJ, Chollet P, Guastalla JP, Serin D. Complete hormonal blockade versus epirubicin-based chemotherapy in premenopausal, one to three node-positive, and hormone-receptor positive, early breast cancer patients: 7-year follow-up results of French Adjuvant Study Group 06 randomised trial. Ann Oncol 2006; 17:1221–1227.
176. Torrisi R, Colleoni M, Veronesi P, Rocca A, Peruzzotti G, Severi G, Medici M, Renne G, Intra M, Luini A, Nole F, Viale G, Goldhirsch A. Primary therapy with ECF in combination with a GnRH analog in premenopausal women with hormone receptor-positive T2-T4 breast cancer. Breast 2007; 16:73–80.
177. Jonat W. Overview of luteinizing hormone-releasing hormone agonists in early breast cancer-benefits of reversible ovarian ablation. Breast Cancer Res Treat 2002; 75:S23–S26.
178. Sverrisdottir A, Fornander T, Jacobsson H, von Schoultz E, Rutqvist LE. Bone mineral density among premenopausal women with early breast cancer in a randomized trial of adjuvant endocrine therapy. J Clin Oncol 2004; 22: 3694–3699.
179. Bianco A, CR, DiLorenzo G. The Mam-1 GOGSI trial: a randomized trial with factorial design of chemoendocrine adjuvant treatment in node positive (N+) early breast cancer (EBC). Proc Natl Acad Clin Oncol 2001; 20:27.
180. Davidson NE, O'Neill AM, Vukov AM, Osborne CK, Martino S, White DR, Abeloff MD. Chemoendocrine therapy for premenopausal women with axillary lymph node-positive, steroid hormone receptor-positive breast cancer: results from INT 0101 (E5188). J Clin Oncol 2005; 23:5973–5982.
181. Arriagada R, Le MG, Spielmann M, Mauriac L, Bonneterre J, Namer M, Delozier T, Hill C, Tursz T. Randomised trial of adjuvant ovarian suppression in 926 premenopausal patients with early breast cancer treated with adjuvant chemotherapy. Ann Oncol 2005; 16:389–396.
182. Baum M, Hackshaw A, Houghton J, Rutqvist, Fornander T, Nordenskjold B, Nicolucci A, Sainsbury R, and ZIPP International Collaborators Group. Adjuvant goserelin in

pre-menopausal patients with early breast cancer: results from the ZIPP study. Eur J Cancer 2006; 42:895–904.

183. Dowsett M, Stein RC, Coombes RC. Aromatization inhibition alone or in combination with GnRH agonists for the treatment of premenopausal breast cancer patients. J Steroid Biochem Mol Biol 1992; 43:155–159.

184. Forward DP, Cheung KL, Jackson L, Robertson JF. Clinical and endocrine data for goserelin plus anastrozole as second-line endocrine therapy for premenopausal advanced breast cancer. 2004; 90, 590–594.

185. Celio L, Martinetti A, Ferrari L, Buzzoni R, Mariani L, Miceli R, Seregni E, Procopio G, Cassata A, Bombardieri E, Bajetta E. Premenopausal breast cancer patients treated with a gonadotropin-releasing hormone analog alone or in combination with an aromatase inhibitor: a comparative endocrine study. Anticancer Res 1999; 19:2261–2268.

186. Recchia F, Saggio G, Amiconi G, Di Blasio A, Cesta A, Candeloro G, Rea S. Gonadotropin-releasing hormone analogues added to adjuvant chemotherapy protect ovarian function and improve clinical outcomes in young women with early breast carcinoma. Cancer 2006; 106:514–523.

187. Del Mastro L, Catzeddu T, Boni L, Bell C, Sertoli MR, Bighin C, Clavarezza M, Testa D, Venturini M. Prevention of chemotherapy-induced menopause by temporary ovarian suppression with goserelin in young, early breast cancer patients. Ann Oncol 2006; 17:74–78.

188. Nystedt M, Berglund G, Bolund C, Fornander T, Rutqvist LE. Side effects of adjuvant endocrine treatment in premenopausal breast cancer patients: a prospective randomized study. J Clin Oncol 2003; 21:1836–1844.

189. Schwartz L, Guichet N, Keiling R. Two partial remissions induced by an LHRH analogue in two postmenopausal women with metastatic breast cancer. Cancer 1988; 62: 2498–2500.

190. Sanchez-Garrido F, Comaru-Schally AM, Sanchez del Cura G, Gonzalez-Enriquez J, Schally AV. Clearance of lung metastases of breast carcinoma after treatment with triptorelin in postmenopausal woman. Lancet 1995; 345:868.

191. Dowsett M, CantWell B, Anshumala L, Jeffcote SL, Harris AL. Suppression of postmenopausal ovarian steroidogenesis with the luteinizing hormone-releasing hormone agonist goserelin. J Clin Endocrinol Metab 1988; 66:672–677.

192. Crighton IL, Dowsett M, Lal A, Man A, Smith IE. Use of luteinizing hormone-releasing hormone agonist (leuprorelin) in advanced post-menopausal breast cancer:clinical and endocrine effects. Br J Cancer 1989; 60:644–648.

193. Korkut E, Comaru-Schally AM, Schally AV, Plowman PM. LH-RH Analogues and Breast Cancer Br J Cancer 1991; 64:1190.

194. Slamon DJ, Leyland-Jones B, Shak S, Fuchs H, Paton V, Bajamonde A, Fleming T, Eiermann W, Wolter J, Pegram M, Baselga J, Norton L. Use of chemotherapy plus a monoclonal antibody against HER2 for metastatic breast cancer that overexpresses HER2. N Engl J Med 2001; 344:783–792.

195. Hurwitz H, Saini S. Related Articles. Bevacizumab in the treatment of metastatic colorectal cancer: safety profile and management of adverse events. Semin Oncol 2006; 33:S26–S34.

196. Hankinson SE, Willett WC, Colditz GA, Hunter DJ, Michaud DS, Deroo B, Rosner B, Speizer FE, Pollak M. Circulating concentrations of insulin-like growth factor-I and risk of breast cancer. Lancet 1998; 351:1393–1396.

197. Bajo AM, Schally AV, Krupa M, Hebert F, Groot K, Szepeshazi K. Bombesin antagonists inhibit growth of MDA-MB-435 estrogen independent breast cancers and decrease the expression of ErbB-2/HER-2 oncoprotein and c-jun and c-fos oncogenes Proc Nat Acad Sci USA 2002; 99:3836–3841.

198. Waters MJ, Conway-Campbell BL. The oncogenic potential of autocrine human growth hormone in breast cancer. Proc Natl Acad Sci USA 2004; 101:14992–14993.

199. Mukhina S, Mertani HC, Guo K, Lee KO, Gluckman PD, Lobie PE. Phenotypic conversion of human mammary carcinoma cells by autocrine human growth hormone. Proc Natl Acad Sci USA 2004; 101:15166–15171.

200. Schally AV, Varga JL. Antagonistic analogs of growth hormone-releasing hormone: new potential antitumor agents. Trends Endocrinol Metabol 1999; 10:383–391.

201. Schally AV, Varga JL. Antagonists of growth hormone-releasing hormone. Comb Chem High Throughput Screen 2006; 9:163–170.

202. Zia H, Hida T, Jakowlew S, Birrer M, Gozes Y, Reubi JC, Fridkin M, Gozes I, Moody TW. Breast cancer growth is inhibited by vasoactive intestinal peptide (VIP) hybrid, a synthetic VIP receptor antagonist. Cancer Res 1996; 56:3486–349.

203. Ingle JN, Suman VJ, Kardinal CG, Krook JE, Mailliard JA, Veeder MH, Loprinzi CL, Dalton RJ, Hartmann LC, Conover CA, Pollak MN. A randomized trial of tamoxifen alone or combined with octreotide in the treatment of women with metastatic breast carcinoma. Cancer 1999; 85:1284–1292.

204. Yano T, Pinski J. Szepeshazi K, Halmos G, Radulovic S, Groot K, Schally AV. Inhibitory effect of bombesin/gastrin releasing peptide antagonist RC-3095 and luteinizing hormone-releasing hormone antagonist SB-75 on growth of MCF-7 MIII human breast cancer xenografts in athymic nude mice cancer 1994; 73:1229–1238.

205. Emons G, Kauffmann M, Gunthert AR, Hamid-Werner M, Grundker C, Loibl S, Schally AV. Phase I study of Zen-008 (AN-152), a targeted cytotoxic LHRH analog in female patients with cancers expressing LHRH receptors. J Clin Oncol 2006 ASCO Annual Meeting Proceedings Part I. Vol 24, No. 18S (June 20 Supplement), 2006; 13146 (abstr).

206. Emons G, Hesse O, Kaufman M, Gunthert M, Hami-Werner M, Grundker C, Loibl S, Schally AV. ZEN-008: eine Phase I Studie mit einem zytotoxischen GnRH-Analogon (AN-152) bei Patientinnen mit fortgeschrittenen, GnRH-Rezeptor I exprimierenden Kariznomen. Annual Meeting of the German Gynecology Society, Berlin, 2006 (abstr).

15

Vitamin D and Breast Cancer

JoELLEN WELSH

*Department of Biomedical Sciences and Gen*NY*Sis Center for Excellence in Cancer Genomics, University at Albany, Rensselaer, New York, U.S.A.*

INTRODUCTION

It is quite clear that estrogen, through interactions with the nuclear estrogen receptor, drives mammary epithelial cell proliferation and contributes to the etiology of human breast cancer. In addition to estrogen receptors (ERs), other nuclear receptors present in mammary cells, such as the progesterone receptor, the retinoid receptors, and the vitamin D receptor (VDR), exert cell regulatory effects in mammary tissue and thus have emerged as promising therapeutic targets for breast cancer. On the basis of the importance of nuclear receptors in mediating expression of genes involved in proliferation, differentiation, and apoptosis, synthetic structural analogs of nuclear receptor ligands that exhibit biological properties distinct from the natural ligands represent a feasible approach to manipulate nuclear receptor activity. It is well established that targeting ER pathways via synthetic ligands such as tamoxifen can effectively treat and prevent breast cancer, and studies with additional nuclear receptor ligands are ongoing.

In the case of the VDR, many synthetic analogs with desirable therapeutic profiles have been developed, and some are in clinical trials for various indications including cancer. However, further development of synthetic VDR ligands for either treatment or prevention of breast cancer requires more accurate understanding of the role of the vitamin D signaling pathway in both normal and transformed mammary cells. This chapter will review the extensive literature documenting the effects of 1,25 $(OH)_2D_3$ (the natural ligand for VDR) and numerous bioactive vitamin D analogs on breast cancer cells and tumors. Emerging data on the role of the vitamin D endocrine system in normal mammary tissue and the possibility that the VDR may represent a target for breast cancer prevention are also discussed.

VITAMIN D: INTERPLAY BETWEEN DIET, GENETICS, AND ENVIRONMENT

Forms, Functions, and Metabolism of Vitamin D

The term vitamin D refers to calciferols, steroid compounds originally identified for their ability to ameliorate the childhood bone disease rickets. Indeed, the best-characterized role of vitamin D is maintenance of extracellular calcium homeostasis, and rickets results from impaired bone mineralization secondary to insufficient calcium availability to the growing skeleton. Normally, low calcium availability induces transient hypocalcemia that stimulates secretion of parathyroid hormone and enhances metabolic activation of vitamin D. Vitamin D in turn promotes absorption of dietary calcium in enterocytes, release of calcium from bone, and reabsorption of calcium in the kidney, processes mediated by the VDR.

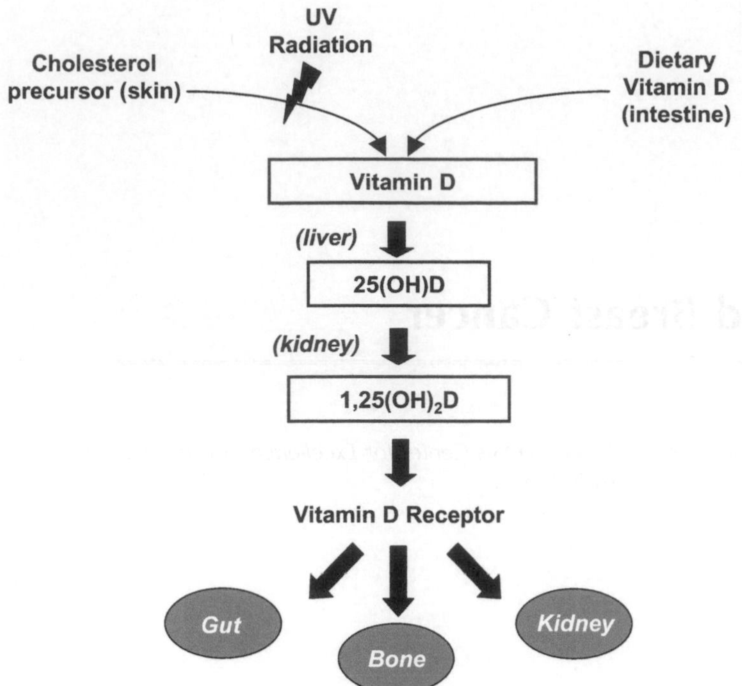

Figure 1 The vitamin D endocrine system. Classical control of extracellular calcium homeostasis is mediated via systemic $1,25(OH)_2D$, which is generated from ingested or endogenously synthesized vitamin D through a series of hydroxylation reactions in liver and kidney. Binding of $1,25(OH)_2D$ to the vitamin D receptor in gut, bone, and kidney enhances calcium uptake and retention to maintain extracellular calcium at levels sufficient for bone mineralization. Production of $1,25(OH)_2D$ for the systemic circulation by the kidney is tightly regulated and geared to the body's calcium needs. See text for additional details.

Once calcium influx restores normocalcemia, parathyroid hormone secretion is diminished in a classic endocrine-negative feedback loop. Under normal circumstances, therefore, this endocrine system maintains extracellular calcium homeostasis and allows for normal bone mineralization as long as sufficient calcium and vitamin D are available.

The two naturally occurring forms of vitamin D are cholecalciferol (vitamin D_3, from animal sources) and ergocalciferol (vitamin D_2, from plant sources), and both forms require metabolism for biological activity. For simplicity, this review focuses on vitamin D_3 (Fig. 1), but the metabolism and functions of vitamin D_2 are similar. Vitamin D_3 can be synthesized from a cholesterol derivative (7-dehydrocholesterol) in the epidermis, a conversion that requires UVB radiation. Vitamin D_3 can also be obtained from natural and fortified foods as well as supplements (discussed in the next section) and is absorbed along with other dietary lipids. Regardless of source (endogenous synthesis or diet), the initial step in metabolism of vitamin D_3 is hepatic hydroxylation at the 25 position, generating 25-hydroxyvitamin D_3 [$25(OH)D_3$]. $25(OH)D_3$ is the major circulating form, which is also stored in adipose tissue and is the most accurate biomarker of overall vitamin D_3 status. Further hydroxylation of $25(OH)D_3$ can generate two metabolites: 24,25-dihydroxyvitamin D_3 ($24,25(OH)_2D_3$) or 1α,25-dihydroxyvitamin D_3 ($1,25(OH)_2D_3$). Production of $24,25(OH)_2D_3$ is catalyzed by the $25(OH)D_3$ 24-hydroxylase (also termed CYP24), an enzyme present in the majority of vitamin D target tissues. The $24,25(OH)_2D_3$ metabolite does not readily bind VDR, and its production is considered the first step in degradation of $25(OH)D_3$. Production of $1,25(OH)_2D_3$, the biologically active vitamin D_3 metabolite, is mediated by the $25(OH)D_3$ 1α-hydroxylase (also termed CYP27B1), an enzyme that is highly expressed in renal proximal tubules. Because the kidney 1α-hydroxylase produces $1,25(OH)_2D_3$ for the systemic circulation, its activity reflects calcium availability. If calcium demand is increased, renal 1α-hydroxlase activity is induced and more $1,25(OH)_2D_3$ is generated (it is this activation step that is enhanced by parathyroid hormone). Elevated circulating $1,25(OH)_2D_3$ subsequently interacts with VDR in target tissues such as kidney, intestine, and bone to mobilize calcium. Conversely, when calcium demands are low, the renal 1α-hydroxlase is suppressed and the 24-hydroxylase is enhanced, leading to formation of $24,25(OH)_2D_3$ and initiation of catabolism. These regulatory concepts of $25(OH)D_3$ hydroxylation are based on the renal enzymes and control of extracellular calcium homeostasis, and are not likely to be applicable to regulation of these enzymes in other tissues. This issue is discussed further in the section "Uptake and Metabolism of Vitamin D Steroids in Target Tissues" in the context of extrarenal hydroxylases and control of epithelial cell turnover by $1,25(OH)_2D_3$.

Diet, Sunlight, and Vitamin D Deficiency

Factors associated with low vitamin D status include limited epidermal synthesis of cholecalciferol (because of infrequent exposure to sunlight, living in geographic areas with low solar radiation, dark pigmentation, and liberal use of sunscreen), liver or kidney disease, certain medications, poor diet, and aging.

Very few natural foods, with the exception of certain fish, contain nutritionally significant amounts of calciferols, and epidermal synthesis of vitamin D is highly variable (Chen et al., 2007). For this reason, milk and other products (orange juice, cereal) are often fortified with vitamin D_3 in the United States, Canada, and many other countries. It should be noted, however, that fortification is voluntary, and the actual vitamin D_3 content of fortified milk is often less than the stated 400 units/quart (Holick et al., 1992).

Despite the fortification of vitamin D_3 in foods and endogenous synthesis, the prevalence of vitamin D insufficiency, as defined by low (<30 nM) circulating 25(OH)D, is surprisingly common, especially in populations living in northern climates and in the elderly (Vieth et al., 2007). Particularly relevant to the possible relationship between vitamin D and breast cancer, vitamin D deficiency has been reported in a high percentage of women, including during adolescence, pregnancy/lactation, and after menopause, even in sunny climates (Lisa et al., 2007; Gonzalez et al., 2007; Siddiqui and Kamfer, 2007).

The increasing number of reports of vitamin D insufficiency has prompted reevaluation of the recommended adequate intake for vitamin D (Vieth et al., 2007), which was directed against prevention of rickets. There is fairly compelling evidence that prolonged subclinical vitamin D deficiency, which may not be associated with hypocalcemia or bone disease but could limit availability of vitamin D metabolites to tissues, contributes to chronic disease in human populations. However, relevant biomarkers of vitamin D status that reflect newly identified actions in target tissues such as colon, prostate, and breast (as discussed below) remain to be identified.

In the majority of cases, overt vitamin D deficiency can be prevented or cured by dietary adjustments or use of a supplement. However, the doses of vitamin D needed to elevate serum $25(OH)D_3$ into the optimal range may be higher than previously thought (Hollis, 2005). There are a number of inherited genetic defects in humans that impair bioactivation or utilization of vitamin D, and these are not cured by increasing vitamin D intake. These vitamin D–resistant syndromes are rare and have been well characterized at the biochemical and molecular levels. Vitamin D–resistant rickets type I is characterized by inability to produce $1,25(OH)_2D_3$ secondary to loss of function mutations in the $25(OH)D_3$ 1α-hydroxylase, whereas vitamin D–resistant rickets type II develops secondary to mutations in the VDR. Mouse models of these hereditary vitamin D–resistant syndromes have become powerful research tools for identification of new functions of vitamin D (Li et al., 1997; Dardenne et al., 2001).

CELLULAR AND MOLECULAR MECHANISMS OF VITAMIN D ACTION

Uptake and Metabolism of Vitamin D Steroids in Target Tissues

Examples of nonrenal cell types that express 25(OH)D 1α-hydroxylase include macrophages and epithelial cells derived from the epidermis, prostate, breast, pancreas, and colon. The presence of 1α-hydroxylase in extrarenal tissues suggests that concentrations of $1,25(OH)_2D_3$ sufficient to elicit local effects could be generated from $25(OH)D_3$. As discussed in more detail in section "Vitamin D Actions on Breast Cancer Cells In Vitro," these tissue-specific effects of vitamin D signaling include control of proliferation, differentiation, and apoptosis. This concept is supported by data demonstrating that mammary epithelial cells that express 1α-hydroxylase are growth inhibited by physiologic concentrations of $25(OH)D_3$ in vitro, presumably due to conversion to $1,25(OH)_2D_3$ (Welsh et al., 2003; Kemmis et al., 2006).

These observations have thus identified two distinct pathways of vitamin D biosynthesis and action: an endocrine pathway geared toward maintenance of calcemia via circulating $1,25(OH)_2D_3$ (Fig. 1), and an autocrine/paracrine pathway (Fig. 2) that mediates tissue-specific cell-regulatory effects via local generation of $1,25(OH)_2D_3$. The implication of the autocrine pathway is that cellular production of $1,25(OH)_2D_3$ would likely be regulated in a tissue-specific fashion independently of systemic calcium homeostasis. Similarly, the actions of locally produced $1,25(OH)_2D_3$ would be confined to the immediate cellular environment and would not necessarily impact on body calcium homeostasis. Existence of the autocrine pathway implies that delivery and uptake of circulating $25(OH)D_3$ to cells that express 25(OH)D 1α-hydroxylase become a critical determinant of cellular vitamin D activity.

Vitamin D metabolites, including $25(OH)D_3$ and $1,25(OH)_2D_3$, circulate in the free form as well as bound to the vitamin D–binding protein (DBP), a member of the albumin gene family. Free steroids, in particular $1,25(OH)_2D_3$, which has relatively low affinity for DBP, are presumed to enter cells via diffusion through the plasma membrane.

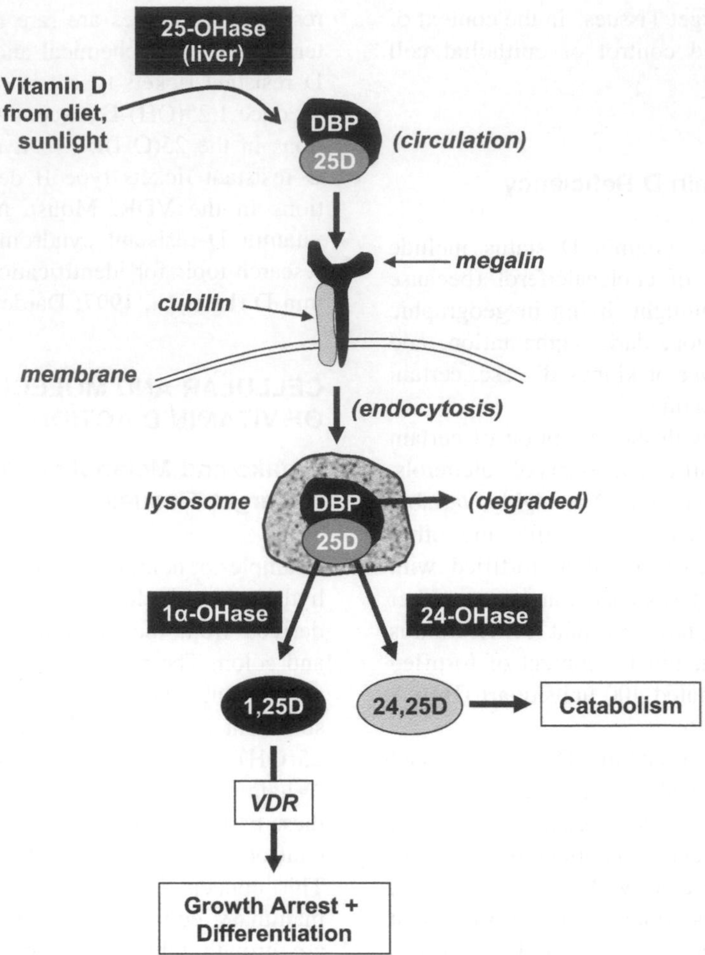

Figure 2 Model for extrarenal vitamin D metabolism and autocrine vitamin D signaling. The presence of vitamin D metabolizing enzymes (1α-OHase and 24-OHase) in extrarenal tissues enables production of $1,25(OH)_2D$ (1,25D) and $24,25(OH)_2D$ (24,25D) from 25(OH)D (25D)], which circulates bound to the DBP. However, only cells expressing the megalin-cubilin coreceptors are able to internalize 25-DBP complexes via receptor-mediated endocytosis. Within lysosomes, DBP is degraded and 25D is released where it traffics to mitochondria and can be metabolized to either 24,25D, a metabolite that is degraded and ultimately excreted, or 1,25D (the VDR ligand). In the autocrine/paracrine pathway, 1,25D can bind to VDR within the same cell (autocrine) or in adjacent cells (paracrine) to mediate negative-growth regulation. See text for additional details. *Abbreviations*: VDR, vitamin D receptor; DBP, vitamin D–binding protein.

In contrast, $25(OH)D_3$ bound to DBP enters renal cells via receptor mediated endocytosis, facilitated by the megalin-cubilin complex (Willnow and Nykjaer, 2002). Recent studies have demonstrated that $25(OH)D_3$ bound to DBP can also be imported into nonrenal cells that express megalin and cubilin, including breast cancer cells (Rowling et al., 2006). These data suggest that the metabolic fate of $25(OH)D_3$ will depend on the relative expression/activity of $25(OH)D_3$ metabolizing enzymes. In cells with high levels of the $25(OH)D_3$ 24-hydroxylase, catabolism would predominate, whereas in cells with functional $25(OH)D_3$ 1α-hydroxylase, activation to $1,25(OH)_2D_3$ would occur. This new concept of tissue-specific vitamin D metabolism and action indicates that the optimal serum levels of $25(OH)D_3$ will need to be redefined in terms of maintenance of local $1,25(OH)_2D_3$ generation.

The VDR

Whether generated in cells from $25(OH)D_3$ or taken up from the circulation, $1,25(OH)_2D_3$ binds to the VDR, a member of the steroid receptor family of ligand-dependent transcription factors that modulate gene expression in a tissue-specific manner (Carlberg and Molnar, 2006). Gene regulation by the liganded VDR requires dimerization, most often with the retinoid X receptor (RXR) family, and binding to specific DNA sequences in target gene promoters. Although a variety of structurally distinct vitamin D responsive elements have been identified, the best characterized is a hexanucleotide direct repeat separated by three variable base pairs (DR3) to which VDR:RXR heterodimers bind. However, the recognition that VDR also functions as a homodimer, or as a heterodimer with partners other than RXR, and can bind diverse DNA sequences suggests enormous flexibility to the genomic pathways regulated by vitamin D. Additional complexity arises through VDR interactions with other transcription factors such as Sp1 and β catenin, activity of the unoccupied receptor, and the possibility that additional physiologic VDR ligands may exist (Shah et al., 2006; Ellison et al., 2007; Makishima et al., 2002). In addition, the VDR is subject to posttranslational modifications, including phosphorylation, which affect its transcriptional activity.

In addition to genomic signaling, $1,25(OH)_2D_3$ can exert rapid effects on signal transduction pathways, leading to biological responses at the plasma membrane or in the cytoplasm (Fig. 2). Identification of an alternative binding pocket in the VDR for ligands that mediate rapid effects (Mizwicki et al., 2004) suggests that the VDR mediates the majority of these nongenomic effects, a suggestion supported by studies with cells from VDR null mice (Erben et al., 2002). Localization of the nuclear VDR protein to caveolae, specialized signaling complexes present in plasma membrane, further supports this concept (Huhtakangas et al., 2004). Examples of nontranscriptional effects of the $1,25(OH)_2D_3$-VDR complex with potential relevance to cancer cell regulation include regulation of intracellular calcium, protein kinase C activation, and modulation of protein phosphatases PP1c and PP2Ac (Palmer et al., 2001; Bettoun et al., 2002; Norman, 2006). The possibility that alternative receptors for vitamin D metabolites that have been linked to rapid responses may contribute to cancer cell regulation by $1,25(OH)_2D_3$ is yet to be thoroughly investigated. Thus, the relative contributions of genomic and nongenomic signaling in mediating the diverse biological effects of $1,25(OH)_2D_3$, particularly in relation to its anticancer properties, remain to be fully clarified.

VITAMIN D ACTIONS ON BREAST CANCER CELLS IN VITRO

Overview

Although originally identified on the basis of its role in calcium and bone metabolism, the VDR is expressed in many tissues that do not contribute to control of extracellular calcium homeostasis, including pancreas, brain, keratinocytes, colon, and mammary gland. In an early study, 23 of 33 established human cancer cell lines surveyed expressed VDR (Frampton et al., 1982). Receptors for $1,25(OH)_2D_3$ have been demonstrated in carcinogen-induced rat mammary tumors, human breast tumors, and established breast cancer cell lines (Eisman et al., 1980; Colston et al., 1986; Buras et al., 1994). In most VDR-positive cells, $1,25(OH)_2D_3$ mediates antiproliferative effects and may subsequently trigger differentiation or apoptosis. Importantly, studies with cells from VDR null mice have demonstrated that the VDR is required for the growth-regulatory effects of $1,25(OH)_2D_3$ in transformed epithelial cells (Zinser et al., 2003). Expression profiling of breast, prostate, colon, and squamous carcinoma cells has identified vitamin D–responsive gene clusters involved in regulation of cell cycle, differentiation, apoptosis, DNA repair, cell adhesion, and immune responses, indicating a diverse and broad range of VDR targets potentially involved in cell regulation (Palmer et al., 2001; Lin et al., 2002; Swami et al., 2003; Krishnan et al., 2004; Lee et al., 2006).

The VDR is expressed in the majority of human breast tumors, thus it represents a potential therapeutic target for established cancer. Extensive research has been directed toward elucidation of the effects of $1,25(OH)_2D_3$ and its synthetic analogs on breast cancer cells, and several reviews on this topic are available (Colston and Mork Hansen, 2001; Mørk-Hansen et al., 2001a; Mehta and Mehta, 2002). In this section, we provide a concise summary of the effects of $1,25(OH)_2D_3$ and several of its structural analogs on proliferation, differentiation, apoptosis, angiogenesis, and invasion of breast cancer cells.

Effects of Vitamin D Signaling on Breast Cancer Cell Cycle

Treatment of MCF-7 breast cancer cells with $1,25(OH)_2D_3$ at nanomolar concentrations induces cell cycle arrest in G_0/G_1, dephosphorylation of the retinoblastoma protein, and increases in the CDK inhibitors p21 and p27 (Fan and Yu, 1995; Wu et al., 1997; Mørk-Hansen et al., 2001b, Flanagan et al., 2003). Vitamin D–responsive elements in the human p21 gene promoter suggest that p21 is a direct transcriptional target of the VDR (Liu et al., 1996; Saramaki et al., 2006). Effects of vitamin D compounds on p27 vary with cell type; in some studies, p27 is unchanged after treatment with VDR agonists (Mørk-Hansen et al., 2001b, Jensen et al., 2001; Wu et al., 1997), whereas in others p27 expression is increased (Wu et al., 1997; Verlinden et al., 1998; Flanagan et al., 2003). Analysis of the p27 gene promoter suggests that the $1,25(OH)_2D_3$-VDR complex induces transcription of this gene through SP1 and NF-Y transcription factors rather than direct DNA binding (Inoue et al., 1999).

Upregulation of p21 and/or p27 by vitamin D compounds is associated with inhibition of CDK activity, including cyclin D1/CDK4 and cyclin A/CDK2 complexes (Wu et al., 1997; Verlinden et al., 1998). In colon cancer cells, VDR interacts with protein phosphatases PP1c and PP2Ac to inactivate the p70 S6 kinase, which is essential for G_1/S phase transition (Bettoun et al., 2002). Thus, the net result of vitamin D signaling is to prevent entry into S phase, leading to accumulation in G_1. In some breast cancer cells, vitamin D–mediated G_1 arrest is associated with induction of differentiation markers such as lipid and casein (Mathiasen et al., 1993; Lazzaro et al., 2000; Wang et al., 2001).

Effects of VDR Agonists on Estrogen and Growth Factor Signaling

VDR agonists downregulate ER and attenuate estrogen-stimulated growth and gene activation (James et al., 1994; Simboli-Campbell et al., 1997; Swami et al., 2000). Sequence analysis of the ERα gene promoter has identified a potential VDR element (VDRE), suggesting a direct regulatory effect of $1{,}25(OH)_2D_3$ on ERα gene transcription (Stoica et al., 1999). Since $1{,}25(OH)_2D_3$ also inhibits growth of estrogen-independent breast cancer cells, downregulation of ER does not appear to be necessary for the antiproliferative effects of vitamin D compounds (Abe et al., 1991; Nolan et al., 1998; Colston et al., 1998; Flanagan et al., 1999, 2003). Furthermore, in some cases, breast cancer cells selected for antiestrogen resistance show increased sensitivity to vitamin D (Larsen et al., 2001).

Vitamin D compounds have been shown to modulate secretion, processing and/or signaling of multiple growth factors in breast cancer cells. VDR agonists attenuate the growth-stimulatory effects of epidermal growth factor (EGF) and repress EGF receptor expression via displacement of Sp1 (Koga et al., 1988; McGaffin and Chrysogelos, 2005). Vitamin D compounds also block the mitogenic effects of insulin-like growth factor (IGF)-I, decrease expression of the IGF-I receptor, and induce inhibitory IGF-binding proteins such as IGFBP-3 and IGFBP-5 (Rozen et al., 1997; Vink-van Wijngaarden et al., 1996; Colston et al., 1998). Other growth factors shown to be regulated by $1{,}25(OH)_2D_3$ in breast cells include fibroblast growth factor (FGF)-8 (Kawata et al., 2006) and amphiregulin (Akutsu et al., 2001).

In breast cancer cells, $1{,}25(OH)_2D_3$ enhances the expression of the TGFβ pathway (Koli and Keski-Oja, 1994; Mercier et al., 1996; Swami et al., 2003), in part through induction of TGFβ2 gene expression via VDR responsive promoter sequences (Wu et al., 1999). The antiproliferative effects of vitamin D compounds are partially abrogated by neutralizing antibodies to TGFβ (Simboli-Campbell and Welsh, 1995; Mercier et al., 1996; Yang et al., 2001), indicating that TGFβ can be functionally linked to the growth-inhibitory effects of vitamin D in vitro.

Induction of Cell Death by Vitamin D Compounds in Breast Cancer Cells

In addition to their antiproliferative effects, $1{,}25(OH)_2D_3$ induces morphologic and biochemical features of apoptosis and autophagy (chromatin condensation, DNA fragmentation, lysosomal activation) in breast cancer cells (Welsh, 1994; James et al., 1995; Simboli-Campbell et al., 1996; 1997; Hoyer-Hansen et al., 2005). In MCF-7 cells, $1{,}25(OH)_2D_3$-mediated cell death is not blocked by caspase inhibitors but can be attenuated by overexpression of Bcl-2 (Mathiasen et al., 1999; Narvaez and Welsh, 2001). Treatment of MCF-7 cells with $1{,}25(OH)_2D_3$ downregulated Bcl-2 and induced redistribution of Bax from cytosol to mitochondria (James et al., 1995; Simboli-Campbell et al., 1997; Narvaez and Welsh, 2001; Narvaez et al., 2003), suggesting that translocation of Bax in conjunction with downregulation of Bcl-2 may facilitate $1{,}25(OH)_2D_3$-mediated apoptosis. Vitamin D–mediated Bax translocation triggers reactive oxygen species generation, dissipation of the mitochondrial membrane potential, and release of cytochrome c into the cytosol (Narvaez and Welsh, 2001; Narvaez et al., 2003). Consistent with an autophagic process, $1{,}25(OH)_2D_3$-mediated apoptosis requires beclin-1 and atg-7 and is associated with protease activation (calpain, cathepsin B) and increased cytosolic calcium (Simboli-Campbell and Welsh, 1995;. Mathiasen et al., 2003; Hoyer-Hansen et al., 2007). While the specific interactions between these apoptotic pathways are yet to be resolved, it appears that signals generated from both the mitochondria and the endoplasmic reticulum may cooperate to induce cell death in response to $1{,}25(OH)_2D_3$.

$1{,}25(OH)_2D_3$ exerts additive or synergistic effects in combination with other triggers of apoptosis, such as antiestrogens, TNFα, radiation, and chemotherapeutic agents (James et al., 1995; Nolan et al., 1998; Wang et al., 2000; Sundaram et al., 2003; Demasters et al., 2006). It is not quite clear whether these synergistic effects result from interactions of $1{,}25(OH)_2D_3$ with agonist-specific signals or whether $1{,}25(OH)_2D_3$ impacts on common cell death pathways.

Interaction Between VDR Signaling and DNA Repair Pathways

The p53 tumor suppressor gene plays a crucial role in regulation of growth arrest and apoptosis in response to DNA damage and other cellular stresses. Recent screening studies to identify p53 target genes have provided evidence that VDR is a transcriptional target of p53 and the related proteins p63 and p73 (Maruyama et al., 2006; Kommagani et al., 2006). These data suggest that induction of vitamin D signaling may contribute to the p53-mediated global cellular damage response. Consistent with this suggestion, $1,25(OH)_2D_3$ induces a number of proteins involved in DNA repair, including GADD45, Rad 23, PCNA, and BRCA1 (Jiang et al., 2003; Abedin et al., 2006; Campbell et al., 2000; Swami et al., 2003). Furthermore, ChIP assays colocalized p53 and VDR on the human p21 gene promoter and demonstrated both independent and cooperative effects of p53 and VDR on p21 gene transcription (Saramaki et al., 2006).

Effects of $1,25(OH)_2D_3$ on Angiogenesis, Invasion, and Metastasis

The antitumor effects of $1,25(OH)_2D_3$ may also involve regulation of angiogenesis, since $1,25(OH)_2D_3$ inhibited angiogenesis in the chorioallantoic membrane assay (Oikawa et al., 1990) and in angiogenesis assays in mice (Majewski et al., 1996). Moreover, vitamin D analogs reduced angiogenesis of MCF-7 breast tumors overexpressing vascular endothelial growth factor (VEGF) and inhibited VEGF expression in MDA-MB-231 xenografts (Matsumoto et al., 1999; Mantell et al., 2000). VDR is expressed in endothelial cells (Merke et al., 1989) and $1,25(OH)_2D_3$ blocked both basal and VEGF induced endothelial cell sprouting, elongation, and proliferation (Mantell et al., 2000). Interestingly, $1,25(OH)_2D_3$ selectively inhibited proliferation and induced apoptosis in tumor-derived endothelial cells (Bernardi et al., 2002; Flynn et al., 2006) Collectively, these studies indicate that vitamin D signaling likely inhibits angiogenesis via VDRs expressed on both the transformed mammary epithelial cells and the endothelial cells within tumors.

Effects of VDR agonists on late stage breast cancer have been studied in ER-negative breast cancer cell lines, such as MDA-MB-231 and SUM159PT cells, which are invasive in vitro and metastatic in vivo. $1,25(OH)_2D_3$ and analogs inhibited invasion of metastatic breast cancer cells as measured by the in vitro Boyden chamber assay (Mørk-Hansen et al., 1994; Flanagan et al., 2003; Sundaram et al., 2006). Inhibition of invasion by vitamin D compounds may be linked to regulation of extracellular proteases (MMP-9, urokinase-type plasminogen activator, tissue-type plasminogen activator), protease inhibitors, and adhesion molecules (Koli and Keski-Oja, 2000; Swami et al., 2003; Pendas-Franco et al., 2006). In experimental metastasis paradigms, the vitamin D analog EB1089 inhibited secondary tumors, blocked skeletal metastases, and improved survival (El Abdaimi et al., 2000; Flanagan et al., 2003).

DETERMINANTS OF BREAST CANCER CELL SENSITIVITY TO VITAMIN D

Uptake and Metabolism of Vitamin D Metabolites in Mammary Cells

As discussed earlier, circulating vitamin D steroids are delivered to cells bound to DBP, but little is known about uptake, metabolism, or trafficking of vitamin D metabolites in mammary cells. Comparative genome hybridization studies have found that CYP24, an enzyme that degrades both $25(OH)D_3$ and $1,25(OH)_2D_3$, is amplified in human breast cancer (Albertson et al., 2001), suggesting that deregulation of vitamin D catabolism may reduce ligand availability to the VDR and contribute to breast cancer development or progression. Although mammary cells also express the $25(OH)D_3$ 1α-hydroxylase which can convert $25(OH)D_3$ to $1,25(OH)_2D_3$ (Zinser and Welsh, 2004a; Townsend et al., 2005; Kemmis et al., 2006), breast cancer cells may lose the ability to internalize $25(OH)D_3$ in the presence of DBP (Rowling et al., 2006). Further studies to assess the uptake and metabolism of both $25(OH)D_3$ and $1,25(OH)_2D_3$ in mammary cells as a function of transformation will be necessary to clarify the role of 1α-hydroxylase in breast cancer.

Expression and Regulation of VDR in Breast Cancer Cells and Tumors

A high proportion (>80%) of breast cancer biopsy specimens contain VDR (Freake et al., 1984; Eisman et al., 1986; Berger et al., 1987), but no significant correlation between VDR expression and ER status, lymph node status, tumor grade, or survival was detected (Berger et al., 1991). However, in a study of 136 patients with primary breast cancer, it was found that women with VDR-negative tumors relapsed significantly earlier than women with VDR-positive tumors (Colston et al., 1989; Berger et al., 1991).

VDR abundance is affected by many physiologic factors and is achieved through a variety of mechanisms, including alterations in transcription and/or mRNA stability, posttranslational effects and ligand-induced stabilization. Expression of the VDR is regulated by many physiologic agents, including $1,25(OH)_2D_3$ itself, estrogens, retinoids, and growth factors. Thus, breast cancer cell sensitivity to $1,25(OH)_2D_3$-mediated growth regulation may in part reflect the activity of other hormone signaling pathways through their impact on VDR expression. Of particular interest with respect to breast cancer is the regulation of VDR expression and activity by estrogens. ER-positive cells tend to express higher levels of VDR than ER-negative cells (Buras et al., 1994; Campbell et al., 2000), and in vitro studies have demonstrated that estrogen upregulates, whereas antiestrogens downregulate VDR in ER-positive breast cancer cells (Narvaez et al., 1996; Byrne et al., 2000; Wietzke and Welsh, 2003). The mechanisms involved in upregulation of VDR by estrogen are incompletely understood, but both Sp1 and extracellular signal-regulated kinase (ERK) have been implicated (Wietzke et al., 2005; Gilad et al., 2005). Demonstration that estrogen and antiestrogens regulate VDR in breast cancer cells has clinical implications arising from the use of selective estrogen receptor modulators (SERMs) for prevention and/or treatment of breast cancer and osteoporosis. Further studies are therefore warranted to determine the degree to which estrogen status influences VDR abundance in different $1,25(OH)_2D_3$ target tissues (i.e., breast, bone, uterus), and whether SERMs or phytoestrogens act as estrogen agonists or antagonists in regulation of VDR expression.

Vitamin D Resistance

Although it is clear that the VDR is required for breast cancer cell responsiveness to vitamin D compounds, a number of established breast cancer cell lines that express VDR fail to respond to the antiproliferative effects of $1,25(OH)_2D_3$. Data from mammary cell lines suggest that oncogenic transformation with SV40 or ras inhibits VDR signaling and induces resistance to the growth-inhibitory effects of $1,25(OH)_2D_3$ (Escaleira and Brentani, 1999; Agadir et al., 1999), raising the possibility that breast cancer progression may be facilitated by deregulation of the vitamin D pathway.

In an effort to understand the cellular basis for insensitivity to vitamin D, Narvaez et al. (1996) selected and characterized $1,25(OH)_2D_3$-resistant subclones of MCF-7 cells. The resulting MCF-7^{DRES} cells express VDR, but do not undergo growth arrest or apoptosis in response to $1,25(OH)_2D_3$. MCF-7^{DRES} cells are selectively resistant to $1,25(OH)_2D_3$ and its structural analogs and respond to other antiproliferative agents (Narvaez et al., 1996; Narvaez and Welsh, 1997; Nolan et al., 1998). Similar results have been obtained in an independently derived $1,25(OH)_2D_3$-resistant subclone of MCF-7 cells, labeled MCF-7/VDR (Mørk-Hansen et al., 2001b). The mechanisms underlying vitamin D resistance in these MCF-7 clones are incompletely understood. Theoretically, selective insensitivity to $1,25(OH)_2D_3$ could be secondary to defective VDR, reduced availability of ligand, or uncoupling of a functional vitamin D signaling pathway from growth arrest/apoptosis. While resistance could be associated with elevated expression of the vitamin D 24-hydroxylase enzyme which inactivates $1,25(OH)_2D_3$, this does not appear to be the case for either of the vitamin D–resistant MCF-7 variants. Both MCF-7^{DRES} and MCF-7/VDR cells contain transcriptionally active VDRs when measured with consensus VDREs; however, basal VDR expression is lower in both resistant cell lines than in parental MCF-7 cells. In MCF-7^{DRES} cells, $1,25(OH)_2D_3$ comparably upregulates the steady state level of the VDR protein in both sensitive and resistant cell lines (Narvaez and Welsh, 1997). MCF-7^{DRES} cells can be sensitized to the growth-inhibitory effects of $1,25(OH)_2D_3$ by cotreatment with low concentrations of the phorbol ester TPA, suggesting that phosphorylation pathways may be altered in this cell line (Narvaez and Welsh, 1997; Narvaez et al., 2003). Further studies with these interesting cell lines will be necessary to resolve the mechanism(s) of vitamin D resistance. Significantly, the MCF-7^{DRES} cell line retains resistance to vitamin D analogs when grown as xenografts in nude mice (VanWeelden et al., 1998), providing an important model system for understanding the basis of vitamin D resistance in vivo.

VITAMIN D ANALOGS: PRECLINICAL AND CLINICAL TRIALS

Natural Ligands Vs. Synthetic Analogs

While the beneficial effects of $1,25(OH)_2D_3$ on cancer cells support its use as a therapeutic agent, natural vitamin D metabolites exert potentially toxic effects on calcium handling at the doses required for antitumor effects. Thus, the metabolite $1\alpha(OH)D_3$, which is converted to $1,25(OH)_2D_3$ in vivo, effectively inhibits tumor growth in vivo, but the therapeutic window is extremely narrow (reviewed in Mørk-Hansen et al., 2001a). Modifications to the parent vitamin D structure, particularly the side chain, generate synthetic analogs with enhanced growth-regulatory effects and limited calcium mobilizing action. Several of these vitamin D analogs have been tested against breast cancer as described below.

Studies on Vitamin D Analogs in Breast Cancer

One of the most extensively studied vitamin D analogs is EB1089 (LEO Pharmaceuticals), which is approximately 50 times more effective than $1,25(OH)_2D_3$ on growth inhibition in vitro yet has reduced calcemic effects in vivo (Colston et al., 1992; Mathiasen et al., 1993; Mørk-Hansen et al., 2000). EB1089 inhibited growth of NMU-induced rat breast tumors as well as human MCF-7 xenografts without increasing serum calcium (Colston et al., 1992; Mackay et al., 1996; VanWeelden et al., 1998). Synergistic effects of EB1089 on breast tumors were demonstrated with paclitaxel (Koshizuka et al., 1999a), retinoic acid (Koshizuka et al., 1999b), tamoxifen (Abe-Hashimoto et al., 1993; McKay et al., 1996), aromatase inhibitors (Andoh and Iino, 1996), and radiation (Sundaram et al., 2003). In both NMU-induced tumors and MCF-7 xenografts, EB1089 inhibited proliferation and induced death of tumor epithelial cells (James et al., 1998; VanWeelden et al., 1998). EB1089 also inhibited skeletal metastases and increased survival of mice inoculated with MDA-MB-231 cells (El Abdaimi et al., 2000).

On the basis of these and other promising animal studies, a phase I trial of oral EB1089 was conducted in patients with advanced breast and colorectal cancer (Gulliford et al., 1998). The data from this study determined a maximum tolerated dose of EB1089 for prolonged administration at approximately 7 μg/m^2/day. Although no clear antitumor effects of EB1089 were documented in this open noncontrolled single-center trial, six patients (two colorectal, four breast cancer) showed disease stabilization for at least three months.

Other vitamin D analogs that have been studied in relation to breast cancer include: Calcipotriol (MC903), 20-epi analogs (CB1093, KH1060), from Leo Pharmaceuticals (Elstner et al., 1995); 22-oxa-1,25(OH)$_2$D$_3$ (OCT), from Chugai Pharmaceutical; several 19-nor analogs and analogs with two side chains ("Gemini" series) from Hoffman LaRoche and Bioxell (Koike et al., 1997; Maehr et al., 2007); 1α-hydroxy-24-ethyl-cholecalciferol [1α(OH)D$_5$], developed by Mehta's group (Mehta et al., 1997), and a series of novel analogs with 19-nor and 14-epi modifications developed by Bouillon and colleagues (Verlinden et al., 2000). Compared with the natural VDR ligand 1,25(OH)$_2$D$_3$, these analogs all display enhanced potency against breast cancer cell proliferation with better therapeutic window in vivo. While it is clear that most, and possibly all, vitamin D analogs mediate growth-inhibitory effects through VDR (Zinser et al., 2003), further mechanistic studies are required to understand the selective actions of these analogs in vivo.

VITAMIN D AND PREVENTION OF BREAST CANCER

Expression and Role of VDR in Normal Mammary Tissue

The VDR is present in rat, mouse, and human mammary glands (Narbaitz et al., 1981; Colston et al., 1988; Zinser et al., 2002), and its expression is developmentally regulated. VDR expression is high throughout puberty, pregnancy and lactation, periods of maximal tissue growth and remodeling (Colston et al., 1988; Zinser et al., 2002; Zinser and Welsh, 2004a). Developmental regulation of VDR in mammary cells implies that vitamin D signaling may be involved in the regulation of glandular function. In vitro, 1,25(OH)$_2$D$_3$ inhibited growth of nontransformed mammary cells, but, in contrast to breast cancer cells, normal mammary cells exhibited markers of differentiation rather than apoptosis (Escaleira and Brentani, 1999; Kanazawa et al., 1999; Lazzaro et al., 2000; Kemmis et al., 2006). In mammary gland organ culture studies, 1,25(OH)$_2$D$_3$ regulated calcium transport, casein expression, and branching morphogenesis (Bhattacharjee et al., 1987; Mezzetti et al., 1988; Zinser et al., 2002). Furthermore, mammary glands from VDR null mice exhibited increased ductal extension and branching morphogenesis in vivo, and enhanced growth in response to estrogen and progesterone compared with glands from control mice (Zinser et al., 2002) (Table 1). Ex vivo, 1,25(OH)$_2$D$_3$ inhibited branching of mammary glands from control mice but had no effect on glands from VDR null mice. These data support the concept that 1,25(OH)$_2$D$_3$ and the VDR induce a program of genes that inhibit proliferation and maintain differentiation in the normal gland.

Table 1 Effects of Vitamin D Signaling on Normal and Transformed Mammary Cells In Vitro and In Vivo. Summary of Effects of Natural and Synthetic Vitamin D Compounds on Breast Cancer Cells In Vitro and In Vivo

In vitro effects of vitamin D signaling on mammary cells

- Normal and transformed human mammary cells express VDR and vitamin D metabolizing enzymes
- VDR agonists inhibit cell cycle progression, maintain differentiation, and/or trigger cell death
- Vitamin D–mediated G1 arrest linked to modulation of cell cycle regulatory proteins, oncogenes, and tumor suppressor genes
- 1,25(OH)$_2$D$_3$ induces cell death via mechanisms that involve mitochondria, lysosomes, and/or endoplasmic reticulum
- 1,25(OH)$_2$D$_3$ and synthetic analogs inhibit angiogenesis and invasion via effects on tumor cells, endothelial cells and, extracellular matrix proteases
- Oncogenes and tumor suppressor genes modulate VDR signaling

Evidence for antitumor effects of vitamin D in animal models of breast cancer

- VDR agonists inhibit growth of carcinogen-induced mammary tumors and human breast cancer xenografts
- Vitamin D analogs inhibit proliferation and induce apoptosis in tumor epithelial cells
- EB1089 exerts antimetastatic effects in vivo
- VDR null mice exhibit accelerated mammary gland development and impaired postlactational involution
- VDR null mice are more sensitive to tumorigenesis in mammary gland, skin, and lymphoid tissue

Abbreviation: VDR, vitamin D receptor.

Prevention of Breast Cancer by Vitamin D: Preclinical Studies

Identification of $1,25(OH)_2D_3$ and the VDR as components of a signaling network that impacts on proliferation and differentiation in the normal mammary gland raises the possibility that optimal vitamin D status may protect against mammary transformation. In support of this suggestion, rats fed diets high in calcium and vitamin D developed fewer mammary tumors in response to the carcinogen DMBA than mice fed diets low in calcium and vitamin D (Jacobson et al., 1989). Prevention of NMU-induced mammary tumors with vitamin D analogs, including Ro24-5531 (1,25-dihydroxy-16-ene-23-yne-26-27-hexafluorocholecalciferol) and $1\alpha(OH)D_5$ provided further support that vitamin D may protect against breast cancer (Anzano et al., 1994; Mehta et al., 2000). A direct effect of $1,25(OH)_2D_3$ and $1\alpha(OH)D_5$ on the sensitivity of the mammary gland to transformation was suggested by studies indicating that both vitamin D compounds prevented DMBA induced preneoplastic lesions in organ culture (Mehta et al., 1997). In vivo, VDR ablation enhanced the development of hyperplasias and hormone independent mammary tumors after DMBA administration and VDR haploinsufficiency sensitized the mammary gland to tumorigenesis driven by the neu oncogene (Zinser and Welsh, 2004b; Zinser et al., 2005).

Epidemiologic Studies on Vitamin D and Breast Cancer

The majority of women who develop breast cancer are of postmenopausal age, and estrogen deficiency and aging are often associated with vitamin D deficiency. However, few epidemiologic studies have examined whether dietary intake of vitamin D per se alters breast cancer incidence in populations. An evaluation of the Nurses Health Study (Knekt et al., 1996) found that intakes of dairy products, dairy calcium, and total vitamin D (as measured by food frequency questionnaires) were inversely associated with breast cancer risk in premenopausal, but not postmenopausal, women. Another study demonstrated that measures of sunlight exposure and dietary vitamin D were associated with a reduced risk of breast cancer; however, the associations were dependent on region of residence (John et al., 1999). Correlations between breast cancer risk and exposure to solar radiation have also been suggested in larger epidemiologic studies (Garland et al., 1990; Freedman et al., 2002). In five studies where vitamin D status was measured in relation to breast cancer, low levels of $25(OH)D_3$ or $1,25(OH)_2D_3$ were found to be associated with increased breast cancer risk or disease progression (Mawer et al., 1997; Janowsky et al., 1999; Lowe et al., 2005; de Lyra et al., 2006; Colston et al., 2006), however, not all studies have supported this association (Bertone-Johnson et al., 2005).

VDR Polymorphisms and Breast Cancer Risk

There are a number of common allelic variants, or polymorphisms, in the human VDR gene that have been examined in relation to breast cancer risk. The best-studied VDR polymorphisms in relation to breast cancer are the Bsm I and Apa I polymorphisms in an intronic region between exons VIII and IX. Two studies reported that allele frequencies of the Apa I polymorphism were correlated with breast cancer risk while the Taq I and Fok 1 polymorphisms were not (Curran et al., 1999; Sillanpää et al., 2004). Four studies reported correlations between the Bsm I polymorphism and breast cancer risk with odds ratio for bb versus BB genotype between two and sevenfold (Yamagata et al., 1997; Bretherton-Watt et al., 2001; Chen et al., 2005; Lowe et al., 2005). However, the data are not entirely consistent, as an increased (rather than decreased) breast cancer risk was associated with the BB genotype among Latina women (Ingles at al., 2000) and with the AA genotype in Taiwanese women (Hou et al., 2002). Some of these inconsistencies may be due to interactions between genotype and environmental factors, for example, dietary calcium (McCullough et al., 2007) or vitamin D status (Lowe et al., 2005). Other studies have demonstrated associations of VDR polymorphisms with breast cancer progression rather than risk (Ruggiero et al., 1998; Lundin et al., 1999; Schondorf et al., 2003).

Although these findings are intriguing, the underlying basis for an association between VDR polymorphisms and breast cancer susceptibility is currently unclear. The VDR polymorphisms that have been most consistently linked to breast cancer susceptibility (Bsm I and Apa I variants) do not alter the amount or structure of the VDR protein produced. Thus, further studies are required to ascertain how these VDR polymorphisms may function, and whether VDR genotype interacts with other risk factors for breast cancer.

SUMMARY AND OUTSTANDING RESEARCH QUESTIONS

VDR and $1,25(OH)_2D_3$, its natural ligand, act through multiple pathways to induce growth arrest, differentiation, and apoptosis in mammary epithelial cells. Synthetic analogs of $1,25(OH)_2D_3$ that have potent growth-inhibitory effects with minimal calcemic activity in vivo provide proof of principle that VDR agonists can inhibit the growth of established tumors in animal models. Studies with VDR null mice indicate a functional role for vitamin D signaling in the normal mammary gland. Clinical studies and epidemiologic approaches have provided evidence that VDR represents a target for breast cancer prevention. Challenges for the future include better understanding of the transport, uptake and metabolism of $1,25(OH)_2D_3$ and bioactive analogs in breast cancer cells, the molecular mechanism of action and specific targets of the VDR in mammary gland, and the influence of genetic differences in the VDR on an individual's response to vitamin D compounds. Such understanding should provide insight into design of vitamin D–based strategies to impact on breast cancer development or therapy.

REFERENCES

Abe-Hashimoto J, Kikuchi T, Matsumoto T, Nishii Y, Ogata E, Ikeda K. Anti-tumor effect of 22-oxa-calcitriol, a non-calcaemic analog of calcitriol in athymic mice implanted with human breast carcinoma and its synergism with tamoxifen. Cancer Res 1993; 53:2534–2537.

Abe J, Nakano T, Nishii Y, Matsumoto T, Ogata E, Ikeda K. A novel vitamin D_3 analog, 22-oxa-1,25-dihydroxyvitamin D_3, inhibits the growth of human breast cancer in vitro and in vivo without causing hypercalcaemia. Endocrinology 1991; 129:832–837.

Abedin SA, Banwell CM, Colston KW, Carlberg C, Cambell MJ. Epigenetic corruption of VDR signaling in malignancy. Anticancer Res 2006; 26:2557–2566.

Agadir A, Lazzara G, Zheng Y, Mehta R. Resistance of HBL100 human breast epithelial cells to vitamin D action. Carcinogenesis 1999; 20:577–582.

Akutsu N, Bastien Y, Lin R, Mader S, White JH. Amphiregulin is a vitamin D_3 target gene in squamous cell and breast carcinoma. Biochem Biophys Res Commun 2001; 281: 1051–1056.

Albertson DG, Ylstra B, Segraves R, Collins C, Dairkee SH, Kowbel D, Kuo WL, Gray JW, Pinkel D. Quantitative mapping of amplicon structure by array CGH identifies CYP24 as a candidate oncogene. Nat Genet 2001; 25: 144–146.

Andoh T, Iino Y. Usefulness of 22-oxa-1,25-dihydroxyvitamin D_3 (OCT) as a single agent or combined therapy with aromatase inhibitor (CGS16949A) on 7,12-dimethylbenzanthracene-induced rat mammary tumors. Int J Oncol 1996; 9:79–82.

Anzano M, Smith J, Uskokovic M, Peer C, Mullen L, Letterio J, Welsh M, Shrader M, Logsdon D, Driver C, Brown C, Roberts A, Sporn M. 1α-Dihydroxy-16-ene-23-yne-26,27-hexafluorocholcalciferol (Ro24-5531), a new deltanoid (vitamin D analog) for prevention of breast cancer of breast cancer in the rat. Cancer Res 1994; 54:1653–1656.

Berger U, McClelland RA, Wilson P, Greene GL, Haussler MR, Pike JW, Colston K, Easton D, Coombes RC. Immunocytochemical detection of 1,25-dihydroxyvitamin D_3 receptor in primary breast cancer. Cancer Res 1987; 47: 6793–6795.

Berger U, Wilson P, McClelland RA, Colston K, Haussler MR, Pike JW, Coombes RC. Immunocytochemical detection of estrogen receptor, progesterone receptor and 1,25-dihydroxyvitamin D_3 receptor in breast cancer and relation to prognosis. Cancer Res 1991; 51:239–244.

Bernardi RJ, Johnson CS, Modzelewski RA, Trump DL. Anti-proliferative effect of 1alpha,25-dihydroxyvitamin D(3) and vitamin D analogs on tumor derived endothelial cells. Endocrinology 2002; 143:2508–2514.

Bertone-Johnson ER, Chen WY, Holick MF, Hollis BW, Colditz GA, Willett WC, Hankinson SE. Plasma 25-hydroxyvitamin D and 1,25-dihydroxyvitamin D and risk of breast cancer. Cancer Epidemiol Biomarkers Prev 2005; 14:1991–1997.

Bettoun DJ, Buck DW II, Lu J, Khalifa B, Chin WW, Nagpal S. A vitamin D receptor-Ser/Thr phosphatase-p70 S6 kinase complex and modulation of its enzymatic activities by the ligand. J Biol Chem 2002; 277:24847–24850.

Bhattacharjee M, Wientroub S, Wonderhaar BK. Milk protein synthesis by mammary glands of vitamin D-deficient mice. Endocrinology 1987; 121:865–874.

Bretherton-Watt D, Given-Wilson R, Mansi JL, Thomas V, Carter N and Colston KW. Vitamin D receptor gene polymorphisms are associated with breast cancer risk in a UK Caucasian population. Br J Cancer 2001; 85:171–176.

Buras RR, Schumaker LM, Davoodi F, Brenner RV, Shabahang M, Nauta RJ, Evans SR. Vitamin D receptors in breast cancer cells. Breast Cancer Res Treat 1994; 31:191–202.

Byrne I, Flanagan L, Tenniswood M, Welsh J. Identification of a hormone responsive promoter immediately upstream of exon 1c in the human vitamin D receptor gene. Endocrinology 2000; 141:2829–2836.

Campbell MJ, Gombart AF, Kwok SH, Park S, Koeffler HP. The anti-proliferative effects of 1alpha,$25(OH)_2D_3$ on breast and prostate cells are associated with induction of BRCA1 gene expression. Oncogene 2000; 19:5091–5097.

Carlberg C, Molnar F. Detailed molecular understanding of agonistic and antagonistic vitamin D receptor ligands. Curr Top Med Chem 2006; 6:1243–1253.

Chen TC, Chimeh F, Lu Z, Mathieu J, Person KS, Zhang A, Kohn N, Martinello S, Berkowitz R, Holick MF. Factors that influence the cutaneous synthesis and dietary sources of vitamin D. Arch Biochem Biophys 2007; 460:213–217; [Epub Jan 8, 2007].

Chen WY, Bertone-Johnson ER, Hunter DJ, Willett WC, Hankinson SE. Associations between polymorphisms in the vitamin D receptor and breast cancer risk. Cancer Epidemiol Biomarkers Prev 2005; 10:2335–2339.

Colston KW, Berger U, Coombes RC. Possible role for vitamin D in controlling breast cancer cell proliferation. Lancet 1989; 1:185–191.

Colston KW, Berger U, Wilson P, Hadcocks L, Naeem I, Earl HM, Coombes RC. Mammary gland 1,25-dihydroxyvitamin D_3 receptor content during pregnancy and lactation. Mol Cell Endocrinology 1988; 60:15–22.

Colston KW, Lowe LC, Mansi JL, Campbell MJ. Vitamin D status and breast cancer risk. Anticancer Res 2006; 26:2573–2580.

Colston KW, Mackay AG, James SY, Binderup L, Chander S, Coombes RC. EB1089: a new vitamin D analogue that inhibits the growth of breast cancer cells *in vivo* and *in vitro*. Biochem Pharmacol 1992; 44: 2273–2280.

Colston KW, Mork Hansen C. Mechanisms implicated in the growth regulatory effects of vitamin D in breast cancer. Endocrine Related Cancer 2001; 9:45–59.

Colston KW, Perks CM, Xie SP, Holly JM. Growth inhibition of both MCF-7 and Hs578T human breast cancer cell lines by vitamin D analogues is associated with increased expression of insulin-like binding protein-3. J Mol Endocrinol 1998; 20:157–162.

Colston KW, Wilkinson JR, Coombes RC. 1,25-Dihydroxyvitamin D_3 binding in estrogen responsive rat breast tumor. Endocrinology 1986; 119:397–403.

Curran JE, Vaughn T, Lea RA, Weinstein SR, Morrison NA, Griffiths LR. Association of a vitamin D receptor polymorphism with sporadic breast cancer development. Int J Cancer 1999; 83:723–726.

Dardenne O, Prud'homme J, Arabian A, Glorieux FH, St-Arnoud R. Targeted inactivation of the 25-hydroxyvitamin D(3)-1 (alpha)-hydroxylase gene (CYP27B1) creates an animal model of pseudovitamin D-deficiency rickets. Endocrinology 2001; 142:3135–3141.

de Lyra EC, da Silva IA, Katayama ML, Brentani MM, Nonogaki S, Goes GC, Folqueira MA. 25(OH)D_3 and 1,25 $(OH)_2D_3$ serum concentration and breast tissue expression of 1alpha-hydroxylase, 24-hydroxylase and Vitamin D receptor in women with and without breast cancer. J Steroid Biochem Mol Biol 2006; 100:184–192.

Demasters G, Di X, Newsham I, Shiu R, Gewirtz DA. Potentiation of radiation sensitivity in breast tumor cells by the vitamin D_3 analogue, EB 1089, through promotion of autophagy and interference with proliferative recovery. Mol Cancer Ther 2006; 5:2786–2797.

Eisman JA, Macintyre I, Martin TJ, Frampton RJ, King RJ. Normal and malignant breast tissue is a target organ for 1,25$(OH)_2$ vitamin D_3. Clin Endocrinol 1980; 13:267–272.

Eisman JA, Suva LJ, Martin TJ. Significance of 1,25-dihydroxyvitamin D_3 receptor in primary breast cancers. Cancer Res 1986; 46:5406–5408.

El Abdaimi K, Dion N, Papavasiliou V, Cardinal PE, Binderup L, Goltzman D, Ste-Marie LG, Kremer R. The vitamin D analog EB1089 prevents skeletal metastasis and prolongs survival time in nude mice transplanted with human breast cancer cells. Cancer Res 2000; 60:4412–4418.

Ellison TI, Eckert RL, Macdonald PN. Evidence for 1,25(OH)-$_2D_3$-independent transactivation by VDR: uncoupling the receptor and ligand in keratinocytes. J Biol Chem 2007; 282:10953–10962.

Elstner E, Linker-Israeli M, Said J, Umiel T, de Vos S, Shintaku IP, Heber D, Binderup L, Uskokovic M, Koeffler HP. 20-epi-vitamin D analogues: a novel class of potent inhibitors of proliferation and inducers of differentiation of human breast cancer cell lines. Cancer Res 1995; 55:2822–2830.

Erben RG, Soegiarto DW, Weber K, Zeitz U, Lieberherr M, Gniadecki R, Moller G, Adamski J, Balling R. Deletion of deoxyribonucleic acid binding domain of the vitamin D receptor abrogates genomic and nongenomic functions of vitamin D. Mol Endocrinol 2002; 16:1524–1537.

Escaleira MT, Brentani MM. Vitamin D_3 receptor (VDR) expression in HC-11 mammary cells: regulation by growth modulatory agents, differentiation and Ha-ras transformation. Breast Cancer Research Treat 1999; 54:123–133.

Fan FS, Yu W. 1,25 dihydroxyvitamin D_3 suppresses cell growth, DNA synthesis and phosphorylaton of retinoblastoma protein in a breast cancer cell line. Cancer Invest 1995; 13:280–286.

Flanagan L, Packman K, Juba B, O'Neill S, Tenniswood M, Welsh J. Efficacy of vitamin D compounds to modulate estrogen receptor negative breast cancer growth and invasion. J Steroid Biochem Mol Biol 2003; 84:181–192.

Flanagan L, VanWeelden K, Ammerman C, Ethier S, Welsh JE. SUM-159PT cells, a novel estrogen independent human breast cancer model system. Breast Cancer Research Treat 1999; 58:193–204.

Flynn G, Chung I, Yu WD, Romano M, Modzelewski RA, Johnson CS, Trump DL. Calcitriol (1,25-dihydroxycholecalciferol) selectively inhibits proliferation of freshly isolated tumor-derived endothelial cells and induces apoptosis. Oncology 2006; 70:447–457.

Frampton RJ, Suva LJ, Eisman JA, Findlay DM, Moore GE, Moseley JM, Martin TJ. Presence of 1,25-dihydroxyvitamin D_3 receptors in established human cancer cell lines in culture. Cancer Res 1982; 42:1116–1119.

Freake H, Abeyasekera G, Iwasaki J, Marcocci C, MacIntyre I, McClelland R, Skilton R, Easton D, Coombes RC. Measurement of 1,25-dihydroxyvitamin D_3 receptors in breast cancer and relationship to biochemical and clinical indices. Cancer Res 1984; 44:1677–1681.

Freedman DM, Dosemeci M, McGlynn K. Sunlight and mortality from breast, ovarian, colon, prostate, and non-melanoma skin cancer: a composite death certificate based case-control study. Occup Environ Med 2002; 59:257–262.

Garland FC, Garland CF, Gorham ED, Miller MR, Brodine SK, Fallon A, Balazs LL. Geographic variation in breast cancer mortality in the United States: a hypothesis involving exposure to solar radiation. Prev Med 1990; 19:614–622.

Gilad LA, Bresler T, Gnainsky J, Smirnoff P, Schwartz B. Regulation of vitamin D receptor expression via estrogen-induced activation of the ERK 1/2 signaling pathway in colon and breast cancer cells. J Endocrinol 2005; 185:577–592.

González G, Alvarado JN, Rojas A, Navarrete C, Velásquez CG, Arteaga E. High prevalence of vitamin D deficiency in Chilean healthy postmenopausal women with normal sun exposure: additional evidence for a worldwide concern. Menopause 2007; 14:455–461.

Gulliford T, English J, Colston IKW, Menday P, Moller S, Coombes RC. A phase I study of the vitamin D analogue EB1089 in patients with advanced breast and colorectal cancer. Br J Cancer 1998; 78:6–13.

Holick MF, Shao Q, Liu WW, Chen TC, Lisa M. Bodnar, Hyagriv N. Simhan. The vitamin D content of fortified milk and infant formula. N Engl J Med 1992; 326: 1178–1181.

Hollis BW. Circulating 25-hydroxyvitamin D levels indicative of vitamin D sufficiency: implications for establishing a new effective dietary intake recommendation for vitamin D. J Nutr 2005; 135:317–322.

Hou MF, Tien YC, Lin GT, Chen CJ, Liu CS, Lin SY, Huang TJ. Association of vitamin D receptor gene polymorphisms with sporadic breast cancer in Taiwanese patients. Breast Cancer Res Treat 2002; 74:1–7.

Hoyer-Hansen M, Bastholm L, Mathiasen IS, Elling F, Jaattela M. Vitamin D analog EB1089 triggers dramatic lysosomal changes and Beclin 1-mediated autophagic cell death. Cell Death Differ 2005; 12:1297–1309.

Hoyer-Hansen M, Bastholm L, Szyniarowski P, Campanella M, Szabadkai G, Farkas T, Bianchi K, Fehrenbacher N, Elling F, Rizzuto R, Mathiasen IS, Jaattela M. Control of macro-autophagy by calcium, calmodulin-dependent kinase kinase-beta, and Bcl-2. Mol Cell 2007; 25:193–205.

Huhtakangas J, Olivera C, Bishop J, Zanello L, Norman A. The vitamin D receptor is present in caveolae-enriched plasma membranes and binds 1 alpha,25(OH)2-vitamin D_3 in vivo and in vitro. Mol Endocrinol 2004; 18:2660–2671.

Ingles SA, Garcia DG, Wang W, Nieters A, Henderson BE, Kolonel LN, Haile RW, Coetzee. Vitamin D receptor genotype and breast cancer in Latinas (United States). Cancer Causes Control 2000; 11:25–30.

Inoue T, Kamiyama J, Sakai T. Sp1 and NF-Y synergistically mediate the effect of vitamin D(3) in the p27(kip1) gene promoter that lacks vitamin D response elements. J Biol Chem 1999; 274:32309–32317.

Jacobson E, James K, Newmark H, Carroll KK. Effects of dietary fat, calcium, and vitamin D on growth and mammary tumorigenesis induced by 7,12-dimethylbenz(a) anthracene in female Sprague-Dawley rats. Cancer Res 1989; 49:6300–6303.

James SY, Mackay AG, Binderup L, Colston KW. Effects of a new synthetic vitamin D analogue, EB1089, on the oestrogen-responsive growth of human breast cancer cells. J Endocrinol 1994; 141:555–546.

James SY, Mackay AG, Colston KW. Vitamin D derivatives in combination with 9-*cis* retinoic acid promote active cell death in breast cancer cells. J Mol Endocrinol 1995; 14: 391–394.

James SY, Mercer E, Brady M, Binderup L, Colston KW. EB1089, a synthetic analogue of vitamin D_3, induces apoptosis in breast cancer cells *in vivo* and *in vitro*. Br J Pharmacol 1998; 125:953–962.

Janowsky EC, Lester GE, Weinberg CR, Millikan RC, Schildkraut JM, Garrett PA, Hulka BS. Association between low levels of 1,25-dihydroxyvitamin D and breast cancer risk. Public Health Nutr 1999; 2:283–291.

Jensen SS, Madsen MW, Lukas J, Binderup L, Bartek J. Inhibitory effects of 1α,25-dihydroxyvitamin D_3 on the G1-S phase controlling machinery. Mol Endocrinol 2001; 15: 1370–1380.

Jiang F, Li P, Fornace AJ, Nicosia SV, Bai W. G2/M arrest by 1,25-dihydroxyvitamin D_3 in ovarian cancer cells mediated through the induction of GADD45 via an exonic enhancer. J Biol Chem 2003; 278:48030–48040.

John EM, Schwartz GG, Dreon DM, Koo J. Vitamin D and breast cancer risk: the NHANES I epidemiologic follow up study, 1971-1975 to 1992. Cancer Epidemiol Biomarkers Prev 1999; 8:399–406.

Kanazawa T, Enami J, Hohmoto K. Effects of 1 alpha, 25-dihydroxy-cholecalciferol and cortisol on the growth and differentiation of primary cultures of mouse mammary epithelial cells in collagen gel. Cell Biol Int 1999; 23: 481–487.

Kawata H, Kamiakito T, Takayashiki N, Tanaaka A. Vitamin D_3 suppresses the androgen-stimulated growth of mouse mammary carcinoma SC-3 cells by transcriptional repression of fibroblast growth factor 8. J Cell Physiol 2006; 207:793–799.

Kemmis CM, Salvador SM, Smith KM, Welsh J. Human mammary epithelial cells express CYP27B1 and are growth inhibited by 25-hydroxyvitamin D-3, the major circulating form of vitamin D-3. J Nutr 2006; 136:887–892.

Knekt P, Jarvinen R, Seppanen R, Pukkala E, Aromaa A. Intake of dairy products and risk of breast cancer. Br J Cancer 1996; 73:687–691.

Koga M, Eisman JA, Sutherland RL. Regulation of epidermal growth factor receptor levels by 1,25-dihydroxyvitamin D_3 in human breast cancer cells. Cancer Res 1988; 48: 2734–2739.

Koike M, Elstner E, Campbell MJ, Asou H, Uskokovic M, Tsuruoka N, Koeffler HP. 19-nor-hexafluoride analogue of vitamin D_3: a novel class of potent inhibitors of proliferation of human breast cell lines. Cancer Res 1997; 57:4545–4550.

Koli K, Keski-Oja J. 1,25-dihydroxyvitamin D_3 has been shown to enhance the expression of transforming growth factor B1 and its latent form binding protein in breast carcinoma cells. Cancer Res 1994; 55:1540–1547.

Koli K, Keski-Oja J. 1,25-dihydroxyvitamin D_3 and its analogues down-regulate cell invasion-associated proteases in cultured malignant cells. Cell Growth Differ 2000; 11: 221–229.

Kommagani R, Caserta TM, Kadakia MP. Identification of vitamin D receptor as a target of p63. Oncogene 2006; 25: 3745–3751.

Koshizuka K, Koike M, Asou H, Cho SK, Stephen T, Rude RK, Binderup L, Uskokovic M, Koeffler HP. Combined effect of vitamin D_3 analogs and paclitaxel on the growth of MCF-7 breast cancer cells in vivo. Breast Cancer Res Treat 1999a; 53:113–120.

Koshizuka K, Koike M, Kubota T, Said J, Binderup L, Koeffler HP. Novel vitamin D_3 analog (CB1093) when combined with paclitaxel and cisplatin inhibit growth of MCF-7 human breast cancer cells *in vivo*. Int J Oncol 1998; 13:421–428.

Koshizuka K, Kubota T, Said J, Koike M, Binderup L, Uskokovic M, Koeffler HP. Combination therapy of a vitamin D analog and all trans retinoic acid. Effect on human breast cancer in nude mice. Anticancer Res 1999b; 19:519–524.

Krishnan AV, Shinghal R, Raghavachari N, Brooks JD, Peehl DM, Feldman D. Analysis of vitamin D-regulated gene expression in LNCaP human prostate cancer cells using cDNA microarrays. Prostate 2004; 59:243–251.

Larsen SS, Heiberg I, Lykkesfeldt AE. Anti-oestrogen resistant human breast cancer cell lines are more sensitive towards treatment with the vitamin D analogue EB1089 than parent MCF-7 cells. Br J Cancer 2001; 84:686–690.

Lazzaro G, Agadir A, Qing W, Poria M, Mehta RR, Moriarty RM, Das Gupta TK, Zhang X-K, Mehta RG. Induction of differentiation by 1alpha-hydroxyvitamin D5 in T47D human breast cancer cells and its interaction with vitamin D receptors. Eur J Cancer 2000; 36:780–786.

Lee HJ, Liu H, Goodman C, Ji Y, Maehr H, Uskokovic M, Notterman D, Reiss M, Suh N. Gene expression profiling changes induced by a novel Gemini Vitamin D derivative during the progression of breast cancer. Biochem Pharmacol 2006; 72:332–343.

Li YC, Pirro AE, Amling M, Delling G, Baron R, Bronson R, Demay MB. Targeted ablation of the vitamin D receptor: an animal model of vitamin D-dependent rickets type II with alopecia. Proc Natl Acad Sci U S A 1997; 94:9831–9835.

Lin R, Nagai Y, Sladek R, Bastien Y, Ho J, Petrecca K, Sotiropoulou G, Diamandis EP, Hudson TJ, White JH. Expression profiling in squamous carcinoma cells reveals pleiotropic effects of vitamin D_3 analog EB1089 signaling on cell proliferation, differentiation, and immune system regulation. Mol Endocrinol 2002; 16:1243–1256.

Lisa MB, Hyagriv NS, Robert WP, Frank MP, Cooperstein E, Roberts JM. High prevalence of vitamin D insufficiency in black and white pregnant women residing in the northern United States and their neonates. J Nutr 2007; 137:447–452.

Liu M, Lee MH, Cohen M, Bommakanti M, Freedman LP. Transcriptional activation of the cdk inhibitor p21 by vitamin D_3 leads to the induced differentiation of the myelocytic cell line U937. Genes Dev 1996; 10:142–153.

Lowe LC, Guy M, Mansi JL, Peckitt C, Bliss J, Wilson RG, Colston KW. Plasma 25-hydroxy vitamin D concentrations, vitamin D receptor genotype and breast cancer risk in a UK Caucasian population. Eur J Cancer 2005; 41:1164–1169.

Lundin AC, Soderkvist P, Eriksson B, Bergman-Jungestrom M, Wingren S. Association of breast cancer progression with a vitamin D receptor polymorphism. Cancer Res 1999; 59: 2332–2334.

Mackay AG, OforiKuragu EA, Lansdown A, Coombes RC, Binderup L, Colston KW. Effects of the synthetic vitamin D analogue EB1089 and tamoxifen on the growth of experimental rat mammary tumors. Endocr Relat Cancer 1996; 3:327–335.

Maehr H, Uskokovic M, Adorini L, Penna G, Mariani R, Panina P, Passini N, Bono E, Perego S, Biffi M, Holick M, Spina C, Suh N. Calcitriol derivatives with two different side chains at C-20 III. An epimeric pair of the gemini family with unprecedented anti-proliferative effects on tumor cells and renin mRNA expression inhibition. J Steroid Biochem Mol Biol 2007; 103:277–281; [Epub Jan 23, 2007].

Majewski S, Skopinska M, Marczak M, Szmurlo A, Bollag W, Jablonska S. Vitamin D_3 is a potent inhibitor of tumor cell-induced angiogenesis. J Investig Dermatol Symp Proc 1996; 1:97–101.

Makishima M, Lu TT, Xie W, Whitfield GK, Domoto H, Evans RM, Haussler MR, Mangelsdorf DJ. Vitamin D receptor as an intestinal bile acid sensor. Science 2002; 296:1313–1316.

Mantell DJ, Owens PE, Bundred NJ, Mawer EB, Canfield AE. 1alpha,25-dihydroxy-vitamin D(3) inhibits angiogenesis in vitro and in vivo. Circ Res 2000; 87:214–220.

Maruyama R, Aoki F, Toyota M, Sasaki Y, Akashi H, Mita H, Suzuki H, Akino K, Ohe-Toyota M, Maruyama Y, Tatsumi H, Imai K, Shinomura Y, Tokino T. Comparative genome analysis identifies the vitamin D receptor gene as a direct target of p53-mediated transcriptional activation. Cancer Res 2006; 66:4574–4583.

Mathiasen IS, Colston KW, Binderup L. EB1089, a novel vitamin D analogue, has strong antiproliferative and differentiation inducing effects on cancer cells. J Steroid Biochem Mol Biol 1993; 46:365–371.

Mathiasen IS, Lademann U, Jäättelä M. Apoptosis induced by vitamin D compounds in breast cancer cells is inhibited by Bcl-2 but does not involve known caspases or p53. Cancer Res 1999; 59:4848–4856.

Mathiasen IS, Sergeev IN, Bastholm L, Elling F, Norman AW, Jaattela M. Calcium and calpain as key mediators of apoptosis like death induced by vitamin D compounds in breast cancer cells. J Biol Chem 2003; 277:30738–30745.

Matsumoto H, Iino Y, Koibuchi Y, Andoh T, Horii Y, Takei H, Horiguchi J, Maemura M, Yokoe T, Morishita Y. Antitumor effect of 22-oxacalcitriol on estrogen receptor negative MDA-MB-231 tumors in athymic mice. Oncol Rep 1999; 6:349–352.

Mawer EB, Walls J, Howell A, Davies M, Ratcliffe W, Bundred J. Serum 1,25-dihydroxy-vitamin D may be related inversely to disease activity in breast cancer patients with bone metastases. J Clin Endocrinol Metab 1997; 82:118–122.

McGaffin KR, Chrysogelos SA. Identification and characterization of a response element in the EGFR promoter that mediates transcriptional repression by 1,25-dihydroxyvitamin D_3 in breast cancer cells. J Mol Endocrinol 2005; 35:117–133.

McCullough ML, Stevens VL, Diver WR, Feigelson HS, Rodriguez C, Bostick RM, Thun MJ, Calle EE. Vitamin D. pathway gene polymorphisms, diet, and risk of postmenopausal breast cancer: a nested case-control study. Breast Cancer Res 2007; 9(1):R9; [Epub ahead of print].

Mehta R, Hawthorne M, Uselding L, Albinescu D, Moriarty R, Christov K, Mehta R. Prevention of N-methyl-N-nitrosourea-induced mammary carcinogenesis in rats by 1α-hydroxyvitamin D_5. J Natl Cancer Inst 2000; 92: 1836–1840.

Mehta RG, Mehta RJ. Vitamin D and cancer. J Nutr Biochem 2002; 13:252–264.

Mehta RG, Moriarty RM, Mehta RR, Penmasta R, Lazzaro G, Constantinou A, Guo L. Prevention of preneoplastic mammary lesion development by a novel vitamin D analogue, 1α hydroxyvitamin D_5. J Natl Cancer Inst 1997; 89:212–218.

Mercier T, Chaumontet C, Gaillard-Sanchez I, Martel P, Heberden C. Calcitriol and Lexicalcitol (KH1060) inhibit the growth of human breast adenocarcinoma cells by enhancing transforming growth factor-β production. Biochem Pharmacol 1996; 52:505–510.

Merke J, Milde P, Lewicka S, Hugel U, Klaus G, Mangelsdorf DJ, Haussler MR, Rauterberg EW, Ritz E. Identification and regulation of 1,25-dihydroxyvitamin D_3 receptor activity and biosynthesis of 1,25-dihydroxyvitamin D_3. Studies in cultured bovine aortic endothelial cells and human dermal capillaries. J Clin Invest 1989; 83:1903–1915.

Mezzetti G, Monti MG, Casolo LP, Piccinini G, Moruzzi MS. 1,25-Dihydroxy-cholecalciferol-dependent calcium uptake by mouse mammary gland in culture. Endocrinology 1988; 122:389–394.

Mizwicki MT, Keidel D, Bula CM, Bishop JE, Zanello LP, Wurtz JM, Moras D, Norman AW. Identification of an alternative ligand-binding pocket in the nuclear vitamin D receptor and its functional importance in 1alpha,25(OH)2-vitamin D_3 signaling. Proc Natl Acad Sci U S A 2004; 101:12876–12881.

Mørk-Hansen CM, Binderup L, Hamberg KJ, Carlberg C. Vitamin D and cancer: effects of $1,25(OH)_2D_3$ and its analogues on growth control and tumorigenesis. Front Biosci 2001a; 6: 820–848.

Mørk-Hansen CM, Frandsen TL, Brunner N, Binderup L. 1,25-Dihydroxyvitamin D_3 inhibits the invasive potential of human breast cancer cells *in vitro*. Clin Exp Metastasis 1994; 12:195–202.

Mørk-Hansen CM, Hamberg KJ, Binderup E, Binderup L. Seocalcitol (EB1089): a vitamin D analogue of anti-cancer potential. Background, design, synthesis, pre-clinical and clinical evaluation. Curr Pharmaceut Des 2000; 6:803–828.

Mørk-Hansen C, Rhode L, Madsen MW, Hansen D, Colston K, Pirianov G, Holm PK, Binderup L. MCF-7/VDR: a new vitamin D resistant cell line. J Cell Biochem 2001b; 82:422–436.

Narbaitz R, Sar M, Stumpf WE, Huang S, DeLuca HF. 1,25-Dihydroxyvitamin D_3 target cells in rat mammary gland. Horm Res 1981; 15:263–269.

Narvaez CJ, Byrne BM, Romu S, Valrance M, Welsh J. Induction of apoptosis by 1,25-Dihydroxyvitamin D_3 in MCF-7 vitamin D_3-resistant variant can be sensitized by TPA. J Steroid Biochem Mol Biol 2003; 84:199–209.

Narvaez CJ, Vanweelden K, Byrne I, Welsh J. Characterization of a Vitamin D_3 resistant MCF-7 cell line. Endocrinology 1996; 137:400–409.

Narvaez CJ, Welsh JE. Differential effects of 1,25-dihydroxyvitamin D_3 and tetradecanoylphorbol acetate on cell cycle and apoptosis of MCF-7 cells and a vitamin D_3 resistant variant. Endocrinology 1997; 138:4690–4698.

Narvaez CJ, Welsh JE. Role of mitochondria and caspases in vitamin D mediated apoptosis of MCF-7 breast cancer cells. J Biol Chem 2001; 276:9101–9107.

Nolan E, Donepudi M, VanWeelden K, Flanagan L, Welsh J. Dissociation of vitamin D_3 and anti-estrogen mediated growth regulation in MCF-7 breast cancer cells. Mol Cell Biochem 1998; 188:13–20.

Norman AW. Minireview: vitamin D receptor: new assignments for an already busy receptor. Endocrinology 2006; 147: 5542–5548.

Oikawa T, Hirotani K, Ogasawara H, Katayama T, Nakamura O, Iwaguchi T, Hiragun A. Inhibition of angiogenesis by vitamin D_3 analogues. Eur J Pharmacol 1990; 178:247–250.

Palmer HG, Gonzalez-Sancho JM, Espada J, Berciano MT, Puig I, Baulida J, Quintanilla M, Cano A, de Herreros AG, Lafarga M, Munoz A. Vitamin D(3) promotes the differentiation of colon carcinoma cells by the induction of E-cadherin and the inhibition of beta-catenin signaling. J Cell Biol 2001; 154:369–387.

Pendas-Franco N, Gonzalez-Sancho JM, Suarez Y, Aguilera O, Steinmeyer A, Gamallo C, Berciano MT, Lafarga M, Munoz A. Vitamin D regulates the phenotype of human breast cancer cells. Differentiation 2007; 75:193–207; [Epub Dec 11, 2006].

Rowling MJ, Kemmis CM, Taffany DA, Welsh J. Megalin-mediated endocytosis of vitamin D binding protein correlates with 25-hydroxycholecalciferol actions in human mammary cells. J Nutr 2006; 136:2754–2759.

Rozen F, Yang XF, Huynh H, Pollak M. Antiproliferative action of vitamin D-related compounds and insulin-like growth factor binding protein 5 accumulation. J Natl Cancer Inst 1997; 89:652–656.

Ruggiero M, Pacini S, Aterini S, Fallai C, Ruggiero C, Pacini P. Vitamin D receptor gene polymorphism is associated with metastatic breast cancer. Oncol Res 1998; 10:43–46.

Saramaki A, Banwell CM, Campbell MJ, Carlberg C. Regulation of the human p21(waf1/cip1) gene promoter via multiple binding sites for p53 and the vitamin D_3 receptor. Nucleic Acids Res 2006; 34:543–554.

Schondorf T, Eisberg C, Wassmer G, Warm M, Becker M, Rein DT, Gohring UJ. Association of the vitamin D receptor genotype with bone metastases in breast cancer patients. Oncology 2003; 64:154–159.

Shah S, Islam MN, Dakshanamurthy S, Rizvi I, Rao M, Herrell R, Zinser G, Valrance M, Aranda A, Moras D, Norman A, Welsh J, Byers SW. The molecular basis of vitamin D receptor and beta-catenin crossregulation. Mol Cell 2006; 21:799–809.

Siddiqui AM, Kamfar HZ. Prevalence of vitamin D deficiency rickets in adolescent school girls in Western region, Saudi Arabia. Saudi Med J 2007; 28:441–444.

Sillanpää P, Hirvonen A, Kataja V, Eskelinen M, Kosma VM, Uusitupa M, Vainio H, Mitrunen K. Vitamin D receptor gene polymorphism as an important modifier of positive family history related breast cancer risk. Pharmacogenetics 2004; 14:239–245.

Simboli-Campbell M, Narvaez CJ, Tenniswood M, Welsh J. 1,25-Dihydroxyvitamin D_3 induces morphological and biochemical markers of apoptosis in MCF-7 breast cancer cells. J Steroid Biochem Mol Biol 1996; 58:367–376.

Simboli-Campbell M, Narvaez CJ, van Weelden K, Tenniswood M, Welsh J. Comparative effects of $1,25(OH)_2D_3$ and EB1089 on cell cycle kinetics and apoptosis in MCF-7 cells. Breast Cancer Res Treat 1997; 42:31–41.

Simboli-Campbell M, Welsh JE. 1,25 Dihydroxyvitamin D_3: coordinate regulator of active cell death and proliferation in MCF-7 breast cancer cells. In: Tenniswood M, Michna H, eds. Schering Foundation Workshop. Vol 14. Heidleberg: Springer Verlag, 1995:191–200.

Stoica A, Saceda M, Fakhro A, Solomon HB, Fenster BD, Martin MB. Regulation of estrogen receptor-α gene expression by 1,25-dihydroxyvitamin D in MCF-7 cells. J Cell Biochem 1999; 75:640–651.

Sundaram S, Beckman MJ, Bajwa A, Wei J, Smith KM, Posner GH, Gewirtz DA. QW-1624F2-2, a synthetic analogue of 1,25-dihydroxyvitamin D_3, enhances the response to other deltanoids and suppresses the invasiveness of human metastatic breast tumor cells. Mol Cancer Ther 2006; 5:2806–2814.

Sundaram S, Sea A, Feldman S, Strawbridge R, Hoopes PJ, Demidenko E, Binderup L, Gewirtz DA. The combination of a potent vitamin D analog, EB1089, with ionizing radiation reduces tumor growth and induces apoptosis of MCF-7 breast tumor xenografts in nude mice. Clin Cancer Res 2003; 9:2350–2356.

Swami S, Krishnan AV, Feldman D. 1,25-Dihydroxyvitamin D_3 down-regulates estrogen receptor abundance and suppresses estrogen action in MCF-7 human breast cancer cells. Clin Cancer Res 2000; 6:3371–3379.

Swami S, Raghavachari N, Muller UR, Bao YP, Feldman D. Vitamin D growth inhibition of breast cancer cells: gene expression patterns assessed by cDNA microarray. Breast Cancer Res Treat 2003; 80:49–62.

Townsend K, Banwell CM, Guy M, Colston KW, Mansi JL, Stewart PM, Campbell MJ, Hewison M. Autocrine metabolism of vitamin D in normal and malignant breast tissue. Clin Cancer Res 2005; 11:3579–3586.

VanWeelden K, Flanagan L, Binderup L, Tenniswood M, Welsh J. Apoptotic regression of MCF-7 xenografts in nude mice treated with the vitamin D analog EB1089. Endocrinology 1998; 139:2102–2110.

Verlinden L, Verstuyf A, Convents R, Marcelis S, Van Camp M, Bouillon R. Action of $1,25(OH)_2D_3$ on the cell cycle genes, cyclin D1, p21 and p27 in MCF-7 cells. Mol Cell Endocrinol 1998; 142:57–65.

Verlinden L, Verstuyf A, Van Camp M, Marcelis S, Sabbe K, Zhao XY, De Clercq P, Vandewalle M, Bouillon R. Two novel 14-Epi-analogues of 1,25-dihydroxyvitamin D_3 inhibit the growth of human breast cancer cells in vitro and in vivo. Cancer Res 2000; 60:2673–2679.

Vieth R, Bischoff-Ferrari H, Boucher BJ, Dawson-Hughes B, Garland CF, Heaney RP, Holick MF, Hollis BW, Lamberg-Allardt C, McGrath JJ, Norman AW, Scragg R, Whiting SJ, Willett WC, Zittermann A. The urgent need to recommend an intake of vitamin D that is effective. Am J Clin Nutr 2007; 85:649–650.

Vink-van Wijngaarden T, Pols HA, Buurman CJ, van den Bemd GJ, Dorssers LC, Birkenhager JC, van Leeuwen JP. Inhibition of breast cancer cell growth by combined treatment with vitamin D analogues and tamoxifen. Cancer Res 1994; 54:5711–5717.

Vink-van Wijngaarden T, Pols HA, Buurman CJ, Birkenhager JC, van Leeuwen JP. Inhibition of insulin- and insulin-like growth factor stimulated growth of human breast cancer cells by 1,25-dihydroxyvitamin D_3 and the vitamin D analogue EB1089. Eur J Cancer 1996; 32A:842–848.

Wang Q, Lee D, Sysounthone V, Chandraratna RAS, Christakos S, Korah R, Wieder R. 1,25-Dihydroxyvitamin D_3 and retinoic acid analogues induce differentiation in breast cancer cells with function and cell specific additive effects. Breast Cancer Res Treat 2001; 67: 157–168.

Wang Q, Yang W, Uytingco MS, Christakos S, Wieder R. 1,25-Dihydroxyvitamin D_3 and all-trans-retinoic acid sensitize breast cancer cells to chemotherapy-induced cell death. Cancer Res 2000; 60:2040–2048.

Welsh JE. Induction of apoptosis in breast cancer cells in response to vitamin D and antiestrogens. Biochem Cell Biol 1994; 72:537–545.

Welsh JE, Wietzke JA, Zinser GM, Byrne B, Smith K, Narvaez C. Vitamin D_3 Receptor as Target for Breast Cancer Prevention. J Nutr 2003; 133: 2425S–2433S.

Wietzke JA, Ward EC, Schneider J, Welsh J. Regulation of the human vitamin D_3 receptor promoter in breast cancer cells is mediated through Sp1 sites. Mol Cell Endocrinol 2005; 230:59–68.

Wietzke JA, Welsh JE. Phytoestrogen regulation of a vitamin D_3 receptor promoter and 1,25-dihydroxyvitamin D_3 actions in human breast cancer cells. J Steroid Biochem Mol Biol 2003; 84:149–157.

Willnow TE, Nykjaer A. Pathways for kidney-specific uptake of the steroid hormone 25-hydroxyvitamin D_3. Curr Opin Lipidol 2002; 13:255–260.

Wu G, Fan RS, Li W, Ko TC, Brattain MG. Modulation of cell cycle by vitamin D_3 and its analogue EB1089 in human breast cancer cells. Oncogene 1997; 15:1555–1563.

Wu Y, Craig TA, Lutz WH, Kumar R. Identification of vitamin D response elements in the human transforming growth factor beta 2 gene. Biochemistry 1999; 38:2654–2660.

Yamagata Z, Zhang Y, Asaka A, Kanamori M, Fukutomi T. Association of breast cancer with vitamin D receptor gene. Am J Hum Genet 1997; 61:388.

Yang L, Yang J, Venkateswarlu S, Ko T, Brattain MG. Autocrine TGFβ signaling mediates vitamin D_3 analog-induced growth inhibition in breast cells. J Cell Physiol 2001; 188: 383–393.

Zinser GM, McEleney K, Welsh JE. Characterization of mammary tumor cell lines from wild type and vitamin D receptor knockout mice. Mol Cell Endocrinol 2003; 200: 67–80.

Zinser GM, Packman K, Welsh JE. Vitamin D_3 receptor ablation alters mammary gland morphogenesis. Development 2002; 129:3067–3076.

Zinser GM, Suckow M, Welsh JE. Vitamin D receptor (VDR) ablation alters carcinogen-induced tumorigenesis in mammary gland, epidermis and lymphoid tissues. J Steroid Biochem Mol Biol 2005; 97:153–164.

Zinser GM, Welsh JE. Accelerated mammary gland development during pregnancy and delayed postlactational involution in vitamin D_3 receptor null mice. Mol Endocrinol 2004a; 18:2208–2223.

Zinser GM, Welsh JE. Vitamin D receptor status alters mammary gland morphology and tumorigenesis in MMTV-neu mice. Carcinogenesis 2004b; 25:2361–2372.

16

Insulin-Like Growth Factor Signaling in Normal Mammary Gland Development and Breast Cancer Progression

ANGELO CASA, BEATE LITZENBURGER, ROBERT DEARTH, and ADRIAN V. LEE
Breast Center, Departments of Medicine and Molecular and Cellular Biology, Baylor College of Medicine, Houston, Texas, U.S.A.

INTRODUCTION

Research over the last 15 years has shown that insulin-like growth factors (IGFs) regulate many critical processes during cancer initiation and progression and that inhibition of IGF action may be a strategy for prevention or blockade of tumor growth. In breast cancer, the IGFs interact at numerous levels with two of the most studied pathways, the estrogen receptor (ER) and ErbB2. This has led many investigators and pharmaceutical companies to test inhibitors of IGF signaling in breast cancer. Proof-of-principle studies have shown that blockade of IGF receptor can block both tumor growth and metastasis. Many pharmaceutical drugs targeting the IGF pathway are now entering clinical trials and thus the next five years promise to be truly exciting for the study of this pathway in human breast cancer.

IGF SYSTEM

The IGF family consists of two ligands (IGF-I and IGF-II), three receptors (IGF-IR, IGF-IIR, and hybrid IGF-IR/insulin receptor), six high-affinity IGF binding proteins (IGFBP 1–6), and other low-affinity IGFBP-related proteins (IGFBPrPs).

IGF Ligands

The IGFs, formerly known as somatomedins, are single-chain polypeptides that were purified and sequenced in 1976 (Rinderknecht and Humbel, 1976), and due to their close homology to proinsulin (~50%) were termed insulin-like growth factors. Initial characterization concentrated on the production of IGF-I in the liver and control of serum IGF-I levels by growth hormone (GH), which was thought to mediate bone elongation in an endocrine manner (Daughaday, 1988). IGF-II, in contrast to IGF-I is minimally GH responsive, and is thought to be involved in fetal growth and development. While early work concentrated on the endocrine function of IGFs, work has highlighted both autocrine and paracrine functions in growth, malignant transformation, and apotosis (Baserga, 1995).

IGF Receptors

IGF-I and IGF-II are single-chain polypeptides that interact with high-affinity receptors. Type I insulin-like growth factor receptor (IGF-IR) is a classical tyrosine kinase receptor normally found as a heterotetramer consisting of two α and two β subunits, which span the plasma membrane (Ullrich et al., 1986). However, the receptor can also be found as hybrid heterodimer with the structurally similar insulin receptor (IR) (discussed in detail in sec. "Insulin Receptor"). Unlike other classical tyrosine kinase receptors such as epidermal growth factor receptor and platelet-derived growth factor receptor, IGF-IR activity is dependent on ligand binding, thus simple overexpression of IGF-IR does not result in ligand-dependent activation (Steele-Perkins et al., 1988). IGF-I and IGF-II have approximately equal affinity for IGF-IR in most systems, and IGF-IR is thought to transduce the effects of both ligands. Type II insulin-like growth factor receptor (IGF-IIR), in contrast to IGF-IR, has no tyrosine kinase activity, and its role in IGF signaling remains unclear. IGF-IIR is a single chain molecule (Morgan, 1987; MacDonald et al., 1988) that is identical to the mannose-6-phosphate (M-6-P) receptor, which is involved in sorting of M-6-P-bearing lysosomal enzymes in the Golgi and endoplasmic reticulum. There are conflicting data concerning a role for IGF-IIR in IGF signaling and detailed mutational analysis of IGF-IIR has failed to find any signaling capability (Korner et al., 1995). Because of the failure to conclusively prove that IGF-IIR has a signaling function, many have been led to hypothesize that it acts as an inactive "sink" by binding and inhibiting IGF-II-mediated action through the IGF-IR. This hypothesis is substantiated by IGF-IIR gene knockouts that had higher circulating IGF-II levels and were born larger than wild-type littermates (Baker et al., 1993) and studies in breast cancer showing that overexpression of IGF-IIR blocks cell proliferation. Of interest in breast cancer is the fact that IGF-IIR can bind transforming growth factor β (TGF-β) and procathepsin D (Mathieu et al., 1990). The binding of this growth factor and protease is competed by IGF-II, providing a complicated scenario of IGF-IIR regulating a growth promoter (IGF-II), a growth inhibitor (TGF-β), and a protease (procathepsin D). The importance of all these factors in breast cancer warrants further analysis of the role of this receptor in breast cancer growth.

IGF Binding Proteins

The IGFBPs provide another level of control of IGF action, by binding the IGFs with higher affinity than IGF-IR (Clemmons et al., 1995). The IGFBPs expressed in a complex tissue-specific pattern, along with the fact that a single IGFBP species is rarely expressed by itself, have hampered assigning specific roles for IGFBPs. The IGFBPs seem to have four main functions: (1) to increase the half-life of bound IGFs by providing storage in the circulation and in the extracellular matrix, (2) to present IGFs to IGFRs and augment IGF action, (3) to sequester IGFs from IGFRs and inhibit IGF action, and (4) IGF-independent effects on other cellular processes, e.g., cell motility via the interaction of IGFBP-1 with α5β1 integrin receptor (Jones et al., 1993). The first role of IGFBPs, increasing IGF half-life, has been clearly shown for IGFBP-3, the binding protein species that binds the majority of IGF-I in human serum.

The role of IGFBPs in inhibiting and potentiating IGF action is less clear and depends upon the biological situation in which they are studied. For example, IGFBP-3 can be both stimulatory and inhibitory to IGF action when added exogenously to the same cell line, simply depending upon whether it is added before or after IGF stimulation (De Mellow and Baxter, 1988).

IGF SIGNALING

Most signal transduction pathways have the ability to activate numerous downstream molecules. Moreover, signaling pathways act like networks and cross talk with other pathways in the cell. The IGF signaling pathway is no exception. This section will highlight some of the important downstream effectors of the IGF signal cascade and will also examine how the IGF system interacts with other signal transduction pathways.

Downstream Elements

IGFs elicit their effects primarily by binding to the IGF-IR. Ligand binding induces a conformational change in receptor subunits, resulting in activation of the intrinsic tyrosine kinase of the cytoplasmic domain of IGF-IR (reviewed in Sachdev and Yee, 2001). The kinase autophosphorylates and transphosphorylates the receptor, which is essential for IGF-IR activation (Tollefsen et al., 1991). This activation results in the recruitment of adaptor proteins (aptly named since they link cell surface receptors to downstream signaling pathways) to the plasma membrane. Tyrosine phosphorylation of these adaptor proteins by the kinase activity of IGF-IR results in the formation of protein complexes that transduce the intracellular signal. Although various cytoplasmic proteins, including Src homologous and collagen (SHC) (Dey et al., 1996), Grb2-associated binder (GAB) (Winnay et al., 2000), and v-crk sarcoma virus CT10 oncogene homolog (CRK) (Koval et al., 1998) can interact with the activated IGF-IR, it is primarily the insulin receptor substrate (IRS) family of adaptor proteins that is responsible for mediating signals downstream of IGF-IR.

The IRS protein family consists of six members: IRS-1, -2, -3, -4, -5, and -6. While IRS-1 and IRS-2 are ubiquitously expressed (Sun et al., 1991; Sun et al., 1995), IRS-3 and IRS-4 exhibit restricted expression patterns; specifically, IRS-3 is predominantly localized to adipose tissue, and IRS-4 is mainly found in the brain (Lavan et al., 1997a; Lavan et al., 1997b). The most recently identified members of the IRS family are IRS-5 and IRS-6 (Cai et al., 2003). This same study showed that IRS-5 transcript levels are highest in kidney and liver, and IRS-6 is most abundant in skeletal muscle. However, physiological roles for these two IRS proteins have not been extensively examined. Each IRS protein contains an amino-terminal pleckstrin homology (PH) domain adjacent to a phosphotyrosine-binding (PTB) domain. Both these domains mediate specific interactions between the IRS proteins and the IGF-IR. While the PTB domain binds to phosphorylated asparagine-proline-any amino acid-tyrosine (NPXY) motifs in the cytoplasmic domain of the receptor (Wolf et al., 1995), the PH domain helps recruit the IRS proteins to the receptor through interactions with phospholipids in the cell membrane (DiNitto and Lambright, 2006). Although the carboxyl termini are less conserved than the amino termini, they contain multiple tyrosine phosphorylation sites that serve as docking sites for Src homology 2 (SH2) domain-containing proteins (Yenush and White, 1997). It is through these protein–protein interactions that IRS proteins couple to downstream signaling components.

The IGF system couples to multiple cell signaling pathways to promote various responses, including proliferation, protection from apoptosis, and transformation. The Ras/mitogen-activated protein kinase (MAPK) cascade involves a series of cytoplasmic phosphorylation reactions that eventually result in activation of transcription factors that function in the nucleus to primarily stimulate cell growth and proliferation. This cascade is activated by IGF-IR-mediated phosphorylation of both IRS-1 and SHC and involves interaction with Grb-2/Sos (Yamauchi and Pessin, 1994). While the proliferative effects of IGF are primarily mediated by the Ras/MAPK cascade, IGF-mediated protection from apoptosis results from activation of phosphatidyl inositol-3 kinase (PI3K) and Akt (Peruzzi et al., 1999).

One major mechanism by which PI3K/Akt signaling promotes cell survival is through phosphorylation and inactivation of the proapoptotic protein BAD (Zha et al., 1996; Datta et al., 1997). In addition to its roles in cell proliferation and survival, IGF-IR is also critical for transformation. Numerous studies have supported this claim. For example, activated Ras (Sell et al., 1994) or SV40 large T antigen (Sell et al., 1993), both of which are transforming oncogenes, fails to malignantly transform mouse embryonic fibroblasts with a targeted disruption of IGF-IR.

Cross Talk with Other Pathways

Like other growth factor signaling pathways, the IGF system is quite complex. It integrates extracellular signals with multiple intracellular responses. These intracellular responses involve multiple docking proteins and kinases that are largely influenced by their phosphorylation status and their subcellular localization. To add to the complexity, the IGF signaling pathway is not a linear cascade. Instead, multiple pathways, including IR, ER, and ErbB family receptors interact with the IGF system in the cell. Understanding this cross talk will lead to better comprehension of the complex nature of IGF signaling within the cell.

Insulin Receptor

IGF-IR and IR use similar downstream signaling intermediates and share significant homology, with the kinase domains showing 84% similarity at the amino acid level. Each receptor can form a heterotetramer consisting of two α and two β subunits (e.g., IGF-IR at right side of Fig. 1). However, hybrid receptors consisting of an IR α/β and an IGFIR α/β subunit also exist (Fig. 1). These hybrid receptors can bind both insulin and IGF-I but are thought to preferentially support IGF-I signaling (Pandini et al., 1999; Slaaby et al., 2006). The formation of hybrid receptors seems to depend on the relative levels of IGF-IR and IR on the cell surface. For example, specific downregulation of IGF-IR results in diminished hybrid receptor formation, enhanced IR homotetramer formation, and insulin sensitivity (Zhang et al., 2007).

In addition, the IR exists in two isoforms. One isoform (IR-A) is generally expressed in fetal tissue, and another (IR-B) is generally expressed in adult tissue (Frasca et al., 1999). Interestingly, IGF-II binds IR-A with a similar affinity as insulin (Frasca et al., 1999), and mouse genetic studies support the concept that IGF-II uses this receptor in fetal development (Louvi et al., 1997).

Estrogen Receptor

Components of the IGF system can interact with the ER pathway at many levels, and this interaction is bidirectional. ERα (one of two genes encoding a specific isoform of ER) can increase expression of multiple IGF signaling components, including IGF-II (Osborne et al., 1989), IGF-IR (Stewart et al., 1990), and IRS-1 (Lee et al., 1999). Estrogen directly increases IRS-1 levels by elevating IRS-1 mRNA levels (Molloy et al., 2000) via an estrogen response element in the promoter (Mauro et al., 2001). As previously stated, interaction between the IGF system and the ER pathway is bidirectional. Thus, IGFs can also enhance ER activity. IGF-I can directly activate ERα in a ligand-independent manner in cell line models (Lee et al., 1997) and in vivo (Molloy et al., 2000). A controversial mechanism of cross talk involves nonnuclear ERα. Some groups have proposed that there is a pool of ERα outside the nucleus, and that this fraction of ERα may interact with components of the IGF signaling pathway, such as IGF-IR (Kahlert et al., 2000) and PI3K (Simoncini et al., 2000).

In addition to the cell culture data, much work has been done in vivo to show the importance of cross talk between

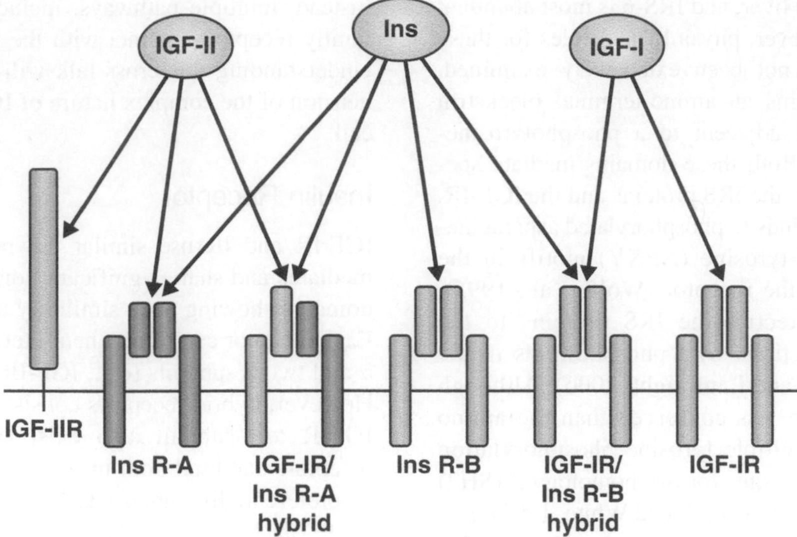

Figure 1 Insulin and IGF signaling. Schematic highlighting the different insulin and IGF receptor isoforms. IR exists as two alternatively spliced isoforms, the fetal IR-A and adult IR-B. IGF-IR and IR can form hybrid heterotetramers. IGF-IIR binds IGF-II with high affinity, but has no signaling capacity, and thus acts as an inhibitor of IGF-II action. *Abbreviations*: IR, insulin receptor; IGF-IR, type I insulin-like growth factor receptor; IGF-IIR, type II insulin-like growth factor receptor; IGF-II, insulin-like growth factor II.

the IGF and ER pathways. For example, the combination of estrogen and IGF-I is critical for normal mammary gland development. ERα-null mice fail to undergo ductal elongation (Bocchinfuso and Korach, 1997; Bocchinfuso et al., 2000). IGF-I-null mice also have severely retarded mammary ductal development and branching, similar to ERα-null mice (Kleinberg et al., 2000). This effect can be reversed by giving back estrogen and IGF-I (Ruan and Kleinberg, 1999). Treatment of the rat with estrogen and progesterone for three weeks results in an increase in the level and phosphorylation of IGF-IR and IRSs, and this is reversed by antiestrogens (Chan et al., 2001). Finally, recent work has also shown that IRSs are hormonally regulated in the mouse mammary gland (Lee et al., 2002).

ErbB Receptors

The human epidermal growth factor (EGF/ErbB) family comprises four receptors (EGFR/ErbB1/HER1, ErbB2/HER2, ErbB3/HER3, ErbB4/HER4) that induce a wide variety of cellular responses (Yarden and Sliwkowski, 2001). Considering that ErbB and IGF-IR signaling pathways share many signaling intermediates, stimulation of either receptor should result in multiple levels of cross talk. Although there is still much to be discovered, many studies have already been carried out that highlight the degree of interaction between the ErbB and IGF-IR pathways.

One potential mechanism for cross talk between these two pathways is direct interaction between epidermal growth factor receptor (EGFR) and IGF-IR, which possibly occurs via IGF-IR-mediated transphosphorylation of EGFR (Gilmore et al., 2002). Interactions between these two pathways also occur downstream of the receptors. For example, a recent study used protein microarrays to identify novel ErbB-interacting proteins (Jones et al., 2006b). The data revealed potential interactions between various ErbB receptors and IRS-1, -4, -5, and -6. IRS-1 had the highest affinity for ErbB2 ($K_d \approx 1$ μM). IRS-2 was not found to interact with any of the ErbB receptors. Another study highlighting the interaction between ErbB receptors and the IGF signaling pathway showed that EGF ligand can induce expression of both IRS-1 and IRS-2 protein levels and that this induction depends on the presence of functional EGFR (Cui et al., 2006). Furthermore, EGF treatment enhances both IGF-I-mediated tyrosine phosphorylation of IRSs and downstream signaling, such as binding of IRS-2 to the p85 regulatory subunit of PI3K.

BIOLOGICAL EFFECTS OF IGF ON BREAST CANCER CELLS

IGF signaling plays a central role in many aspects of tumorigenesis. This section will summarize the effects of IGF on breast cancer cells with focus on the requirement of IGF-IR in proliferation, survival, and migration of breast cancer. Disruptions in the balance of the IGF components leading to excessive proliferation and survival signals have been implicated in the development of breast cancer and suggest IGF-IR as a promising anticancer target.

Proliferation

Several lines of evidence implicate IGF signaling in the growth of breast cancer cells. Breast cancer cell lines show increased expression of IGF-IR (Cullen et al., 1990) as well as increased IGF-I and IGF-II levels (Peyrat et al., 1988). Overexpression of IGF-IR in MCF-7 breast cancer cell lines showed enhanced proliferation under serum-free medium conditions (Surmacz, 2000). In contrast, inhibition of the IGF-IR function by dominant negative mutants, antibodies against IGF-IR, or antisense-IGF-IR resulted in growth inhibition. Furthermore, downstream adaptor signals are important for IGF-IR-mediated cell growth. MCF-7 breast cancer cells expressing antisense RNA for IRS-1 or SHC, show inhibition of growth. Consistent with this, MCF-7 cells overexpressing IRS-1 exhibited enhanced proliferation in serum-free medium as well as in complete growth medium (Surmacz, 2000).

Survival

Among all growth factor receptors described, IGF-IR has one of the most potent antiapoptotic abilities and, therefore, confers cells the capacity to survive, an essential feature of cancer cells (Resnicoff et al., 1995). In breast cancer cells, activated IGF-IR protects cells from apoptosis induced by various therapeutic agents (Dunn et al., 1997a). In contrast, inhibition of IGF-IR action via antisense-based technology, anti-IGF-IR antibodies, or dominant negative receptor induces apoptosis (Pollak et al., 2004). Supporting this observation, downregulation of IRS-1 in MCF-7 cells shows induction of apoptosis and suggests that IRS and PI-3 kinase pathway are required for IGF-IR-mediated survival (Surmacz, 2000). An interesting characteristic of the IGFIR is that the receptor is not an essential requirement for monolayer growth (10–15% growth inhibition) (Resnik et al., 1998), however, IGF is a strict requirement for anchorage-independent growth (Baserga et al., 2003). This differential effect on monolayer cultures and abnormal anchorage-independent growth indicates that targeting of the IGF-IR is a promising candidate for use in cancer therapy.

Migration

The mitogenicity of IGF-I is widely recognized, however evidence has also demonstrated the involvement of IGF-I in migration. IGF-I has been shown to induce migration in various cancer cell types including breast cancer cells (Dunn et al., 1998). A truncated dominant-negative IGF-IR was introduced in MDA-MB-435 breast cancer cells and inhibited the motility and metastatic potential in these breast cancer cells (Sachdev et al., 2004). However, the truncated receptor did not affect growth of the primary tumor suggesting that IGF-IR may regulate the metastatic phenotype independent of tumor growth.

The migration response requires the activation of the downstream adaptor IRS-2 that seems to be an important mediator of mammary tumor metastasis. IRS-1 and IRS-2 were expressed in T47D-YA cells, which lack IRS-1 and IRS-2 but retain functional IGF-IR. Expression of IRS-2-enhanced IGF-I stimulated migration while expression of IRS-1 mediated proliferation. Furthermore, cell migration is associated with cytoskeletal rearrangements. Downstream of IRS-2, IGF-I causes a redistribution of FAK (Focal adhesion kinase) away from the focal adhesion plaques in MDA-231-BO breast cancer cell lines. Stimulation of this breast cancer cell line with IGF-I caused activation of RhoA, which regulates a wide range of biological processes including the reorganization of cytoskeleton, adhesion, and metastasis (Zhang et al., 2005).

IGFs IN NORMAL MAMMARY GLAND DEVELOPMENT

Defined by its ability to change form and function, the development and maturation of the murine mammary gland is one of the most physiologically impressive events, next to pregnancy, in a female's life cycle. Embryonically, the mammary gland ductal structure is rather quiescent, as a rudimentary ductal structure is formed in the mammary fat pad between embryonic days 10 to 17, with no further development until after parturition. After birth, the mammary ducts elongate at the pace of the growing animal. Interestingly, the majority of mammary development occurs postnatally and starts at the onset of puberty (3–6 weeks in the mouse). During postnatal development the mammary gland goes through a series of key events that restructure the mammary gland: ductal growth and primary alveolar development (virgin); increased proliferation, differentiation, and lobuloalveolar development (pregnancy and lactation); apoptosis and tissue remodeling (involution); for review see Richert et al. (2000). Importantly, postnatal growth and differentiation of the mammary gland is critically dependent upon the synergistic actions of ovarian hormones (estrogen and progesterone), pituitary hormones (GH and prolactin), and locally acting growth factors, most notably IGFs (Hennighausen and Robinson, 1998; Kleinberg, 1998; Kleinberg et al., 2000; Hadsell et al., 2002).

IGFs in Ductal Development

Ductal development is marked by the puberty-induced proliferation of epithelial cells within primary mammary structures called terminal end buds (TEBs). TEBs mediate ductal elongation and primary alveolar differentiation until 10 to 12 weeks (mature virgin) when the TEBs reach the limit of the mammary fat pad and regress. Kleinberg and others have shown that IGF-I, induced by GH, is required for TEB formation and ductal morphogenesis (Kleinberg et al., 2000). Importantly, TEBs themselves express IGF-I, IGF-IR and IRS signaling adaptors (Richert and Wood, 1999; Lee et al., 2003), and GH has been shown to increase expression of IGF-I mRNA in mammary stromal cells (Richert and Wood, 1999). Thus, the suggested scenario is that IGF-I works in a paracrine fashion, being released from GH-regulated mammary stromal cells to stimulate proliferation and differentiation of TEB epithelial cells resulting in the virgin mammary ductal structure. Supporting this, Yee et al. (1989) showed that paracrine IGF-I action influences the growth of human breast cancers in situ. Perhaps the best evidence for this comes from gene-targeted deletion of these growth factors or their receptors. GH receptor null mice have retarded ductal development in part because of a lack of stromal GH receptors (Gallego et al., 2001) and an indirect result of reduced IGF-I signaling in the mammary gland (Ruan and Kleinberg, 1999). Consistent with this, IGF-I null mice have severely retarded mammary ductal development and branching (Kleinberg et al., 2000; Stull et al., 2000). Furthermore, IGF-IR null mice exhibit perinatal lethality (Baker et al., 1993), but by grafting of IGF-IR null embryonic anlage into cleared fat pads of syngeneic female hosts, Hadsell's group showed very limited growth of IGF-IR null epithelium compared with wild type (Bonnette and Hadsell, 2001).

Although IGF-I alone can stimulate moderate ductal growth (Kleinberg et al., 2000), the synergism between the mammary GH/IGF-I axis and the peripubertal surge of estrogen (and estrogen release in subsequent cycles) has been shown to be a key factor in regulating ductal development(Bocchinfuso and Korach, 1997; Bocchinfuso et al., 2000). Similar to IGF-I null mice (Kleinberg et al., 2000; Stull et al., 2000), ERα null mice (ERKO) fail to undergo ductal elongation (Bocchinfuso and Korach, 1997; Bocchinfuso et al., 2000), and further transplantation studies have implicated stromal ERα as the major mediator of ductal morphogenesis (Cunha et al., 1997). In fact, GH has been shown to increase mammary gland ER concentrations and estradiol (E2) has been shown to increase the GH stimulation of IGF-I mRNA expression. Not to downplay the role of estrogen, but GH and/or E2 replacement in IGF-I null mice cannot induce mammary development (Kleinberg et al., 2000).

IGFs in Pregnancy and Lactation

During pregnancy the primary alveolar structures proliferate and differentiate, cleaving into lobuloalveolar sacs featuring numerous individual alveoli that produce and secrete copious quantities of milk after birth (during lactation) (Richert et al., 2000). Unfortunately, there are limited studies focusing on the role of IGF after mammary gland maturation, however IGF-I mRNA expression is present in stromal and epithelial cells of pregnant mice and IGF-I mRNA (and IGF-I protein) has been found to be associated with milk proteins in alveolar epithelium during pregnancy (Richert and Wood, 1999). The increase in IGF-I during pregnancy directly relates to our own studies showing that levels of critical down-stream IGF-IR signaling adaptors IRS-1 and IRS-2 are increased dramatically (10- to 20-fold) during pregnancy and increased further (another 10- to 20-fold) during lactation (Lee et al., 2003). In addition, both IRS-1 null and IRS-2 null mice show diminished lactational capacity (Hadsell et al., 2007). It is also important to note that progesterone receptor (PgR) null mice (PRKO) have normal ductal development but fail to undergo pregnancy-induced lobuloalveolar development (Humphreys et al., 1997)—an action thought to be mediated by epithelial PgR (Gallego et al., 2001) working in a juxtacrine manner, possibly via IGF-II (Seagroves et al., 2000).

IGFs in Involution

At weaning, milk stasis in the mammary gland initiates dramatic tissue remodeling that causes regression of the mammary gland structures back to the prepregnant state (involution). While the role of IGF-I during pubertal gland development is to drive proliferation, it seems that reduced IGF-I during late-lactation/involution induces apoptosis (Hadsell et al., 2002). Supporting this, involution results in significant decreases in IRS-1, IRS-2 and Akt signaling in the mammary gland (Hadsell et al., 2002; Lee et al., 2003). Furthermore, Hadsell et al., (1996) and others have shown that forced overexpression of IGF-I in the mammary gland during lactation inhibits involution (Neuenschwander et al., 1996). However, increased levels of IGF-I cannot protect mammary cells from apoptosis if the mammary gland undergoes forced involution (Hadsell et al., 2002).

The studies mentioned above represent only a fraction of the work on the importance of hormone receptors and growth factors in mammary development but clearly show that IGFs and their signaling intermediates are critical for normal mammary development.

IGFs IN MAMMARY TRANSFORMATION

Transformation of Mouse Fibroblasts

The role of IGF-IR in transformation has mainly been studied in mouse fibroblasts. The first evidence that IGF-IR is an oncogene was first reported in 1990. NIH-3T3, a fibroblast cell line, overexpressing the human IGF-IR showed full transformation and tumor growth in vivo (Kaleko et al., 1990). Furthermore, IGF-IR is actually required for transformation (Sell et al., 1993). Fibroblasts derived from IGF-IR null mice (R-cells) were resistant to transformation with the oncogene SV40T-antigen. It has also been found that numerous other oncogenes, such as H-ras, c-src, the human papilloma virus E7, overexpressed IRS-1 and other overexpressed growth factors failed to transform R-cells. This is an important observation because normally mouse embryonic fibroblasts (MEFs) are susceptible to spontaneous transformation by oncogenes in culture. The protection against transformation could be reversed by reintroduction of the IGF-IR into R-cells (Baserga, 2000).

Specific tyrosine residues of the receptor have been shown to be required for the ability of IGF-IR to cooperate with oncogenes (Li et al., 1996) indicating that specific signal transduction pathways engaged by IGF-IR are associated with transformation. A dominant negative IGF-IR lacking the C-terminus (truncated at either residue 1229 or 1245) lost the ability to transform fibroblasts as well as breast tumor cells (Surmacz, 2000). However, the dominant negative IGF-IR is still mitogenic and also protects cells from apoptosis (Baserga, 2000).

Furthermore, downregulation of the IGF-IR in malignant cells reverses the transformed phenotype. Introducing siRNA or dominant negative mutants in tumor cells resulted in enhanced apoptosis and inhibits tumorigenesis and metastasis in vitro and in vivo (Valentinis and Baserga, 2001). These data suggest that IGF-IR is critically involved in malignant transformation and that IGF-IR is necessary to maintain a transformed phenotype. It also suggests that IGF-IR is an important target in cancer therapy.

Transformation of Human Mammary Epithelial Cells

MCF-10A is a spontaneously immortalized, but nontransformed, human mammary epithelial cell line (Debnath and Brugge, 2005). In 3D matrigel culture, MCF-10A cells undergo proliferation, apicobasal polarization, apoptosis of cells in the luminal space, and finally growth arrest, to form functional acini. This model has proven useful for determining the effects of oncogenes on proliferation, polarity, and apoptosis in cell culture. For example, oncogenes such as ErbB2 reinduce proliferation of growth-arrested acini, directly disrupt polarity, and also inhibit apoptosis, thus filling the luminal space (Muthuswamy et al., 2001). In contrast, inhibition of apoptosis (e.g., Bcl-2) or increased proliferation alone (e.g., cyclinD1 or HPV E7) results in large acini with open lumens (Debnath and Brugge, 2005).

Two studies have used the human MCF-10A immortalized mammary epithelial cell line to examine the effect of elevated IGF-IR levels on mammary acini formation in 3D culture (Irie et al., 2005; Yanochko and Eckhart, 2006). Both groups found that overexpressed IGF-IR remained ligand-dependent, but when stimulated by IGF-I caused hyperproliferation, decreased apoptosis, and altered polarity, resulting in large complex disrupted acini. Blockade of PI3K or ERK1/2 blocked the formation of disrupted acini by MCF-10A-IGF-IR (Yanochko and Eckhart, 2006).

We examined whether overexpressing a constitutively active IGF-IR (CD8-IGF-IR) would similarly disrupt normal mammary acinar morphogenesis of MCF-10A cells, but also cause transformation. Indeed, CD8-IGF-IR caused hyper-proliferation, disruption of polarity, and decreased apoptosis, resulting in the generation of large and misshapen acini. More importantly, CD8-IGF-IR caused transformation of MCF-10A cells, as measured by lack of contact inhibition, foci formation, and growth in soft agar.

Numerous oncogenes are able to disrupt MCF-10A acini formation and transform MCF-10A cells in vitro. However, oncogenes such as ErbB2 disrupt acini formation (Debnath and Brugge, 2005), but fail to convey in vivo xenograft growth (Giunciuglio et al., 1995). In contrast, we observed that CD8-IGF-IR caused cells to grow in immunocompromised mice. Taken together, these data indicate that overexpression of a single oncogene (CD8-IGF-IR) in MCF-10A cells is sufficient to cause transformation.

Transformation in Mouse Models

Despite extensive knowledge regarding a role for IGF-IR in transformation in vitro, until 2005 there were no reports of IGF-IR induced transformation in vivo. We then reported that overexpression of a constitutive active IGF-IR in the mouse mammary gland resulted in transformation in vitro and rapid mammary tumorigenesis in vivo (Carboni et al., 2005). This was subsequently supported by a similar observation using inducible overexpression of wild-type IGF-IR (Jones et al., 2006a).

IGFs IN BREAST CANCER

The IGF system plays multiple roles in many tissues, including the mammary gland. While IGFs are clearly essential for normal mammary gland development, dysregulation of the IGF axis can lead to cancer. The importance of the IGF signaling pathway in breast tumorigenesis is directly related to the cellular processes it regulates, including proliferation, survival, migration, and transformation. This section will consider the evidence that the IGF system plays a role in breast cancer.

IGF Ligands: Autocrine/Paracrine Signaling

In breast cancer, both IGF-I mRNA and IGF-II mRNA have higher expression in stromal cells compared with epithelial cells (Yee et al., 1989; Giani et al., 1996). The presence of IGF-IR on the surface of mammary epithelial cells (Pollack et al., 1987) results in paracrine signaling between the breast epithelium and the stromal compartment. Autocrine signaling has also been shown to play a role in breast cancer progression. In fact, numerous data obtained with both cultured cells and animal models provide evidence that implicates the IGF ligands in breast cancer.

IGF-I signaling enhances proliferation and prolongs survival of cells in culture (Jones and Clemmons, 1995), and IGF-I has also been shown to influence breast cancer cell motility through regulation of cell adhesion to the extracellular matrix (Lynch et al., 2005). Transgenic mice expressing either IGF-I or IGF-II specifically in the mammary gland display increased tumor incidence. For example, 53% of mice expressing amino-terminally truncated IGF-I, des(1-3) IGF-I, develop mammary adenocarcinomas by 23 months of age (Hadsell et al., 2000). Mice overexpressing IGF-II in the mammary gland have also been generated, and these mice have higher incidence of mammary tumor development (Bates et al., 1995). IGF-II is parentally imprinted; only the paternal allele is expressed. In many cancers, there is loss of imprinting, which leads to increased expression of IGF-II. This would likely confer a growth advantage.

Circulating IGF Ligands: Endocrine Action

In addition to functioning as local growth factors, IGF ligands also act as circulating hormones. IGF-I is synthesized in the liver (where its synthesis is regulated by GH) and released into the circulation where it can affect distant tissues, including the breast. While little experimental data exist on the role of serum IGF-I levels in breast cancer, it has been shown that *little* (lit/lit) mice, which have only 10% of circulating IGF-I levels, display a significant reduction of growth of human MCF-7 breast cancer cell xenografts (Yang et al., 1996).

Supporting this, our lab has recently reported that the GH antagonist pegvisomant can also lower serum IGF-I levels in mice and block MCF-7 xenograft growth (Divisova et al., 2006a). Similarly, T-antigen-induced mammary tumors are decreased in mice with low serum IGF-I levels (Yakar et al., 2001). Another study showed that mice with a liver-specific deficiency of IGF-I have approximately a 75% reduction of circulating IGF-I levels and a decreased incidence of both chemically and genetically induced mammary tumors (Wu et al., 2003). Despite the progress that is being made to understand the role of circulating IGF-I in breast cancer, there is still much that is unknown about the endocrine role of IGF-II in humans. However, recent evidence suggests that increased circulating IGF-II levels are associated with increased cancer risk perhaps due to an increased chance of developing or propagating mutations in stem/progenitor cells (Sakatani et al., 2005).

IGF Receptors

All breast cancer cell lines express IGF-IR (Cullen et al., 1990). Amplification and overexpression of IGF-IR in cancer seem to be less common than amplification and overexpression of other oncogenes, such as ErbB2. Furthermore, in clinical breast cancer specimens, IGF-IR is detected at very high frequency and is overexpressed compared with normal breast cancer (Papa et al., 1993). Additionally, it has been shown that IGF-IR levels, and their activity, are elevated in human breast tumors (Resnik et al., 1998).

The IGF-IIR binds IGF-II but lacks tyrosine kinase activity. Thus, IGF-IIR appears to act as a sink for IGF-II by failing to transduce intracellular signals. IGF-IIR has properties of a tumor-suppressor gene. Loss of heterozygosity (LOH) at the IGF-IIR gene locus occurs in about 30% of invasive and in situ breast cancers (Hankins et al., 1996).

IGF Activity and Breast Cancer Risk

Although many studies have been carried out to understand the relationship between IGF activity and breast cancer risk, there is still much that is unknown. However, it is clear that IGF ligands, IGF receptors, and proteins that modify IGF action can all influence a woman's likelihood of developing breast cancer and her prognosis.

Circulating levels of IGF-I vary considerably in normal individuals. It was previously believed that there was no biological significance for individuals whose serum IGF-I levels fell within this broad normal range. However, new evidence suggests that premenopausal women possessing circulating IGF-I levels at the high-normal end of the spectrum are at greater risk for developing breast cancer (Hankinson et al., 1998). However, in assessing the risk of circulating IGF-I, the bioavailability of the ligand must also be considered. Insulin-like growth factor binding protein-3 (IGFBP-3) can bind to circulating IGF-I and prevent it from binding its receptor. Thus, an increased ratio of IGF-I to IGFBP-3 is associated with increased breast cancer risk (Li et al., 2001). Furthermore, mammographic density is strongly related to breast cancer risk (Boyd et al., 1998), and evidence supports a positive correlation between circulating IGF-I levels and mammographic density (Byrne et al., 2000).

In addition to IGF ligands, receptors and downstream adaptor proteins may also serve as good prognostic markers in breast cancer. Early studies hinted that high levels of IGF-IR might confer a good prognosis for breast cancer patients (Papa et al., 1993), but more recent findings show that IGF-IR overexpression leads to radioresistance and a poor outcome (Turner et al., 1997). IRS-1 is also more active (phosphorylated) in breast tumors than in normal breast (Chang et al., 2002). We have found by immunoblotting that high levels of IRS-1 are associated with a poor prognosis in breast cancer (Lee et al., 1999).

Cross Talk Between IGF and ER Pathways

The IGF system has a strong positive interaction with the ER pathway not only during normal mammary gland development as previously discussed but also in breast cancer. Estrogen and IGF-I are both potent mitogens for breast cancer cells, and many laboratories have documented synergistic responses. We have shown that estrogen and IGF-I increase MCF-7 breast cancer cell proliferation (Lee et al., 1999). However, there also seems to be synergistic changes in survival, migration, and cell motility. Thus, it appears that cross talk between the IGF and ER pathways has the potential to regulate breast cancer progression on multiple levels. While estrogen can sensitize breast cancer cells to IGFs, it is possible that antiestrogen-inhibition of MCF-7 growth involves downregulation of IGF signaling. We have shown that antiestrogens strongly downregulate IRS-1 expression (Lee et al., 1999) in MCF-7 xenografts. Furthermore, antiestrogens can downregulate serum IGF-I levels (Pollak, 1998), and MCF-7 xenograft growth is reduced in mice that have low circulating levels of IGF-I (Yang et al., 1996). In breast cancer specimens, we have demonstrated a correlation between IRS-1 and ER expression (Lee et al., 1999), and others have shown similar results for IGF-IR (Surmacz et al., 1998).

TARGETING IGF-IR IN BREAST CANCER

The IGF-IR has become a promising anticancer target because it is frequently overexpressed in tumors where it mediates enhanced proliferation and reduced apoptosis. Elevated IGF-IR content in breast tumors was found to be nearly 14-fold higher than the normal breast tissue indicating a prognostic factor in breast cancer. In addition to being present at higher levels, increased IGF-IR kinase activity (2- to 4-fold) was observed in these tumors accounting for up to 40-fold hyperactivation of IGF-IR in breast cancer (Resnik et al., 1998). In short, it can be concluded that IGF-IR plays an important role in carcinogenesis and that this knowledge can be used to design new anticancer therapies. Multiple strategies have been employed to block IGF-I receptor signaling and these can occur at multiple levels by blocking GH/IGF axis, by inhibition of the transmembrane IGF-IR, and by inhibition of the intracellular IGF-IR tyrosinekinase domain. Strategies of IGF-I manipulation are summarized in Figure 2.

Proof-of-principle studies have shown that blockade of IGF-IR action can block breast cancer growth and metastasis (Sachdev and Yee, 2006). IGF-IR levels have been lowered by antisense IGF-IR (Resnicoff et al., 1995), and this strategy was actually tested and showed some success in a phase 1 clinical trial in glioblastoma multiforme (Andrews et al., 2001; Schillaci et al., 2006). Another potential therapeutic approach is the use of soluble IGF-IR molecules. A C-terminal truncated IGF-IR was constructed that contains the ligand-binding site but lacks the tyrosine kinase domain in the C-terminus. The truncated receptor behaved in a dominant-negative manner and inhibited endogenous IGF-IR activation and signaling. Furthermore, it was shown that the dominant negative receptor inhibits metastasis (Sachdev et al., 2004). Truncated IGF-IR mutants are soluble and bind circulating IGF. This dominant negative IGF-IR showed complete blockade of metastasis of MDA-MB-435 breast cancer cells, despite no change in the growth of the primary tumor (Sachdev et al., 2004). Pharmaceutical companies have attempted to inhibit IGF-IR function by two main strategies—small molecule inhibitors that block the tyrosine kinase domain and humanized monoclonal blocking antibodies (Table 1).

Several problems arise when targeting the IGF-IR. One important aspect to consider is the cross-reactivity with the IR because the two receptors share 70% homology. Therefore, glucose metabolism must be carefully analyzed during IGF-IR blockade when treating patients. Another worry is that IGF-IR is ubiquitously expressed throughout the body. Blocking the receptor may cause toxicity or other unwanted effects in multiple tissues. During childhood, IGF plays an important role in development and growth making IGF-IR blockade in children not a suitable strategy. Blocking IGF signaling could have toxic effects on the central and peripheral nervous systems. In addition, disruption of the IGF-IR signaling in the heart may affect cardiac myocyte survival (Miller and Yee, 2005).

Studies have shown an added benefit by combining IGF-IR targeting strategies with conventional cytotoxic chemotherapies, irradiation, or with other growth factor receptor inhibitors. For instance, a preclinical study

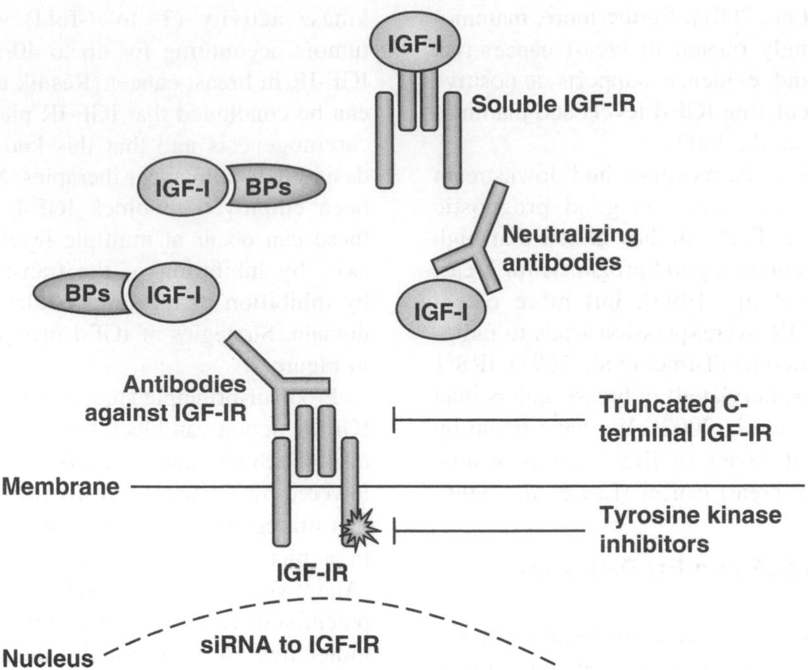

Figure 2 Therapeutic approaches to target circulating IGF ligands and IGF-IR. On the extracellular level, IGF ligands can be blocked by neutralizing antibodies, soluble IGF-IRs, and IGFBPs. The IGF-IR can also be targeted by multiple strategies including antibodies against the extracellular domain of IGF-IR and truncated C-terminal IGF-IR. On the intracellular level, IGF-IR can be blocked by small molecule TKIs and siRNA to IGF-IR. *Abbreviations*: IGF, insulin-like growth factor; IGF-IRs, type I insulin-like growth factor receptors; IGFBPs, IGF binding proteins; TKIs, tyrosine kinase inhibitors.

Table 1 Clinical Development of IGF-IR Inhibitors[a]

Tyrosine kinase inhibitors	Company	Development
Insm-18 (NDGA)	Insmed	Phase I
BMS-536924, BMS-554417	Bristol Myers Squibb	Preclinical
NVP-AEW541, NVP-AEW742	Novartis	Preclinical
EXEL-2280	Exelixis	Preclinical
Compound 1	Oncogene Science Inc.	Preclinical
Cycololigans	Karolinska University Hospital, Stockholm, Sweden	Preclinical
Monoclonal antibodies	Company	Development
CP 751,871	Pfizer	Phase I/II
scFv-Fc	Fujita-Yamaguchi, Sachdev, Yee	Preclinical
A12	ImClone	Phase I/II
AVE-1642	Sanofi-Aventis	Phase I
MK0646	Merck	Phase I
AMG479	Amgen	Phase I
RO4858696	Roche	Phase I
19D12	Schering	Preclinical

[a]The table summarizes agents targeting IGF-IR that are either at the end of preclinical development or already in clinical trials. Of note, several of the tyrosine kinase inhibitors are expected to enter clinical trials in 2007.

showed that an anti-IGF-IR antibody sensitizes cells to chemotherapy (Goetsch et al., 2005). Lowering the chemotherapy agent doses may significantly prolong the patient's life span due to reduced side effects (LeRoith and Helman, 2004). In addition, IGF-IR blockade enhanced radiation-induced apoptosis of different breast cancer cell lines suggesting that interruption of IGF-IR signaling may be combined with radiation therapy (Allen et al., 2007). The combination of an anti-IGF-IR antibody with other growth factor receptor inhibitors, such as the epidermal growth factor receptor inhibitor, gefitinib, has shown a great potential for cancer therapy (Goetsch et al., 2005).

Lowering or Neutralization of Ligands

Supporting the notion that circulating IGF-I regulates somatic cell turnover and susceptibility to oncogenes, downregulation of IGF-I level reduces cancer incidence (Yakar et al., 2005). Reduction of IGF levels is an effective strategy for the prevention and treatment of breast cancer. Energy-restricted diets led to a significant reduction in circulating IGF-I levels (Thissen et al., 1994). Liver-specific IGF-I gene deleted (LID) mice showed a 25% reduction of circulating IGF-I and exhibited delayed mammary tumor development in response to carcinogens (Wu et al., 2003). Similarly, dwarf animals, which are deficient in GH and IGF-I production, showed resistance to DMBA-induced carcinogenesis (Ramsey et al., 2002). Application of GH to these animals was sufficient to raise IGF-I levels, and increased tumor incidence was observed. On the basis of these preliminary data, disruption of the GH/IGF axis could inhibit IGF-IR signaling. For instance, pegvisomant (Pfizer, New York, U.S.), a GH antagonist, is a Food and Drug Administration (FDA) approved drug that lowers serum IGF-I level. Pegvisomant was able to block growth of MCF-7 xenografts and completely blocked GH and IGF-IR signaling in the mammary gland (Divisova et al., 2006b).

Furthermore, anti-IGF-I strategy involves ligand neutralization. This can be achieved by IGFBP-1 or antibodies against IGF-I. IGFBPs have higher affinity for IGF-I and IGF-II than the receptors resulting in inhibition of monolayer growth of MCF-7 breast cancer cells and reduction of cell motility (Sachdev et al., 2006). However, a short protein half-life makes it difficult in its therapeutic application. Furthermore, novel antibody against IGF-I, KM1468, successfully inhibited bone metastasis of prostate cancer, but was not applied in breast cancer (Goya et al., 2004).

Inhibiting IGF-IR

Two main strategies have been employed to target the IGF-IR. Inhibition of the IGF-IR can be achieved by monoclonal antibodies blocking the ligand-binding domain or by small molecule inhibitors targeting the intracellular tyrosine domain.

Blocking Antibodies

Antibodies are promising agents to achieve inhibition of IGF-IR function. Importantly, none of the monoclonal antibodies target the IR disrupting insulin–IR interaction (Miller and Yee, 2005).

Single-chain antibodies against human IGF-IR (αIGF-IR, scFvs) were constructed and expressed. Administration of these antibodies such as AVE-1642 and h7C10 inhibited IGF-dependent growth and inhibited tumor growth of MCF7 cells in xenografts (Li et al., 2000). Pfizer used XenoMouse technology to generate a fully human IgG2 antibody (CP-751,871) that has a very high affinity ($K_d = 1.5$ nmol/L) for human IGF-IR and little or no cross-reactivity with IR. CP-751,871 blocks binding of IGF-I to IGF-IR, inhibits IGF-I-induced IGF-IR autophosphorylation, and causes the downregulation of IGF-IR in vitro and in tumor xenografts (Cohen et al., 2005). CP-751,871 showed significant antitumor activity both as a single agent and in combination with Adriamycin, 5-fluorouracil, or tamoxifen in multiple tumor models. A first human Phase 1 study in multiple myeloma showed little toxicity from the antibody. There was one near-complete response (CR) and two partial responses (PR) in patients treated with CP-751,871 and dexamethasone (Lacy et al., 2006). A phase 1b study of CP-751,871 in combination with docetaxel in advanced solid tumors again showed little toxicity attributed to CP-751,871 (Attard et al., 2006). Of 18 hormone-refractory prostate cancer patients, 4 had a confirmed PR, 2 had unconfirmed PR, and 2 had stable disease (SD) for more than 6 months. Five patients maintained SD with CP-751,871 alone for two to seven courses (Attard et al., 2006).

Tyrosine Kinase Inhibitors

Small molecule inhibitors function as ATP-competitive inhibitors of the IGF-IR kinase domain. In contrast to the monoclonal antibodies, the development of small molecule inhibitors targeting the kinase domain of IGF-IR has historically been hindered by the high similarity between IGF-IR and IR kinase domains, and the inability of any companies to develop tyrosine kinase inhibitors (TKIs) that show selectivity for IGF-IR over IR. The ATP-binding cleft is 100% homologous between the IGF-IR and IR, but the whole kinase domains in the two receptors share only 84% sequence similarity (Garcia-Echeverria et al., 2004). Besides blocking the IGF-IR kinase domain, these inhibitors also block the IR kinase domain to a degree creating problems of insulin resistance when given in high doses. Insulin resistance is characterized by hyperglycemia, a condition in which there is too much circulating glucose in the blood (Pollak et al., 2004). Therefore, a major challenge has been the development of specific IGF-IR kinase domain inhibitors. The combination of computer technology and crystallography has made it possible to characterize the 3D structures of the IGF-IR and IR. These studies showed that the phosphorylated forms of these receptors are conformationally different allowing the design of specific

IGF-IR inhibitors such as derivatives of podophyllotoxin and pyrimidine that were patented and entered preclinical trials. Other advantages of these agents are that they can be administered orally and have low toxicity (Surmacz, 2003). Thus far, no fully selective IGF-IR inhibitor has been found. Only one group reported a potent and selective small molecule inhibitor, called cycloligans. They bind to 2 tyrosine residues in the kinase domain that has a different 3D structure compared with the IR. Thus, cycloligans did not affect the IR. Cycloligans successfully inhibited IGF-IR phosphorylation and malignant cell growth in vitro and in vivo (Girnita et al., 2004).

Another class of small molecule inhibitors are the pyrrolo[2,3-d]pyrimidine derivatives. These compounds have some increased activity against IGF-IR versus IR, either in cell free-kinase assays or in cells (generally fibroblasts) that overexpress artificially high levels of either IGF-IR or IR alone (Garcia-Echeverria et al., 2004). However, most of these TKIs show little selectivity against endogenous IGF-IR or IR in breast cancer cells (Sachdev and Yee, 2006). Another TKI was developed by Bristol-Myers Squibb (BMS-536924). BMS-536924 is an ATP-competitive inhibitor that has a nanomolar IC50 against IGF-IR (Wittman et al., 2005). It can reverse IGF-IR-induced transformation of immortalized mammary epithelial cells and can block cancer xenograft growth (Carboni et al., 2005). However, like other TKIs, this inhibitor has an equal affinity for IR, and when given in vivo causes both hyperinsulinemia and hyperglycemia (Wittman et al., 2005). As blocking IR seems to be a predictable side effect of targeting IGF-IR, investigators are testing whether intermittent inhibition of IR may reduce the toxicity, but may require addition of chemotherapy or other therapies that act synergistically with IGF-IR/IR inhibition for maximum therapeutic effect. These studies have the potential to greatly enhance the clinical development of IGF-IR inhibitors for the treatment of breast cancer.

IGF-IR IN RESISTANCE TO BREAST CANCER THERAPY

Many patients experience resistance to anticancer therapy either de novo (at the beginning of the therapy) or acquired (after prolonged use). The IGF-IR has received increased attention as the antiapoptotic effect of the IGF-IR may mediate decreased sensitivity to anticancer therapy. Thus, targeting the IGF-IR could serve as an approach to overcome clinical drug resistance.

Antiestrogens

The antiestrogen tamoxifen is commonly used as a therapy for ER-positive breast cancer patients. Unfortunately, many patients experience resistance to this endocrine therapy, and this development includes the cross talk between ER and the IGF-IR. Tamoxifen-resistant MCF-7 breast cancer cells show increased proliferation upon stimulation with IGFs (Knowlden et al., 2005). Moreover, IGF-IR activates the PI3K pathway and mediates activation of ERα (Campbell et al., 2001). Exposure to an IGF-IR inhibitor AG1024 reduces ER phosphorylation and diminishes tumor cell growth of tamoxifen resistant cells. These data suggest that combination therapy of targeting IGF-IR and ER may reduce tamoxifen resistance in breast cancer (Nicholson et al., 2005).

HER2 Inhibitors

The humanized anti-HER2 monoclonal antibody trastuzumab (Herceptin) inhibits growth of ErbB2-overexpressing breast cancers, but its efficiency is limited because of the development of resistance. There are several studies reporting that elevation of IGF-IR signaling interferes with the action of trastuzumab. For instance, in SKBR3 breast cancer cells that overexpress HER2/neu, trastuzumab inhibited cell growth. However, when these cells overexpress IGF-IR and HER2/neu, trastuzumab lost its efficacy (Lu et al., 2001). Herceptin resistance was overcome by blocking IGF-IR signaling through co-treatment with recombinant IGFBP-3 and trastuzumab (Lu et al., 2001). The underlying mechanism of trastuzumab resistance is not clear. However, it is suggested that IGF-IR and HER-2 form heterodimers and that IGF-I causes phosphorylation of HER-2 in trastuzumab resistant cells. Furthermore, p27kip1, a critical mediator of responsiveness to trastuzumab is downregulated and confers trastuzumab resistance in these cells. These observations support the concept to simultaneously co-target IGF-IR in combination with HER2 targeting strategies in anticancer therapy.

EGFR Inhibitors

Gefitinib (ZD1839; Iressa) is a specific TKI targeting the EGFR. Overexpression of EGFR is seen in a variety of tumors including breast cancer and it is associated with poor prognosis. Breast cancer cell lines that are resistant to gefitinib have high levels of IGF-IR and also elevated levels of activated AKT and protein kinase C (PKC). Treatment with IGF-IR inhibitor leads to downregulation of AKT and PKC. Such findings indicate that IGF-IR is an important therapeutic target in acquired gefitinib resistance in breast cancer, and strategies that target this receptor may increase the efficacy and duration of response to gefitinib (Jones et al., 2004).

Radioresistance and Chemoresistance

In ER-positive breast tumors, the levels of the IGF-IR and IRS-1 are often elevated, and these characteristics have been linked with increased radioresistance and cancer recurrence. The blockade of IGF-IR signaling by a monoclonal antibody enhanced radiation-induced apoptosis. This effect may be mediated by enhanced double-stranded DNA damage. IGF-IR is known to modulate double-stranded DNA break repair and blockade of IGF-IR was shown to downregulate ATM kinase activation. Blockade of IGF-IR may therefore delay radiation induced double-stranded DNA break repair (Allen et al., 2007).

Several evidences suggest a role for IGF-IR signaling in chemoresistance. Most cytostatic drugs kill cancer cells via apoptosis (Eastman, 1990). Therefore, chemotherapy depends on cellular responses to apoptotic signals within a cell. Stimulation of IGF-IR shows a protective effect against apoptosis-inducing agents in breast cancer (Dunn et al., 1997a). In contrast, blockade of IGF-IR sensitizes cells to chemotherapy (Warshamana-Greene et al., 2005).

TARGETING IGFs FOR PREVENTION OF BREAST CANCER

The IGF family and its upstream regulator GH are clearly involved in many aspects of breast cancer. This leads to the question of whether inhibition of GH or IGF action may actually be a strategy for prevention of breast cancer. Thus far there have been limited experiments to address this.

Diet restriction (DR) of mice lowers serum IGF-I levels and can reduce growth of chemically induced bladder cancer (Dunn et al., 1997b). Furthermore, administration of IGF-I to these DR mice promotes cancer progression. Mice that have the liver IGF-I gene deleted (using Cre-lox technology) have a 75% reduction in serum IGF-I levels and this is associated with decreased growth of colon cancer xenografts and metastases in these mice (Wu et al., 2002). Again, readminstration of IGF-I increases both xenograft growth and metastasis. MCF-7 xenograft growth is reduced in mice that have low levels of circulating IGF-I (Yang et al., 1996).

These data suggest that lowering of serum IGF-I levels may be a potential mechanism for blockade of tumor growth. This was first tested clinically using somatostatin analogues, but many of the trials, particularly in breast cancer, were performed in small numbers of patients that had previously failed multiple therapies (14 trials had a total of 210 patients). Despite this, a recent meta-analysis of all trials from 1989 to 1999 showed that a positive tumor response occurred in 41.4% of patients (4.3% complete response, 14.8% partial response, and 22.4% stable disease) (Dolan et al., 2001). Serum IGF-I levels were not decreased in all of the patients, suggesting that a better response could be achieved with more potent suppressors of serum IGF-I levels. However, two large randomized trials showed no benefit of adding somatostatin analogues to tamoxifen in the treatment of advanced breast cancer (Ingle et al., 1999; Bajetta et al., 2002), however one trial did not measure serum IGF-I levels (Bajetta et al., 2002), and the other only achieved a 39% reduction with the combination of tamoxifen and somatostatin analogue, whereas tamoxifen alone caused a 16.5% decline (suggesting that the somatostatin analogue only lowered serum IGF-I levels by 23%). Pegvisomant, a recently developed GH antagonist, is much more potent at lowering serum IGF-I levels; 20 mg/day in humans can lower serum IGF-I by 62.5% (Trainer et al., 2000) and does not cause an increase in GH levels, which may be one of the negative features of somatostatin analogues. We have shown that pegvisomant can lower serum IGF-I levels by up to 80% in mice, and that it can block the growth of MCF-7 xenografts. As pegvisomant is already FDA approved for the treatment of acromegaly, and has relatively few side effects, this would make this drug an attractive candidate to test as a preventative agent in breast cancer.

SUMMARY AND CONCLUSION

Substantial evidence indicates that the IGF family regulates both mammary gland development and function and also mammary tumorigenesis and metastasis. This has led to the IGF pathway becoming a very attractive target for therapeutic intervention, and numerous pharmaceutical agents are currently being developed and tested. One interesting aspect of the IGF family is its ability to interact with pathways we already know to be critical in breast cancer, e.g., ER and ErbB2. It is likely that these critical signaling networks are essential for normal mammary gland development and become deregulated during the earliest stages of breast cancer initiation. It is with this knowledge that we believe the IGF pathway is a very attractive candidate for not only therapeutic intervention but also breast cancer prevention. The next five to ten years will see the testing of multiple inhibitors of IGF signaling in breast cancer and will finally place the clinical significance of this pathway in breast cancer.

ACKNOWLEDGMENTS

This work was supported in part by Public Health Service grants R01CA94118 (AVL) and P01CA30195 (CKO/AVL). AVL is a recipient of a T.T. Chao Scholar Award (Department of Medicine, Baylor College of Medicine). Dr. Dearth was supported in part by a Training

Program in Molecular Endocrinology (DK07696) and a Training Program in Translational Breast Cancer Research (CA90221). Angelo Casa is supported by a Department of Defense Predoctoral Fellowship Award (W81XWH-06-1-0714).

REFERENCES

Allen GW, Saba C, Armstrong EA, Huang SM, Benavente S, Ludwig DL, Hicklin DJ, Harari PM. Insulin-like Growth Factor-I Receptor Signaling Blockade Combined with Radiation. Cancer Res 2007; 67(3):1155–1162.

Andrews DW, Resnicoff M, Flanders AE, Kenyon L, Curtis M, Merli G, Baserga R, Iliakis G, Aiken RD. Results of a pilot study involving the use of an antisense oligodeoxynucleotide directed against the insulin-like growth factor type I receptor in malignant astrocytomas. J Clin Oncol 2001; 19(8):2189–2200.

Attard G, Fong PC, Molife R, Reade S, Shaw II, Reid A, Spicer J, Hamlin J, Gualberto A, De Bono JS. Phase I trial involving the pharmacodynamic (PD) study of circulating tumour cells, of CP-751,871 (C), a monoclonal antibody against the insulin-like growth factor 1 receptor (IGF-1R), with docetaxel (D) in patients (p) with advanced cancer. 2006 ASCO Annual Meeting Proceedings Part I, June 20 supplement. J Clin Oncol 2006; 24(18S):3023.

Bajetta E, Procopio G, Ferrari L, Martinetti A, Zilembo N, Catena L, Alu M, Della TS, Alberti D, Buzzoni R. A randomized, multicenter prospective trial assessing long-acting release octreotide pamoate plus tamoxifen as a first line therapy for advanced breast carcinoma. Cancer 2002; 94(2):299–304.

Baker J, Liu J-P, Robertson EJ, Efstratiadis A. Role of insulin-like growth factors in embryonic and postnatal growth. Cell 1993; 75:73–82.

Baserga R. The insulin-like growth factor I receptor: a key to tumor growth? Cancer Res 1995; 55(2):249–252.

Baserga R. The contradictions of the insulin-like growth factor 1 receptor. Oncogene 2000; 19(49):5574–5581.

Baserga R, Peruzzi F, Reiss K. The IGF-1 receptor in cancer biology. Int J Cancer 2003; 107(6):873–877.

Bates P, Fisher R, Ward A, Richardson L, Hill DJ, Graham CF. Mammary cancer in transgenic mice overexpressing insulin-like growth factor II (IGF-II). Br J Cancer 1995; 72:1189–1193.

Bocchinfuso WP, Korach KS. Mammary gland development and tumorigenesis in estrogen receptor knockout mice. J Mammary Gland Biol Neoplasia 1997; 2(4):323–334.

Bocchinfuso WP, Lindzey JK, Hewitt SC, Clark JA, Myers PH, Cooper R, Korach KS. Induction of mammary gland development in estrogen receptor-alpha knockout mice. Endocrinology 2000; 141(8):2982–2994.

Bonnette SG, Hadsell DL. Targeted disruption of the IGF-I receptor gene decreases cellular proliferation in mammary terminal end buds. Endocrinology 2001; 142(11):4937–4945.

Boyd NF, Lockwood GA, Martin LJ, Knight JA, Byng JW, Yaffe MJ, Tritchler DL. Mammographic densities and breast cancer risk. Breast Dis 1998; 10(3–4):113–126.

Byrne C, Hankinson SE, Pollak M, Willett WC, Colditz GA, Speizer FE. Insulin-like growth factors and mammographic density. Growth Horm IGF Res 2000; 10(suppl A):S24–S25.

Cai D, Dhe-Paganon S, Melendez PA, Lee J, Shoelson SE. Two new substrates in insulin signaling, IRS5/DOK4 and IRS6/DOK5. J Biol Chem 2003; 278(28):25323–25330.

Campbell RA, Bhat-Nakshatri P, Patel NM, Constantinidou D, Ali S, Nakshatri H. Phosphatidylinositol 3-kinase/AKT-mediated activation of estrogen receptor alpha: a new model for anti-estrogen resistance. J Biol Chem 2001; 276 (13):9817–9824.

Carboni JM, Lee AV, Hadsell DL, Rowley BR, Lee FY, Bol DK, Camuso AE, Gottardis M, Greer AF, Ho CP, Hurlburt W, Li A, Saulnier M, Velaparthi U, Wang C, Wen ML, Westhouse RA, Wittman M, Zimmermann K, Rupnow BA, Wong TW. Tumor development by transgenic expression of a constitutively active insulin-like growth factor I receptor. Cancer Res 2005; 65(9):3781–3787.

Chan TW, Pollak M, Huynh H. Inhibition of insulin-like growth factor signaling pathways in mammary gland by pure anti-estrogen ICI 182,780. Clin Cancer Res 2001; 7(8):2545–2554.

Chang Q, Li Y, White MF, Fletcher JA, Xiao S. Constitutive activation of insulin receptor substrate 1 is a frequent event in human tumors: therapeutic implications. Cancer Res 2002; 62(21):6035–6038.

Clemmons DR, Busby WH, Arai T, Nam TJ, Clark JB, Jones JI, Ankrapp DK. Role of insulin-like growth factor binding proteins in the control of IGF action. Prog Growth Factor Res 1995; 6:357–366.

Cohen BD, Baker DA, Soderstrom C, Tkalcevic G, Rossi AM, Miller PE, Tengowski MW, Wang F, Gualberto A, Beebe JS, Moyer JD. Combination therapy enhances the inhibition of tumor growth with the fully human anti-type 1 insulin-like growth factor receptor monoclonal antibody CP-751,871. Clin Cancer Res 2005; 11(5):2063–2073.

Cui X, Kim HJ, Kuiatse I, Kim H, Brown PH, Lee AV. Epidermal growth factor induces insulin receptor substrate-2 in breast cancer cells via c-Jun NH(2)-terminal kinase/activator protein-1 signaling to regulate cell migration. Cancer Res 2006; 66(10):5304–5313.

Cullen KJ, Yee D, Sly WS, Perdue J, Hampton B, Lippman ME, Rosen N. Insulin-like growth factor receptor expression and function in human breast cancer. Cancer Res 1990; 50(1): 48–53.

Cunha GR, Young P, Hom YK, Cooke PS, Taylor JA, Lubahn DB. Elucidation of a role for stromal steroid hormone receptors in mammary gland growth and development using tissue recombinants. J Mammary Gland Biol Neoplasia 1997; 2(4):393–402.

Datta SR, Dudek H, Tao X, Masters S, Fu H, Gotoh Y, Greenberg ME. Akt phosphorylation of BAD couples survival signals to the cell-intrinsic death machinery. Cell 1997; 91(2):231–241.

Daughaday W. Insulin-like growth factors I and II. Peptide, messenger ribonucleic acid and gene structures, serum, and tissue concentrations. Endocr Rev 1988; 10:68–91.

Debnath J, Brugge JS. Modelling glandular epithelial cancers in three-dimensional cultures. Nat Rev Cancer 2005; 5(9): 675–688.

De Mellow JS, Baxter RC. Growth hormone-dependent insulin-like growth factor (IGF) binding protein both inhibits and potentiates IGF-stimulated DNA synthesis in human skin fibroblasts. Biochem Biophys Res Commun 1988; 156: 199–204.

Dey BR, Frick K, Lopaczynski W, Nissley SP, Furlanetto RW Evidence for the direct interaction of the insulin-like growth factor I receptor with IRS-1, Shc, and Grb10. Mol Endocrinol 1996; 10(6):631–641.

DiNitto JP, Lambright DG. Membrane and juxtamembrane targeting by PH and PTB domains. Biochim Biophys Acta 2006; 1761(8):850–867.

Divisova J, Kuiatse I, Lazard Z, Weiss H, Vreeland F, Hadsell DL, Schiff R, Osborne CK, Lee AV. The growth hormone receptor antagonist pegvisomant blocks both mammary gland development and MCF-7 breast cancer xenograft growth. Breast Cancer Res Treat 2006a; 98(3):315–327.

Divisova J, Kuiatse I, Lazard Z, Weiss H, Vreeland F, Hadsell DL, Schiff R, Osborne CK, Lee AV. The growth hormone receptor antagonist pegvisomant blocks both mammary gland development and MCF-7 breast cancer xenograft growth. Breast Cancer Res Treat 2006b; 98(3):315–327.

Dolan JT, Miltenburg DM, Granchi TS, Miller CC III, Brunicardi FC. Treatment of metastatic breast cancer with somatostatin analogues—a meta-analysis. Ann Surg Oncol 2001; 8(3):227–233.

Dunn SE, Ehrlich M, Sharp NJ, Reiss K, Solomon G, Hawkins R, Baserga R, Barrett JC. A dominant negative mutant of the insulin-like growth factor-I receptor inhibits the adhesion, invasion, and metastasis of breast cancer. Cancer Res 1998; 58(15):3353–3361.

Dunn SE, Hardman RA, Kari FW, Barrett JC. Insulin-like Growth Factor 1 (IGF-1) Alters Drug Sensitivity of HBL100 Human Breast Cancer Cells by Inhibition of Apoptosis Induced by Diverse Anticancer Drugs. Cancer Res 1997a; 57(13):2687–2693.

Dunn SE, Kari FW, French J, Leininger JR, Travlos G, Wilson R, Barrett JC Dietary restriction reduces insulin-like growth factor I levels, which modulates apoptosis, cell proliferation, and tumor progression in p53-deficient mice. Cancer Res 1997b; 57(21):4667–4672.

Eastman A. Activation of programmed cell death by anticancer agents: cisplatin as a model system. Cancer Cell 1990; 2(8–9):275–280.

Frasca F, Pandini G, Scalia P, Sciacca L, Mineo R, Costantino A, Goldfine ID, Belfiore A, Vigneri R. Insulin receptor isoform A, a newly recognized, high-affinity insulin-like growth factor II receptor in fetal and cancer cells. Mol Cell Biol 1999; 19(5):3278–3288.

Gallego MI, Binart N, Robinson GW, Okagaki R, Coschigano KT, Perry J, Kopchick JJ, Oka T, Kelly PA, Hennighausen L. Prolactin, Growth Hormone, and Epidermal Growth Factor Activate Stat5 in Different Compartments of Mammary Tissue and Exert Different and Overlapping Developmental Effects. Dev Biol 2001; 229(1):163–175.

Garcia-Echeverria C, Pearson MA, Marti A, Meyer T, Mestan J, Zimmermann J, Gao J, Brueggen J, Capraro HG, Cozens R, Evans DB, Fabbro D, Furet P, Porta DG, Liebetanz J, Martiny-Baron G, Ruetz S, Hofmann F. In vivo antitumor activity of NVP-AEW541-A novel, potent, and selective inhibitor of the IGF-IR kinase. Cancer Cell 2004; 5(3): 231–239.

Giani C, Cullen KJ, Campani D, Rasmussen A. IGF-II mRNA and protein are expressed in the stroma of invasive breast cancers: an in situ hybridization and immunohitochemistry study. Breast Cancer Res Treat 1996; 41(1):43–50.

Gilmore AP, Valentijn AJ, Wang P, Ranger AM, Bundred N, O'Hare MJ, Wakeling A, Korsmeyer SJ, Streuli CH. Activation of BAD by therapeutic inhibition of epidermal growth factor receptor and transactivation by insulin-like growth factor receptor. J Biol Chem 2002; 277(31): 27643–27650.

Girnita A, Girnita L, del Prete F, Bartolazzi A, Larsson O, Axelson M. Cyclolignans as inhibitors of the insulin-like growth factor-1 receptor and malignant cell growth. Cancer Res 2004; 64(1):236–242.

Giunciuglio D, Culty M, Fassina G, Masiello L, Melchiori A, Paglialunga G, Arand G, Ciardiello F, Basolo F, Thompson EW, et al. Invasive phenotype of MCF10A cells overexpressing c-Ha-ras and c-erbB-2 oncogenes. Int J Cancer 1995; 63(6):815–822.

Goetsch L, Gonzalez A, Leger O, Beck A, Pauwels PJ, Haeuw JF, Corvaia N. A recombinant humanized anti-insulin-like growth factor receptor type I antibody (h7C10) enhances the antitumor activity of vinorelbine and anti-epidermal growth factor receptor therapy against human cancer xenografts. Int J Cancer 2005; 113(2):316–328.

Goya M, Miyamoto S, Nagai K, Ohki Y, Nakamura K, Shitara K, Maeda H, Sangai T, Kodama K, Endoh Y, Ishii G, Hasebe T, Yonou H, Hatano T, Ogawa Y, Ochiai A. Growth inhibition of human prostate cancer cells in human adult bone implanted into nonobese diabetic/severe combined immunodeficient mice by a ligandspecific antibody to human insulin-like growth factors. Cancer Res 2004; 64(17):6252–6258.

Hadsell DL, Bonnette SG, Lee AV. Genetic manipulation of the IGF-I axis to regulate mammary gland development and function. J Dairy Sci 2002; 85(2):365–377.

Hadsell DL, Greenberg NM, Fligger JM, Baumrucker CR, Rosen JM. Targeted expression of des(1-3) human insulin-like growth factor I in transgenic mice influences mammary gland development and IGF-binding protein expression [see comments]. Endocrinology 1996; 137(1):321–330.

Hadsell DL, Murphy KL, Bonnette SG, Reece N, Laucirica R, Rosen JM. Cooperative interaction between mutant p53 and des(1-3)IGF-I accelerates mammary tumorigenesis. Oncogene 2000; 19(7):889–898.

Hadsell DL, Olea W, Lawrence N, George J, Torres D, Kadowaki T, Lee AV. Decreased lactation capacity and altered milk composition in insulin receptor substrate null mice is associated with decreased maternal body mass and reduced insulin-dependent phosphorylation of mammary Akt. J Endocrinol 2007; 194(2):327–336.

Hankins GR, De Souza AT, Bentley RC, Patel MR, Marks JR, Iglehart JD, Jirtle RL. M6P/IGF2 receptor: a candidate breast tumor supressor gene. Oncogene 1996; 12: 2003–2009.

Hankinson SE, Willett WC, Colditz GA, Hunter DJ, Michaud DS, Deroo B, Rosner B, Speizer FE, Pollak M. Circulating concentrations of insulin-like growth factor-I and risk of breast cancer. Lancet 1998; 351(9113):1393–1396.

Hennighausen L, Robinson GW. Think globally, act locally: the making of a mouse mammary gland. Genes Dev 1998; 12 (4):449–455.

Humphreys RC, Lydon J, O'Malley BW, Rosen JM. Mammary gland development is mediated by both stromal and epithelial progesterone receptors. Mol Endocrinol 1997; 11(6):801–811.

Ingle JN, Suman VJ, Kardinal CG, Krook JE, Mailliard JA, Veeder MH, Loprinzi CL, Dalton RJ, Hartmann LC, Conover CA, Pollak MN. A randomized trial of tamoxifen alone or combined with octreotide in the treatment of women with metastatic breast carcinoma. Cancer 1999; 85(6): 1284–1292.

Irie HY, Pearline RV, Grueneberg D, Hsia M, Ravichandran P, Kothari N, Natesan S, Brugge JS. Distinct roles of Akt1 and Akt2 in regulating cell migration and epithelial-mesenchymal transition. J Cell Biol 2005; 171(6): 1023–1034.

Jones RA, Campbell CI, Gunther EJ, Chodosh LA, Petrik JJ, Khokha R, Moorehead RA. Transgenic overexpression of IGF-IR disrupts mammary ductal morphogenesis and induces tumor formation. Oncogene 2006a.

Jones JI, Clemmons DR. Insulin-like growth factors and their binding proteins: biological actions. Endocr Rev 1995; 16(1): 3–34.

Jones JI, Gockerman A, Busby WH Jr., Wright G, Clemmons DR Insulin-like growth factor binding protein 1 stimulates cell migration and binds to the alpha 5 beta 1 integrin by means of its Arg-Gly-Asp sequence. Proc Natl Acad Sci U S A 1993; 90(22):10553–10557.

Jones HE, Goddard L, Gee JM, Hiscox S, Rubini M, Barrow D, Knowlden JM, Williams S, Wakeling AE, Nicholson RI. Insulin-like growth factor-I receptor signalling and acquired resistance to gefitinib (ZD1839; Iressa) in human breast and prostate cancer cells. Endocr Relat Cancer 2004; 11(4): 793–814.

Jones RB, Gordus A, Krall JA, MacBeath G A quantitative protein interaction network for the ErbB receptors using protein microarrays. Nature 2006b; 439(7073):168–174.

Kahlert S, Nuedling S, van Eickels M, Vetter H, Meyer R, and Grohe C. Estrogen receptor alpha rapidly activates the IGF-1 receptor pathway. J Biol Chem 2000; 275(24): 18447–18453.

Kaleko M, Rutter WJ, Miller AD. Overexpression of the human insulinlike growth factor I receptor promotes ligand-dependent neoplastic transformation. Mol Cell Biol 1990; 10(2):464–473.

Kleinberg DL. Role of IGF-I in normal mammary development. Breast Cancer Res Treat 1998; 47(3):201–208.

Kleinberg DL, Feldman M, Ruan W. IGF-I: an essential factor in terminal end bud formation and ductal morphogenesis. J Mammary Gland Biol Neoplasia 2000; 5(1):7–17.

Knowlden JM, Hutcheson IR, Barrow D, Gee JM, Nicholson RI. Insulin-like growth factor-I receptor signaling in tamoxifen-resistant breast cancer: a supporting role to the epidermal growth factor receptor. Endocrinology 2005; 146(11): 4609–4618.

Korner C, Nurnberg B, Uhde M, Braulke T. Mannose-6-phosphate/insulin-like growth factor II receptor fails to interact with G-proteins. J Biol Chem 1995; 270(1):287–295.

Koval AP, Blakesley VA, Roberts CT Jr., Zick Y, Leroith D. Interaction in vitro of the product of the c-Crk-II proto-oncogene with the insulin-like growth factor I receptor. Biochem J 1998; 330(pt 2):923–932.

Lacy M, Alsina M, Melvin CL, Roberts L, D., Y., Petersen JF, Birgin A, Poutney S, Sharma A, Gualberto A. Phase 1 first-in-human dose escalation study of cp- 751,871, a specific monoclonal antibody against the insulin like growth factor 1 receptor. ASCO Annual Meeting Proceedings Part I. J Clin Oncol 2006; 24(18S):7609.

Lavan BE, Fantin VR, Chang ET, Lane WS, Keller SR, Lienhard GE A novel 160-kDa phosphotyrosine protein in insulin-treated embryonic kidney cells is a new member of the insulin receptor substrate family. J Biol Chem 1997a; 272 (34):21403–21407.

Lavan BE, Lane WS, Lienhard GE. The 60-kDa phosphotyrosine protein in insulin-treated adipocytes is a new member of the insulin receptor substrate family. J Biol Chem 1997b; 272 (17):11439–11443.

Lee A, Zhang P, Ivanova M, Bonnette SG, Oesterreich S, Rosen JM, Grimm SL, Hovey RC, Vonderhaar BK, Kahn CR, Torres D, George J, Mohsin S, Allred DC, Hadsell DL. Developmental and hormonal signals dramatically alter the localization and abundance of insulin receptor substrate proteins in the mammary gland. Proceeding of the 84th Annual Endocrine Society Meeting, 2002.

Lee AV, Jackson JG, Gooch JL, Hilsenbeck SG, Coronado-Heinsohn E, Osborne CK, and Yee D. Enhancement of insulin-like growth factor signaling in human breast cancer: estrogen regulation of insulin receptor substrate-1 expression in vitro and in vivo. Mol Endocrinol 1999; 13(5): 787–796.

Lee AV, Weng CN, Jackson JG, Yee D. Activation of estrogen receptormediated gene transcription by IGF-I in human breast cancer cells. J Endocrinol 1997; 152(1):39–47.

Lee AV, Zhang P, Ivanova M, Bonnette S, Oesterreich S, Rosen JM, Grimm S, Hovey RC, Vonderhaar BK, Kahn CR, Torres D, George J, Mohsin S, Allred DC, Hadsell DL. Developmental and hormonal signals dramatically alter the localization and abundance of insulin receptor substrate proteins in the mammary gland. Endocrinology 2003; 144 (6):2683–2694.

LeRoith D, Helman L. The new kid on the block(ade) of the IGF-1 receptor. Cancer Cell 2004; 5(3):201–202.

Li BD, Khosravi MJ, Berkel HJ, Diamandi A, Dayton MA, Smith M, Yu H. Free insulin-like growth factor-I and breast cancer risk. Int J Cancer 2001; 91(5):736–739.

Li SL, Liang SJ, Guo N, Wu AM, Fujita-Yamaguchi Y. Single-chain antibodies against human insulin-like growth factor I receptor: expression, purification, and effect on tumor growth. Cancer Immunol Immunother 2000; 49(4–5): 243–252.

Li S, Resnicoff M, Baserga R. Effect of mutations at serines 1280-1283 on the mitogenic and transforming activities of the insulin-like growth factor I receptor. J Biol Chem 1996; 271(21):12254–12260.

Louvi A, Accili D, Efstratiadis A. Growth-promoting interaction of IGF-II with the insulin receptor during mouse embryonic development. Dev Biol 1997; 189(1):33–48.

Lu Y, Zi X, Zhao Y, Mascarenhas D, Pollak M. Insulin-Like Growth Factor-I Receptor Signaling and Resistance to Trastuzumab (Herceptin). J Natl Cancer Inst 2001; 93 (24):1852–1857.

Lynch L, Vodyanik PI, Boettiger D, Guvakova MA. Insulin-like growth factor I controls adhesion strength mediated by alpha5beta1 integrins in motile carcinoma cells. Mol Biol Cell 2005; 16(1):51–63.

MacDonald RG, Pfeffer S, Coussens L, Tepper M, Brocklebank C, Mole J, Anderson J, Chen E, Czech M, Ullrich A. A single receptor binds both insulin-like growth factor II and mannose-6-phosphate. Science 1988; 239:1134–1137.

Mathieu M, Rochefort H, Barenton B, Prebois C, Vignon F. Interactions of cathepsin-D and insulin-like growth factor-II (IGF-II) on the IGF-II/mannose-6-phosphate receptor in human breast cancer cells and possible consequences on mitogenic activity of IGF-II. Mol Endocrinol 1990; 4 (9):1327–1335.

Mauro L, Salerno M, Panno ML, Bellizzi D, Sisci D, Miglietta A, Surmacz E, Ando S. Estradiol increases IRS-1 gene expression and insulin signaling in breast cancer cells. Biochem Biophys Res Commun 2001; 288(3):685–689.

Miller BS, Yee D. Type I insulin-like growth factor receptor as a therapeutic target in cancer. Cancer Res 2005; 65 (22):10123–10127.

Molloy CA, May FE, Westley BR. Insulin receptor substrate-1 expression is regulated by estrogen in the MCF-7 human breast cancer cell line. J Biol Chem 2000; 275(17): 12565–12571.

Morgan DO. Insulin-like growth factor II receptor as a multi-functional binding protein. Nature 1987; 326:300–307.

Muthuswamy SK, Li D, Lelievre S, Bissell MJ, Brugge JS. ErbB2, but not ErbB1, reinitiates proliferation and induces luminal repopulation in epithelial acini. Nat Cell Biol 2001; 3(9):785–792.

Neuenschwander S, Schwartz A, Wood TL, Roberts CT Jr., Henninghausen L, LeRoith D. Involution of the lactating mammary gland is inhibited by the IGF system in a transgenic mouse model. J Clin Invest 1996; 97(10): 2225–2232.

Nicholson RI, Hutcheson IR, Britton D, Knowlden JM, Jones HE, Harper ME, Hiscox SE, Barrow D, Gee JMW. Growth factor signalling networks in breast cancer and resistance to endocrine agents: new therapeutic strategies. J Steroid Biochem Mol Biol 2005; 93(2–5):257.

Osborne CK, Coronado EB, Kitten LJ, Arteaga CR, Fuqua SAW, Ramasharma K, Marshall M, Li CH. Insulin-like growth factor-II (IGF-II): A potential autocrine/paracrine growth factor for human breast cancer acting via the IGF-I receptor. Mol Endocrinol 1989; 3(11):1701–1709.

Pandini G, Vigneri R, Costantino A, Frasca F, Ippolito A, Fujita-Yamaguchi Y, Siddle K, Goldfine ID, Belfiore A Insulin and insulin-like growth factor-I (IGF-I) receptor overexpression in breast cancers leads to insulin/IGF-I hybrid receptor overexpression: evidence for a second mechanism of IGF-I signaling. Clin Cancer Res 1999; 5(7):1935–1944.

Papa V, Gliozzo B, Clark G, McGuire W, Moore D, Fujita-Yamaguchi Y, Vigneri R, Goldfine I, Pezzino V. Insulin-like growth factor-I receptors are overexpressed and predict a low risk in human breast cancer. Cancer Res 1993; 53:3736–3740.

Peruzzi F, Prisco M, Dews M, Salomoni P, Grassilli E, Romano G, Calabretta B, Baserga R. Multiple signaling pathways of the insulin-like growth factor 1 receptor in protection from apoptosis. Mol Cell Biol 1999; 19(10):7203–7215.

Peyrat JP, Bonneterre J, Beuscart R, Djiane J, Demaille A. Insulin-like growth factor 1 receptors in human breast cancer and their relation to estradiol and progesterone receptors. Cancer Res 1988; 48(22):6429–6433.

Pollak MN. Endocrine effects of IGF-I on normal and transformed breast epithelial cells: potential relevance to strategies for breast cancer treatment and prevention. Breast Cancer Res Treat 1998; 47(3):209–217.

Pollack MN, Perdue JF, Margolese RG, Baer K, Richard M. Presence of somatomedin receptors on human breast and colon carcinoma. Cancer Lett 1987; 38:223–230.

Pollak MN, Schernhammer ES, Hankinson SE. Insulin-like growth factors and neoplasia. Nat Rev Cancer 2004; 4(7):505–518.

Ramsey MM, Ingram RL, Cashion AB, Ng AH, Cline JM, Parlow AF, Sonntag WE. Growth hormone-deficient dwarf animals are resistant to dimethylbenzanthracine (DMBA)-induced mammary carcinogenesis. Endocrinology 2002; 143(10):4139–4142.

Resnicoff M, Burgaud JL, Rotman HL, Abraham D, Baserga R. Correlation between apoptosis, tumorigenesis, and levels of insulin-like growth factor I receptors. Cancer Res 1995; 55(17):3739–3741.

Resnik JL, Reichart DB, Huey K, Webster NJ, Seely BL. Elevated insulin-like growth factor I receptor autophosphorylation and kinase activity in human breast cancer. Cancer Res 1998; 58(6):1159–1164.

Richert MM, Schwertfeger KL, Ryder JW, Anderson SM. An atlas of mouse mammary galnd development. J Mammary Gland Biol Neoplasia 2000; 5:227–241.

Richert MM, Wood TL. The insulin-like growth factors (IGF) and IGF type I receptor during postnatal growth of the murine mammary gland: sites of messenger ribonucleic acid expression and potential functions. Endocrinology 1999; 140(1):454–461.

Rinderknecht E, Humbel RE. Polypeptides with nonsuppressible insulin-like and cell-growth promoting activities in human serum: isolation, chemical characterization, and some biological properties of forms I and II. Proc Natl Acad Sci USA 1976; 73(7):2365–2369.

Ruan W, Kleinberg DL. Insulin-like growth factor I is essential for terminal end bud formation and ductal morphogenesis during mammary development. Endocrinology 1999; 140 (11):5075–5081.

Sachdev D, Hartell JS, Lee AV, Zhang X, Yee D. A dominant negative type I insulin-like growth factor receptor inhibits metastasis of human cancer cells. J Biol Chem 2004; 279 (6):5017–5024.

Sachdev D, Singh R, Fujita-Yamaguchi Y, Yee D. Down-regulation of insulin receptor by antibodies against the type I insulin-like growth factor receptor: implications for anti-insulin-like growth factor therapy in breast cancer. Cancer Res 2006; 66(4):2391–2402.

Sachdev D, Yee D. The IGF system and breast cancer. Endocr Relat Cancer 2001; 8(3):197–209.

Sachdev D, Yee D. Inhibitors of insulin-like growth factor signaling: a therapeutic approach for breast cancer. J Mammary Gland Biol Neoplasia 2006; 11(1):27–39.

Sakatani T, Kaneda A, Iacobuzio-Donahue CA, Carter MG, de Boom Witzel S, Okano H, Ko MS, Ohlsson R, Longo DL, Feinberg AP. Loss of imprinting of Igf2 alters intestinal maturation and tumorigenesis in mice. Science 2005; 307 (5717):1976–1978.

Schillaci R, Salatino M, Cassataro J, Proietti CJ, Giambartolomei GH, Rivas MA, Carnevale RP, Charreau EH, Elizalde PV. Immunization with murine breast cancer cells treated with antisense oligodeoxynucleotides to type I insulin-like growth factor receptor induced an antitumoral effect mediated by a CD8+ response involving Fas/Fas ligand cytotoxic pathway. J Immunol 2006; 176(6):3426–3437.

Seagroves TN, Lydon JP, Hovey RC, Vonderhaar BK, Rosen JM. C/EBPbeta (CCAAT/enhancer binding protein) controls cell fate determination during mammary gland development. Mol Endocrinol 2000; 14(3):359–368.

Sell C, Dumenil G, Deveaud C, Miura M, Coppola D, DeAngelis T, Rubin R, Efstratiadis A, Baserga R. Effect of a null mutation of the insulin-like growth factor I receptor gene on growth and transformation of mouse embryo fibroblasts. Mol Cell Biol 1994; 14(6):3604–3612.

Sell C, Rubini M, Rubin R, Liu JP, Efstratiadis A, Baserga R. Simian virus 40 large tumor antigen is unable to transform mouse embryonic fibroblasts lacking type 1 insulin-like growth factor receptor. Proc Natl Acad Sci U S A 1993; 90(23):11217–11221.

Simoncini T, Hafezi-Moghadam A, Brazil DP, Ley K, Chin WW, Liao JK. Interaction of oestrogen receptor with the regulatory subunit of phosphatidylinositol-3-OH kinase. Nature 2000; 407(6803):538–541.

Slaaby R, Schaffer L, Lautrup-Larsen I, Andersen AS, Shaw AC, Mathiasen IS, Brandt J. Hybrid receptors formed by insulin receptor (IR) and insulin-like growth factor I receptor (IGF-IR) have low insulin and high IGF-1 affinity irrespective of the IR splice variant. J Biol Chem 2006; 281(36):25869–25874.

Steele-Perkins G, Turner J, Edman J, Hari J, Pierce S, Stover C, Rutter W, Roth R. Expression and characterisation of a functional human insulin-like growth factor I receptor. J Biol Chem 1988; 23:11486–11492.

Stewart AJ, Johnson MD, May FE, Westley BR. Role of insulin-like growth factors and the type I insulin-like growth factor receptor in the estrogen-stimulated proliferation of human breast cancer cells. J Biol Chem 1990; 265(34):21172–21178.

Stull M, Richert M, Wood T. IGF-mediated growth of mammary epithelium during ductal development in the mouse. Growth Horm IGF Res 2000; 9(5):320.

Sun XJ, Rothenberg P, Kahn CR, Backer JM, Araki E, Wilden PA, Cahill DA, Goldstein BJ, White MF. Structure of the insulin receptor substrate IRS-1 defines a unique signal transduction protein. Nature 1991; 352 (6330):73–77.

Sun XJ, Wang LM, Zhang Y, Yenush L, Myers MG Jr., Glasheen E, Lane WS, Pierce JH, White MF. Role of IRS-2 in insulin and cytokine signalling. Nature 1995; 377 (6545):173–177.

Surmacz E. Function of the IGF-I receptor in breast cancer. J Mammary Gland Biol Neoplasia 2000; 5(1):95–105.

Surmacz E. Growth factor receptors as therapeutic targets: strategies to inhibit the insulin-like growth factor I receptor. Oncogene 2003; 22(42):6589–6597.

Surmacz E, Guvakova MA, Nolan MK, Nicosia RF, Sciacca L. Type I insulin-like growth factor receptor function in breast cancer. Breast Cancer Res Treat 1998; 47(3):255–267.

Thissen JP, Ketelslegers JM, Underwood LE. Nutritional regulation of the insulin-like growth factors. Endocr Rev 1994; 15(1):80–101.

Tollefsen SE, Stoszek RM, Thompson K. Interaction of the alpha beta dimers of the insulin-like growth factor I receptor is required for receptor autophosphorylation. Biochemistry 1991; 30(1):48–54.

Trainer PJ, Drake WM, Katznelson L, Freda PU, Herman-Bonert V, van der Lely AJ, Dimaraki EV, Stewart PM, Friend KE, Vance ML, Besser GM, Scarlett JA, Thorner MO, Parkinson C, Klibanski A, Powell JS, Barkan AL, Sheppard MC, Malsonado M, Rose DR, Clemmons DR, Johannsson G, Bengtsson BA, Stavrou S, Kleinberg DL, Cook DM, Phillips LS, Bidlingmaier M, Strasburger CJ, Hackett S, Zib K, Bennett WF, Davis RJ. Treatment of acromegaly with the growth hormone-receptor antagonist pegvisomant (see comments). N Engl J Med 2000; 342(16):1171–1177.

Turner BC, Haffty BG, Narayanan L, Yuan J, Havre PA, Gumbs AA, Kaplan L, Burgaud JL, Carter D, Baserga R, Glazer PM. Insulin-like growth factor-I receptor overexpression mediates cellular radioresistance and local breast cancer recurrence after lumpectomy and radiation. Cancer Res 1997; 57(15):3079–3083.

Ullrich A, Gray A, Tam A, Yang-Feng T, Tsubokawa M, Collins C, Henzel W, Le Bon T, Kathuria S, Chen E, Jacobs S, Francke U, Ramachandran J, Fujita-Yamaguchi Y. Insulin-like growth factor I receptor primary structure: comparison with insulin receptor suggests structural determinants that define functional specificity. EMBO J 1986; 5(10): 2503–2512.

Valentinis B, Baserga R. IGF-I receptor signalling in transformation and differentiation. Mol Pathol 2001; 54(3): 133–137.

Warshamana-Greene GS, Litz J, Buchdunger E, Garcia-Echeverria C, Hofmann F, Krystal GW. The Insulin-Like Growth Factor-I Receptor Kinase Inhibitor, NVPADW742, Sensitizes Small Cell Lung Cancer Cell Lines to the Effects of Chemotherapy. Clin Cancer Res 2005; 11(4):1563–1571.

Winnay JN, Bruning JC, Burks DJ, Kahn CR. Gab-1-mediated IGF-1 signaling in IRS-1-deficient 3T3 fibroblasts. J Biol Chem 2000; 275(14):10545–10550.

Wittman M, Carboni J, Attar R, Balasubramanian B, Balimane P, Brassil P, Beaulieu F, Chang C, Clarke W, Dell J, Eummer J, Frennesson D, Gottardis M, Greer A, Hansel S, Hurlburt W, Jacobson B, Krishnananthan S, Lee FY, Li A, Lin TA, Liu P, Ouellet C, Sang X, Saulnier MG, Stoffan K, Sun Y, Velaparthi U, Wong H, Yang Z, Zimmermann K,

Zoeckler M, Vyas D. Discovery of a (1H-benzoimidazol-2-yl)-1H-pyridin-2-one (BMS-536924) inhibitor of insulin-like growth factor I receptor kinase with in vivo antitumor activity. J Med Chem 2005; 48(18):5639–5643.

Wolf G, Trub T, Ottinger E, Groninga L, Lynch A, White MF, Miyazaki M, Lee J, Shoelson SE. PTB domains of IRS-1 and Shc have distinct but overlapping binding specificities. J Biol Chem 1995; 270(46):27407–27410.

Wu Y, Cui K, Miyoshi K, Hennighausen L, Green JE, Setser J, LeRoith D, Yakar S. Reduced circulating insulin-like growth factor I levels delay the onset of chemically and genetically induced mammary tumors. Cancer Res 2003; 63 (15):4384–4388.

Wu Y, Yakar S, Zhao L, Hennighausen L, LeRoith D. Circulating insulin-like growth factor-I levels regulate colon cancer growth and metastasis. Cancer Res 2002; 62 (4):1030–1035.

Yakar S, Green JE, LeRoith D. Serum IGF-I levels as a risk marker in mammary tumors. Proceeding of the 83rd Annual Endocrine Society Meeting. 2001.

Yakar S, LeRoith D, Brodt P. The role of the growth hormone/insulin-like growth factor axis in tumor growth and progression: Lessons from animal models. Cytokine Growth Factor Rev 2005; 16(4–5):407.

Yamauchi K, Pessin JE. Insulin receptor substrate-1 (IRS1) and Shc compete for a limited pool of Grb2 in mediating insulin downstream signaling. J Biol Chem 1994; 269(49): 31107–31114.

Yang XF, Beamer WG, Huynh H, Pollak M. Reduced growth of human breast cancer xenografts in hosts homozygous for the lit mutation. Cancer Res 1996; 56(7):1509–1511.

Yanochko GM, Eckhart W. Type I insulin-like growth factor receptor overexpression induces proliferation and anti-apoptotic signaling in a three-dimensional culture model of breast epithelial cells. Breast Cancer Res 2006; 8(2):R18.

Yarden Y, Sliwkowski MX. Untangling the ErbB signalling network. Nat Rev Mol Cell Biol 2001; 2(2):127–137.

Yee D, Paik S, Lebovic GS, Marcus RR, Favoni RE, Cullen KJ, Lippman ME, Rosen N. Analysis of IGF-I gene expression in human malignancy: evidence for a paracrine role in human breast cancer. Mol Endocrinol 1989; 3:509–517.

Yenush L, White MF. The IRS-signalling system during insulin and cytokine action. Bioessays 1997; 19(6):491–500.

Zha J, Harada H, Yang E, Jockel J, Korsmeyer SJ. Serine phosphorylation of death agonist BAD in response to survival factor results in binding to 14-3-3 not BCLX(L). Cell 1996; 87(4):619–628.

Zhang X, Lin M, van Golen KL, Yoshioka K, Itoh K, Yee D. Multiple signaling pathways are activated during insulin-like growth factor-I (IGF-I) stimulated breast cancer cell migration. Breast Cancer Res Treat 2005; 93(2):159–168.

Zhang H, Pelzer AM, Kiang DT, Yee D. Down-regulation of type I insulin-like growth factor receptor increases sensitivity of breast cancer cells to insulin. Cancer Res 2007; 67(1): 391–397.

17

Insulin-Like Growth Factor-I and Breast Cancer: Epidemiological and Clinical Data

CARLO CAMPAGNOLI and CLEMENTINA PERIS
S.C. Ginecologia Endocrinologica, Ospedale Ginecologico Sant'Anna, Torino, Italy

PATRIZIA PASANISI and FRANCO BERRINO
Dipartimento di Medicina Preventiva e Predittiva, Fondazione IRCCS Istituto Nazionale dei Tumori, Milano, Italy

INTRODUCTION

Insulin-like growth factor-I (IGF-I) has powerful mitogenic and antiapoptotic effects on many cell types, including normal and transformed breast epithelial cells (see chap. 16). The proliferative effects of IGF-I on breast cancer (BC) cells are synergistic with those of estrogens (see chap. 16).

IGF-I production is present in many tissues and is responsive to growth hormone (GH) (Le Roith et al., 2001). Locally produced IGF-I is present also in mammary tissue, particularly in stromal cells clustered around intra- and interlobular ducts (Yee et al., 1989; Cullen et al., 1992; Ng et al., 1997) and in adjacent nonneoplastic tissue in case of BC (Chong et al., 2006). In the breast, IGF-I production is stimulated not only by GH (Ng et al., 1997; Pollak, 1998), but also by estrogens (Veldhuis et al., 2006a). Despite the importance of paracrine effects of locally produced IGF-I (Le Roith et al., 2001), circulating IGF-I could also act on BC (Hecquet and Peyrat, 1990; Westley and May, 1994; Wu et al., 2003).

Circulating IGF-I is mainly of hepatic derivation (Veldhuis et al., 2006a). The production of IGF-I by the hepatocites is stimulated by GH, the secretion of which is influenced by circulating IGF-I level through a negative feedback mechanism. There is tremendous heterogeneity in serum IGF-I concentrations among healthy adults: normal levels of IGF-I can range from 100 to 300 ng/mL, and although GH remains the major regulatory factor controlling serum levels, there are clearly other determinants (Rosen, 2000). Among these, nutritional factors and insulin level have a relevant role, because they modulate the liver responsivity to GH and, consequently, the relationship between GH stimulation and hepatic IGF-I synthesis. Fasting and nutrient deprivation cause a decrease in IGF-I production and serum level with a reactive increase of GH level (Counts et al., 1992; Thissen et al., 1994; Veldhuis et al., 2006a).

A number of epidemiological studies suggest that relatively high levels of circulating IGF-I are associated with clinical conditions that reflect a high degree of tissue proliferation, for instance, a reduced risk of postmenopausal osteoporosis (Rosen, 2000; Garnero et al., 2000; Muñoz-Torres et al., 2001) and an increased risk of some types of cancer, including BC (Renehan et al., 2004; Sugumar et al., 2004; Shi et al., 2004).

Approximately 99% of IGF-I circulates bound to specific proteins (insulin-like growth factor binding proteins, IGFBPs) (Rajaram et al., 1997; Hwa et al., 1999). The most important of these proteins is IGFBP-3, which is synthesized in Kupffer cells of the liver under GH stimulation. More than 75% of circulating IGF-I is carried in a 150-kDa ternary complex composed of IGF-I, IGFBP-3, and an acid-labile subunit (ALS), produced, as the IGF-I, by the hepatocytes. This ternary complex prevalently acts as a reservoir of IGF-I, prolonging the half-life of IGFs and possibly facilitating their endocrine actions (Yakar et al., 2002; Boonen et al., 2002; Veldhuis et al., 2006a). Insulin enhances GH-stimulated synthesis of both IGF-I and IGFBP-3 by increasing levels of GH receptors (Kaaks and Lukanova, 2001). Conversely, insulin inhibits the hepatic synthesis of other non-GH-dependent IGFBPs, the IGFBP-1 and IGFBP-2, that decrease the bioactivity of IGF-I (Rajaram et al., 1997; Veldhuis et al., 2006a). Epidemiological data, even if not consistently, suggest that IGFBP levels can be associated with the risk of developing some kinds of cancer, including BC (Renehan et al., 2004; Sugumar et al., 2004; Shi et al., 2004).

Aim of this chapter is to review the endocrine effects of IGF-I, the epidemiological data on IGF-I/IGFBP system and BC, the regulation of circulating IGF-I levels, and the therapies that influence, increasing or decreasing, blood levels and bioavailability of IGF-I.

ENDOCRINE EFFECTS OF IGF-I

Systemic Metabolic Effects

IGF-I has systemic effects on the whole-body anabolism and also on glucose homeostasis (Gluckmann et al., 1991; Iranmanesh and Veldhuis, 1992; Veldhuis et al., 2006a). The latter effect is partially due to the binding of IGF-I to insulin receptor (IR) or to hybrid insulin/IGF-I receptors. Actually, IGF-I is highly homologous to insulin. The IGF-I receptor (IGF-1R) shares 55% homology with IR. Activation of IGF-1R by IGF-I activates the same proteins and pathways that are activated by insulin and IR (Wolf et al., 2005). Moreover, IGF-I improves insulin sensitivity (contrasting insulin resistance) by both GH dependent and independent mechanisms (O'Connell and Clemmons, 2002). Epidemiological studies have shown that individuals with low serum IGF-I have a twofold increased risk of developing glucose intolerance or type 2 diabetes (Sandhu et al., 2002). This metabolic effect could contribute to explain (together with other potential, more direct mechanisms) the epidemiological findings of an association between low levels of circulating IGF-I and an increased risk of cardiovascular problems, like ischemic heart disease (Juul et al., 2002; Laughlin et al., 2004), hypertension (Hunt et al., 2006), and fatal stroke (van Rijn et al., 2006).

Proliferative Effects on the Tissues

Regarding the mitogenic and antiapoptotic effetcs on the tissues, the levels of circulating IGF-I could have a double significance. Being a marker of the activity of the GH/IGF-I axis, they could reflect the GH-induced expression of the IGF-I at the tissue level (Pollak, 1998). However, several findings do suggest an endocrine GH-independent role of serum IGF-I on some tissues, e.g., bone, muscle, and even the breast.

Bone and Muscle

Liver IGF-I deficient and ALS knockout mice have a sharp decrease (by 85–90%) in circulating IGF-I and a 15-fold reactive increase in serum GH levels. These mice have a significant reduction in growth and in bone mineral density (Yakar et al., 2002). Though this finding does demonstrate that circulating IGF-I is essential for normal bone growth, it must be remembered that this model involves very large variations in IGF-I levels, compared with the more subtle variations in IGF-I physiology that exist among humans (Jenkins et al., 2006). However, even some findings in women support the endocrine action of IGF-I.

1. In young women with anorexia nervosa (AN), the level of circulating IGF-I is significantly decreased and its bioactivity is further reduced by the sharp increase of IGFBP-1 and IGFBP-2 (Kaaks et al., 2003), with very high reactive levels of GH (Counts et al., 1992). The reduction in circulating IGF-I level and activity contributes to the loss of bone tissue, due to reduced tissue formation (Grinspoon et al., 1996). Studies of physiologic doses of recombinant IGF-I (rhIGF-I) in women with AN demonstrate a potent effect of IGF-I to increase indices of bone formation, in spite of a 40% reduction of GH levels (Grinspoon et al., 1996), and also an effect to increase spinal bone density and lean body mass (Grinspoon et al., 2002).
2. The administration of a rhIGF-I/IGFBP-3 complex in patients with femoral fracture contrasts the decrease in hip bone density and increases the muscle strength (Boonen et al., 2002).
3. As estrogen affects GH action at the level of receptor expression and signaling (Leung et al., 2004), high estrogen level in the liver, as obtained by oral estrogen administration, causes a decrease in circulating IGF-I (see sec. "Sex Hormone Therapies"). In a study of menopausal women, markers of connective and bone tissue formation, and even lean body mass, fell in parallel with IGF-I during oral estrogen administration despite a threefold reactive increase in circulating GH levels, and rose during estrogen transdermal treatment in concert with an increase in IGF-I (Leung et al., 2004). The finding provides

indirect evidence that endocrine IGF-I is a more important determinant of peripheral tissue growth in adult humans than local, GH-induced, IGF-I (Leung et al., 2004).

4. Relatively high levels of circulating IGF-I are associated with bone mineral density in young women (Soot et al., 2006) and with reduced risk of osteoporosis and fractures in postmenopausal women (Rosen, 2000; Garnero et al., 2000; Muñoz-Torres et al., 2001).

Breast

1. Liver IGF-I-deficient mice have a 75% reduction in circulating IGF-I, a fourfold reactive increase in serum GH, normal levels of IGF-I mRNA in nonhepatic tissues, and normal body growth and development (Le Roith et al., 2001). However, the reduction in circulating IGF-I in these mice is associated with a marked delay in the onset of chemically and genetically induced mammary tumors (Wu et al., 2003).
2. The administration of IGF-I caused epithelial proliferation in the breast of aging primates, despite relatively suppressed GH levels; the mitogenic effects were apparent even at serum IGF-I concentrations considered physiological for young adults (Ng et al., 1997).
3. Most epidemiological studies suggest that the circulating IGF-I level is associated with BC risk, particularly in premenopausal women (see next section).

CIRCULATING INSULIN-LIKE GROWTH FACTOR-I AND BREAST CANCER RISK: EPIDEMIOLOGICAL DATA

The first case-control study suggesting an association between circulating IGF-I levels and BC risk was published in 1993 (Peyrat et al., 1993). Over 30 papers were subsequently published, most of which reported also on the association of BC with IGFBP-3 and a few with IGFBP-1 and IGFBP-2 also. Several case-control studies were based on small numbers and opportunistically recruited subjects and the results were largely inconsistent. We systematically review here only the results of prospective studies on healthy volunteers who donated a blood sample at recruitment, all of which were analysed comparing prediagnostic circulating levels of incident cases with those of a suitable sample of control subjects who did not develop the disease, with a nested case-control design (Table 1 and Table 2).

The first results of a prospective study were published in 1998 from the Nurses' Health Study cohort (Hankinson et al., 1998) and suggested a strong positive association confined to premenopausal women. All the subsequent studies presented separate results for pre and postmenopausal women. Out of 12 publications on premenopausal women from 10 different studies (Table 1), only one which combined the results of two Swedish cohorts found a relative risk (RR) of BC lower than one, comparing the upper and the lower quartile of the IGF-I distribution

Table 1 Nested Case-Control Analyses of Prospective Cohort Studies of Serum IGF-I and IGFBP-3 Levels and Subsequent BC. Risks of Women in the Upper Quantile of the Distribution Relative to Those in the Lower Quantile

References	Cases	Controls	IGF-I	IGFBP-3
Premenopausal women at recruitment				
Hankinson et al., 1998	76	105	2.3 (1.1–5.2)	
<50 yr at recruitment	60	78	4.6 (1.8–12)	
Schernhammer et al., 2005	218	281	1.6 (1.0–2.5)	1.2 (0.8–1.9)
<50 yr at recruitment (Hankinson et al., 1998)	155	193	2.5 (1.4–4.5)	1.4 (0.8–2.4)
Toniolo et al., 2000	172	486	1.6 (0.9–2.81)	1.2 (0.7–2.1)
≤50 yr at recruitment	96	280	2.3 (1.1–4.9)	2.2 (1.0–4.8)
Rinaldi et al., 2005, Age ≤50 yr (Toniolo et al., 2000)	138	259	1.93 (1.00–3.72)[a]	2.0 (1.1–3.8)[a] functional[b] 1.0 (0.4–2.1)
Muti et al., 2002	69	265	3.1 (1.1–8.6)[a]	2.3 (1.0–5.5)
Krajcik et al., 2000	66	66	3.5 (0.7–18)	5.3 (1.1–24)[a] (adj for IGF-I)
Kaaks et al., 2002	116	330	0.6 (0.3–1.4)	1.4 (0.7–2.9)
Decensi et al., 2003 (second BC in BC patients)	45	220	1.9 (0.9–4.3)	0.4 (0.2–0.9)
Allen et al., 2005	70	209	1.7 (0.7–4.0)	0.5 (0.2–1.1)[a]
Rollison et al., 2006 (post-menopausal at incidence)	175	175	1.4 (0.8–2.4)	0.9 (0.5–1.5)
Lukanova et al., 2006 IGF-I in pregnancy	212	369	1.7 (1.1–2.7)[a]	
Rinaldi et al., 2006 (age at diagnosis ≤50 yr)	250	491	1.0 (0.6–1.8)	0.9 (0.5–1.7)

[a] p trend < 0.05.
[b] Functional IGFBP-3 includes total IGFBP-3 and fragments that can bind IGF-I.

Table 2 Nested Case-Control Analyses of Prospective Cohort Studies of Serum IGF-I and IGFBP-3 Levels and Subsequent BC. Risks of Women in the Upper Quantile of the Distribution Relative to Those in the Lower Quantile

References	Cases	Controls	IGF-I	IGFBP-3
Postmenopausal women				
Hankinson et al., 1998	305	220	0.9 (0.5–1.4)	
Schernhammer et al., 2005 (includes Hankinson et al., 1998)	514	754	1.0 (0.7–1.4)	0.8 (0.6–1.1)
Toniolo et al., 2000	115	220	1.0 (0.5–1.9)	1.1 (0.5–2.2)
Muti et al., 2002	64	238	0.6 (0.2–1.4)	0.7 (0.3–1.7)
Krajcik et al., 2000	60	60	0.8 (0.2–2.6)	0.3 (0.1–1.4) (adj for IGF-I)
Kaaks et al., 2002	392	519	1.3 (0.8–2.1)	1.3 (0.8–2.1)
Keinan-Boker et al., 2003	143	333	1.1 (0.6–2.1)	1.6 (0.7–3.5)
Grønbæk et al., 2004	411	397	1.0 (1.0–1.1)	1.1 (1.0–1.2)
Allen, 2005	47	141	0.8 (0.3–1.7)	0.99 (0.4–2.5)
Rollison, 2006	91	91	1.7 (0.8–3.6)	1.5 (0.8–3.1)
Rinaldi et al., 2006	715	1440	1.4(1.02–1.86)	1.4 (1.0–2.0)[a]

[a] p trend < 0.05.

(Kaaks et al., 2002). The recent extension of the analysis of the Nurses' Health Study did not confirm such a strong association as in the first study, but the overall results remained statistically significant, especially in the young women (Schernhammer et al., 2005). The Northern Sweden Maternity Cohort (Lukanova et al., 2006) confirmed the importance of IGF-I in premenopausal BC by measuring IGF-I during pregnancy. The study showed that BC risk increased significantly with increasing IGF-I. The overall pattern of positive association emerging from the cohort studies, however, was not confirmed by recent analysis of the large European Prospective Investigation into Cancer and Nutrition (EPIC) cohort, which was confined to premenopausal women who developed BC within the age of 50 and did not show any association, except in a subgroup analysis that excluded the cases occurred in the first two years of follow-up (Rinaldi et al., 2006). RR shown in Table 1 are adjusted for age and several potential confounding factors, but not for circulating levels of IGFBPs. Several studies also presented results adjusted for IGFBP-3 and the effect of IGF-I was strengthened after this adjustment in one study (Hankinson et al., 1998) but not in the others. Three of the studies that examined the effect of premenopausal IGFBP-3 levels on BC risk reported a significantly increased RR of the order of 2 or more but the confidence intervals (CI) were wide and several other studies reported no or negative associations (Table 1). In conclusion, the association of circulating IGF-I with increased BC risk in premenopausal women is largely confirmed, but may not be as strong as suggested by earlier studies, possibly with RRs of the order of 2 instead of 3 or 4. One must consider, however, that commercial kits for measuring IGF-I were developed for the diagnosis of GH disorders and not for the investigation of relatively small inter-individual variations within normal populations. For the latter purpose, the performance of these assays may be far from optimal (Fletcher et al., 2005). For IGFBP-3 the picture is more complex, as the original hypothesis was that high circulating levels of IGFBP-3 would be protective, and the results of epidemiological studies are highly heterogeneous. Actually, IGFBP-3 would protect against BC by sequestrating IGF-I and preventing it from interacting with cell receptors, but could also increase the half-life of IGF-I, protecting it from degradation and hence increasing the amount that can reach local tissues (Yakar et al., 2002; Boonen et al., 2002; Veldhuis et al., 2006a). Moreover, the function of the binding proteins, may be modified by the presence of specific proteases and protease inhibitors (Maile et al., 1998).

Epidemiological prospective data on the association of serum IGF-I and postmenopausal BC (Table 2) suggest substantially a lack of association. Only the EPIC study reported a significant positive association with BC risk (Rinaldi et al., 2006). The ORDET cohort suggested a positive but nonsignificant relationship between serum IGF-I and BC only in overweight women (Muti et al., 2002), and the Swedish cohorts in women under hormone replacement therapy (HRT) treatment (Kaaks et al., 2002). These results suggested that IGF-I may increase BC risk only in presence of a sufficient concentration of estrogens, as in postmenopausal overweight women, but have not been replicated. An alternative explanation of the effect modification by menopausal status could be the insulin sensitizing effect of IGF-I (Sandhu et al., 2002). After menopause, in fact, type 2 diabetes (Wolf et al., 2005), overweight (Lahmann et al., 2004), and other markers of insulin resistance, such as high levels of circulating C-peptide (Verheus et al., 2006) are associated with increased BC risk. IGF-I, therefore, might have opposing effects on BC risk in postmenopausal, frequently overweight, women. On one hand it stimulates breast epithelial cell proliferation (at least in overweight women who have higher circulating levels of sex hormones), on the other hand it stimulates insulin sensitivity, which could reduce the elevated BC risk of overweight women.

As for the relationship between circulating IGFBP-3 and BC in postmenopausal women, most studies did not find any association, although the EPIC study (Rinaldi et al., 2006) suggested a positive association and one large case-control study carried out in China reported a statistically significant linear trend (Yu et al., 2002). In this study the risk of both IGF-I and IGFBP-3 were high—of the order of 2 to 3—if also circulating sex hormones, either testosterone or estradiol, were high (Yu et al., 2003).

Plasma IGF-I levels may also have prognostic significance in BC patients. In premenopausal patients, an analysis of the control arm of the Italian Fenretinide Phase III trial (Decensi et al., 2003), which randomised BC patients to test whether fenretinide prevents second BC, showed that high serum IGF-I levels were associated with significantly increased risk of second BC. In postmenopausal patients we have recently shown that serum IGF-I levels are associated with BC recurrences when also serum platelet derived growth factor (PDGF) is elevated (Pasanisi et al., 2008, submitted for publication). PDGF, in fact, activates the expression of IGF-I and other growth factors receptors (Baserga et al., 1994).

Few studies have examined the association of circulating levels of IGFBP-1 and IGFBP-2 with BC risk (Kaaks et al., 2002; Krajcik et al., 2002; Muti et al., 2002; Keinan-Boker et al., 2003). The single statistically significant result was for IGFBP-2 in postmenopausal women (RR = 0.29, with 95% CI, 0.09–0.92, for the upper quartile vs. the bottom one, P for linear trend 0.007) (Krajcik et al., 2002); this association, however, was not replicated either by Muti et al. (2002) or by Keinan-Boker et al. (2003).

REGULATION OF CIRCULATING IGF-I

Circulating IGF-I is mainly regulated by GH stimulation on the liver. However the activity of the GH/IGF-I axis is strongly influenced by other factors—e.g., sex hormones, genetic, and, particularly, nutritional factors—that interfere with the neuroendocrine control of GH output and/or with the response of the liver to the GH stimulation.

The GH/IGF-I Axis

Pituitary secretion of GH is mainly regulated by the interaction of two hypothalamic peptides, the stimulatory GH-releasing hormone (GHRH) and the inhibitory somatostatin (SS). Another GH-releasing peptide, ghrelin, is synthesized in the hypothalamus and pituitary gland and also in other organs like pancreas and stomach: it induces GH secretion via combined hypothalamo-hypophyseal mechanisms (Veldhuis et al., 2006a). SS, GHRH, and ghrelin jointly govern GH and thereby IGF-I secretion via independent and interactive mechanisms (Veldhuis et al., 2006a). On its part, circulating IGF-I has a negative feedback activity on GH secretion. This negative feedback operates via hypothalamic mechanisms, probably by increasing SS action; in addition, IGF-I could also inhibit GH synthesis and secretion at the pituitary level (Veldhuis, 1996; Veldhuis et al., 2006a). However, in subjects with normal nutritional conditions and weight, the regulatory actions of hypothalamus and CNS have a prevailing role. For instance, the peak of GH secretion is reached at puberty, with consequent, and in spite of, very high circulating IGF-I level (Corpas et al., 1993). After puberty the GH secretion presents a progressive decrease, mainly due to the increase of hypothalamic somatostatinergic tone (Iranmanesh and Veldhuis, 1992; Corpas et al., 2003). As a consequence of the reduced GH stimulation, levels of IGF-I progressively decrease with age in both men and women. The mean serum IGF-I concentration in subjects in the seventh decade is approximately one-half that of persons in the third decade (Corpas et al., 2003).

Endogenous Sex Hormones

Sex hormones, particularly estrogens, influence the GH/IGF-I axis at various levels. This topic has been recently reviewed by Leung et al. (2004) and Veldhuis et al. (2006a).

Estrogens and androgens stimulate GH secretion. The effect of testosterone is probably dependent on prior aromatization to estrogen (Veldhuis, 1996; Leung et al., 2004). GH and estrogen levels show positive correlations both in girls and boys, and there is ample evidence that GH secretion is regulated by estrogens in adult life: GH secretion and IGF-I levels are higher in young women than in menopausal women or in young men, and are highest during the periovulatory phase of the menstrual cycle when estrogen concentrations are maximal (Veldhuis, 1996; Leung et al., 2004). Administration of GnRH agonist to block ovarian function reduces basal serum GH and IGF-I concentrations and attenuates the effect of GHRH administration. This suggests that estrogen withdrawal may increase inhibitory tone of SS (Veldhuis, 1996). The reduction in estrogen levels because of menopause could contribute to the decline in IGF-I level, and the difference in levels of GH and IGF-I between men and women is lost after menopause (Leung et al., 2004).

Besides the estrogen stimulatory effects on GH secretion at the hypothalamic and pituitary level, estrogen can contrast GH action on the liver, causing a reduction in the synthesis of IGF-I (Leung et al., 2004). This is particularly evident in the case of oral estrogen administration, as a consequence of the supraphysiological concentrations of estrogen in the liver, due to the hepatic first pass (see sec. "Sex Hormone Therapies").

Nutritional Factors

As reviewed by Clemmons and Underwood (1991), the role of nutrition in the regulation of IGFs was first demonstrated by Grant et al. (1973), who reported that serum somatomedins (IGFs) bioactivity was low in children with protein-calorie malnutrition, despite high GH values. Subsequently the development of reliable radioimmunassay (RIA) methods to measure IGF-I concentrations made it possible to study the effect of fasting in normal subjects. Five to ten days of fasting decreased IGF-I plasma concentrations by about 70% (Clemmons et al., 1981; Isley et al., 1983; Isley et al., 1984), and the injection of GH in fasting subjects did not increase plasma IGF-I (Merimee et al., 1982), proving that the effect of fasting was due to GH resistance. In fasting rats the decline in GH binding is accompanied by a decrease in hepatic GH receptor mRNA expression (Straus & Takemoto, 1990), indicating that regulation occurs at the transcriptional level. Protein restriction, on the contrary, seems to cause a postreceptor resistance to the action of GH. Protein restricted rats, in fact, have low IGF-I levels and low IGF-I response to GH treatment even if the reduction of GH binding is modest (Maes et al., 1988). It has been suggested, however, that severe protein-calorie restriction may also induce IGF-I resistance (Clemmons & Underwood, 1991).

To define the requirement of specific calorie-providing nutrients to maintain normal serum IGF-I concentrations, several fasting/refeeding experiments have been carried out in normal human volunteers (Isley et al., 1983, 1984). Approximately eight days of refeeding were required to revert IGF-I concentration to the levels of control subjects. Refeeding with adequate energy but low protein (0.4 g/kg) attenuated the IGF-I response. Refeeding with adequate protein but low total calorie (11 kcal/kg), however, did not increase IGF-I levels, suggesting that a threshold quantity of energy must be provided for normal subjects to maintain normal IGF-I concentrations. Interestingly, a refeeding diet rich in essential amino acids (80% of total amino acids) produced significantly higher serum IGF-I levels than a diet poor of essential amino acids (20% of total) (Clemmons et al., 1985).

Nutritional factors and body weight influence the GH output. In general, obesity and food ingestion decrease GH secretion, while the opposite effect is seen in underweight and undernourished subjects. Several mechanisms can be involved in the decrease of GH release in the case of overnutrition and obesity: an increase in IGF-I bioactivity (Corpas et al., 1993) because of insulin-driven reduction in the hepatic synthesis of IGFBP-1 and IGFBP-2 (Kaaks and Lukanova, 2001), but also somatic inputs to the CNS by adipocyte-derived factors, such as leptin (elevated in obesity) and adiponectin (reduced in obesity), and suppression of ghrelin output (Veldhuis et al., 2006a). The increase of GH production in the cases of underweight and/or food deprivation can be due to opposite mechanisms, e.g., ghrelin concentrations increase during fasting and anorexia nervosa (Veldhuis et al., 2006b). However, the most relevant mechanism seems to be the strong reduction in IGF-I level (due to reduced sensitivity of the liver to GH effects) and bioactivity (due to the sharp increase in IGFBP-1 and IGFBP-2 level), and hence of the IGF-I inhibitory feedback, as seen in anorectic girls (Counts et al., 1992).

Several studies have shown that the relationship of circulating IGF-I levels and body mass index (BMI) is not linear (Lukanova et al., 2002; Lukanova et al., 2004). In a cross-sectional analysis of women participating to the EPIC study, mean serum IGF-I values were significantly lower in women with BMI <22.5 kg/m^2 or BMI $>$ 29.2 kg/m^2 compared with women with BMI in this range, and were not related to waist to hip ratio (WHR) after adjustment for BMI (Gram et al., 2006). IGFBP-3, on the other hand, was positively related to waist and WHR, so that the molar ratio IGF-I/IGFBP-3 showed a linear inverse relationship with WHR.

Besides the experimental studies on human volunteers carried out in the 1980s and 1990s, showing that fasting or calorie restriction dramatically decreased circulating IGF-I levels (Clemmons et al., 1981, 1985; Isley et al., 1983, 1984; Smith et al., 1995; Thissen et al., 1994), several cross-sectional studies addressed the relationship of calorie intake and IGF-I levels. Among the largest studies a significant positive association was reported by Holmes et al. (2002), Giovannucci et al. (2003), Heald et al. (2003), but not by DeLellis et al. (2004), Larsson et al. (2005) and Norat et al. (2007), where the association was a minor one. As for the intake of specific nutrients, the single calorie-providing nutrient that consistently showed a positive association was protein (Holmes et al., 2002; Giovannucci et al., 2003; Heald et al., 2003; Larsson et al., 2005; Norat et al., 2007), and, particularly animal protein (Giovannucci et al., 2003; Holmes et al., 2002). Allen et al. (2000) showed lower IGF-I levels in vegans than in vegetarians and Fontana et al. (2006) in men and women who had been eating a low-protein and low-calorie diet for several years. In the latter group of mainly vegetarian raw food eaters, the daily intake of protein was 0.73 g per kg per day (9.3% of total energy) and average serum IGF-I was 139 ng/mL against 201 ng/mL in a western diet comparison group. People voluntarily decreasing calorie intake showed a dramatic decrease in cardiovascular risk factors (Fontana et al., 2004) but only those who also substantially decreased protein intake showed a significant reduction in circulating IGF-I (Fontana et al., 2006). As for protein rich animal food, the strongest association was for cow milk (Ma et al., 2001, Holmes et al., 2002; DeLellis et al., 2004; Norat et al., 2007), and only occasionally a significant association was reported for meat or cheese. In the EPIC study, the IGF-I concentration increased from 216 ng/mL to 234 ng/mL with increasing quintiles of milk consumption ($p < 0.007$), and from 225 ng/mL to 252 ng/mL for increasing quintiles of total protein consumption ($p < 0.001$) (Norat et al., 2007).

The DIANA (Diet and Androgens) dietary intervention trials (Berrino et al., 2001; Kaaks et al., 2003) showed that a diet low in refined carbohydrates and animal products, which obtains a moderate calorie restriction through its highly satiating effect, increased SHBG, IGFBP1, and IGFBP2 levels and decreased insulin and testosterone, but did not affect significantly circulating levels of IGF-I. In these trials, however, total protein intake (15% of total calorie intake) did not change but only shifted from mostly animal to mostly vegetable sources. Further studies with moderate calorie/protein restriction are needed.

As for the intake of non-calorie-providing nutrients, a significant positive association with circulating IGF-I values has been reported for Zinc (Devine et al., 1998; Larsson et al., 2005; Holmes et al., 2002), Potassium, and Magnesium (Norat et al., 2007; Larsson et al., 2005).

Many cross-sectional analyses looked also at the relationship between diet and circulating levels of IGFBP-3. Apart from alcool consumption, occasionally found positively associated with increased IGFBP-3 levels (Holmes et al., 2002; DeLellis et al., 2004), no other consistent association was reported. In animal experiments, prolonged fasting and/or protein deficiency resulted in significant reduction of IGFBP-3 concentrations (Clemmons et al., 1989). Among cross-sectional epidemiological studies on diet and IGFBP-3, however, only Giovannucci et al. (2003) reported a significant positive association between protein intake and IGFBP-3 levels.

Only a few studies considered the relationship of diet with IGFBP-1 and IGFBP-2 levels. A fasting experiment (Smith et al., 1995) and a randomized study on 104 postmenopausal women with an insulin lowering diet (Kaaks et al., 2003) showed a significant increase of both proteins.

Genetic Factors

A series of twin studies have shown that serum levels of IGF-I and IGFBP-3 are determined by a combination of genetic and environmental factors (Hong et al., 1996). For IGF-I, estimates of the proportion of variance that is explained by genetic effects range from over 80% in children and newborns (Kao et al., 1994; Verhaeghe et al., 1996) to 38% in adults (Harrela et al., 1996). In adults the intrapair correlations for IGF-I levels were $r = 0.41$ for monozygotic twins and $r = 0.12$ for dizygotic twins, suggesting that nongenetic age-related factors may affect the expression of the gene. In the same study the intrapair correlations were much higher for IGFBP-3 ($r = 0.65$ for monozygotic twins and $r = 0.23$ for dizygotic twins), suggesting that a greater genetic component is responsible for the variation of serum IGFBP-3. No genetic component was detected for serum IGFBP-1 levels (Harrela et al., 1996).

More recently, several epidemiological studies have examined the role of genetic polymorphism within or around the structural genes for IGF-I and IGFBPs. As reviewed by Fletcher et al. (2005), 10 studies reported on a simple tandem repeat (STR) that lies 1 kb 5' to the IGF-I gene transcriptional start site. A first report suggested that the most frequent allele (the 19 CA repeat allele, present in about 60% to 70% of normal Caucasian populations) was associated with decreased levels of serum IGF-I. Among subsequent publications, two showed a significant association in the same direction, two in the opposite direction and five did not find any genotype effect. Evidence of an effect of this polymorphism, therefore, remains inconsistent.

Recent studies have thoroughly characterized common genetic variations in IGF-I and IGFBP-3 and examined this in relation to BC risk (Setiawan et al., 2006) and to serum IGF-I levels (Canzian et al., 2006; Al Zahrani et al., 2006) using a combination of direct (resequencing) and indirect (haplotype based) methods. The c-allele of IGF-1 SNPrs1520220 was reported to be associated both with increased BC risk and with increased circulating IGF-I, but it accounted only for 2% of the total variance of IGF-I levels (Al Zahrani et al., 2006).

Several studies reported that an A/C polymorphism at −202 bp relative to the transcriptional start site of the IGFBP-3 is associated with lower circulating levels of IGFBP-3, which decrease as the number of copies of the A allele decreased (AA > AC > CC) (Canzian et al., 2006; Al Zahrani et al., 2006; Fletcher et al., 2005). Results of studies on the effect of this SNP on BC risk have, however, been inconsistent (Ren et al., 2004; Al Zahrani et al., 2006; Cheng et al., 2006; Canzian et al., 2006; Shernhammer et al., 2003).

Results produced up to now suggest that common germ line variations in IGF-I and IGFBPs are not major contributors to serum concentrations of these peptides nor to BC risk. A study examining several SNPs of genes involved in the GH synthesis pathway, including GH, GHRH, its receptor, somatostatin and its receptor, also concluded that they are not major determinants of IGF-I and IGFBP-3 circulating levels and do not play a major role in BC causation (Canzian et al., 2005). Whether other genes, or the combined effect of several modest associations within the GH/IGF-I pathway, or interactive effects between gene and environment may have greater cumulative effect, remains to be determined.

THERAPIES INFLUENCING IGF-I

Sex Hormone Therapies

Estrogens

Exogenous estrogens can cause differential effects on the GH/IGF-I axis depending on route of administration, estrogen concentrations reached in the blood, and, particularly, estrogen concentrations in the liver. This is due to the fact that depending on these variants, one or the other of two opposite effects prevails: the enhancement of GH secretion (with consequent increase in IGF-I synthesis) on one hand, and the reduction of GH action at the level of receptor expression and signal in the liver (with reduction in IGF-I synthesis) (Leung et al., 2004), on the other hand.

Actually, both oral contraceptives (Mah et al., 2005) and estrogen replacement therapy (ERT) in menopausal women reduces circulating IGF-I levels via a hepatocellular effect (Leung et al., 2004). This decrease is more abrupt and more constant when oral ERT is used, as a consequence of the supraphysiological estrogen concentrations in the liver, due to hepatic first pass effect. Several studies have consistently shown a 20% to 40% decrease in IGF-I levels in women on oral ERT. Most of these are longitudinal studies of small size (as reviewed, Campagnoli et al., 1998a); however, a reduction in IGF-I has been confirmed in a large cross-sectional study (Goodman-Gruen et al., 1996). Transdermal estradiol at the currently used doses, in general, does not cause variations in IGF-I levels (as reviewed, Campagnoli et al., 1998a), while it can reduce IGF-I level when administered at uncommon high doses (Friend et al., 1996; Veldhuis et al., 2006b). Possibly, the IGF-I modifications induced by estrogen administration depend on basal IGF-I values. When oral estrogens are used, the decrease in IGF-I is greater in women with higher basal levels (Campagnoli et al., 1998b); with transdermal estradiol, women with higher basal levels tend to show a decrease in IGF-I, while women with lower basal levels tend to have an increase (Campagnoli et al., 1998a).

According to some studies (Carmina et al., 1996; Kam et al., 2000; Heald et al., 2005; Gibney et al., 2005), oral ERT also decreases IGFBP-3 levels, and this could happen either directly (via inhibition of IGFBP-3 synthesis by Kupffer cells) or indirectly (faster clearance due to the reduction in IGF-I levels) (Kam et al., 2000). However, data on the effect of oral ERT on IGFBP-3 levels are not consistent: some other studies reported no variations (Bellantoni et al., 1996; Garnero et al., 1999; Cardim et al., 2001; Decensi et al., 2004; Duschek et al., 2004) or even an increase (Kim and Lee, 2001). This is in contrast to an approximately 30% decrease of IGF-I seen in all the studies. The different sites of production of IGF-I and IGFBP-3, the hepatocytes and the Kupffer cells respectively, possibly account for this different impact of estrogen administration.

Oral ERT, through hepatocellular action (amplified by the hepatic first pass) causes a two to threefold increase in IGFBP-1 levels (Carmina et al., 1996; Helle et al., 1996a; Cardim et al., 2001; Heald et al., 2005; Veldhuis et al., 2005, 2006b), which results in a reduction in IGF-I bioavailability.

Oral estrogen administration is followed by a sharp increase (50–250%) in GH levels, while with transdermal estradiol the GH increase is lower and less constant (as reviewed, Campagnoli et al., 1998a). Most of the GH increase during oral ERT occurs as a result of reduced negative feedback inhibition of IGF-I on GH secretion (Ho et al., 1996; Leung et al., 2004). This strongly suggests that the modifications in the IGF-I system induced by oral ERT cause a decrease in bioactivity of circulating IGF-I.

The increase in GH levels, reactive to the IGF-I reduction in women treated with oral estrogens, could theoretically increase BC risk through a paracrine effect due to IGF-I production in the adjacent nonneoplastic tissue. However, most epidemiological studies indicate that administration of oral estrogens alone (particularly, conjugated equine estrogens, CEE) does not increase BC risk (Viscoli et al., 2001; Ross et al., 2000; Moorman et al., 2000; Porch et al., 2002; Chen et al., 2002; Li et al., 2003; Olsson et al., 2003; Stefanick et al., 2006), or does so only modestly (Schairer et al., 2000; Newcomb et al., 2002; Beral, 2003; Chen et al., 2006; Rosenberg et al., 2006; Lee et al., 2006). The most important randomized controlled trial, the CEE-only study of the Women's Health Initiative, even suggests a decrease in BC risk (Stefanick et al., 2006). It has been hypothesized that this may be because BC cells are susceptible to estrogen fluctuations (Stefanick et al., 2006). Another reason could be that some components of the CEE mixture have a nonestrogenic or even an antiestrogenic effect on breast tissue (Campagnoli et al., 1999). However, the sharp reduction in IGF-I level and bioactivity induced by oral estrogen could give an important contribution to the protective activity (Campagnoli et al., 1995).

The possibility that the IGF-I reduction induced by oral ERT has other clinical effects, e.g., on the risk of stroke, cannot be discarded. However, while oral estrogens are associated with an increased risk of ischemic stroke, prevalently due to an increase in trombophilia (Glueck et al., 2002), they are associated with increased mortality from stroke only among women with a recent history of cerebrovascular problems (Viscoli et al., 2001) and not in normal women (Bushnell, 2005). Conversely, a spontaneous reduction in IGF-I levels because of genetic variant is associated with an increased mortality from stroke (van Rijn et al., 2006). Probably this is due to a reduction in the protective effect that IGF-I exerts on neurons (Bondanelli et al., 2006). Estrogen also, by their part, has protective effects on neurons (Bushnell, 2005), and this could minimize the consequences of the IGF-I reduction in the CNS.

Androgens

Androgen administration increases basal GH secretion without decreasing, or even increasing, IGF-I levels (Veldhuis, 1996; Veldhuis et al., 2006a). The action at the level of the GH regulatory system is prevalently obtained via aromatization to estrogen (Veldhuis, 1996). Actually, the administration of the nonaromatizable oxandrolone is without effect on the GH secretion both in hypogonadal men and in older women (Veldhuis, 1996; Sheffield-Mooreat et al., 2006). Data referring to androgen administration in women, however, are scanty. In female to male transsexual, high doses of oral testosterone undecanoate increased IGF-I levels, without affecting IGFBP-3 (Duschek et al., 2005). DHEA administration, 25 to 100 mg/day, also increases IGF-I levels (Casson et al., 1998; Morales et al., 1998; Villareal and Holloszy, 2006) without affecting IGFBP-3 level.

No data on the effect of estrogen plus androgens coadministration on IGF-I level are available. According to one study, oral estrogen plus androgen coadministration increased BC risk more than the estrogen alone (Tamimi et al., 2006).

Progestins

The various progestins used in hormone therapy (HT) for menopausal women have differential effects on circulating IGF-I levels. This was suggested for the first time by one of our studies (Campagnoli et al., 2004). In this longitudinal study of menopausal women treated with CEE 0.625 mg, sequential addition of the androgenic progestin norethisterone acetate (NETA) 5 mg completely reversed the 25% decrease in IGF-I levels observed with the addition of the nonandrogenic dydrogesterone 10 mg (Campagnoli et al., 1994). We suggested that the androgenic progestin interferes with the estrogenic hepatocellular effect of reducing IGF-I synthesis, as it does with other estrogenic hepatocellular effects [e.g., increase in sex hormone binding globulin (SHBG)]. Although NETA 5 mg is a relatively high dose, even the use of 1 mg NETA, continuously combined with oral estradiol 2 mg, was associated, in longitudinal studies, with only a slight (10%) decrease (Raudaskoski et al., 1998; Hofling et al., 2005), or even with a 10% increase (Ravn et al., 1995) in IGF-I levels. In a larger longitudinal study, the same combined preparation caused a 65% increase in IGF-I in women with basal IGF-I levels below the median and a slight, nonsignificant decrease (9%) in women with high basal levels (Posaci et al., 2001).

A differential effect of progestins, depending on their androgenicity, has also been observed in a cross-over study of two contraceptive pills containing ethinylestradiol 0.03 mg (Balogh et al., 2000). The preparation containing the nonandrogenic dienogest 2 mg caused a 30% reduction in mean IGF-I concentrations, while the pill containing the androgenic levonorgestrel 0.125 mg caused only a 12% reduction.

The best evidence for the interference of androgenic progestins on the estrogen-induced decrease in IGF-I levels comes from two randomized cross-over studies. In the study by Heald et al. (2005), the IGF-I decrease observed with CEE 0.625 mg was partially reversed by the sequential addition of the slightly androgenic medroxyprogesterone acetate (MPA) 10 mg, but it was counteracted to a greater extent by the addition of the more androgenic desogestrel 0.075 mg, and almost halved with the addition of the androgenic norethisterone 1 mg. In the second randomized cross-over study (Nugent et al., 2003), contrarily to the two nonandrogenic progestins cyproterone acetate and dydrogesterone, NETA 2.5 mg counteracted the IGF-I decrease in women treated with CEE, and both NETA and MPA 10 mg caused a significant increase in IGF-I levels in women given transdermal estradiol. The fact that the slightly androgenic MPA is able to partially interfere with the estrogen-induced IGF-I decrease was also confirmed by a large cross-sectional study (Goodman-Gruen et al., 1996) and by a longitudinal study comparing women treated with either CEE alone or CEE combined with MPA (Malarkey et al., 1997). Chlormadinone acetate, although nonandrogenic, seems to have a similar effect; it has been used in two longitudinal studies in which an increase (not a decrease) in IGF-I levels was observed during HRT (Slowinska-Srzednicka et al., 1992; Fonseca et al., 1999). Conversely, our recent studies have confirmed that dydrogesterone does not interfere with the IGF-I decrease induced by oral estrogens (Campagnoli et al., 2002; 2003). In a longitudinal study of 45 menopausal women given oral estradiol 2 mg with the sequential addition of dydrogesterone 10 mg, IGF-I levels determined during the progestogenic phase of the 6th cycle showed a 15% decrease in women with basal levels below the median and a 40% decrease in women with high basal levels (Campagnoli et al., 2002).

In the cross-over study by Heald et al. (2005), administration of estrogen alone caused a 15% decrease in

IGFBP-3 levels and a threefold increase in IGFBP-1 levels. Both effects were opposed by MPA, desogestrel, and norethisterone, in a manner proportional to their androgenicity. For IGFBP-1, a reversal of the increase induced by oral estrogen was also observed with NETA 1 mg (Helle et al., 1996a). This effect probably contributes to the increase in IGF-I bioavailability.

In summary, some synthetic progestins reverse the reduction in IGF-I bioactivity, due either to the decrease in IGF-I or the IGFBP-1 increase, induced by oral estrogens.

Regarding the consequences on BC risk of progestin addition in HT, the available data up to 2005 refered only to MPA and 19-nortestosterone derivatives. These data indicated an increase in risk, which was greater with the latter (as reviewed, Campagnoli et al., 2005). This was attributed to the effect of androgenic progestins on the favorable modifications induced by oral estrogens on metabolic risk factors, particularly the IGF-I reduction (Campagnoli et al., 2005). New important data on the consequences of progestogen addition come from the French study based on the E3N-EPIC cohort. This cohort included approximately 55,000 postmenopausal teachers followed up with periodic questionnaires. The first results were published in 2005 (Fournier et al., 2005). Further results with longer follow-up and more detailed data are now available (Fournier et al., 2007). The relative risks were 1.4 with unopposed estrogen (mainly transdermal estradiol), 1.0 with the addition of natural progesterone, 1.3 with the addition of dydrogesterone, and 1.8 with the addition of other synthetic progestins. The finding that progesterone addition does not increase the risk is consistent with the in vivo data suggesting that natural progesterone does not have detrimental effects on breast tissue (as reviewed, Campagnoli et al., 2005), and with epidemiological findings showing that high levels of endogenous progesterone do not increase (Eliassen et al., 2006), or may even reduce (Micheli et al., 2004; Kaaks et al., 2005), BC risk in premenopausal women. The activities of dydrogesterone are very similar to those of natural progesterone (Schindler et al., 2003), so it is not surprising that it also does not cause an increase in risk, in contrast to the other synthetic progestins. In France, androgenic progestins were used in only a minority of women (Fournier et al., 2005), while the most used synthetic progestins were nonandrogenic (progesterone-derivatives or 19-norprogesterone-derivatives) or even antiandrogenic (e.g., cyproterone acetate). It is possible that preferential prescribing of antiandrogenic HRT to women with signs of hyperandrogenism, who are at higher BC risk (Muti et al., 2000), partly explain these findings. However, a real association between the use of most synthetic progestins and BC risk has to be considered. It is possible that different mechanisms are involved for different progestins. For some progestins, possible differences from progesterone could be relevant in relation to pharmacokinetics, potency, nongenomic actions, binding to other steroid receptors, and interaction with the two isoforms of the progesterone receptor (PRA and PRB). Differences in the activation of the two progesterone receptors could be particularly relevant; while PRB acts as an activator of transcription, PRA may act as a repressor not only of the activity of the PRB, but also of that of the estrogen, androgen, and glucocorticoid receptors (Kuhl, 2005). However, for the time being, these are theoretical speculations. In the uncertainty surrounding this issue, the possibility that progestins endowed with androgenic activity prevalently increase BC risk through their influence on IGF-I level cannot be discarded (Campagnoli et al., 1995; McCarty, 2001).

Tibolone

Tibolone has weak estrogenic, progestogenic, and androgenic properties. Tibolone, at the currently used dose of 2.5 mg/day, does not modify circulating IGF-I levels (Hopkins et al., 1995; Hofling et al., 2005); conversely, when the uncommon dose of 5 mg/day was used, an increase in IGF-I level was observed (Porcile et al., 2003).

Therapies for Breast Cancer Prevention and Treatment

Given the potential relevance of the IGF-I level and bioactivity, the influence on the IGF system of the drugs currently used in the prevention and treatment of BC has been evaluated by many studies. Other therapeutical approaches specifically oriented in decreasing IGF-I level and bioactivity have been, and are being, suggested.

Selective Estrogen Receptor Modulators

Tamoxifen (TAM) can interfere in various ways on the IGF-I activity at the level of BC cells, and this could contribute to its therapeutic action (Winston et al., 1994; Guvakova and Surmacz, 1997). Moreover, TAM, like other selective estrogen receptor modulators (SERMS), can influence the GH/IGF-I axis. Actually, TAM, droloxifene, and raloxifene reduce circulating IGF-I, probably through an estrogen agonistic effect on the liver (Helle, 2004). TAM, at the current used doses in BC treatment, reduces IGF-I levels by 15% to 30% (Ho et al., 1998; Ingle et al., 1999; Helle, 2004). A similar reduction was observed with the lower TAM doses of 10 mg daily or on alternate days (Decensi et al., 1998). The raloxifene-induced reduction in IGF-I level is lower than that observed with oral estrogen (Duschek et al., 2004; Gibney et al., 2005).

Contrarily to what happens with oral estrogen, the reduction in the level of IGF-I is not accompanied by reactive increase in GH secretion. Actually, TAM administration does not cause any effect, or even show inhibitory action, on GH secretion (Corsello et al., 1998; De Marinis et al., 2000). This is probably because of an antiestrogenic effect on the hypothalamic regulatory system of GH secretion.

IGFBP-3 protease activity is increased in patients with advanced BC, as observed in other cancers and other serious conditions (Helle, 2004). In these cases, TAM has no significant effect on total IGFBP-3 levels, but patients responding to treatment had a reduction in fragmentation of IGFBP-3 (Helle et al., 1996b). In patients with nonadvanced BC TAM causes an increase in IGFBP-3 levels (Ho et al., 1998). An increase of IGFBP-3 is observed also in healthy women treated with raloxifene (Duschek et al., 2004; Gibney et al., 2005).

Several studies consistently show that TAM, droloxifene, and raloxifene, through an estrogen-like effect on the liver, cause a sharp increase in IGFBP-1 levels (Helle, 2004) and, hence, a decrease in IGF-I bioactivity.

Epidemiological and clinical data on the association between IGF-I level and the outcome of stroke (van Rijn et al., 2006; Bondanelli et al., 2006) suggest that the reduction in IGF-I induced by raloxifene could contribute to the increased risk of fatal stroke observed in the Raloxifene Use for The Heart (RUTH) study on the use of raloxifene in women at high cardiovascular risk (Barrett-Connor et al., 2006).

Aromatase Inhibitors

Specific aromatase inhibitors—formestane (4-hydroxy androstenedione), at the high dose of 500 mg, and letrozole—significantly increase IGF-I level (by 25–50%), without affecting IGFBP-3 (Ferrari et al., 1994; Bajetta et al., 1997). It is possible that the almost total estrogen deprivation, induced by these drugs, increases the responsivity of the hepatocytes to GH stimulation. The clinical importance of this effect is probably minor (Helle, 2004).

Somatostatin Analog

Preclinical data suggested that somatostatin analogs, like octreotide, could have an anticancer activity by both direct (trough somatostatin receptors in cancer cells) and indirect (through the influence on the GH/IGF-I axis) effects (Pollak and Schally, 1998). Octreotide reduced the blood IGF-I level by 33% (Vennin et al., 1989). Adding octreotide to TAM an IGF-I reduction by 39% was observed, compared with the 16% reduction with TAM alone (Ingle et al., 1999). However, octreotide had no clinical effects (Ingle at al, 1999), and the combination of TAM plus octreotide was no more efficacious than TAM alone in the treatment of postmenopausal women with metastatic BC (Ingle et al., 1999; Bajetta et al., 2002).

Sex Hormone Therapies

High dose estrogen diethylstilbestrol, when used in patients with metastatic BC, affects all components of the IGF system. It decreases IGF-I and IGF-II, and also IGFBP-2 and IGFBP-3, in spite of a decrease of IGFBP-3 protease activity. It also sharply increases IGFBP-1 (by 250%) causing a 65% to 75% decrease in free IGF-I (Helle, 2004).

High dose of the progestin MPA (500 mg/day), when used in women with advanced BC, caused a doubling of IGF-I level and a significant reduction in IGFBP-I concentrations (Reed et al., 1992). Another progestin, megestrol acetate 160 mg/day, caused an 80% increase in IGF-I levels, no variations in IGFBP-1, a moderate elevation in IGFBP-3, and a significant reduction in IGFBP-3 protease activity (Helle, 2004).

Other Therapies

- GnRH analogs, when used in premenopausal women with BC, cause a decrease in IGF-I level (Lien et al., 1992), probably by decreasing the estrogen stimulatory effect on GH secretion.
- Adjuvant anthracycline-containg chemotherapy does not cause significant changes in IGF-1 and IGFBP-3 serum concentration (Furstenberger et al., 2006).
- Retinoids inhibit BC cells in vitro, possibly by affecting IGF-I activity (Fontana et al., 1991; Adamo et al., 1992). When used as a chemopreventive agent for controlateral cancer in early BC patients, the synthetic retinoid fenretinide caused a decrease in IGF-I level, particularly pronounced in premenopausal women, and in IGFBP-3 level (Torrisi et al., 1998; Decensi et al., 2003). However, a recent trial from the same group found no activity of fenretinide on IGF-I level and no synergistic interaction with low dose TAM on the IGF-I reduction (Guerrieri-Gonzaga et al., 2006).

Possible Future Approaches

A number of new therapeutic approaches, with the aim of reducing IGF-I level and bioactivity are on study.

Several natural agents interfere with IGF signaling and could be used as cancer chemoprevention (Friend, 2001; Adhami et al., 2006).

The clinically available competitive GH receptor antagonist, Pegvisomant, normalizes IGF-I concentrations in 95% of patients with acromegaly (Veldhuis et al., 2006a). Preliminary reports on several model systems suggest that it could have antitumor effects (Ibrahim and Yee, 2005).

Another strategy points to inhibit IGF activity, ranging from the use of polyethilene glycol-conjugated IGFBP-1 to neutralize IGFs, to the block of IGF receptor activation (dominant negative IGF-1R, IGF-1R antisense, IGF-1R antibodies, and IGF-1R tyrosine kinase inhibitors) (Ibrahim and Yee, 2005; Haddad and Yee, 2006). Actually, disrupting type 1 IGF-1R function in vitro and in vivo results in antitumor effect in several model systems (Haddad and Yee, 2006).

However, anti-IGF-1 and anti-IGF-1R therapies raise theoretical concerns for the possible development of metabolic and cardiovascular side effects (Haddad and Yee, 2006). Actually, as already discussed (see sec. "Systemic Metabolic Effects"), epidemiological and clinical data suggest that individuals with low serum IGF-I have an increased risk of diabetes and vascular problems (Sandhu et al., 2002; Juul et al., 2002; Laughlin et al., 2004; Hunt et al., 2006; van Rijn et al., 2006). Possibly, the best way to decrease IGF-I bioactivity with the aim of reducing BC risk and BC recurrence is the nutritional approach. A moderate calorie restriction, based on the widely accepted dietary recommendation of choosing predominantly plant based diets, rich in a variety of vegetable and fruits, pulses, and minimally processed starchy staple foods, has been recommended both for the prevention of cancer (WCRF, 1997) and as adjuvant diet to improve BC prognosis (Berrino et al., 2006). With this approach, other metabolic factors of BC are also contrasted (Berrino et al., 2006), while cardiovascular risk is reduced.

SUMMARY

IGF-I has powerful mitogenic and antiapoptotic effects on many cell types, including normal and transformed breast epithelial cells. The proliferative effects of IGF-I on BC cells are synergistic with those of estrogens.

IGF-I production is present in many tissues and is responsive to GH. Locally produced IGF-I is present also in mammary tissue, particularly in stromal cells clustered around intra- and interlobular ducts and in adjacent non-neoplastic tissue in case of BC. Despite the importance of paracrine effects of locally produced IGF-I, also circulating IGF-I could have a role in stimulating breast tissue and BC cells. This is suggested by several reports proving the endocrine effects of IGF-I on bone, muscle, and also the breast. Moreover, most epidemiological studies suggest that circulating IGF-I levels are associated with breast cancer risk, particularly in premenopausal women.

Circulating IGF-I is mainly of hepatic derivation. The production of IGF-I by the hepatocites is stimulated by GH, the secretion of which is influenced by circulating IGF-I level through a negative feedback mechanism. In healthy adults, normal levels of IGF-I can range from 100 to 300 ng/mL, and although GH remains the major regulatory factor, there are clearly other determinants. Among these, nutritional conditions and insulin level have a relevant role, because they modulate the liver responsivity to GH. Fasting and nutrient deprivation cause a decrease in IGF-I production and serum level. Another determinant of serum IGF-I level are genetic factors.

Approximately 99% of IGF-I circulates bound to specific proteins (IGFBPs). The most important of these proteins is IGFBP-3, which is synthesized in Kupffer cells of the liver under GH stimulation. More than 75% of circulating IGF-I is carried in a ternary complex composed of IGF-I, IGFBP-3, and an acid-labile subunit. This ternary complex prevalently acts as a reservoir of IGF-I, prolonging the half-life of IGFs and, possibly, facilitating their endocrine actions.

Insulin enhances GH-stimulated synthesis of IGFBP-3 by increasing levels of GH. Conversely, insulin inhibits the hepatic synthesis of other IGFBPs, the IGFBP-1 and IGFBP-2, that decrease the bioactivity of IGF-I.

Sex hormones, particularly estrogens, influence the GH/IGF-I axis at various levels. Estrogens and androgens stimulate GH secretion. However, estrogen can contrast GH action on the liver, causing a reduction in the synthesis of IGF-I. This is particularly evident in the case of oral estrogen administration, as a consequence of the supraphysiological concentrations of estrogen in the liver, due to the hepatic first pass. Oral estrogens of contraceptive pill or of preparations used in HT in menopausal women, cause a decrease in IGF-I level and a reactive increase in GH level. They also increase IGFBP-1 level, while the data on IGFBP-3 modification are not consistent. Transdermal estrogens, at the doses currently used in HT, on average, do not cause variations in IGF-I levels. The effect of oral androgen administration is opposite to that of estrogens, because they increase IGF-I level. Contrarily to nonandrogenic progestins that are without effects, androgenic progestins (if orally administered) contrast the estrogen hepatocellular effect of reducing IGF-I synthesis. Tibolone, at the currently used dose of 2.5 mg/day, does not modify circulating IGF-I levels.

Some therapies for BC prevention and treatment affect IGF-I level. For instance, tamoxifen, droloxifene, and raloxifene reduce circulating IGF-I and increase IGFBP-1 through estrogen agonistic effects on the liver, without causing a reactive increase in GH secretion. Conversely, specific aromatase inhibitors significantly increase IGF-I level.

A number of new therapeutic approaches, with the aim of reducing IGF-I level and bioactivity are on study. One approach could be the use of competitive GH receptor antagonist Pegvisomant. Another strategy points to inhibit IGF activity, ranging from the use of polyethilene glycol-conjugated IGFBP-1 to the block of IGF receptor (dominant negative IGF-1R, IGF-1R antisense, IGF-1R antibodies, IGF-1R tyrosine kinase inhibitors). However, anti-IGF-1 and anti-IGF-1R therapies raise theoretical concerns for the development of metabolic and cardiovascular side effects. Actually, epidemiological and clinical data suggest that individuals with low serum IGF-I have an increased risk of diabetes and vascular problems. Possibly, the best way to decrease IGF-I level and bioactivity with the aim of reducing BC risk and BC recurrence is the nutritional approach. Actually, with this approach, other metabolic factors of BC are contrasted, while cardiovascular risk is reduced.

ACKNOWLEDGMENTS

The authors thank Dr. Emanuela Arvat, Dept. of Endocrinology, University of Torino, for her precious suggestions, and Ms Maria Grazia Guerrini and Ms Saveria Battaglia for their skilled secretarial work.

REFERENCES

Adamo ML, Shao ZM, Lanau F, Chen JC, Clemmons DR, Roberts CT Jr., LeRoith D, Fontana JA. Insulin-like growth factor-I (IGF-I) and retinoic acid modulation of IGF-binding proteins (IGFBPs): IGFBP-2, -3, and -4 gene expression and protein secretion in a breast cancer cell line. Endocrinology 1992; 131(4):1858–1866.

Adhami VM, Afaq F, Mukhtar H. Insulin-like growth factor-I axis as a pathway for cancer chemoprevention. Clin Cancer Res 2006; 12(19):5611–5614.

Al Zahrani A, Sandhu MS, Luben RN, Thompson D, Baynes C, Pooley KA, Luccarini C, Munday H, Perkins B, Smith P, Pharoah PD, Wareham NJ, Easton DF, Ponder BA, Dunning AM IGF1 and IGFBP3 tagging polymorphisms are associated with circulating levels of IGF1, IGFBP3 and risk of breast cancer. Hum Mol Genet 2006; 15(1): 1–10.

Allen NE, Appleby PN, Davey GK. Hormones and diet: low insulin-like growth factor-I but normal bioavailable androgens in vegan men. Br J Cancer 2000; 83(1):95–97.

Allen NE, Roddam AW, Allen DS, Fentiman IS, Dos SS, I, Peto J, Holly JM, Key TJ. A prospective study of serum insulin-like growth factor-I (IGF-I), IGF-II, IGF-binding protein-3 and breast cancer risk. Br J Cancer 2005; 92:1283–1287.

Bajetta E, Ferrari L, Celio L, Mariani L, Miceli R, Di Leo A, Zilembo N, Buzzoni R, Spagnoli I, Martinetti A, Bichisao E, Seregni E. The aromatase inhibitor letrozole in advanced breast cancer: effects on serum insulin-like growth factor (IGF)-I and IGF-binding protein-3 levels. J Steroid Biochem Mol Biol 1997; 63(4–6):261–267.

Bajetta E, Procopio G, Ferrari L, Martinetti A, Zilembo N, Catena L, Alu M, Della TS, Alberti D, Buzzoni R. A randomized, multicenter prospective trial assessing long-acting release octreotide pamoate plus tamoxifen as a first line therapy for advanced breast carcinoma. Cancer 2002; 94(2):299–304.

Balogh A, Kauf E, Vollanth R, Graser G, Klinger G, Oettel M. Effects of two oral contraceptives on plasma levels of insulin-like growth factor I (IGF-I) and growth hormone (hGH). Contraception 2000; 62(5):259–269.

Barrett-Connor E, Mosca L, Collins P, Geiger MJ, Grady D, Kornitzer M, McNabb MA, Wenger NK. Effects of raloxifene on cardiovascular events and breast cancer in postmenopausal women. N Engl J Med 2006; 355(2): 125–137.

Baserga R, Sell C, Porcu P, Rubini M. The role of the IGF-I receptor in the growth and transformation of mammalian cells. Cell Prolif 1994; 27(2):63–71.

Bellantoni MF, Vittone J, Campfield AT, Bass KM, Harman SM, Blackman MR. Effects of oral versus transdermal estrogen on the growth hormone/insulin-like growth factor I axis in younger and older postmenopausal women: a clinical research center study. J Clin Endocrinol Metab 1996; 81(8):2848–2853.

Beral V. Breast cancer and hormone-replacement therapy in the Million Women Study. Lancet 2003; 362(9382):419–427.

Berrino F, Bellati C, Secreto G, Camerini E, Pala V, Panico S, Allegro G, Kaaks R. Reducing bioavailable sex hormones through a comprehensive change in diet: the diet and androgens (DIANA) randomized trial. Cancer Epidemiol Biomarkers Prev 2001; 10(1):25 33.

Berrino F, Villarini A, De Petris M, Raimondi M, Pasanisi P. Adjuvant diet to improve hormonal and metabolic factors affecting breast cancer prognosis. Ann N Y Acad Sci 2006; 1089:110–118.

Bondanelli M, Ambrosio MR, Onofri A, Bergonzoni A, Lavezzi S, Zatelli MC, Valle D, Basaglia N, degli Uberti EC. Predictive value of circulating insulin-like growth factor I levels in ischemic stroke outcome. J Clin Endocrinol Metab 2006; 91(10):3928–3934.

Boonen S, Rosen C, Bouillon R, Sommer A, McKay M, Rosen D, Adams S, Broos P, Lenaerts J, Raus J, Vanderschueren D, Geusens P. Musculoskeletal effects of the recombinant human IGF-I/IGF binding protein-3 complex in osteoporotic patients with proximal femoral fracture: a double-blind, placebo-controlled pilot study. J Clin Endocrinol Metab 2002; 87(4):1593–1599.

Bushnell CD. Oestrogen and stroke in women: assessment of risk. Lancet Neurol 2005; 4(11):743–751.

Campagnoli C, Abba C, Ambroggio S, Peris C. Differential effects of progestins on the circulating IGF-I system. Maturitas 2003; 46(suppl 1):S39–S44.

Campagnoli C, Ambroggio S, Biglia N, Peris C, Sismondi P. Insulin-like growth factor-I and risk of breast cancer. Lancet 1998b; 352(9126):488–489.

Campagnoli C, Ambroggio S, Biglia N, Sismondi P. Conjugated estrogens and breast cancer risk. Gynecol Endocrinol 1999; 13(suppl 6):13–19.

Campagnoli C, Biglia N, Cantamessa C, Lesca L, Lotano MR, Sismondi P. Insulin-like growth factor I (IGF-I) serum level modifications during transdermal estradiol treatment in postmenopausal women: a possible bimodal effect depending on basal IGF-I values. Gynecol Endocrinol 1998a; 12(4):259–266.

Campagnoli C, Biglia N, Lanza MG, Lesca L, Peris C, Sismondi P. Androgenic progestogens oppose the decrease of insulin-like growth factor I serum level induced by conjugated oestrogens in postmenopausal women. Preliminary report. Maturitas 1994; 19(1):25–31.

Campagnoli C, Biglia N, Peris C, Sismondi P. Potential impact on breast cancer risk of circulating insulin-like growth factor I modifications induced by oral HRT in menopause. Gynecol Endocrinol 1995; 9(1):67–74.

Campagnoli C, Clavel-Chapelon F, Kaaks R, Peris C, Berrino F. Progestins and progesterone in hormone replacement therapy and the risk of breast cancer. J Steroid Biochem Mol Biol 2005; 96(2):95–108.

Campagnoli C, Colombo P, De Aloysio D, Gambacciani M, Grazioli I, Nappi C, Serra GB, Genazzani AR. Positive effects on cardiovascular and breast metabolic markers of oral estradiol and dydrogesterone in comparison with transdermal estradiol and norethisterone acetate. Maturitas 2002; 41(4):299–311.

Canzian F, McKay JD, Cleveland RJ, Dossus L, Biessy C, Boillot C, Rinaldi S, Llewellyn M, Chajes V, Clavel-Chapelon F, Tehard B, Chang-Claude J, Linseisen J, Lahmann PH, Pischon T, Trichopoulos D, Trichopoulou A, Zilis D, Palli D, Tumino R, Vineis P, Berrino F, Bueno-de-Mesquita HB, van Gils CH, Peeters PH, Pera G, Barricarte A, Chirlaque MD, Quiros JR, Larranaga N, Martinez-Garcia C, Allen NE, Key TJ, Bingham SA, Khaw KT, Slimani N, Norat T, Riboli E, Kaaks R. Genetic variation in the growth hormone synthesis pathway in relation to circulating insulin-like growth factor-I, insulin-like growth factor binding protein-3, and breast cancer risk: results from the European prospective investigation into cancer and nutrition study. Cancer Epidemiol Biomarkers Prev 2005; 14(10):2316–2325.

Canzian F, McKay JD, Cleveland RJ, Dossus L, Biessy C, Rinaldi S, Landi S, Boillot C, Monnier S, Chajes V, Clavel-Chapelon F, Tehard B, Chang-Claude J, Linseisen J, Lahmann PH, Pischon T, Trichopoulos D, Trichopoulou A, Zilis D, Palli D, Tumino R, Vineis P, Berrino F, Bueno-de-Mesquita HB, van Gils CH, Peeters PH, Pera G, Ardanaz E, Chirlaque MD, Quiros JR et al. Polymorphisms of genes coding for insulin-like growth factor 1 and its major binding proteins, circulating levels of IGF-I and IGFBP-3 and breast cancer risk: results from the EPIC study. Br J Cancer 2006; 94(2):299–307.

Cardim HJ, Lopes CM, Giannella-Neto D, da Fonseca AM, Pinotti JA. The insulin-like growth factor-I system and hormone replacement therapy. Fertil Steril 2001; 75(2):282–287.

Carmina E, Lo Dico G, Carollo F, Stanczyk FZ, Lobo RA. Serum IGF-I binding proteins 1 and 3 in postmenopausal women and the effect of estrogens. Menopause 1996; 3:85–89.

Casson PR, Santoro N, Elkind-Hirsch K, Carson SA, Hornsby PJ, Abraham G, Buster JE. Postmenopausal dehydroepiandrosterone administration increases free insulin-like growth factor-I and decreases high-density lipoprotein: a six-month trial. Fertil Steril 1998; 70(1):107–110.

Chen CL, Weiss NS, Newcomb P, Barlow W, White E. Hormone replacement therapy in relation to breast cancer. JAMA 2002; 287(6):734–741.

Chen WY, Manson JE, Hankinson SE, Rosner B, Holmes MD, Willett WC, Colditz GA. Unopposed estrogen therapy and the risk of invasive breast cancer. Arch Intern Med 2006; 166(9):1027–1032.

Cheng I, Penney KL, Stram DO, Le Marchand L, Giorgi E, Haiman CA, Kolonel LN, Pike M, Hirschhorn J, Henderson BE, Freedman ML. Haplotype-based association studies of IGFBP1 and IGFBP3 with prostate and breast cancer risk: the multiethnic cohort. Cancer Epidemiol Biomarkers Prev 2006; 15(10):1993–1997.

Chong YM, Williams SL, Elkak A, Sharma AK, Mokbel K. Insulin-like growth factor 1 (IGF-1) and its receptor mRNA levels in breast cancer and adjacent non-neoplastic tissue. Anticancer Res 2006; 26(1A):167–173.

Clemmons DR, Klibanski A, Underwood LE, McArthur JW, Ridgway EC, Beitins IZ, Van Wyk JJ. Reduction of plasma immunoreactive somatomedin C during fasting in humans. J Clin Endocrinol Metab 1981; 53(6):1247–1250.

Clemmons DR, Seek MM, Underwood LE. Supplemental essential amino acids augment the somatomedin-C/insulin-like growth factor I response to refeeding after fasting. Metabolism 1985; 34(4):391–395.

Clemmons DR, Thissen JP, Maes M, Ketelslegers JM, Underwood LE. Insulin-like growth factor-I (IGF-I) infusion into hypophysectomized or protein-deprived rats induces specific IGF-binding proteins in serum. Endocrinology 1989; 125(6):2967–2972.

Clemmons DR, Underwood LE. Nutritional regulation of IGF-I and IGF binding proteins. Annu Rev Nutr 1991; 11:393–412.

Corpas E, Harman SM, Blackman MR. Human growth hormone and human aging. Endocr Rev 1993; 14(1):20–39.

Corsello SM, Rota CA, Putignano P, Della CS, Barnabei A, Migneco MG, Vangeli V, Barini A, Mandala M, Barone C, Barbarino A. Effect of acute and chronic administration of tamoxifen on GH response to GHRH and on IGF-I serum levels in women with breast cancer. Eur J Endocrinol 1998; 139(3):309–313.

Counts DR, Gwirtsman H, Carlsson LM, Lesem M, Cutler GB Jr. The effect of anorexia nervosa and refeeding on growth hormone-binding protein, the insulin-like growth factors (IGFs), and the IGF-binding proteins. J Clin Endocrinol Metab 1992; 75(3):762–767.

Cullen KJ, Allison A, Martire I, Ellis M, Singer C. Insulin-like growth factor expression in breast cancer epithelium and stroma. Breast Cancer Res Treat 1992; 22(1):21–29.

De Marinis L, Mancini A, Izzi D, Bianchi A, Giampietro A, Fusco A, Liberale I, Rossi S, Valle D. Inhibitory action on GHRH-induced GH secretion of chronic tamoxifen treatment in breast cancer. Clin Endocrinol (Oxf) 2000; 52(6):681–685.

Decensi A, Bonanni B, Baglietto L, Guerrieri-Gonzaga A, Ramazzotto F, Johansson H, Robertson C, Marinucci I,

Mariette F, Sandri MT, Daldoss C, Bianco V, Buttarelli M, Cazzaniga M, Franchi D, Cassano E, Omodei U. A two-by-two factorial trial comparing oral with transdermal estrogen therapy and fenretinide with placebo on breast cancer biomarkers. Clin Cancer Res 2004; 10(13):4389–4397.

Decensi A, Bonanni B, Guerrieri-Gonzaga A, Gandini S, Robertson C, Johansson H, Travaglini R, Sandri MT, Tessadrelli A, Farante G, Salinaro F, Bettega D, Barreca A, Boyle P, Costa A, Veronesi U. Biologic activity of tamoxifen at low doses in healthy women. J Natl Cancer Inst 1998; 90(19):1461–1467.

Decensi A, Veronesi U, Miceli R, Johansson H, Mariani L, Camerini T, Di Mauro MG, Cavadini E, De Palo G, Costa A, Perloff M, Malone WF, Formelli F. Relationships between plasma insulin-like growth factor-I and insulin-like growth factor binding protein-3 and second breast cancer risk in a prevention trial of fenretinide. Clin Cancer Res 2003; 9(13):4722–4729.

DeLellis K, Rinaldi S, Kaaks RJ, Kolonel LN, Henderson B, Le Marchand L. Dietary and lifestyle correlates of plasma insulin-like growth factor-I (IGF-I) and IGF binding protein-3 (IGFBP-3): the multiethnic cohort. Cancer Epidemiol Biomarkers Prev 2004; 13(9):1444–1451.

Devine A, Rosen C, Mohan S, Baylink D, Prince RL. Effects of zinc and other nutritional factors on insulin-like growth factor I and insulin-like growth factor binding proteins in postmenopausal women. Am J Clin Nutr 1998; 68 (1):200–206.

Duschek EJ, de Valk-de Roo GW, Gooren LJ, Netelenbos C. Effects of conjugated equine estrogen vs. raloxifene on serum insulin-like growth factor-i and insulin-like growth factor binding protein-3: a 2-year, double-blind, placebo-controlled study. Fertil Steril 2004; 82(2):384–390.

Duschek EJ, Gooren LJ, Netelenbos C. Comparison of effects of the rise in serum testosterone by raloxifene and oral testosterone on serum insulin-like growth factor-1 and insulin-like growth factor binding protein-3. Maturitas 2005; 51(3):286–293.

Eliassen AH, Missmer SA, Tworoger SS, Spiegelman D, Barbieri RL, Dowsett M, Hankinson SE. Endogenous steroid hormone concentrations and risk of breast cancer among premenopausal women. J Natl Cancer Inst 2006; 98(19):1406–1415.

Ferrari L, Zilembo N, Bajetta E, Buzzoni R, Noberasco C, Martinetti A, Celio L, Galante E, Orefice S, Cerrotta AM. Effect of two-4-hydroxyandrostenedione doses on serum insulin-like growth factor I levels in advanced breast cancer. Breast Cancer Res Treat 1994; 30(2): 127–132.

Fletcher O, Gibson L, Johnson N, Altmann DR, Holly JM, Ashworth A, Peto J, Silva IS. Polymorphisms and circulating levels in the insulin-like growth factor system and risk of breast cancer: a systematic review. Cancer Epidemiol Biomarkers Prev 2005; 14(1):2–19.

Fonseca E, Ochoa R, Galvan R, Hernandez M, Mercado M, Zarate A. Increased serum levels of growth hormone and insulin-like growth factor-I associated with simultaneous decrease of circulating insulin in postmenopausal women receiving hormone replacement therapy. Menopause 1999; 6(1):56–60.

Fontana JA, Burrows-Mezu A, Clemmons DR, LeRoith D. Retinoid modulation of insulin-like growth factor-binding proteins and inhibition of breast carcinoma proliferation. Endocrinology 1991; 128(2):1115–1122.

Fontana L, Klein S, Holloszy JO. Long-term low-protein, low-calorie diet and endurance exercise modulate metabolic factors associated with cancer risk. Am J Clin Nutr 2006; 84(6):1456–1462.

Fontana L, Meyer TE, Klein S, Holloszy JO. Long-term calorie restriction is highly effective in reducing the risk for atherosclerosis in humans. Proc Natl Acad Sci U S A 2004; 101(17):6659–6663.

Fournier A, Berrino F, Clavel-Chapelon F. Unequal risks for breast cancer associated with different hormone replacement therapies: results from the E3N cohort study. Breast Cancer Res Treat 2007; 107(1):103–111.

Fournier A, Berrino F, Riboli E, Avenel V, Clavel-Chapelon F. Breast cancer risk in relation to different types of hormone replacement therapy in the E3N-EPIC cohort. Int J Cancer 2005; 114(3):448–454.

Friend KE. Cancer and the potential place for growth hormone receptor antagonist therapy. Growth Horm IGF Res 2001; 11(suppl A):S121–S123.

Friend KE, Hartman ML, Pezzoli SS, Clasey JL, Thorner MO. Both oral and transdermal estrogen increase growth hormone release in postmenopausal women—a clinical research center study. J Clin Endocrinol Metab 1996; 81(6):2250–2256.

Furstenberger G, Senn E, Morant R, Bolliger B, Senn HJ. Serum levels of IGF-1 and IGFBP-3 during adjuvant chemotherapy for primary breast cancer. Breast 2006; 15(1):64–68.

Garnero P, Sornay-Rendu E, Delmas PD. Low serum IGF-1 and occurrence of osteoporotic fractures in postmenopausal women. Lancet 2000; 355(9207):898–899.

Garnero P, Tsouderos Y, Marton I, Pelissier C, Varin C, Delmas PD. Effects of intranasal 17beta-estradiol on bone turnover and serum insulin-like growth factor I in postmenopausal women. J Clin Endocrinol Metab 1999; 84(7):2390–2397.

Gibney J, Johannsson G, Leung KC,. Ho KK. Comparison of the metabolic effects of raloxifene and oral estrogen in post-menopausal and growth hormone-deficient women. J Clin Endocrinol Metab 2005; 90(7):3897–3903.

Giovannucci E, Pollak M, Liu Y, Platz EA, Majeed N, Rimm EB, Willett WC. Nutritional predictors of insulin-like growth factor I and their relationships to cancer in men. Cancer Epidemiol Biomarkers Prev 2003; 12(2):84–89.

Gluckman PD, Douglas RG, Ambler GR, Breier BH, Hodgkinson SC, Koea JB, Shaw JH. The endocrine role of insulin-like growth factor I. Acta Paediatr Scand Suppl 1991; 372:97–105; discussion 106.

Glueck CJ, Wang P, Fontaine RN, Sieve-Smith L, Lang JE. Estrogen replacement therapy, thrombophilia, and atherothrombosis. Metabolism 2002; 51(6):724–732.

Goodman-Gruen D, Barrett-Connor E. Effect of replacement estrogen on insulin-like growth factor-I in postmenopausal women: the Rancho Bernardo Study. J Clin Endocrinol Metab 1996; 81(12):4268–4271.

Gram IT, Norat T, Rinaldi S, Dossus L, Lukanova A, Tehard B, Clavel-Chapelon F, van Gils CH, Van Noord PA, Peeters PH, Bueno-de-Mesquita HB, Nagel G, Linseisen J, Lahmann PH, Boeing H, Palli D, Sacerdote C, Panico S, Tumino R, Sieri S, Dorronsoro M, Quiros JR, Navarro CA, Barricarte A, Tormo MJ, Gonzalez CA, Overvad K, Paaske JS, Olsen A, Tjonneland A et al. Body mass index, waist circumference and waist-hip ratio and serum levels of IGF-I and IGFBP-3 in European women. Int J Obes (Lond) 2006; 30(11):1623–1631.

Grant DB, Hambley J, Becker D, Pimstone BL. Reduced sulphation factor in undernourished children. Arch Dis Child 1973; 48(8):596–600.

Grinspoon S, Baum H, Lee K, Anderson E, Herzog D, Klibanski A. Effects of short-term recombinant human insulin-like growth factor I administration on bone turnover in osteopenic women with anorexia nervosa. J Clin Endocrinol Metab 1996; 81(11):3864–3870.

Grinspoon S, Thomas L, Miller K, Herzog D, Klibanski A. Effects of recombinant human IGF-I and oral contraceptive administration on bone density in anorexia nervosa. J Clin Endocrinol Metab 2002; 87(6):2883–2891.

Gronbaek H, Flyvbjerg A, Mellemkjaer L, Tjonneland A, Christensen J, Sorensen HT, Overvad K. Serum insulin-like growth factors, insulin-like growth factor binding proteins, and breast cancer risk in postmenopausal women. Cancer Epidemiol Biomarkers Prev 2004; 13:1759–1764.

Guerrieri-Gonzaga A, Robertson C, Bonanni B, Serrano D, Cazzaniga M, Mora S, Gulisano M, Johansson H, Formelli F, Intra M, Latronico A, Franchi D, Pelosi G, Johnson K, Decensi A. Preliminary results on safety and activity of a randomized, double-blind, 2 × 2 trial of low-dose tamoxifen and fenretinide for breast cancer prevention in premenopausal women. J Clin Oncol 2006; 24(1):129–135.

Guvakova MA, Surmacz E. Tamoxifen interferes with the insulin-like growth factor I receptor (IGF-IR) signaling pathway in breast cancer cells. Cancer Res 1997; 57 (13):2606–2610.

Haddad T, Yee D. Targeting the insulin-like growth factor axis as a cancer therapy. Future Oncol 2006; 2(1):101–110.

Hankinson SE, Willett WC, Colditz GA, Hunter DJ, Michaud DS, Deroo B, Rosner B, Speizer FE, Pollak M. Circulating concentrations of insulin-like growth factor-I and risk of breast cancer. Lancet 1998; 351(9113):1393–1396.

Harrela M, Koistinen H, Kaprio J, Lehtovirta M, Tuomilehto J, Eriksson J, Toivanen L, Koskenvuo M, Leinonen P, Koistinen R, Seppala M. Genetic and environmental components of interindividual variation in circulating levels of IGF-I, IGF-II, IGFBP-1, and IGFBP-3. J Clin Invest 1996; 98(11):2612–2615.

Heald AH, Cade JE, Cruickshank JK, Anderson S, White A, Gibson JM. The influence of dietary intake on the insulin-like growth factor (IGF) system across three ethnic groups: a population-based study. Public Health Nutr 2003; 6 (2):175–180.

Heald A, Kaushal K, Anderson S, Redpath M, Durrington PN, Selby PL, Gibson MJ. Effects of hormone replacement therapy on insulin-like growth factor (IGF)-I, IGF-II and IGF binding protein (IGFBP)-1 to IGFBP-4: implications for cardiovascular risk. Gynecol Endocrinol 2005; 20 (3):176–182.

Hecquet B, Peyrat JP. Diffusion of insulin-like growth factor 1 in human breast cancer explants. Cancer Lett 1990; 54(1–2):29–36.

Helle SI. The insulin-like growth factor system in advanced breast cancer. Best Pract Res Clin Endocrinol Metab 2004; 18(1):67–79.

Helle SI, Omsjo IH, Hughes SC, Botta L, Huls G, Holly JM, Lonning PE. Effects of oral and transdermal oestrogen replacement therapy on plasma levels of insulin-like growth factors and IGF binding proteins 1 and 3: a cross-over study. Clin Endocrinol (Oxf) 1996a; 45(6):727–732.

Helle SI, Holly JM, Tally M, et al. Influence of treatment with tamoxifen and change in tumor burden on the IGF-system in breast cancer patients. Int J Cancer 1996b; 69(4): 335–339.

Ho GH, Ji CY, Phang BH. Tamoxifen alters levels of serum insulin-like growth factors and binding proteins in postmenopausal breast cancer patients: a prospective paired cohort study. Ann Surg Oncol 1998; 5(4):361–367.

Ho KK, O'Sullivan AJ, Weissberger AJ, Kelly JJ. Sex steroid regulation of growth hormone secretion and action. Horm Res 1996; 45(1–2):67–73.

Hofling M, Carlstrom K, Svane G, Azavedo E, Kloosterboer H, Von Schoultz B. Different effects of tibolone and continuous combined estrogen plus progestogen hormone therapy on sex hormone binding globulin and free testosterone levels–an association with mammographic density. Gynecol Endocrinol 2005; 20(2):110–115.

Holmes MD, Pollak MN, Willett WC, Hankinson SE Dietary correlates of plasma insulin-like growth factor I and insulin-like growth factor binding protein 3 concentrations. Cancer Epidemiol Biomarkers Prev 2002; 11(9):852–861.

Hong Y, Pedersen NL, Brismar K, Hall K, de Faire U. Quantitative genetic analyses of insulin-like growth factor I (IGF-I), IGF-binding protein-1, and insulin levels in middle-aged and elderly twins. J Clin Endocrinol Metab 1996; 81(5):1791–1797.

Hopkins KD, Parker JR, Lehmann ED, Rymer J, Holly JM, Fogelman I, Cwyfan-Hughes S, Teale JD, Gosling RG. Insulin-like growth factor (IGF)-I levels in postmenopausal women receiving tibolone. Horm Metab Res 1995; 27 (8):387–388.

Hunt KJ, Lukanova A, Rinaldi S, Lundin E, Norat T, Palmqvist R, Stattin P, Riboli E, Hallmans G, Kaaks R. A potential inverse association between insulin-like growth factor I and hypertension in a cross-sectional study. Ann Epidemiol 2006; 16(7):563–571.

Hwa V, Oh Y, Rosenfeld RG. The insulin-like growth factor-binding protein (IGFBP) superfamily. Endocr Rev 1999; 20(6):761–787.

Ibrahim YH, Yee D. Insulin-like growth factor-I and breast cancer therapy. Clin Cancer Res 2005; 11(2): 944s–950s.

Ingle JN, Suman VJ, Kardinal CG, Krook JE, Mailliard JA, Veeder MH, Loprinzi CL, Dalton RJ, Hartmann LC, Conover CA, Pollak MN. A randomized trial of tamoxifen alone or combined with octreotide in the treatment of women with metastatic breast carcinoma. Cancer 1999; 85(6):1284–1292.

Iranmanesh A, Veldhuis JD. Clinical pathophysiology of the somatotropic (GH) axis in adults. Endocrinol Metab Clin North Am 1992; 21(4):783–816.

Isley WL, Underwood LE, Clemmons DR. Dietary components that regulate serum somatomedin-C concentrations in humans. J Clin Invest 1983; 71(2):175–182.

Isley WL, Underwood LE, Clemmons DR. Changes in plasma somatomedin-C in response to ingestion of diets with variable protein and energy content. JPEN J Parenter Enteral Nutr 1984; 8(4):407–411.

Jenkins PJ, Mukherjee A, Shalet SM. Does growth hormone cause cancer? Clin Endocrinol (Oxf) 2006; 64(2):115–121.

Juul A, Scheike T, Davidsen M, Gyllenborg J, Jorgensen T. Low serum insulin-like growth factor I is associated with increased risk of ischemic heart disease: a population-based case-control study. Circulation 2002; 106(8):939–944.

Kaaks R, Bellati C, Venturelli E, Rinaldi S, Secreto G, Biessy C, Pala V, Sieri S, Berrino F. Effects of dietary intervention on IGF-I and IGF-binding proteins, and related alterations in sex steroid metabolism: the Diet and Androgens (DIANA) Randomised Trial. Eur J Clin Nutr 2003; 57(9):1079–1088.

Kaaks R, Berrino F, Key T, Rinaldi S, Dossus L, Biessy C, Secreto G, Amiano P, Bingham S, Boeing H, Bueno De Mesquita HB, Chang-Claude J, Clavel-Chapelon F, Fournier A, van Gils CH, Gonzalez CA, Gurrea AB, Critselis E, Khaw KT, Krogh V, Lahmann PH, Nagel G, Olsen A, Onland-Moret NC, Overvad K, Palli D, Panico S, Peeters P, Quiros JR, Roddam A. Serum sex steroids in premenopausal women and breast cancer risk within the European Prospective Investigation into Cancer and Nutrition (EPIC). J Natl Cancer Inst 2005; 97(10):755–765.

Kaaks R, Lukanova A. Energy balance and cancer: the role of insulin and insulin-like growth factor-I. Proc Nutr Soc 2001; 60(1):91–106.

Kaaks R, Lundin E, Rinaldi S, Manjer J, Biessy C, Soderberg S, Lenner P, Janzon L, Riboli E, Berglund G, Hallmans G. Prospective study of IGF-I, IGF-binding proteins, and breast cancer risk, in northern and southern Sweden. Cancer Causes Control 2002; 13(4):307–316.

Kam GY, Leung KC, Baxter RC, Ho KK. Estrogens exert route- and dose-dependent effects on insulin-like growth factor (IGF)-binding protein-3 and the acid-labile subunit of the IGF ternary complex. J Clin Endocrinol Metab 2000; 85(5):1918–1922.

Kao PC, Matheny AP Jr., Lang CA. Insulin-like growth factor-I comparisons in healthy twin children. J Clin Endocrinol Metab 1994; 78(2):310–312.

Keinan-Boker L, Bueno De Mesquita HB, Kaaks R, van Gils CH, Van Noord PA, Rinaldi S, Riboli E, Seidell JC, Grobbee DE, Peeters PH. Circulating levels of insulin-like growth factor I, its binding proteins -1,-2, -3, C-peptide and risk of postmenopausal breast cancer. Int J Cancer 2003; 106(1):90–95.

Kim JG, Lee JY. Changes in profiles of circulating insulin-like growth factor components during hormone replacement therapy according to the responsiveness to therapy in postmenopausal women. Am J Obstet Gynecol 2001; 184(6):1139–1144.

Krajcik RA, Borofsky ND, Massardo S, Orentreich N. Insulin-like growth factor I (IGF-I), IGF-binding proteins, and breast cancer. Cancer Epidemiol Biomarkers Prev 2002; 11(12):1566–1573.

Kuhl H. Pharmacology of estrogens and progestogens: influence of different routes of administration. Climacteric 2005; 8(suppl 1):3–63.

Lahmann PH, Hoffmann K, Allen N, van Gils CH, Khaw KT, Tehard B, Berrino F, Tjonneland A, Bigaard J, Olsen A, Overvad K, Clavel-Chapelon F, Nagel G, Boeing H, Trichopoulos D, Economou G, Bellos G, Palli D, Tumino R, Panico S, Sacerdote C, Krogh V, Peeters PH, Bueno-de-Mesquita HB, Lund E, Ardanaz E, Amiano P, Pera G, Quiros JR, Martinez C, et al. Body size and breast cancer risk: findings from the European Prospective Investigation into Cancer And Nutrition (EPIC). Int J Cancer 2004; 111 (5):762–771.

Larsson SC, Wolk K, Brismar K, Wolk A. Association of diet with serum insulin-like growth factor I in middle-aged and elderly men. Am J Clin Nutr 2005; 81(5):1163–1167.

Laughlin GA, Barrett-Connor E, Criqui MH, Kritz-Silverstein D. The prospective association of serum insulin-like growth factor I (IGF-I) and IGF-binding protein-1 levels with all cause and cardiovascular disease mortality in older adults: the Rancho Bernardo Study. J Clin Endocrinol Metab 2004; 89(1):114–120.

Le Roith D, Bondy C, Yakar S, Liu JL, Butler A. The somatomedin hypothesis: 2001. Endocr Rev 2001; 22(1):53–74.

Lee S, Kolonel L, Wilkens L, Wan P, Henderson B, Pike M. Postmenopausal hormone therapy and breast cancer risk: the Multiethnic Cohort. Int J Cancer 2006; 118(5):1285–1291.

Leung KC, Johannsson G, Leong GM, Ho KK. Estrogen regulation of growth hormone action. Endocr Rev 2004; 25(5):693–721.

Li CI, Malone KE, Porter PL, Weiss NS, Tang MT, Cushing-Haugen KL, Daling JR. Relationship between long durations and different regimens of hormone therapy and risk of breast cancer. JAMA 2003; 289(24):3254–3263.

Lien EA, Johannessen DC, Aakvaag A, Lonning PE. Influence of tamoxifen, aminoglutethimide and goserelin on human plasma IGF-I levels in breast cancer patients. J Steroid Biochem Mol Biol 1992; 41(3–8):541–543.

Lukanova A, Lundin E, Zeleniuch-Jacquotte A, et al. Body mass index, circulating levels of sex-steroid hormones, IGF-I and IGF-binding protein-3: a cross-sectional study in healthy women. Eur J Endocrinol 2004; 150(2):161–171.

Lukanova A, Soderberg S, Stattin P, Palmqvist R, Lundin E, Biessy C, Rinaldi S, Riboli E, Hallmans G, Kaaks R. Nonlinear relationship of insulin-like growth factor (IGF)-I and IGF-I/IGF-binding protein-3 ratio with indices of adiposity and plasma insulin concentrations (Sweden). Cancer Causes Control 2002; 13(6):509–516.

Lukanova A, Toniolo P, Zeleniuch-Jacquotte A, Grankvist K, Wulff M, Arslan AA, Afanasyeva Y, Johansson R, Lenner P, Hallmans G, Wadell G, Lundin E. Insulin-like growth factor I in pregnancy and maternal risk of breast cancer. Cancer Epidemiol Biomarkers Prev 2006; 15 (12):2489–2493.

Ma J, Giovannucci E, Pollak M, Chan JM, Gaziano JM, Willett W, Stampfer MJ. Milk intake, circulating levels of insulin-like growth factor-I, and risk of colorectal cancer in men. J Natl Cancer Inst 2001; 93(17):1330–1336.

Maes M, Amand Y, Underwood LE, Maiter D, Ketelslegers JM. Decreased serum insulin-like growth factor I response to growth hormone in hypophysectomized rats fed a low protein diet: evidence for a postreceptor defect. Acta Endocrinol (Copenh) 1988; 117(3):320–326.

Mah PM, Webster J, Jonsson P, Feldt-Rasmussen U, Koltowska-Haggstrom M, Ross RJ. Estrogen replacement in women of fertile years with hypopituitarism. J Clin Endocrinol Metab 2005; 90(11):5964–5969.

Maile LA, Xu S, Cwyfan-Hughes SC, Fernihough JK, Pell JM, Holly JM. Active and inhibitory components of the insulin-like growth factor binding protein-3 protease system in adult serum, interstitial, and synovial fluid. Endocrinology 1998; 139(12):4772–4781.

Malarkey WB, Burleson M, Cacioppo JT, Poehlmann K, Glaser R, Kiecolt-Glaser JK. Differential effects of estrogen and medroxyprogesterone on basal and stress-induced growth hormone release, IGF-1 levels, and cellular immunity in postmenopausal women. Endocrine 1997; 7(2):227–233.

McCarty MF. Androgenic progestins amplify the breast cancer risk associated with hormone replacement therapy by boosting IGF-I activity. Med Hypotheses 2001; 56(2):213–216.

Merimee TJ, Zapf J, Froesch ER. Insulin-like growth factors in the fed and fasted states. J Clin Endocrinol Metab 1982; 55 (5):999–1002.

Micheli A, Muti P, Secreto G, Krogh V, Meneghini E, Venturelli E, Sieri S, Pala V, Berrino F. Endogenous sex hormones and subsequent breast cancer in premenopausal women. Int J Cancer 2004; 112(2):312–318.

Moorman PG, Kuwabara H, Millikan RC, Newman B. Menopausal hormones and breast cancer in a biracial population. Am J Public Health 2000; 90(6):966–971.

Morales AJ, Haubrich RH, Hwang JY, Asakura H, Yen SS. The effect of six months treatment with a 100 mg daily dose of dehydroepiandrosterone (DHEA) on circulating sex steroids, body composition and muscle strength in age-advanced men and women. Clin Endocrinol (Oxf) 1998; 49(4):421–432.

Muñoz-Torres M, Mezquita-Raya P, Lopez-Rodriguez F, Torres-Vela E, de Dios LJ, Escobar-Jimenez F. The contribution of IGF-I to skeletal integrity in postmenopausal women. Clin Endocrinol (Oxf) 2001; 55(6):759–766.

Muti P, Quattrin T, Grant BJ, Krogh V, Micheli A, Schunemann HJ, Ram M, Freudenheim JL, Sieri S, Trevisan M, Berrino F. Fasting glucose is a risk factor for breast cancer: a prospective study. Cancer Epidemiol Biomarkers Prev 2002; 11(11):1361–1368.

Muti P, Stanulla M, Micheli A, Krogh V, Freudenheim JL, Yang J, Schunemann HJ, Trevisan M, Berrino F. Markers of insulin resistance and sex steroid hormone activity in relation to breast cancer risk: a prospective analysis of abdominal adiposity, sebum production, and hirsutism (Italy). Cancer Causes Control 2000; 11(8):721–730.

Newcomb PA, Titus-Ernstoff L, Egan KM, Trentham-Dietz A, Baron JA, Storer BE, Willett WC, Stampfer MJ. Postmenopausal estrogen and progestin use in relation to breast cancer risk. Cancer Epidemiol Biomarkers Prev 2002; 11(7):593–600.

Ng ST, Zhou J, Adesanya OO, Wang J, LeRoith D, Bondy CA. Growth hormone treatment induces mammary gland hyperplasia in aging primates. Nat Med 1997; 3(10):1141–1144.

Norat T, Dossus L, Rinaldi S, Overvad K, Gronbaek H, Tjonneland A, Olsen A, Clavel-Chapelon F, Boutron-Ruault MC, Boeing H, Lahmann PH, Linseisen J, Nagel G, Trichopoulou A, Trichopoulos D, Kalapothaki V, Sieri S, Palli D, Panico S, Tumino R, Sacerdote C, Bueno-de-Mesquita HB, Peeters PH, van Gils CH, Agudo A, Amiano P, Ardanoz E, Martinez C, Quiros R, Tormo MJ et al. Diet, serum insulin-like growth factor-I and IGF-binding protein-3 in European women. Eur J Clin Nutr 2007; 61(1):91–98.

Nugent AG, Leung KC, Sullivan D, Reutens AT, Ho KK. Modulation by progestogens of the effects of oestrogen on hepatic endocrine function in postmenopausal women. Clin Endocrinol (Oxf) 2003; 59(6):690–698.

O'Connell T, Clemmons DR. IGF-I/IGF-binding protein-3 combination improves insulin resistance by GH-dependent and independent mechanisms. J Clin Endocrinol Metab 2002; 87(9):4356–4360.

Olsson HL, Ingvar C, Bladstrom A. Hormone replacement therapy containing progestins and given continuously increases breast carcinoma risk in Sweden. Cancer 2003; 97(6):1387–1392.

Pasanisi P, Venturelli E, Morelli D, Fontana L, Secreto G, Berrino F. Serum insulin-like growth factor I and platelet-derived growth factor as biomarkers of breast cancer prognosis. Cancer Epidemiol Biomarkers Prev 2008 (submitted for publication)

Peyrat JP, Bonneterre J, Hecquet B, Vennin P, Louchez MM, Fournier C, Lefebvre J, Demaille A. Plasma insulin-like growth factor-1 (IGF-1) concentrations in human breast cancer. Eur J Cancer 1993; 29A(4):492–497.

Pollak MN. Endocrine effects of IGF-I on normal and transformed breast epithelial cells: potential relevance to strategies for breast cancer treatment and prevention. Breast Cancer Res Treat 1998; 47(3):209–217.

Pollak MN, Schally AV. Mechanisms of antineoplastic action of somatostatin analogs. Proc Soc Exp Biol Med 1998; 217 (2):143–152.

Porch JV, Lee IM, Cook NR, Rexrode KM, Burin JE. Estrogen-progestin replacement therapy and breast cancer risk: the Women's Health Study (United States). Cancer Causes Control 2002; 13(9):847–854.

Porcile A, Gallardo E, Duarte P, Aedo S. [Differential effects on serum IGF-1 of tibolone (5 mg/day) vs combined continuous estrogen/progestagen in post menopausal women]. Rev Med Chil 2003; 131(10):1151–1156.

Posaci C, Altunyurt S, Islekel H, Onvural A. Effects of HRT on serum levels of IGF-I in postmenopausal women. Maturitas 2001; 40(1):69–74.

Rajaram S, Baylink DJ, Mohan S. Insulin-like growth factor-binding proteins in serum and other biological fluids: regulation and functions. Endocr Rev 1997; 18(6):801–831.

Raudaskoski T, Knip M, Laatikainen T. Plasma insulin-like growth factor-I and its binding proteins 1 and 3 during continuous nonoral and oral combined hormone replacement therapy. Menopause 1998; 5(4):217–222.

Ravn P, Overgaard K, Spencer EM, Christiansen C. Insulin-like growth factors I and II in healthy women with and without established osteoporosis. Eur J Endocrinol 1995; 132 (3):313–319.

Reed MJ, Christodoulides A, Koistinen R, Seppala M, Teale JD, Ghilchik MW. The effect of endocrine therapy with medroxyprogesterone acetate, 4-hydroxyandrostenedione or tamoxifen on plasma concentrations of insulin-like growth factor (IGF)-I, IGF-II and IGFBP-1 in women with advanced breast cancer. Int J Cancer 1992; 52(2): 208–212.

Ren Z, Cai Q, Shu XO, Cai H, Li C, Yu H, Gao YT, Zheng W. Genetic polymorphisms in the IGFBP3 gene: association with breast cancer risk and blood IGFBP-3 protein levels among Chinese women. Cancer Epidemiol Biomarkers Prev 2004; 13(8):1290–1295.

Renehan AG, Zwahlen M, Minder C, O'Dwyer ST, Shalet SM, Egger M. Insulin-like growth factor (IGF)-I, IGF binding protein-3, and cancer risk: systematic review and meta-regression analysis. Lancet 2004; 363(9418):1346–1353.

Rinaldi S, Kaaks R, Zeleniuch-Jacquotte A, Arslan AA, Shore RE, Koenig KL, Dossus L, Riboli E, Stattin P, Lukanova A, Toniolo P. Insulin-like growth factor-I, IGF binding protein-3, and breast cancer in young women: a comparison of risk estimates using different peptide assays. Cancer Epidemiol Biomarkers Prev 2005; 14:48–52.

Rinaldi S, Peeters PH, Berrino F, Dossus L, Biessy C, Olsen A, Tjonneland A, Overvad K, Clavel-Chapelon F, Boutron-Ruault MC, Tehard B, Nagel G, Linseisen J, Boeing H, Lahmann PH, Trichopoulou A, Trichopoulos D, Koliva M, Palli D, Panico S, Tumino R, Sacerdote C, van Gils CH, van Noord P, Grobbee DE, Bueno-de-Mesquita HB, Gonzalez CA, Agudo A, Chirlaque MD, Barricarte A, et al. IGF-I, IGFBP-3 and breast cancer risk in women: The European Prospective Investigation into Cancer and Nutrition (EPIC). Endocr Relat Cancer 2006; 13(2):593–605.

Rollison DE, Newschaffer CJ, Tao Y, Pollak M, Helzlsouer KJ. Premenopausal levels of circulating insulin-like growth factor I and the risk of postmenopausal breast cancer. Int J Cancer 2006; 118:1279–1284.

Rosen CJ. IGF-I and osteoporosis. Clin Lab Med 2000; 20(3): 591–602.

Rosenberg L, Palmer JR, Wise LA, Adams-Campbell LL. A prospective study of female hormone use and breast cancer among black women. Arch Intern Med 2006; 166(7): 760–765.

Ross RK, Paganini-Hill A, Wan PC, Effect of hormone replacement therapy on breast cancer risk: estrogen versus estrogen plus progestin. J Natl Cancer Inst 2000; 92(4): 328–332.

Sandhu MS, Heald AH, Gibson JM, Cruickshank JK, Dunger DB, Wareham NJ. Circulating concentrations of insulin-like growth factor-I and development of glucose intolerance: a prospective observational study. Lancet 2002; 359 (9319):1740–1745.

Schairer C, Lubin J, Troisi R, Sturgeon S, Brinton L, Hoover R. Menopausal estrogen and estrogen-progestin replacement therapy and breast cancer risk. JAMA 2000; 283(4): 485–491.

Schernhammer ES, Hankinson SE, Hunter DJ, Blouin MJ, Pollak MN. Polymorphic variation at the -202 locus in IGFBP3: Influence on serum levels of insulin-like growth factors, interaction with plasma retinol and vitamin D and breast cancer risk. Int J Cancer 2003; 107(1):60–64.

Schernhammer ES, Holly JM, Pollak MN, Hankinson SE. Circulating levels of insulin-like growth factors, their binding proteins, and breast cancer risk. Cancer Epidemiol Biomarkers Prev 2005; 14(3):699–704.

Schindler AE, Campagnoli C, Druckmann R, Huber J, Pasqualini JR, Schweppe KW, Thijssen JHH. Classification and pharmacology of progestins. Maturitas 2003; 46:S7–S16.

Setiawan VW, Cheng I, Stram DO, Penney KL, Le Marchand L, Altshuler D, Kolonel LN, Hirschhorn J, Henderson BE, Freedman ML. Igf-I genetic variation and breast cancer: the multiethnic cohort. Cancer Epidemiol Biomarkers Prev 2006; 15(1):172–174.

Sheffield-Moore M, Paddon-Jones D, Casperson SL, Gilkison C, Volpi E, Wolf SE, Jiang J, Rosenblatt JI, Urban RJ. Androgen therapy induces muscle protein anabolism in older women. J Clin Endocrinol Metab 2006; 91(10): 3844–3849.

Shi R, Yu H, McLarty J, Glass J. IGF-I and breast cancer: a meta-analysis. Int J Cancer 2004; 111(3):418–423.

Slowinska-Srzednicka J, Zgliczynski S, Jeske W, Stopinska-Gluszak U, Srzednicki M, Brzezinska A, Zgliczynski W, Sadowski Z. Transdermal 17 beta-estradiol combined with oral progestogen increases plasma levels of insulin-like growth factor-I in postmenopausal women. J Endocrinol Invest 1992; 15(7):533–538.

Smith WJ, Underwood LE, Clemmons DR. Effects of caloric or protein restriction on insulin-like growth factor-I (IGF-I) and IGF-binding proteins in children and adults. J Clin Endocrinol Metab 1995; 80(2):443–449.

Soot T, Jurimae T, Jurimae J. Relationships between bone mineral density, insulin-like growth factor-1 and sex hormones in young females with different physical activity. J Sports Med Phys Fitness 2006; 46(2):293–297.

Stefanick ML, Anderson GL, Margolis KL, Hendrix SL, Rodabough RJ, Paskett ED, Lane DS, Hubbell FA, Assaf AR, Sarto GE, Schenken RS, Yasmeen S, Lessin L, Chlebowski RT. Effects of conjugated equine estrogens on breast cancer and mammography screening in postmenopausal women with hysterectomy. JAMA 2006; 295(14):1647–1657.

Straus DS, Takemoto CD. Effect of dietary protein deprivation on insulin-like growth factor (IGF)-I and -II, IGF binding protein-2, and serum albumin gene expression in rat. Endocrinology 1990; 127(4):1849–1860.

Sugumar A, Liu YC, Xia Q. Insulin-like growth factor (IGF)-I and IGF-binding protein 3 and the risk of premenopausal breast cancer: a meta-analysis of literature. Int J Cancer 2004; 111(2):293–297.

Tamimi RM, Hankinson SE, Chen WY, Rosner B, Colditz GA. Combined estrogen and testosterone use and risk of breast cancer in postmenopausal women. Arch Intern Med 2006; 166(14):1483–1489.

Thissen JP, Ketelslegers JM, Underwood LE. Nutritional regulation of the insulin-like growth factors. Endocr Rev 1994; 15(1):80–101.

Toniolo P, Bruning PF, Akhmedkhanov A, Bonfrer JM, Koenig KL, Lukanova A, Shore RE, Zeleniuch-Jacquotte A. Serum insulin-like growth factor-I and breast cancer. Int J Cancer 2000; 88:828–832.

Torrisi R, Parodi S, Fontana V, Pensa F, Casella C, Barreca A, De Palo G, Costa A, Decensi A. Effect of fenretinide on plasma IGF-I and IGFBP-3 in early breast cancer patients. Int J Cancer 1998; 76(6):787–790.

van Rijn MJ, Slooter AJ, Bos MJ, Catarino CF, Koudstaal PJ, Hofman A, Breteler MM, van Duijn CM. Insulin-like growth factor I promoter polymorphism, risk of stroke, and survival after stroke: the Rotterdam study. J Neurol Neurosurg Psychiatry 2006; 77(1):24–27.

Veldhuis JD. Gender differences in secretory activity of the human somatotropic (growth hormone) axis. Eur J Endocrinol 1996; 134(3):287–295.

Veldhuis JD, Frystyk J, Iranmanesh A, Orskov H. Testosterone and estradiol regulate free insulin-like growth factor I (IGF-I), IGF binding protein 1 (IGFBP-1), and dimeric IGF-I/IGFBP-1 concentrations. J Clin Endocrinol Metab 2005; 90(5):2941–2947.

Veldhuis JD, Roemmich JN, Richmond EJ, Bowers CY. Somatotropic and gonadotropic axes linkages in infancy, childhood, and the puberty-adult transition. Endocr Rev 2006a; 27(2):101–140.

Veldhuis JD, Keenan DM, Iranmanesh A, Mielke K, Miles JM, Bowers CY. Estradiol potentiates ghrelin-stimulated pulsatile growth hormone secretion in postmenopausal women. J Clin Endocrinol Metab 2006b; 91(9):3559–3565.

Vennin P, Peyrat JP, Bonneterre J, Louchez MM, Harris AG, Demaille A. Effect of the long-acting somatostatin analogue SMS 201–995 (Sandostatin) in advanced breast cancer. Anticancer Res 1989; 9(1):153–155.

Verhaeghe J, Loos R, Vlietinck R, Herck EV, van Bree R, Schutter AM. C-peptide, insulin-like growth factors I and II, and insulin-like growth factor binding protein-1 in cord serum of twins: genetic versus environmental regulation. Am J Obstet Gynecol 1996; 175(5):1180–1188.

Verheus M, Peeters PH, Rinaldi S, Dossus L, Biessy C, Olsen A, Tjonneland A, Overvad K, Jeppesen M, Clavel-Chapelon F, Tehard B, Nagel G, Linseisen J, Boeing H, Lahmann PH, Arvaniti A, Psaltopoulou T, Trichopoulou A, Palli D, Tumino R, Panico S, Sacerdote C, Sieri S, van Gils CH, Bueno-de-Mesquita BH, Gonzalez CA, Ardanaz E, Larranaga N, Garcia CM, Navarro C et al. Serum C-peptide levels and breast cancer risk: results from the European Prospective Investigation into Cancer and Nutrition (EPIC). Int J Cancer 2006; 119(3):659–667.

Villareal DT, Holloszy JO. DHEA enhances effects of weight training on muscle mass and strength in elderly women and men. Am J Physiol Endocrinol Metab 2006; 291(5): E1003–E1008.

Viscoli CM, Brass LM, Kernan WN, Sarrel PM, Suissa S, Horwitz RI. A clinical trial of estrogen-replacement therapy after ischemic stroke. N Engl J Med 2001; 345 (17):1243–1249.

Westley BR, May FE. Role of insulin-like growth factors in steroid modulated proliferation. J Steroid Biochem Mol Biol 1994; 51(1–2):1–9.

Winston R, Kao PC, Kiang DT. Regulation of insulin-like growth factors by antiestrogen. Breast Cancer Res Treat 1994; 31(1):107–115.

Wolf I, Sadetzki S, Catane R, Karasik A, Kaufman B. Diabetes mellitus and breast cancer. Lancet Oncol 2005; 6(2): 103–111.

World Cancer Research Fund, American Institute for Cancer Research. Food, nutrition and the prevention of cancer: A global perspective. Washington: WCRF/AICR; 1997.

Wu Y, Cui K, Miyoshi K, Hennighausen L, Green JE, Setser J, LeRoith D, Yakar S. Reduced circulating insulin-like growth factor I levels delay the onset of chemically and genetically induced mammary tumors. Cancer Res 2003; 63 (15):4384–4388.

Yakar S, Rosen CJ, Beamer WG, Ackert-Bicknell CL, Wu Y, Liu JL, Ooi GT, Setser J, Frystyk J, Boisclair YR, LeRoith D. Circulating levels of IGF-1 directly regulate bone growth and density. J Clin Invest 2002; 110(6):771–781.

Yee D, Paik S, Lebovic GS, Marcus RR, Favoni RE, Cullen KJ, Lippman ME, Rosen N. Analysis of insulin-like growth factor I gene expression in malignancy: evidence for a paracrine role in human breast cancer. Mol Endocrinol 1989; 3(3):509–517.

Yu H, Jin F, Shu XO, Li BD, Dai Q, Cheng JR, Berkel HJ, Zheng W. Insulin-like growth factors and breast cancer risk in Chinese women. Cancer Epidemiol Biomarkers Prev 2002; 11(8):705–712.

Yu H, Shu XO, Li BD, Dai Q, Gao YT, Jin F, Zheng W. Joint effect of insulin-like growth factors and sex steroids on breast cancer risk. Cancer Epidemiol Biomarkers Prev 2003; 12(10):1067–1073.

18

Proliferation of Breast Cells by Steroid Hormones and Their Metabolites

HELENIUS J. KLOOSTERBOER
KC2, Oss, The Netherlands

WILLEM G. E. J. SCHOONEN and HERMAN A. M. VERHEUL
Research and Development, Organon, a part of Schering-Plough Corporation, Oss, The Netherlands

INTRODUCTION

Estradiol (E_2) and progesterone (P_4) play a pivotal role in the development of normal breast tissue (Ismail et al., 2003; Russo and Russo, 2004; Tekmal et al., 2005; Couse and Korach, 1999; Vandenberg et al., 2006). Both hormones are also associated with a modest increase in breast cancer. Oral contraceptives (OCs) are related with a small increase in the risk of breast cancer, as was found by the Collaborative Group on Hormonal Factors in Breast Cancer (Beral et al., 1996), when they reanalyzed the individual data of 54 studies. No difference was found between low-dose, medium-dose, and high-dose preparations. Information about OCs with 20 μg of ethinylestradiol or OCs with newly introduced progestagens is not yet available. Hormonal Treatment (HT) in postmenopausal women also shows an increased risk for the prognosis of breast cancer (Beral et al., 1997). However, it is important to note that the available data of these epidemiological studies are coming for 80% from estrogen-only trials. A few years later Bush et al. (2001) concluded in a qualitative review from largely the same data set that little consistency is seen in the outcome of these studies. They found little support for the hypothesis that HT increased the risk of breast cancer.

Recently the results of two large studies on HT and breast cancer risk in postmenopausal women were published. These two studies differ in design, which is most likely the cause of the difference in outcome. In the Women's Health Initiative (WHI) study, a prospective randomized controlled trial with either conjugated equine estrogens (CEE) alone or in combination with medroxyprogesterone acetate (MPA), it was found that the combined treatment showed an increased risk of breast cancer in elderly postmenopausal women (Chlebowski et al., 2003), whereas the treatment of CEE alone did not show such an increased risk (Anderson et al., 2004). These results point to an adverse side effect of MPA, which is often generalized to the same adverse effect for all progestagens used in HT. The results of the observational Million Women Study (MWS) show a similar tendency with respect to the increased risk of breast cancer for the various estrogen and progestagen combinations (Beral et al., 2003). These hormonal combinations showed again a higher risk than the estrogen-only preparations. The calculated risk appears to be higher in the MWS than in the WHI study for the estrogen-only arm as well as for the estrogen and progestagen combinations, which confirmed findings from others (Newcomb et al., 2002). The occurrence of the cancers in these studies was relatively fast (5.2 years in the WHI and 1.2 years in the MWS, after start of HT). When the exogenous steroids would be the cancer initiators, one would expect a latency period of about 7 to 10 years from initiation to detection (Tilanus-Linthorst et al., 2005; Dietel et al., 2005; Kopans et al., 2003; Wertheimer et al., 1986), assuming a volume doubling time of 100 days. It is, therefore, more likely that the steroids are promoters of the growth of existing (dormant) hormone-dependent tumors that were apparently already present and undetectable by the existing screening methods applied just prior to the start of HT.

The increased breast tumor risk may thus be due to the stimulation of proliferation. It has been hypothesized in the 1980s that increased cell multiplication by endogenous and exogenous hormones may be associated with an increased risk of breast cancer (Preston-Martin et al., 1990). An increase in cell division may increase the chance of genetic defects as seen in cancers. Both E_2 and P_4 are capable of stimulating breast cell proliferation, and this might enhance the risk of mutations. This together with a few inherited or randomly acquired mutations in cell cycle control factors and factors involved in DNA repair mechanisms may disturb the balance between proliferation and apoptosis in the breast tissue and may finally result in pathology (Zhang and Powell, 2005; Tutt and Ashworth, 2002).

In addition, E_2 has also been classified as tumor initiator because of the formation of DNA adducts (Cavalieri et al., 2006; Yager and Davidson, 2006). This may cause mutations, and if DNA repair mechanisms are not optimally functional, this may lead to breast cancer. Whether the concentrations of E_2 in breast tissue are sufficient for tumor initiation is not yet known. The debate whether estrogens are tumor initiators or promoters is still not concluded.

Breast cancer risk of estrogens and progestagens is often assessed by determination of proliferation of breast tumor cell lines. Cell lines may originate from the same source, but at the time of publication of data the cells have a different history (different passage number, period of steroid deprivation) and the experimental conditions may vary (steroid-free interval, growth medium, source of fetal calf serum, duration of treatment, concentration range). Consequently, receptor expression and steroid metabolizing enzymes may show remarkable differences. In addition, the methodology for estimation of proliferation differs among research groups (Rasmussen and Nielsen, 2002). When interpreting in vitro effects, it should be realized that in addition to the above aspects other factors may influence the result, such as

1. a steroid may act via more than one steroid receptor and may possess different receptor affinity levels,
2. a steroid may have antagonistic effects on its receptor,
3. a steroid may down- or upregulate its own or other receptors (Hackenberg et al., 1990),
4. a steroid concentration can be physiological ($<10^{-7}$M) or supraphysiological ($>10^{-7}$M),
5. a steroid may operate via nonclassical steroid receptor pathways.

Where relevant, these aspects will be addressed in this review.

Here we review the effects of (natural) estrogens and P_4, as well as their metabolites, on the proliferation of breast cells, both normal breast cells and cancer cell lines. In OCs, ethinyl estradiol (EE) is used as estrogen, while in HT in postmenopausal women E_2 (esters) or CEE is mainly used. The available data about EE and CEE on proliferation are included in this review. Many progestagens used in OCs and HT are either derived from P_4 or from 19-nortestosterone (see for review Stanczyck, 2002). Especially, the last class of compounds may have residual binding to the androgen receptor. Androgenic activity may antagonize estrogenic activity. We have evaluated whether there is a difference in effect on proliferation of these two classes of progestagens. Progestagens derived from 19-nortestosterone also influence circulating levels of sex hormone–binding globulin (SHBG) (Van der Vange et al., 1990), which binds androgens. Since these progestagens have an indirect effect on circulating and tissue levels of androgens, we also evaluated the effect of the most prevalent androgens and their metabolites on the proliferation of breast cancer cells. Tibolone, a 19-nortestosterone derivative, is used in postmenopausal women as a single compound for the treatment of climacteric complaints and prevention of osteoporosis. It does not stimulate the endometrium (Archer et al., 2007) and the breast (Conner et al., 2004). The tissue selective action of tibolone is explained by its site-specific metabolism (Kloosterboer, 2001), and we have included in our evaluation the effect of tibolone and its metabolites on the proliferation of breast cells. We have limited our review to those in vitro studies in which the growth was studied in a concentration range. The results of the in vitro studies were compared with in vivo studies in which proliferation markers or tumor growth was studied. Finally, the results are compared with the outcome of findings in some large observational and prospective clinical trials.

EFFECT OF ESTRADIOL AND METABOLITES ON BREAST CELL PROLIFERATION

The role of E_2 and estrogen receptor α (ERα) in normal breast development is well established (Russo and Russo, 2004) and confirmed by studies with estrogen receptor knockout (ERKO) mice (Tekmal et al., 2005; Couse and Korach, 1999). In the ERα knockout mice, breast tissue is

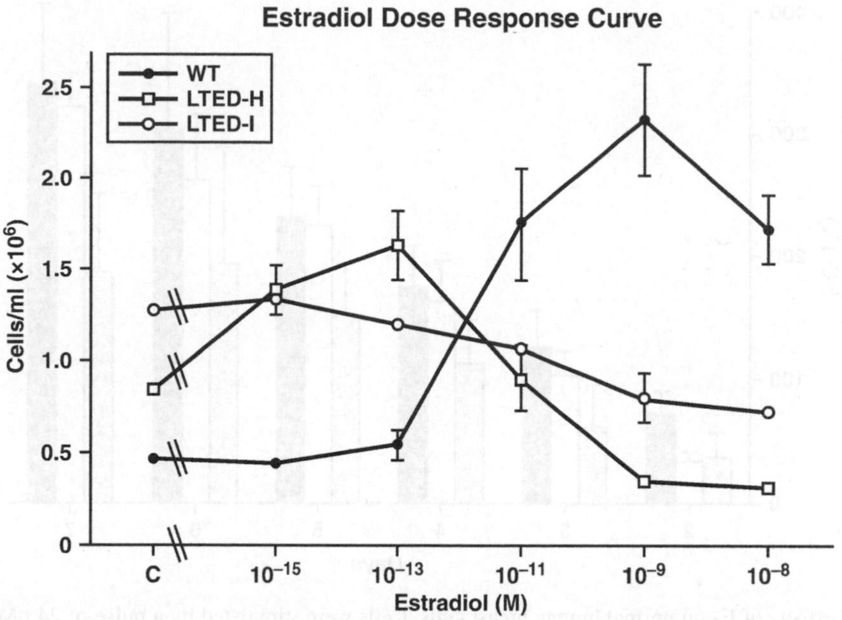

Figure 1 E_2 dose-response curves in human breast tumor MCF-7 cells, being WT or being LTED for 90 weeks, in which one cell line became hypersensitive (H) and another insensitive (I) for E_2; cell counts were performed after 6 days growth in 12-well plates. All experiments were performed in triplicate. Representative dose-response curves are shown. Data are presented as mean ± SD. *Abbreviations*: E_2, estradiol; WT, wild type; LTED, long-term estrogen deprived; SD, standard deviation. *Source*: From Chan et al. (2002).

poorly developed and lobular end buds do not develop in the presence of E_2. ERβ does not play a role in this process. On the other hand, estrogens play a role in the pathogenesis of breast cancer by stimulating proliferation and therefore increasing the chance of DNA mismatches, leading to mutations (Preston-Martin et al., 1990). Alternatively, estrogen metabolites can form DNA adducts and may increase the chance of mutations (Cavalieri et al., 2006; Yager and Davidson, 2006; Russo and Russo, 2006). Breast cancer cell lines are frequently used for studying the molecular mechanisms of steroids on proliferation, apoptosis, and breast safety of newly selected steroidal compounds. Breast cancer cell lines are readily available, but their characteristics may not be the same as those of normal breast cells. We review here the effects of E_2 on the proliferation of breast cancer cell lines and normal breast cells.

In Vitro

Growth Curve Characteristics of Breast Cancer Cell Lines Stimulated by E_2

The effects of E_2 on growth of breast cancer cell lines have been studied for decades (Katzenellenbogen et al., 1987; Reddel and Sutherland, 1987; Schatz et al., 1985; Chalbos et al., 1982; Kendra and Katzenellenbogen, 1987). The responses with the same cell line can be quite different, when the results of various research groups are compared. This may indicate that the growth characteristics may change due to different handlings. In our laboratory, we have compared subclones of MCF-7 cells (originating from McGrath, Litton, and Hubrecht Laboratory) and T47D cells [from American Type of Culture Collections (ATCC) and Sutherland] and found large differences in growth curves between the subclones of the two cell line types (Kloosterboer et al., 1994; Schoonen et al., 1995a,b). The reasons for these differences are difficult to identify, but are certainly not handling or treatment related. Genetic differences between the subclones and cell types are likely. Another explanation may be adaptation to certain culture conditions in the past. Steroid deprivation, for instance, can have a major impact on the growth stimulation by E_2. Estrogen sensitivity can be increased easily by four log-units or more (Masamura et al., 1995; Chan et al., 2002) (Fig. 1). This effect may be explained, at least partly, by a 100-fold higher level of ER(s) (Zajchowski et al., 1993), but coactivator sensitivity as well as the degree of phosphorylation of transactivation factors (TAF-1 and/or TAF-2) may also be crucial. High supraphysiological E_2 concentrations may inhibit cell growth, which leads to a bell-shaped growth curve. This inhibition is stronger in long-term estrogen-deprived (LTED) cells than in wild-type (WT) cells. On the other hand, estrogen withdrawal in vitro may lead to spontaneous growth of MCF-7 cells (Schafer and Jordan, 2006). ER-negative breast cancer cells are not stimulated by estrogens using a medium without growth factors (Cavaillès et al., 2002).

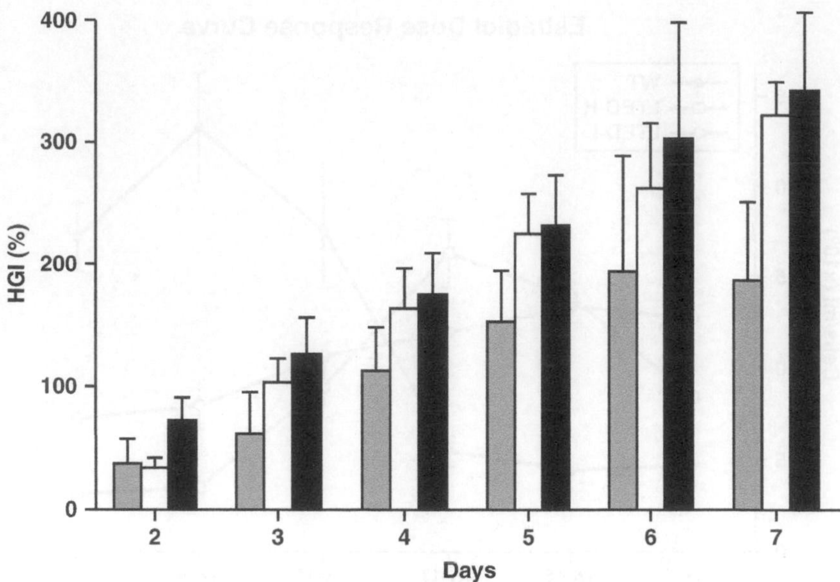

Figure 2 Proliferative effects of E_2 on normal human breast cells. Cells were stimulated by a pulse of 24 nM E_2 for 1 hr (*open bars*) and with continuous 1 nM E_2 (*solid bars*) for 24 hour for a treatment period of 7 days. Control cells (*gray bars*) received no hormone. Proliferation was measured every day using a histomorphic method. Results are expressed as histomorphometric growth index (HGI, for calculation see Gompel et al., 2002) and present means ± SEM of five experiments in which each sample was run in triplicate. *Abbreviations*: E_2, estradiol; SEM, standard error of mean. *Source*: From Cavaillès et al. (2002).

Normal Breast Cells and the Effects of E_2 on Growth

E_2 is required for the normal growth of mammary glands. The effects of E_2 on breast tumor cell proliferation may not reflect the ideal conditions for assessing the tumor risk of an estrogen. The growth effects on human breast epithelial cells may be more relevant, although the cell-cell interactions are lacking. Furthermore, steroid receptor levels and activity of steroid metabolizing enzymes may differ. In isolated (immortalized) human mammary epithelial cells (HMEC), ER was undetectable and the cells did not respond to estrogens, but when these cells were stably transfected with ER and treated with estrogens, growth inhibition was observed (Zajchowski et al., 1993). This growth inhibition could be blocked by a pure antiestrogen. Normal human breast epithelial cells in primary culture are not stimulated by E_2 in a serum-free medium (Gabelman and Emerman, 1992). The absence of proliferation in ER-positive cells is also seen in normal breast tissue (Clarke et al., 1997a). However, mitosis was seen in ER-negative cells, which suggest that paracrine growth factors may be involved. In contrast, ER-positive tumor cells become proliferative by E_2. Gompel et al. (1986, 2002) used a medium supplemented with 1% serum and growth factors and found an increase in proliferation of normal breast cells. This was not observed in the absence of growth factors, despite that these cells contain ER (Malet et al., 1991, 2000). As is shown in Figure 2 (Cavaillès et al., 2002), the increase in proliferation of normal breast cells compared with controls is small and is far less pronounced than is seen in general with ER-positive breast tumor cell lines.

MCF-10F is a normal, immortalized, nontransformed human breast epithelial cell line (Singhal et al., 1999) and these cells cannot be stimulated by E_2, because it is an ER-negative cell line. Surprisingly, Calaf (2006) found a bell-shaped growth curve with these cells (90th passage) with a significant increase in proliferation at 10 nM E_2 after 10 days of culture. This may imply that cell growth activation is mediated via pathways, which do not involve the classical ER.

Effect of Estrogen Metabolites and Synthetic Estrogens on Breast Cell Proliferation

Figure 3 shows the structure of the metabolites of E_2 and the metabolism by the various steroid metabolizing enzymes. The ER affinity of these metabolites is far lower than that of E_2, but when they are continuously present in sufficiently high amounts in cell culture they can increase the proliferation of cells to the same maximal level as that of E_2 (Katzenellenbogen, 1984). Estriol (E_3), which binds weakly to ER, is only slightly less potent than E_2. However, Jozan et al. (1981) found that E_3 and estrone (E_1) were 10 and 50 times weaker than E_2 in MCF-7 cell proliferation. Certain E_2 metabolites, such as 4-hydroxy-E_2 and 16α-hydroxy-E_1,

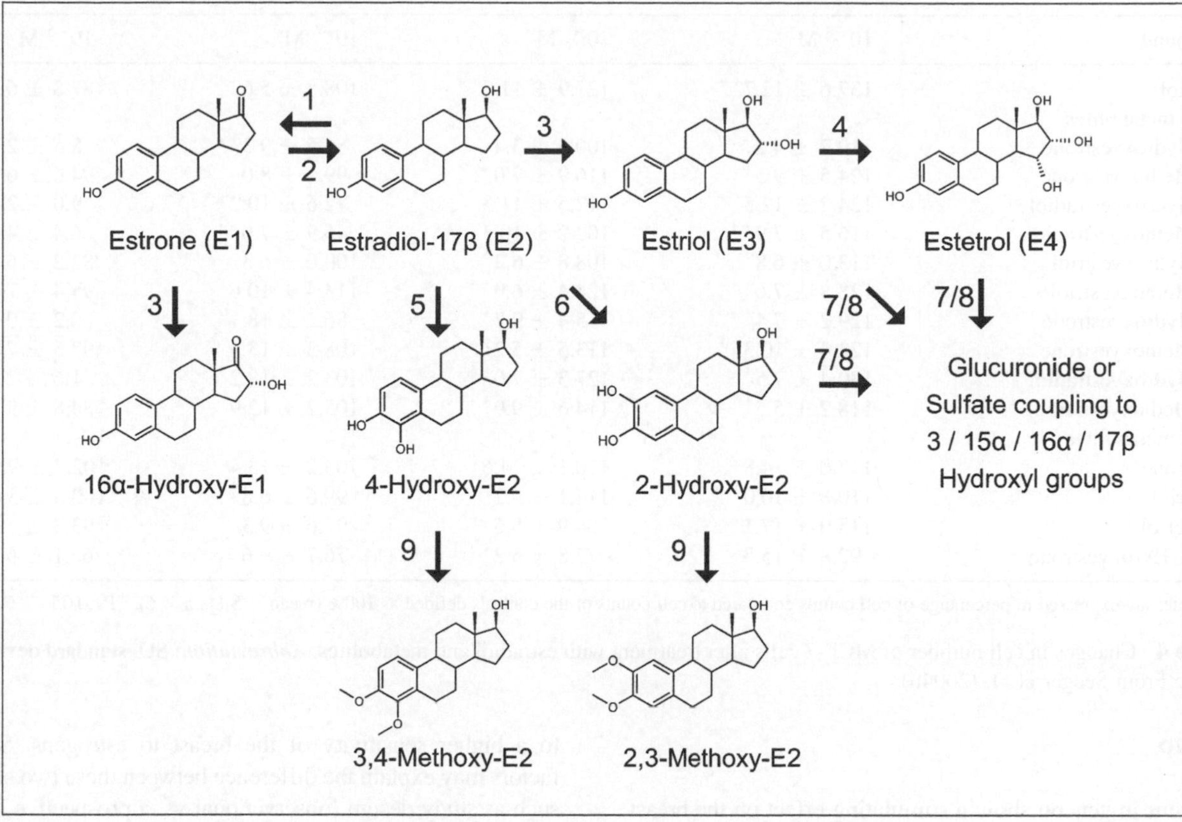

Figure 3 Metabolism pattern of estradiol by the enzymes 17β-oxidoreductase (1), 17β-hydroxysteroid-dehydrogenase (2), 16α-hydroxylase (3), 15α-hydroxylase (4), 4-hydroxylase (5), 2-hydroxylase (6), UDP-glucuronosyl-transferase (7), sulfotransferase (8), and catechol-*O*-methyltransferase (9). The structures of the individual sulfated and glucuronidated steroids are not displayed.

may play a role in breast carcinogenesis (Russo and Russo, 2003; Yager et al., 2006; Cavalieri et al., 2006; Yue et al., 2003). The group of Mueck (Seeger et al., 2004a, 2004b, 2006; Lippert et al., 2003) extensively tested the various E_2 metabolites on proliferation of ER-positive MCF-7 cells (Fig. 4) (Seeger et al., 2004b). In Figure 4, it is shown that the A-ring metabolites have a bell-shaped dose-response curve just as seen for E_2. Many metabolites have inhibitory activity at high pharmacological concentrations (10 μM). 2-Methoxy-E_2, the most potent inhibitor is still a strong inhibitor at 10 times lower concentrations. LaVallee et al. (2002) have confirmed inhibitory effects of 2-methoxy-E_2, but they showed that its action is independent of ER. Reddel and Sutherland (1987) have studied the mechanism of this antiproliferative effect and on the basis of the findings with ER-positive and ER-negative breast cancer cells suggest that this is due to a cell cycle–specific interaction and/or cell cycle–independent cytotoxicity. The weakest stimulatory effect is seen with 2-hydroxy-E_1, 2-methoxy-E_1, and 4-methoxy-E_2, while the highest stimulation is seen with 4-hydroxy-E_2. Schneider et al. (1984) explained that the minor response of 2-hydroxy-E_1 was due to the fast O-methylation of this E_2 metabolite. The D-ring metabolites, except 16α-hydroxy-E_1, maintain (some) stimulatory activity at high concentrations. Gupta et al. (1998) have compared the effect of 2-hydroxy-E_2, 2-hydroxy-E_1, 16α-hydroxy-E_2, and 16α-hydroxy-E_1 to that of E_2 in both T47D cells and MCF-7 cells. The order of potencies is not the same in both cells and the potency of 16α-hydroxy-E_2 was even greater in T47D cells than that of E_2. Surprisingly, the ER-negative MCF-10F cells are stimulated by 16α-hydroxy-E_1 and E_3 (Singhal et al., 1999).

The Mueck group tested two components of CEE, equilin and 17α-dihydroequilin, both of which showed a weaker proliferative effect in MCF-7 cells than E_2 (Mueck et al., 2003b).

Lippert et al. (2002b) showed that EE had a stronger inhibitory activity than E_2 at high concentrations. Reddel and Sutherland (1987) also found an inhibitory activity of diethylstilbestrol (DES). Sulfated metabolites may also stimulate cell proliferation in MCF-7 cells, if they are desulfated by sulfatases present in the tumor cells (Santner et al., 1993a; Billich et al., 2000).

Compound	10^{-8} M	10^{-7} M	10^{-6} M	10^{-5} M
Estradiol	$137.6 \pm 12.7^{++}$	$127.9 \pm 11.5^{++}$	$108.8 \pm 5.6^{+}$	$87.8 \pm 6.7^{++}$
A-ring metabolites				
2-Hydroxyestrone	$110.7 \pm 4.2^{+}$	100.3 ± 3.4	$86.5 \pm 9.3^{++}$	$8.5 \pm 2.2^{++}$
2-Methoxyestrone	$124.5 \pm 9.5^{++}$	$116.9 \pm 7.0^{+}$	99.1 ± 8.0	94.6 ± 6.0
2-Hydroxyestradiol	$124.2 \pm 12.5^{++}$	$112.5 \pm 11.3^{+}$	$72.6 \pm 10.2^{++}$	$9.0 \pm 2.7^{++}$
2-Methoxyestradiol	$116.5 \pm 7.9^{++}$	102.2 ± 10.3	$46.9 \pm 7.0^{++}$	$6.4 \pm 4.0^{++}$
2-Hydroxyestriol	$113.0 \pm 6.8^{+}$	$108.8 \pm 6.2^{+}$	100.0 ± 6.3	$83.2 \pm 6.1^{++}$
2-Methoxyestriol	$128.8 \pm 7.6^{++}$	$124.4 \pm 6.9^{++}$	113.4 ± 10.6	95.4 ± 7.0
4-Hydroxyestrone	$129.2 \pm 7.4^{++}$	$115.4 \pm 9.7^{+}$	86.2 ± 18.1	$0.2 \pm 0.6^{++}$
4-Methoxyestrone	$124.4 \pm 10.3^{++}$	$113.5 \pm 5.2^{+}$	108.3 ± 13.5	97.5 ± 7.7
4-Hydroxyestradiol	$130.4 \pm 7.5^{++}$	$127.3 \pm 7.0^{++}$	103.2 ± 18.2	$1.6 \pm 2.4^{++}$
4-Methoxyestradiol	$118.2 \pm 5.5^{++}$	$114.6 \pm 9.9^{+}$	105.2 ± 12.9	$84.8 \pm 9.3^{++}$
D-ring metabolites				
Estrone	$117.0 \pm 14.8^{+}$	$120.1 \pm 14.6^{+}$	103.2 ± 13.4	102.7 ± 9.7
Estriol	$110.8 \pm 10.0^{+}$	114.1 ± 4.2	99.6 ± 6.8	100.3 ± 3.0
Estetrol	$115.0 \pm 17.1^{+}$	104.9 ± 5.6	97.6 ± 9.3	93.8 ± 7.7
16α-Hyroxyestrone	92.8 ± 15.3	$77.8 \pm 5.2^{++}$	$76.7 \pm 9.6^{+}$	$66.1 \pm 6.9^{++}$

The values are expressed in percentage of cell counts compared to cell counts of the controls defined as 100% (mean ± S.D., n = 6). $^{+}P<0.05$; $^{++}P < 0.01$.

Figure 4 Changes in cell number of MCF-7 cells after treatment with estradiol and metabolites. *Abbreviation*: SD, standard deviation. *Source*: From Seeger et al. (2004b).

In Vivo

Estrogens in general show a stimulating effect on the breast. In tumor models, estrogens have a stimulating effect on the growth of the tumors in ovariectomized (ovx) animals (rat DMBA model and nude mice) (Callejo et al., 2005; Shafie and Grantham, 1981). High doses of E_2 can also inhibit DMBA-induced tumors (Ohi and Yoshida, 1992). Surprisingly, intermittent administration of E_3 prevents 80% to 90% of the DMBA-induced cancers during life span of intact Sprague Dawley rats (Lemon, 1977). In ovx monkeys (Cline et al., 2007; Dimitrakakis et al., 2003; Wood et al., 2007) and humans (Hofseth et al., 1999), estrogens (CEE and E_2) show an increase of the proliferation marker Ki-67 in the breast. Some estrogen metabolites show an inhibitory effect in vitro on proliferation of breast tumor cell lines (see above). Surprisingly, 2-methoxy-E_2, which has been developed as a novel antitumor agent on the basis of its inhibitory effects in in vitro studies, has no antitumor effect in vivo in specific tumor models (Sutherland et al., 2005). E_2 induces proliferation of normal human breast tissue xenografted in nude mice (Clarke et al., 1997b). This study also shows that higher E_2 doses are required for proliferation than for PR induction. In the MWS (Beral et al., 2003), estrogen treatment results in an increased breast cancer risk, and this becomes enhanced with duration of use. This is in contrast with the observation in the WHI study (Stefanick et al., 2006) in which no significant increase is seen in the estrogen-only treatment (using CEE) and even a lower risk was found for ductal carcinoma. In the WHI study, the participants were deprived of estrogens for many years and apparently this does not lead to a higher sensitivity of the breast to estrogens. Several factors may explain the difference between these two studies: such as study design (observational vs. a prospective study), type of progestagen and estrogen, difference in inclusion/exclusion criteria, selection bias, and other factors. It is quite remarkable that the tumors in the MWS appear very soon after treatment started, while in the Nurses Health Study, a prospective cohort study, a significant increase was observed only after 20 years of estrogen use (Chen et al., 2006). Santen and Allred (2007) recently discussed the differences between the study outcomes and possible explanations.

Conclusion

ER-positive breast cancer cell lines respond without exception to E_2, but the dose-response curves of different cell lines and their individual subclones markedly differ in profile. Normal breast cells respond weakly to E_2 and growth factors are often required in appropriate concentrations to achieve a response. High concentrations of E_2 may inhibit growth, as do many of its metabolites. These high pharmacological concentrations may give nonspecific effects leading to growth inhibition. In vivo E_2 has a growth promoting effect on ER-positive tumors in models using ovx animals. Weak estrogens may inhibit tumor growth in intact animals. In ovx monkeys, E_2 has a weak stimulating effect on normal breast tissue (measured as Ki-67 expression). The effects of estrogen-only treatment in large clinical trials with postmenopausal women on breast tumor risk are inconclusive and may depend on the design of the study and age after menopause. In the WHI

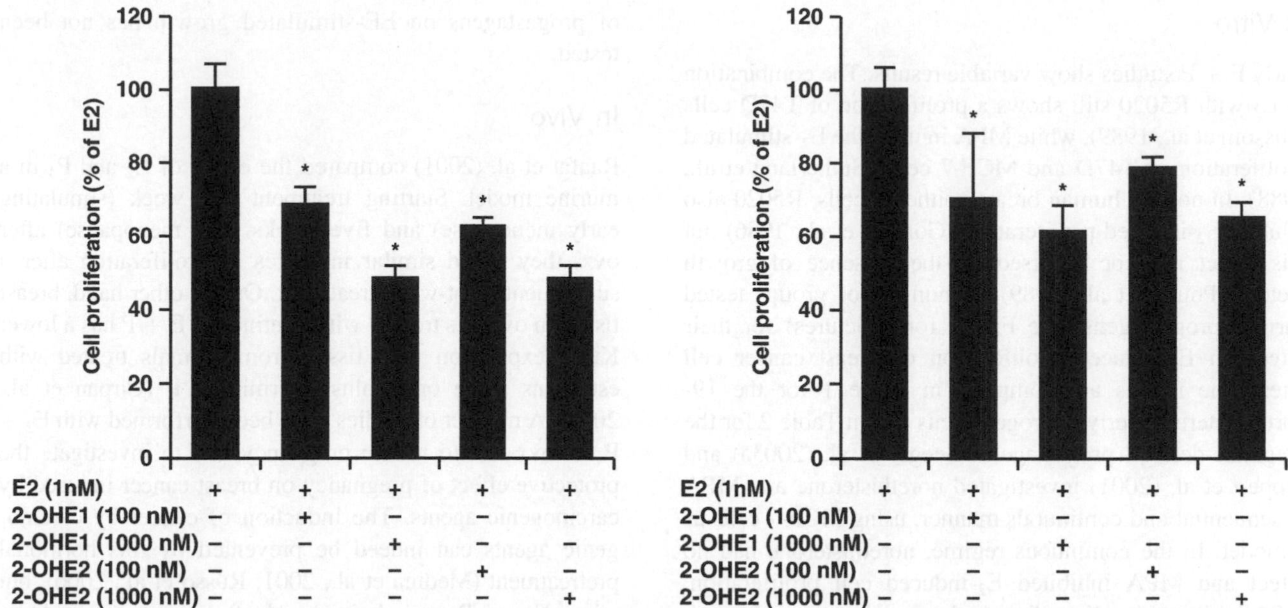

Figure 5 Inhibition of the E_2-induced proliferation of T47D (*left*) and MCF-7 (*right*) cells by 2-catecholestrogens. Significant inhibition ($p < 0.05$) of the E_2-induced proliferation is indicated with an asterix. *Abbreviation*: E_2, estradiol. *Source*: From Gupta et al. (1998).

study (2006), a prospective study with a randomized design, using late postmenopausal women, the risk for breast cancer did not increase with CEE.

EFFECT OF PROGESTAGENS AND WEAK ESTROGENS ON E_2-INDUCED PROLIFERATION

E_2-induced proliferation can be antagonized by antiestrogens and reduced by progestagens, but a weak estrogen, like E_3, can also inhibit E_2-stimulated proliferation. Here we will not discuss the action of antiestrogens (see reviews: Clarke et al., 2001; MacGregor and Jordan, 1998).

Inhibition by Weak Estrogens

In Vitro

Weak estrogens may show antagonistic or inhibitory properties on E_2-induced proliferation, due to a fast dissociation of the receptor complex, which leads to depletion of ER (Clark et al., 1977). Figure 5 shows that the weak estrogenic metabolites, 2-hydroxy-E_1 and 2-hydroxy-E_2, have antagonistic or inhibitory effects on E_2-induced proliferation of MCF-7 and T47D cells (Gupta et al., 1998). Sasson and Notides (1983) have shown that E_3 and E_1 can inhibit the cooperative binding of E_2 to ER.

In Vivo

E_3 is a weak estrogen on the uterus after a single dose administration to ovx rats, but becomes a full agonist after frequent dosing. However, when it is coadministered with E_2 it acts as an antagonist or inhibitor (Clark and Markaverich, 1984; Melamed et al., 1997). Similar effects are seen on breast. In the DMBA model using intact animals, treatment with E_3 induces a lower tumor incidence than in controls (Wotiz et al., 1984), indicating that it antagonizes or inhibits the effect of endogenous E_2. It has even been postulated that the high levels of E_3 during pregnancy may play a role in the protection against carcinogenesis (Melamed et al., 1997; Cole et al., 1976).

Effect of Progestagens on Estrogen Response

OC and HT preparations in postmenopausal women consist mainly of continuous treatment with an estrogen (E) and a progestagen (P), which is needed for good cycle control and/or to achieve an atrophic endometrium. For the breast, E + P shows a different clinical outcome: a stimulating effect on proliferation of epithelial cells in the breast, which may after long-term treatment lead to pathology. Apparently, the progestagen does not have an antiproliferative effect on estrogen action in the breast, but instead it has even an additional stimulatory effect. It is therefore surprising that the number of in vitro studies in which the effect on proliferation by the E + P combination is investigated is very limited. Studies combining E + P are highly relevant because the two components regulate the ER and PR content in breast cells (Berkenstam et al., 1989; Savoldi et al., 1995) as well as the activity of steroid metabolizing enzymes (Xu et al., 2007; Pasqualini, 2004).

In Vitro

Early E + P studies show variable results. The combination of E_2 with R5020 still shows a proliferation of T47D cells (Hissom et al., 1989), while MPA inhibits the E_2-stimulated proliferation of T47D and MCF-7 cells (Sutherland et al., 1988). In normal human breast epithelial cells, R5020 also inhibits E_2-induced proliferation (Gompel et al., 1986) but this effect may be reversed by the presence of growth factors (Poulin et al., 1989). A number of groups tested various progestagens (see Fig. 6 for structures) for their effect on E_2-induced proliferation of breast cancer cell lines. The results are compiled in Table 1 for the 19-nortestosterone-derived progestagens and in Table 2 for the pregnane-derived progestagens. Seeger et al. (2003a) and Lippert et al. (2001) investigated norethisterone and MPA in sequential and continuous manner, using MCF-7 cells as a model. In the continuous regime, norethisterone had no effect and MPA inhibited E_2-induced cell proliferation. MPA inhibited in all studies, with one exception, although the magnitude of inhibition differed (Table 2). In the sequential mode, MPA was more potent than in the continuous mode. What is striking is that P_4 (not presented in Table 2) had the strongest inhibition of all progestagens in the continuous E + P regime, while no inhibitory effects were observed in the sequential mode (Lippert et al., 2001). Van der Burg et al. (1992) studied in MCF-7 cells the effect of a few 19-nortestosterone derivatives (gestodene, etonogestrel, and levonorgestrel) in combination with E_2 and did not find any significant effect (Table 1). Schoonen et al. (1995a) also did not observe any effect for the Litton MCF-7 and the ATCC T47D cell lines, but an inhibitory effect on the E_2-induced proliferation was observed in the Hubrecht Laboratory MCF-7 and the Sutherland T47D subclones for the same 19-nortestosterone-derived progestagens as used by the Van der Burg group. Seeger et al. (2003a) also found an inhibition in MCF-7 cells with these three compounds. Norethisterone showed only an inhibitory effect in the Sutherland T47D subclone (Schoonen et al., 1995a) and ZR-75-1 cell line (Poulin et al., 1990). For the pregnanes tested (Table 2), all pregnanes showed an inhibition of E_2-stimulated proliferation, except for the Litton MCF-7 and the ATCC T47D subclones. These subclones were also an exception with the 19-nortestosteron-derived progestagens. The concentrations at which significantly inhibitory effects were seen differ for the various progestagens, but differences are also seen among groups. Krämer et al. (2006b) reported similar results as shown in Tables 1 and 2 with a less common breast cancer cell line (HCC1500). The type of the estrogen component may also play a role because different effects are found between CEE and E_2 in the presence of various progestagens. Some progestagens enhance the CEE but not the E_2-induced proliferation (Mueck et al., 2003b). The effect of progestagens on EE-stimulated growth has not been tested.

In Vivo

Raafat et al. (2001) compared the effect of E_2 and P_4 in a murine model. Starting treatment one week (simulating early menopause) and five weeks (late menopause) after ovx, they found similar increases in proliferation after a subsequent eight-week treatment. On the other hand, breast tissue in ovx rats treated with continuous E + P has a lower Ki-67 expression than tissue from animals treated with estrogens alone or E plus intermittent P (Cirpan et al., 2006). A number of studies have been performed with E_2 + P_4 in ovx rats to mimic pregnancy and to investigate the protective effect of pregnancy on breast cancer induced by carcinogenic agents. The induction of cancer by carcinogenic agents can indeed be prevented by this hormonal pretreatment (Medina et al., 2001; Russo et al., 2006), but when E and P are administered after the tumor inducer (DMBA) the tumor growth is accelerated. Treatment with E + P soon after the tumor inducer is partly protective (Ohi and Yoshida, 1992). This treatment appears to be dependent on the dose of E_2 used (Sakamoto et al., 1997). Normal human breast tissue xenografted subcutaneously in athymic nude mice and treated with E_2 + P_4 shows an increased proliferation (Clarke, 2006). Transplanted tissue from HT users and nonusers show the same proliferation rate in nude mice (Hargreaves et al., 1998). This is in contrast with the observation of Hofseth et al. (1999), who demonstrated that epithelial proliferation was increased in tissue of HT users. Apparently, this difference is lost after transplantation of the tissue in mice. In ovx monkeys, E_2 or CEE + MPA increase significantly Ki-67 expression in epithelial cells, which is not seen with E_2 + P_4 (Wood et al., 2007; Cline et al., 2002; Cline, 2007). In postmenopausal women treated with E_2 + NETA (norethisterone acetate) and E_2V (valerate) + DNG (dienogest) for six months, Conner et al. (2003; 2004) have shown a significant increase in Ki-67 expression in breast cells. The positive cells for Ki-67 expression increased from 2.25% to 9.1%. In contrast, topical P_4 reduces the E_2-induced proliferation already after 14 days of treatment (Foidart et al., 1998). Chang et al. (1995) also found that topical P_4 applied to the breast decreases the number of proliferating cells as induced by E_2.

In women, combined OCs and HT show a small increase in the risk for breast cancer (Beral et al., 1996, 1997). In a recent evaluation of the data of the Royal College of General Practitioners, no significant effect of OCs was seen on breast cancer risk (Hannaford et al., 2007). Both in the MWS (Beral et al., 2003) and the WHI study (Chlebowski et al., 2003), the E + P combinations show a significant increase in breast cancer risk compared

19-Nortestosterone derivatives

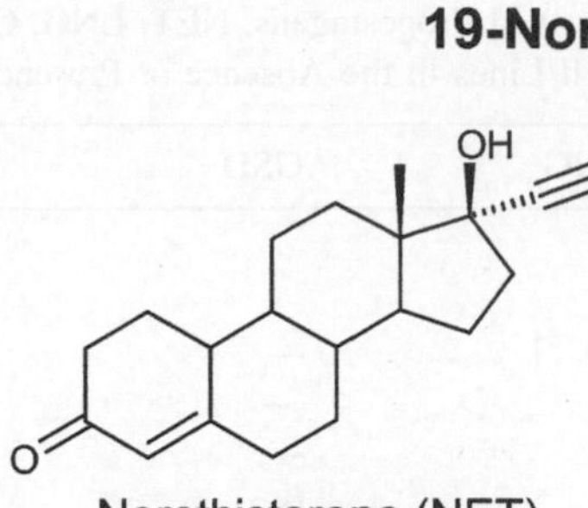

Norethisterone (NET)

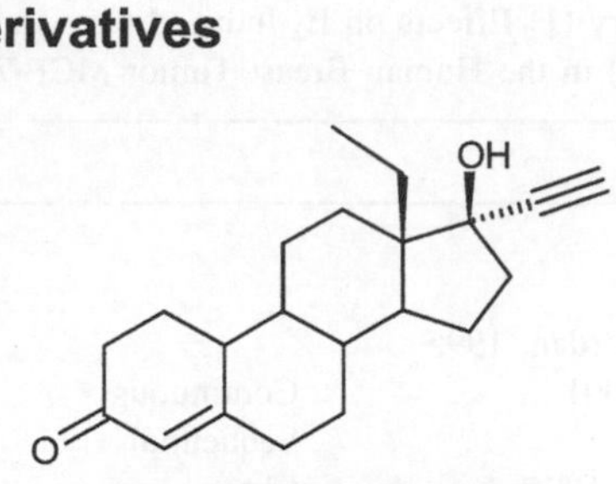

Levonorgestrel (LNG)

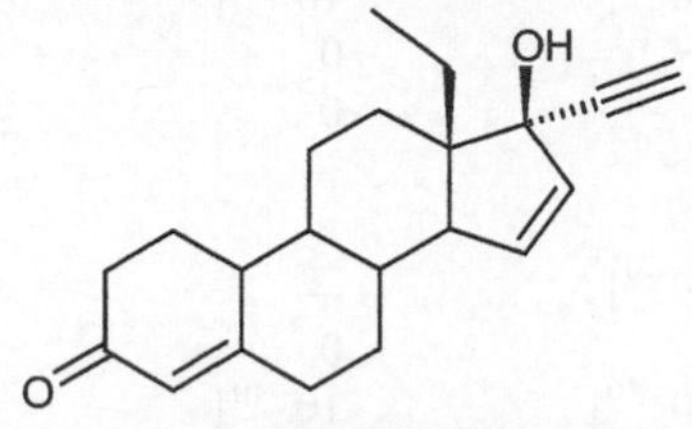

Gestodene (GSD)

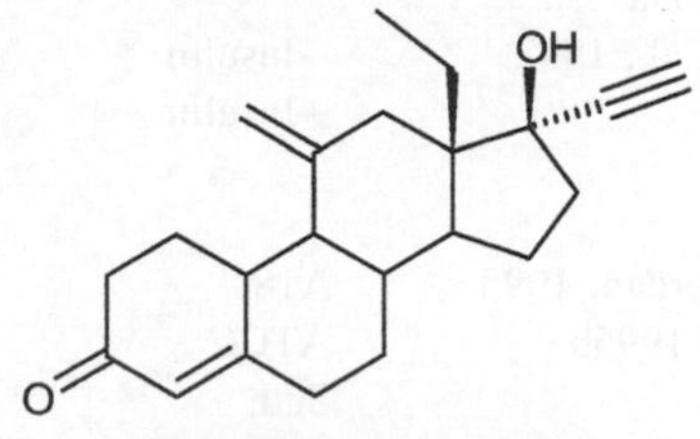

Etonogestrel (ENG)

Pregnane derivatives

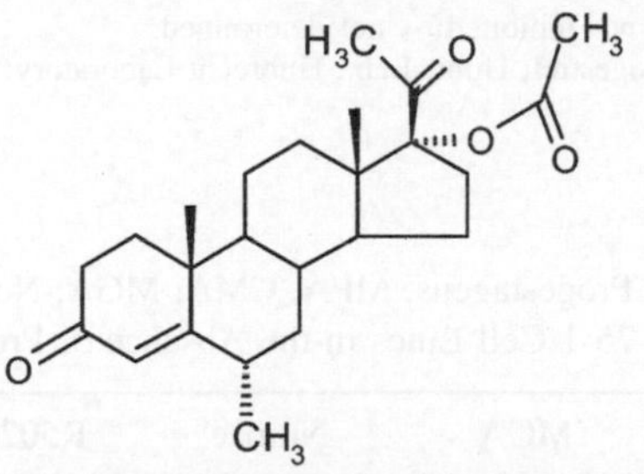

Medroxyprogesterone acetate (MPA)

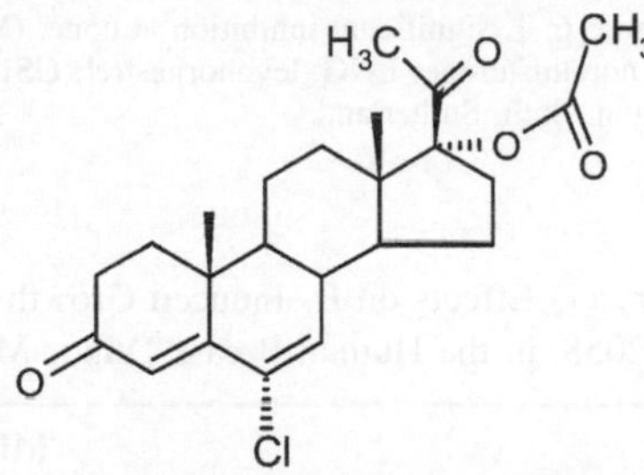

Chlormadinone acetate (CMA)

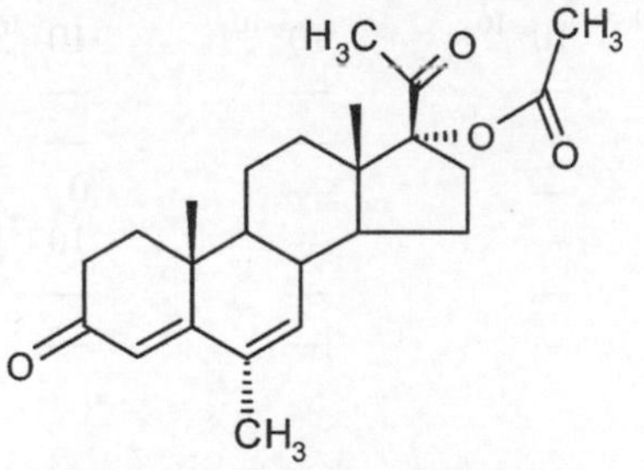

Megestrol acetate (MGA)

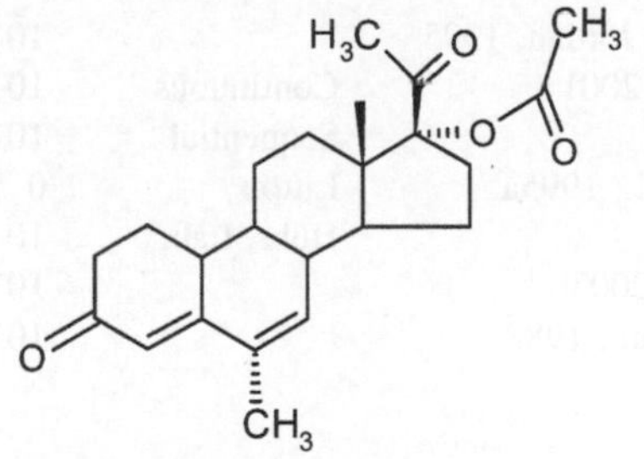

Nomegestrol acetate (Nomac)

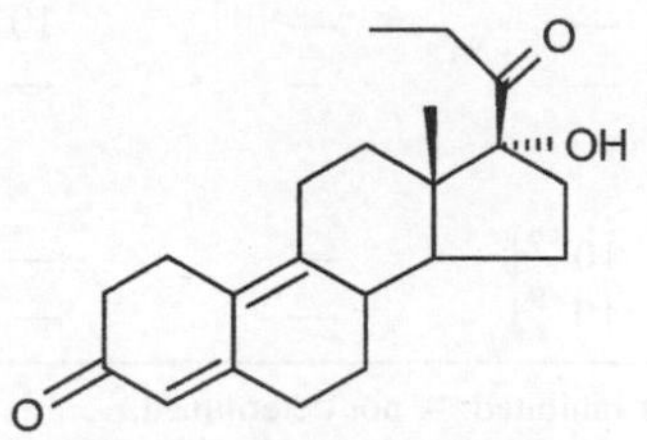

Promegestone (R5020)

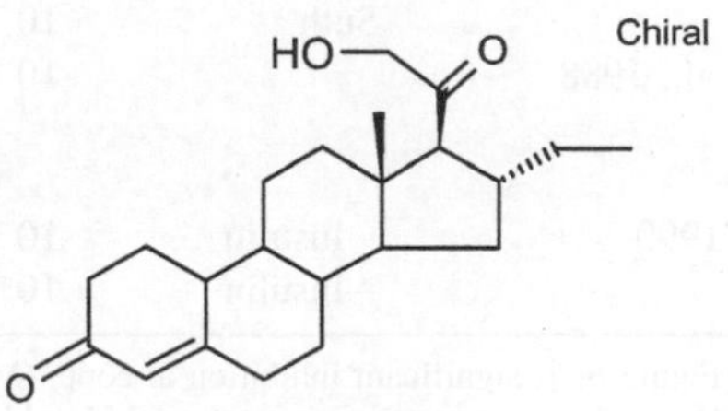

Org 2058

Figure 6 Structures of progestagens.

Table 1 Inhibitory (↓) Effects on E_2-Induced Growth by 19-Nortestosterone-Derived Progestagens, NET, LNG, GSD, and ENG (3-Ketodesogestrel) in the Human Breast Tumor MCF-7, T47D, and ZR-75-1 Cell Lines in the Absence or Presence of Insulin

		NET	LNG	GSD	ENG
MCF-7					
E2 (10^{-10} M)					
Catherino and Jordan, 1995		—	10^{-8}↓	—	—
Lippert et al., 2001	Continuous	0	—	—	—
	Sequential	0	—	—	—
Schoonen et al., 1995a	Litton	0	0	0	0
	Hubr. Lab.	0	10^{-9}↓	10^{-9}↓	10^{-9}↓
Seeger et al., 2003a		0	10^{-9}↓	10^{-11}↓	10^{-9}↓
Van der Burg et al., 1992	−Insulin	—	0	0	0
	+Insulin	—	0	0	0
T47D					
E2 (10^{-10} M)					
Catherino and Jordan, 1995	A18	—	10^{-9}↓	—	—
Schoonen et al., 1995b	ATCC	0	0	0	0
	Suth	10^{-8}↓	10^{-10}↓	10^{-10}↓	10^{-10}↓
ZR 75-1					
E2 (10^{-9} M)					
Poulin et al., 1990	−Insulin	10^{-9}↓	10^{-10}↓	—	—
	+Insulin	10^{-9}↓	10^{-10}↓	—	—

For structures see Figure 6; ↓, significant inhibition at conc. (M); 0, neither stimulated nor inhibited; –, not determined.
Abbreviations: NET, norethisterone; LNG, levonorgestrel; GSD, gestodene; ENG, etonogestrel; Hubr. Lab., Hubrecht Laboratory; ATCC, American Type Culture Collection; Suth, Sutherland.

Table 2 Inhibitory (↓) Effects on E_2-Induced Growth by Pregnane-Derived Progestagens, MPA, CMA, MGA, Nomac, Promegestone (R5020), and Org 2058, in the Human Breast Tumor MCF-7, T47D, and ZR-75-1 Cell Lines in the Absence or Presence of Insulin

		MPA	CMA	MGA	Nomac	R5020	Org 2058
MCF-7							
E2 (10^{-10} M)							
Catherino and Jordan, 1995		10^{-10}↓	—	10^{-10}↓	10^{-10}↓	10^{-10}↓	—
Lippert et al., 2001	Continuous	10^{-8}↓	—	—	—	—	—
	Sequential	10^{-10}↓	—	—	—	—	—
Schoonen et al., 1995a	Litton	0	—	—	—	0	0
	Hubr. Lab.	10^{-9}↓	—	—	—	10^{-7}↓	0
Seeger et al., 2003b		10^{-5}↓	10^{-9}↓	—	—	—	—
Sutherland et al., 1988		10^{-6}↓	—	—	—	—	—
T47D							
E2 (10^{-10} M)							
Catherino and Jordan, 1995		—	—	10^{-10}↓	10^{-10}↓	—	—
Schoonen et al., 1995b	ATCC	0	—	—	—	0	0
	Suth	10^{-10}↓	—	—	—	10^{-8}↓	10^{-10}↓
Sutherland et al., 1988		10^{-8}↓	—	—	—	—	—
ZR 75-1							
E2 (10^{-9} M)							
Poulin et al., 1990	−Insulin	10^{-10}↓	10^{-10}↓	10^{-9}↓	—	—	—
	+Insulin	10^{-10}↓	10^{-10}↓	10^{-9}↓	—	—	—

For structures see Figure 6; ↓, significant inhibition at conc. (M); 0, neither stimulated nor inhibited; –, not determined.
Abbreviations: MPA, medroxyprogesterone acetate; CMA, chlormadinone acetate; MGA, megestrol acetate; Nomac, nomegestrol acetate; Hubr. Lab., Hubrecht Laboratory; ATCC, American Type Culture Collection; Suth, Sutherland.

with nonusers. The effect in the MWS is stronger than in the WHI study, which may be due to a difference in study design. In a French cohort study (de Lignières et al., 2002) in postmenopausal women using HT of which the majority of the women used transdermal E_2 gel (83%) and oral P_4 (58%) no increase in breast cancer risk was seen indicating that route of administration as well as the type of progestagen are important.

Conclusion

Weak estrogens can inhibit E_2-induced proliferation of breast cancer cells and there is strong evidence that this may also occur in vivo. However, there is no clinical evidence to support that this may also be the case in humans.

In vitro studies with E + P combinations show variable results; a few studies show no effect or even a stimulation of the E_2-induced proliferation, but the majority of the experiments show an inhibitory effect both with 19-nortestosterone and pregnane-derived progestagens. Animal experiments with carcinogenic agents show that the effect on tumor development is highly dependent on the timing of the HT, and in treatment before or shortly after the tumors are induced, an E + P treatment may have (some) protective effect, while a stimulation is seen when tumors are more developed. Nude mice studies show variable results on the growth effect of E + P combinations on normal human breast tissue. Clinical studies show an increase in breast cancer risk for E + P combinations, apparently with an exception for P_4 when combined with a low exposure of E_2. It is concluded that in vitro studies do not seem to be predictive for clinical outcomes. The increased proliferation in breast tissue of ovx monkeys as seen with E + P combinations may be indicative for the increased breast cancer risk observed in clinical studies.

EFFECT OF PROGESTERONE AND METABOLITES ON BREAST CELL PROLIFERATION

In the progesterone receptor knockout (PRKO) mice (Conneely et al., 2001), ductal structures in the breast cannot be formed on treatment with E + P, as is seen during normal pregnancy. During the luteal phase of the menstrual cycle of fertile women a higher mitotic index is seen in breast tissue than during the follicular phase (Going et al., 1988; Anderson et al., 1989). Pregnancy protects against breast cancer (Chie et al., 2000; Campagnoli et al., 2005) but not in BRCA1 and 2 carriers (Jernström et al., 1999). Thus, P_4 seems to have a dual action in the breast: both proliferating and differentiating effects. Differentiation will result in an inhibition of proliferation by P_4. A number of research groups tried to reveal the molecular mechanisms (Musgrove et al., 1991; Lange et al., 1999).

In Vitro

Calaf (2006) has recently shown that natural P_4 stimulates proliferation in normal breast cells (MCF-10A), but Krämer et al. (2006b) found no effect with the same cell line. In contrast, Wiebe et al. (2000) observed in MCF-10A (and MCF-7) cells an inhibitory effect of P_4 on proliferation. Similar observations were done by Schoonen et al. (1995a,b) using various subclones of MCF-7 and T47D cells. Also, in primary breast cells, Malet et al. (2000) found a dose-dependent decrease in proliferation by P_4 (added twice daily due to strong metabolism). No studies on proliferation have been done with pregnenolone or 17α-hydroxy-P_4. Wiebe et al. (2000) studied the effects of P_4 metabolites (see Fig. 7 for metabolism of progesterone) formed in normal and tumor tissues for their effects on proliferation of breast cells (MCF-7, MCF-10A, and ZR-75-1). They found opposite effects for the 3α-hydroxy-Δ^4-pregnenes (3α-HP; inhibition) and the 5α-pregnanes (5α-pregnane-3,20-dione) (5α-DHP; stimulation) on proliferation (Fig. 8). The 3β-hydroxy- and 5β-DHP metabolites have no effect. The concentration of the 3α-hydroxy-Δ^4-pregnanes is higher in normal tissue than in breast tumor tissue (Wiebe et al., 2005), and the opposite is true for the 5α-pregnanes. Most of the mechanistic studies are done with synthetic progestagens of the pregnane series (Musgrove et al., 1991; Lange et al., 1999), which are not or less susceptible to intracellular metabolism than P_4.

In Table 3, the effect of 19-nortestosterone derivatives (see Fig. 6 for structures) on proliferation by a number of research groups has been compiled. The majority of the studies show that norethisterone, levonorgestrel, gestodene, and etonogestrel showed a stimulation of growth of MCF-7, T47D, and ZR-75-1 cell lines, but in some subclones no effect was seen. Also, the absence or presence of growth factors may result in a different effect. Botella et al. (1994) found with norethisterone acetate an inhibition of T47D cells, while in Table 3, almost exclusively, stimulation is observed. In most studies significant effects were found at high concentrations (10^{-7} M). Schoonen et al. (1995a,b) and Catherino et al. (1993) used antihormones to determine whether the effects were mediated through the PR or ER. Surprisingly, the stimulatory effect of 19-nortestosterone-derived progestagens could be blocked by an antiestrogen. Jeng et al. (1992) and Krämer et al. (2006b) found that the stimulatory effect was not seen in ER-negative cells (MDA-MB-231 and MCF10A). Later, estrogenic metabolites were identified for levonorgestrel (Santillán et al., 2001; Lemus et al., 1992), norethisterone (Larrea et al., 1987), and gestodene (Lemus et al., 2000) after incubation with these progestagens. Whether the ER-positive cell lines, which are not

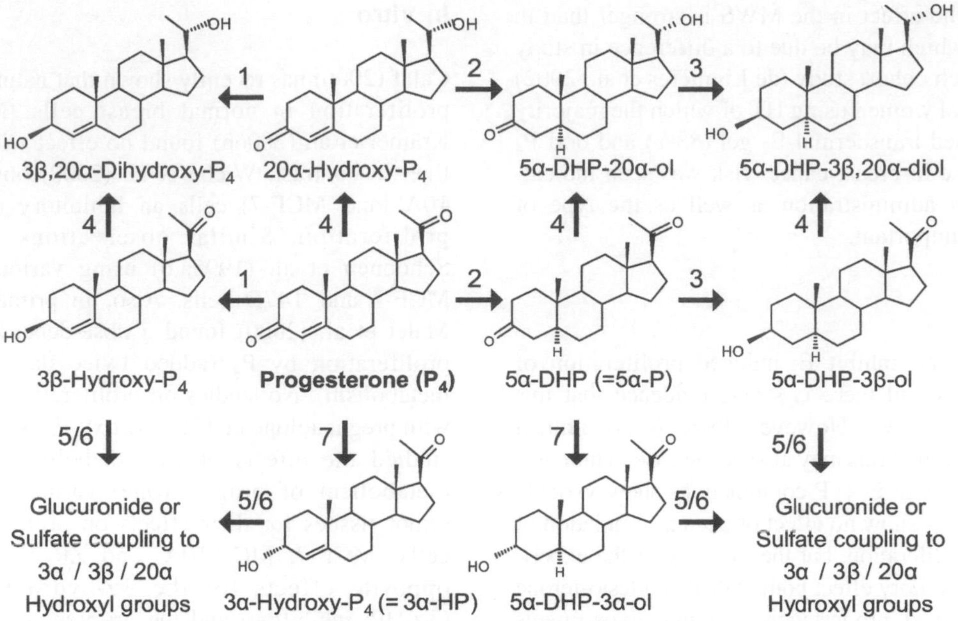

3β,20α-Dihydroxy-P_4 ← 1 — 20α-Hydroxy-P_4 — 2 → 5α-DHP-20α-ol — 3 → 5α-DHP-3β,20α-diol

4 ↑ 4 ↑ 4 ↑ 4 ↑

3β-Hydroxy-P_4 ← 1 — Progesterone (P_4) — 2 → 5α-DHP (=5α-P) — 3 → 5α-DHP-3β-ol

5/6 ↓ 7 ↓ 7 ↓ 5/6 ↓

Glucuronide or Sulfate coupling to 3α / 3β / 20α Hydroxyl groups ← 5/6 — 3α-Hydroxy-P_4 (= 3α-HP) 5α-DHP-3α-ol — 5/6 → Glucuronide or Sulfate coupling to 3α / 3β / 20α Hydroxyl groups

Figure 7 Metabolism pattern of progesterone (P_4) by the enzymes 3β-hydroxysteroid-dehydrogenase (1,3), 5α-reductase (2), 20α-hydroxysteroid-dehydrogenase (4), UDP-glucuronosyl-transferase (5), sulfotransferase (6), and 3α-hydroxysteroid-dehydrogenase (7). The structures of the individual sulfated and glucuronidated steroids are not displayed. *Abbreviations*: P_4, progesterone; 5α-DHP (5α-P), 5α-dihydroprogesterone or 5α-pregnane-3,20-dione; 3α-HP, 3α-hydroxy-P_4 or 3α-hydroxy-4-pregnen-20-one.

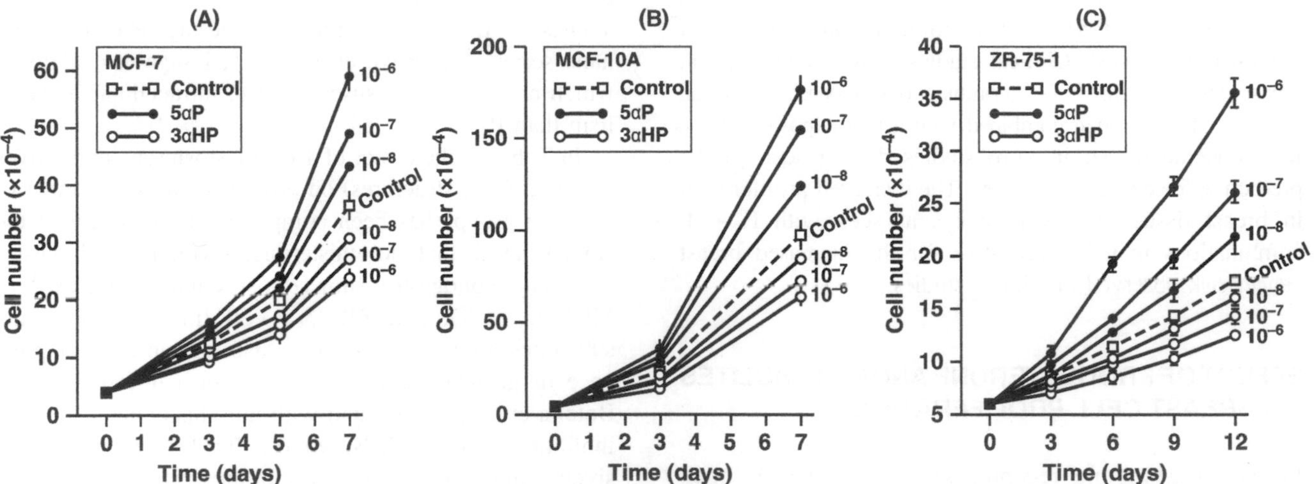

Figure 8 The dose and time dependent stimulatory and inhibitory effects of 5α-progesterone (5α-P, 5α-pregnane-3,20-dione) and 3α-hydroxyprogesterone (3α-HP, 3α-hydroxy-4-pregnen-20-one), respectively, on proliferation of MCF-7 (**A**), MCF-7-10A (**B**), and ZR-75-1 (**C**) breast cell lines. Data are the mean of six separate experiments for **A** and **B** and one of two experiments for ZR-75-1 cells (**C**). Each point in an experiment had 5 to 6 replicates; bars, SE. The number of cells seeded per dish was 40,000 for (**A**) and (**B**) and 60,000 for (**C**). Cells were exposed, for the time given, to the steroid (control) or to 10^{-8}–10^{-6} M 5α-P or 3α-HP. *Abbreviations*: 5α-DHP (= 5α-P), 5α-dihydroprogesterone or 5α-pregnane-3,20-dione; 3α-HP, 3α-hydroxy-P_4 or 3α-hydroxy-4-pregnen-20-one. *Source*: From Wiebe et al. (2000).

responding to the 19-nor-testosterone-derived progestagens, lack a specific metabolic enzyme requires further investigations.

In Table 4, the effects of pregnane-derived progestagens (see Fig. 6 for structures) on proliferation of breast cell clones are summarized. The results with the various pregnanes are far more variable than seen with the 19-nortestosterone derivatives. Clear differences are found among various pregnanes, but differences are also seen among groups with the same progestagen. For both

Table 3 Growth Stimulatory (↑) and Inhibitory (↓) Effects of 19-Nortestosterone-Derived Progestagens, NET, LNG, GSD, and ENG (3-Ketodesogestrel), in the Human Breast Tumor MCF-7, T47D, and ZR-75-1 Cell Lines in the Absence or Presence of Insulin

		NET	LNG	GSD	ENG
MCF-7					
Catherino et al., 1993		—	10^{-7}↑	10^{-7}↑	—
Catherino and Jordan, 1995		—	10^{-7}↑	—	—
Jeng et al., 1992		10^{-8}↑	10^{-7}↑	10^{-7}↑	—
Kalkhoven et al., 1994		—	—	10^{-7}↑	10^{-7}↑
Krämer et al., 2006a	+GF mix	0	10^{-7}↓	0	10^{-7}↓
Schoonen et al., 1995a	McGrath	10^{-7}↑	10^{-7}↑	10^{-7}↑	10^{-7}↑
	Litton	10^{-7}↑	10^{-6}↑	10^{-7}↑	10^{-7}↑
	Hubr. Lab.	10^{-7}↑	10^{-7}↑	10^{-7}↑	10^{-7}↑
Seeger et al., 2003b		10^{-7}↑	0	10^{-7}↑	10^{-7}↑
Van der Burg et al., 1992	−Insulin	—	0	0	0
	+Insulin	—	10^{-6}↑	10^{-6}↑	10^{-6}↑
T47D					
Catherino and Jordan, 1995		—	10^{-6}↑	—	—
Jeng et al., 1992		10^{-8}↑	10^{-7}↑	—	—
Kalkhoven et al., 1994		—	—	10^{-6}↑	10^{-6}↑
Schoonen et al., 1995b	ATCC	10^{-8}↑	10^{-8}↑	10^{-8}↑	10^{-8}↑
	Suth	0	0	0	0
ZR 75-1					
Poulin et al., 1990	−Insulin	10^{-7}↑	10^{-6}↑	—	—
	+Insulin	10^{-7}↑	10^{-6}↑	—	—

For structures see Figure 6; ↑, significant stimulation at conc. (M); ↓, significant inhibition; 0, neither stimulated nor inhibited; –, not determined.
Abbreviations: NET, norethisterone; LNG, levonorgestrel; GSD, gestodene; ENG, etonogestrel; GF, Growth factor; Hubr. Lab., Hubrecht Laboratory; ATCC, American Type Culture Collection; Suth, Sutherland.

Table 4 Growth Stimulatory (↑) and Inhibitory (↓) Effects of Pregnane-Derived Progestagens, MPA, CMA, MGA, Nomac, Promegestone (R5020), and Org 2058, in the Human Breast Tumor MCF-7, T47D, and ZR-75-1 Cell Lines in the Absencc or Presence of Insulin

		MPA	CMA	MGA	Nomac	R5020	Org 2058
MCF-7							
Catherino et al., 1993		0	—	—	—	—	—
Catherino and Jordan, 1995		0	—	0	0	0	—
Jeng et al., 1992		0	—	—	—	3 × 10^{-6}↑	—
Krämer et al., 2006a		10^{-7}↑	10^{-6}↑	—	—	—	—
Schoonen et al., 1995a	McGrath	0	—	—	—	0	10^{-6}↑
	Litton	0	—	—	—	0	0
	Hubr. Lab.	0	—	—	—	0	10^{-6}↑
Seeger et al., 2003b		10^{-5}↑	10^{-5}↑	—	—	—	—
Sutherland et al., 1988		10^{-8}↓	—	—	—	—	—
Van der Burg et al., 1992	+Insulin	0	—	—	—	—	0
T47D							
Botella et al., 1994	+Insulin	10^{-9}↓	—	—	10^{-9}↓	10^{-9}↓	—
Catherino and Jordan, 1995	A18	—	—	0	0	—	—
Jeng et al., 1992		10^{-6}↑	—	—	—	3 × 10^{-6}↑	—
Kalkhoven et al., 1994		—	—	—	—		0
Musgrove et al., 1991	+Insulin	10^{-9}↓	—	—	—	—	10^{-9}↓
Schoonen et al., 1995b	ATCC	10^{-8}↑	—	—	—	10^{-9}↓	10^{-6}↑
	Suth	0	—	—	—	10^{-6}↑	0
Sutherland et al., 1988		10^{-10}↓	—	—	—	0	10^{-10}↓
ZR 75-1							
Poulin et al., 1990	−Insulin	10^{-9}↓	0	0	—	—	—
	+Insulin	10^{-9}↓	0	0	—	—	—
Sutherland et al., 1988		10^{-7}↓	—	—	—	—	—

For structures see Figure 6; ↑, significant stimulation at conc. (M); ↓, significant inhibition; 0, neither stimulated nor inhibited; –, not determined.
Abbreviations: MPA, Medroxyprogesterone Acetate; CMA, chlormadinone acetate; MGA, megestrol acetate; Nomac, nomegestrol acetate; Hubr. Lab., Hubrecht Laboratory; ATCC, American Type Culture Collection; Suth, Sutherland.

the 19-norpregnanes (Nomac, R5020 and Org 2058) and the other pregnanes with a 19-angular methyl group (MPA, CMA, and MGA), the results vary within the same cell line, indicating that the history of the cell line is of great influence. In addition, the presence of growth factors may determine the effect in some but not in all cell lines.

In Vivo

Sartorius et al. (2005) showed that WT T47D tumor growth can be inhibited in ovx nude mice by P_4 implants. MPA administered shortly after the tumor inducer (DMBA) is protective, but the opposite is seen when tumors are more progressed (Benakanakere et al., 2006). Etonogestrel (or 3-ketodesogestrel) and gestodene inhibit tumor growth in the DMBA model (Kloosterboer et al., 1994). In ovx monkeys, after long-term treatment, MPA and P_4 do not increase proliferation, as measured by Ki-67 expression (Cline and Wood, 2005, 2006; Cline et al., 1996). Depot MPA (Chilvers, 1996) is used as a contraceptive and reassuring breast tumor risk data are obtained. In the reanalysis of 54 epidemiological studies with OC users (Beral et al., 1996), it appeared that the number of P-alone users was low, but the results show a similar, small increase in breast cancer risk as seen with combined OCs. This was also observed in a more recent study in the French population (Fabre et al., 2007).

Conclusion

Most in vitro studies show a growth-inhibitory effect of P_4 on normal and breast cancer cells, likely caused by 3α-hydroxy-Δ^4-pregnene, a metabolite of progesterone. In contrast, the 19-nortestosterone-derived progestagens show a stimulation of breast cancer cell lines. This effect can be blocked by antiestrogens, and metabolites of these progestagenes are shown to possess affinity for ER. In tumor models, P_4 and both classes of progestagens inhibit tumor growth, although this seems to be dependent on whether it is administered before the carcinogenic agent, the interval between the two treatments is also important. In ovx monkeys, breast tissue is not stimulated by progestagens. Results from epidemiological studies show that progestagen-only preparations show a slight increase in breast cancer risk.

EFFECT OF ANDROGENS ON BREAST CELL PROLIFERATION

Androgens do not seem to play a direct role in normal breast development, but certainly have an indirect role as precursor for estrogens. However, an excess of androgens may disturb the growth and differentiation of breast tissue (Zhang et al., 2004). Polycystic ovary syndrome (PCOS) patients, who have high circulating androgens, do not show an increased risk for breast cancer (Gadducci et al., 2005). Some progestagens are derived of 19-nortestosterone and possess residual androgenic activity. This may also result in a reduced synthesis in the liver of SHBG. SHBG binds testosterone and a reduction may lead to a higher percentage of free testosterone and consequently tissue levels of testosterone in the breast will increase. In women, androgens originate from adrenals and ovaries. The metabolism of androgens is presented in Figure 9. We evaluate here the effects of various androgens on breast cells and tissue.

In Vitro

In an excellent review (Somboonporn and Davies, 2004), two studies showed inhibition of testosterone on proliferation of breast cells in four different cell lines, while in four other studies the results with the more active and non-aromatizable androgen, 5α-DHT, were variable and both stimulatory (Maggiolini et al., 1999) and inhibitory (Greeve et al., 2004) effects were found. It has been suggested that the stimulatory effects of 5α-DHT may be due to a direct interaction with ER (Aspinall et al., 2004); on the other hand, it has been shown that 5α-DHT is able to inhibit E_2-stimulated growth of MCF-7 and T47D cells. Ortmann et al. (2002) showed clear inhibition by testosterone and 5α-DHT (Fig. 10) in four different cell lines. The inhibitory activity seems to be dose and time dependent, but differs in different cell lines and the more potent androgen, 5α-DHT, does not always show the largest inhibition (Ortmann et al., 2002). In a recent study (Sonne-Hansen and Lykkesfeldt, 2005), it was shown that testosterone could stimulate MCF-7 cells when cultured in a low estrogen milieu. This effect could be inhibited by aromatase inhibitors, suggesting that in these experiments testosterone was converted into E_2.

The adrenal androgens, androst-5-ene-3β,17β-diol (Adiol), dehydroepiandrosterone (DHEA), and DHEA-sulfate (DHEAS), stimulated ER-positive MCF-7 cells, but not ER-negative BT-20 cells. However, the investigators did not find any E_2 formation in these MCF-7 cells (Najid and Habrioux, 1990). Schmitt et al. (2001) observed stimulation of MCF-7 cells by DHEA. Similar results on proliferation were found by Poulin and Labrie (1986) using ER-positive or ER-negative ZR-75-1 cells. These data seem to indicate that the androgens act through the ER, but without the manifestation of conversion into E_2 (Najid and Habrioux, 1990). On the other hand, other studies showed that androstenedione, the substrate for aromatase, did not stimulate MCF-7 cells (Santner et al., 1993b). However, when these cells were transfected with aromatase (thus allowing conversion to estrogens) growth was enhanced, suggesting that in vitro conversion to

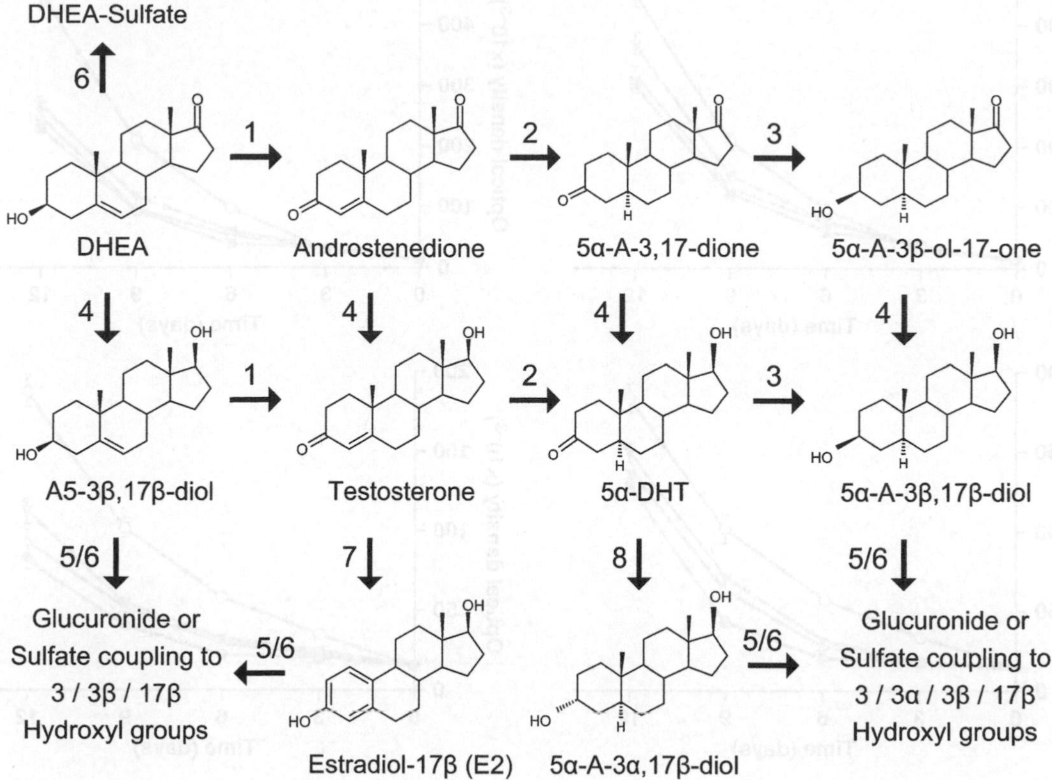

Figure 9 Metabolism pattern of testosterone by the enzymes 3β-hydroxysteroid-Δ^4-isomerase-dehydrogenase (1), 5α-reductase (2), 3β-hydroxysteroid-dehydrogenase (3), 17β-hydroxysteroid-dehydrogenase (3), UDP-glucuronosyl-transferase (5), sulfotransferase (6), aromatase (7), and 3α-hydroxysteroid-dehydrogenase (8). The structures of the individual sulfated and glucuronidated steroids are not displayed. *Abbreviations*: DHEA, dehydroepiandrosterone; DHEA-S, dehydroepiandrosterone-sulfate; A, androstane, A5, androst-5-ene; 5α-DHT, 5α-dihydrotestosterone.

estrogens does play a role in this system. Calhoun et al. (2003) found stimulatory effects with DHEAS, which persisted in the presence of the antiestrogen, fulvestrant. This implies that the effect is not mediated through the ER. Gayosso et al. (2006) also found a stimulatory effect in MCF-7 cells at physiological concentrations of DHEA, but at supraphysiological concentrations an inhibition was observed. In contrast, DHEAS was inactive at all concentrations in this system. In the presence of E_2, DHEA and Adiol partly antagonized the stimulatory effect of E_2. The inhibition by Adiol of E_2-stimulated proliferation of MCF-7 and T47D cells has been confirmed by other groups (Aspinall et al., 2004). The in vitro effect of androgens on breast cell lines thus widely varies and differs between cell lines. The observed effects may be due to in vitro conversion to E_2, E_2-independent ER-mediated effects and non-ER-mediated effects.

In Vivo

Labrie (2006) reviewed the effect of DHEA and androgens on the mammary gland. The work of his group shows that 5α-DHT and DHEA prevent tumor growth in various animal tumor models. In ovx monkeys (Dimitrakakis et al., 2003; Zhou et al., 2000), testosterone was able to inhibit Ki-67 expression by 40% to 50% after a three-day treatment.

A retrospective observational study in postmenopausal women who received testosterone in addition to HT showed that there was no increased breast cancer risk (Dimitrakakis et al., 2004). In a six-month prospective randomized double-blind placebo-controlled study, in which a testosterone patch was given to a group of women receiving continuous combined E_2 2 mg /NETA 1 mg, it was shown that testosterone prevented the increase in mammographic density and breast cell proliferation marker (Ki-67) that was seen with E + P treatment (Hofling et al., 2007a,b). Liao and Dickson (2002) were less convinced about the coadministration of androgens because concomitant increase in androgens as well as estrogens may be a greater risk for breast cancer.

Conclusion

Testosterone shows variable results on proliferation of breast cells. In low estrogen milieu and when aromatase activity is present growth stimulation is seen, but in the

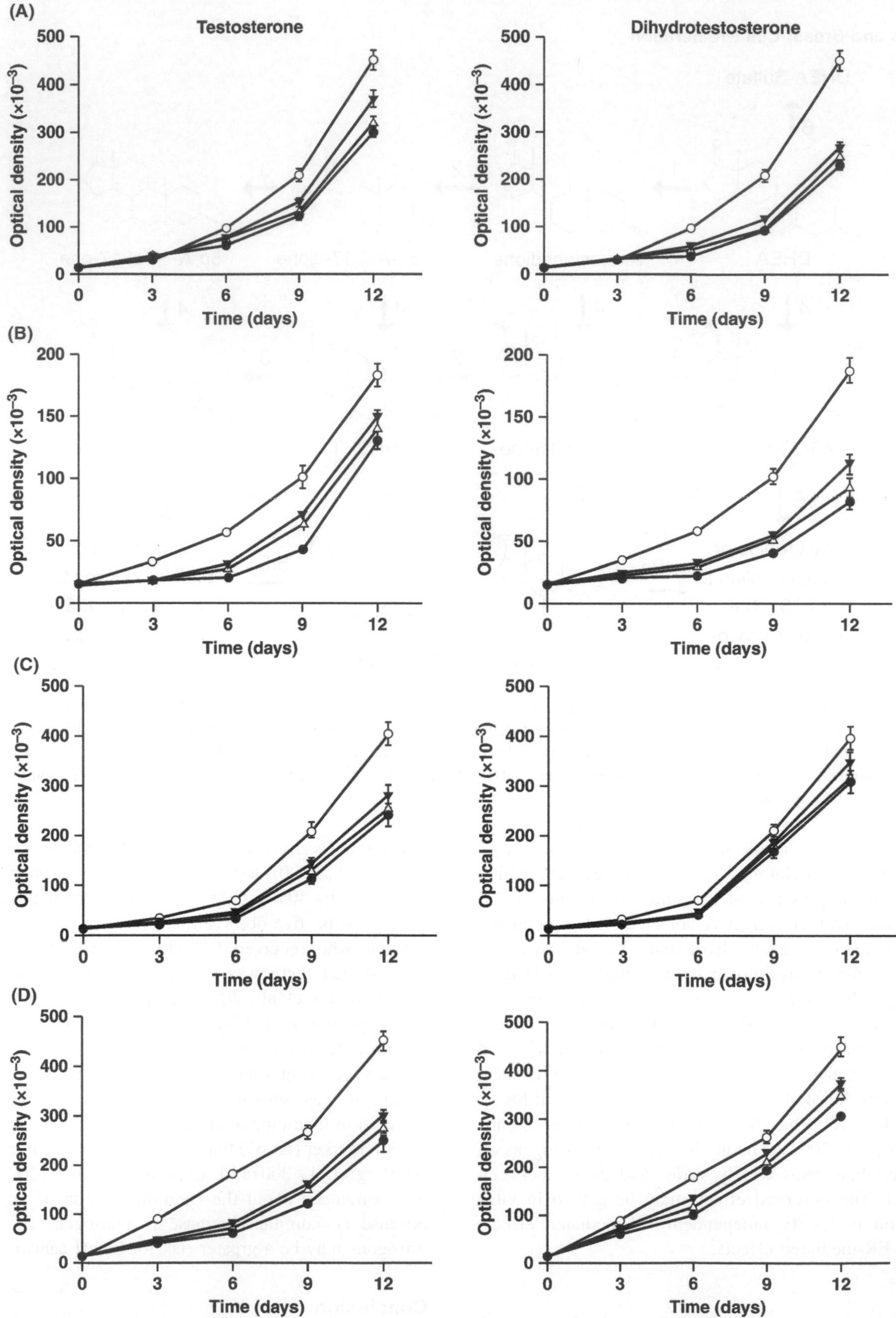

Figure 10 Dose dependence of proliferation of (**A**) MCF-7, (**B**) T47D, (**C**) MDA-MB 4355, and (**D**) BT-20 after treatment with 10^{-7} M (*black squares*), 10^{-8} M (*open triangles*), and 10^{-9} M (*closed triangles*) testosterone (*left side*) and 10^{-7} M (*black squares*), 10^{-8} M (*open triangles*), and 10^{-9} M (*closed triangles*) dihydrotestosterone (*right side*). Untreated cells served as controls (*open circles*). After cell incubation in serum-free medium, analysis with MTT was used for the determination of cell proliferation on days 0, 3, 6, 9, and 12. Results are expressed as mean ± SD. *Abbreviations*: MTT, methylthiazoletetrazolium; SD, standard deviation. *Source*: From Ortmann et al. (2002).

absence of aromatase inhibitory effects are observed. The nonaromatizable androgen, 5α-DHT, inhibits growth in the majority of studies, but whether stimulating effects as occasionally observed can be explained by binding to ER remains questionable. Similarly, it remains unexplained why in some cell lines stimulatory effects are seen without detectable amounts of estrogenic metabolites, although insufficient sensitivity of the detection method cannot be excluded. Apparently, the effects of androgens in in vitro studies depend on the system used; no overall clear picture has been found. Animal studies and clinical studies clearly show an inhibitory effect on proliferation of breast tissue.

EFFECTS OF TIBOLONE AND ITS METABOLITES ON PROLIFERATION

Tibolone is used for treatment of climacteric complaints and prevention of bone loss, whereas it does not stimulate the breast and the endometrium. Tibolone is a 19-nortestosterone derivative, with estrogenic effects on brain, vagina, and bone, but not on the endometrium. This tissue-selective action of tibolone is determined by its site-selective conversion to estrogenic metabolites and subsequent inactivation to sulfated metabolites. In addition, a small amount of tibolone is converted to the Δ^4-metabolite. See Figure 11 for tibolone's metabolism. The effects of tibolone on breast will be discussed here. For clinical effects on other tissues we refer to review articles (Modelska and Cummings, 2002; Kloosterboer, 2004).

In Vitro

The effect of tibolone on proliferation of breast cancer cells is quite different in various subclones of MCF-7 and T47D cells (Kloosterboer et al., 1994). Differences in potency and maximal responses are observed in different cell lines. The potency of tibolone was never larger than 1% of that of E_2. Lippert et al. (2002a) and Mueck et al. (2003a) reported a significant effect on MCF-7 cell proliferation with tibolone (10 nM to μM), comparable with that of 0.1 nM E_2. Schoonen et al. (2000) found a negligible growth effect of the Δ^4-metabolite on MCF-7 cells compared with E_2. Studies with different concentrations of the 3-hydroxytibolone metabolites in breast cancer cell lines have not been reported. Gompel et al. (2002) studied tibolone and its metabolites in normal breast cells. Tibolone and the Δ^4-metabolite showed antiproliferative effects, while in a slightly different medium with low growth factors, the 3α-hydroxy-metabolite showed at a 10^{-6} M concentration the same growth stimulation as 10 nM E_2. The 3β-hydroxytibolone did not stimulate, which may be due to back conversion of this 3β-hydroxymetabolite into tibolone and/or the Δ^4-metabolite (Figure 11).

In Vivo

Neutral effects of tibolone were found on xenograft transplants in the nude mice using either implanted MCF-7 cells (Desreux et al., 2007) or normal breast tissue (Dobson et al., 2001). The growth of DMBA induced

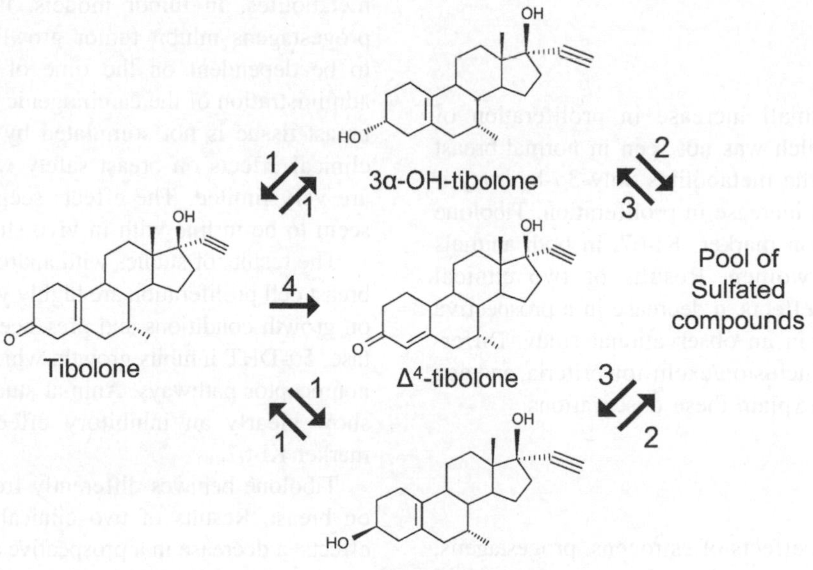

Figure 11 Metabolism pattern of tibolone by the enzymes aldo-keto reductases AKR1C-family (1), sulfotransferase (2), sulfatase (3), and isomerase or non-enzymatic conversion (4). The structures of the individual sulphated metabolites are not displayed.

tumors in intact rats was inhibited by tibolone and its metabolites (Kloosterboer et al., 1994; Kloosterboer and Deckers, 1997). Also, no effect was seen on the incidence of DMBA-induced tumors in ovx, prepubertal rats (Callejo et al., 2005). However, in GnRH antagonist treated, ovarian suppressed rats, tibolone stimulated the growth of established DMBA tumors (Kloosterboer and Deckers, 1999). In contrast, the proliferation marker Ki-67 is not significantly increased in breast tissue of ovx monkeys after two years of treatment with tibolone (Cline et al., 2002).

Comparative randomized clinical studies have shown that tibolone (2.5 mg) does not increase mammographic density (Lundström et al., 2002; Valdivia et al., 2004) and expression of the proliferation marker Ki-67 (Valdivia et al., 2004; Conner et al., 2004).

Despite these neutral effects of tibolone (2.5 mg) on breast, the observational MWS showed an increased risk of breast cancer in the U.K. population (Beral et al., 2003). Recently, the Long-Term Intervention on Fractures with Tibolone (LIFT) study (Cummings et al., 2007), which is a prospective randomized, placebo-controlled, double-blind fracture study in elderly postmenopausal women, showed a protective effect of tibolone (1.25 mg) against invasive breast cancer with a relative hazard of 0.32 (95% CI, 0.13–0.80; $p = 0.015$). Dimitrakakis et al. (2005) have shown in an observational study that in cancer patients after five years of tamoxifen treatment, which was followed with a three-year tibolone treatment, no increase in tumor recurrence was seen compared with untreated women.

Conclusion

Tibolone showed a small increase in proliferation of breast cancer cells, which was not seen in normal breast epithelial cells. From the metabolites only 3α-hydroxytibolone showed a small increase in proliferation. Tibolone reduced the proliferation marker, Ki-67, in both animals and postmenopausal women. Results of two clinical studies show opposite effects, a decrease in a prospective study and an increase in an observational study. Differences in study design, inclusion/exclusion criteria, and age after menopause may explain these observations.

SUMMARY

We have evaluated the effects of estrogens, progestagens, and their combinations and also of androgens on cell proliferation of breast (cancer) cells and on breast tissue growth in preclinical (tumor) models and compared the results with outcomes of large clinical trials. The main question we wanted to address was: "How relevant are preclinical studies for the outcome in animal studies and in clinical use?"

Estrogens are stimulating breast (cancer) cell lines and breast tissue almost without exception. Large concentrations or doses of estrogens may have an inhibitory effect. Observational clinical trials show a small increase in breast tumor risk by estrogens, which increases with duration of use. However, the prospective WHI study did not show an increase with CEE. Difference in age of the study population, study design, and inclusion/exclusion criteria may explain this.

The majority of in vitro experiments show an inhibitory effect of progestagens, both with 19-nortestosterone and pregnane-derived progestagens, on E_2-induced cell proliferation. In breast tumor models, E + P combination may have either a protective or stimulating effect dependent on whether the treatment is given before or after the carcinogenic agent. The in vitro studies are not predictive of the effects seen in studies with monkey and in clinical studies in which an increase in proliferation of breast tissue is found for E + P combinations. Both observational and prospective studies show an increased breast cancer risk for E + P combinations, although the effects in prospective studies are less pronounced. Also, weak estrogens can inhibit the action of E_2, although the clinical evidence is lacking.

P_4 has a growth-inhibitory effect on normal and breast cancer cells, which is likely due to its metabolite 3α-hydroxy-Δ^4-pregnene. In contrast, the 19-nortestosterone-derived progestagens show a stimulation of breast cancer cell lines, which is due to the formation of estrogenic metabolites. In tumor models, P_4 and both classes of progestagens inhibit tumor growth, although this seems to be dependent on the time of HT in relation to the administration of the carcinogenic agent. In ovx monkeys, breast tissue is not stimulated by progestagens. Data on clinical effects on breast safety with progestagens alone are very limited. The effects seen in breast cells do not seem to be in line with in vivo studies in animals.

The results of studies with androgens on proliferation of breast cell proliferation are highly variable and may depend on growth conditions and presence of the enzyme, aromatase. 5α-DHT inhibits growth, which may be mediated via nonreceptor pathways. Animal studies and clinical studies show clearly an inhibitory effect on the proliferation marker Ki-67.

Tibolone behaves differently from an E + P treatment on breast. Results of two clinical studies show opposite effects, a decrease in a prospective study and an increase in an observational study. Similar results were seen with CEE.

It is concluded that the results obtained in in vitro studies have to be interpreted with caution, since many factors influence the result. Therefore, the correlation between in vitro results and in vivo observations is not always straightforward and depends on steroid type, doses, timing, and many host factors.

REFERENCES

Anderson TJ, Battersby S, King RJ, McPherson K, Going JJ. Oral contraceptive use influences resting breast proliferation. Hum Pathol 1989; 20:1139–1144.

Anderson GL, Limacher M, Assaf AR, Bassford T, Beresford SA, Black H, Bonds D, Brunner R, Brzyski R, Caan B, Chlebowski R, Curb D, Gass M, Hays J, Heiss G, Hendrix S, Howard BV, Hsia J, Hubbell A, Jackson R, Johnson KC, Judd H, Kotchen JM, Kuller L, LaCroix AZ, Lane D, Langer RD, Lasser N, Lewis CE, Manson J, Margolis K, Ockene J, O'Sullivan MJ, Phillips L, Prentice RL, Ritenbaugh C, Robbins J, Rossouw JE, Sarto G, Stefanick ML, Van Horn L, Wactawski-Wende J, Wallace R, Wassertheil-Smoller S; Women's Health Initiative Steering Committee. Effects of conjugated equine estrogen in postmenopausal women with hysterectomy: the Women's Health Initiative randomized controlled trial. JAMA 2004; 291:1701–1712.

Archer DF, Hendrix S, Gallagher JC, Rymer J, Skouby S, Ferenczy A, den Hollander W, Stathopoulos V, Helmond FA. Endometrial effects of tibolone. J Clin Endocrinol Metab 2007; 92:911–918.

Aspinall SR, Stamp S, Davison A, Shenton BK, Lennard TW. The proliferative effects of 5-androstene-3 beta,17 beta-diol and 5 alpha-dihydrotestosterone on cell cycle analysis and cell proliferation in MCF7, T47D and MDAMB231 breast cancer cell lines. J Steroid Biochem Mol Biol 2004; 88:37–51.

Benakanakere I, Besch-Williford C, Schnell J, Brandt S, Ellersieck MR, Molinolo A, Hyder SM. Natural and synthetic progestins accelerate 7,12-dimethylbenz[a] anthracene-initiated mammary tumors and increase angiogenesis in Sprague-Dawley rats. Clin Cancer Res 2006; 12:4062–4071.

Beral V. Collaborative Group on Hormonal Factors in Breast Cancers. Breast cancer and hormonal contraceptives: collaborative reanalysis of individual data on 53 297 women with breast cancer and 100 239 women without breast cancer from 54 epidemiological studies. Collaborative Group on Hormonal Factors in Breast Cancer. Lancet 1996; 347:1713–1727.

Beral V. Collaborative Group on Hormonal Factors in Breast Cancers. Breast cancer and hormone replacement therapy: collaborative reanalysis of data from 51 epidemiological studies of 52,705 women with breast cancer and 108,411 women without breast cancer. Collaborative Group on Hormonal Factors in Breast Cancer. Lancet 1997; 350:1047–1059.

Beral V. Million Women Study Collaborators. Breast cancer and hormone-replacement therapy in the Million Women Study. Lancet 2003; 362:419–427.

Berkenstam A, Glaumann H, Martin M, Gustafsson JA, Norstedt G. Hormonal regulation of estrogen receptor messenger ribonucleic acid in T47Dco and MCF-7 breast cancer cells. Mol Endocrinol 1989; 3:22–28.

Billich A, Nussbaumer P, Lehr P. Stimulation of MCF-7 breast cancer cell proliferation by estrone sulfate and dehydroepiandrosterone sulfate: inhibition by novel non-steroidal steroid sulfatase inhibitors. J Steroid Biochem Mol Biol 2000; 73:225–235.

Botella J, Duranti E, Duc I, Cognet AM, Delansorne R, Paris J. Inhibition by nomegestrol acetate and other synthetic progestins on proliferation and progesterone receptor content of T47-D human breast cancer cells. J Steroid Biochem Mol Biol 1994; 50:41–47.

Bush TL, Whiteman M, Flaws JA. Hormone replacement therapy and breast cancer: a qualitative review. Obstet Gynecol 2001; 98:498–508.

Calaf GM. Susceptibility of human breast epithelial cells in vitro to hormones and drugs. Int J Oncol 2006; 28:285–295.

Calhoun KE, Pommier RF, Muller P, Fletcher WS, Toth-Fejel S. Dehydroepiandrosterone sulfate causes proliferation of estrogen receptor-positive breast cancer cells despite treatment with fulvestrant. Arch Surg 2003; 138:879–883.

Callejo J, Cano A, Medina M, Villaronga M, Gonzalez-Bosquet E, Sabria J, Lailla JM. Hormonal environment in the induction of breast cancer in castrated rats using dimethylbenzanthracene: influence of the presence or absence of ovarian activity and of treatment with estradiol, tibolone, and raloxifene. Menopause 2005; 12:601–608.

Campagnoli C, den Abbà C, Ambroggio S, Peris C. Pregnancy, progesterone and progestins in relation to breast cancer risk. J Steroid Biochem Mol Biol 2005; 97:441–450.

Catherino WH, Jeng MH, Jordan VC. Norgestrel and gestodene stimulate breast cancer cell growth through an oestrogen receptor mediated mechanism. Br J Cancer 1993; 67: 945–952.

Catherino WH, Jordan VC. Nomegestrol acetate, a clinically useful 19-norprogesterone derivative which lacks estrogenic activity. J Steroid Biochem Mol Biol 1995; 55:239–246.

Cavaillès V, Gompel A, Portois MC, Thénot S, Mabon N, Vignon F. Comparative activity of pulsed or continuous estradiol exposure on gene expression and proliferation of normal and tumoral human breast cells. J Mol Endocrinol 2002; 28:165–175.

Cavalieri E, Chakravarti D, Guttenplan J, Hart E, Ingle J, Jankowiak R, Muti P, Rogan E, Russo J, Santen R, Sutter T. Catechol estrogen quinones as initiators of breast and other human cancers: implications for biomarkers of susceptibility and cancer prevention. Biochem Biophys Acta 2006; 1766:63–78.

Chalbos D, Vignon F, Keydar I, Rochefort H. Estrogens stimulate cell proliferation and induce secretory proteins in a human breast cancer cell line (T47D). J Clin Endocrinol Metab 1982; 55:276–283.

Chan CM, Martin LA, Johnston SR, Ali S. Dowsett M. Molecular changes associated with the acquisition of oestrogen hypersensitivity in MCF-7 breast cancer cells on long-term oestrogen deprivation. J Steroid Biochem Mol Biol 2002; 81:333–341.

Chang KJ, Lee TT, Linares-Cruz G, Fournier S, de Ligniéres B. Influences of percutaneous administration of estradiol and progesterone on human breast epithelial cell cycle in vivo. Fertil Steril 1995; 63:785–791.

Chen WY, Manson JE, Hankinson SE, Rosner B, Holmes MD, Willett WC, Colditz GA. Unopposed estrogen therapy and the risk of invasive breast cancer. Arch Intern Med 2006; 166:1027–1032.

Chie WC, Hsieh C, Newcomb PA, Longnecker MP, Mittendorf R, Greenberg ER, Clapp RW, Burke KP, Titus-Ernstoff L, Trentham-Dietz A, MacMahon B. Age at any full-term pregnancy and breast cancer risk. Am J Epidemiol 2000; 151:715–722.

Chilvers CE. Depot medroxyprogesterone acetate and breast cancer. A review of current knowledge. Drug Saf 1996; 15:212–218.

Chlebowski RT, Hendrix SL, Langer RD, Stefanick ML, Gass M, Lane D, Rodabough RJ, Gilligan MA, Cyr MG, Thomson CA, Khandekar J, Petrovitch H, McTiernan A. WHI Investigators. Influence of estrogen plus progestin on breast cancer and mammography in healthy postmenopausal women: the Women's Health Initiative Randomized Trial. JAMA 2003; 289:3243–3253.

Cirpan T, Iscan O, Terek MC, Ozsener S, Kanit L, Pogun S, Zekioglu O, Yucebilgin S. Proliferative effects of different hormone regimens on mammary glands in ovariectomized rats. Eur J Gynaecol Oncol 2006; 27:256–261.

Clark JH, Markaverich BM. The agonistic and antagonistic actions of estriol. J Steroid Biochem 1984; 20:1005–1013.

Clark JH, Paszko Z, Peck EJ Jr. Nuclear binding and retention of the receptor estrogen complex: relation to the agonistic and antagonistic properties of estriol. Endocrinology 1977; 100:91–96.

Clarke RB. Ovarian steroids and the human breast: regulation of stem cells and cell proliferation. Maturitas 2006; 54: 327–334.

Clarke RB, Howell A, Anderson E. Estrogen sensitivity of normal human breast tissue in vivo and implanted into athymic nude mice: analysis of the relationship between estrogen-induced proliferation and progesterone receptor expression. Breast Cancer Res Treat 1997a; 45:121–133.

Clarke RB, Howell A, Potten CS, Anderson E. Dissociation between steroid receptor expression and cell proliferation in the human breast. Cancer Res 1997b; 57:4987–4991.

Clarke R, Leonessa F, Welch JN, Skaar TC. Cellular and molecular pharmacology of antiestrogen action and resistance. Pharmacol Rev 2001; 53:25–71.

Cline JM. Assessing the mammary gland of nonhuman primates: effects of endogenous hormones and exogenous hormonal agents and growth factors. Birth Defects Res B Dev Reprod Toxicol 2007; 80:126–146.

Cline JM, Register TC, Clarkson TB. Effects of tibolone and hormone replacement therapy on the breast of cynomolgus monkeys. Menopause 2002; 9:422–429.

Cline JM, Soderqvist G, von Schoultz E, Skoog L, von Schoultz B. Effects of hormone replacement therapy on the mammary gland of surgically postmenopausal cynomolgus macaques. Am J Obstet Gynecol 1996; 174:93–100.

Cline JM, Wood CE. Hormonal effects on the mammary gland of postmenopausal nonhuman primates. Breast Dis 2005–2006; 24:59–70.

Cole P, MacMahon B, Brown JB. Oestrogen profiles of parous and nulliparous women. Lancet 1976; 2:596–599.

Conneely OM, Mulac-Jericevic B, Lydon JP, De Mayo FJ. Reproductive functions of the progesterone receptor isoforms: lessons from knock-out mice. Mol Cell Endocrinol 2001; 179:97–103.

Conner P, Christow A, Kersemaekers W, Söderqvist G, Skoog L, Carlström K, Tani E, Mol-Arts M, von Schoultz B. A comparative study of breast cell proliferation during hormone replacement therapy: effects of tibolone and continuous combined estrogen-progestogen treatment. Climacteric 2004; 7:50–58.

Conner P, Söderqvist G, Skoog L, Gräser T, Walter F, Tani E, Carlström K, von Schoultz B. Breast cell proliferation in postmenopausal women during HRT evaluated through fine needle aspiration cytology. Breast Cancer Res Treat 2003; 78:159–165.

Couse JF, Korach KS. Estrogen receptor null mice: what have we learned and where will they lead us? Endocr Rev 1999; 20:358–417.

Cummings SR, Bilezikian JP, Christiansen C, Eastell R, Ettinger B, Delmas P, Grobbee DE, Johnson S, Kenemans P, Mosca, Amari N, Seifert W, Verweij P, Stathopoulos V, Mol-Arts M. The effects of tibolone in older women: results of the LIFT trial. 34th Eur Symp on calcified tissues 2007; abst LB3.

de Lignières B, de Vathaire F, Fournier S, Urbinelli R, Allaert F, Le MG, Kuttenn F. Combined hormone replacement therapy and risk of breast cancer in a French cohort study of 3175 women. Climacteric 2002; 5:332–340.

Desreux J, Kloosterboer H, Noël A, Frankenne F, Lemaire M, Putman M, Foidart JM. Effects of tibolone on sulfatase pathway of estrogens metabolism and on growth of MCF-7 human breast tumors implanted in ovariectomized nude mice. Gynecol Obstet Invest 2007; 63:31–38.

Dietel M, Lewis MA, Shapiro S. Hormone replacement therapy: pathobiological aspects of hormone-sensitive cancers in women relevant to epidemiological studies on HRT: a mini-review. Hum Reprod 2005; 20:2052–2060.

Dimitrakakis C, Jones RA, Liu A, Bondy CA. Breast cancer incidence in postmenopausal women using testosterone in addition to usual hormone therapy. Menopause 2004; 11:531–535.

Dimitrakakis C, Keramopoulos D, Vourli G, Gaki V, Bredakis N, Keramopoulos A. Clinical effects of tibolone in postmenopausal women after 5 years of tamoxifen therapy for breast cancer. Climacteric 2005; 8:342–351.

Dimitrakakis C, Zhou J, Wang J, Belanger A, LaBrie F, Cheng C, Powell D, Bondy C. A physiologic role for testosterone in limiting estrogenic stimulation of the breast. Menopause 2003; 10:292–298.

Dobson R, Chan K, Knox WF, Potten C, Kloosterboer HJ, Bundred NJ. Tibolone does not stimulate epithelial proliferation in the breast. Breast Cancer Res Treat 2001; 69:292.

Fabre A, Fournier A, Mesrine S, Desreux J, Gompel A, Boutron-Ruault MC, Clavel-Chapelon F. Oral progestagens before menopause and breast cancer risk. Br J Cancer 2007; 96:841–844.

Foidart JM, Colin C, Denoo X, Desreux J, Béliard A, Fournier S, de Lignières B. Estradiol and progesterone regulate the proliferation of human breast epithelial cells. Fertil Steril 1998; 69:963–969.

Gabelman BM, Emerman JT. Effects of estrogen, epidermal growth factor, and transforming growth factor-alpha on the growth of human breast epithelial cells in primary culture. Exp Cell Res 1992; 201:113–118.

Gadducci A, Gargini A, Palla E, Fanucchi A, Genazzani AR. Polycystic ovary syndrome and gynecological cancers: is there a link? Gynecol Endocrinol 2005; 20:200–208.

Gayosso V, Montano LF, López-Marure R. DHEA-induced antiproliferative effect in MCF-7 cells is androgen- and estrogen receptor-independent. Cancer J 2006; 12:160–165.

Going JJ, Anderson TJ, Battersby S, MacIntyre CC. Proliferative and secretory activity in human breast during natural and artificial menstrual cycles. Am J Pathol 1988; 130:193–204.

Gompel A, Chaouat M, Jacob D, Perrot JY, Kloosterboer HJ, Rostene W. In vitro studies of tibolone in breast cells. Fertil Steril 2002; 78:351–359.

Gompel A, Malet C, Spritzer P, Lalardrie JP, Kuttenn F, Mauvais-Jarvis P. Progestin effect on cell proliferation and 17 beta-hydroxysteroid dehydrogenase activity in normal human breast cells in culture. J Clin Endocrinol Metab 1986; 63:1174–1180.

Greeve MA, Allan RK, Harvey JM, Bentel JM. Inhibition of MCF-7 breast cancer cell proliferation by 5alpha-dihydrotestosterone; a role for p21(Cip1/Waf1). J Mol Endocrinol 2004; 32:793–810.

Gupta M, McDougal A, Safe S. Estrogenic and antiestrogenic activities of 16alpha- and 2-hydroxy metabolites of 17beta-estradiol in MCF-7 and T47D human breast cancer cells. J Steroid Biochem Mol Biol 1998; 67:413–419.

Hackenberg R, Hofmann J, Wolff G, Hölzel F, Schulz KD. Down-regulation of androgen receptor by progestins and interference with estrogenic or androgenic stimulation of mammary carcinoma cell growth. J Cancer Res Clin Oncol 1990; 116:492–498.

Hannaford PC, Selvaraj S, Elliott AM, Angus V, Iversen L, Lee AJ. Cancer risk among users of oral contraceptives: cohort data from the Royal College of General Practitioner's oral contraception study. BMJ 2007; 335:651; [Epub Sep 11, 2007].

Hargreaves DF, Knox F, Swindell R, Potten CS, Bundred NJ. Epithelial proliferation and hormone receptor status in the normal post-menopausal breast and the effects of hormone replacement therapy. Br J Cancer 1998; 78:945–949.

Hissom JR, Bowden RT, Moore MR. Effects of progestins, estrogens, and antihormones on growth and lactate dehydrogenase in the human breast cancer cell line T47D. Endocrinology 1989; 125:418–423.

Hofling M, Hirschberg AL, Skoog L, Tani E, Hägerström T, von Schoultz B. Testosterone inhibits estrogen/progestogen-induced breast cell proliferation in postmenopausal women. Menopause 2007b; 14:183–190.

Hofling M, Lundström E, Azavedo E, Svane G, Hirschberg AL, von Schoultz B. Testosterone addition during menopausal hormone therapy: effects on mammographic breast density. Climacteric 2007a; 10:155–163.

Hofseth LJ, Raafat AM, Osuch JR, Pathak DR, Slomski CA, Haslam SZ. Hormone replacement therapy with estrogen or estrogen plus medroxyprogesterone acetate is associated with increased epithelial proliferation in the normal post-menopausal breast. J Clin Endocrinol Metab 1999; 84:4559–4565.

Ismail PM, Amato P, Soyal SM, DeMayo FJ, Conneely OM, O'Malley BW, Lydon JP. Progesterone involvement in breast development and tumorigenesis–as revealed by progesterone receptor "knockout" and "knockin" mouse models. Steroids 2003; 68:779–787.

Jeng MH, Parker CJ, Jordan VC. Estrogenic potential of progestins in oral contraceptives to stimulate human breast cancer cell proliferation. Cancer Res 1992; 52:6539–6546.

Jernström H, Lerman C, Ghadirian P, Lynch HT, Weber B, Garber J, Daly M, Olopade OI, Foulkes WD, Warner E, Brunet JS, Narod SA. Pregnancy and risk of early breast cancer in carriers of BRCA1 and BRCA2. Lancet 1999; 354:1846–1850.

Jozan S, Kreitmann B, Bayard F. Different effects of oestradiol, oestriol, oestetrol and of oestrone on human breast cancer cells (MCF-7) in long term tissue culture. Acta Endocrinol (Copenh) 1981; 98:73–80.

Kalkhoven E, Kwakkenbos-Isbrücker L, de Laat SW, van der Saag PT, van der Burg B. Synthetic progestins induce proliferation of breast tumor cell lines via the progesterone or estrogen receptor. Mol Cell Endocrinol 1994; 102:45–52.

Katzenellenbogen BS. Biology and receptor interactions of estriol and estriol derivatives in vitro and in vivo. J Steroid Biochem 1984; 20:1033–1037.

Katzenellenbogen BS, Kendra KL, Norman MJ, Berthois Y. Proliferation, hormonal responsiveness, and estrogen receptor content of MCF-7 human breast cancer cells grown in the short-term and long-term absence of estrogens. Cancer Res 1987; 47:4355–4360.

Kendra KL, Katzenellenbogen BS. An evaluation of the involvement of polyamines in modulating MCF-7 human breast cancer cell proliferation and progesterone receptor levels by estrogen and antiestrogen. J Steroid Biochem 1987; 28:123–128.

Kloosterboer HJ. Tibolone: a steroid with a tissue-specific mode of action. J Steroid Biochem Mol Biol 2001; 76:231–238.

Kloosterboer HJ. Tissue-selective effects of tibolone on the breast. Maturitas 2004; 49:S5–S15.

Kloosterboer HJ, Deckers GH. Effects of tibolone (Livial®) and metabolites on the growth of DMBA induced tumors in rats. Acta Obstet Gynecol Scand 1997; 76(suppl 167):59.

Kloosterboer HJ, Deckers GH. Effects of tibolone and/or tamoxifen on DMBA induced breast tumors in ovarian suppressed rats. Breast Cancer Res Treat 1999; 57:136.

Kloosterboer HJ, Schoonen WG, Deckers GH, Klijn JG. Effects of progestagens and Org OD14 in in vitro and in vivo tumor models. J Steroid Biochem Mol Biol 1994; 49:311–318.

Kopans DB, Rafferty E, Georgian-Smith D, Yeh E, D'Alessandro H, Moore R, Hughes K, Halpern E. A simple model of breast carcinoma growth may provide explanations for observations of apparently complex phenomena. Cancer 2003; 97:2951–2959.

Krämer EA, Seeger H, Krämer B, Wallwiener D, Mueck AO. Characterization of the stimulatory effect of medroxyprogesterone acetate and chlormadinone acetate on growth factor treated normal human breast epithelial cells. J Steroid Biochem Mol Biol 2006a; 98:174–178.

Krämer EA, Seeger H, Krämer B, Wallwiener D, Mueck AO. The effect of progesterone, testosterone and synthetic progestogens on growth factor- and estradiol-treated human cancerous and benign breast cells. Eur J Obstet Gynecol Reprod Biol 2006b; 129:77–83.

Labrie F. Dehydroepiandrosterone, androgens and the mammary gland. Gynecol Endocrinol 2006; 22:118–130.

Lange CA, Richer JK, Horwitz KB. Hypothesis: progesterone primes breast cancer cells for cross-talk with proliferative or antiproliferative signals. Mol Endocrinol 1999; 13:829–836.

Larrea F, Vilchis F, Chávez B, Pérez AE, Garza-Flores J, Pérez-Palacios G. The metabolism of 19-nor contraceptive progestins modulates their biological activity at the neuroendocrine level. J Steroid Biochem 1987; 27:657–663.

LaVallee TM, Zhan XH, Herbstritt CJ, Kough EC, Green SJ, Pribluda VS. 2-Methoxyestradiol inhibits proliferation and induces apoptosis independently of estrogen receptors alpha and beta. Cancer Res 2002; 62:3691–3697.

Lemon HM. Clinical and experimental aspects of the anti-mammary carcinogenic activity of estriol. Front Horm Res 1977; 5:155–173.

Lemus AE, Vilchis F, Damsky R, Chávez BA, García GA, Grillasca I, Pérez-Palacios G. Mechanism of action of levonorgestrel: in vitro metabolism and specific interactions with steroid receptors in target organs. J Steroid Biochem Mol Biol 1992; 41:881–890.

Lemus AE, Zaga V, Santillán R, García GA, Grillasca I, Damián-Matsumura P, Jackson KJ, Cooney AJ, Larrea F, Pérez-Palacios G. The oestrogenic effects of gestodene, a potent contraceptive progestin, are mediated by its A-ring reduced metabolites. J Endocrinol 2000; 165:693–702.

Liao DJ, Dickson RB. Roles of androgens in the development, growth, and carcinogenesis of the mammary gland. J Steroid Biochem Mol Biol 2002; 80:175–189.

Lippert C, Seeger H, Mueck AO. The effect of endogenous estradiol metabolites on the proliferation of human breast cancer cells. Life Sci 2003; 72:877–883.

Lippert C, Seeger H, Wallwiener D, Mueck AO. The effect of medroxyprogesterone acetate and norethisterone on the estradiol stimulated proliferation in MCF-7 cells: comparison of continuous combined versus sequential combined estradiol/progestin treatment. Eur J Gynaecol Oncol 2001; 22:331–335.

Lippert C, Seeger H, Wallwiener D, Mueck AO. Tibolone versus 17beta-estradiol/norethisterone: effects on the proliferation of human breast cancer cells. Eur J Gynaecol Oncol 2002a; 23:127–130.

Lippert C, Seeger H, Wallwiener D, Mueck AO. Comparison of the effects of 17alpha-ethinylestradiol and 17beta-estradiol on the proliferation of human breast cancer cells and human umbilical vein endothelial cells. Clin Exp Obstet Gynecol 2002b; 29:87–90.

Lundström E, Christow A, Kersemaekers W, Svane G, Azavedo E, Söderqvist G, Mol-Arts M, Barkfeldt J, von Schoultz B. Effects of tibolone and continuous combined hormone replacement therapy on mammographic breast density. Am J Obstet Gynecol 2002; 186:717–722.

MacGregor JI, Jordan VC. Basic guide to the mechanisms of antiestrogen action. Pharmacol Rev 1998; 50:151–196.

Maggiolini M, Donzé O, Jeannin E, Andò S, Picard D. Adrenal androgens stimulate the proliferation of breast cancer cells as direct activators of estrogen receptor alpha. Cancer Res 1999; 59:4864–4869.

Malet C, Gompel A, Yaneva H, Cren H, Fidji N, Mowszowicz I, Kuttenn F, Mauvais-Jarvis P. Estradiol and progesterone receptors in cultured normal human breast epithelial cells and fibroblasts: immunocytochemical studies. J Clin Endocrinol Metab 1991; 73:8–17.

Malet C, Spritzer P, Guillaumin D, Kuttenn F. Progesterone effect on cell growth, ultrastructural aspect and estradiol receptors of normal human breast epithelial (HBE) cells in culture. J Steroid Biochem Mol Biol 2000; 73:171–181.

Masamura S, Santner SJ, Heitjan DF, Santen RJ. Estrogen deprivation causes estradiol hypersensitivity in human breast cancer cells. J Clin Endocrinol Metab 1995; 80:2918–2925.

Medina D, Peterson LE, Moraes R, Gay J. Short-term exposure to estrogen and progesterone induces partial protection against N-nitroso-N-methylurea-induced mammary tumorigenesis in Wistar–Furth rats. Cancer Lett 2001; 169:1–6.

Melamed M, Castaño E, Notides AC, Sasson S. Molecular and kinetic basis for the mixed agonist/antagonist activity of estriol. Mol Endocrinol 1997; 11:1868–1878.

Modelska K, Cummings S. Tibolone for postmenopausal women: systematic review of randomized trials. J Clin Endocrinol Metab 2002; 87:16–23.

Mueck AO, Lippert C, Seeger H, Wallwiener D. Effects of tibolone on human breast cancer cells and human vascular coronary cells. Arch Gynecol Obstet. 2003a 267; 139–144.

Mueck AO, Seeger H, Wallwiener D. Comparison of the proliferative effects of estradiol and conjugated equine estrogens on human breast cancer cells and impact of continuous combined progestogen addition. Climacteric 2003b; 6:221–227.

Musgrove EA, Lee CS, Sutherland RL. Progestins both stimulate and inhibit breast cancer cell cycle progression while increasing expression of transforming growth factor alpha, epidermal growth factor receptor, c-fos, and c-myc genes. Mol Cell Biol 1991; 11:5032–5043.

Najid A, Habrioux G. Biological effects of adrenal androgens on MCF-7 and BT-20 human breast cancer cells. Oncology 1990; 47:269–274.

Newcomb PA, Titus-Ernstoff L, Egan KM, Trentham-Dietz A, Baron JA, Storer BE, Willett WC, Stampfer MJ. Postmenopausal estrogen and progestin use in relation to breast cancer risk. Cancer Epidemiol Biomarkers Prev 2002; 11:593–600.

Ohi Y, Yoshida H. Influence of estrogen and progesterone on the induction of mammary carcinomas by 7,12-dimethylbenz(a) anthracene in ovariectomized rats. Virchows Arch B Cell Pathol Incl Mol Pathol 1992; 62:365–370.

Ortmann J, Prifti S, Bohlmann MK, Rehberger-Schneider S, Strowitzki T, Rabe T. Testosterone and 5 α-dihydrotestosterone inhibit in vitro growth of human breast cancer cell lines. Gynecol Endocrinol 2002; 16: 113–120.

Pasqualini JR. The selective estrogen enzyme modulators in breast cancer: a review. Biochim Biophys Acta 2004; 1654:123–43.

Poulin R, Baker D, Poirier D, Labrie F. Multiple actions of synthetic 'progestins' on the growth of ZR-75-1 human breast cancer cells: an in vitro model for the simultaneous assay of androgen, progestin, estrogen, and glucocorticoid agonistic and antagonistic activities of steroids. Breast Cancer Res Treat 1990; 17:197–210.

Poulin R, Dufour JM, Labrie F. Progestin inhibition of estrogen-dependent proliferation in ZR-75-1 human breast cancer cells: antagonism by insulin. Breast Cancer Res Treat 1989; 13:265–276.

Poulin R, Labrie F. Stimulation of cell proliferation and estrogenic response by adrenal C19-delta 5-steroids in the ZR-75-1 human breast cancer cell line. Cancer Res 1986; 46:4933–4937.

Preston-Martin S, Pike MC, Ross RK, Jones PA, Henderson BE. Increased cell division as a cause of human cancer. Cancer Res 1990; 50:415–421.

Raafat AM, Hofseth LJ, Haslam SZ. Proliferative effects of combination estrogen and progesterone replacement therapy on the normal postmenopausal mammary gland in a murine model. Am J Obstet Gynecol 2001; 184: 340–349.

Rasmussen TH, Nielsen JB. Critical parameters in the MCF-7 cell proliferation bioassay (E-Screen). Biomarkers 2002; 7:322–336.

Reddel RR, Sutherland RL. Effects of pharmacological concentrations of estrogens on proliferation and cell cycle kinetics of human breast cancer cell lines in vitro. Cancer Res 1987; 47:5323–5329.

Russo J, Balogh GA, Heulings R, Mailo DA, Moral R, Russo PA, Sheriff F, Vanegas J, Russo IH. Molecular basis of pregnancy-induced breast cancer protection. Eur J Cancer Prev 2006; 15:306–342.

Russo J, Russo IH. Development of the human breast. Maturitas 2004; 49:2–15.

Russo J, Russo IH. The role of estrogen in the initiation of breast cancer. J Steroid Biochem Mol Biol 2006; 102:89–96.

Sakamoto S, Kudo H, Suzuki S, Mitamura T, Sassa S, Kuwa K, Chun Z, Yoshimura S, Maemura M, Nakayama T, Shinoda H. Additional effects of medroxyprogesterone acetate on mammary tumors in oophorectomized, estrogenized, DMBA-treated rats. Anticancer Res 1997; 17:4583–4587.

Santen RJ, Allred DC. The estrogen paradox. Nat Clin Pract Endocrinol Metab 2007; 3:496–497.

Santillán R, Pérez-Palacios G, Reyes M, Damián-Matsumura P, García GA, Grillasca I, Lemus AE. Assessment of the oestrogenic activity of the contraceptive progestin levonorgestrel and its non-phenolic metabolites. Eur J Pharmacol 2001; 427:167–174.

Santner SJ, Chen S, Zhou D, Korsunsky Z, Martel J, Santen RJ. Effect of androstenedione on growth of untransfected and aromatase-transfected MCF-7 cells in culture. J Steroid Biochem Mol Biol 1993b; 44:611–616.

Santner SJ, Ohlsson-Wilhelm B, Santen RJ. Estrone sulfate promotes human breast cancer cell replication and nuclear uptake of estradiol in MCF-7 cell cultures. Int J Cancer 1993a; 54:119–124.

Sartorius CA, Harvell DM, Shen T, Horwitz KB. Progestins initiate a luminal to myoepithelial switch in estrogen-dependent human breast tumors without altering growth. Cancer Res 2005; 65:9779–9788.

Sasson S, Notides AC. Estriol and estrone interaction with the estrogen receptor II. Estriol and estrone-induced inhibition of the cooperative binding of [3H] estradiol to the estrogen receptor. J Biol Chem 1983; 258: 8118–8122.

Savoldi G, Ferrari F, Ruggeri G, Sobek L, Albertini A, Di Lorenzo D. Progesterone agonists and antagonists induce down- and up-regulation of estrogen receptors and estrogen inducible genes in human breast cancer cell lines. Int J Biol Markers 1995; 10:47–54.

Schafer JM, Jordan VC. Models of hormone resistance in vitro and in vivo. Methods Mol Med 2006; 120:453–464.

Schatz RW, Soto AM, Sonnenschein C. Effects of interaction between estradiol-17 beta and progesterone on the proliferation of cloned breast tumor cells (MCF-7 and T47D). J Cell Physiol 1985; 124:386–390.

Schmitt M, Klinga K, Schnarr B, Morfin R, Mayer D. Dehydroepiandrosterone stimulates proliferation and gene expression in MCF-7 cells after conversion to estradiol. Mol Cell Endocrinol 2001; 173:1–13.

Schneider J, Huh MM, Bradlow HL, Fishman J. Antiestrogen action of 2-hydroxyestrone on MCF-7 human breast cancer cells. J Biol Chem 1984; 259:4840–4845.

Schoonen WG, Deckers GH, de Gooijer ME, de Ries R, Kloosterboer HJ. Hormonal properties of norethisterone, 7alpha-methyl-norethisterone and their derivatives. J Steroid Biochem Mol Biol 2000; 74:213–222.

Schoonen WG, Joosten JW, Kloosterboer HJ. Effects of two classes of progestagens, pregnane and 19-nortestosterone derivatives, on cell growth of human breast tumor cells: I. MCF-7 cell lines. J Steroid Biochem Mol Biol 1995a; 55:423–437.

Schoonen WG, Joosten JW, Kloosterboer HJ. Effects of two classes of progestagens, pregnane and 19-nortestosterone derivatives, on cell growth of human breast tumor cells: II. T47D cell lines. J Steroid Biochem Mol Biol 1995b; 55:439–444.

Seeger H, Deuringer FU, Wallwiener D, Mueck AO. Breast cancer risk during HRT: influence of estradiol metabolites on breast cancer and endothelial cell proliferation. Maturitas 2004b; 49:235–240.

Seeger H, Huober J, Wallwiener D, Mueck AO. Inhibition of human breast cancer cell proliferation with estradiol metabolites is as effective as with tamoxifen. Horm Metab Res 2004a; 36:277–280.

Seeger H, Wallwiener D, Kraemer E, Mueck AO. Comparison of possible carcinogenic estradiol metabolites: effects on proliferation, apoptosis and metastasis of human breast cancer cells. Maturitas 2006; 54:72–77.

Seeger H, Wallwiener D, Mueck AO. The effect of progesterone and synthetic progestins on serum- and estradiol-stimulated proliferation of human breast cancer cells. Horm Metab Res 2003a; 35:76–80.

Seeger H, Wallwiener D, Mueck AO. Comparison of the effect of progesterone, medroxyprogesterone acetate and norethisterone on the proliferation of human breast cancer cells. J Br Menopause Soc 2003b; 9:36–38.

Shafie SM, Grantham FH. Role of hormones in the growth and regression of human breast cancer cells (MCF-7) transplanted into athymic nude mice. J Natl Cancer Inst 1981; 67:51–56.

Singhal H, Guo L, Bradlow HL, Mittelman A, Tiwari RK. Endocrine characteristics of human breast epithelial cells, MCF-10F. Horm Res 1999; 52:171–177.

Somboonporn W, Davis SR. Postmenopausal testosterone therapy and breast cancer risk. Maturitas 2004; 49:267–275.

Sonne-Hansen K, Lykkesfeldt AE. Endogenous aromatization of testosterone results in growth stimulation of the human MCF-7 breast cancer cell line. J Steroid Biochem Mol Biol 2005; 93:25–34.

Stanczyk FZ. Pharmacokinetics and potency of progestins used for hormone replacement therapy and contraception. Rev Endocr Metab Disord 2002; 3:211–224.

Stefanick ML, Anderson GL, Margolis KL, Hendrix SL, Rodabough RJ, Paskett ED, Lane DS, Hubbell FA, Assaf AR, Sarto GE, Schenken RS, Yasmeen S, Lessin L, Chlebowski RT; WHI Investigators. Effects of conjugated equine estrogens on breast cancer and mammography screening in postmenopausal women with hysterectomy. JAMA 2006; 295:1647–1657.

Sutherland RL, Hall RE, Pang GY, Musgrove EA, Clarke CL. Effect of medroxyprogesterone acetate on proliferation and cell cycle kinetics of human mammary carcinoma cells. Cancer Res. 1988; 48:5084–5091.

Sutherland TE, Schuliga M, Harris T, Eckhardt BL, Anderson RL, Quan L, Stewart AG. 2-methoxyestradiol is an estrogen receptor agonist that supports tumor growth in murine xenograft models of breast cancer. Clin Cancer Res 2005; 11:1722–1732.

Tekmal RR, Liu YG, Nair HB, Jones J, Perla RP, Lubahn DB, Korach KS, Kirma N. Estrogen receptor alpha is required for mammary development and the induction of mammary hyperplasia and epigenetic alterations in the aromatase transgenic mice. J Steroid Biochem Mol Biol 2005; 95:9–15.

Tilanus-Linthorst MM, Kriege M, Boetes C, Hop WC, Obdeijn IM, Oosterwijk JC, Peterse HL, Zonderland HM, Meijer S, Eggermont AM, de Koning HJ, Klijn JG, Brekelmans CT. Hereditary breast cancer growth rates and its impact on screening policy. Eur J Cancer 2005; 41:1610–1617.

Tutt A, Ashworth A. The relationship between the roles of BRCA genes in DNA repair and cancer predisposition. Trends Mol Med 2002; 8:571–576.

Valdivia I, Campodónico I, Tapia A, Capetillo M, Espinoza A, Lavín P. Effects of tibolone and continuous combined hormone therapy on mammographic breast density and breast histochemical markers in postmenopausal women. Fertil Steril 2004; 81:617–623.

Vandenberg LN, Wadia PR, Schaeberle CM, Rubin BS, Sonnenschein C, Soto AM. The mammary gland response to estradiol: monotonic at the cellular level, non-monotonic at the tissue-level of organization? J Steroid Biochem Mol Biol 2006; 101:263–274.

Van der Burg B, Kalkhoven E, Isbrücker L, de Laat SW. Effects of progestins on the proliferation of estrogen-dependent human breast cancer cells under growth factor-defined conditions. J Steroid Biochem Mol Biol 1992; 42:457–465.

Van der Vange N, Blankenstein MA, Kloosterboer HJ, Haspels AA, Thijssen JH. Effects of seven low-dose combined oral contraceptives on sex hormone binding globulin, corticosteroid binding globulin, total and free testosterone. Contraception 1990; 41:345–352.

Wertheimer MD, Costanza ME, Dodson TF, D'Orsi C, Pastides H, Zapka JG. Increasing the effort toward breast cancer detection. JAMA 1986; 255:1311–1315.

WHI Investigators. Effects of conjugated equine estrogens on breast cancer and mammography screening in postmenopausal women with hysterectomy. JAMA 2006; 295:1647–1657.

Wiebe JP, Lewis MJ, Cialacu V, Pawlak KJ, Zhang G. The role of progesterone metabolites in breast cancer: potential for new diagnostics and therapeutics. J Steroid Biochem Mol Biol 2005; 93:201–208.

Wiebe JP, Muzia D, Hu J, Szwajcer D, Hill SA, Seachrist JL. The 4-pregnene and 5alpha-pregnane progesterone metabolites formed in nontumorous and tumorous breast tissue have opposite effects on breast cell proliferation and adhesion. Cancer Res 2000; 60:936–943.

Wood CE, Register TC, Lees CJ, Chen H, Kimrey S, Cline JM. Effects of estradiol with micronized progesterone or medroxyprogesterone acetate on risk markers for breast cancer in postmenopausal monkeys. Breast Cancer Res Treat 2007; 101:125–134.

Wotiz HH, Beebe DR, Müller E. Effect of estrogens on DMBA induced breast tumors. J Steroid Biochem 1984; 20:1067–1075.

Xu B, Kitawaki J, Koshiba H, Ishihara H, Kiyomizu M, Teramoto M, Kitaoka Y, Honjo H. Differential effects of progestogens, by type and regimen, on estrogen-metabolizing enzymes in human breast cancer cells. Maturitas 2007; 56:142–152.

Yager JD, Davidson NE. Estrogen carcinogenesis in breast cancer. N Engl J Med 2006; 354:270–282.

Yue W, Santen RJ, Wang JP, Li Y, Verderame MF, Bocchinfuso WP, Korach KS, Devanesan P, Todorovic R, Rogan EG, Cavalieri EL. Genotoxic metabolites of estradiol in breast: potential mechanism of estradiol induced carcinogenesis. J Steroid Biochem Mol Biol 2003; 86:477–486.

Zajchowski DA, Sager R, Webster L. Estrogen inhibits the growth of estrogen receptor-negative, but not estrogen receptor-positive, human mammary epithelial cells expressing a recombinant estrogen receptor. Cancer Res 1993; 53:5004–5011.

Zhang J, Powell SN. The role of the BRCA1 tumor suppressor in DNA double-strand break repair. Mol Cancer Res 2005; 3:531–539.

Zhang J, Sun Y, Liu Y, Sun Y, Liao DJ. Synergistic effects of androgen and estrogen on the mouse uterus and mammary gland. Oncol Rep 2004; 12:709–716.

Zhou J, Ng S, Adesanya-Famuiya O, Anderson K, Bondy CA. Testosterone inhibits estrogen-induced mammary epithelial proliferation and suppresses estrogen receptor expression. FASEB J 2000; 14:1725–1730.

19

Lignans and Breast Cancer

HERMAN ADLERCREUTZ
Folkhälsan Research Center and Division of Clinical Chemistry, Biomedicum, University of Helsinki, Helsinki, Finland

PLANT AND ENTEROLIGNANS AND THEIR METABOLISM

The lignans were first detected in human beings in 1979 (Setchell and Adlercreutz, 1979) and identified independently by two groups describing their work in the same number of Nature (Setchell et al., 1980b, 1980c; Stitch et al., 1980). The original observation was made in urine of the female green monkey (Setchell et al., 1980a) who showed urinary peak excretion in the luteal phase during the menstrual cycle which we soon also found in women (Setchell et al., 1980c). This has never been explained, but unpublished results from our laboratory suggests that the luteal peak may be due to stimulation of the enterolactone (ENL) formation in the gut by estrogens in the bile reaching the colon during enterohepatic circulation (Adlercreutz, 1962). The reason for this hypothesis was that in connection with stimulation of ovaries by follicle-stimulating hormone (FSH) in infertile women both estrogens and lignans in urine increased steadily until ovulation, at which time both decreased rapidly.

The mammalian lignans (also called enterolignans) enterodiol (END) and ENL are formed from plant lignan glycoside precursors by the activity of the gut microflora in the proximal colon (Borriello et al., 1985; Glitsø et al., 2000; Setchell et al., 1981). The structure of the main plant and enterolignans and the present view of the metabolism of lignans in the gut are presented in Figure 1. The upper part of the scheme also corresponds to a part of the biosynthetic pathway of lignans in plants. Pinoresinol (PIN) is converted to lariciresinol (LAR) and further metabolized to secoisolariciresinol (SEC) and matairesinol (MAT), which are converted to END and ENL, respectively. END is oxidized to ENL. Syringaresinol (SYR), particularly abundant in rye bran, is also converted to enterolignans (Heinonen et al., 2001). The in vitro studies carried out with human feces suggested that only a small portion of SYR is converted, in vivo this may not be the case. Such studies are being carried out in collaboration with Dr. Bach Knudsen's group. The conversion of medioresinol (MED) to END and ENL is not known, but we anticipate that it is similar to that of SYR. Until a few years ago only two plant enterolignan precursors, SEC and MAT were known (Axelson et al., 1982; Borriello et al., 1985). In addition to the new precursors described above, 7-hydroxymatairesinol (HMR) and arctiin are converted to enterolignans by colon microflora (Nose et al., 1992; Saarinen et al., 2000; Xie et al., 2003). In addition, isolariciresinol (isoLAR) [also called cyclolariciresinol (cLAR)] has been found, but this lignan seems not to be converted to enterolignans in the gut (Heinonen et al., 2001) and may be easily formed from LAR during acid treatment of samples. Recently, very comprehensive and important studies on the intestinal bacteria involved in the formation of ENL from secoisolariciresinol diglucoside (SDG) were published. The conclusion was that activation of SDG involved

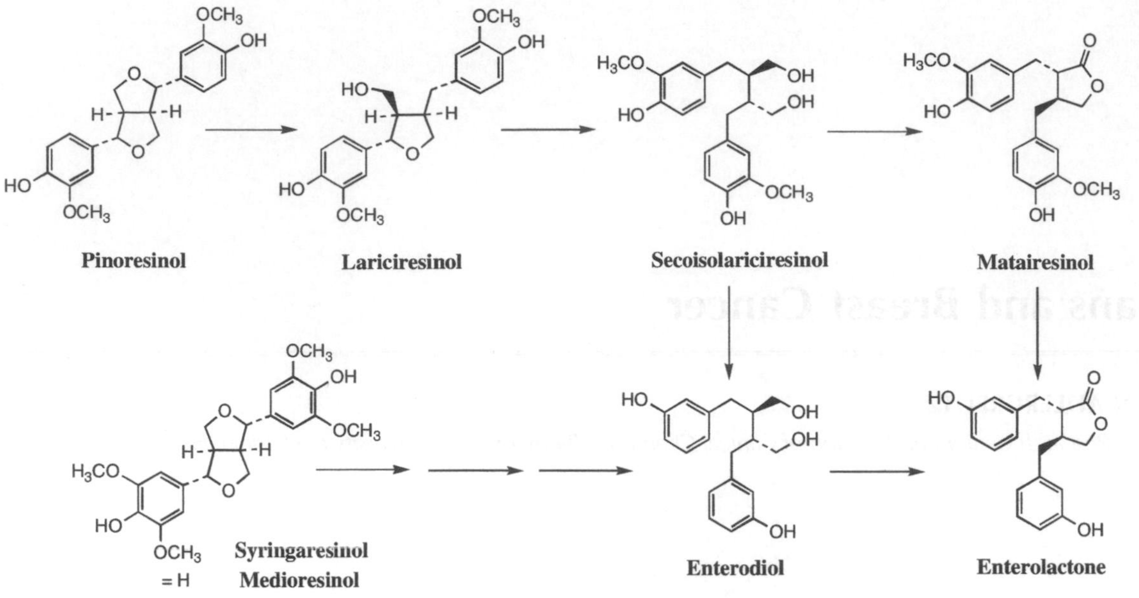

Figure 1 Proposed metabolism of lignans in the gut.

phylogenetically diverse bacteria, most of which are members of the dominant human intestinal microbiota and need anaerobic conditions (Clavel et al., 2005; Clavel et al., 2006).

FOOD SOURCES OF LIGNANS

Because only two plant precursors, SEC and MAT, were known during about two decades, only values for them in foods have been available until recently. Lignans occur particularly in seeds like flaxseed (mainly SEC) and sesame seed [mainly lignan precursor sesamin (SES)], but in the Western hemisphere most of the lignans consumed derive from whole-grain cereals, beans, including soybeans (Penalvo et al., 2004a), and other vegetables and some fruits, fruit juice, and berries, and also from wines, particularly red wine (Mazur, 1998a; Nurmi et al., 2003), tea and coffee (Mazur et al., 1998b). Olive oil does not contain SEC and MAT, but it contains PIN and acetoxy-PIN (Bonoli et al., 2004; Christophoridou et al., 2005), LAR, and small amounts of MED. A considerable part of the SEC and MAT values published derive from the work by Mazur et al. using an isotope dilution gas chromatography-mass spectrometry method (ID-GC-MS-SIM) utilizing deuterated internal standards (Mazur et al., 1996). The overall values with our new method (Penalvo et al., 2005a) are close to the values for MAT and SEC obtained with the old method. The earlier values have all been published (Mazur, 1998a; Mazur and Adlercreutz, 1998). Another GC-MS method has also been published (Liggins et al., 2000) and values for a number of foods presented. Furthermore, values for MAT and SEC have been obtained by liquid chromatography-mass spectrometry (LC-MS) (Horn-Ross et al., 2000) in 112 American food items and a phytoestrogen database including lignan values in 180 Finnish foods has been published (Valsta et al., 2003). Using the method giving values of ENL and END production after fermentation with intestinal bacteria and developed by Thompson et al. (1991), a database was developed (Pillow et al., 1999). The Vegetal Estrogens in Nutrition and the Skeleton (VENUS) database contains data for SEC and MAT in 158 foods (Kiely et al., 2003) and another recently developed database gives values for SEC and MAT for a total of 1332 individual foods (Blitz et al., 2007). However, recently a method was developed including food values for four plant lignans previously identified in whole-grain products by Heinonen et al. (Heinonen et al., 2001) based on liquid chromatography with double quadrupole mass spectrometers (LC-MS-MS) (Milder et al., 2004, 2005) and another measuring the six most common plant lignans in food by isotope dilution gas chromatography in selected ion mode (ID-GC-MS-SIM) using ^{13}C-lignans as internal standards (Penalvo et al., 2005a). In the latter publication also values for seven common cereals as well as for 10 fruits and vegetables are presented. Kale, broccoli, white and red cabbage, Brussels sprouts, sauerkraut, and cauliflower contain relatively high amounts as well as some fruits but the most common vegetables are relatively poor in lignans (Milder et al., 2005; Penalvo et al., 2005a). Phytoestrogen content including four lignans (SEC, MAT, PIN, and LAR) in 121 Canadian foods were also recently published (Thompson et al., 2006). Even soybeans contain lignans (Penalvo et al., 2004a). We have also analyzed 120 Japanese food samples (manuscript in preparation) and more Finnish food samples are being analyzed.

FACTORS INFLUENCING ENL LEVELS

In a study in 2383 Finnish men and women, living in different parts of Finland, the determinants of plasma ENL were assessed. The values varied considerably between subjects and the factors influencing plasma concentrations of ENL differed also between sexes. Smoking in both sexes and obesity and thinness in women were negatively associated with plasma ENL. In women with constipation, intake of vegetables and age were positively associated with plasma ENL (Kilkkinen et al., 2001); in men with constipation, intake of whole-grain products (rye bread) and fruit and berries were positively associated with plasma ENL. Recently it was found that in American women intake of coffee, fruit juices, and alcohol correlated positively with plasma ENL (Horner et al., 2002). Tea and wine contain substantial amounts of lignans, and coffee contributes to lignan level in the body. In a Dutch study wine drinking was also associated with plasma ENL (Keinan-Boker et al., 2002). We showed that during preparation of the tea in the British way the lignans are quantitatively extracted from the leaves. The proportion of lignans obtained from tea and coffee consumption show very large variations in different studies and it has been suggested that calculation errors may be involved (Hollman et al., 2006).

However, a generally "healthy lifestyle" and diet seem to explain only a small part of the variation in the population. Therefore, gut microflora and its activity is likely the major determinant of plasma ENL. Administration of antibiotics drastically reduce plasma and urinary ENL concentrations (Adlercreutz et al., 1986; Setchell et al., 1981), and this effect may persist for a long time even for more than one year (Kilkkinen et al., 2002). It is of interest that the between individual variation in recovery time of the ENL production after a course of antibiotics varies to a great extent. The production of ENL parallels the production of butyrate and both depend on the fermentation in the gut (Bach Knudsen et al., 2007, 2003). It is possible that those consuming fiber have a better fermentation because of a healthy diet and recover more quickly from the negative effects of antibiotics.

In the Finnish diet, particularly if it is relatively healthy, about 40% to 50% of ENL in plasma derives from whole-grain cereals, particularly rye bread and the other half from vegetables, fruits, and berries (Kilkkinen et al., 2001; Linko et al., 2005). Men consume more rye bread and less vegetables and fruits than women but more berries. In Danish women whole grains and vegetables determine the plasma ENL concentration (Johnsen et al., 2004). Recently Danish scientists found that eight weeks intake of rye-bran products did not increase plasma ENL levels in 16 young healthy male volunteers (Bach Kristensen et al., 2005). They explained the results, which are in contradiction to all previous results (Adlercreutz et al., 1982, 1986, 1987; Horner et al., 2002; Jacobs et al., 2002; Juntunen et al., 2000; Kilkkinen et al., 2001, 2003; Lampe et al., 1999; McIntosh et al., 2003) by a decrease in transit time due to the high-fiber intake. It has been shown that constipation lengthening transit time increases ENL production (Kilkkinen et al., 2001) perhaps by giving more time for the fermentation process and ENL production.

Studying plasma ENL concentrations in various countries in epidemiological studies need information of the dietary habits and life style of the subjects. Because this has been unknown in most investigations the very discrepant results obtained with regard to the association of plasma ENL with cancer risk are understandable. ENL assays were originally thought to reflect intake of lignin and grain fiber, (Adlercreutz et al., 1981, 1982, 1984) and the hypothesis on the role of fiber and lignans in breast and colon cancer was based on this assumption. After reading the literature the impression obtained is that when in epidemiological studies a significant part of the lignans and fiber derives from cereals and fiber-rich vegetables and berries negative associations with disease risk are found (see below). Drinking fruit juice, wine, tea, and coffee increases ENL in plasma but does not add any fiber to the diet. However, the decrease in cancer risk may depend more on the fiber and its other components than on the lignans and intake of wine, and other alcoholic beverages may have the opposite effect because alcohol increases breast and colon cancer risk.

SUGGESTED MECHANISMS OF ACTION OF LIGNANS AT THE CELLULAR LEVEL

In early studies in mice no in vivo detectable estrogenic activity of the lignans could be observed (Setchell et al., 1981). However, in vitro in four sensitive assays in tissue culture, including breast cancer cell lines, lignans showed estrogenic activity and were stimulatory with regard to breast cancer cells, and the effect could be blocked by the antiestrogen tamoxifen. No antiestrogenic properties could be observed (Jordan et al., 1985; Welshons et al., 1987). This is in agreement with results obtained for ENL showing that it is a very weak estrogen receptor (ER) agonist and binds to the ERs (Pettersson and Gustafsson, 2001). ENL and its metabolite 6-hydroxy-ENL bind weakly and preferably to ERα and very little to ERβ (Mueller et al., 2004). We also observed stimulatory effect of ENL on MCF-7 breast cancer cell proliferation in the absence of estradiol, but a slightly stimulatory or non-stimulatory concentration of estradiol combined with a slightly stimulatory concentration of ENL did not cause any stimulation or a tendency to inhibition (Mousavi and Adlercreutz, 1992). The ENL concentration was 1 μM that can be regarded as physiological because such levels have been observed in vegetarians (Adlercreutz et al., 1993b, 1994a). ENL, but not END, was shown to stimulate pS2 expression in MCF-7 cells (Mäkelä et al., 1994; Sathyamoorthy et al., 1994). These diverging results are difficult to explain but it has been suggested (Adlercreutz, 1990; Adlercreutz et al., 1998b; Whitten and Naftolin, 1991) that the effect of exogenous weak estrogens may be either agonistic or antagonistic depending on the level of endogenous estrogens, and this has been experimentally confirmed with regard to coumestrol (Whitten and Naftolin, 1991). Furthermore biphasic effects of ENL have been demonstrated using human breast cancer cells showing that low concentrations stimulate DNA synthesis but high concentrations inhibit it (Mousavi and Adlercreutz, 1992; Whitten and Naftolin, 1991). Many studies showing weak stimulation of MCF-7 cells by the enterolignans are contrast to the result recently obtained in MCF-7 cell tumors in ovariectomized nude mice because no stimulation was found after injection of ENL or END but an enhanced apoptosis was recorded (Bergman-Jungestrom et al., 2007). It was also shown that both injected lignans as well as 10% flaxseed in the diet inhibited estradiol-induced growth of these xenografts. These results clearly show the anticarcinogenic activity of the lignans administered both orally and parenterally.

A controversial issue has been the physiological and pathological role of the binding of bioflavonoids as well as lignans and other phytoestrogens, to the estradiol-binding nuclear type II binding sites. We found that MAT, isoLAR, ENL, and END bind to these sites. Other lignans have not been investigated. The most effective binder of these was MAT, which displaces 50% of estradiol bound to these sites at a concentration of 1 μM (Adlercreutz et al., 1992). The type II estrogen-binding sites were originally discovered by Jim Clarks group (Clark et al., 1978). Dr Markaverich, a member of his group, has continued the work until today.

The nuclear type II estrogen-binding sites have been suggested to constitute a component of the genome which regulates estrogen-stimulated growth (Markaverich and Clark, 1979; Markaverich et al., 1981). It was suggested that some bioflavonoids bind to these sites that by this mechanism may be cell growth-regulating agents (Markaverich et al., 1988, 1992). Therefore, we postulated that the antiproliferative and antiestrogenic effect of phytoestrogens could be mediated via these binding sites (Adlercreutz et al., 1992).

Type II binding sites have also been found in MCF-7 human breast cancer cells (Markaverich et al., 1984). Markaverich and coworkers' extensive work with the aim to identify the binding site finally succeeded and they were identified as histone H4 (Shoulars et al., 2002). They found two binding sites that bind to a histone H4 antibody. The larger one occurred in very small amounts and was found to be a histone H3-H4 complex (Shoulars et al., 2005). The authors concluded that it is possible that type II site ligands "may control histone-dependent gene transcription and cellular proliferation via binding to and modulating core histone/nucleosome function." The group further reconstituted the type II estradiol-binding site with recombinant histone H4 (Shoulars et al., 2006). Further evidence has been obtained indicating that ligands for the type II binding site regulate malignant cell proliferation (Attalla et al., 1997; Markaverich et al., 1992, 2006). In our studies with 2,6-bis[(3,4-dihydroxyphenyl)-methylene] cyclohexanone (BDHPC) the growth inhibition of various malignant ER-positive or ER-negative breast cancer cells was due to accumulation of cells in the G1 phase and apoptosis (Attalla et al., 1997). In a recent study Markaverich (Markaverich et al., 2006) using new synthesized ligands for the type II sites found an inhibition of both ER-positive and ER-negative breast cancer cells by blocking estradiol stimulation of c-Myc and cyclin D1 gene expression. It was also shown that the type II binding sites are much smaller than the ERα and ERβ receptors separating them clearly from these (Markaverich et al., 2001, 2006).

As mentioned above, the tested lignans, particularly MAT, bind to the type II sites. Some MAT is not converted to ENL in the gut and occurs in urine (Nurmi and Adlercreutz, 1999). Other lignans should be tested as to their binding to these sites and its relation to inhibition of malignant cell proliferation. The findings by the group of Markaverich are of great interest because no specific receptor has been found for lignans (they bind very weakly to ERα) but it must be remembered that the type II binding sites have low affinity and high capacity, differentiating them from the ERs, ERα and ERβ, and consequently not regarded as true receptors. But we must be open to the possibility that the nuclear type II estrogen-binding sites may mediate the anticancer action of lignans.

Urinary ENL in women is positively and significantly associated with serum sex hormone–binding globulin (SHBG) and negatively with plasma percentage-free estradiol and free testosterone (SHBG adjusted for BMI) (Adlercreutz et al., 1987). If the small amounts of isoflavones in urine are added to the ENL values, the correlation with BMI-adjusted SHBG values is even better. In the same study in women we found a significant negative correlation between urinary ENL and plasma-free testosterone and free estradiol (E2) and urinary END correlated negatively with plasma-free E2. In our study, the assays of ENL and SHBG were on the basis of a total of two to four 72-hour urines and 12 plasma samples, respectively, obtained on different days for each individual and collected with three to six months intervals during one year. Recently, it was found that in a study in New York on

ENL and breast cancer plasma, ENL correlated positively with SHBG (Zeleniuch-Jacquotte et al., 2004). In another study in the United States, ENL correlated positively with plasma SHBG in 242 old Mexican–American women (Monroe et al., 2007). The SHBG level was 27% higher in the highest quintile of plasma ENL concentration compared with the lowest. The large material and the wide range of fiber intake make this study important. Increase in SHBG inevitably leads to lowering of free (unbound) estradiol and increases free testosterone that is an additional risk factor for breast cancer. The described association of lignans with hormonal changes reduces breast cancer risk. It is of interest that some lignans including ENL and END bind to SHBG and interferes with 5α-dihydrotestosterone binding (Schöttner et al., 1998). In in vitro HepG2 cell studies with ENL (Adlercreutz et al., 1992) a significant stimulation of SHBG production was found at lower physiological concentrations but inhibition at higher concentrations. An increase of SHBG results in addition to the above-described hormonal changes in a reduction of both the albumin-bound and free fraction of the sex hormones. This reduces the metabolic clearance rate of the steroids and in this way their biological activity. An important finding is that SHBG interacts with a cell-membrane receptor when no steroids are bound to it, but when steroids are bound to SHBG they may activate cellular enzymes (Hammond, 1995; Rosner et al., 1991). Consequently SHBG has an important role as a regulator of cell function, and the stimulatory effect of lignans on SHBG production becomes even more important.

On the other hand, three studies of flaxseed containing very high amounts of SEC to human subjects showed no increase in SHBG (Hutchins et al., 2001; Phipps et al., 1993; Shultz et al., 1991) despite that SEC is converted to a great extent to END and ENL. As mentioned above high concentrations of ENL in our in vitro studies in fact inhibited SHBG production in hepG2 cells (Adlercreutz et al., 1992) and after intake of flaxseed the ENL concentrations are very high. If the original level of SHBG is relatively high, it is likely that no significant effect is seen as observed for isoflavones (Adlercreutz, 1998b; Pino et al., 2000). The controversial results could consequently be due to the fact that a stimulating effect may be obtained only in women with relatively low SHBG with moderate intake of lignans. In one of the studies, the original SHBG level was 60.2 nmol/L, which is relatively high for postmenopausal women not using HRT (Phipps et al., 1993) or having a vegetarian diet or trying to slim and can probably not be increased by a very weak estrogen. In one study the number of subjects was small ($N = 7$) and all were men (Shultz et al., 1991). The third study was a randomized crossover study in 28 postmenopausal women. In this study the mean SHBG level was 38.9 nmol/L, which is normal, and the result is in disagreement with our results. The existing large between- and within-individual variability of SHBG level and known methodological problems with the assays could also have caused the differences in results. It is also known that SHBG levels decreases in stored samples (Adlercreutz et al., 1989b), which influences studies with frozen samples. A dimerization of the molecule occurs. More studies in women with low SHBG (<30 nmol/L) could clarify these discrepancies.

In a recent study sesame seeds were ingested by postmenopausal women resulting in a significant increase of SHBG level (15%) (Wu et al., 2006). Sesame contains very high amounts of SES, which is converted to ENL by the gut microflora (Liu et al., 2006; Penalvo et al., 2005b). In Table 1, in the latter publication, our most recent lignan results in organic sesame seeds using the new method (Penalvo et al., 2005a) are shown. The increase of SHBG caused by sesame seed (Wu et al., 2006) is in agreement with our view, but because intake of sesame seeds results in similar excretion of lignans in urine (Coulman et al., 2005), the flaxseed results do not agree with this result. Other confounding factors are the effect of different diets on hormone metabolism and SHBG (Adlercreutz, 1991a; Adlercreutz et al., 1994b; Monroe et al., 2007). It should be remembered that usually only one assay of ENL and SHBG has been carried out in all except our early study (Adlercreutz et al., 1987, 1989a).

The conversion of androgens to estrogens in breast cells is thought to be important in the etiology of breast cancer (Brodie et al., 1997; Miller, 1991), but there is no evidence indicating that lignans affect enzymes involved in this conversion except for a possible effect on aromatase (Adlercreutz et al., 1993a) (see below). Possible other mechanisms, which could be involved are alteration of growth factor action (Adlercreutz, 2002; Boccardo et al., 2003), and inhibition of phenol sulfatases (Adlercreutz, 1998a) but there is little evidence that these effects occur in vivo in human subjects. It has also been shown that SEC (but not the diglucoside), END and ENL have antioxidant activity which could be one mechanism of action, but the activity is moderate (Prasad, 2000).

In rats, flaxseed reduces insulin-like growth factor-1 (IGF-1) levels (Rickard et al., 2000) and higher lignan intake is associated with higher plasma insulin-like growth factor binding protein-1 (IGFBP-1) concentrations (Vrieling et al., 2004). However, a mixture of soy, rye, and linseed administered to 10 healthy women caused an increase of plasma IGF-1 and IGFBP-3 (Woodside et al., 2006) but the composition of the supplement prohibits further evaluation of these results. There is a significant negative correlation between SHBG and insulin and a positive correlation between SHBG and IGFBP-1 in postmenopausal breast cancer patients (Lönning et al., 1995). It is important to remember that estrogen and insulin are

Table 1 Association Between Enl Levels in Plasma or Urine or Lignan Intake with Breast Cancer in Epidemiological Studies

Reference	Method	Design	Results
Adlercreutz et al., 1982, 1986	GC (urine) ENL and END	Case control	ENL significantly lower in postmenopausal breast cancer women compared to omnivores and vegetarians. Small number of women studied during all four seasons
Adlercreutz et al., 1988	GC-MS (urine) ENL and END	Case control	Total lignans lower in premenopausal breast cancer women compared to vegetarians but not significantly lower than in omnivores. Similar study as above
Ingram et al., 1997	GC-MS (urine) ENL and END	Case control	High ENL protective.
Pietinen et al., 2001	TR-FIA (ENL) Stumpf, 2004	Case control	High plasma ENL protective. 60% reduction in risk. Taking into account the intra-individual variation high plasma ENL concentrations reduced risk by 70%
Den Tonkelaar et al., 2001	TR-FIA (ENL) (urine)	Prospective	No association. Nonsignificant tendency to higher risk at high ENL concentrations
Horn-Ross et al., 2001	Food records (MAT and SEC)	Prospective	No association. Dietary intake recorded during the year prior to diagnosis. Multiethnic population
Horn-Ross et al., 2002	Food records (MAT and SEC)	Prospective	No association. California Teachers study.
McCann et al., 2002	Food records ENL and END production Calculated according to (Pillow et al., 1999)	Case control	Only significantly lower risk when associated with one A2 of CYP 17
Hultén et al., 2002	TR-FIA (ENL)	Prospective	Very low level associated with increased risk. Very high levels in premenopausal women tended to have increased risk (not significant).
Dai et al., 2002	LC-MS (urine) (ENL and END)	Case control	Reduced risk with increasing lignan excretion (Chinese women).
Grace et al., 2004	GC-MS (urine and serum) using ^{13}C- labeled internal standards. EPIC study (Dutch part)	Prospective study.	No association Spot urine ENL and END ($n = 114$ cases) and serum ENL ($n = 97$ cases).
McCann et al., 2004	Food records (MAT and SECO)	Case control	Reduced breast cancer risk in premenopausal women with high intake of lignans.
Linseisen et al., 2004	Food records ENL and END production calculated		Premenopausal women. High intake of MAT and high calculated production of ENL and END was associated with low breast cancer risk.
Keinan-Boker et al., 2004	Food records. ENL and END production calculated according to (Pillow et al., 1999)	Prospective	Tendency to lower risk with higher lignan production values but not significant. Lignan intake correlated to wine intake
Olsen et al., 2004	TR-FIA (ENL)	Prospective	Lower risk with higher levels of ENL in ERα-negative breast cancer.
Zeleniuch-Jacquotte et al., 2004	TR-FIA (ENL)	Prospective	No association in postmenopausal women.
Kilkkinen et al., 2004	TR-FIA (ENL)	Prospective	No association in postmenopausal women, a nonsignificant inverse association was found for premenopausal women.
dos Santos Silva et al., 2004	Food records	Case control	Inverse association of lignan intake with breast cancer risk, but significant only at 10% level.
Piller et al., 2006b	TR-FIA (ENL)	Case control	Strong inverse association between plasma ENL and premenopausal breast cancer risk. However, very low lignan values.

(Continued)

Table 1 Association Between Enl Levels in Plasma or Urine or Lignan Intake with Breast Cancer in Epidemiological Studies (*Continued*)

Reference	Method	Design	Results
Piller et al., 2006a	TR-FIA (ENL)	Case control	Plasma ENL in premenopausal women was significantly inversely related to breast risk only in P450c17α (CYP 17) A2A2 carriers. The association was found also for calculated enterolignan production as well as for MAT intake.
Suzuki, 2006	Food records (SEC, MAT, LAR, PIN)	Prospective	No overall association. Higher intake of lignans reduced risk for women with hormone replacement therapy (HRT). No association with receptors
McCann et al., 2006	Food records MAT and SEC intake calculated from food records	Case control	Reduced risk of ER- breast cancer in premenopausal women
Touillaud et al., 2006	Food records. PIN, LAR, SEC and MAT calculated Also END and ENL calculated	Prospective	No association in premenopausal women
Ha et al., 2006	ENL and END production Calculated according to Thompson et al. (1991) from food records	Prospective	Lignan intake prior to diagnosis may improve breast cancer prognosis
Thanos et al., 2006	Food records	Prospective	Higher lignan intake during adolescence was associated with a reduced breast cancer risk with a significant trend.
Touillaud et al., 2007	As in Touillaud et al. 2006	Prospective	High dietary plant intake and high exposure to enterolignans were associated with reduced risk of ER+, PR+ postmenopausal breast cancer. Intake of LAR was significantly negatively correlated with breast cancer risk
Fink et al., 2007	Food records	Case control	Decreased risk in postmenopausal women associated with high intake of lignans.
Verheus et al., 2007	ID-LC-MS-MS	Prospective	No association with lignans. Geometric mean values of plasma ENL <10 nmol/L.

Abbreviations: END, enterodiol; ENL, enterolactone; SEC, secoisolariciresinol; LAR, laricresinol; PIN, Pinoresinol; MAT, matairesinol.

major mitogens for breast epithelial cells and stimulate them cooperatively but with a slightly different mode of action (Mawson et al., 2005). Vegetarian diet rich in both lignans and isoflavones and shown to reduce risk of Western diseases is associated with low plasma concentration of the two potent mitogens, insulin, and IGF-1, and higher levels of IGFBP-1. A lower level of IGF-1 and a higher level of its binding proteins (and SHBG) reduce breast cancer risk in premenopausal women. (Giovannucci, 1999). It is possible that the phytoestrogen effects are mediated via their action on growth factors and growth factor–binding proteins in vegetarians consuming phytoestrogen-rich food. Based on rat experiments it was suggested that the anticancer effect of flaxseed and SDG may in part be related to reductions in plasma IGF-1 (Rickard et al., 2000).

ENL and to a lesser degree END were found to inhibit 5α-reductase converting testosterone to 5α-dihydrotestosterone, the biologically most active androgen. ENL and END inhibit in genital skin fibroblasts 17β-hydroxysteroid dehydrogenase. A concentration of 100 μmol/L resulted in an almost 100% inhibition of both enzymes by ENL. These lignans also inhibited 5α-reductase in prostate tissue homogenates (Evans et al., 1995). A cocktail of seven compounds including both isoflavones and lignans, each at 10 μM concentration, inhibited 5α-reductase by 77% and 17β-hydroxysteroid dehydrogenase by 94% in human genital skin monolayers. The inhibition of 5α-reductase by the phytoestrogen cocktail was of the same magnitude as that caused by 10 μM concentration of Finasteride, a potent drug used for the inhibition of 5α-reductase in benign prostatic hyperplasia. ENL was recently found to be associated with plasma androstanediol glucuronide levels in men and an interaction with CYP19 gene may be involved (Low et al., 2005). The mechanism could theoretically be that the lignans displace 5α-dihydrotestosterone from SHBG (Schöttner et al., 1998) which then may be converted to androstanediol glucuronide in the skin or liver.

ENL, the most abundant enterolignan, is a moderate inhibitor of placental aromatase and competes with the natural substrate androstenedione for the enzyme (Adlercreutz et al., 1993a). A theoretical intermediate between MAT and ENL, 4,4′-dihydroxy-ENL, showed the strongest inhibition. Other experiments with a choriocarcinoma cell line (JEG-3) showed that ENL is very readily transferred from cell culture media into the cells and inhibits the aromatase (Adlercreutz et al., 1993a). Recently it was found that both ENL and END inhibited the production of estrone and estradiol in MCF-7 breast cancer cells and reduced the proliferation of the cells (Brooks and Thompson, 2005). In earlier similar studies with isoflavones and coumestrol such an antiproliferative effect could not be observed probably because of the estrogenicity of the isoflavones competing with a possible inhibition of the 17β-hydroxysteroid dehydrogenase type 1 reducing formation of estrogens (Mäkelä et al., 1995). For ENL and END this is not a problem as they are very weak estrogens. SEC, a precursor of END, showed no activity with regard to the aromatase (Gansser and Spiteller, 1995). Studies in human preadipocytes show inhibition of the aromatase enzyme to various degrees by lignans, the most effective being didemethoxy-MAT (also 4,4′dihydroxy-ENL) (Campbell and Kurzer, 1993; Wang et al., 1994). Most of the lignans are only weak inhibitors. However, a diet rich in vegetables, fruits, and berries may, due to the abundance of these compounds and flavonoids, lead to sufficient concentrations, e.g., in fat and other cells or cancer cells to reduce conversion of androstenedione to estrone, lowering risk for estrogen-dependent cancer (Henderson et al., 1988). There is no evidence that enterolignans reduce estrogen levels in the body and in vivo studies in human subjects are indicated.

ENL has a moderate activating effect on the pregnane X receptor (PXR) which mediates the induction of enzymes involved in steroid metabolism and xenobiotic detoxification (Jacobs et al., 2005). Sesamin ingestion in rats regulates the transcription level of hepatic metabolizing enzymes for alcohol and lipids (Wu et al., 2006).

LIGNANS AND BREAST CANCER

General Aspects

The possible favorable effects of lignans on breast cancer risk may be mediated via many different mechanisms of which some have been discussed above. In a situation when we do not even know whether the effect of unrefined cereal products or lignan-containing food in general are due to their content of lignans or to dietary fiber or to other compounds or to a combined action of fiber and lignans or many different compounds, a causal relationship in human subjects between lignans and disease prevention is hypothetical. With two exceptions (Bylund et al., 2003; Thompson et al., 2005) only in animal experiments flaxseed, pure lignans, rye bran, or purified SEC diglycoside (SDG) have been shown to be anticarcinogenic in vivo (Bylund et al., 2005; Chen and Thompson, 2003; Chen et al., 2002; Dabrosin et al., 2002; Li et al., 1999; Rickard et al., 1999; Saarinen et al., 2000, 2002; Wang et al., 2005; Yan et al., 1998). Intervention trials with pure compounds in human subjects have not been done because only HMR is available in such amounts that human trials are possible. On the other hand a considerable part of HMR is converted to ENL both in rats and mice (Bylund et al., 2005; Saarinen et al., 2000, 2005; Smeds et al., 2004) and both this metabolite and HMR are anticarcinogenic in rodents (Saarinen et al., 2000, 2002).

For decades only the two enterolignans ENL and END have been measured. ENL is the main metabolite of plant lignans followed by END, but END is the main metabolite in experiments with high doses of flaxseed or SDG. Values for ENL have been reported for Finnish, Japanese, United States, Dutch, Chinese, and Korean populations. A table showing most of the urinary assays carried out was recently published (Valentin-Blasini et al., 2005). Diet has a pronounced effect on the results, omnivorous women and men having the lowest values and extreme vegetarians like macrobiotics have the highest and the lactovegetarians are in between (Adlercreutz et al., 1986). The main diet of the studied populations has also a great influence on the results. Japanese have low lignan levels in urine (Adlercreutz et al., 1991b) but in plasma the concentrations of free and sulfate-conjugated lignans are higher than in Finnish subjects despite the fact that the Finnish subjects have much higher urinary and plasma concentrations (Adlercreutz et al., 1993c). Plant lignans occur also in whole soybeans (Penalvo et al., 2004a), a common food in Japan, and contributes to the formation of ENL.

Thoroughly evaluated plasma methods for lignans (and isoflavonoids) appeared first in the beginning of the 1990s (Adlercreutz et al., 1993b, 1994a) and in these methods isotope dilution GC-MS-SIM was used. HPLC could be used for urinary lignans, but when high-performance liquid chromatography with a coulometric electrode array detector (HPLC-CEAD) became available, more convenient methods for plant lignans in plasma and urine could be developed (Nurmi and Adlercreutz, 1999; Penalvo et al., 2004b, 2005b).

Recently the potential role of lignans in human health and cancer prevention has been reviewed (Boccardo et al., 2006; Cornwell et al., 2004; Magee and Rowland, 2004; Wang, 2002; Webb and McCullough, 2005). Two reviews also include comprehensive summaries of animal experimental studies (Power and Thompson, 2005; Thompson, 2003). I also reviewed relatively recently the topic "Phytoestrogens and cancer" (Adlercreutz, 2002).

Comments on the Role of Fiber and Fat in Breast Cancer

In very early studies in the beginning of the 1980s we measured urinary ENL in 72-hour urines during four seasons in small groups of postmenopausal omnivorous and vegetarian Boston women as well as in healthy breast cancer patients after surgical removal of small breast tumors. The diet of the subjects was recorded for three days at the same time as the urine collections. We found in these Boston breast cancer patients a significantly lower excretion of lignans in urine. The ENL values were significantly lower compared with those of the control omnivores but particularly from those of the vegetarians (Adlercreutz et al., 1982). The number of subjects in each group was very low but, because of the follow-up during one year, each subject was very well characterized. The Finnish groups of women, both pre- and postmenopausal omnivorous and vegetarian women and women with breast cancer, were included later into the study (Adlercreutz, et al., 1987; Adlercreutz, 1988, 1989a, 1989b). In the Boston study there was a highly significant correlation between urinary ENL and grain fiber as well as grain calorie intake (Adlercreutz et al., 1982; Adlercreutz, 1986). The intake of cereal fiber was only about 3.5 g/day in the postmenopausal breast cancer cases living in Boston (Adlercreutz et al., 1982). These are extremely low values because at that time nobody was advocating for higher intake of whole-grain cereals. The low urinary excretion of ENL in breast cancer was confirmed 15 years later in an Australian material (Ingram et al., 1997). In our Finnish study, grain fiber intake measured during five consecutive days with about three months' intervals during one year also correlated with urinary ENL excretion in 72-hour urines in a long-term study in 12 young women (Adlercreutz et al., 1988, 2002). The original early observations in 1982 paved the way for research on lignans and cancer and were formulated in a hypothesis (Adlercreutz, 1984). It was suggested that both fiber and lignans may be involved in reducing breast and colon cancer risk and presented as an extension of the Burkitts original fiber hypothesis (Burkitt, 1978). The mechanism of the effect of insoluble fiber itself, mainly cereal fiber, on breast cancer risk is probably a reduction of the enterohepatic circulation of estrogens and their plasma concentration and urinary excretion particularly in combination with low fat intake (Goldin et al., 1982; Adlercreutz et al., 1987, 1989a, 1989b, 1991a, 1994b; Rock et al., 2004) (and others). Estrogens are the most important hormones involved in breast cancer. Because fat intake has the opposite effect compared with fiber on the enterohepatic circulation of estrogens and it is common that those with high fiber intake have a low fat intake, it is difficult to separate these effects from one another. We concluded in one study with subjects having a relatively low fiber intake that fat intake has a greater effect on estrogen metabolism than fiber intake (Adlercreutz et al., 1994b), but in other situations the fiber intake seems to be of more importance. Because of the close relationship between total or cereal fiber intake and lignan levels, the role of lignans in breast cancer and their mechanism of action has since then been investigated by many groups.

During the last 15 to 20 years there has been an intense discussion on the role of fat and fiber for the risk of breast and colon cancer (Adlercreutz, 1990; Beresford et al., 2006; Prentice et al., 2006; Willett et al., 1992, 1994; (World Cancer Research Fund and American Institute for Cancer Research, 1997). In this connection only, the possible role of whole-grain fiber, and other "insoluble fiber," lignans and their plant lignan precursors and lignin (Begum et al., 2004), as well as the role of the intestinal microflora for breast cancer risk will be discussed.

Role of Intestinal Microflora and Fermentation

The effect of cereal fiber and fat on estrogen and bile acid metabolism (Adlercreutz, 1990, 1991a; Korpela et al., 1988, 1992) is mediated by the intestinal microflora, particularly in the colon. The controversial findings regarding the role of dietary fat and fiber for breast cancer risk could perhaps be explained by both their effect on estrogen metabolism and lignan bioavailability and metabolism and production of ENL and END in the gut. In both rats and human subjects an increase in dietary fat decreases the urinary excretion of lignans despite identical grain fiber intake (Hallmans et al., 1998, 1999). Obesity is negatively associated with plasma ENL in women (Kilkkinen et al., 2001). Thus if high ENL lowers breast cancer risk, the effect of fat intake may be an indirect one via reduction of the production of enterolignans. If the food contains little lignans or if the intestinal microflora is destroyed with antibiotics, the amount of dietary fat will not have any effect on risk, if we postulate that this is related to production of ENL in the gut. Consumption of fiber-rich whole-grain cereal products stimulates the production of ENL (Jacobs et al., 2002; Juntunen et al., 2000) and intake of whole-grain rye stimulates the formation of butyrate in the gut simultaneously with an increase in ENL production. Butyric acid is a short chain fatty acid with anticancer activity (Avivi-Green et al., 2000) and may contribute to an anticancer effect of the cereal fiber complex. If ENL is protective, changes in fat and grain fiber intake definitely alters its formation, plasma concentration, and urinary excretion provided that the intestinal microflora is normal and may in this way reduce or increase the postulated protective effect of lignans.

The observation that women with infections treated with antibiotics have higher risk of breast cancer is an indication of a possibly important role of the intestinal microflora in this disease (Knekt et al., 2000). There are experimental and other observations suggesting that the intestinal microflora, influenced by diet and other factors, may play an important role in disease etiology. The observation that intake of antibiotics may increase breast cancer risk was confirmed in one (Velicer et al., 2004a), but not in two other epidemiological studies (Rodriguez and Gonzalez-Perez, 2005; Sørensen et al., 2005). Recently (Friedman et al., 2006) a slightly increased risk in women treated with antibiotics was found but there was little, if any dose response. We suggested that the risk increase could be due to reduced ENL levels in the body. This reduction may continue for more than one year after one course of antibiotic treatment (Kilkkinen et al., 2002). If this is the factor influenced by antibiotics, one cannot expect any dose response because the effect on ENL production depends so much on the original diet and intestinal microflora. The concentrations of phytoestrogens, also including ENL, in hormone-dependent tissues are frequently higher than in plasma (Boccardo et al., 2003; Dehennin et al., 1982; Hong et al., 2002; Rannikko et al., 2006). The studies have evoked a lively discussion on all the numerous factors that may be involved and causing confounding results (Harpe, 2004; Lyman et al., 2004; Ness and Cauley, 2004; Shear et al., 2004; Velicer et al., 2004b). A recent study in proto-*neu*-transgenic mice with spontaneous mammary carcinomas showed a more than three times higher occurrence of cancer in metronidazole/ciprofloxacin-treated mice compared with controls (Rossini et al., 2006) supporting the view that antibiotics may play a role in breast cancer development. It should be emphasized that the contribution of low lignan intake and low formation of ENL to breast cancer risk is probably relatively small compared with all other known factors affecting risk. Our primary observation on the relation between intake of antibiotics and breast cancer risk (Knekt et al., 2000) cannot yet be abandoned as impossible even if our suggested mechanism may not be the correct one. More mechanistic and epidemiological studies are warranted.

Breast Cancer Studies in Rodents

Flaxseed (linseed) contains very high amounts of SEC diglucoside (SDG), which is converted in the gut to END and ENL. Flaxseed and particularly the purified SDG seem to inhibit the growth of mammary tumors in experimental rat studies both in the initiation and promotional phase of the disease. Both tumor size and multiplicity were influenced. Also the oil component of flaxseed containing unsaturated fatty acids contributed to the effect (Dabrosin et al., 2002; Rickard et al., 1999; Serraino and Thompson, 1992; Thompson et al., 1996a, 1996b; Tou and Thompson, 1999; Ward et al., 2000). The earlier results have been reviewed (Thompson, 1995, 1998) and more recent ones too (Thompson, 2003; Power and Thompson, 2005). Interestingly flaxseed seems to inhibit both growth and metastasis of ER-negative human breast cancer xenografts in mice (Wang et al., 2005) in concordance with studies on the reduction of ER-negative breast cancer risk associated with high plasma ENL level (McCann et al., 2006; Olsen et al., 2004). I am aware of another study with the same results, but it has not yet been published because it is being extended. Other evidence indicates that flaxseed components reduce metastasis also in an animal melanoma model (Yan et al., 1998).

Some interesting recent results in rodents suggest that flaxseed or purified lignans may have the same effect on the mammary gland as isoflavones when administered neonatally or prepubertally by enhancing differentiation of highly proliferative terminal end bud structures (Thompson, 1998). In addition, it was shown that the effect on differentiation also occurred during pregnancy and lactation (Chen et al., 2003; Tan et al., 2004; Tou and Thompson, 1999; Ward et al., 2000). As for isoflavones intake of lignans before puberty may be beneficial because the increase of differentiation of the mammary end bud cells observed in rats seems to reduce breast cancer risk. This is in agreement with the interesting results of a recent large Canadian study in adolescent girls (Thanos et al., 2006). They studied more than 3000 cases and the same number of controls and found that high lignan or isoflavones or total phytoestrogen intake during adolescence was highly protective.

Furthermore, another lignan, the glycoside of arctigenin, called arctiin, found in burdock seeds was found to inhibit chemically induced rat mammary carcinogenesis by reducing the multiplicity of the cancers (Hirose et al., 2000). Pure HMR isolated from Norway spruce and fed to rats is converted to ENL in the gut and has been found to inhibit mammary carcinogenesis in 7, 12-dimethylbenzanthracene (DMBA)-treated rats (Saarinen et al., 2000). It is possible that both HMR itself and its metabolite ENL play a role for this effect. Pure ENL inhibited the growth of 7, 12-DMBA-induced mammary carcinomas in rats but plasma concentrations at least 10 times (400 nmol/L) the basal levels (15–40 nmol/L) in normal women were needed (Saarinen et al., 2002). However, the levels observed can easily be achieved by consuming sesame or flaxseed in relatively small amounts. It is likely that the metabolism of ENL is different when administered in the unconjugated form compared with administration as glycoside in the food. The free ENL will probably not reach the large bowel as do the glycosides, because like other free estrogens, ENL will most likely be rapidly absorbed, conjugated, and excreted into the bile and urine. Whether these different metabolic pathways change the biological activity and bioavailability of ENL is not known.

Human Epidemiological Studies

Fifteen prospective and 12 case-control epidemiological studies on lignan intake or plasma or urinary ENL and breast cancer risk have been identified. Most of the case-control studies show a negative association between ENL concentration and breast cancer risk, but all were not significant. Most prospective studies show no effect and a few times an opposite but nonsignificant effect or a negative but nonsignificant association. The studies are presented in Table 1. The reasons for the variable results are difficult to sort out and explain because it is likely that the differences are due to many factors. The establishment of a person's ENL level needs three different blood samples or 24-hour urine collections or five spot urines corrected for creatinine excretion (Stumpf and Adlercreutz, 2003). In practically all studies only one sample has been obtained. In addition to the numerous factors affecting ENL production in the gut or its plasma concentration (antibiotics, smoking, obesity, fat intake) the dietary source of the plant lignan precursors may play an important role as it is likely that other phytochemicals, vitamins, and minerals in the food are also playing a role in cancer prevention. The lignan intake calculated from databases they have until now included only about 10% of the plant lignans (MAT and SEC) that contribute to ENL production in the colon. Even if we would know the content of plant lignans in all foods, we do not know exactly how much is converted to enterolignans from certain foods and from which food source the lignans derive. Therefore, the assay of more specific biomarkers for lignan intake would be preferable, because at present we cannot separate ENL formed from fruits or vegetables from that formed from cereals. This would theoretically be important because other components contained in food, being the main source of the lignans, may contribute to risk reduction. According to our original hypothesis (Adlercreutz, 1984, 1990), it is mainly but not exclusively the cereal fiber (now cereal fiber complex) including the associated lignans (and perhaps other phytochemicals) that is protective. We suggest that the usual concentrations of lignans in blood are not sufficient without additional fibers to diminish breast cancer risk. This may be one explanation for the fact that despite similar lignan levels, results are controversial.

In our early studies (Adlercreutz et al., 1982, 1986, 1988) (Table 1) the urinary excretion of lignans in the breast cancer patients was significantly lower than in the omnivorous and/or in the vegetarian subjects. Most case-control studies show a negative association between lignan intake or plasma concentrations of ENL but all are not significant. Of the prospective studies one showed a decreased risk of ERα-negative breast cancers associated with high ENL concentrations (Olsen et al., 2004), and another showed high risk at very low ENL levels but a tendency to higher risk also in women in the highest 12.5% of the values. In this group, however, relatively more premenopausal subjects occurred (Hultén et al., 2002). In a prospective study from the Netherlands, a tendency to negative association of risk and plasma level of ENL was found, though not significant (Keinan-Boker et al., 2004), but the lignan levels were associated with consumption of wine. In an earlier also prospective Dutch study measuring ENL twice in overnight urines (correcting for creatinine values) with about one year interval in 268 controls and in 88 breast cancer cases one to nine years before the cancer no association between urinary ENL and breast cancer risk was detected (den Tonkelaar et al., 2001). There was a tendency to higher ENL values in the subjects who developed breast cancer. No association between lignan levels and breast cancer risk was obtained in a third Dutch prospective study (Grace et al., 2004) and also in a fourth Dutch prospective study (Verheus et al., 2007). In the second study no information was given on intake of wine and other alcoholic drinks frequently consumed on a daily basis in this country. In the third study no data on alcoholic beverage consumption was presented and in the fourth study the alcohol intake was very low and may be unrealistic low. Red wine and other alcoholic drinks contain considerable amounts of lignans, the alcohol increasing risk for breast cancer. A possible positive effect of lignans on breast cancer risk may be abolished by the alcohol intake. It must also be pointed out that the ENL values in the second study (den Tonkelaar et al., 2001) depend on two variables influenced by diet (ENL and creatinine), which may cause errors. Five such samples are needed to assess a subject's ENL level. In the studies by Grace et al. (2004) and Verheus et al. (2007), good GC-MS methodology was used. In one of the studies (Grace et al., 2004) fiber intake correlated signif-icantly with the lignan values. When discussing various studies the main problem is that usually only one blood or urine sample has been obtained. Plasma analyses need three samples and three 72-hour urines must be collected to establish a person's ENL level (Stumpf and Adlercreutz, 2003). However, repeated measurements with one-year interval in women in the New York Women Health Study showed that the serum ENL values are reasonably stable within individuals because the intraclass correlation was 0.6 (Zeleniuch-Jacquotte et al., 1998). However, in prospective studies we deal with much longer periods of time.

As previously indicated an explanation for these controversial results may be confounding because of wine and tea. Intake of coffee and fruit juice (Horner et al., 2002) increases lignan consumption without increasing total or cereal fiber intake. We believe that protective effect of lignans on breast cancer risk is only found if the amount of fiber consumed is sufficiently high and that the decreased risk is due to the combined effect of fiber and lignans derived from the fiber. The two studies by Horn-Ross (Horn-Ross et al., 2001, 2002), of which the latter was prospective, did not find any association between lignan intake and breast cancer risk and they represent the largest studies with highest number of cases. However, they were carried out at a time when all the new lignans in foods were not known and consequently only about 10% of the lignans consumed were measured. Later it was found that in the United States intake of alcoholic beverages is an important confounding factor (Horner et al., 2002) because it increases ENL levels considerably and at the same time breast cancer risk due to the alcohol (Hankinson et al., 1995). The intake of whole-grain bread in the United States is also very low, which may contribute to the negative results, if we think that in addition to the lignans an additional fiber component is needed to reduce the risk of breast cancer (Adlercreutz, 1984).

The study by Ingram et al. (1997) confirmed our early studies measuring ENL in urine as we did. In a Finnish case-control study comprising 194 breast cancer cases and 208 community-based controls the mean serum ENL concentration was 20 nmol/L for the cases and 26 nmol/L for the controls. The odds ratio (OR) in the highest quintile of ENL values compared with the lowest quintile adjusted for all the known risk factors for breast cancer was 0.38 (Pietinen et al., 2001; Stumpf, 2004). However, when later corrected for individual variations the risk decreased further to an OR of 0.28 (Stumpf, 2004). Low risk was associated with high intake of rye products, fiber, tea, and vitamin E. In Finland rye bread commonly consumed on a daily basis contains high amounts of fiber and Vitamin E (www.rye.VTT.fi). Judged from these studies a plasma level of about 20 to 60 nmol/L of ENL may protect against breast cancer (Stumpf et al., 2001; Stumpf, 2004) in analogy with results in men showing that this level protects against acute coronary events (Vanharanta et al., 1999). The minimum ENL level we regard as showing a relatively healthy lifestyle is 15 to 20 nmol/L, but the optimum level is likely to be higher (>30 nmol/L).

In an American study (Zeleniuch-Jacquotte et al., 2004) subjects were excluded if they had taken antibiotics within four weeks before the sampling. Finally, 417 cases were included. Nine participants became cases after being selected as controls and were included both as cases and controls in the appropriately matched sets. The overall median lag time between blood donation and diagnosis was 5.1 years (range 0.5–9.5 years). Among the premenopausal women cases reported more often a family history of breast cancer ($p < 0.001$) and had higher median level of ENL (13.9 nmol/L) than their matched controls (10.9 nmol/L). In the postmenopausal women the median values were similar in cases (14.3 nmol/L) and controls (14.5 nmol/L). These values are, however, quite low. The OR for the highest versus the lowest quintile of ENL concentration in the premenopausal women group for the highest versus the lowest quintile of ENL was 1.7 and adjusted for known risk factors it was 1.6, but the trend was not significant. All median values are below the minimum level of ENL, which we regard as showing a healthy lifestyle (15–20 nmol/L) (Stumpf et al., 2001; Stumpf, 2004). Recent intake of antibiotics may play a role for the results as subjects treated with antibiotics were excluded only if they had taken the drugs within four weeks before the study. Fiber intake was lower than in the Finnish subjects (Pietinen et al., 2001), but there was a positive association between plasma ENL and SHBG. The main difference between the American and Finnish studies was that the New York study was prospective and included more cases. However, the relatively low levels of plasma ENL both in cases and controls and the lower fiber intake in the American study compared with the Finnish study may be the reasons for the discrepant results. In the Finnish study, there was a correlation between fiber intake and plasma ENL. However, the results are difficult to compare as the Finnish study reports mean values and the American study reports median values after log transformation. Another point that we know is about half of the Finnish women were abstainers of alcohol but alcohol intake in the American women was not shown; however, it is probably higher than in the Finnish women.

The Finnish second breast cancer–ENL study that was prospective involved 206 cases and 215 controls within a cohort of more than 15,000 women and the follow-up time was eight years (Kilkkinen et al., 2004). Pre- and postmenopausal women were separated by age; those older than 51 were regarded as postmenopausal. A total of 322 cases were eligible for the study but samples were available only for 206 cases and 215 controls. Antibiotic intake and diet or alcohol consumption were not recorded. There was no consistent trend in the four cohorts studied and there were no differences in the mean ENL level (cases 25.2, controls 24.0 nmol/L) between the four five-year cohorts studied but the range was large (0.6–155.2 nmol/L). There was a marginal inverse association with regard to premenopausal breast cancer. The values are higher than those found in New York with the same method but because the American values are median values after log transformation the values are difficult to compare. Based on the results of an earlier study of the Finnish population (Kilkkinen et al., 2003) the identical values in cases and controls would imply that the cases and controls had the same intake of lignan-rich foods, in Finnish women mainly cereals and vegetables. However, nothing is known about the food intake in these subjects. The main difference between the two Finnish studies was that the first one was a case-control study and the latter a prospective study and that the diet was unknown in the prospective study. The participants in the prospective study were mainly from other regions (western and southern parts of Finland) compared with exclusively northeast Finland in the case-control study. The consumption of whole-grain rye bread is higher in northeast Finland compared with southwest Finland where vegetable consumption is higher.

Recently it has also been found that vegetable and fruit consumption has no or only a very weak protective effect in women with regard to breast cancer (Hung et al., 2004; Olsen et al., 2005; Smith-Warner et al., 2001; van Gils et al., 2005). This indirectly points to a more important role of whole-grain cereals in breast cancer prevention.

In 14 studies (Table 1) food records were used and from them the intake of SEC and MAT was calculated on the basis of published values or the production of ENL and END calculated from published results (Thompson et al., 1991). In two studies (Touilland et al., 2006; Suzuki et al., 2006, 2007a) four lignans were investigated because at that time values for PIN and LAR were available. Both are prospective studies and found no overall association between lignans and breast cancer risk.

In an interesting study the women who had a genotype with one A2 allele of CYP 17, resulting in elevated androgen and estrogen levels, and high lignan levels reduced risk highly significantly (McCann et al., 2002). In another study (McCann et al., 2004) it was found that high lignan intake is associated with lower risk of breast cancer and concluded "that dietary lignans may be important in the etiology of breast cancer, particularly among premenopausal women." The first-mentioned study results were confirmed in a recent German study in premenopausal women showing that the genotype with one CYP 17 A2 allele was associated with lower breast cancer risk not only with regard to plasma ENL, but also for calculated ENL production, and MAT intake (Piller et al., 2006a). The same group found that in premenopausal women high intake of MAT and also that high calculated production of ENL and END were associated with less risk for breast cancer (Linseisen et al., 2004). Later they confirmed their observation by measuring plasma ENL (Piller et al., 2006b).

Recently some other highly interesting results were obtained both in Denmark and in the United States. It was found that lower risk with higher levels of ENL occurred mainly for ER-negative breast cancer (McCann et al., 2006; Olsen et al., 2004). A third unpublished study carried out in Umea by Hallmans group (personal communication) is being extended but shows the same result. This is one likely explanation for the very controversial results obtained in breast cancer studies. ER-negative breast cancer is likely to be stimulated by growth factors, and not by estrogens and there is indication that in such situations ENL may be protective (Boccardo et al., 2003; Boccardo et al., 2004, 2006) in agreement with the results of the above mentioned studies. However, recently two large studies showed that lignan intake and breast cancer risk are not associated with ER status (Touillaud et al., 2007; Suzuki, 2006; Suzuki et al., 2007a). The difference between the studies is that in the study in Denmark (Olsen et al., 2004) and Sweden plasma ENL was measured but in the last-mentioned studies and in the study by McCann et al., the intake was calculated from food-frequency questionnaires. To solve the problem we have to wait until we have more data on lignan values in food and also on their metabolism in the gut or better we have to use more assays of lignans in plasma and urine with good methods.

Very recently some results, to date only published in a thesis (Suzuki, 2006; Suzuki et al., 2007a), support the view that lignan-rich food intake may be protective in situations when the woman has increased estrogen levels when being on hormone replacement therapy which is known to increase breast cancer risk (Lee et al., 2006). This latter group of women showed a significant inverse association between cereal fiber intake and breast cancer risk (Suzuki, 2006; Suzuki et al., 2007b) but there was no association with other types of fiber. Lignan intake was also negatively correlated with fat intake ($r = -0.4$). In another study high total lignan intake adjusted for total energy intake and breast cancer risk factors was associated with a reduced risk (OR 0.66) but the reverse trend in the odds of breast cancer risk was only statistically significant at the 10% level ($p = 0.09$) (dos Santos Silva et al., 2004).

Lignan intake prior to breast cancer diagnosis seems to affect the prognosis (Ha et al., 2006). A higher intake gives a better prognosis.

A very important randomized placebo-controlled intervention study in postmenopausal women on the effect of intake of 25 g flaxseed/day on tumor biological markers showed very favorable effects by reducing Ki-67 labeling index (34.2%), c-erbB2 (HER2) expression (71.0%) and increasing apoptosis (30.7%), all highly significant. Similar changes were seen in a few of the placebo patients, but they were very small and not significant (Thompson et al., 2005). As pointed out earlier the effect may be partly due to the unsaturated fatty acid content of flaxseed. However, 25 g of flaxseed contains relatively much fiber, which also could have had an effect.

It is difficult to draw any conclusion from all these controversial studies, at least no definitive ones. Lignan intake or plasma ENL concentrations have been studied in breast cancer to a larger extent than in connection with any other diseases. Case-control studies frequently showing a reduced risk with high lignan intake or lignan plasma levels around 20 (15) to 60 nmol/L usually means that the subjects have consumed fiber-rich whole-grain bread and lignan-rich vegetables and fruits. The perfect epidemiological study has still to be carried out. Subjects with very high levels have consumed flax or sesame seeds and should not be included (ENL levels above 100 nmol/L) in the statistics in epidemiological studies because the fiber intake does not correspond to the levels of lignans and the intake is usually occasional. We believe that in diets without flaxseed or sesame seeds the lignans must be associated with fiber intake to be protective because additional factors must be involved otherwise the results would not be so controversial. In epidemiological studies negative associations between lignans and breast cancer risk seem to be found mainly in regions with traditional at least reasonable intake of whole-grain products like in Finland (Pietinen et al., 2001), Sweden (Hultén et al., 2002; Suzuki, 2006), Denmark (Olsen et al., 2004), Germany (Linseisen et al., 2004; Piller et al., 2006b) and perhaps Australia (Ha et al., 2006). When wine intake is a determinant of ENL (Horner et al., 2002; Keinan-Boker, 2004) no association may be expected as wine increases lignan levels and simultaneously increases risk of breast cancer because alcohol intake increases estrogen levels. However in many studies no adjustment is made for alcohol intake or alcohol intake is not known and in no study the nature of the alcohol beverages used is known. Different types of beverages have also very different contents of lignans and measuring only amount of alcohol is not sufficiently exact. For example, white wine contains much less lignans than red wine (Nurmi et al., 2003). Because both tea and coffee contain lignans (Mazur et al., 1998a,b), but do not contain fiber, they may influence the outcome in epidemiological studies. However, tea, due to its content of antioxidants, may also contribute positively to the protective effect of diet. This does not mean that the effect of flaxseed or sesame seed in sufficiently high doses in human subjects, or used as supplement to the diet, may not be protective. In fact the already mentioned recent very important study would suggest that intake of 25 g of flax seed per day could be tried as an adjuvant therapy in breast cancer (Thompson et al., 2005), because the effects on breast cancer cell proliferation and apoptosis in vivo are remarkable and unsurpassed by any other food today.

CONCLUSION

Despite much evidence indicating that treatment with flaxseed, SDG, or pure lignans of breast tumors in animals definitely inhibits breast cancer growth, causes apoptosis of the malignant cells, and reduces metastasis, prospective epidemiological studies have usually not shown any significant association between lignan intake or lignan levels in the body and breast cancer risk. However, case-control studies frequently show an association. As pointed out single assays do not characterize a lignan intake status very well and it is possible that this is one reason for the variable results. One problem is the time frame; breast cancer development is a long-term process and in most studies the samples have been taken less than 10 years before and sometimes the food records were obtained only a few years or even less than one year before the cancer appeared. We also need to know more about the diet of the participants because it seems that the lignan intake should be associated with fiber and whole-grain intake because the fiber intake also reduces risk and the combination may be effective. Particularly dietary insoluble fiber (European Cancer Prevention [ECP] consensus panel on cereals and cancer), preferably in combination with low fat intake, reduces estrogen levels in the body. If the main source of lignans is fruit juice, tea, coffee, wine, and other alcoholic beverages, the lignan levels do not seem to be associated with breast cancer risk. Other compounds of the fiber complex are also likely to be involved. High intake of flaxseed or sesame seed may protect as such, but the probably high amounts needed may not be feasible during a whole life. This has to be studied in a prospective investigation by adding lower amounts of flaxseed to the diet during a long follow-up period and also tried as adjuvant therapy in breast cancer. It also seems that only certain groups of women benefit from lignans (those with CYP 17 A2 alleles, those on hormone treatment and perhaps those who are at risk to develop ER-negative breast cancer) and that the good habits with regard to lignan-rich diet should start already before puberty. This may be the most important preventive measure. The results indicate that the problem of the association of lignans with breast cancer is very complex and needs further studies.

REFERENCES

Consensus meeting on cereals, fibre and colorectal and breast cancers. ECP consensus panel on cereals and cancer. Eur J Cancer Prev 1997; 6:512–514; [published erratum appears in Eur J Cancer Prev 1998; 7(1):83].

Adlercreutz H. Studies on oestrogen excretion in human bile. Acta Endocrinol (Copenh) 1962; 42(suppl 72):1–220.

Adlercreutz H, Fotsis T, Heikkinen R, Dwyer JT, Goldin BR, Gorbach SL, Lawson AM, Setchell KDR. Diet and urinary excretion of lignans in female subjects. Med Biol 1981; 59:259–261.

Adlercreutz H, Fotsis T, Heikkinen R, Dwyer JT, Woods M, Goldin BR, Gorbach SL. Excretion of the lignans enterolactone and enterodiol and of equol in omnivorous and vegetarian women and in women with breast cancer. Lancet 1982; 2:1295–1299.

Adlercreutz H. Does fiber-rich food containing animal lignan precursors protect against both colon and breast cancer? An extension of the "fiber hypothesis". Gastroenterology 1984; 86:761–764.

Adlercreutz H, Fotsis T, Bannwart C, Wähälä K, Mäkelä T, Brunow G, Hase T. Determination of urinary lignans and phytoestrogen metabolites, potential antiestrogens and anticarcinogens, in urine of women on various habitual diets. J Steroid Biochem 1986; 25:791–797.

Adlercreutz H, Höckerstedt K, Bannwart C, Bloigu S, Hämäläinen E, Fotsis T, Ollus A. Effect of dietary components, including lignans and phytoestrogens, on enterohepatic circulation and liver metabolism of estrogens, and on sex hormone binding globulin (SHBG). J Steroid Biochem 1987; 27:1135–1144.

Adlercreutz H. Lignans and phytoestrogens. Possible preventive role in cancer. In: Horwitz C, Rozen P, Karger S, eds. Progress in Diet and Nutrition. 1988:165–176.

Adlercreutz H, Höckerstedt K, Bannwart C, Hämäläinen E, Fotsis T, Bloigu S. Association between dietary fiber, urinary excretion of lignans and isoflavonic phytoestrogens, and plasma non-protein bound sex hormones in relation to breast cancer. In: Bresciani F, King RJB, Lippman ME, Raynaud J-P, eds. Progress in Cancer Research and Therapy. Vol 35: Hormones and Cancer 3. New York: Raven Press, 1988:409–412.

Adlercreutz H, Fotsis T, Höckerstedt K, Hämäläinen E, Bannwart C, Bloigu S, Valtonen A, Ollus A. Diet and urinary estrogen profile in premenopausal omnivorous and vegetarian women and in premenopausal women with breast cancer. J Steroid Biochem 1989a; 34:527–530.

Adlercreutz H, Hämäläinen E, Gorbach SL, Goldin BR, Woods MN, Dwyer JT. Diet and plasma androgens in postmenopausal vegetarian and omnivorous women and postmenopausal women with breast cancer. Am J Clin Nutr 1989b; 49:433–442.

Adlercreutz H. Western diet and Western diseases: some hormonal and biochemical mechanisms and associations. Scand J Clin Lab Invest 1990; 50(suppl 201):3–23.

Adlercreutz H. Diet and sex hormone metabolism. In: Rowland IR, ed. Nutrition, Toxicity, and Cancer. Boca Raton: CRC Press, 1991a:137–195.

Adlercreutz H, Honjo H, Higashi A, Fotsis T, Hämäläinen E, Hasegawa T, Okada H. Urinary excretion of lignans and isoflavonoid phytoestrogens in Japanese men and women consuming traditional Japanese diet. Am J Clin Nutr 1991b; 54:1093–1100.

Adlercreutz H, Mousavi Y, Clark J, Höckerstedt K, Hämäläinen E, Wähälä K, Mäkelä T, Hase T. Dietary phytoestrogens and cancer: in vitro and in vivo studies. J Steroid Biochem Molec Biol 1992; 41:331–337.

Adlercreutz H, Bannwart C, Wähälä K, Mäkelä T, Brunow G, Hase T, Arosemena PJ, Kellis JT Jr., Vickery LE. Inhibition of human aromatase by mammalian lignans and isoflavonoid phytoestrogens. J Steroid Biochem Mol Biol 1993a; 44:147–153.

Adlercreutz H, Fotsis T, Lampe J, Wähälä K, Mäkelä T, Brunow G, Hase T. Quantitative determination of lignans and isoflavonoids in plasma of omnivorous and vegetarian women by isotope dilution gas-chromatography mass-spectrometry. Scand J Clin Lab Invest 1993b; 53:5–18.

Adlercreutz H, Markkanen H, Watanabe S. Plasma concentrations of phytooestrogens in Japanese men. Lancet 1993c; 342:1209–1210.

Adlercreutz H, Fotsis T, Watanabe S, Lampe J, Wähälä K, Mäkelä T, Hase T. Determination of lignans and isoflavonoids in plasma by isotope dilution gas chromatography-mass spectrometry. Cancer Detect Prev 1994a; 18:259–271.

Adlercreutz H, Gorbach SL, Goldin BR, Woods MN, Dwyer JT, Hämäläinen E. Estrogen metabolism and excretion in oriental and caucasian women. J Natl Cancer Inst 1994b; 86:1076–1082.

Adlercreutz H. Evolution, nutrition, intestinal microflora, and prevention of cancer: a hypothesis. Proc Soc Exp Biol Med 1998a; 217:241–246.

Adlercreutz H. Human health and phytoestrogens. In: Reproductive and Developmental Toxicology Korach KS, ed. New York: Marcel Dekker, Inc. 1998b:299–371.

Adlercreutz H. Phyto-oestrogens and cancer. Lancet Oncol 2002; 3:32–41.

Attalla H, Mäkelä TP, Wähälä K, Rasku S, Andersson LC, Adlercreutz H. 2,6-bis((3,4-dihydroxyphenyl)-methylene) cyclohexanone (BDHPC)-induced apoptosis and p53-independent growth inhibition: synergism with genistein. Biochem Biophys Res Commun 1997; 239:467–472.

Avivi-Green C, Polak-Charcon S, Madar Z, Schwartz B. Apoptosis cascade proteins are regulated in vivo by high intracolonic butyrate concentration: Correlation with colon cancer inhibition. Oncol Res 2000; 12:83–95.

Axelson M, Sjövall J, Gustafsson BE, Setchell KDR. Origin of lignans in mammals and identification of a precursor from plants. Nature 1982; 298:659–660.

Bach Knudsen KE, Serena A, Adlercreutz H. Cereal fibre sources that enhance the production and plasma concentrations of enterolignans and butyrate. AgroFood Industry Hi-Tech 2007; 18:46–48.

Bach Knudsen KE, Serena A, Kjaer AKB, Tetens I, Heinonen SM, Nurmi T, Adlercreutz H. Rye bread in the diet of pigs enhances the formation of enterolactone and increases its levels in plasma, urine and feces. J Nutr 2003; 133: 1368–1375.

Bach Kristensen M, Hels O, Tetens I. No changes in serum enterolactone levels after eight weeks intake of rye-bran products in healthy young men. Scand J Nutr 2005; 49:62–67.

Begum AN, Nicolle C, Mila I, Lapierre C, Nagano K, Fukushima K, Heinonen SM, Adlercreutz H, Remesy C, Scalbert A.

Dietary lignins are precursors of mammalian lignans in rats. J Nutr 2004; 134:120–127.

Beresford SA, Johnson KC, Ritenbaugh C, Lasser NL, Snetselaar LG, Black HR, Anderson GL, Assaf AR, Bassford T, Bowen D, Brunner RL, Brzyski RG, Caan B, Chlebowski RT, Gass M, Harrigan RC, Hays J, Heber D, Heiss G, Hendrix SL, Howard BV, Hsia J, Hubbell FA, Jackson RD, Kotchen JM, Kuller LH, LaCroix AZ, Lane DS, Langer RD, Lewis CE, Manson JE, Margolis KL, Mossavar-Rahmani Y, Ockene JK, Parker LM, Perri MG, Phillips L, Prentice RL, Robbins J, Rossouw JE, Sarto GE, Stefanick ML, Van Horn L, Vitolins MZ, Wactawski-Wende J, Wallace RB, Whitlock E. Low-fat dietary pattern and risk of colorectal cancer: the Women's Health Initiative Randomized Controlled Dietary Modification Trial. JAMA 2006; 295:643–54.

Bergman-Jungestrom M, Thompson LU, Dabrosin C. Flaxseed and its lignans inhibit estradiol-induced growth, angiogenesis, and secretion of vascular endothelial growth factor in human breast cancer xenografts in vivo. Clin Cancer Res 2007; 13:1061–1067.

Blitz CL, Murphy SP, Donna LM. Adding lignan values to a food composition database. J Food Compost Anal 2007; 20:99–105.

Boccardo F, Lunardi GL, Petti AR, Rubagotti A. Enterolactone in breast cyst fluid: correlation with EGF and breast cancer risk. Breast Cancer Res Treat 2003; 79:17–23.

Boccardo F, Lunardi G, Guglielmini P, Parodi M, Murialdo R, Schettini G, Rubagotti A. Serum enterolactone levels and the risk of breast cancer in women with palpable cysts. Eur J Cancer 2004; 40:84–89.

Boccardo F, Puntoni M, Guglielmini P, Rubagotti A. Enterolactone as a risk factor for breast cancer: a review of the published evidence. Clin Chim Acta 2006; 365: 58–67.

Bonoli M, Bendini A, Cerretani L, Lercker G, Toschi TG. Qualitative and semiquantitative analysis of phenolic compounds in extra virgin olive oil as a function of the ripening degree of olive fruits by different analytical techniques. J Agr Food Chem 2004; 52:7026 7032.

Borriello SP, Setchell KDR, Axelson M, Lawson AM. Production and metabolism of lignans by the human faecal flora. J Appl Bacteriol 1985; 58:37–43.

Brodie A, Lu Q, Nakamura J. Aromatase in the normal breast and breast cancer. J Steroid Biochem Mol Biol 1997; 61:281–286.

Brooks JD, Thompson LU. Mammalian lignans and genistein decrease the activities of aromatase and 17 beta-hydroxy steroid dehydrogenase in MCF-7 cells. J Steroid Biochem Mol Biol 2005; 94:461–467.

Burkitt DP. Colonic-rectal cancer: fiber and other dietary factors. Am J Clin Nutr 1978; 31:S58–S64.

Bylund A, Lundin E, Zhang JX, Nordin A, Kaaks R, Stenman U-H, Åman P, Adlercreutz H, Nilsson TK, Hallmans G, Bergh A, Stattin P. Randomized controlled short-term intervention pilot study on rye bran bread in prostate cancer. Eur J Cancer Prev 2003; 12:407–415.

Bylund A, Saarinen N, Zhang JX, Bergh A, Widmark A, Johansson A, Lundin E, Adlercreutz H, Hallmans G, Stattin P, Mäkelä S. Anticancer effects of a plant lignan 7-hydroxymatairesinol on a prostate cancer model in vivo. Exp Biol Med 2005; 230:217–223.

Campbell DR, Kurzer MS. Flavonoid inhibition of aromatase enzyme activity in human preadipocytes. J Steroid Biochem Mol Biol 1993; 46:381–388.

Chen J, Thompson LU. Lignans and tamoxifen, alone or in combination, reduce human breast cancer cell adhesion, invasion and migration in vitro. Breast Cancer Res Treat 2003; 80:163–170.

Chen JM, Stavro PM, Thompson LU. Dietary flaxseed inhibits human breast cancer growth and metastasis and down-regulates expression of insulin-like growth factor and epidermal growth factor receptor. Nutr Cancer 2002; 43:187–192.

Chen JM, Tan KP, Ward WE, Thompson LU. Exposure to flaxseed or its purified lignan during suckling inhibits chemically induced rat mammary tumorigenesis. Exp Biol Med 2003; 228:951–958.

Christophoridou S, Dais P, Tseng LH, Spraul M. Separation and identification of phenolic compounds in olive oil by coupling high-performance liquid chromatography with postcolumn solid-phase extraction to nuclear magnetic resonance spectroscopy (LC-SPE-NMR). J Agric Food Chem 2005; 53:4667–4679.

Clark JH, Hardin JW, Upchurch S. Heterogeneity of estrogen binding sites in the cytosol of the rat uterus. J Biol Chem 1978; 253:7630–7634.

Clavel T, Henderson G, Alpert CA, Philippe C, RigottierGois L, Dore J, Blaut M. Intestinal bacterial communities that produce active estrogen-like compounds enterodiol and enterolactone in humans. Appl Environ Microbiol 2005; 71:6077–6085.

Clavel T, Henderson G, Engst W, Dore J, Blaut M. Phylogeny of human intestinal bacteria that activate the dietary lignan secoisolariciresinol diglucoside. FEMS Microbiol Ecol 2006; 55:471–478.

Cornwell T, Cohick W, Raskin I. Dietary phytoestrogens and health. Phytochemistry 2004; 65:995–1016.

Coulman KD, Liu Z, Hum WQ, Michaelides J, Thompson LU. Whole sesame seed is as rich a source of mammalian lignan precursors as whole flaxseed. Nutr Cancer 2005; 52: 156–165.

Dabrosin C, Chen JM, Wang L, Thompson LU. Flaxseed inhibits metastasis and decreases extracellular vascular endothelial growth factor in human breast cancer xenografts. Cancer Lett 2002; 185:31–37.

Dai Q, Franke AA, Yin F, Shu XO, Herbert JR, Gai YT, Zheng W. Urinary excretion of phytoestrogens and risk of breast cancer among Chinese women in Shanghai. Cancer Epidemiol Biomark Prev 2002; 11:815–821.

Dehennin L, Reiffsteck A, Joudet M, Thibier M. Identification and quantitative estimation of a lignan in human and bovine semen. J Reprod Fertil 1982; 66:305–309.

den Tonkelaar I, Keinan-Boker L, Van't Veer P, Arts CJM, Adlercreutz H, Thijssen JHH, Peeters PHM. Urinary phyto-oestrogens and breast cancer risk in a Western population. Cancer Epidemiol Biomarkers Prev 2001; 10:223–228.

dos Santos Silva I, Mangtani P, McCormack V, Bhakta D, McMichael AJ, Sevak L. Phyto-oestrogen intake and breast cancer risk in South Asian women in England: findings from a population-based case-control study. Cancer Causes Control 2004; 15:805–818.

Evans BAJ, Griffiths K, Morton MS. Inhibition of 5α-reductase in genital skin fibroblasts and prostate tissue by dietary lignans and isoflavonoids. J Endocrin 1995; 147:295–302.

Fink BN, Steck BE, Wolf MS, Britton JA, Kabat GC, Schroeder JC, Teitelbann SL, Neugut AI, Gammon MD. Dietary flavonoid intake and breast cancer risk among women on Long Island. Am J Epidemiol 2007; 185:514–523.

Friedman GD, Oestreicher N, Chan J, Quesenberry CP Jr., Udaltsova N, Habel LA. Antibiotics and risk of breast cancer: up to 9 years of follow-up of 2.1 million women. Cancer Epidemiol Biomarkers Prev 2006; 15:2102–2106.

Gansser D, Spiteller G. Aromatase inhibitors from urtica dioica roots. Planta Med 1995; 61:138–140.

Giovannucci E. Insulin-like growth factor-1 and binding protein-3 and risk of cancer. Horm Res 1999; 51:34–41.

Glitsø LV, Mazur WM, Adlercreutz H, Wähälä K, Mäkelä T, Sandströom B, Bach Knudsen KE. Intestinal metabolism of rye lignans in pigs. Br J Nutr 2000; 84:429–437.

Grace PB, Taylor JI, Low Y-L, Luben RN, Mulligan AA, Botting NP, Dowsett M, Welch AA, Khaw K-T, Wareham NJ, Day NE, Bingham SA. Phytoestrogen concentrations in serum and spot urine as biomarkers for dietary phytoestrogen intake and their relation to breast cancer risk in European prospective investigation of cancer and nutrition-norfolk. Cancer Epidemiol Biomarkers Prev 2004; 13:698–708.

Goldin BR, Adlercreutz H, Gorbach SL, Warram JH, Dwyer JT, Swenson L, Woods MN. Estrogen excretion patterns and plasma levels in vegetarian and omnivorous women. N Engl J Med 1982; 307:1542–1547.

Ha TC, Lyons-Wall PM, Moore DE, Tattam BN, Boyages J, Ung OA, Taylor RJ. Phytoestrogens and indicators of breast cancer prognosis. Nutr Cancer 2006; 56:3–10.

Hallmans G, Zhang J-X, Lundin E, Bergh A, Landström M, Sylvan A, Bylund A, Widmark A, Damber J-E, Åman P, Johansson A, Adlercreutz H. Metabolism of lignans and their relation to experimental prostate cancer. In: Bausch-Goldbohm S, Kardinaal A, Serra F, eds. Cost 916. Bioactive Plant Cell Wall Components in Nutrition and Health. Phytoestrogens: Exposure, Bioavailability, Health Benefits and Safety Concerns. Doorwerth, The Netherlands: European Communities, 1999:65–72.

Hammond GL. Potential functions of plasma steroid-binding proteins. Trends Endocrinol Metab 1995; 6:298–304.

Hankinson SE, Willett WC, Manson JE, Hunter DJ, Colditz GA, Stampfer MJ, Longcope C, Speizer FE. Alcohol, height, and adiposity in relation to estrogen and prolactin levels in postmenopausal women. J Natl Cancer Inst 1995; 87:1297–1302.

Harpe SE. Use of antibiotics and risk of cancer. JAMA 2004; 291:2699.

Heinonen S, Nurmi T, Liukkonen K, Poutanen K, Rafaelli B, Wähälä K, Deyama T, Nishibe S, Adlercreutz H. In vitro metabolism of plant lignans: new precursors of mammalian lignans enterolactone and enterodiol. J Agric Food Chem 2001; 49:3178–3186.

Henderson BE, Ross R, Bernstein L. Estrogens as a cause of human cancer: the Richard and Hinda Rosenthal foundation award lecture. Cancer Res 1988; 48:246–253.

Hirose M, Yamaguchi T, Lin C, Kimoto N, Futakuchi M, Kono T, Nishibe S, Shirai T. Effects of arctiin on PhIP-induced mammary, colon and pancreatic carcinogenesis in female Sprague-Dawley rats and MeIQx-induced hepatocarcinogenesis in male F344 rats. Cancer Lett 2000; 155:79–88.

Hollman PC, Milder IE, Arts IC, Feskens EJ, Bueno de Mesquita HB, Kromhout D. Phytoestrogens and risk of lung cancer. JAMA 2006; 295:755 (author reply 755–756).

Hong SJ, Kim SI, Kwon SM, Lee JR, Chung BC. Comparative study of concentration of isoflavones and lignans in plasma and prostatic tissues of normal control and benign prostatic hyperplasia. Yonsei Med J 2002; 43:236–241.

Horn-Ross PL, Barnes S, Lee M, Coward L, Mandel JE, Koo J, John EM, Smith M. Assessing phytoestrogen exposure in epidemiologic studies: development of a database (United States). Cancer Causes Control 2000; 11:289–298.

Horn-Ross PL, John EM, Lee M, Stewart SL, Koo J, Sakoda LC, Shiau AG, Goldstein J, Davis P, Perez-Stable EJ. Phytoestrogen consumption and breast cancer risk in a multiethnic population: the Bay Area Breast Cancer Study. Am J Epidemiol 2001; 154:434–441.

Horn-Ross PL, Hoggatt KJ, West DW, Krone MR, Stewart SL, Anton H, Bernstei CL, Deapen D, Peel D, Pinder R, Reynolds P, Ross RK, Wright W, Ziogas A. Recent diet and breast cancer risk: the California Teachers Study (USA). Cancer Causes Control 2002; 13:407–415.

Horner NK, Kristal AR, Prunty J, Skor HE, Potter JD, Lampe JW. Dietary determinants of plasma enterolactone. Cancer Epidemiol Biomarkers Prev 2002; 11:121–126.

Hultén K, Winkvist A, Lenner P, Johansson R, Adlercreutz H, Hallmans G. An incident case-referent study on the lignan enterolactone and breast cancer. Eur J Nutr 2002; 41:168–176.

Hung HC, Joshipura KJ, Jiang R, Hu FB, Hunter D, SmithWarner SA, Colditz GA, Rosner B, Spiegelman D, Willett WC. Fruit and vegetable intake and risk of major chronic disease. J Natl Cancer Inst 2004; 96:1577–1584.

Hutchins AM, Martini MC, Olson BA, Thomas W, Slavin JL. Flaxseed consumption influences endogenous hormone concentrations in postmenopausal women. Nutr Cancer 2001; 39:58–65.

Ingram D, Sanders K, Kolybaba M, Lopez D. Case-control study of phyto-oestrogens and breast cancer. Lancet 1997; 350:990–994.

Jacobs DR, Pereira MA, Stumpf K, Pins JJ, Adlercreutz H. Whole grain food intake elevates serum enterolactone. Br J Nutr 2002; 88:111–116.

Jacobs MN, Nolan GT, Hood SR. Lignans, bacteriocides and organochlorine compounds activate the human pregnane X receptor (PXR). Toxicol Appl Pharmacol 2005; 209: 123–133.

Johnsen NF, Hausner H, Olsen A, Tetens I, Christensen J, Knudsen KEB, Overvad K, Tjonneland A. Intake of whole grains and vegetables determines the plasma enterolactone concentration of Danish women. J Nutr 2004; 134:2691–2697.

Jordan VC, Koch R, Bain RR. Prolactin synthesis by cultured rat pituitary cells: An assay to study estrogens, antiestrogens and their metabolites in vitro. Estrogens in the Environment II. Influences on Development. McLachlan JA, ed. New York: Elsevier, 1985:221–234.

Juntunen KS, Mazur WM, Liukkonen KH, Uehara M, Poutanen KS, Adlercreutz HCT, Mykkänen HM, Consumption of wholemeal rye bread increases serum concentrations and urinary excretion of enterolactone compared with consumption of white wheat bread in healthy Finnish men and women. Br J Nutr 2000; 84:839–846.

Keinan-Boker LK, van der Schouw YT, de Kleijn MJJ, Jacques PF, Grobbee DE, Peeters PHM. Intake of dietary phytoestrogens by Dutch women. J Nutr 2002; 132: 1319–1328.

Keinan-Boker L, van der Schouw YT, Grobbee DE, Peeters PH. Dietary phytoestrogens and breast cancer risk. Am J Clin Nutr 2004; 79:282–288.

Kiely M, Faughnan M, Wähälä K, Brants H, Mulligan A. Phyto-oestrogen levels in foods: the design and construction of the VENUS database. Br J Nutr 2003; 89:S19–S23.

Kilkkinen A, Stumpf K, Pietinen P, Valsta LM, Tapanainen H, Adlercreutz H. Determinants of serum enterolactone concentration. Am J Clin Nutr 2001; 73:1094–1100.

Kilkkinen A, Pietinen P, Klaukka T, Virtamo J, Korhonen P, Adlercreutz H. Use of oral antimicrobials decreases serum enterolactone concentration. Am J Epidemiol 2002; 155:472–477.

Kilkkinen A, Valsta LM, Virtamo J, Stumpf K, Adlercreutz H, Pietinen P. Intake of lignans is associated with serum enterolactone concentration in Finnish men and women. J Nutr 2003; 133:1830–1833.

Kilkkinen A, Virtamo J, Vartiamen E, Sankila R, Virtanen MJ, Adlercreutz H, Pietinen P. Serum enterolactone concentration is not associated with breast cancer risk in a nested case-control study. Int J Cancer 2004; 108:277–280.

Knekt P, Adlercreutz H, Rissanen H, Aromaa A, Teppo L, Heliövaara M. Does antibacterial treatment for urinary tract infection contribute to the risk of breast cancer? Br J Cancer 2000; 82:1107–1110.

Korpela JT, Adlercreutz H, Turunen MJ. Fecal free and conjugated bile acids and neutral sterols in vegetarians, omnivores, and in patients with colorectal cancer. Scand J Gastroenterol 1988; 23:277–283.

Korpela JT, Korpela R, Adlercreutz H. Fecal bile acid metabolic pattern after administration of different types of bread. Gastroenterol 1992; 103:1246–1253.

Lampe JW, Gustafson DR, Hutchins AM, Martini MC, Li S, Wähälä K, Grandits GA, Potter JD, Slavin JL. Urinary isoflavonoid and lignan excretion on a Western diet: relation to soy, vegetable, and fruit intake. Cancer Epidemiol Biomarkers Prev 1999; 8:699–707.

Lee S, Kolonel L, Wilkens L, Wan P, Henderson B, Pike M. Postmenopausal hormone therapy and breast cancer risk: the Multiethnic Cohort. Int J Cancer 2006; 118: 1285–1291.

Li DH, Yee JA, Thompson LU, Yan L. Dietary supplementation with secoisolariciresinol diglycoside (SDG) reduces experimental metastasis of melanoma cells in mice. Cancer Lett 1999; 142:91–96.

Liggins J, Grimwood R, Bingham SA. Extraction and quantification of lignan phytoestrogens in food and human samples. Anal Biochem 2000; 287:102–109.

Linko A-M, Juntunen KS, Mykkänen HM, Adlercreutz H. Whole grain rye bread consumption by women correlates with plasma alkylresorcinols and increases their concentration compared with low-fiber wheat bread. J Nutr 2005; 135:580–583.

Linseisen J, Piller R, Hermann S, ChangClaude J. Dietary phytoestrogen intake and premenopausal breast cancer risk in a German case-control study. Int J Cancer 2004; 110:284–290.

Liu Z, Saarinen NM, Thompson LU. Sesamin is one of the major precursors of mammalian lignans in sesame seed (Sesamum indicum) as observed in vitro and in rats. J Nutr 2006; 136:906–912.

Lönning PE, Helle SI, Johannessen DC, Adlercreutz H, Lien EA, Tally M, Ekse D, Fotsis T, Anker GB, Hall K. Relations between sex hormones, sex hormone binding globulin, insulin-like growth factor-I and insulin-like growth factor binding protein-1 in post-menopausal breast cancer patients. Clin Endocrinol 1995; 42:23–30.

Low YL, Taylor JI, Grace PB, Dowsett M, Folkerd E, Doody D, Dunning AM, Scollen S, Mulligan AA, Welch AA, Luben RN, Khaw KT, Day NE, Wareham NJ, Bingham SA. Polymorphisms in the CYP19 gene may affect the positive correlations between serum and urine phytoestrogen metabolites and plasma androgen concentrations in men. J Nutr 2005; 135:2680–2686.

Lyman GH, Culakova E, Griggs J. Use of antiobiotics and risk of cancer. JAMA 2004; 291:2700.

Magee PJ, Rowland IR. Phyto-oestrogens, their mechanism of action: current evidence for a role in breast and prostate cancer. Br J Nutr 2004; 91:513–531.

Mäkelä S, Davis VL, Tally WC, Korkman J, Salo L, Vihko R, Santti R, Korach KS. Dietary estrogens act through estrogen receptor-mediated processes and show no antiestrogenicity in cultured breast cancer cells. Environ Health Perspect 1994; 102:572–578.

Mäkelä S, Poutanen M, Lehtimäki J, Kostian ML, Santti R, Vihko R. Estrogen-specific 17β-hydroxysteroid oxidoreductase type 1 (EC 1.1.1.62) as a possible target for the action of phytoestrogens. Proc Soc Exp Biol Med 1995; 208:51–59.

Markaverich BM, Clark JH. Two binding sites for estradiol in rat uterine nuclei: relationship to uterotropic response. Endocrinology 1979; 105:1458–1462.

Markaverich BM, Upchurch S, Clark JH. Progesterone and dexamethasone antagonism of uterine growth: a role for a second nuclear binding site for estradiol in estrogen action. J Steroid Biochem 1981; 14:125–132.

Markaverich BM, Roberts RR, Alejandro MA, Clark JH. An endogenous inhibitor of [^{3}H]estradiol binding to nuclear type II estrogen binding sites in normal and malignant tissues. Cancer Research 1984; 44: 1515–1519.

Markaverich BM, Roberts RR, Alejandro M, Johnson GA, Middleditch BS, Clark JH. Bioflavonoid interaction with rat uterine type II binding sites and cell growth inhibition. J Steroid Biochem 1988; 30:71–78.

Markaverich BM, Schauweker TH, Gregory RR, Varma M, Kittrell FS, Medina D, Varma RS. Nuclear type-II sites and malignant cell proliferation: inhibition by 2,6-bis-benzylidenecyclohexanones. Cancer Res 1992; 52:2482–2488.

Markaverich BM, Shoulars K, Brown MAT. Purification and characterization of nuclear type II[^{3}H] estradiol binding sites from the rat uterus: covalent labeling with [$^{-3}$H] luteolin. Steroids 2001; 66:707–719.

Markaverich BM, Shoulars K, Alejandro MA. Nuclear type II [^{3}H]estradiol binding site ligands: inhibition of ER-positive and ER-negative cell proliferation and c-Myc and cyclin D1 gene expression. Steroids 2006; 71:865–874.

Mawson A, Lai A, Carroll JS, Sergio CM, Mitchell CJ, Sarcevic B. Estrogen and insulin/IGF-1 cooperatively stimulate cell cycle progression in MCF-7 breast cancer cells through differential regulation of c-Myc and cyclin D1. Mol Cell Endocrinol 2005; 229:161–173.

Mazur W, Fotsis T, Wähälä K, Ojala S, Salakka A, Adlercreutz H. Isotope dilution gas chromatographic-mass spectrometric method for the determination of isoflavonoids, coumestrol, and lignans in food samples. Anal Biochem 1996; 233:169–180.

Mazur W. Phytoestrogen content in foods. In: Adlercreutz H, ed. Phytoestrogens. London: Baillière Tindall, 12(4),1998a: 729–742.

Mazur W, Adlercreutz H. Natural and anthropogenic environmental oestrogens: the scientific basis for risk assessment. Naturally occurring oestrogens in food. Pure Appl Chem 1998; 70:1759–1776.

Mazur WM, Wähälä K, Rasku S, Salakka A, Hase T, Adlercreutz H. Lignan and isoflavonoid concentrations in tea and coffee. Br J Nutr 1998b; 79:37–45.

McCann SE, Moysich KB, Freudenheim JL, Ambrosone CB, Shields PG. The risk of breast cancer associated with dietary lignans differs by CYP17 genotype in women. J Nutr 2002; 132:3036–3041.

McCann SE, Muti P, Vito D, Edge SB, Trevisan M, Freudenheim JL. Dietary Lignan intakes and risk of pre- and postmenopausal breast cancer. Int J Cancer 2004; 111:440–443.

McCann SE, Kulkarni S, Trevisan M, Vito D, Nie J, Edge SB, Muti P, Freudenheim JL. Dietary lignan intakes and risk of breast cancer by tumor estrogen receptor status. Breast Cancer Res Treat 2006; 99:309–311.

McIntosh GH, Noakes M, Royle PJ, Foster PR. Whole-grain rye and wheat foods and markers of bowel health in overweight middle-aged men. Am J Clin Nutr 2003; 77:967–974.

Milder IE, Arts IC, Venema DP, Lasaroms JJP, Wähälä K, Hollman PCH. Optimization of a liquid chromatography-tandem mass spectrometry method for quantification of the plant lignans secoisolariciresinol, matairesinol, lariciresinol, and pinoresinol in foods. J Agric Food Chem 2004; 52:4643–4651.

Milder IE, Arts IC, van de Putte B, Venema DP, Hollman PCH. Lignan contents of Dutch plant foods: a database including lariciresinol, pinoresinol, secoisolariciresinol and matairesinol. Br J Nutr 2005; 93:393–402.

Miller WR. Aromatase activity in breast tissue. J Steroid Biochem Mol Biol 1991; 39:783–790.

Monroe KR, Murphy SP, Henderson BE, Kolonel LN, Stanczyk FZ, Adlercreutz H, Pike MC. Dietary fiber intake and endogenous serum hormone levels in naturally postmenopausal Mexican-American women: the multiethnic cohort study. Nutr Cancer 2007; 58:127–135.

Mousavi Y, Adlercreutz H. Enterolactone and estradiol inhibit each other's proliferative effect on MCF-7 breast cancer cells in culture. J Steroid Biochem Mol Biol 1992; 41: 615–619.

Mueller SO, Simon S, Chae K, Metzler M, Korach KS. Phytoestrogens and their human metabolites show distinct agonistic and antagonistic properties on estrogen receptor alpha (ERalpha) and ERbeta in human cells. Toxicol Sci 2004; 80:14–25.

Ness RB, Cauley JA. Antibiotics and breast cancer—What's the meaning of this? JAMA 2004; 291:880–881.

Nose M, Fujimoto T, Takeda T, Nishibe S, Ogihara Y. Structural transformation of lignan compounds in rat gastrointestinal tract. Planta Med 1992; 58:520–523.

Nurmi T, Adlercreutz H. Sensitive high-performance liquid chromatographic method for profiling plasma phytoestrogens using coulometric electrode array detection. Application to plasma analysis. Anal Biochem 1999; 274:110–117.

Nurmi T, Heinonen S, Mazur W, Deyama T, Nishibe S, Adlercreutz H. Lignans in selected wines. Food Chem 2003; 83:303–309.

Olsen A, Knudsen KE, Thomsen BL, Loft S, Stripp C, Overvad K, Moller S, Tjonneland A. Plasma enterolactone and breast cancer incidence by estrogen receptor status. Cancer Epidemiol Biomarkers Prev 2004; 13:2084–2089.

Olsen A, Stripp C, Christense J, Thomsen BL, Overvad K, Tjonneland A. Re: Fruit and vegetable intake and risk of major chronic disease. J Natl Cancer Inst 2005; 97: 1307–1308.

Penalvo JL, Heinonen SM, Nurmi T, Deyama T, Nishibe S, Adlercreutz H. Plant lignans in soy-based health supplements. J Agr Food Chem 2004a; 52:4133–4138.

Penalvo JL, Nurmi T, Haajanen K, Al-Maharik N, Botting N, Adlercreutz H. Determination of lignans in human plasma by liquid chromatography with coulometric electrode array detection. Anal Biochem 2004b; 332:384–393.

Penalvo JL, Haajanen KM, Botting NP, Adlercreutz H. Quantification of lignan in food using isotope dilution gas chromatography-mass spectrometry. J Agric Food Chem 2005a; 53:9342–9347.

Penalvo JL, Heinonen SM, Aura AM, Adlercreutz H. Dietary sesamin is converted to enterolactone in humans. J Nutr 2005b; 135:1056–1062.

Pettersson K, Gustafsson JA. Role of estrogen receptor beta in estrogen action. Annu Rev Physiol 2001; 63:165–192.

Phipps WR, Martini MC, Lampe JW, Slavin JL, Kurzer MS. Effect of flax seed ingestion on the menstrual cycle. J Clin Endocrinol Metab 1993; 77:1215–1219.

Pietinen P, Stumpf K, Männistö S, Kataja V, Adlercreutz H. Serum enterolactone and risk of breast cancer: a case-control study in eastern Finland. Cancer Epidemiol Biomarkers Prev 2001; 70:339–344.

Piller R, Verla-Tebit E, Wang-Gohrke S, Linseisen J, Chang-Claude J. CYP17 genotypes modifies the association between lignan supply and premenopausal breast cancer risk in humans. J Nutr 2006a; 136:1596–1603.

Piller RA, Chang-Claude JB, Linseisen JAB. Plasma enterolactone and genistein and the risk of premenopausal breast cancer. Eur J Cancer Prev 2006b; 15:225–232.

Pillow PC, Duphorne CM, Chang S, Contois JH, Strom SS, Spitz MR, Hursting SD. Development of a database for assessing dietary phytoestrogen intake. Nutr Cancer 1999; 33:3–19.

Pino AM, Valladares LE, Palma MA, Mancilla AM, Yanez M, Albala C. Dietary isoflavones affect sex hormone-binding globulin levels in postmenopausal women. J Clin Endocrinol Metab 2000; 85:2797–2800.

Power KA, Thompson LU. Flaxseed and lignans: Effects on breast cancer. In: Atif A, Bradford P, eds. Nutrition and Cancer Prevention. New York: Marcel Dekker Inc., 2005:385–410.

Prasad K. Antioxidant Activity of Secoisolariciresinol Diglucoside-derived Metabolites, Secoisolariciresinol, Enterodiol, and Enterolactone. Int J Angiol 2000; 9:220–225.

Prentice RL, Caan B, Chlebowski RT, Patterson R, Kuller LH, Ockene JK, Margolis KL, Limacher MC, Manson JE, Parker LM, Paskett E, Phillips L, Robbins J, Rossouw JE, Sarto GE, Shikany JM, Stefanick ML, Thomson CA, Van Horn L, Vitolins MZ, Wactawski-Wende J, Wallace RB, Wassertheil-Smoller S, Whitlock E, Yano K, Adams-Campbell L, Anderson GL, Assaf AR, Beresford SA, Black HR, Brunner RL, Brzyski RG, Ford L, Gass M, Hays J, Heber D, Heiss G, Hendrix SL, Hsia J, Hubbell FA, Jackson RD, Johnson KC, Kotchen JM, LaCroix AZ, Lane DS, Langer RD, Lasser NL, Henderson MM. Low-fat dietary pattern and risk of invasive breast cancer: the Women's Health Initiative Randomized Controlled Dietary Modification Trial. JAMA 2006; 295:629–642.

Rannikko A, Petas A, Rannikko S, Adlercreutz H. Plasma and prostate phytoestrogen concentrations in prostate cancer patients after oral phytoestrogen supplementation. Prostate 2006; 66:82–87.

Rickard SE, Yuan YV, Chen J, Thompson LU. Dose effects of flaxseed and its lignan on N-methyl-N-nitrosourea-induced mammary tumorigenesis in rats. Nutr Cancer 1999; 35: 50–57.

Rickard SE, Yuan YV, Thompson LU. Plasma insulin-like growth factor I levels in rats are reduced by dietary supplementation of flaxseed or its lignan secoisolariciresinol diglycoside. Cancer Lett 2000; 161:47–55.

Rock CL, Flatt SW, Thomson CA, Stefanick ML, Newman VA, Jones LA, Natarajan L, Ritenbaugh C, Hollenbach KA, Pierce JP, Chang RJ. Effects of a high-fiber, low-fat diet intervention on serum concentrations of reproductive steroid hormones in women with a history of breast cancer. J Clin Oncol 2004; 22:2379–2387.

Rodriguez LAG, Gonzalez-Perez A. Use of antibiotics and risk of breast cancer. Am J Epidemiol 2005; 161:616–619.

Rosner W, Hryb DJ, Khan MS, Nakhla AM, Romas NA. Sex hormone-binding globulin:anatomy and physiology of a new regulatory system. J Steroid Biochem Mol Biol 1991; 40:813–820.

Rossini A, Rumio C, Sfondrini L, Tagliabue E, Morelli D, Miceli R, Mariani L, Palazzo M, Menard S, Balsari A. Influence of antibiotic treatment on breast carcinoma development in proto-neu transgenic mice. Cancer Res 2006; 66: 6219–6224.

Saarinen NM, Wärri A, Mäkelä SI, Eckerman C, Reunanen M, Ahotupa M, Salmi SM, Franke AA, Kangas L, Santti R. Hydroxymatairesinol, a novel enterolactone precursor with antitumor properties from coniferous tree (Picea abies). Nutr Cancer 2000; 36:207–216.

Saarinen NM, Huovinen R, Warri A, Mäkelä SI, Valentin-Blasini L, Sjöholm R, Ämmälä J, Lehtilä R, Eckerman C, Collan YU, Santti RS. Enterolactone inhibits the growth of 7,12-dimethylbenz(a) anthracene-induced mammary carcinomas in the rat. Mol Cancer Ther 2002; 1:869–876.

Saarinen NM, Penttinen PE, Smeds AI, Hurmerinta TT, Mäkelä SI, Structural determinants of plant lignans for growth of mammary tumors and hormonal responses in vivo. J Steroid Biochem Mol Biol 2005; 93:209–219.

Sathyamoorthy N, Wang TTY, Phang JM. Stimulation of pS2 expression by diet-derived compounds. Cancer Res 1994; 54:957–961.

Schöttner M, Spiteller G, Gansser D. Lignans interfering with 5α-dihydrotestosterone binding to human sex hormone-binding globulin. J Nat Prod 1998; 61:119–121.

Serraino M, Thompson LU. The effect of flaxseed supplementation on the initiation and promotional stages of mammary tumorigenesis. Nutr and Cancer 1992; 17:153–159.

Setchell KDR, Adlercreutz H. The excretion of two new phenolic compounds (180/442 and 180/410) during the human menstrual cycle and in pregnancy. J Steroid Biochem 1979; 11:xv–xvi.

Setchell KDR, Bull R, Adlercreutz H. Steroid excretion during the reproductive cycle and in pregnancy of the vervet monkey (*Cercopithecus aethiopus pygerythrus*). J Steroid Biochem 1980a; 12:375–384.

Setchell KDR, Lawson AM, Axelson M, Adlercreutz H. The excretion of two new phenolic compounds during the menstrual cycle and in pregnancy. In: Adlercreutz H, Bulbrook R, van der Molen H, Vermeulen A and Sciarra F, eds. Endocrinological Cancer, Ovarian Function and Disease. Amsterdam: Excerpta Medica, 1980b:297–315.

Setchell KDR, Lawson AM, Mitchell FL, Adlercreutz H, Kirk DN, Axelson M. Lignans in man and in animal species. Nature 1980c; 287:740–742.

Setchell KDR, Lawson AM, Borriello SP, Harkness R, Gordon H, Morgan DML, Kirk DN, Adlercreutz H, Anderson LC, Axelson M. Lignan formation in man—microbial involvement and possible roles in relation to cancer. Lancet 1981; 2:4–7.

Shear NH, Redelmeyer DA, Callen JP. Ad Hoc Task Force of the American Academy of Dermatology. Use of antibiotics and risk of cancer. JAMA 2004; 291:2699.

Shoulars K, Brown T, Alejandro MA, Crowley J, Markaverich BM. Identification of nuclear type II [^{3}H]estradiol binding sites as histone H4. Biochem Biophys Res Commun 2002; 296:1083–1090.

Shoulars K, Rodrigues MA, Crowley JR, Turk J, Thompson T, Markaverich BM. Nuclear type II [3H]estradiol binding sites: a histone H3-H4 complex. J Steroid Biochem Molec Biol 2005; 96:19–30.

Shoulars K, Rodriguez MA, Crowley J, Turk J, Thompson T, Markaverich BM. Reconstitution of the type II [^{3}H]estradiol binding site with recombinant histone H4. J Steroid Biochem Molec Biol 2006; 99:1–8.

Shultz TD, Bonorden WR, Seaman WR. Effect of short-term flaxseed consumption on lignan and sex hormone metabolism in men. Nutr Res 1991; 11:1089–1100.

Smeds AI, Saarinen NM, Hurmerinta TT, Penttinen PE, Sjoholm RE, Makela SI. Urinary excretion of lignans after administration of isolated plant lignans to rats: the effect of single dose and ten-day exposures. J Chromatogr B Analyt Technol Biomed Life Sci 2004; 813:303–312.

Smith-Warner SA, Spiegelman D, Yaun SS, Adami HO, Beeson WL, van den Brandt PA, Folsom AR, Fraser GE, Freudenheim JL, Goldbohm RA, Graham S, Miller AB, Potter JD, Rohan TE, Speizer FE, Toniolo P, Willett WC, Wolk A, Zeleniuch-Jacquotte A, Hunter DJ. Intake of fruits and vegetables and risk of breast cancer:a pooled analysis of cohort studies. JAMA 2001; 285:769–776.

Sørensen HT, Skriver MV, Friis S, McLaughlin J, Blot WJ, Baron JA. Use of antibiotics and risk of breast cancer: a population-based case-control study. Br J Cancer 2005; 92:594–596.

Stitch SR, Toumba JK, Groen MB, Funke CW, Leemhuis J, Vink J, Woods GF. Excretion, isolation and structure of a phenolic constituent of female urine. Nature 1980; 287: 738–740.

Stumpf K, Pietinen P, Puska P, Wang G, Adlercreutz H. Determination of serum enterolactone, genistein and daidzein in samples from the North Karelian intervention study. Cancer Epidemiol Biomarkers Prev 2001; 9:1369–1372.

Stumpf K, Adlercreutz H. Short-term variations in enterolactone in serum, 24-hour urine, and spot urine and relationship with enterolactone concentrations. Clin Chem 2003; 49:178–181.

Stumpf K. Serum enterolactone as a biological marker and in breast cancer: from laboratory to epidemiological studies. Folkhälsan Research Center, Institute for Preventive Medicine, Nutrition and Cancer, and Division of Clinical Chemistry, University of Helsinki. Helsinki: University of Helsinki, 2004:157.

Suzuki R. Hormone-Related Dietary Factors and Estrogen/ Progesterone-Receptor Defined Postmenopausal Breast Cancer [PhD thesis]. Stockholm, Sweden: The National Institute of Environmental Medicine, Karolinska Institutet., 2006:112.

Suzuki R, Rylander-Rudqvist T, Saji S, Bergkvist L, Adlercreutz H, Wolk A. Dietary lignans and postmenopausal breast cancer risk defined by estrogen and progesterone receptor status:a prospective cohort study of Swedish women. 2007a; [Epub ahead of print].

Suzuki R, Rylander-Rudqvist T, Weimin J, Saji S, Bergkvist L, Adlercreutz H, Wolk A. Dietary fiber intake and postmenopausal breast cancer risk defined by estrogen and progesterone receptor status:a prospective cohort study among Swedish women. 2007b; (Epub ahead of print).

Tan KP, Chen JM, Ward WE, Thompson LU. Mammary gland morphogenesis is enhanced by exposure to flaxseed or its major lignan during suckling in rats. Exp Biol Med 2004; 229:147–157.

Thanos J, Cotterchio M, Boucher BA, Kreiger N, Thompson LU. Adolescent dietary phytoestrogen intake and breast cancer risk (Canada). Cancer Causes Control 2006; 17:1253–1261.

Thompson LU, Robb P, Serraino M, Cheung F. Mammalian lignan production from various foods. Nutr Cancer 1991; 16:43–52.

Thompson LU. Flaxseed, lignans, and cancer. Cunnane SC, Thompson LU, eds. Champaign, IL: AOCS Press, 1995:219–36.

Thompson LU, Rickard SE, Orcheson LJ, Seidl MM. Flaxseed and its lignan and oil components reduce mammary tumor growth at a late stage of carcinogenesis. Carcinogenesis 1996a; 17:1373–1376.

Thompson LU, Seidl MM, Rickard SE, Orcheson LJ, Fong HHS. Antitumorigenic effect of a mammalian lignan precursor from flaxseed. Nutr Cancer 1996b; 26:159–165.

Thompson LU. Experimental studies on lignans and cancer. In: Adlercreutz H, ed. Bailliere's Clin Endocrinol Met England: Bailliere Tindall, 1998; 12:691–705.

Thompson LU. Flaxseed, lignans, cancer. Thompson LU and Cunnane SC, eds. Flaxseed in Human Nutrition. Champaign, IL: AOCS Press, 2003:Chapter 9.

Thompson LU, Chen JM, Li T, Strasser-Weippl K, Goss PE. Dietary flaxseed alters tumor biological markers in postmenopausal breast cancer. Clin Cancer Res 2005; 11:3828–3835.

Thompson LU, Boucher BA, Liu Z, Cotterchio M, Kreiger N. Phytoestrogen content of foods consumed in Canada, including isoflavones, lignans, and coumestan. Nutr Cancer 2006; 54:184–201.

Tou JCL, Thompson LU. Exposure to flaxseed or its lignan component during different developmental stages influences rat mammary gland structures. Carcinogenesis 1999; 20:1831–1835.

Touillaud MS, Pillow PC, Jakovljevic J, Bondy ML, Singletary SE, Li DH, Chang SN. Effect of dietary intake of phytoestrogens on estrogen receptor status in premenopausal women with breast cancer. Nutr Cancer 2005; 51:162–169.

Touillaud MS, Thiébaut AC, Niravong M, Boutron-Ruault MC, Clavel-Chapelon E. No association between dietary phytoestrogens and risk of premenopausal breast cancer in a french cohort study. Cancer Epidemiol Biomark Prev 2006; 15:2574–2576.

Touillaud MS, Thiébaut ACM, Fournier A, Niravong M, Boutron-Ruault M-C, Clavel-Chapelon F. Dietary lignan intake and postmenopausal breast cancer risk by estrogen and progesterone receptor status. J Natl Cancer Inst 2007; 99:475–486.

Valentin-Blasini L, Sadowski MA, Walden D, Caltabiano L, Needham LL, Barr DB. Urinary phytoestrogen concentration in the U.S. population (1999–2000). J Expo Anal Environ Epidemiol 2005; 15:509–523.

Valsta LM, Kilkkinen A, Mazur W, Nurmi T, Lampi AM, Ovaskainen ML, Korhonen T, Adlercreutz H, Pietinen P. Phyto-oestrogen database of foods and average intake in Finland. Br J Nutr 2003; 89:S31–S38.

van Gils CH, Peeters PHT, Bueno-De-Mesquita HB, Boshuizen HC, Lahmann PH, ClavelChapelon F, Thiebaut A, Kesse E, Sieri S, Palli D, Tumino R, Panico S, Vineis P, Gonzalez CA, Ardanaz E, Sanchez MJ, Amiano P, Navarro C, Quiros JR, Key TJ, Allen N, Khaw KT, Bingham SA, Psaltopoulou T, Koliva M, Trichopoulou A, Nagel G, Linseisen J, Boeing H, Berglund G, Wirfalt E, Hallmans G, Lenner P, Overvad K, Tjonneland A, Olsen A, Lund E, Engeset D, Alsaker E, Norat TA, Kaaks R, Slimani N, Riboli E. Consumption of vegetables and fruits and risk of breast cancer. JAMA 2005; 293:183–193.

Vanharanta M, Voutilainen S, Lakka TA, van der Lee M, Adlercreutz H, Salonen JT. Risk of acute coronary events according to serum concentrations of enterolactone: a prospective population-based case-control study. Lancet 1999; 354:2112–2115.

Velicer CM, Heckbert SR, Lampe JW, Potter JD, Robertson CA, Taplin SH. Antibiotic use in relation to the risk of breast cancer. JAMA 2004a; 291:827–835.

Velicer CM, Heckbert SR, Potter JD, Taplin SH. Use of antibiotics and risk of cancer. JAMA 2004b; 291:2700.

Verheus M, van Gils CH, Keinan-Boker L, Grace PB, Bingham SA, Peeters PHM. Plasma phytoestrogens and subsequent breast cancer risk. J Clin Oncol 2007; 25:648–655.

Vrieling A, Voskuil DW, Bueno de Mesquita HB, Kaaks R, van Noord PA, Keinan-Boker L, van Gils CH, Peeters PH. Dietary determinants of circulating insulin-like growth factor (IGF)-I and IGF binding proteins 1, -2 and -3 in women in the Netherlands. Cancer Causes Control 2004; 15:787–796.

Wang CF, Mäkelä T, Hase T, Adlercreutz H, Kurzer MS. Lignans and flavonoids inhibit aromatase enzyme in human preadipocytes. J Steroid Biochem Mol Biol 1994; 50: 205–212.

Wang L, Chen JM, Thompson LU. The inhibitory effect of flaxseed on the growth and metastasis of estrogen receptor negative human breast cancer xenografts is attributed to both its lignan and oil components. Int J Cancer 2005; 116:793–798.

Wang LQ. Mammalian phytoestrogens: enterodiol and enterolactone. J Chromatogr B Analyt Technol Biomed Life Sci 2002; 777:289–309.

Ward WE, Jiang FO, Thompson LU. Exposure to flaxseed or purified lignan during lactation influences rat mammary gland structures. Nutr Cancer 2000; 37:187–192.

Webb AL, McCullough ML. Dietary lignans: potential role in cancer prevention. Nutr Cancer 2005; 51:117–131.

Welshons WV, Murphy CS, Koch R, Calaf G, Jordan VC. Stimulation of breast cancer cells in vitro by the environmental estrogen enterolactone and the phytoestrogen equol. Breast Cancer Res Treat 1987; 10:169–175.

Whitten PL, Naftolin F. Dietary estrogens: a biologically active background for estrogen action. Hochberg RB, Naftolin F, eds. New Biology of Steroid Hormones. New York: Raven Press, 1991:155–167.

Willett WC, Hunter DJ, Stampfer MJ, Colditz G, Manson JE, Spiegelman D, Rosner B, Hennekens CH, Speizer FE. Dietary fat and fiber in relation to risk of breast cancer. JAMA 1992; 21:2037–2044.

Willett WC. Dietary fat and risk of breast and colon cancer. Proc Nutr Soc 1994; 53:25–26.

Woodside JV, Campbell MJ, Denholm EE, Newton L, Honour JW, Morton MS, Young IS, Leathem AJC. Short-term phytoestrogen supplementation alters insulin-like growth factor profile but not lipid or antioxidant status. J Nutr Biochem 2006; 17:211–215.

World Cancer Research Fund and American Institute for Cancer Research. Food, Nutrition and the Prevention of Cancer: A Global Perspective. Washington: American Institute for Cancer Research, 1997.

Wu WH, Kang YP, Wang NH, Jou HJ, Wang TA. Sesame ingestion affects sex hormones, antioxidant status, and blood lipids in postmenopausal women. J Nutr 2006; 136:1270–1275.

Xie LH, Ahn EM, Akao T, AbdelHafez AAM, Nakamura N, Hattori M. Transformation of arctiin to estrogenic and antiestrogenic substances by human intestinal bacteria. Chem Pharm Bull (Tokyo) 2003; 51:378–384.

Yan L, Yee JA, Li DH, Mcguire MH, Thompson LU. Dietary flaxseed supplementation and experimental metastasis of melanoma cells in mice. Cancer Lett 1998; 124:181–186.

Zeleniuch-Jacquotte A, Adlercreutz H, Akhmedkhanov A, Toniolo P. Reliability of serum measurements of lignans and isoflavonoid phytoestrogens over a two-year period. Cancer Epidemiol Biomarkers Prev 1998; 7:885–889.

Zeleniuch-Jacquotte A, Adlercreutz H, Shore RE, Koenig KL, Kato I, Arslan AA, Toniolo P. Circulating enterolactone and risk of breast cancer: a prospective study in New York. Br J Cancer 2004; 91:99–105.

20

Breast Cancer Risk, Soyfood Intake, and Isoflavone Exposure: A Review of the In Vitro, Animal, Epidemiologic, and Clinical Literature

MARK MESSINA

Department of Nutrition, School of Public Health, Loma Linda University, Loma Linda, California, U.S.A.

INTRODUCTION

Soyfoods have played an important role in the diets of many Southeast Asian countries for centuries and have been consumed by vegetarians and other health-conscious individuals for decades in non-Asian countries. But during the past 15 years foods made from the soybean have been embraced by a broad spectrum of the population in many Western countries. The increased popularity of soyfoods can be attributed to research suggesting that soyfood intake may be associated with a number of health benefits. For example, soyfoods have been posited to reduce the risk of osteoporosis (1) and coronary heart disease (2–7). Notable in this regard, in 1999, the U.S. Food and Drug Administration approved a health claim for soy protein and coronary heart disease based on the hypocholesterolemic effects of soy protein (8).

There is also an enormous amount of interest in the role of soyfoods in reducing the risk of cancer. This possibility first attracted widespread attention in 1990 when participants at a workshop sponsored by the U.S. National Cancer Institute concluded that there were several putative chemopreventive agents in soybeans and recommended funding research in this area (9). Unquestionably though, most cancer research has focused on just one group of compounds in soybeans, the isoflavones. Of the more than 700 papers published annually on these soybean constituents, about 25% involve cancer investigations.

Isoflavones exert both hormonal (10) and nonhormonal (11) effects under a variety of experimental conditions relevant to the cancer process and have been classified as selective estrogen receptor modulators (SERMs) (12–14). Parenthetically, because the soybean is one of the few commonly consumed foods to contain nutritionally relevant amounts of isoflavones, soyfoods are often mentioned as possible alternatives to conventional menopausal hormone therapy. More than 40 clinical trials have examined the effects of soyfoods and isoflavone supplements on the alleviation of hot flashes (15–18).

There is evidence suggesting that soyfoods and isoflavones may be protective against a wide range of cancers but most focus has been on cancer of the breast (11,19–21). Initial focus on this particular cancer can be attributed to the historically low breast cancer incidence rates in Asia (22), early research demonstrating the potential for soybean isoflavones to exert antiestrogenic effects (23) and early epidemiologic (24) and rodent (25) studies showing soy intake was protective against breast and mammary cancer, respectively. However, as discussed below, despite the impressive amount of research conducted during the past 15 years, no clear consensus on whether adult soy intake reduces breast cancer risk has emerged (26–44).

This having been said, one of the most intriguing hypotheses in the diet-cancer field is that soy intake during childhood and/or adolescence reduces the likelihood of developing breast cancer during adulthood (45). If early soy intake does in fact reduce breast cancer risk than expectations are for the already markedly increasing breast cancer rates in Japan to continue to rise because soy intake is not only lower among younger in comparison to older Japanese people, but it is decreasing among the former (46).

Somewhat ironically though, despite the continued interest in the anticancer effects, in recent years concern has emerged that soyfoods, because they contain isoflavones, may stimulate the growth of estrogen receptor–positive (ER+) tumors in vivo (for review see reference) (47). For this reason, the oncological community generally recommends that their ER+ breast cancer patients avoid or at least limit soy intake although there are varying opinions on this subject (28), and the American Cancer Society (48,49) has stated that when consumed at levels consistent with the Asian diet soyfoods are not contraindicated for breast cancer patients. They do however recommend against the consumption of more concentrated sources of isoflavones. Determining the impact of soyfood intake on the survival of ER+ breast cancer patients is a critically important public health need (47).

The purpose of this review is to examine the evidence relating to the impact of soyfoods and isoflavones on the development of breast cancer in healthy women and on breast cancer recurrence in breast cancer patients. Before approaching these subjects, background information on isoflavones is presented.

OVERVIEW OF ISOFLAVONES

Isoflavone Structure and Content in Soyfoods

Isoflavones are a subclass of flavonoids that have a very limited distribution in nature. Among commonly consumed foods they are found in significant amounts, primarily only in the soybean. Not surprisingly, therefore, daily per capita isoflavone intake is quite low in the United States (50–53) and in Europe (54–56)—typically less than 3 mg. Furthermore, much of that intake comes from ingesting foods to which small amounts of soy protein have been added for functional (hydration, whitening, etc.) purposes rather than from soyfoods per se (57).

There are three soybean isoflavone aglycones: genistein (4′,5,7-trihydroxyisoflavone), daidzein (4′,7-dihydroxyisoflavone), and glycitein (7,4′-dihydroxy-6-methoxyisoflavone). However, isoflavones are naturally present in the soybean and nonfermented soyfoods primarily in their beta glycoside form (genistin, daidzin, and glycitin). Typically, more genist(e)in exists in soybeans and soyfoods than daidz(e)in, while glycit(e)in comprises less than 10% of the total isoflavone content of the soybean (58).

Soybeans contain $\approx$1.2 to 3.3 mg isoflavones/g dry weight (expressed as the aglycone weight), and every gram of protein in traditional Asian soyfoods is associated with $\sim$3.5 mg isoflavones (59). Note though that soybean varieties differ markedly in isoflavone content and that isoflavone content is also affected by growing conditions (60–65). More importantly, processing can dramatically reduce isoflavone content, especially in the making of alcohol-extracted soy protein concentrate and isolate (66). Consequently, it is difficult to predict the isoflavone content of soy protein without knowledge about the process used to make the specific product.

Heating at extreme temperatures can cause some loss of isoflavones (67), especially at very low pH (68), but temperatures to which soy protein is more commonly exposed causes little loss of isoflavone, although decarboxylation will occur; this results in the conversion of malonyl isoflavone glycosides into acetyl glycosides (69). Storage for up to one year at temperatures from $-18°C$ to $42°C$ also has no effect on the total isoflavone content (70). Finally, isoflavones in soymilk appear to be quite stable over prolonged storage times (71).

Physiologic Attributes

Isoflavones have a chemical structure similar to the hormone estrogen, so it is not surprising that they bind to ERs and exert some estrogen-like effects in cells (72,73). However, despite sharing some properties with estrogen, isoflavones and estrogen are quite different molecules (74). Importantly, in clinical studies, often neither soyfoods nor isoflavones affect biological parameters known to be affected by estrogen (14,75,76).

As noted previously, isoflavones have been classified as SERMs (12,13). The selectivity of isoflavones may stem in part from their preferential binding to and activation of ERβ in comparison to ERα (77–79). This preferential binding may have implications related to breast cancer risk as some evidence suggests that, when activated by certain ligands, this ER isoform inhibits mammary cancer cell growth as well as the stimulatory effects of ERα (80). But not all evidence indicates that ERβ activation is beneficial and its precise role in cancer is unclear (81). Furthermore, there is conflicting evidence about the selectivity of genistein (82). Finally, as also noted previously, isoflavones, and especially genistein, have a variety of nonhormonal properties that are especially relevant to cancer prevention and treatment (11,83).

Isoflavone Absorption and Metabolism

Isoflavone glycosides are not absorbed intact, but hydrolysis (from the acid pH of the stomach, endogenous enzymes, and microflora) does readily occur in vivo primarily in the intestinal mucosa such that there appears to be little difference in bioavailability between the glycoside and aglycone forms of isoflavones (84). In fact, recent data suggest that saliva, perhaps from the contribution of both oral bacteria and oral epithelial cells, can hydrolyze genistin to genistein (85). However, due to the relatively small residence time of isoflavones in the mouth, the contribution of saliva to the overall hydrolysis of isoflavone glycosides is unclear. In any event, after the ingestion of soyfoods, there is a small peak in serum levels approximately one to two hours later, but the major serum peak occurs four to six hours post ingestion. Most work estimates the half-life of isoflavones to be between four and eight hours; 24 hours after the consumption of soyfoods, nearly all of the isoflavones are excreted (84). Serum isoflavone levels increase in a dose-dependent fashion in response to soyfood consumption (86,87). Plasma levels in free-living Asians are around 500 nmol/L when measured after an overnight fast (88–90). However, isoflavones circulate in plasma primarily in the conjugated form, mostly bound to glucuronic acid; less than 3% circulates in the free form (91,92).

Finally, it is important to note that there is considerable interindividual variation in the metabolism of isoflavones (93–95). In this regard, an intriguing hypothesis is that individuals who possess the intestinal bacteria capable of converting the isoflavone daidzein into equol are more likely to benefit from isoflavone exposure than those who do not (94). Approximately 30% of subjects make equol (94), although evidence suggests that this varies among populations and that the percentage of equol producers is higher among the Japanese (96–98) and vegetarians (99) than among the Western omnivores.

Asian Soy Intake and Serum Isoflavone Levels

Widely varying estimates of Asian soy intake have been reported in the literature, but within the past seven years many large surveys of soy protein and isoflavone consumption by Asian adults have been published. These surveys, which often include as many as nine different questions related to soyfood intake, provide a very accurate picture of Asian isoflavone intake. As recently reviewed by Messina et al. (59), it is clear from these data that early estimates of soy intake were greatly exaggerated. Surveys suggest that older ($\geq$50 years) Japanese adults typically consume from 7 to 11 g soy protein and 30- to 50-mg isoflavones/day (100–103). Intake in Hong Kong and Singapore is lower than in Japan, whereas significant regional intake differences exist for China. Evidence suggests $\leq$10% of the Asian population consumes as much as 25-g soy protein or 100-mg isoflavones/day.

IN VITRO EFFECTS OF ISOFLAVONES ON CANCER CELLS

Growth Inhibition

Early on, genistein was recognized as a potential chemopreventive agent because of its ability to inhibit the activity of tyrosine protein kinase (104,105), an enzyme overexpressed in many different cancer cell lines (106). Subsequent research has, in fact, demonstrated that genistein inhibits the growth of a wide range of cancer cells in vitro, including both hormone-dependent and hormone-independent breast cancer cells, with IC_{50} values ranging approximately from 10 to 50 μmol/L (83,107–110). Whether phosphorylation inhibition plays a role in this in vitro growth suppression is uncertain (111); however, as more recent research has revealed numerous other molecular mechanisms by which genistein inhibits cancer cell growth (112–126). Interestingly, in vitro work also shows that BRCA1 mutant cells are more sensitive to genistein than some other types of cancer cells, highlighting the possible therapeutic potential of genistein for BRCA1-associated breast cancer (116).

However, it is also well established that genistein exhibits a biphasic effect on the growth of ER+ mammary cancer cells (126–129). At relatively low (<1 μM) concentrations, genistein stimulates (77,126–128,130,131) growth, whereas at higher (>10 μM) concentrations MCF-7 cell growth is inhibited (32,109,127,128,132–139). The MCF-7 cell line is the first estrogen-sensitive stable cell line of human breast tumor epithelial cells and was created in 1972 by Soule et al. (140). Genistein does not stimulate the growth of ER− breast cancer cells (131,141) and only stimulates those ER+ cells that contain ERα (142). Current thinking is that growth stimulation and inhibition occur through estrogen-dependent and independent mechanisms, respectively.

Although initially overlooked, the in vitro growth stimulatory effects of genistein have not surprisingly contributed to concern about soyfoods, and especially isoflavone supplements, stimulating the growth of existing breast tumors in women (142). There is, however, much debate about the potential in vivo implications of in vitro data, although in vitro growth suppression is often cited in support of the anticancer effects of isoflavones and soyfoods. A potentially important consideration when evaluating the in vitro genistein data is the impact of adding estrogen to the culture medium. Some studies show that in a high-estrogenic environment, no growth stimulation occurs or growth is inhibited (143,144), whereas others still show a modest increase in growth (32,130,131,145). The hormonal milieu may also be an important factor determining the in vivo effects of isoflavones. Interestingly, despite reduced serum levels, breast tissue estrogen concentrations are similar in pre- and postmenopausal women (146,147)

The high in vitro genistein concentrations required to inhibit the growth of breast cancer cells led Barnes (148) to suggest that more attention should be given to the effects of genistein on the growth of normal breast cells. Genistein inhibits the growth of primary human epithelial cells (124,149) and initial research by Peterson et al. (149) reported that the IC_{50} was considerably lower than for the transformed cells. In agreement, Singletary et al. (121) recently found that at concentrations of only 0.5 μM, genistein inhibited the proliferation of nonneoplastic, immortalized human breast epithelial MCF-10F cells by as much as 20%. Also, unlike transformed cells, the growth of primary human mammary epithelial cells (these cells express both ERα and ERβ) is not stimulated by genistein at any concentration and the stimulatory effects of 17β-estradiol on these cells are inhibited by this isoflavone (150). However, Nguyen et al. (151) recently found that higher (3–30 μM) genistein concentrations were required to inhibit the growth of normal (MCF-10A) compared with tumorigenic (T47D) breast cells and that the difference in sensitivity could be attributed to differences in genistein metabolism between the two cell lines. Finally, in contrast to both Peterson et al. (149) and Nguyen et al. (151), Frey et al. (124) found normal and transformed breast cells were similarly sensitive to genistein.

Angiogenesis and Metastasis

In addition to cell growth, it is important to consider the effects of genistein on angiogenesis and metastasis, since most often death due to cancer results from tumor cells in the tissue of origin migrating to a vital organ. Angiogenesis is required for the growth as well as expansion of solid tumors, especially those at 1 to 2 mm in diameter (152). The progression of breast cancer is largely affected by an imbalance that exists between angiogenic and angiostatic mediators, favoring the expression and activities of the angiogenic factors (153–158).

In 1993, Fotsis et al. (159) were the first to show that genistein inhibited endothelial cell proliferation and in vitro angiogenesis with concentrations of 5 and 150 μmol/L, respectively, giving half-maximal inhibition. However, Fotsis et al. (160) later determined that the genistein concentration for the half-maximal inhibitory effect on angiogenesis was only 10 μmol/L, the higher value in the previous report being due to the poor solubility of genistein in sodium bicarbonate compared to dimethyl sulfoxide. Recently, Piao et al. (161) using human umbilical vein endothelial cells found that at this concentration (10 μM) genistein inhibited angiogenesis partially by downregulating cell adhesion–related genes and impairing cell adhesion. The reader is directed toward the reference for an interesting discussion on the antiangiogenesis effects of genistein (162).

In 1994, Scholar et al. (163) showed that genistein inhibited the invasion of BALB/c mammary carcinoma 410.4 cells with an EC_{50} of only ~1 μM, whereas much higher concentrations were required to inhibit cell growth. Similarly, Magee et al. (164) noted some inhibition of the invasive properties of MDA-MB-231 breast cancer cells in vitro by several isoflavones at concentrations as low as 2.5 μM. Shao et al. (32) also found that genistein inhibited the invasion of MCF-7 and MDA-MB-231 cells, although concentrations of approximately 18 μM were needed. This inhibition was characterized by the downregulation of matrix metalloproteinase (MMP)-9 and upregulation of tissue inhibitor of metalloproteinase-1, the former of which was transcriptionally regulated at activation protein-1 sites in the MMP-9 promoter. Results by Li et al. (136) also suggest that genistein inhibits breast cancer cell invasion. They found that genistein upregulated Bax and p21WAF1 expression and downregulated the expression of Bcl-2 and c-erbB-2 and inhibited the secretion of MMP.

Progression of breast cancer requires the degradation of extracellular matrix (ECM) by MMPs, and in this regard, Kousidou et al. (165) found that the addition of genistein to the culture medium resulted in downregulation of the transcription of all MMP genes in MDA-MB-231 (a highly invasive ER− breast cancer line) cells and most of the MMPs in MCF-7 cells (a less invasive ER+ breast cancer line) and that this downregulation was correlated with significant inhibition of the invasive properties of the cancer cells in vitro.

Finally, Valachovicova et al. (161) found that genistein suppresses cell adhesion and migration by inhibiting the constitutively active transcription factors NF-κB and AP-1, resulting in suppression of the secretion of urokinase-type plasminogen activator in MDA-MB-231 cells.

Perspectives on the In Vitro Findings

There are several considerations that may help to put into perspective the in vitro results discussed above. First, additive and even synergistic effects between isoflavones and other chemopreventive agents (114,166–173), and among different isoflavones (174), on the growth of cancer cells and various growth and differentiation-related processes in normal (175) and cancer cells (115,170) have been noted. Thus, because humans consuming a mixed diet are regularly exposed to a variety of chemopreventive agents, the high genistein concentrations required to inhibit cancer cell growth when used alone may actually underestimate the potential chemopreventive properties of this isoflavone. In fact, as discussed in the next section, Kim et al. (176) found that background diet determined the efficacy of genistein to inhibit chemically induced tumors in rodents. Furthermore, lycopene and other carotenoids were found to inhibit the stimulatory effect of phytoestrogens on breast cell proliferation (177). Thus, both the inhibitory and stimulatory effects of isoflavones on breast cancer cells may be influenced by background diet.

Second, there is evidence, at least in regard to prostate cancer, that the longer genistein is exposed to cells in the media the lower is the concentration required to inhibit growth (178,179). Greater exposure time may mimic chronic isoflavone ingestion, which is reflective of individuals who have been long-term consumers of soyfoods. Also of potential relevance is the finding that the IC_{50} for unstimulated prostate cancer cells was about threefold higher than for epidermal growth factor-stimulated cells (180). Finally, Dalu et al. (181) found that dietary genistein downregulated epidermal growth factor receptor levels in the dorsolateral prostate of Lobund-Wistar rats despite free genistein concentrations in serum and prostate tissue of only 18.4 nmol/L and 17.5 pmol/g, respectively. These concentrations are below that needed for the inhibition of prostate cancer cell growth in vitro. Perhaps a similar situation exists for breast cancer, i.e., the in vitro data underestimates the potential in vivo chemopreventive effects of isoflavones.

EFFECTS OF ISOFLAVONES IN ANIMAL STUDIES

Prevention Models

Summarizing the results from the more than 40 animal studies in which the effects of isoflavones or soy protein on experimentally induced mammary cancer have been examined is complicated by the large number of different models and dietary products that have been used. The text below does not include every published study but rather attempts to provide a general overview of the literature.

Early research by Carroll (182) and Gridley et al. (183) failed to find that isolated soy protein (ISP, by definition ISP is ~90% soy protein) inhibited carcinogenesis; in the former case, the indirect-acting breast carcinogen 7,12-dimethylbenz(α)anthracene (DMBA) was used to initiate tumors, whereas tumors developed spontaneously in the latter study. However, no information about the isoflavone content of the ISP used in these studies was provided. Barnes et al. (25) can be credited as the first to focus specifically on isoflavones, although in their work two different types of soy protein, not isolated isoflavones, were used. In two separate experiments, they found that different soy proteins inhibited tumors initiated either by *N*-methyl-*N*-nitrosourea (MNU) or DMBA and attributed this inhibition to isoflavones since a protein from which the isoflavones were extracted was without effect. Unfortunately, the description of the experimental designs of these studies was woefully lacking in details.

The inhibition of DMBA-induced mammary tumors in Sprague-Dawley (SD) rats observed by Barnes et al. (25) concurs with older research by Baggott et al. (184) and very recent research by Mukhopadhyay et al. (185) and Gallo et al. (186). The products used in these three studies were miso, ISP, and isoflavone extracts, respectively. In contrast, no inhibition was observed in Big Blue® transgenic rats in response to dietary additions of genistein or daidzein or the combination of both the isoflavones, although in this case, the basal diet was the NIH-31C diet and not the AIN-76 diet used in the previously cited studies (187).

As already noted, dietary background may be a factor in the efficacy of isoflavones to prevent chemically induced cancer. Kim et al. (176) found that in SD rats genistein administered as part of the AIN-76A diet failed to show chemopreventive activity against MNU-induced tumors; however, when administered at the same dose in the Teklad 4% rodent diet, tumor development was inhibited from 44% to 61%. This being said, Constantinou et al. (31,188) found only very modest reductions in DMBA-induced tumors using the AIN diet to which genistein or daidzein was added.

In 1991, Hawrylewicz et al. (189) found that ISP inhibited MNU-induced mammary tumors by ~50% although when the amino acid methionine was added to the soy-containing diet, this reduction was mitigated. Relative to the control protein casein, ISP is lower in methionine and some data indicate cancer cells have a higher requirement for methionine than nontransformed cells (190). These results agree with those from the above cited study by Kim et al. (176) and two studies by Gotoh et al. (191,192), who examined the effects of miso, soybeans, and biochanin-A [an isoflavone not present in soybean but which is converted to genistein (149)]. However, no such protection was noted in studies by Cohen et al. (35) and Kijkuokool (193) in response to dietary soy and injected genistein, respectively. In fact, in the latter study, tumor multiplicity and size were actually increased.

Semi-Prevention and Treatment Models

In addition to the prevention models, soy products have been examined in models attempting to reflect the treatment setting and also in models that fall somewhere between prevention and treatment. In regard to treatment, in 1995, Hawrylewicz et al. (194) were the first to examine the impact of ISP on tumor recurrence. In their model, when the first MNU-induced tumor grew to between 0.3 and 0.5 cm in diameter, it was excised and diets were begun. In comparison to the control diet, the incidence of secondary tumors was lower and tumors developed significantly later in rats fed with the ISP-containing diet. Similarly, when Imrhan et al. (195) delayed the administration of the ISP-containing diet for five weeks after MNU injection, tumor incidence and weight were decreased and tumor development delayed. In contrast, when Ueda et al. (196) delayed the administration of diets containing 25 or 250 ppm genistein until 12 weeks after the second of two DMBA injections there was no reduction in tumorigenesis.

One of the most impressive studies in terms of tumor inhibition was conducted by Zhou et al. (33). Diets were fed two weeks prior to the implantation of 17β-estradiol (90-day release) and MCF-7 cells, which were implanted orthotopically into mammary fat pads. There was a dose-dependent decrease in tumor growth in response to diets containing isolated genistein or soy phytochemical concentrate, which contained a mixture of isoflavones. There was also a synergistic inhibitory effect on tumor development when genistein was combined with tea extracts. Genistein was also effective when begun five days post s.c. injection of F3II cells in Balb/c mice (197). Finally, Shao et al. (32) was able to demonstrate impressive tumor inhibition in response to s.c. injections of genistein even though treatment administration began six weeks postbilateral injections of either MDA-MB-231 or MCF-7 cells into nude mice.

Tumor Stimulation

As already noted, there are concerns that isoflavones may be contraindicated for some women because of the possible stimulatory effects of these soybean constituents on mammary tumor growth. This concern is based primarily on the research conducted by Helferich and colleagues from the University of Illinois. In their basic model, ovariectomized athymic nude mice are injected s.c. with MCF-7 cells and implanted with estradiol. When tumors reach approximately 35 to 40 mm^2 the estradiol implants are removed from all mice except those in the positive control and dietary treatments are begun. Results repeatedly show that in this basic model tumors typically undergo initial regression (except in mice in the positive control) but then in response to diets containing genistein (127), genistin (198), ISP (199), and mixed isoflavones (200) tumors begin to grow in size (relative to the negative control fed the standard AIN-76 diet) in a dose-dependent fashion.

Interestingly, in this model, unprocessed soy flour does not stimulate tumor growth (although tumors do not fully regress as they do in the negative control) (200) and isolated daidzin has only a slight stimulatory effect, whereas equol leads to tumor regression similar to the negative control (201). Importantly, equol failed to stimulate tumor growth in vivo despite stimulating the proliferation of MCF-7 cell in vitro. Recent work has also shown that equol does not stimulate breast cell proliferation in ovariectomized monkeys (202).

It is evident that tumor stimulation noted in the above experiments is due to genistein but why unprocessed soy flour, which contained sufficient genistein to stimulate tumor growth, does not cause tumor stimulation is unclear although two explanations have been proposed: one is that processing causes greater increases in the serum levels of free genistein (203); and the other is that compounds removed during processing inhibit the tumor-stimulatory effects of isoflavones and/or directly inhibit mammary tumor growth (204).

The model used by Helferich and colleagues as described above has been criticized because of the very low estrogen levels that exist in ovariectomized mice. It has been suggested that this hypoestrogenic environment does not reflect conditions in postmenopausal women and that only under these conditions will isoflavones exert tumor-stimulatory effects. The claim that this low-estrogen environment is not reflective of postmenopausal women has merit since estrogen-sensitive tumors are able to grow even in postmenopausal women because of the production of estrogen within breast tissue, whereas in ovariectomized mice not exposed to a source of estrogen, this is not the case. Although serum estrogen levels decrease in postmenopausal women, breast tissue estrogen levels (which determine tumor growth) are similar between pre- and postmenopausal women (146,147). However, tumor-stimulatory effects of genistein have also been observed by Helferich and colleagues in a model similar to that described above but wherein the mice are continually given small amounts of estradiol to maintain estrogen levels (205).

Finally, Canadian researchers have in essence repeated the findings by Helferich and colleagues, although the tumor-stimulatory effects were not as pronounced (206). Interestingly, the addition of flaxseed to the ISP-containing diet caused tumor regression that was similar to the regression that occurred in response to the basal diet (206,207). Similarly, although injected genistein caused tumor stimulation, when combined with enterolignans, enterolactone, and enterodiol, tumor stimulation was inhibited (207).

Metastasis

It is important to consider the effects of isoflavones on tumor metastases and angiogenesis in animals since, as noted previously, death due to breast cancer results from tumor cells in the tissue of origin migrating to a vital organ. Unfortunately, MCF-7 cells are thought not to produce tumors that metastasize so ER− cell lines are typically used, although a new model that may allow detection of metastasis of ER+ breast cancer cells has been developed (208). To study metastasis, Vantyghem et al. (209) established tumors by implanting MDA-MB-435/HAL cells into the mammary fat pad of female nude mice. Primary tumors were left to grow for five weeks before being surgically removed. Mice were then randomized into the control or genistein (750 ppm)-containing diets and metastatic burden was assessed five weeks later. Genistein reduced the percent metastatic burden in the lungs by 10-fold.

In agreement, Yan et al. (30) found that ISP markedly reduced tumor metastasis of primary mammary tumors to the lungs. Animals were fed the experimental diets for three weeks prior to the orthotopic injection of 4526 murine mammary carcinoma cells in female BALB/c mice. The primary tumors were excised when they reached a size of 1.0 cm in diameter. After surgery, mice were maintained on their respective diets for another three weeks.

In contrast to the findings from the previous two studies (30,209), Charland et al. (210) found that a soybean extract actually increased metastasis. In their study, 60 Lewis rats were injected s.c. with mammary tumor (MAC-33) and randomized to receive i.p. injections of a soybean extract or saline five times per week for 30 days. When comparing the soybean extract with controls, there was a significant increase in the number of lung metastases in the animals receiving the extract. Finally, although Farina et al. (211) did not study metastasis, they found that i.p. administration of genistein at a dose of 10 mg/kg/day reduced tumor-induced angiogenesis in syngeneic mice implanted with F3II cells. Several researchers have also found evidence that genistein reduces angiogenesis in primary mammary tumors (32,33).

SOY AND ISOFLAVONES INTAKE AND BREAST CANCER RISK: EPIDEMIOLOGIC STUDIES

The historically low incidence rates of breast cancer in soyfood-consuming countries greatly contributed to the interest in the role of soy in reducing breast cancer risk (22). Of course, gross ecological comparisons provide little insight into specific factors that might account for differences in disease rates among countries. However, in 1991, a case-control study conducted in Singapore found that the consumption of a modest (~3.4 g/day) amount of soy protein was associated with an approximate 50% reduction in premenopausal (postmenopausal risk was unaffected) breast cancer risk (24). Support for this observation came a few years later from a Japanese case-control study that also found that soy intake was modestly protective against premenopausal, but not postmenopausal, breast cancer (212). However, a large case-control study involving women from two locations in China published in the same year failed to find that soy intake was associated with a reduction in the risk of either type of breast cancer (213). Thus, from the beginning, the epidemiologic literature provided only modest support for the hypothesis that soy intake is associated protection against breast cancer.

In 2006, Trock et al. (27) published a meta-analysis of epidemiologic studies investigating the relationship between soy exposure (based on soy protein and isoflavone intake and urinary isoflavone excretion) and breast cancer risk. Their analysis included 18 studies, 12 of which were case control and six of which were cohort or nested case control. The pooled relative risk estimates were based on either the original soy exposure measure defined in each study or on an estimate of daily soy protein intake. To permit comparison of exposure across studies using a common measure, soy or isoflavone exposure in each study was converted to an estimate of grams of soy protein consumed daily. To convert urinary isoflavones to soy protein, linear regression–derived estimates of mean urinary genistein and daidzein for levels of soy protein intake were used.

In a pooled analysis, among all women, high soy intake was modestly associated with reduced breast cancer risk [odds ratio (OR) = 0.86, 95% confidence interval (CI) = 0.75–0.99]; however, the association was not statistically significant among women in Asian countries (OR = 0.89, 95% CI, 0.71–1.12). Among the 10 studies stratified by menopausal status, the inverse association between soy exposure and breast cancer risk was somewhat stronger in premenopausal women (OR = 0.70, 95% CI, 0.58–0.85) than in postmenopausal women (OR = 0.77, 95% CI, 0.60–0.98); however, eight studies did not provide menopause-specific results, six of which did not support an association.

When exposure was analyzed by soy protein intake in grams per day, a statistically significant association with breast cancer risk was seen only among premenopausal women (OR = 0.94, 95% CI, 0.92–0.97). Trock et al. (27) concluded that soy intake may be associated with a small reduction in breast cancer risk but emphasized that the findings should be viewed with caution because of potential exposure misclassification, confounding, and lack of a dose response.

The overall results from this analysis are relatively unimpressive. Furthermore, the OR of 0.94 for pre- and postmenopausal women, respectively, was associated with a soy protein intake of only about 1 g/day. There is considerable doubt as to whether such a low soy intake is sufficient to exert physiological effects (214). In addition, these epidemiologic studies were not designed to control the confounding effects of early soy consumption. That is, protective effects observed in Asian studies may simply have been a reflection of the fact that adult soy intake tracks with childhood and adolescent intake and because, as discussed later, there is evidence that early soy intake is protective against breast cancer.

EFFECT OF SOY/ISOFLAVONES ON MARKERS OF BREAST CANCER RISK

One of the more difficult challenges to understanding the relationship between diet and cancer is the lack of well-accepted, noninvasive, intermediary markers. There is, however, little evidence from studies that have examined the impact of soy or isoflavone intake on routinely-used markers of breast cancer risk that adult soy intake is protective. In fact, one of the first clinical studies found that the consumption of ISP led to a two- to sixfold increase in nipple aspirate fluid volume in premenopausal women (215). Of much greater concern was the detection of epithelial hyperplasia in 7 of 24 women while consuming soy. However, this was a pilot study that did not include a control group.

Two years later, an interim analysis reported that a two-week soy intervention increased breast cell proliferation in premenopausal women undergoing breast reductions (216). However, when the entire cohort was analyzed, this effect disappeared (217), although levels of pS2, a protein that is upregulated in response to estrogen, were increased (218). The lack of effect on cell proliferation was recently confirmed by Cheng et al. (219) in a three-month intervention trial involving healthy postmenopausal women and by Palomares et al. (43) in a pilot one-year study in which biopsies were taken from the healthy breast of postmenopausal breast cancer patients. Parenthetically, in contrast to isoflavones, conventional hormone therapy markedly increases breast cell proliferation within just a 12-week period (220).

There is also little evidence to suggest that either soyfoods or isoflavones affect serum estrogen levels (41,42,221), although there is some indication that estrogen metabolism may be favorably affected (44). That is, soy may cause estrogen to be metabolized through the 2-hydroxylation, rather than the 16-hydroxylation pathway; however, there are conflicting data regarding the relative importance of differences in this pathway on breast cancer risk (222). Menstrual cycle length is often studied in relation to breast cancer risk—longer cycles are associated with protection against this disease (223). Generally, longer cycle length results from an increase in the luteal phase, and early research found that soy intake led to an increase menstrual cycle length (224). However, the effects of soy on menstrual cycle length appear to be fairly modest, on average, length is increased by about one day (41).

Finally, several studies have examined the effect of soy or isoflavones on breast tissue density but none have shown changes in this parameter (39,40,225). Differences in the parenchymal pattern of the breast on mammography reflect differences in the amounts of stromal, epithelial, and fat tissue present in the breast (226). Stroma and epithelium are radiologically dense, whereas fat is lucent. Extensive areas of mammographically dense breast tissue are strongly associated with the risk of breast cancer, four to six times that of women with little or no density (227,228).

EARLY SOY/ISOFLAVONE EXPOSURE

Introduction

With few exceptions, convincingly identifying adult lifestyle factors that markedly influence breast cancer risk has proven difficult. Excessive alcohol intake (229), postmenopausal obesity (230), and long-term use of combined hormone therapy (231), are thought to increase risk but increasingly, it appears that early life events markedly influence later risk of developing breast cancer. This may be one reason that results from epidemiologic studies, which primarily focus on adult characteristics, are often so inconsistent. Evidence in support of the importance of early life events includes the observations that parity, lactation, age at menses, and birth weight impact risk of developing breast cancer (232–243). Studies of migrants suggest that the first 20 years of life have an especially profound impact on risk (243–245).

Early pregnancy appears to be particularly protective against breast cancer (246). According to Russo et al. (247) the hormonal milieu of an early full-term pregnancy induces lobular development, completing the cycle of differentiation of the breast. This process induces a specific genomic signature in the mammary gland that results in the production of a type of stem cell that is permanently more refractory to carcinogenesis. There is evidence, as discussed below, that early exposure to isoflavones produces similar effects as early pregnancy, and possibly, through a similar mechanism.

Animal Studies

In 1995, Lamartiniere et al. (248) demonstrated that neonatal genistein markedly suppressed mammary carcinogenesis. In this model, genistein (5 mg) was subcutaneously injected on postnatal days 2, 4, and 6, and DMBA (80 μg/g b.w.) was administered via oral gavage on postnatal day 50, and tumors assessed on day 230 or until animals became moribund. Tumor number (6.4 ± 0.7 vs. 3.7 ± 0.4, $p < 0.001$) was significantly decreased and tumor latency (mean number of days to detection of first palpable tumor; 87 ± 37 vs. 124 ± 33, $p < 0.001$) significantly increased in the genistein group. One year later in a similarly designed study, but in which rats were injected (500 μg/g bw) with genistein on postnatal days 16, 18, and 20, there was also a reduction in tumor number (7.36 ± 0.95 vs. 3.93 ± 0.69, $p < 0.01$), although tumor incidence was only modestly (92% vs. 85%) reduced; however, unlike the previous study, tumor latency was not affected (249). The results from these two studies clearly demonstrate that pharmacological amounts of genistein administered prior to puberty markedly reduce mammary carcinogenesis.

In agreement with these results, Hilakivi-Clarke et al. (250), who used physiologic, rather than pharmacologic, levels of genistein also noted tumor inhibition in response to early genistein exposure. Specifically, rats were injected with genistein [the dose ranged from 2 (day 7) to 0.7 mg/kg b.w. (day 20)] on postnatal days 7, 10, 14, 17, and 20, and DMBA (10 mg, ≈50 mg/kg b.w.) was administered by oral gavage on day 45 (250). Tumors were assessed at week 18. The DMBA dose, which is slightly more than half the amount used by Lamartiniere and colleagues (248), is a suboptimal dose that according to the authors allows assessments of both increases and decreases in tumorigenicity. The number of rats per tumor-bearing rat and the percentage of proliferating tumors was 1.8 and 1.1 ($p < 0.01$), and 94% and 60% ($p < 0.001$), respectively, in the control and genistein groups. Also, 100% of the tumors in the control but only 40% in the genistein group were malignant. Tumor incidence in the genistein group was only modestly (57% vs. 43%) and nonsignificantly reduced. This study demonstrates that physiologic levels of genistein are efficacious; however, in all three studies discussed thus far genistein was subcutaneously injected.

To test the effects of dietary genistein, Lamartiniere and colleagues fed seven-week old female SD CD rats an AIN-76 (soy-free) diet supplemented with 0-, 25-, or 250-mg genistein/kg diet (251). Two weeks later females were bred. Offspring were sexed at birth and liters reduced so that each dam had 10 offspring (4–6 females/dam). At day 21 postpartum, all offspring were weaned and fed the AIN-76A diet for the remainder of the experiment. As in the previous experiments DMBA was administered on day 50, and tumors assessed on day 200, when animals became moribund, or when tumor size reached 2.5 cm. In addition to receiving genistein via mammary milk, on postpartum day 14, the offspring began eating the powdered diet containing the same amount of genistein fed to the respective dams. Tumor number in the 0, 25, or 250-mg genistein/kg diet groups was 8.8 ± 0.8, 7.1 ± 0.8, and 4.4 ± 0.6 ($p < 0.001$), respectively. There were no differences in tumor latency.

An additional observation of importance by Lamartiniere and colleagues is that even though in their laboratory adult genistein exposure alone has no impact on DMBA-induced tumorigenesis, adult exposure enhances the protective effects of neonatal and prepubertal genistein. They have reported that tumor number in the control rats, rats exposed to genistein during the prenatal (in utero) period, during adulthood only (postnatal days 100–180), neonatal and prepubertal period (postnatal days 1–21), or neonatal and prepubertal and adulthood was 8.9, 8.8, 8.2, 4.3, and 2.8, respectively (252).

Finally, in contrast to the above, Yang et al (253) found that when SD CD rats received 12.5 mg genistein s.c. on neonatal days 15 and 18 and given 50 mg/kg MNU i.p., there was no effect on the incidence of mammary tumors >1 cm or latency, and the number of mammary cancer lesions actually increased. And Pei et al. (254) in a similarly designed experiment also failed to find that genistein affected tumor multiplicity although they did find that the incidence of mammary carcinomas ≥1 cm was suppressed.

Epidemiology

The limited epidemiologic data are quite supportive of the hypothesis that early soy intake reduces later risk of developing breast cancer. For example, a large Chinese case-control study involving 1459 breast cancer cases and 1556 age-matched controls from Shanghai found that soy protein intake during adolescence (13–15 years) was associated with a 50% reduction (trend test $p < 0.01$) in risk when comparing the fifth versus the first intake quintile (255). Dietary intake data were obtained by interview from all study participants and, in addition, from mothers of subjects less than 45 years of age (296 cases and 359 controls). The soy protein intake cutoff for the fifth quintile was only 11.01 g/day.

Also in support of the importance of early soy intake are findings from a U.S. case-control study involving Asian Americans that found high soy consumption throughout life was associated with a one-third reduction in risk of breast cancer (256). This was a population-based case-control study involving 501 cases and 594 controls. Women were stratified into four different categories according to their tofu intake (low or high) during both adolescence and adulthood. Low and high tofu intake during adolescence was defined as monthly or less, and weekly or more, respectively, whereas low and high intake during adulthood was defined as 0 to 3×/month and ≥1×/week, respectively. The adjusted ORs (adolescence is listed first, adulthood second) for the low-low, low-high, high-low, and high-high categories were 1.00, 1.02,

0.88, and 0.65 (trend test $p < 0.03$), respectively. These results differ from the Chinese study discussed previously in that although high adolescent intake alone was marginally protective, maximum protectiveness was achieved only with high tofu intake throughout life.

A recently presented subanalysis of this cohort provides additional insight into the critical soy exposure period for protection against breast cancer. This analysis involved 99 cases and 156 controls (257). Soy intake was examined during three stages of life; childhood (5–11 years of age), adolescence (12–19 years of age), and adulthood ($\geq$20 years of age). The ORs (95% CI) when comparing the third versus the first intake tertiles were 0.42 (0.20–0.90), 0.77 (0.57–1.04), and 0.71 (0.53–0.95), respectively. Finally, a large Canadian case-control study involving over 6000 cases and controls found both isoflavones and lignan intake was associated with protection against breast cancer (258). Adolescent phytoestrogen intake was obtained using a brief food frequency questionnaire. The ORs (95% CI) for the first through fourth isoflavone intake quartiles were 1.0, 0.95 (0.83–1.09), 0.89 (0.77–1.09), and 0.81 (0.71–0.94), respectively. However, it should be noted that as expected, isoflavone intake was quite low and in fact, fewer than 5% of the participants reported consuming any soyfoods. As commented previously, there is considerable uncertainty as to whether such low isoflavone exposure is sufficient to exert physiological effects (214).

Proposed Mechanism of Action

The evidence strongly suggests that early genistein exposure reduces mammary tumorigenesis by increasing mammary tissue differentiation thereby leading to a reduction in the number of terminal end buds (TEB) and an increase in the number of lobules (252,259). TEBs are located in the growing fringe of the mammary gland. With maturation, TEBs regress to terminal ducts, or differentiate in response to each estrus cycle, giving rise to alveolar buds that comprise type 1 and type II lobules.

The TEBs are terminal ductal structures found primarily in young animals and contain many undifferentiated epithelial cells. As a result they are the structures most susceptible to chemical carcinogens. Corresponding structures in the human breast (terminal ductal lobular units) are the sites in which most breast tumors are initiated (260). In contrast, lobules are the terminal ductal structure most differentiated and least susceptible to chemical carcinogens. The lobules respond to the hormones of pregnancy by differentiating further to lobules III that form functional units of the lactating gland.

The means by which genistein stimulates breast tissue differentiation is not entirely clear although one possibility is through an estrogen-like effect on mammary tissue. In rats, pregnancy (which increases estrogen levels) (261), estrogen (262), and chorionic gonadotrophin (263) all decrease carcinogenesis. However, Lamartiniere et al. (264,265) reported that early exposure to the soybean isoflavone daidzein, which in the rat is converted to the highly estrogenic isoflavonoid equol, does not protect against mammary carcinogenesis and does not stimulate mammary tissue differentiation (266). In contrast, an unpublished report indicates that equol does in fact increase breast tissue differentiation (KD Setchell, personal communication). The discrepancy between these two studies may be due to lower equol levels in the former study.

Other possible mechanisms for the breast tissue differentiating effects of genistein include downregulation of epidermal growth factor receptor expression (267) and upregulation of mammary gland BRCA1 mRNA expression (268). Finally, recently Rowell et al. (269) found that in rats injected subcutaneously with 500 μg genistein/g body weight on days 16, 18, and 20 postpartum, GTP-cyclohydrolase 1 (GTP-CH1) in mammary glands was significantly upregulated at day 21. This change appeared to lead to an upregulation in tyrosine hydroxylase and a downregulation in vascular endothelial growth factor receptor 2 (VEGFR2) in the mammary glands of 50-days rats. Rowell et al. (269) concluded that this unique developmental maturation leads to a new biochemical blueprint, whereby the mammary cells have reduced EGF signaling and VEGFR2, which renders the mature mammary gland less proliferative and less susceptible to cancer.

IS SOY CONTRAINDICATED FOR CERTAIN WOMEN?

Concern over the effects of isoflavones on breast cancer risk is based in part on the role of estrogen in the etiology of this disease and on data suggesting conventional hormone therapy increases risk (270). It is important to point out however that although epidemiologic and clinical trial (271) data show the combination of estrogen plus progestin increase risk, by itself estrogen has either no effect or only very slightly increases risk (231,272–275). The differing effects of estrogen and estrogen plus progestin may be relevant to soy isoflavones since they do not possess progestin activity (276).

Undoubtedly, the major finding cited in support of the concern that isoflavones are contraindicated for certain women is the previously discussed research showing that genistein stimulates the growth of existing mammary tumors in ovariectomized athymic mice implanted with MCF-7 cells (127,205,207). In contrast to the animal studies however, the human evidence does not support these findings.

Unlike conventional hormone therapy (277) neither soyfoods nor isoflavones increase breast tissue density (39,40,225), and four studies have found that isoflavones do not affect breast cell proliferation; these studies were conducted in healthy pre- (217) and postmenopausal (219) women and breast cancer patients (43,278). In addition, over a five-year period, neither soy protein nor isoflavone intake was associated with the disease-free survival of Chinese breast cancer patients, the majority of whom were estrogen-receptor positive (279).

Nevertheless, because the existing human data cannot be used to definitively refute the animal studies breast cancer patients should discuss any dietary changes involving soyfoods or isoflavone supplements with their primary health care practitioner. This having been said, the animal studies do indicate that any theoretical concern can be avoided by consuming unprocessed soyfoods (as opposed to processed soy) (200) or combining soy/isoflavones with flax (206) or lignans (207). Also, the isoflavonoid equol does not stimulate tumor growth in mice (201); thus, equol-containing foods, which are being developed, would also appear to avoid any theoretical concern (280).

OVERALL SUMMARY AND CONCLUSION

An impressive number of studies investigating the effects of soyfoods, soy protein, and isolated isoflavones on breast cancer risk have been conducted. The in vitro data clearly show that high concentrations of the isoflavone genistein inhibit the growth of hormone-dependent and independent breast cancer cells but there is considerable uncertainty as to whether such high concentrations are physiological relevant. The animal data generally suggest that when given prior to the administration of chemical carcinogens isoflavones inhibit mammary tumor development. In contrast, the epidemiologic data at best are only mildly supportive of soy intake being protective against breast cancer. And there is little to no evidence that soy intake favorably affects markers of breast cancer risk including serum estrogen levels, breast cell proliferation, and breast tissue density. Thus, when all of the evidence is considered it is not possible to conclude that adult soy intake reduces breast cancer risk. Further, given the number of studies already conducted, it is unlikely that in the foreseeable future, new research will be able to alter the current assessment.

While the evidence does not permit concluding that adult soy intake is protective against breast cancer there are intriguing animal and epidemiologic data indicating soy/isoflavone exposure during adolescence is markedly protective against breast cancer later in life. This hypothesis is consistent with evidence highlighting the important role of early life events in the etiology of breast cancer. Clearly, more research investigating the effects of early soy intake on breast cancer risk is warranted.

Finally, there is concern that isoflavones are contraindicated for breast cancer patients or women at high risk of this disease. This concern is based on work in mice showing that isoflavones and ISP stimulates the growth of existing tumors in ovariectomized nude mice. However, the available human data do not concur with these findings. Furthermore, to avoid any theoretical concern, women can use unprocessed soy products or combine flaxseed with soy or lignans with isoflavones.

REFERENCES

1. Messina M, Ho S, Alekel DL. Skeletal benefits of soy isoflavones: a review of the clinical trial and epidemiologic data. Curr Opin Clin Nutr Metab Care 2004; 7: 649–658.
2. Zhan S, Ho SC. Meta-analysis of the effects of soy protein containing isoflavones on the lipid profile. Am J Clin Nutr 2005; 81:397–408.
3. Desroches S, Mauger JF, Ausman LM, Lichtenstein AH, Lamarche B. Soy protein favorably affects LDL size independently of isoflavones in hypercholesterolemic men and women. J Nutr 2004; 134:574–579.
4. Steinberg FM, Guthrie NL, Villablanca AC, Kumar K, Murray MJ. Soy protein with isoflavones has favorable effects on endothelial function that are independent of lipid and antioxidant effects in healthy postmenopausal women. Am J Clin Nutr 2003; 78:123–130.
5. Cuevas AM, Irribarra VL, Castillo OA, Yanez MD, Germain AM. Isolated soy protein improves endothelial function in postmenopausal hypercholesterolemic women. Eur J Clin Nutr 2003; 57:889–894.
6. Wiseman H, O'Reilly JD, Adlercreutz H, Mallet AI, Bowey EA, Rowland IR, Sanders TA. Isoflavone phytoestrogens consumed in soy decrease F(2)-isoprostane concentrations and increase resistance of low-density lipoprotein to oxidation in humans. Am J Clin Nutr 2000; 72:395–400.
7. Zhang X, Shu XO, Gao YT, Yang G, Li Q, Li H, Jin F, Zheng W. Soy food consumption is associated with lower risk of coronary heart disease in Chinese women. J Nutr 2003; 133:2874–2878.
8. Food and Drug Administration. Food labeling, health claims, soy protein, and coronary heart disease. Fed Regist 1999; 57:699–733.
9. Messina M, Barnes S. The role of soy products in reducing risk of cancer. J Natl Cancer Inst 1991; 83:541–546.
10. Thomsen AR, Almstrup K, Nielsen JE, Sorensen IK, Petersen OW, Leffers H, Breinholt VM. Estrogenic effect of soy isoflavones on mammary gland morphogenesis and gene expression profile. Toxicol Sci 2006; 93: 357–368.
11. Sarkar FH, Li Y. Soy isoflavones and cancer prevention. Cancer Invest 2003; 21:744–757.

12. Brzezinski A, Adlercreutz H, Shaoul R, Rösler R, Shmueli A, Tanos V, Schenker JG. Short-term effect of phytoestrogen-rich diet on postmenopausal women. Menopause 1997; 4:89–94.
13. Diel P, Geis RB, Caldarelli A, Schmidt S, Leschowsky UL, Voss A, Vollmer G. The differential ability of the phytoestrogen genistein and of estradiol to induce uterine weight and proliferation in the rat is associated with a substance specific modulation of uterine gene expression. Mol Cell Endocrinol 2004; 221:21–32.
14. Yildiz MF, Kumru S, Godekmerdan A, Kutlu S. Effects of raloxifene, hormone therapy, and soy isoflavone on serum high-sensitive C-reactive protein in postmenopausal women. Int J Gynaecol Obstet 2005; 90:128–133.
15. Nelson HD, Vesco KK, Haney E, Fu R, Nedrow A, Miller J, Nicolaidis C, Walker M, Humphrey L. Nonhormonal therapies for menopausal hot flashes: systematic review and meta-analysis. JAMA 2006; 295:2057–2071.
16. Messina M, Hughes C. Efficacy of soyfoods and soybean isoflavone supplements for alleviating menopausal symptoms is positively related to initial hot flush frequency. J Med Food 2003; 6:1–11.
17. Williamson-Hughes PS, Flickinger BD, Messina MJ, Empie MW. Isoflavone supplements containing predominantly genistein reduce hot flash symptoms: a critical review of published studies. Menopause 2006; 13:831–839.
18. Howes LG, Howes JB, Knight DC. Isoflavone therapy for menopausal flushes: a systematic review and meta-analysis. Maturitas 2006; 55:203–211.
19. Zhou JR, Mukherjee P, Gugger ET, Tanaka T, Blackburn GL, Clinton SK. Inhibition of murine bladder tumorigenesis by soy isoflavones via alterations in the cell cycle, apoptosis, and angiogenesis. Cancer Res 1998; 58:5231–5238.
20. Zhou JR, Yu L, Zhong Y, Blackburn GL. Soy phytochemicals and tea bioactive components synergistically inhibit androgen-sensitive human prostate tumors in mice. J Nutr 2003; 133:516–521.
21. Hillman GG, Wang Y, Che M, Raffoul JJ, Yudelev M, Kucuk O, Sarkar FH. Progression of renal cell carcinoma is inhibited by genistein and radiation in an orthotopic model. BMC Cancer 2007; 7:4.
22. Pisani P, Bray F, Parkin DM. Estimates of the world-wide prevalence of cancer for 25 sites in the adult population. Int J Cancer 2002; 97:72–81.
23. Folman Y, Pope GS. The interaction in the immature mouse of potent oestrogens with coumestrol, genistein and other utero-vaginotrophic compounds of low potency. J Endocrinol 1966; 34:215–225.
24. Lee HP, Gourley L, Duffy SW, Esteve J, Lee J, Day NE. Dietary effects on breast-cancer risk in Singapore. Lancet 1991; 337:1197–2000.
25. Barnes S, Grubbs C, Setchell KD, Carlson J. Soybeans inhibit mammary tumors in models of breast cancer. Prog Clin Biol Res 1990; 347:239–253.
26. Yan L, Spitznagel E. A meta-analysis of soyfoods and risk of breast cancer in women. Int J Can Prev 2005; 1:281–293.
27. Trock BJ, Hilakivi-Clarke L, Clarke R. Meta-analysis of soy intake and breast cancer risk. J Natl Cancer Inst 2006; 98:459–471.
28. Messina MJ, Loprinzi CL. Soy for breast cancer survivors: a critical review of the literature. J Nutr 2001; 131:3095S–108S.
29. Magee PJ, Rowland IR. Phyto-oestrogens, their mechanism of action: current evidence for a role in breast and prostate cancer. Br J Nutr 2004; 91:513–531.
30. Yan L, Li D, Yee JA. Dietary supplementation with isolated soy protein reduces metastasis of mammary carcinoma cells in mice. Clin Exp Metastasis 2002; 19: 535–540.
31. Constantinou AI, Lantvit D, Hawthorne M, Xu X, van Breemen RB, Pezzuto JM. Chemopreventive effects of soy protein and purified soy isoflavones on DMBA-induced mammary tumors in female Sprague-Dawley rats. Nutr Cancer 2001; 41:75–81.
32. Shao ZM, Wu J, Shen ZZ, Barsky SH. Genistein exerts multiple suppressive effects on human breast carcinoma cells. Cancer Res 1998; 58:4851–4857.
33. Zhou JR, Yu L, Mai Z, Blackburn GL. Combined inhibition of estrogen-dependent human breast carcinoma by soy and tea bioactive components in mice. Int J Cancer 2004; 108:8–14.
34. Gallo D, Ferlini C, Fabrizi M, Prislei S, Scambia G. Lack of stimulatory activity of a phytoestrogen-containing soy extract on the growth of breast cancer tumors in mice. Carcinogenesis 2006; 27:1404–1409.
35. Cohen LA, Zhao Z, Pittman B, Scimeca JA. Effect of intact and isoflavone-depleted soy protein on NMU-induced rat mammary tumorigenesis. Carcinogenesis 2000; 21: 929–935.
36. Day JK, Besch-Williford C, McMann TR, Hufford MG, Lubahn DB, MacDonald RS. Dietary genistein increased DMBA-induced mammary adenocarcinoma in wild-type, but not ER alpha KO, mice. Nutr Cancer 2001; 39:226–232.
37. Thomsen AR, Mortensen A, Breinholt VM, Lindecrona RH, Penalvo JL, Sorensen IK. Influence of Prevastein(R), an Isoflavone-Rich Soy Product, on Mammary Gland Development and Tumorigenesis in Tg.NK (MMTV/c-neu) Mice. Nutr Cancer 2005; 52:176–188.
38. Allred CD, Allred KF, Ju YH, Clausen LM, Doerge DR, Schantz SL, Korol DL, Wallig MA, Helferich WG. Dietary genistein results in larger MNU-induced, estrogen-dependent mammary tumors following ovariectomy of Sprague-Dawley rats. Carcinogenesis 2004; 25: 211–218.
39. Atkinson C, Warren RM, Sala E, Dowsett M, Dunning AM, Healey CS, Runswick S, Day NE, Bingham SA. Red-clover-derived isoflavones and mammographic breast density: a double-blind, randomized, placebo-controlled trial. Breast Cancer Res 2004; 6:R170–R179.
40. Maskarinec G, Takata Y, Franke AA, Williams AE, Murphy SP. A 2-year soy intervention in premenopausal women does not change mammographic densities. J Nutr 2004; 134:3089–3094.
41. Kurzer MS. Hormonal effects of soy in premenopausal women and men. J Nutr 2002; 132:570S–573S.
42. Maskarinec G, Franke AA, Williams AE, Hebshi S, Oshiro C, Murphy S, Stanczyk FZ. Effects of a 2-year randomized soy intervention on sex hormone levels in premenopausal women. Cancer Epidemiol Biomarkers Prev 2004; 13:1736–1744.

43. Palomares MR, Hopper L, Goldstein L, Lehman CD, Storer BE, Gralow JR. Effect of soy isoflavones on breast proliferation in postmenopausal breast cancer survivors. Breast Cancer Res Treat 2004; 88(suppl 1):4002.
44. Brown BD, Thomas W, Hutchins A, Martini MC, Slavin JL. Types of dietary fat and soy minimally affect hormones and biomarkers associated with breast cancer risk in premenopausal women. Nutr Cancer 2002; 43:22–30.
45. Whitsett TG Jr., Lamartiniere CA. Genistein and resveratrol: mammary cancer chemoprevention and mechanisms of action in the rat. Expert Rev Anticancer Ther 2006; 6:1699–1706.
46. Ajiki W, Tsukuma H, Oshima A. Cancer incidence and incidence rates in Japan in 1999: estimates based on data from 11 population-based cancer registries. Jpn J Clin Oncol 2004; 34:352–356.
47. Messina M, McCaskill-Stevens W, Lampe JW. Addressing the soy and breast cancer relationship: review, commentary, and workshop proceedings. J Natl Cancer Inst 2006; 98: 1275–1284.
48. Kushi LH, Byers T, Doyle C, Bandera EV, McCullough M, Gansler T, Andrews KS, Thun MJ. American Cancer Society Guidelines on nutrition and physical activity for cancer prevention: reducing the risk of cancer with healthy food choices and physical activity. CA Cancer J Clin 2006; 56:254–281; quiz 313–314.
49. Doyle C, Kushi LH, Byers T, Courneya KS, Demark-Wahnefried W, Grant B, McTiernan A, Rock CL, Thompson C, Gansler T, Andrews KS. Nutrition and physical activity during and after cancer treatment: an American Cancer Society guide for informed choices. CA Cancer J Clin 2006; 56:323–353.
50. Horn-Ross PL, John EM, Canchola AJ, Stewart SL, Lee MM. Phytoestrogen intake and endometrial cancer risk. J Natl Cancer Inst 2003; 95:1158–1164.
51. Goodman-Gruen D, Kritz-Silverstein D. Usual dietary isoflavone intake is associated with cardiovascular disease risk factors in postmenopausal women. J Nutr 2001; 131: 1202–1206.
52. FDA. 2004Q-0151: Qualified Health Claim (QHC): Soy Protein and Cancer. Available at: http://www.fda.gov/ohrms/dockets/dockets/04q0151/04q0151.htm.
53. de Kleijn MJ, van der Schouw YT, Wilson PW, Adlercreutz H, Mazur W, Grobbee DE, Jacques PF. Intake of dietary phytoestrogens is low in postmenopausal women in the United States: the Framingham study (1-4). J Nutr 2001; 131:1826–1832.
54. van Erp-Baart MA, Brants HA, Kiely M, Mulligan A, Turrini A, Sermoneta C, Kilkkinen A, Valsta LM. Isoflavone intake in four different European countries: the VENUS approach. Br J Nutr 2003; 89(suppl 1):S25–S30.
55. van der Schouw YT, Kreijkamp-Kaspers S, Peeters PH, Keinan-Boker L, Rimm EB, Grobbee DE. Prospective study on usual dietary phytoestrogen intake and cardiovascular disease risk in Western women. Circulation 2005; 111:465–471.
56. Boker LK, Van der Schouw YT, De Kleijn MJ, Jacques PF, Grobbee DE, Peeters PH. Intake of dietary phytoestrogens by Dutch women. J Nutr 2002; 132:1319–1328.
57. Umpress ST, Murphy SP, Franke AA, Custer LJ, Blitz CL. Isoflavone content of foods with soy additives. J Food Compost Anal 2005; 18:533–550.
58. Murphy PA, Song T, Buseman G, Barua K, Beecher GR, Trainer D, Holden J. Isoflavones in retail and institutional soy foods. J Agric Food Chem 1999; 47:2697–2704.
59. Messina M, Nagata C, Wu AH. Estimated Asian adult soy protein and isoflavone intakes. Nutr Cancer 2006; 55: 1–12.
60. Wang H-J, Murphy PA. Isoflavone composition of American and Japanese soybeans in Iowa: effects of variety, crop year, and location. J Agric Food Chem 1994; 42:1674–1677.
61. Eldridge AC, Kwolek WF. Soybean isoflavones: effects of environment and variety on composition. J Agric Food Chem 1983; 31:394–396.
62. Tsukamoto C, Shimada S, Igita K, Kudou S, Kokubun M, Okubo K, Kitamura K. Factors affecting isoflavone content in soybean seeds: changes in isoflavones, saponins, and composition of fatty acids at different temperatures during seed development. J Agric Food Chem 1995; 43:1184–1192.
63. Carrão-Panizzi MC, Kitamura K. Isoflavone content in Brazilian soybean cultivars. Breed Sci 1995; 45: 295–300.
64. Setchell KD, Cole SJ. Variations in isoflavone levels in soy foods and soy protein isolates and issues related to isoflavone databases and food labeling. J Agric Food Chem 2003; 51:4146–4155.
65. Ribeiro MLL, Mandarino JMG, Carrao-Panizzi MC, de Oliveira MCN, Campo CBH, Nepomuceno AL, Ida EI. Isoflavone content and B-glucosidase activity in soybean cultivars of different maturity groups. J Food Compost Anal 2007; 20:19–24.
66. Wang H-J, Murphy PA. Mass balance study of isoflavones during soybean processing. J Agric Food Chem 1996; 44: 2377–2383.
67. Mathias K, Ismail B, Corvalan CM, Hayes KD. Heat and pH effects on the conjugated forms of genistin and daidzin isoflavones. J Agric Food Chem 2006; 54:7495–7502.
68. Stintzing FC, Hoffmann M, Carle R. Thermal degradation kinetics of isoflavone aglycones from soy and red clover. Mol Nutr Food Res 2006; 50:373–377.
69. Coward L, Smith M, Kirk M, Barnes S. Chemical modification of isoflavones in soyfoods during cooking and processing. Am J Clin Nutr 1998; 68:1486S–1491S.
70. Pinto Mda S, Lajolo FM, Genovese MI. Effect of storage temperature and water activity on the content and profile of isoflavones, antioxidant activity, and in vitro protein digestibility of soy protein isolates and defatted soy flours. J Agric Food Chem 2005; 53:6340–6346.
71. Eisenstein J, Roberts SB, Dallal G, Saltzman E. High-protein weight-loss diets: are they safe and do they work? A review of the experimental and epidemiologic data. Nutr Rev 2002; 60:189–200.
72. Kuiper GG, Carlsson B, Grandien K, Enmark E, Haggblad J, Nilsson S, Gustafsson JA. Comparison of the ligand binding specificity and transcript tissue distribution of estrogen receptors alpha and beta. Endocrinology 1997; 138:863–870.

73. Kuiper GG, Lemmen JG, Carlsson B, Corton JC, Safe SH, van der Saag PT, van der Burg B, Gustafsson JA. Interaction of estrogenic chemicals and phytoestrogens with estrogen receptor beta. Endocrinology 1998; 139:4252–4263.
74. Naciff JM, Jump ML, Torontali SM, Carr GJ, Tiesman JP, Overmann GJ, Daston GP. Gene expression profile induced by 17alpha-ethynyl estradiol, bisphenol A, and genistein in the developing female reproductive system of the rat. Toxicol Sci 2002; 68:184–199.
75. Teede HJ, Dalais FS, McGrath BP. Dietary soy containing phytoestrogens does not have detectable estrogenic effects on hepatic protein synthesis in postmenopausal women. Am J Clin Nutr 2004; 79:396–401.
76. D'Anna R, Baviera G, Corrado F, Cancellieri F, Crisafulli A, Squadrito F. The effect of the phytoestrogen genistein and hormone replacement therapy on homocysteine and C-reactive protein level in postmenopausal women. Acta Obstet Gynecol Scand 2005; 84:474–477.
77. An J, Tzagarakis-Foster C, Scharschmidt TC, Lomri N, Leitman DC. Estrogen receptor beta-selective transcriptional activity and recruitment of coregulators by phytoestrogens. J Biol Chem 2001; 276:17808–17814.
78. Margeat E, Bourdoncle A, Margueron R, Poujol N, Cavailles V, Royer C. Ligands differentially modulate the protein interactions of the human estrogen receptors alpha and beta. J Mol Biol 2003; 326:77–92.
79. Kostelac D, Rechkemmer G, Briviba K. Phytoestrogens modulate binding response of estrogen receptors alpha and beta to the estrogen response element. J Agric Food Chem 2003; 51:7632–7635.
80. Strom A, Hartman J, Foster JS, Kietz S, Wimalasena J, Gustafsson JA. Estrogen receptor β inhibits 17β-estradiol-stimulated proliferation of the breast cancer cell line T47D. Proc Natl Acad Sci U S A 2004; 101: 1566–1571.
81. Park BW, Kim KS, Heo MK, Ko SS, Hong SW, Yang WI, Kim JH, Kim GE, Lee KS. Expression of estrogen receptor-beta in normal mammary and tumor tissues: is it protective in breast carcinogenesis? Breast Cancer Res Treat 2003; 80:79–85.
82. Mak P, Leung YK, Tang WY, Harwood C, Ho SM. Apigenin suppresses cancer cell growth through ERbeta. Neoplasia 2006; 8:896–904.
83. Constantinou A, Huberman E. Genistein as an inducer of tumor cell differentiation: possible mechanisms of action. Proc Soc Exp Biol Med 1995; 208:109–115.
84. Rowland I, Faughnan M, Hoey L, Wahala K, Williamson G, Cassidy A. Bioavailability of phyto-oestrogens. Br J Nutr 2003; 89(suppl 1):S45–S58.
85. Walle T, Browning AM, Steed LL, Reed SG, Walle UK. Flavonoid glucosides are hydrolyzed and thus activated in the oral cavity in humans. J Nutr 2005; 135:48–52.
86. Xu X, Harris KS, Wang HJ, Murphy PA, Hendrich S. Bioavailability of soybean isoflavones depends upon gut microflora in women. J Nutr 1995; 125:2307–2315.
87. Xu X, Wang HJ, Murphy PA, Cook L, Hendrich S. Daidzein is a more bioavailable soymilk isoflavone than is genistein in adult women. J Nutr 1994; 124:825–832.
88. Adlercreutz H, Fotsis T, Lampe J, Wahala K, Makela T, Brunow G, Hase T. Quantitative determination of lignans and isoflavonoids in plasma of omnivorous and vegetarian women by isotope dilution gas chromatography-mass spectrometry. Scand J Clin Lab Invest Suppl 1993; 215:5–18.
89. Griffiths K, Denis L, Turkes A, Morton MS. Phytoestrogens and diseases of the prostate gland. Baillieres Clin Endocrinol Metab 1998; 12:625–647.
90. Yamada T, Strong JP, Ishii T, Ueno T, Koyama M, Wagayama H, Shimizu A, Sakai T, Malcom GT, Guzman MA. Atherosclerosis and w-3 fatty acids in the populations of a fishing village and a farming village in Japan. Atherosclerosis 2000; 153:469–481.
91. Setchell KD, Brown NM, Desai P, Zimmer-Nechemias L, Wolfe BE, Brashear WT, Kirschner AS, Cassidy A, Heubi JE. Bioavailability of pure isoflavones in healthy humans and analysis of commercial soy isoflavone supplements. J Nutr 2001; 131:1362S–1375S.
92. Gu L, House SE, Prior RL, Fang N, Ronis MJ, Clarkson TB, Wilson ME, Badger TM. Metabolic phenotype of isoflavones differ among female rats, pigs, monkeys, and women. J Nutr 2006; 136:1215–1221.
93. Wiseman H, Casey K, Bowey EA, Duffy R, Davies M, Rowland IR, Lloyd AS, Murray A, Thompson R, Clarke DB. Influence of 10 wk of soy consumption on plasma concentrations and excretion of isoflavonoids and on gut microflora metabolism in healthy adults. Am J Clin Nutr 2004; 80:692–699.
94. Setchell KD, Brown NM, Lydeking-Olsen E. The clinical importance of the metabolite equol-a clue to the effectiveness of soy and its isoflavones. J Nutr 2002; 132: 3577–3584.
95. Lampe JW. Isoflavonoid and lignan phytoestrogens as dietary biomarkers. J Nutr 2003; 133(suppl 3):956S–964S.
96. Watanabe S, Yamaguchi M, Sobue T, Takahashi T, Miura T, Arai Y, Mazur W, Wahala K, Adlercreutz H. Pharmacokinetics of soybean isoflavones in plasma, urine and feces of men after ingestion of 60 g baked soybean powder (kinako). J Nutr 1998; 128:1710–1715.
97. Arai Y, Uehara M, Sato Y, Kimira M, Eboshida A, Adlercreutz H, Watanabe S. Comparison of isoflavones among dietary intake, plasma concentration and urinary excretion for accurate estimation of phytoestrogen intake. J Epidemiol 2000; 10:127–135.
98. Akaza H, Miyanaga N, Takashima N, Naito S, Hirao Y, Tsukamoto T, Fujioka T, Mori M, Kim WJ, Song JM, Pantuck AJ. Comparisons of percent equol producers between prostate cancer patients and controls: case-controlled studies of isoflavones in Japanese, Korean and American residents. Jpn J Clin Oncol 2004; 34:86–89.
99. Setchell KD, Cole SJ. Method of defining equol-producer status and its frequency among vegetarians. J Nutr 2006; 136:2188–2193.
100. Nagata C, Shimizu H, Takami R, Hayashi M, Takeda N, Yasuda K. Soy product intake is inversely associated with serum homocysteine level in premenopausal Japanese women. J Nutr 2003; 133:797–800.

101. Nagata C, Takatsuka N, Kurisu Y, Shimizu H. Decreased serum total cholesterol concentration is associated with high intake of soy products in Japanese men and women. J Nutr 1998; 128:209–213.
102. Nagata C, Takatsuka N, Kawakami N, Shimizu H. Association of diet with the onset of menopause in Japanese women. Am J Epidemiol 2000; 152:863–867.
103. Nagata C, Takatsuka N, Kawakami N, Shimizu H. A prospective cohort study of soy product intake and stomach cancer death. Br J Cancer 2002; 87:31–36.
104. Akiyama T, Ishida J, Nakagawa S, Ogawara H, Watanabe S, Itoh N, Shibuya M, Fukami Y. Genistein, a specific inhibitor of tyrosine-specific protein kinases. J Biol Chem 1987; 262:5592–5595.
105. Akiyama T, Ogawara H. Use and specificity of genistein as inhibitor of protein-tyrosine kinases. Methods Enzymol 1991; 201:362–370.
106. Hunter T, Cooper JA. Protein-tyrosine kinases. Annu Rev Biochem 1985; 54:897–930.
107. Messina MJ, Persky V, Setchell KD, Barnes S. Soy intake and cancer risk: a review of the in vitro and in vivo data. Nutr Cancer 1994; 21:113–131.
108. Adlercreutz H, Mazur W. Phyto-oestrogens and Western diseases. Ann Med 1997; 29:95–120.
109. Peterson G, Barnes S. Genistein inhibition of the growth of human breast cancer cells: independence from estrogen receptors and the multi-drug resistance gene. Biochem Biophys Res Commun 1991; 179:661–667.
110. Pagliacci MC, Spinozzi F, Migliorati G, Fumi G, Smacchia M, Grignani F, Riccardi C, Nicoletti I. Genistein inhibits tumour cell growth in vitro but enhances mitochondrial reduction of tetrazolium salts: a further pitfall in the use of the MTT assay for evaluating cell growth and survival. Eur J Cancer 1993; 29A:1573–1577.
111. Barnes S, Peterson TG. Biochemical targets of the isoflavone genistein in tumor cell lines. Proc Soc Exp Biol Med 1995; 208:103–108.
112. Constantinou A, Kiguchi K, Huberman E. Induction of differentiation and DNA strand breakage in human HL-60 and K-562 leukemia cells by genistein. Cancer Res 1990; 50:2618–2624.
113. Kim H, Peterson TG, Barnes S. Mechanisms of action of the soy isoflavone genistein: emerging role for its effects via transforming growth factor beta signaling pathways. Am J Clin Nutr 1998; 68:1418S–1425S.
114. Conklin CM, Bechberger JF, Macfabe D, Guthrie N, Kurowska EM, Naus CC. Genistein and quercetin increase connexin43 and suppress growth of breast cancer cells. Carcinogenesis 2007; 28:93–100.
115. Lau TY, Leung LK. Soya isoflavones suppress phorbol 12-myristate 13-acetate-induced COX-2 expression in MCF-7 cells. Br J Nutr 2006; 96:169–176.
116. Tominaga Y, Wang A, Wang RH, Wang X, Cao L, Deng CX. Genistein inhibits Brca1 mutant tumor growth through activation of DNA damage checkpoints, cell cycle arrest, and mitotic catastrophe. Cell Death Differ 2007; 14(3):472–479.
117. Duncan RE, El-Sohemy A, Archer MC. Regulation of HMG-CoA reductase in MCF-7 cells by genistein, EPA, and DHA, alone and in combination with mevastatin. Cancer Lett 2005; 224:221–228.
118. Chen WF, Huang MH, Tzang CH, Yang M, Wong MS. Inhibitory actions of genistein in human breast cancer (MCF-7) cells. Biochim Biophys Acta 2003; 1638:187–196.
119. Chinni SR, Alhasan SA, Multani AS, Pathak S, Sarkar FH. Pleotropic effects of genistein on MCF-7 breast cancer cells. Int J Mol Med 2003; 12:29–34.
120. Li Y, Ahmed F, Ali S, Philip PA, Kucuk O, Sarkar FH. Inactivation of nuclear factor κB by soy isoflavone genistein contributes to increased apoptosis induced by chemotherapeutic agents in human cancer cells. Cancer Res 2005; 65:6934–6942.
121. Singletary K, Ellington A. Genistein suppresses proliferation and MET oncogene expression and induces EGR-1 tumor suppressor expression in immortalized human breast epithelial cells. Anticancer Res 2006; 26:1039–1048.
122. Mitropoulou TN, Tzanakakis GN, Nikitovic D, Tsatsakis A, Karamanos NK. In vitro effects of genistein on the synthesis and distribution of glycosaminoglycans/proteoglycans by estrogen receptor-positive and -negative human breast cancer epithelial cells. Anticancer Res 2002; 22:2841–2846.
123. Po LS, Wang TT, Chen ZY, Leung LK. Genistein-induced apoptosis in MCF-7 cells involves changes in Bak and Bcl-x without evidence of anti-oestrogenic effects. Br J Nutr 2002; 88:463–469.
124. Frey RS, Li J, Singletary KW. Effects of genistein on cell proliferation and cell cycle arrest in nonneoplastic human mammary epithelial cells: involvement of Cdc2, p21(waf/cip1), p27(kip1), and Cdc25C expression. Biochem Pharmacol 2001; 61:979–989.
125. Upadhyay S, Neburi M, Chinni SR, Alhasan S, Miller F, Sarkar FH. Differential sensitivity of normal and malignant breast epithelial cells to genistein is partly mediated by p21 (WAF1). Clin Cancer Res 2001; 7:1782–1789.
126. Fioravanti L, Cappelletti V, Miodini P, Ronchi E, Brivio M, Di Fronzo G. Genistein in the control of breast cancer cell growth: insights into the mechanism of action in vitro. Cancer Lett 1998; 130:143–152.
127. Hsieh CY, Santell RC, Haslam SZ, Helferich WG. Estrogenic effects of genistein on the growth of estrogen receptor-positive human breast cancer (MCF-7) cells in vitro and in vivo. Cancer Res 1998; 58:3833–3838.
128. Le Bail JC, Champavier Y, Chulia AJ, Habrioux G. Effects of phytoestrogens on aromatase, 3beta and 17beta-hydroxysteroid dehydrogenase activities and human breast cancer cells. Life Sci 2000; 66:1281–1291.
129. Power KA, Thompson LU. Ligand-induced regulation of ERalpha and ERbeta is indicative of human breast cancer cell proliferation. Breast Cancer Res Treat 2003; 81:209–221.
130. Miodini P, Fioravanti L, Di Fronzo G, Cappelletti V. The two phyto-oestrogens genistein and quercetin exert different effects on oestrogen receptor function. Br J Cancer 1999; 80:1150–1155.
131. Zava DT, Duwe G. Estrogenic and antiproliferative properties of genistein and other flavonoids in human breast cancer cells in vitro. Nutr Cancer 1997; 27:31–40.
132. Pagliacci MC, Smacchia M, Migliorati G, Grignani F, Riccardi C, Nicoletti I. Growth-inhibitory effects of the

natural phyto-oestrogen genistein in MCF-7 human breast cancer cells. Eur J Cancer 1994; 11:1675–1682.

133. Peterson G, Barnes S. Genistein inhibits both estrogen and growth factor-stimulated proliferation of human breast cancer cells. Cell Growth Differ 1996; 7:1345–1351.

134. Shao ZM, Shen ZZ, Fontana JA, Barsky SH. Genistein's "ER-dependent and independent" actions are mediated through ER pathways in ER-positive breast carcinoma cell lines. Anticancer Res 2000; 20:2409–2416.

135. Twaddle GM, Turbov J, Liu N, Murthy S. Tyrosine kinase inhibitors as antiproliferative agents against an estrogen-dependent breast cancer cell line in vitro. J Surg Oncol 1999; 70:83–90.

136. Li Y, Bhuiyan M, Sarkar FH. Induction of apoptosis and inhibition of c-erbB-2 in MDA-MB-435 cells by genistein. Int J Oncol 1999; 15:525–533.

137. Shen F, Xue X, Weber G. Tamoxifen and genistein synergistically downregulate signal transduction and proliferation in estrogen receptor-negative human breast carcinoma MDA-MB-435 cells. Anticancer Res 1999; 19:1657–1662.

138. Leung LK, Wang TT. Bcl-2 is not reduced in the death of MCF-7 cells at low genistein concentration. J Nutr 2000; 130:2922–2926.

139. Lin HM, Moon BK, Yu F, Kim HR. Galectin-3 mediates genistein-induced G(2)/M arrest and inhibits apoptosis. Carcinogenesis 2000; 21:1941–1945.

140. Soule HD, Vazguez J, Long A, Albert S, Brennan M. A human cell line from a pleural effusion derived from a breast carcinoma. J Natl Cancer Inst 1973; 51:1409–1416.

141. Santell RC, Kieu N, Helferich WG. Genistein inhibits growth of estrogen-independent human breast cancer cells in culture but not in athymic mice. J Nutr 2000; 130:1665–1669.

142. Seo HS, DeNardo DG, Jacquot Y, Laios I, Vidal DS, Zambrana CR, Leclercq G, Brown PH. Stimulatory effect of genistein and apigenin on the growth of breast cancer cells correlates with their ability to activate ER alpha. Breast Cancer Res Treat 2006; 99:121–134.

143. Han D, Tachibana H, Yamada K. Inhibition of environmental estrogen-induced proliferation of human breast carcinoma MCF-7 cells by flavonoids. In Vitro Cell Dev Biol Anim 2001; 37:275–282.

144. Han DH, Denison MS, Tachibana H, Yamada K. Relationship between estrogen receptor-binding and estrogenic activities of environmental estrogens and suppression by flavonoids. Biosci Biotechnol Biochem 2002; 66:1479–1487.

145. Wang C, Kurzer MS. Effects of phytoestrogens on DNA synthesis in MCF-7 cells in the presence of estradiol or growth factors. Nutr Cancer 1998; 31:90–100.

146. Geisler J, Detre S, Berntsen H, Ottestad L, Lindtjorn B, Dowsett M, Einstein Lonning P. Influence of neoadjuvant anastrozole (Arimidex) on intratumoral estrogen levels and proliferation markers in patients with locally advanced breast cancer. Clin Cancer Res 2001; 7:1230–1236.

147. Geisler J. Breast cancer tissue estrogens and their manipulation with aromatase inhibitors and inactivators. J Steroid Biochem Mol Biol 2003; 86:245–253.

148. Barnes S. Effect of genistein on in vitro and in vivo models of cancer. J Nutr 1995; 125:777S–783S.

149. Peterson TG, Coward L, Kirk M, Falany CN, Barnes S. The role of metabolism in mammary epithelial cell growth inhibition by the isoflavones genistein and biochanin A. Carcinogenesis 1996; 17:1861–1869.

150. Nebe B, Peters A, Duske K, Richter DU, Briese V. Influence of phytoestrogens on the proliferation and expression of adhesion receptors in human mammary epithelial cells in vitro. Eur J Cancer Prev 2006; 15:405–415.

151. Nguyen DT, Hernandez-Montes E, Vauzour D, Schonthal AH, Rice-Evans C, Cadenas E, Spencer JP. The intracellular genistein metabolite 5,7,3′,4′-tetrahydroxy-isoflavone mediates G2-M cell cycle arrest in cancer cells via modulation of the p38 signaling pathway. Free Radic Biol Med 2006; 41:1225–1239.

152. Folkman J. Role of angiogenesis in tumor growth and metastasis. Semin Oncol 2002; 29:15–18.

153. Belperio JA, Keane MP, Arenberg DA, Addison CL, Ehlert JE, Burdick MD, Strieter RM. CXC chemokines in angiogenesis. J Leukoc Biol 2000; 68:1–8.

154. Crowther M, Brown NJ, Bishop ET, Lewis CE. Microenvironmental influence on macrophage regulation of angiogenesis in wounds and malignant tumors. J Leukoc Biol 2001; 70:478–490.

155. Toi M, Bando H, Ogawa T, Muta M, Hornig C, Weich HA. Significance of vascular endothelial growth factor (VEGF)/soluble VEGF receptor-1 relationship in breast cancer. Int J Cancer 2002; 98:14–18.

156. Gasparini G. Prognostic value of vascular endothelial growth factor in breast cancer. Oncologist 2000; 5(suppl 1):37–44.

157. Linderholm B, Lindh B, Tavelin B, Grankvist K, Henriksson R. p53 and vascular-endothelial-growth-factor (VEGF) expression predicts outcome in 833 patients with primary breast carcinoma. Int J Cancer 2000; 89:51–62.

158. Eppenberger U, Kueng W, Schlaeppi JM, Roesel JL, Benz C, Mueller H, Matter A, Zuber M, Luescher K, Litschgi M, Schmitt M, Foekens JA, Eppenberger-Castori S. Markers of tumor angiogenesis and proteolysis independently define high- and low-risk subsets of node-negative breast cancer patients. J Clin Oncol 1998; 16:3129–3136.

159. Fotsis T, Pepper M, Adlercreutz H, Fleischmann G, Hase T, Montesano R, Schweigerer L. Genistein, a dietary-derived inhibitor of in vitro angiogenesis. Proc Natl Acad Sci U S A 1993; 90:2690–2694.

160. Fotsis T, Pepper MS, Aktas E, Breit S, Rasku S, Adlercreutz H, Wahala K, Montesano R, Schweigerer L. Flavonoids, dietary-derived inhibitors of cell proliferation and in vitro angiogenesis. Cancer Res 1997; 57:2916–2921.

161. Piao M, Mori D, Satoh T, Sugita Y, Tokunaga O. Inhibition of endothelial cell proliferation, in vitro angiogenesis, and the downregulation of cell adhesion-related genes by genistein. Combined with a cDNA microarray analysis. Endothelium 2006; 13:249–266.

162. Su SJ, Yeh TM, Chuang WJ, Ho CL, Chang KL, Cheng HL, Liu HS, Hsu PY, Chow NH. The novel targets for anti-angiogenesis of genistein on human cancer cells. Biochem Pharmacol 2005; 69:307–318.

163. Scholar EM, Toews ML. Inhibition of invasion of murine mammary carcinoma cells by the tyrosine kinase inhibitor genistein. Cancer Lett 1994; 87:159–162.
164. Magee PJ, McGlynn H, Rowland IR. Differential effects of isoflavones and lignans on invasiveness of MDA-MB-231 breast cancer cells in vitro. Cancer Lett 2004; 208: 35–41.
165. Kousidou OC, Mitropoulou TN, Roussidis AE, Kletsas D, Theocharis AD, Karamanos NK. Genistein suppresses the invasive potential of human breast cancer cells through transcriptional regulation of metalloproteinases and their tissue inhibitors. Int J Oncol 2005; 26:1101–1109.
166. Nakagawa H, Yamamoto D, Kiyozuka Y, Tsuta K, Uemura Y, Hioki K, Tsutsui Y, Tsubura A. Effects of genistein and synergistic action in combination with eicosapentaenoic acid on the growth of breast cancer cell lines. J Cancer Res Clin Oncol 2000; 126:448–454.
167. Sakamoto K. Synergistic effects of thearubigin and genistein on human prostate tumor cell (PC-3) growth via cell cycle arrest. Cancer Lett 2000; 151:103–109.
168. Mouria M, Gukovskaya AS, Jung Y, Buechler P, Hines OJ, Reber HA, Pandol SJ. Food-derived polyphenols inhibit pancreatic cancer growth through mitochondrial cytochrome C release and apoptosis. Int J Cancer 2002; 98:761–769.
169. Rao A, Woodruff RD, Wade WN, Kute TE, Cramer SD. Genistein and vitamin d synergistically inhibit human prostatic epithelial cell growth. J Nutr 2002; 132:3191–3194.
170. Fan S, Meng Q, Auborn K, Carter T, Rosen EM. BRCA1 and BRCA2 as molecular targets for phytochemicals indole-3-carbinol and genistein in breast and prostate cancer cells. Br J Cancer 2006; 94:407–426.
171. Swami S, Krishnan AV, Moreno J, Bhattacharyya RB, Peehl DM, Feldman D. Calcitriol and genistein actions to inhibit the prostaglandin pathway: potential combination therapy to treat prostate cancer. J Nutr 2007; 137:205S–210S.
172. Swami S, Krishnan AV, Peehl DM, Feldman D. Genistein potentiates the growth inhibitory effects of 1,25-dihydroxyvitamin D3 in DU145 human prostate cancer cells: role of the direct inhibition of CYP24 enzyme activity. Mol Cell Endocrinol 2005; 241:49–61.
173. So FV, Guthrie N, Chambers AF, Moussa M, Carroll KK. Inhibition of human breast cancer cell proliferation and delay of mammary tumorigenesis by flavonoids and citrus juices. Nutr Cancer 1996; 26:167–181.
174. Su SJ, Chow NH, Kung ML, Hung TC, Chang KL. Effects of soy isoflavones on apoptosis induction and G2-M arrest in human hepatoma cells involvement of caspase-3 activation, Bcl-2 and Bcl-XL downregulation, and Cdc2 kinase activity. Nutr Cancer 2003; 45:113–123.
175. Rice S, Mason HD, Whitehead SA. Phytoestrogens and their low dose combinations inhibit mRNA expression and activity of aromatase in human granulosa-luteal cells. J Steroid Biochem Mol Biol 2006; 101:216–225.
176. Kim H, Hall P, Smith M, Kirk M, Prasain JK, Barnes S, Grubbs C. Chemoprevention by grape seed extract and genistein in carcinogen-induced mammary cancer in rats is diet dependent. J Nutr 2004; 134: 3445S–3452S.
177. Hirsch K, Atzmon A, Danilenko M, Levy J, Sharoni Y. Lycopene and other carotenoids inhibit estrogenic activity of 17beta-estradiol and genistein in cancer cells. Breast Cancer Res Treat 2007; 104:221–230.
178. Kyle E, Neckers L, Takimoto C, Curt G, Bergan R. Genistein-induced apoptosis of prostate cancer cells is preceded by a specific decrease in focal adhesion kinase activity. Mol Pharmacol 1997; 51:193–200.
179. Mitchell JH, Duthie SJ, Collins AR. Effects of phytoestrogens on growth and DNA integrity in human prostate tumor cell lines: PC-3 and LNCaP. Nutr Cancer 2000; 38:223–228.
180. Peterson G, Barnes S. Genistein and biochanin A inhibit the growth of human prostate cancer cells but not epidermal growth factor receptor tyrosine autophosphorylation. Prostate 1993; 22:335–345.
181. Dalu A, Haskell JF, Coward L, Lamartiniere CA. Genistein, a component of soy, inhibits the expression of the EGF and ErbB2/Neu receptors in the rat dorsolateral prostate. Prostate 1998; 37:36–43.
182. Carroll KK. Experimental evidence of dietary factors and hormone-dependent cancers. Cancer Res 1975; 35:3374–3383.
183. Gridley DS, Kettering JD, Slater JM, Nutter RL. Modification of spontaneous mammary tumors in mice fed different sources of protein, fat and carbohydrate. Cancer Lett 1983; 19:133–146.
184. Baggott JE, Ha T, Vaughn WH, Juliana MM, Hardin JM, Grubbs CJ. Effect of miso (Japanese soybean paste) and NaCl on DMBA-induced rat mammary tumors. Nutr Cancer 1990; 14:103–109.
185. Mukhopadhyay S, Ballard BR, Mukherjee S, Kabir SM, Das SK. Beneficial effects of soy protein in the initiation and progression against dimethylbenz [a] anthracene-induced breast tumors in female rats. Mol Cell Biochem 2006; 290:169–176.
186. Gallo D, Giacomelli S, Cantelmo F, Zannoni GF, Ferrandina G, Fruscella E, Riva A, Morazzoni P, Bombardelli E, Mancuso S, Scambia G. Chemoprevention of DMBA-induced mammary cancer in rats by dietary soy. Breast Cancer Res Treat 2001; 69:153–164.
187. Manjanatha MG, Shelton S, Bishop ME, Lyn-Cook LE, Aidoo A. Dietary effects of soy isoflavones daidzein and genistein on 7,12-dimethylbenz[a]anthracene-induced mammary mutagenesis and carcinogenesis in ovariectomized Big Blue(R) transgenic rats. Carcinogenesis 2006; 27:2555–2564.
188. Constantinou AI, White BE, Tonetti D, Yang Y, Liang W, Li W, van Breemen RB. The soy isoflavone daidzein improves the capacity of tamoxifen to prevent mammary tumours. Eur J Cancer 2005; 41:647–654.
189. Hawrylewicz EJ, Huang HH, Blair WH. Dietary soybean isolate and methionine supplementation affect mammary tumor progression in rats. J Nutr 1991; 121:1693–1698.
190. Miki K, Al-Refaie W, Xu M, Jiang P, Tan Y, Bouvet M, Zhao M, Gupta A, Chishima T, Shimada H, Makuuchi M, Moossa AR, Hoffman RM. Methioninase gene therapy of human cancer cells is synergistic with recombinant methioninase treatment. Cancer Res 2000; 60:2696–2702.

191. Gotoh T, Yamada K, Ito A, Yin H, Kataoka T, Dohi K. Chemoprevention of N-nitroso-N-methylurea-induced rat mammary cancer by miso and tamoxifen, alone and in combination. Jpn J Cancer Res 1998; 89:487–495.
192. Gotoh T, Yamada K, Yin H, Ito A, Kataoka T, Dohi K. Chemoprevention of N-nitroso-N-methylurea-induced rat mammary carcinogenesis by soy foods or biochanin A. Jpn J Cancer Res 1998; 89:137–142.
193. Kijkuokool P, Parhar IS, Malaivijitnond S. Genistein enhances N-nitrosomethylurea-induced rat mammary tumorigenesis. Cancer Lett 2006; 242:53–59.
194. Hawrylewicz EJ, Zapata JJ, Blair WH. Soy and experimental cancer: animal studies. J Nutr 1995; 125:698S–708S.
195. Imrhan VL, Garner E, Radcliffe JD, Hsueh AM, Czajka-Narins D. Effects of two types of protein supplemented with retinyl acetate on mammary carcinogenesis in rats. Nutr Res 2000; 20:721–730.
196. Ueda M, Niho N, Imai T, Shibutani M, Mitsumori K, Matsui T, Hirose M. Lack of significant effects of genistein on the progression of 7,12-dimethylbenz(a)anthracene-induced mammary tumors in ovariectomized Sprague-Dawley rats. Nutr Cancer 2003; 47:141–147.
197. Hewitt AL, Singletary KW. Soy extract inhibits mammary adenocarcinoma growth in a syngeneic mouse model. Cancer Lett 2003; 192:133–143.
198. Allred CD, Ju YH, Allred KF, Chang J, Helferich WG. Dietary genistin stimulates growth of estrogen-dependent breast cancer tumors similar to that observed with genistein. Carcinogenesis 2001; 22:1667–1673.
199. Allred CD, Allred KF, Ju YH, Virant SM, Helferich WG. Soy diets containing varying amounts of genistein stimulate growth of estrogen-dependent (MCF-7) tumors in a dose-dependent manner. Cancer Res 2001; 61:5045–5050.
200. Allred CD, Allred KF, Ju YH, Goeppinger TS, Doerge DR, Helferich WG. Soy processing influences growth of estrogen-dependent breast cancer tumors. Carcinogenesis 2004; 25:1649–1657.
201. Ju YH, Fultz J, Allred KF, Doerge DR, Helferich WG. Effects of dietary daidzein and its metabolite, equol, at? physiological concentrations on the growth of estrogen-dependent human breast cancer (MCF-7) tumors implanted in ovariectomized athymic mice. Carcinogenesis 2006; 27:856–863.
202. Wood CE, Appt SE, Clarkson TB, Franke AA, Lees CJ, Doerge DR, Cline JM. Effects of high-dose soy isoflavones and equol on reproductive tissues in female cynomolgus monkeys. Biol Reprod 2006; 75(3): 477–486; [Epub May 24, 2006].
203. Allred CD, Twaddle NC, Allred KF, Goeppinger TS, Churchwell MI, Ju YH, Helferich WG, Doerge DR. Soy processing affects metabolism and disposition of dietary isoflavones in ovariectomized BALB/c mice. J Agric Food Chem 2005; 53:8542–8550.
204. Ju YH, Clausen LM, Allred KF, Almada AL, Helferich WG. beta-Sitosterol, beta-Sitosterol Glucoside, and a Mixture of beta-Sitosterol and beta-Sitosterol Glucoside Modulate the Growth of Estrogen-Responsive Breast Cancer Cells In Vitro and in Ovariectomized Athymic Mice. J Nutr 2004; 134:1145–1151.
205. Ju YH, Allred KF, Allred CD, Helferich WG. Genistein stimulates growth of human breast cancer cells in a novel, postmenopausal animal model, with low plasma estradiol concentrations. Carcinogenesis 2006; 27:1292–1299.
206. Saarinen NM, Power K, Chen J, Thompson LU. Flaxseed attenuates the tumor growth stimulating effect of soy protein in ovariectomized athymic mice with MCF-7 human breast cancer xenografts. Int J Cancer 2006; 119:925–931.
207. Power KA, Saarinen NM, Chen JM, Thompson LU. Mammalian lignans enterolactone and enterodiol, alone and in combination with the isoflavone genistein, do not promote the growth of MCF-7 xenografts in ovariectomized athymic nude mice. Int J Cancer 2006; 118:1316–1320.
208. Harrell JC, Dye WW, Allred DC, Jedlicka P, Spoelstra NS, Sartorius CA, Horwitz KB. Estrogen receptor positive breast cancer metastasis: altered hormonal sensitivity and tumor aggressiveness in lymphatic vessels and lymph nodes. Cancer Res 2006; 66:9308–9315.
209. Vantyghem SA, Wilson SM, Postenka CO, Al-Katib W, Tuck AB, Chambers AF. Dietary genistein reduces metastasis in a postsurgical orthotopic breast cancer model. Cancer Res 2005; 65:3396–3403.
210. Charland SL, Hui JW, Torosian MH. The effects of a soybean extract on tumor growth and metastasis. Int J Mol Med 1998; 2:225–228.
211. Farina HG, Pomies M, Alonso DF, Gomez DE. Antitumor and antiangiogenic activity of soy isoflavone genistein in mouse models of melanoma and breast cancer. Oncol Rep 2006; 16:885–891.
212. Hirose K, Tajima K, Hamajima N, Inoue M, Takezaki T, Kuroishi T, Yoshida M, Tokudome S. A large-scale, hospital-based case-control study of risk factors of breast cancer according to menopausal status. Jpn J Cancer Res 1995; 86:146–154.
213. Yuan JM, Wang QS, Ross RK, Henderson BE, Yu MC. Diet and breast cancer in Shanghai and Tianjin, China. Br J Cancer 1995; 71:1353–1358.
214. Messina M. Western soy intake is too low to produce health effects. Am J Clin Nutr 2004; 80:528–529.
215. Petrakis NL, Barnes S, King EB, Lowenstein J, Wiencke J, Lee MM, Miike R, Kirk M, Coward L. Stimulatory influence of soy protein isolate on breast secretion in pre- and postmenopausal women. Cancer Epidemiol Biomarkers Prev 1996; 5:785–794.
216. McMichael-Phillips DF, Harding C, Morton M, Roberts SA, Howell A, Potten CS, Bundred NJ. Effects of soy-protein supplementation on epithelial proliferation in the histologically normal human breast. Am J Clin Nutr 1998; 68:1431S–1435S.
217. Hargreaves DF, Potten CS, Harding C, Shaw LE, Morton MS, Roberts SA, Howell A, Bundred NJ. Two-week dietary soy supplementation has an estrogenic effect on normal premenopausal breast. J Clin Endocrinol Metab 1999; 84:4017–4024.
218. Kim J, Petz LN, Ziegler YS, Wood JR, Potthoff SJ, Nardulli AM. Regulation of the estrogen-responsive pS2 gene in MCF-7 human breast cancer cells. J Steroid Biochem Mol Biol 2000; 74:157–168.

219. Cheng G, Wilczek B, Warner M, Gustafsson JA, Landgren BM. Isoflavone treatment for acute menopausal symptoms. Menopause 2007; 14:468–471 (3 pt 1).
220. Conner P, Soderqvist G, Skoog L, Graser T, Walter F, Tani E, Carlstrom K, von Schoultz B. Breast cell proliferation in postmenopausal women during HRT evaluated through fine needle aspiration cytology. Breast Cancer Res Treat 2003; 78:159–165.
221. Balk E, Chung M, Chew P, Ip S, Raman G, Kuplenick B, Tatsioni A, Sun Y, Wolk B, DeVine D, Lua J. Effects of soy on health outcomes. Evidence report/technology assessment No. 126 (prepared by Tufts-New England Medical Center Evidence-based Practice Center under Contract No. 290-02-0022.) AHRQ Publication No. 05-E024-2. Rockville, MD Agency for Healthcare Research and Quality, July 2005.
222. Riza E, dos Santos Silva I, De Stavola B, Bradlow HL, Sepkovic DW, Linos D, Linos A. Urinary estrogen metabolites and mammographic parenchymal patterns in postmenopausal women. Cancer Epidemiol Biomarkers Prev 2001; 10:627–634.
223. Whelan EA, Sandler DP, Root JL, Smith KR, Weinberg CR. Menstrual cycle patterns and risk of breast cancer. Am J Epidemiol 1994; 140:1081–1090.
224. Cassidy A, Bingham S, Setchell KD. Biological effects of a diet of soy protein rich in isoflavones on the menstrual cycle of premenopausal women. Am J Clin Nutr 1994; 60:333–340.
225. Maskarinec G, Williams AE, Carlin L. Mammographic densities in a one-year isoflavone intervention. Eur J Cancer Prev 2003; 12:165–169.
226. Boyd NF, Martin LJ, Stone J, Greenberg C, Minkin S, Yaffe MJ. Mammographic densities as a marker of human breast cancer risk and their use in chemoprevention. Curr Oncol Rep 2001; 3:314–321.
227. Boyd NF, Rommens JM, Vogt K, Lee V, Hopper JL, Yaffe MJ, Paterson AD. Mammographic breast density as an intermediate phenotype for breast cancer. Lancet Oncol 2005; 6:798–808.
228. Boyd NF, Guo H, Martin LJ, Sun L, Stone J, Fishell E, Jong RA, Hislop G, Chiarelli A, Minkin S, Yaffe MJ. Mammographic density and the risk and detection of breast cancer. N Engl J Med 2007; 356:227–236.
229. Tjonneland A, Christensen J, Thomsen BL, Olsen A, Stripp C, Overvad K, Olsen JH. Lifetime alcohol consumption and postmenopausal breast cancer rate in Denmark: a prospective cohort study. J Nutr 2004; 134:173–178.
230. Carmichael AR. Obesity as a risk factor for development and poor prognosis of breast cancer. BJOG 2006; 113:1160–1166.
231. Colditz GA. Estrogen, estrogen plus progestin therapy, and risk of breast cancer. Clin Cancer Res 2005; 11:909s–917s.
232. Russo J, Lareef H, Tahin Q, Russo IH. Pathways of carcinogenesis and prevention in the human breast. Eur J Cancer 2002; 38(suppl 6):S31–S32.
233. Hamilton AS, Mack TM. Puberty and genetic susceptibility to breast cancer in a case-control study in twins. N? Engl J Med 2003; 348:2313–2322.
234. Elias SG, Peeters PH, Grobbee DE, van Noord PA. Breast cancer risk after caloric restriction during the 1944-1945 Dutch famine. J Natl Cancer Inst 2004; 96:539–546.
235. Michels KB, Ekbom A. Caloric restriction and incidence of breast cancer. JAMA 2004; 291:1226–1230.
236. Lee SY, Kim MT, Kim SW, Song MS, Yoon SJ. Effect of lifetime lactation on breast cancer risk: a Korean women's cohort study. Int J Cancer 2003; 105:390–393.
237. Leon DA, Carpenter LM, Broeders MJ, Gunnarskog J, Murphy MF. Breast cancer in Swedish women before age 50: evidence of a dual effect of completed pregnancy. Cancer Causes Control 1995; 6:283–291.
238. Zheng T, Duan L, Liu Y, Zhang B, Wang Y, Chen Y, Zhang Y, Owens PH. Lactation reduces breast cancer risk in Shandong Province, China. Am J Epidemiol 2000; 152:1129–1135.
239. Zheng T, Holford TR, Mayne ST, Owens PH, Zhang Y, Zhang B, Boyle P, Zahm SH. Lactation and breast cancer risk: a case-control study in Connecticut. Br J Cancer 2001; 84:1472–1476.
240. Vatten L. Can prenatal factors influence future breast cancer risk? Lancet 1996; 348:1531.
241. Michels KB, Trichopoulos D, Robins JM, Rosner BA, Manson JE, Hunter DJ, Colditz GA, Hankinson SE, Speizer FE, Willett WC. Birthweight as a risk factor for breast cancer. Lancet 1996; 348:1542–1546.
242. Freudenheim JL, Marshall JR, Vena JE, Moysich KB, Muti P, Laughlin R, Nemoto T, Graham S. Lactation history and breast cancer risk. Am J Epidemiol 1997; 146:932–938.
243. Hemminki K, Li X. Cancer risks in second-generation immigrants to Sweden. Int J Cancer 2002; 99:229–237.
244. Shimizu H, Ross RK, Bernstein L, Yatani R, Henderson BE, Mack TM. Cancers of the prostate and breast among Japanese and white immigrants in Los Angeles County. Br J Cancer 1991; 63:963–966.
245. Hemminki K, Li X, Czene K. Cancer risks in first-generation immigrants to Sweden. Int J Cancer 2002; 99:218–228.
246. Lambe M, Hsieh CC, Chan HW, Ekbom A, Trichopoulos D, Adami HO. Parity, age at first and last birth, and risk of breast cancer: a population-based study in Sweden. Breast Cancer Res Treat 1996; 38:305–311.
247. Russo J, Mailo D, Hu YF, Balogh G, Sheriff F, Russo IH. Breast differentiation and its implication in cancer prevention. Clin Cancer Res 2005; 11:931s–936s.
248. Lamartiniere CA, Moore JB, Brown NM, Thompson R, Hardin MJ, Barnes S. Genistein suppresses mammary cancer in rats. Carcinogenesis 1995; 16:2833–2840.
249. Murrill WB, Brown NM, Zhang JX, Manzolillo PA, Barnes S, Lamartiniere CA. Prepubertal genistein exposure suppresses mammary cancer and enhances gland differentiation in rats. Carcinogenesis 1996; 17:1451–1457.
250. Hilakivi-Clarke L, Onojafe I, Raygada M, Cho E, Skaar T, Russo I, Clarke R. Prepubertal exposure to zearalenone or genistein reduces mammary tumorigenesis. Br J Cancer 1999; 80:1682–1688.
251. Fritz WA, Coward L, Wang J, Lamartiniere CA. Dietary genistein: perinatal mammary cancer prevention,

bioavailability and toxicity testing in the rat. Carcinogenesis 1998; 19:2151–2158.

252. Lamartiniere CA, Cotroneo MS, Fritz WA, Wang J, Mentor-Marcel R, Elgavish A. Genistein chemoprevention: timing and mechanisms of action in murine mammary and prostate. J Nutr 2002; 132:552S–558S.
253. Yang J, Nakagawa H, Tsuta K, Tsubura A. Influence of perinatal genistein exposure on the development of MNU-induced mammary carcinoma in female Sprague-Dawley rats. Cancer Lett 2000; 149:171–179.
254. Pei RJ, Sato M, Yuri T, Danbara N, Nikaido Y, Tsubura A. Effect of prenatal and prepubertal genistein exposure on N-methyl-N-nitrosourea-induced mammary tumorigenesis in female Sprague-Dawley rats. In Vivo 2003; 17:349–357.
255. Shu XO, Jin F, Dai Q, Wen W, Potter JD, Kushi LH, Ruan Z, Gao YT, Zheng W. Soyfood intake during adolescence and subsequent risk of breast cancer among chinese women. Cancer Epidemiol Biomarkers Prev 2001; 10:483–488.
256. Wu AH, Wan P, Hankin J, Tseng CC, Yu MC, Pike MC. Adolescent and adult soy intake and risk of breast cancer in Asian-Americans. Carcinogenesis 2002; 23: 1491–1496.
257. Korde LA, Wu AH, Fears T, Nomura AM, West DW, Kolonel LN, Pike MC, However RN, Ziegler RG. Childhood soy intake and breast cancer risk in Asian-American women. American Association for Cancer Research Annual Meeting 2006 (abstr, 06-AB-667-AACRCPR).
258. Thanos J, Cotterchio M, Boucher BA, Kreiger N, Thompson LU. Adolescent dietary phytoestrogen intake and breast cancer risk (Canada). Cancer Causes Control 2006; 17:1253–1261.
259. Lamartiniere CA, Zhang JX, Cotroneo MS. Genistein studies in rats: potential for breast cancer prevention and reproductive and developmental toxicity. Am J Clin Nutr 1998; 68:1400S–1405S.
260. Russo J, Gusterson BA, Rogers AE, Russo IH, Wellings SR, van Zwieten MJ. Comparative study of human and rat mammary tumorigenesis. Lab Invest 1990; 62:244–278.
261. Grubbs CJ, Hill DL, McDonough KC, Peckham JC. N-nitroso-N-methylurea-induced mammary carcinogenesis: effect of pregnancy on preneoplastic cells. J Natl Cancer Inst 1983; 71:625–628.
262. Hilakivi-Clarke L, Cho E, Cabanes A, DeAssis S, Olivo S, Helferich W, Lippman ME, Clarke R. Dietary modulation of pregnancy estrogen levels and breast cancer risk among female rat offspring. Clin Cancer Res 2002; 8:3601–3610.
263. Russo IH, Koszalka M, Russo J. Effect of human chorionic gonadotropin on mammary gland differentiation and carcinogenesis. Carcinogenesis 1990; 11:1849–1855.
264. Schmitt E, Dekant W, Stopper H. Assaying the estrogenicity of phytoestrogens in cells of different estrogen sensitive tissues. Toxicol In Vitro 2001; 15:433–439.
265. Breinholt V, Hossaini A, Svendsen GW, Brouwer C, Nielsen E. Estrogenic activity of flavonoids in mice. The importance of estrogen receptor distribution, metabolism and bioavailability. Food Chem Toxicol 2000; 38: 555–564.
266. Lamartiniere CA, Wang J, Smith-Johnson M, Eltoum IE. Daidzein: bioavailability, potential for reproductive toxicity, and breast cancer chemoprevention in female rats. Toxicol Sci 2002; 65:228–238.
267. Brown NM, Wang J, Cotroneo MS, Zhao YX, Lamartiniere CA. Prepubertal genistein treatment modulates TGF-alpha, EGF and EGF-receptor mRNAs and proteins in the rat mammary gland. Mol Cell Endocrinol 1998; 144: 149–165.
268. Cabanes A, Wang M, Olivo S, DeAssis S, Gustafsson JA, Khan G, Hilakivi-Clarke L. Prepubertal estradiol and genistein exposures up-regulate BRCA1 mRNA and reduce mammary tumorigenesis. Carcinogenesis 2004; 25:741–748.
269. Rowell C, Carpenter DM, Lamartiniere CA. Chemoprevention of breast cancer, proteomic discovery of genistein action in the rat mammary gland. J Nutr 2005; 135:2953S–2959S.
270. Wren BG. Do female sex hormones initiate breast cancer? A review of the evidence. Climacteric 2004; 7:120–128.
271. Writing Group for the Women's Health Initiative Investigators. Risks and benefits of estrogen plus progestin in healthy postmenopausal women: principal results From the Women's Health Initiative randomized controlled trial. JAMA 2002; 288:321–333.
272. Anderson GL, Limacher M, Assaf AR, et al. Effects of conjugated equine estrogen in postmenopausal women with hysterectomy: the Women's Health Initiative randomized controlled trial. JAMA 2004; 291:1701–1712.
273. Beral V. Breast cancer and hormone-replacement therapy in the Million Women Study. Lancet 2003; 362:419–427.
274. Shah NR, Borenstein J, Dubois RW. Postmenopausal hormone therapy and breast cancer: a systematic review and meta-analysis. Menopause 2005; 12:668–678.
275. Zhang SM, Manson JE, Rexrode KM, Cook NR, Buring JE, Lee IM. Use of Oral Conjugated Estrogen Alone and Risk of Breast Cancer. Am J Epidemiol 2007; 165:524–529.
276. Zava DT, Dollbaum CM, Blen M. Estrogen and progestin bioactivity of foods, herbs, and spices. Proc Soc Exp Biol Med 1998; 217:369–378.
277. Greendale GA, Reboussin BA, Slone S, Wasilauskas C, Pike MC, Ursin G. Postmenopausal hormone therapy and change in mammographic density. J Natl Cancer Inst 2003; 95:30–37.
278. Sartippour MR, Rao JY, Apple S, Wu D, Henning S, Wang H, Elashoff R, Rubio R, Heber D, Brooks MN. A pilot clinical study of short-term isoflavone supplements in breast cancer patients. Nutr Cancer 2004; 49:59–65.
279. Boyapati SM, Shu XO, Ruan ZX, Dai Q, Cai Q, Gao YT, Zheng W. Soyfood intake and breast cancer survival: a follow-up of the Shanghai Breast Cancer Study. Breast Cancer Res Treat 2005; 92: 11–17.
280. Ishiwata N, Ueno T, Uschiyama S, Watanabe H. A randomized placebo-controlled trial of oral supplement for treatment of menopausal symptoms among Japanese women. Soy and Health Conference 2006, Dusseldorf, Germany (abstr).

21

Body Size and Breast Cancer

LING YANG

Clinical Trial Service Unit & Epidemiological Studies Unit, University of Oxford, Oxford, U.K.; Department of Medical Epidemiology and Biostatistics, Karolinska Institutet, Stockholm, Sweden; and Samfundet Folkhälsan (NGO), Helsingfors, Finland

MARIE LÖF

Department of Medical Epidemiology and Biostatistics, Karolinska Institutet, Stockholm, Sweden

ELISABETE WEIDERPASS

Department of Medical Epidemiology and Biostatistics, Karolinska Institutet, Stockholm, Sweden; Cancer Registry of Norway, Oslo, Norway; and Samfundet Folkhälsan (NGO), Helsingfors, Finland

INTRODUCTION

The prevalence of overweight and obesity in adults and children has increased rapidly over the last two decades in most countries. In many developed countries, half or more of the adult population is now overweight or obese, and similar prevalence rates have been reached in urban areas of some developing countries. This is of great concern since being overweight or obese is associated with an increased risk for morbidity and mortality. Obesity is a well-established risk factor for cardiovascular diseases and type 2 diabetes mellitus, and also associated with the development of postmenopausal breast cancer (Huang et al., 1997). Epidemiological evidence suggests that body size at birth may influence breast cancer development (Michels and Xue, 2006). In this chapter we review the currently available epidemiological evidence for the association between body size during different periods of life and the risk of breast cancer in terms of cancer incidence, mortality, diagnosis, treatment, and prognosis, along with the related biological mechanism hypotheses. Finally, we propose strategies for breast cancer research related to body size and recommendations for public health action aiming for prevention of obesity-related conditions as well as breast cancer.

Body size can be assessed by means of anthropometric measures such as body weight, height, waist, and hip circumferences, and indices of their combinations. The most widely used indicator of overweight and obesity in adults is the body mass index (BMI); other anthropometric indicators of abdominal obesity, such as waist-hip ratio (WHR) or waist circumference have been proposed recently.

Body Weight, Height, and Birth Weight

Weight and height are often self-reported in epidemiological studies. It is well established that self-reported weight is often slightly lower while height is higher than the real values. On average, women have been reported to underestimate their weight by approximately 1 kg and overestimate their height by 0.7 cm (Rowland, 1990; Roberts, 1995). Nevertheless, epidemiological studies measuring association between

Table 1 WHO Classification of Overweight in Adults Using BMI

Classification	BMI (kg/m^2)
Underweight	<18.50
Normal range	18.50–24.99
Overweight	≥25.00
Pre-obese	25.00–29.99
Obese class I	30.00–34.99
Obese class II	35.00–39.99
Obese class III	≥40

Abbreviation: BMI, body mass index.
Source: From WHO (2000).

weight, height, or BMI and disease are not substantially affected by this degree of measurement error (IARC, 2002). Birth weight information can be obtained from the birth records (more preferable) or by self-reported questionnaires answered by the study subjects or their mothers (Troy et al., 1996; Andersson et al., 2000).

Body Mass Index

BMI is calculated as weight (kg) divided by height squared (m^2). The cutoff points of BMI for the classification of overweight presented by the World Health Organization in 2000 have been widely adopted (Table 1) (WHO, 2000). Briefly, subjects with a BMI of 25 to 30 kg/m^2 are classified as overweight, while subjects with a BMI ≥30 kg/m^2 are classified as obese. BMI has many advantages as a body size measurement: it is easy to measure, noninvasive, and has a relatively high correlation with body fatness (Gibson, 2005). However, BMI cannot distinguish whether weight is associated with muscle or body fat, and BMI does not indicate where the body fat is located. Furthermore, the relationship between BMI and body fat is age and sex dependent. For comparable BMIs, older women tend to have relatively greater percentage of body fat than younger women, and women have significantly greater amounts of total body fat than men have (Larsson et al., 2004; Gibson, 2005). It was also suggested that BMI was an approximately poor predictor of total body fat in overweight and obese women (Heymsfield et al., 1998), and BMI was proportional to percent body fatness in normal-weight subjects but not in severely obese subjects (Larsson et al., 2006). Nevertheless, BMI has been used in a large number of studies to assess disease risk and increasing BMI is clearly associated with increased total morbidity and mortality (WHO, 2000; Hjartaker et al., 2005).

Waist Circumference and WHR

WHR is calculated as the waist circumference divided by the hip circumference. It is a simple method for distinguishing between fatness in the lower trunk and fatness in the upper trunk. Use of WHR has increased since central obesity has been identified as a risk factor for coronary heart disease, stroke, and diabetes mellitus type 2 (IARC, 2002). WHR strongly correlates with total body fatness (Gibson, 2005). One advantage of using WHR is that it provides information about location of body fatness (abdominal in relation to hip). Epidemiological studies often have to rely on self-reported circumference measurements. However, such measurements have been found to be of high validity and reproducibility (Gibson, 2005). The internationally used cutoff points of WHR for abdominal fat accumulation are WHR >1.0 for men and >0.85 for women.

Several studies have shown that waist circumference alone is a better correlate of abdominal fat as well as of total body fat content than WHR (Gibson, 2005). Compared with WHR, waist circumference is more closely related to potential atherogenic metabolic disturbances which are associated with abdominal obesity (Gibson, 2005). As suggested by WHO (WHO, 2000), the general cutoff points for waist circumference to identify the increased risk associated with excess abdominal fat in adults are ≥102 cm for men and ≥88 cm for women. However, the waist circumference varies by age and ethnicity. Lower cutoffs for urban Asians (>90 cm for men and >80 cm for women) have been recommended because these populations have higher rate of obesity-related disorders and are more prone to central adiposity than other ethnic groups (Gibson, 2005).

BODY SIZE AND THE INCIDENCE AND MORTALITY OF BREAST CANCER

Body size, weight changes, and fat distribution patterns among different periods of life may separately or in combination play a role in the development of breast cancer. On the basis of systematical reviews of current available observational studies, the evidence for those anthropometric factors influencing breast cancer incidence and mortality is consolidating. However, the relationships are not straightforward and are strongly modified by menopausal status (Friedenreich, 2001b; IARC, 2002; Carmichael and Bates, 2004; Carmichael, 2006). Studies of body size and breast cancer risk are summarized in Table 2.

Adult Body Size

An inverse relationship has been found between body weight or BMI and breast cancer among premenopausal women in most, but not all, case control and more significantly in cohort or nested case-control studies within cohorts (Paffenbarger et al., 1980; Lubin et al., 1985; Willett et al., 1985; Hislop et al., 1986; Le Marchand et al., 1988; London et al., 1989; Swanson et al., 1989; Tretli, 1989; Hsieh et al., 1990; Chu et al., 1991; Brinton

(*text continues on page 423*)

Table 2 Studies of Body Size and Breast Cancer Risk

Reference, study location	Study dates	Number of cases	Measurement	Contrasts (number of categories)	Relative risk (95% CI)	Adjustment for confounding
Premenopausal breast cancer						
Cohort studies						
Le Marchand et al. (1988), United States	1972–1983	289	BMI	Age 30–44 yr: tertiles Age 45–49 yr: tertiles	0.78 (0.46–1.3) 1.1 (0.63–1.8)	Age, age at first birth, socioeconomic status
			Weight change	Age 30–44 yr: tertiles Age 45–49 yr: tertiles	0.67 (0.39–1.2) 1.1 (0.64–1.8)	
Tretli (1989), Norway	1963–1981	3305	BMI	RR given for 1 unit increase	0.84 (0.74–0.95)	
Vatten and Kvinnsland (1992), Norway	1974–1988	291	BMI	≥27 vs. 22 (4)	0.78 (0.65–0.94)	Age, reproductive risk factors, occupation, county of residence
Tornberg and Carstensen (1994), Sweden	1963–1987	373	BMI	≥28 vs. <22 (5)	0.41	Age
Huang et al. (1997), London et al. (1989), United States	1976–1992	598	BMI at age 18–25 yr	≥25 vs. <20.0 (5)	0.6 (0.5–0.8), age 18 yr	London: Age, height, history of benign breast disease, family history, reproductive factors, smoking
			BMI	>31.0 vs. ≤20.0 (10)	0.62 (0.45–0.86)	Huang: Age, height, history of benign breast disease, family history, reproductive factors
			Weight change	Gain >25 kg vs. loss or gain ≤2.0 kg (6)	0.74 (0.54–1.0)	Weight gain data adjusted for BMI at age 18 yr
Kaaks et al. (1998), Netherlands	1984–1996	147	WHR Waist	>0.80 vs. ≤0.73 (4) >83.5 cm vs. ≤71 cm (4)	0.96 (0.60–1.5) 0.92 (0.57–1.5)	Age, reproductive factors, height, weight
Huang et al. (1999), United States	1976–1994	197	WHR Hip Waist	≥0.84 vs. <0.73 (5) ≥43.0 vs. <36.9 (5) ≥36.0 vs. <27.9 (5)	1.43 (0.86–2.37) 0.56 (0.26–1.21) 1.74 (0.74–4.07)	Age, height, personal history of benign breast disease, family history of breast cancer, age at menarche, physical activity, age at first birth and parity BMI
Borugian et al. (2003), Canada	1991–2002	603	WHR	Highest quartile vs. lowest	1.2 (0.4–3.4)	Age, body mass index, family history, estrogen receptor (ER) status, tumor stage at diagnosis, and systemic treatment

(Continued)

Table 2 Studies of Body Size and Breast Cancer Risk (*Continued*)

Reference, study location	Study dates	Number of cases	Measurement	Contrasts (number of categories)	Relative risk (95% CI)	Adjustment for confounding
Weiderpass et al. (2004), Norway and Sweden	1991–1999	733	Adult BMI	25–30 vs.<20 kg/m^2	0.79 (0.63–0.99)	Age at enrolment, parity, age at first birth, oral contraceptive use, age at menarche, family history of breast cancer, total duration of breast-feeding, and country of residence.
			Body shape at age 7 yr	Fat vs very thin	0.69 (0.50–0.93)	
			BMI at age 18 yr	≥25 vs. <20 kg/m^2	0.74 (0.59–0.91)	
			Height	≥175 vs. <160 m	0.90 (0.67–1.21)	
			Difference in body shape	Increasing weight vs. remain weight	0.87 (0.73–1.03)	
			Adult BMI change	Increased >4.0 vs. increased 0	0.76 (0.60–0.95)	
Lahmann et al. (2004b), 9 of the EPIC countries		474	Height	Increment per 5 cm	1.05 (1.00–1.16)	Age, educational attainment, smoking status, alcohol consumption, parity, age at first pregnancy, age at menarche and current pill use (pre-menopausal)
			Weight (kg)	Per 1 kg increase	1.00 (0.99–1.01)	
			BMI (kg/m^2)	Continues variable	0.98 (0.96–1.00)	
			Waist circ. (cm)	Per 1 cm increase	1.01 (0.99–1.03)	
			Hip circ. (cm)	Per 1 cm increase	1.02 (1.01–1.05)	
			WHR	continues variable	0.99 (0.98–1.01)	
Baer et al. (2005), United States	1989–2000	1318	Childhood body fatness	Most overweight vs. most lean in childhood	0.48 (0.35–0.55)	Age, time period, birth weight, height, recent alcohol consumption, parity and age at first birth, oral contraceptive use, history of benign breast disease and first-degree family history of breast cancer
			adolescent body fatness	Most overweight vs. most lean in childhood	0.57 (0.39–0.83)	
McCormack et al. (2005), Sweden	1960–2001	367	Birth weight	4	1.40 (1.08–1.81)	Birth order and socioeconomic factors
Michels (2006), United States	1991–2002	3140	Birth weight	<5.5 lbs vs. ≥8.5 lbs	0.66 (0.47–0.93)	Age, premature birth, age at menarche, BMI at age 18 yr, current BMI, family history of breast cancer, history of benign breast disease, age at first birth, parity, oral contraceptive use, physical activity and alcohol consumption
Troisi et al., (2006), United States	1978–2001	24	Birth weight	>3.5 kg vs. <3 kg	2.19 (0.83–5.7)	Age

Tehard and Clavel-Chapelon (2006), France	1995–2000	275	Height (cm)	Highest quartile vs. lowest	1.26 (0.80–1.98)	Family history of breast cancer, age at menarche, age at first birth, history of benign breast disease, alcohol consumption, education, marital status and physical activity
			Weight (kg)	Highest quartile vs. lowest	0.57 (0.42–0.98)	
			BMI (kg/m^2)	≥30 vs. 18.5–25	0.26 (0.06–1.00)	
			Waist circ. (cm)	Highest quartile vs. lowest	0.58 (0.38–0.88)	
			Hip circ. (cm)	Highest quartile vs. lowest	0.88 (0.43–1.31)	
			WHR	Highest quartile vs. lowest	0.60 (0.39–0.91)	
Lukanova et al. (2006), Sweden	1985–2003	109	BMI (age<49)	Highest quartile vs. lowest	0.58 (0.29–1.11)	Age, calendar year and smoking
			BMI (age>49)	Highest quartile vs. lowest	1.04 (0.80–1.36)	
Baer et al. (2006), United States	1989–2001	1041	Adult height	>1.75m vs. <1.60m	1.57 (1.23–2.01)	Age, birth weight, childhood body fatness, family history of breast cancer, parity/age at first birth, recency/duration of oral contraceptive use, alcohol consumption, history of benign breast disease, current BMI, age at menarche, and either age at attained height
Lahmann et al. (2005), 6 of the EPIC countries	1992–2004	264	Weight gain	Gained 15–20 kg vs. stable weight	1.00 (0.59, 1.71)	Weight at age 20 yr, age at menarche, age at first birth/ parity, education, height, alcohol intake, smoking status, and leisure physical activity.
Lof M et al. (2007), Sweden	1991–2003	557	Birth weight	<2.5 kg vs. >3 kg	0.65 (0.43–0.99)	Parity, age at first birth, total months of breastfeeding and family history of breast cancer (mother or sister)
Case-control studies						
Paffenbarger et al. (1980), United States	1970–1977	374	BMI	≥24.5 vs. 21.5 (3)	0.65	Age, ethnicity, parity
			BMI at age 18–25 yr	≥22.0 vs. >19.0 (3)	0.70, age 20 yr	Age, ethnicity, parity
Lubin et al. (1985), Israel	1975–1978	363	BMI	Comparison of mean BMI	*p* not significant	Age, ethnic origin
Hislop et al. (1986), Canada	1980–1982	306	BMI	≥27 vs. ≤21 (4)	0.84 (0.52–1.4)	Age
Hsieh et al. (1990), International	NS	3993 pre and post	BMI	Normal BMI not defined; obese defined as+4 kg/m^2	1.0 (0.98–1.1)	Age, centre, reproductive factors
Chu et al. (1991), United States	1980–1982	2053	BMI	Sextiles—cutpoints not stated by menopausal status	1.3 (0.9–2.0)	Age, reproductive risk factors, family history, surgical biopsy for benign breast disease
			BMI at age 18–25 yr	Sextiles—cutpoints not stated by menopausal status	0.6 (0.2–0.9), age 18 yr	Age, reproductive factors, family history, surgical biopsy for benign breast disease

(*Continued*)

Table 2 Studies of Body Size and Breast Cancer Risk (*Continued*)

Reference, study location	Study dates	Number of cases	Measurement	Contrasts (number of categories)	Relative risk (95% CI)	Adjustment for confounding
Brinton and Swanson (1992), United States	1973–1980	414	BMI	≥26 vs. 20 (5)	0.65 (0.4–1.0)	Age, age at menarche, Education
			BMI at age 18–25 yr	>25 vs. <19 (5)	0.58	
			Weight change	Gain 6.0 + BMI vs. no change (5)	0.47	
Franceschi et al. (1996), Italy	1991–1994	988	BMI	>28.8 vs. <21.7 (5)	0.7 (0.5–0.9)	Age, centre, education, parity, total energy and alcohol intake
			WHR	>0.88 vs. <0.78 (5)	0.7 (0.5–1.0)	Age, BMI, centre, education, parity, total energy and alcohol intake
Swanson et al. (1996), United States	1990–1992	1588	WHR	>0.858 vs. 0.753 (4)	0.95 (0.8–1.2)	Age, BMI, centre, reproductive factors, oral contraceptive use, alcohol
			BMI	>28.8 vs. <22.0 (4)	0.65 (0.5–0.8)	Age, centre, ethnicity, reproductive factors, alcohol, oral contraceptive use
Yong et al. (1996), United States	1973–1981	226	BMI	≥34.7 vs. <26.8 (5)	0.9 (0.6–1.4)	Age, education, reproductive risk factors, history of benign breast disease, family history
Ziegler et al. (1996), Asia	1983–1987	421	BMI	>31.3 vs. <22.9	1.6 (0.87–2.9)	Age, ethnicity, centre, reproductive risk factors, history of benign breast disease, family history
Chie et al. (1998), Taiwan	1993–1994	334	BMI	≥25 vs. <20 (4)	0.5 (0.2–1.2)	Age, education, family history, reproductive factors, oral contraceptive use
Coates et al. (1999), United States	1990–1992	1590	BMI at age 18–25 yr	>22.8 vs. >18.5 (5)	0.75 (0.59–0.95), age 20 yr	Age, centre, ethnicity, family history of breast biopsy, education, reproductive factors, history of mammograms, alcohol, height, oral contraceptive use. Weight gain adjusted for BMI at age 20 yr
			BMI	>30.4 vs. >21.5 (5)	0.69 (0.54–0.88)	
			Weight change	Gained ≥ 21 kg vs. gained or lost ± 2 kg	0.72 (0.54–0.95)	

Peacock et al. (1999), United States	1983–1990	845	BMI	≥27.1 vs. ≤19.9 (5)	0.67 (0.49–0.91)	Age, age at menarche
			BMI at age 18–25 yr	≥27.1 vs. ≤19.9 (5)	0.71 (0.53–0.96), age 18 yr	Age at menarche
			Weight change	Average annual BMI change of ≥0.25 units	0.70 (0.54–0.90)	
Enger et al. (2000), United States	1983–1989	714	BMI	≥27.1 vs. <21.7 (4)	ER+/PgR+: 1.11 (0.70–1.8)	Age, socioeconomic status, reproductive risk factors, family history, physical activity
				≥27.1 vs. <21.7 (4)	ER+/PgR–: 0.92 (0.34–2.5)	
				≥27.1 vs. <21.7 (4)	ER–/PgR–: 1.1 (0.56–1.7)	
				≥27.1 vs. <21.7 (4)	Unknown: 0.80 (0.53–1.2)	
Hall et al. (2000), United States	1993–1996	389	BMI	>30.1 vs. <24.6 (3)	Black: 0.89 (0.38–2.1)	Age, reproductive risk factors, education
				>30.1 vs. <24.6 (3)	White: 0.46 (0.26–0.80)	
			WHR	>0.86 vs. <0.77 (3)	Black: 2.5 (1.1–5.7)	Age, BMI, reproductive factors, education
				>0.86 vs. <0.77 (3)	White: 2.4 (1.2–5.1)	
Friedenreich et al. (2002), Canada	1995–1997	462	Height (m)	Highest quartile vs. lowest	1.28 (0.87–1.87)	Current age, total caloric intake, total lifetime physical activity, educational level (in quintiles), ever use of hormone replacement therapy, ever diagnosed with benign breast disease, first-degree family history of breast cancer, ever alcohol consumption, current smoker
			Weight (kg)	Highest quartile vs. lowest	0.81 (0.55–1.19)	
			Body mass index	Highest quartile vs. lowest	0.69 (0.47–1.02)	
			Waist	Highest quartile vs. lowest	0.89 (0.61–1.31)	
			Hip	Highest quartile vs. lowest	0.76 (0.52–1.11)	
			WHR	Highest quartile vs. lowest	1.22 (0.84–1.79)	
			Weight at age 20 yr (kg)	Highest quartile vs. lowest	1.02 (0.68–1.52)	
			Weight gain since age 20 yr (kg)	Highest quartile vs. lowest	0.79 (0.54–1.15)	
			Weight gain over life	Highest quartile vs. lowest	0.92 (0.62–1.37)	
			Ref., min. weight since age 20 yr	Highest quartile vs. lowest	0.94 (0.63–1.38)	
Magnusson et al. (2005), United Kingdom	1982–1991	1560	body fatness	Perceived plump vs. thin at age 10 yr	0.83 (0.69–0.99)	Parity, age at first birth, height, use of oral contraceptives and alcohol consumption.
Verla-Tebit et al. (2005), Germany	1992–1995	558	Weight gain	Highest quartile vs. lowest	0.56 (0.34, 0.94)	
Barba et al. (2006), United States	1996–2001	845	Birth weight	>8.5 lb vs. <5.5 lb	1.84 (1.12–3.02)	Age (yr), education (yr), race, BMI, history of breast benign disease, family history of breast cancer, lactation (mo), age at menarche (yr), age at first full term pregnancy (yr), age at menopause (yr), parity

(Continued)

Table 2 Studies of Body Size and Breast Cancer Risk (*Continued*)

Reference, study location	Study dates	Number of cases	Measurement	Contrasts (number of categories)	Relative risk (95% CI)	Adjustment for confounding
Park et al. (2006), Poland	2000–2003	2386	Birth weight	>4 kg vs. <2.5 kg	1.14 (0.61–2.12)	Age, education, age at menarche, menopausal status and age at menopause, age at first full-term pregnancy, number of full-term pregnancies, family history of breast cancer among first degree relatives, mammography screening and current BMI
Postmenopausal breast cancer						
Cohort studies						
Le Marchand et al. (1988), United States	1972–1983	280	BMI	Age 50–54 yr: tertiles Age 55–65 yr, tertiles	1.2 (0.70–2.0), 1.2 (0.74–2.1)	Age, age at first birth, socioeconomic status
			Weight change	Age 50–54 yr: tertiles Age 55–65 yr: tertiles	1.1 (0.66–1.8) 2.3 (1.4–3.7)	
Tretli (1989), Norway	1963–1981	5122	BMI	RR given for 1 unit increase	1.2 (1.1–1.2)	
Folsom et al. (1990), Sellers et al. (1992), United States	1985–1986	382	BMI at age 18–25 yr	≥24.6 vs. ≤20.0 (5), age 18 yr	Family history –ve: 0.64 (0.45–0.91)	Age. weight gain data adjusted for BMI at age 18 yr
				≥24.6 vs. ≤20.0 (5), age 19 yr	Family history +ve: 0.88 (0.46–1.7)	
			BMI	≥30.7 vs. ≤22.9 (5)	Family history –ve: 1.5 (1.1–2.1)	
				≥30.7 vs. ≤22.9 (5)	Family history +ve: 2.2 (1.4–3.6)	
			Weight change	Current weight at age 18 yr >17.3 vs. <8.2 kg (3)	1.6 (1.1–2.3) (data on 225 women)	
Sellers et al. (1992), United States	1986	469	BMI	≥30.7 vs. ≤22.9	No family history: 1.5 (1.1–2.1)	Age
				≥30.7 vs. ≤22.9	Family history: 2.2 (1.4–3.6)	
			WHR	>0.91 vs. <0.76 (5)	No family history 1.2 (0.87–1.7)	
				>0.91 vs. <0.76 (5)	Family history 3.2 (2.1–5.0)	

Törnberg and Carstensen (1994), Sweden	1963–1987	1093	BMI	≥28 vs. <22 (5)	1.1	Age
Huang et al. (1997), London et al. (1989), United States	1976–1992	384	BMI at age 18–25 yr	≥25 vs. <20.0 (5)	0.8 (0.6–1.2) age 18 yr	London: Age, height, history of benign breast disease, family history, reproductive factors, smoking
			BMI	>31.0 vs. ≤20.0 (10)	1.1 (0.87–1.5)	Huang: Age, height, history of benign breast disease, family history, reproductive factors
			Weight change	Gain > 25 kg vs. loss or gain < 2 kg (6)	1.4 (1.1–1.8)	Weight gain data adjusted for BMI at age 18 yr
Huang et al. (1999), United States	1976–1994	840	WHR	>0.84 vs. <0.73 (5)	1.22 (0.96–1.65)	Age, height, personal history of benign breast disease, family history of breast cancer, age at menarche, physical activity, age at first birth and parity, BMI
			Hip	>43.0 vs. <36.9 (5)	1.07 (0.76–1.51)	
			Waist	>36.0 vs. <27.9 (5)	1.26 (0.88–1.81)	
Hilakivi-Clarke et al. (2001), Finland	1971–1995	177 cases, 49 deaths	Weight, height during childhood	Every kilogram increase in birth weight	1.27 (0.97–1.78)	
				Every kg/m^2 decrease in body mass index at 7.	1.21 (1.06–1.38)	
Petrelli et al. (2002), United States	1982–1996	2852 deaths	BMI	BMI > 40.0 vs. 18.5–20.49	3.08 (2.09–4.51)	Age, height, race, family history of breast cancer, breast cysts, number of live births, age at first live birth, age at menarche, age at menopause, menopausal status, oral contraceptive use, estrogen replacement therapy, education, exercise, smoking, alcohol, and menopausal status
			Height	>66 vs. <66 inches	1.64 (1.23–2.18)	Age, body mass index, race, family history of breast cancer, breast cysts, number of live births, age at first live birth, age at menarche, age at menopause, menopausal status, oral contraceptive use, estrogen replacement therapy, education, exercise, smoking, alcohol, and menopausal status
Okasha et al. (2002), United Kingdom	1948–1999	32 deaths	BMI	Quartile	3.61 (1.00–12.94).	Height, childhood social class, birth order; number of siblings; smoking; pulse rate; age at menarche
Borugian et al. (2003), Canada	1991–2002	603	WHR	Highest quartile vs. lowest	3.3 (1.1, 10.4)	Age, body mass index, family history, estrogen receptor (ER) status, tumor stage at diagnosis, and systemic treatment

(Continued)

Table 2 Studies of Body Size and Breast Cancer Risk (*Continued*)

Reference, study location	Study dates	Number of cases	Measurement	Contrasts (number of categories)	Relative risk (95% CI)	Adjustment for confounding
Lahmann et al. (2003), Sweden	1991–1999	246	Weight	Highest vs. lowest quintile	1.53 (0.97–2.41)	Age, height,, occupation, marital status, smoking status, alcohol consumption, parity/age at first pregnancy, age at menarche and current hormone use.
			Height	Highest vs. lowest quintile	1.41(0.92–2.17)	
			BMI	>28.5 vs. <22.0	1.54 (1.01–2.35)	
			WHR	Highest vs. lowest quintile	1.23 (0.79–1.92)	
			Waist circumference	>86 vs. <70	1.14 (0.62–2.12)	
			Percent body fat	Highest vs. lowest quintile	2.01 (1.26–3.21)	
			Weight gain	>21kg vs. 5.0–9.9kg	1.75 (1.11–2.77)	
Parker and Folsom (2003), United States	1993–2000	772	Weight loss	Intentional weight loss ≥20 vs. never ≥20 lb loss	0.81 (0.66–1.00)	Age, body mass index, waist-to-hip ratio, physical activity, education, marital status, smoking status, pack-years of cigarettes, current estrogen use, alcohol use, parity, and multivitamin use
Lahmann et al. (2004b), 9 of the EPIC countries	1992–2000	1405	Height (cm)	Increment per 5 cm	1.10 (1.05–1.16)	Age, educational attainment, smoking status, alcohol consumption, parity, age at first pregnancy, age at menarche
			Weight (kg) Non-HRT user	Per 1 kg increase	1.02 (1.01–1.02)	
			Weight (kg) HRT user	Per 1 kg increase	1.00 (0.99–1.01)	
			BMI (kg/m^2) Non-HRT user	Continues variable	1.03 (1.01–1.05)	
			BMI (kg/m^2) HRT user	Continues variable	0.99 (0.96–1.01)	
			Waist circ. (cm) Non-HRT user	Per 1 cm increase	1.01 (1.00–1.02)	
			Waist circ. (cm) HRT user	Per 1 cm increase	1.00 (0.97–1.03)	
			Hip circ. (cm) Non-HRT user	Per 1 cm increase	1.03 (1.01–1.04)	
			Hip circ. (cm) HRT user	Per 1 cm increase	1.00 (0.98–1.02)	
			WHR Non-HRT user	Continues variable	0.99 (0.98–1.01)	
			WHR HRT user	Continues variable	1.00 (0.97–1.03)	
Radimer et al. (2004), United States	1948–1996	206	Adult lifetime weight gain	Weight loss from ages 45 to 55 yr	0.5 (0.3–0.9)	Height, BMI at start of age period, hormone use, age at first birth, parity, alcohol use, and smoking.
Lahmann et al. (2005), 6 of the EPIC countries	1992–2004	1094	Weight gain (Non-HRT user)	Gained 15–20 kg vs. stable weight	1.50 (1.06, 2.13)	Weight at age 20 yr, age at menarche, age at first birth/parity, education, height, alcohol intake, smoking status, and leisure physical activity.
			Weight gain (HRT user)	Gained 15–20 kg vs. stable weight	0.76 (0.51, 1.13)	

Harvie et al. (2005), United States	1986–2000	1987	Weight change	Maintained or lost weight age 18–30 yr, then lost weight age 30 yr menopause	0.36 (0.22–0.60)	Age at baseline, BMI at age 18 yr, age at menopause, education, age at menarche, oral contraceptive use, HRT, number of live births, age at first live birth, smoking status, and alcohol consumption.
				Maintained or lost weight age 30 menopause then lost weight after	0.48 (0.22–0.65)	
				Gained weight age 30 menopause then lost weight after	0.77 (0.64–0.92)	
				Gained weight age 18–30 then lost weight age 30 menopause	0.61 (0.46–0.8)	
Rapp et al. (2005), Austria	1985–2001	6241	BMI	30–35 vs. 18.5–25kg/m^2	1.48 (1.12–1.95)	Smoking and occupation
Eliassen, Colditz et al. (2006), United States	1976–2002	4393	Adult weight change since age 18 yr	Gained ≥25.0 kg vs. maintenance	1.45 (1.27–1.66)	Age in months, age at menarche, parity, and age at first birth, height, weight at age 18 yr, first-degree family history of breast cancer, benign breast disease, alcohol consumption, use of PMH and age at menopause
			Adult weight change since menopause	Gained 10.0 kg vs. maintenance	1.18 (1.03–1.35)	
Michels (2006), United States	1991–2002	3140	Birth weight	<5.5 lbs vs. ≥8.5 lbs	0.97 (0.80–1.16)	Age, premature birth, age at menarche, BMI at age 18 yr, current BMI, family history of breast cancer, history of benign breast disease, age at first birth, parity, oral contraceptive use, physical activity, alcohol consumption, age at menopause and postmenopausal hormone use
Rinaldi et al. (2006b), 7 of the EPIC countries		613	BMI	Per 5 kg/m^2 increase in BMI	1.11 (0.99–1.25)	Number of full-term pregnancies and age at first full-term pregnancy
			Waist circ. (cm)	Per 10 cm increase	1.12 (1.02–1.24)	
			Hip circ. (cm)	Per 10 cm increase	1.14 (1.02–1.27)	
Troisi et al. (2006), United States	1978–2001	73	Birth weight	>3.5 kg vs. <3 kg	0.84 (0.46 –1.5)	Age
Tehard et al. (2006), France	1995–2000	860	Height (cm)	Highest quartile vs. lowest	1.06 (0.83–1.34)	Family history of breast cancer, age at menarche, age at first birth, history of benign breast disease, alcohol consumption, education, marital status and physical activity
			Weight (kg)	highest quartile vs. lowest	1.23 (0.97–1.57)	
			BMI (kg/m^2)	≥30 vs. 18.5–25	1.44 (1.04–1.99)	
			Waist circ. (cm)	Highest quartile vs. lowest	1.21 (0.95–1.54)	
			Hip circ. (cm)	Highest quartile vs. lowest	1.20 (0.96–1.50)	
			WHR	Highest quartile vs. lowest	1.03 (0.83–1.28)	

(Continued)

Table 2 Studies of Body Size and Breast Cancer Risk (*Continued*)

Reference, study location	Study dates	Number of cases	Measurement	Contrasts (number of categories)	Relative risk (95% CI)	Adjustment for confounding
Case-control studies						
Paffenbarger et al. (1980), United States	1970–1977	1029	BMI	≥24.5 vs. <21.5 (3)	1.4	Age, ethnicity, parity
		991	BMI at age 18–25 yr	≥22.0 vs. <19.0 (3)	1.0, age 20 yr	Age, ethnicity, parity
Lubin et al. (1985), Israel	1975–1978	664	BMI	≥27.1 vs. ≤19 (4)	2.5	Age, ethnic origin, education, reproductive factors, history of benign breast disease, family history
Hislop et al. (1986), Canada	1980–1982	517	BMI	≥27 vs. ≤21 (4)	0.88 (0.59–1.3)	Age
Kolonel et al. (1986)	1975–1980	272	BMI	highest vs. lowest quartile highest vs. lowest quartile	Japanese:1.6 (0.8–3.1) White: 1.7 (0.8–3.4)	Age, reproductive risk factors, history of benign breast disease, family history
Bouchardy et al. (1990), France	NS	584	BMI	>27+ vs. 23(3) >27+ vs. 23(3)	Age 55–64 yr: 0.9 Age 65–92 yr: 1.0	Socioeconomic status, reproductive risk factors, prior breast biopsy, family history
Hsieh et al. (1990), Japan	NS	3993 Pre and post	BMI	Normal BMI not defined; obese defined as +4 kg/m^2	1.1 (1.1–1.2)	Age, centre, reproductive factors
Chu et al. (1991), United States	1980–1982	547	BMI at age 18–25 yr	Sextiles—cutpoints not stated by menopausal status	0.3 (0.03–2.2), age 18 yr	Age, reproductive factors, family history, surgical biopsy for benign breast disease
			BMI	Sextiles—cutpoints not stated by menopausal status	2.7 (1.4–5.4)	
Brinton and Swanson (1992), United States	1973–1980	1114	BMI	≥26 vs. <20 (5)	0.98 (0.7–1.3)	Age, age at menarche, education
			BMI at age 18–25 yr	≥25 vs. <19 (5), age 18 yr	0.60 (0.4–0.9)	
			Weight change	BMI gain 6.0+ vs. no change (5)	1.5 (1.1–2.2)	
Harris et al. (1992), United States	1987–1989	412	BMI	>27 vs. <22 (3)	1.5 (1.0–2.3)	Age. Education, parity, family history
Franceschi et al. (1996), Italy	1991–1994	1574	BMI	>28.8 vs. <21.7 (5)	1.4 (1.1–1.8)	Age, centre, education, parity, total energy and alcohol intake
			WHR	>0.88 vs. <0.78 (5)	1.0 (0.8–1.3)	Age, BMI, centre, education, parity, total energy and alcohol intake

Yong et al. (1996), United States	1973–1981	1198	BMI	≥34.7 vs. 26.8 (5)	1.3 (1.1–1.6)	Age, education, reproductive risk factors, history of benign breast disease, family history
Chie et al. (1998), Taiwan	1993–1994	216	BMI	≥25 vs. <20 (4)	1.9 (0.5–7.3)	Age, education, family history, reproductive factors, oral contraceptive use
Galanis et al. (1998), United States	1975–1994	292	BMI	>26 vs. <19.6 (5)	1.5 (1.0–2.3)	Age, education, ethnicity and drinking status
Magnusson et al. (1998), Sweden	1993–1995	2904	BMI	≥28.3 vs. <22.2 (5)	1.6 (1.4–2.0)	Age, reproductive factors, use of hormone replacement therapy
			BMI at age 18–25 yr	≥22.7 vs. <18.7 (5)	0.83 (0.69–1.0) age 18 yr	Age, reproductive factors, use of hormone replacement therapy
			Weight change	≥30 kg vs. <0 kg (5)	1.4 (1.1–1.9)	
Enger et al. (2000), United States	1987–1989	1091	BMI at age 18–25 yr	≥27.1 vs. <21.7 (4), age 18 yr	ER+/PgR+: 0.75 (0.38–1.5)	Age, socioeconomic status, reproductive risk factors, family history, alcohol, physical activity
				≥27.1 vs. <21.7 (4), age 19 yr	ER+PgR–: 0.53 (0.16–1.8)	
				≥27.1 vs. <21.7 (4), age 20 yr	ER–/PgR–: 0.79 (0.27–2.3)	
				≥27.1 vs. <21.7 (4), age 21 yr	Unknown: 0.77 (0.38–1.6)	
			BMI	≥27.1 vs. <21.7 (4)	ER+/PgR+: 2.4 (1.7–3.5)	
				≥27.1 vs. <21.7 (4)	ER+/PgR–: 1.3 (0.78–2.2)	
				≥27.1 vs. <21.7 (4)	ER–/PgR–: 1.2 (0.70–2.0)	
				≥27.1 vs. <21.7 (4)	Unknown: 1.6 (1.1–2.2)	
			Weight change	% change age 18 yr to reference age, >29.2 vs. ≤0 (4)	ER+/PgR+: 2.3 (1.6–3.4)	
				% change age 18 yr to reference age, >29.2 vs. ≤0 (4)	ER–/PgR–: 0.99 (0.58–1.8)	
				% change age 18 yr to reference age, >29.2 vs. ≤0 (4)	ER–/PgR–: 1.8 (0.91–3.4)	
				% change age 18 yr to reference age, >29.2 vs. ≤0 (4)	Unknown: 1.7 (1.2–2.5)	
Hall et al. (2000), United States	1993–1996	391	BMI	>30.1 vs. <24.6 (3)	Black: 0.68 (0.33–1.4)	Age, reproductive risk factors, education
				>30.1 vs. <24.6 (3)	White: 1.1 (0.58–2.0)	
			WHR	>0.86 vs. <0.77 (3)	Black: 1.6 (0.70–3.8)	Age, BMI, reproductive risk factors, education
				>0.86 vs. <0.77 (3)	White: 1.6 (0.88–3.1)	

(Continued)

Table 2 Studies of Body Size and Breast Cancer Risk (*Continued*)

Reference, study location	Study dates	Number of cases	Measurement	Contrasts (number of categories)	Relative risk (95% CI)	Adjustment for confounding
Friedenreich et al (2002), Canada	1995–1997	771	Height (m)	Highest quartile vs. lowest	1.15 (0.86–1.54)	Current age, total caloric intake, total lifetime physical activity, educational level (in quintiles), ever use of hormone replacement therapy, ever diagnosed with benign breast disease, first-degree family history of breast cancer, ever alcohol consumption, current smoker
			Weight (kg)	Highest quartile vs. lowest	1.11 (0.83–1.49)	
			Body mass index	Highest quartile vs. lowest	0.99 (0.74–1.32)	
			Waist	Highest quartile vs. lowest	1.30 (0.97–1.73)	
			Hip	Highest quartile vs. lowest	1.00 (0.74–1.33)	
			WHR	Highest quartile vs.. lowest	1.43 (1.07–1.93)	
			Weight at age 20 yr (kg)	Highest quartile vs. lowest	0.76 (0.57–1.03)	
			Weight gain since age 20 yr (kg)	Highest quartile vs. lowest	1.35 (1.01–1.81)	
			Weight gain over life	Highest quartile vs. lowest	1.56 (1.16–2.08)	
			Ref.—min. weight since age 20 yr	Highest quartile vs. lowest	1.47 (1.10–1.97)	
Lahmann et al. (2004a), Sweden	1991–2001	89	Birth weight	Per 100 g increase	1.06 (1.00–1.12)	Socioeconomic status (SES) of origin and adulthood, as well as adult body mass index (BMI) measured prior to diagnosis.
				>4000g vs. <3000 g birth weight	2.66 (0.96–7.41)	
Barba et al. (2006), United States	1996–2001	845	Birth weight	>8.5 vs. <5.5 lb	1.03 (0.74–1.44)	Age, education, race, BMI, history of breast benign disease, family history of breast cancer, lactation, age at menarche, age at first full term pregnancy, age at menopause, parity
Park et al. (2006), Poland	2000–2003	2386	Birth weight	>4 kg vs. <2.5 kg	1.84 (1.19–2.85)	Age, education, age at menarche, menopausal status and age at menopause, age at first full-term pregnancy, number of full-term pregnancies, family history of breast cancer among first degree relatives, mammography screening and current BMI

Abbreviations: NA, not analyzed; NE, not estimated; ER, estrogen receptor; PgR, progesterone receptor; WHR, waist-hip ratio.

and Swanson, 1992; Pathak and Whittemore, 1992; Vatten and Kvinnsland, 1992; Katoh et al., 1994; Tornberg and Carstensen, 1994; Franceschi et al., 1996; Swanson et al., 1996; Yong et al., 1996; Ziegler et al., 1996; Huang et al., 1997; Chie et al., 1998; Coates et al., 1999; Peacock et al., 1999; Enger et al., 2000; Hall et al., 2000; van den Brandt et al., 2000; Lahmann et al., 2004b; Weiderpass et al., 2004; Magnusson et al., 2005; McCormack et al., 2005; Lukanova et al., 2006; Tehard and Clavel-Chapelon, 2006). A meta-analysis based on 23 studies reported a significant trend for a decreased risk for premenopausal breast cancer associated with increasing BMI, with relative risk (RR) of 0.70 (95% CI, 0.54–0.91) from four cohort studies and 0.88 (95% CI, 0.76–1.02) from 19 case-control studies (Ursin et al., 1995). In a pooled analysis from seven prospective cohort studies including 337,819 women and 4385 incident invasive breast cancer cases, the reported RR for premenopausal breast cancer was 0.54 (95% CI, 0.34–0.85) in women with BMI $\geq$31 kg/m^2 compared to those with BMI <21 kg/m^2 (van den Brandt et al., 2000). Nevertheless, a limited number of case-control studies showed no association or a nonsignificant positive risk (Hsieh et al., 1990; Chu et al., 1991; Ziegler et al., 1996; Enger et al., 2000; Hall et al., 2000; Friedenreich et al., 2002).

In contrast to premenopausal breast cancer, overweight or obese postmenopausal women are at increased risk of developing breast cancer, as demonstrated in several large epidemiological studies (Paffenbarger et al., 1980; Lubin et al., 1985; Kolonel et al., 1986; Le Marchand et al., 1988; Tretli, 1989; Folsom et al., 1990; Hsieh et al., 1990; Chu et al., 1991; Harris et al., 1992; Sellers et al., 1992; Tornberg and Carstensen, 1994; Ballard-Barbash and Swanson, 1996; Franceschi al., 1996; Yong et al., 1996; Huang et al., 1997; Chie et al., 1998; Galanis et al., 1998; Magnusson et al., 1998; Enger et al., 2000; Li et al., 2000; Morimoto et al., 2002; Okasha et al., 2002; Petrelli et al., 2002; Lahmann et al., 2003, 2004b, 2004c; Rapp et al., 2005; Rinaldi et al., 2006a, 2006b; Tehard and Clavel-Chapelon, 2006). It was estimated in a meta-analysis that per unit increase in BMI increased the risk of postmenopausal breast cancer by 2% (Bergstrom et al., 2001). For a postmenopausal woman with BMI $\geq$30 kg/m^2, the estimated RR for developing breast cancer ranged from 1.23 (95% CI, 1.00–1.59) to 2.52 (95% CI, 1.62–3.93) (Morimoto et al., 2002; Tehard et al., 2004). The pooled analysis by van den Brandt et al. showed that the RR for postmenopausal breast cancer was 1.26 (95% CI, 1.09–1.46) in women with BMI $\geq$28 kg/m^2 compared to those with BMI <21 kg/m^2, but the risk did not increase further with increasing BMI (van den Brandt et al., 2000). Several large-scale studies have confirmed this positive association (de Waard, 1975; London et al., 1989; Tretli, 1989; Tretli et al., 1990; Vatten and Kvinnsland, 1990b; Le Marchand, 1991; Tornberg and Carstensen, 1994; Swanson et al., 1996; Yong et al., 1996; Li et al., 2000; Okasha et al., 2002; Petrelli et al., 2002; Lahmann et al., 2003, 2004b, 2004c; Rapp et al., 2005; Rinaldi et al., 2006a; Tehard and Clavel-Chapelon, 2006). A large prospective cohort study in Sweden found that obesity and percent body fat are positively associated with breast cancer risk (p for trend = 0.02) in which the percent body fat showed the strongest association (RR = 2.01, 95% CI, 1.26–3.21) for the highest versus lowest quintile (Lahmann et al., 2003). In many case-control studies, overweight or obese women have been reported to be at 10% to 60% increased risk of breast cancer (Paffenbarger et al., 1980; Kolonel et al., 1986; Hsieh et al., 1990; Harris et al., 1992; Franceschi et al., 1996; Yong et al., 1996; Galanis et al., 1998; Magnusson et al., 1998) and at more than twofold increased risk in some other studies (Lubin et al., 1985; Chu et al., 1991; Chie et al., 1998; Enger et al., 2000). However no increased risk was reported in a few studies (Hislop et al., 1986; Bouchardy et al., 1990; Brinton and Swanson, 1992; Hall et al., 2000; Friedenreich et al., 2002). The risks for breast cancer associated with overweight and obesity increased with age at diagnosis from 10% to 30% among women younger than 60 years to 60% to 190% among women older than 65 or 70 years (Franceschi et al., 1996; Yong et al., 1996; La Vecchia et al., 1997). In terms of population attributable risk, 20% of all postmenopausal breast cancer patients were attributable to overweight and obesity in a pooled analysis of three Italian case-control studies (La Vecchia et al., 1997). Several large-scale cohort studies have also indicated a positive association between obesity and mortality from breast cancer (Goodwin and Boyd, 1990; Senie et al., 1992; Jain and Miller, 1994; Galanis et al., 1998; Daling et al., 2001; Petrelli et al., 2002; Berclaz et al., 2004; Kroenke et al., 2005; Whiteman et al., 2005). The USA Cancer Prevention II (CPS-II) study (Petrelli et al., 2002) reported a RR for breast cancer mortality of 3.08 (95% CI, 2.09–4.51) for BMI >40.0 versus 18.5 to 20.49 kg/m^2. About 30% to 50% of breast cancer deaths among postmenopausal women in the US population have been suggested to be attributable to overweight (Petrelli et al., 2002).

The significant inverse and positive associations between BMI and breast cancer among pre- and postmenopausal women, respectively, were also confirmed in some large prospective cohort studies which involving both pre- and postmenopausal women, such as a recent published French longitudinal cohort study with 69,116 women (with 275 premenopausal and 860 postmenopausal incident invasive breast cancers) (Tehard and Clavel-Chapelon, 2006). More precise estimates were reported from two large cohorts of registered female nurses in United States—the Nurses' Health Study (NHS) (initiated in 1976 with 121,700 nurses aged 30 to 55) and the

National Health Survey II study (NHS-II) (begun in 1989 with 116,671 nurses aged 25 to 42) (Willett et al., 1985; London et al., 1989; Swanson et al., 1989; Huang et al., 1997, 1999; Baer et al., 2005, 2006; Eliassen et al., 2006; Michels et al., 2006; Tworoger et al., 2006). Two early NHS studies suggested that the protective effect among heavier premenopausal women was limited to early stage disease due to poorer detection of small tumors (Willett et al., 1985; Swanson et al., 1989). On the basis of follow-up data until 1992 in NHS study, the risk estimate for the top decile of recent BMI (>31 kg/m^2) was 0.62 for premenopausal breast cancer. The risks for the 2nd to 7th deciles were essentially null and then decreased to 0.86 and 0.80 for the 8th and 9th deciles, suggesting that the protective effect for premenopausal breast cancer was limited to very high BMI. Among postmenopausal women, current use of hormone replacement therapy (HRT) modified the association between body size and breast cancer. A significant increased risk only appeared for postmenopausal women who never used HRT with a RR of 1.59 (95% CI, 1.09–2.32, p for trend < 0.001) for women with BMI >31 kg/m^2 versus ≤ 20 kg/m^2 (Huang et al., 1997). Data from the European Prospective Investigation into Cancer and Nutrition (EPIC) Study showed that obese women have a 31% increased risk of developing breast cancer compared with nonobese women (Lahmann et al., 2004a). Using this large cohort study in Europe, more estimates were reported for the association between body size and breast cancer risk, usually including several anthropometric measurement effects and covered both pre- and postmenopausal women in different European countries. On the basis of a substudy from nine countries of the EPIC cohort, with 73,542 premenopausal and 103,344 postmenopausal women, the effects of weight, height, waist, and hip circumferences were examined. Among premenopausal women, weight and BMI showed nonsignificant inverse associations with breast cancer. For postmenopausal breast cancer, similar as found in the NHS study, the positive association between weight, BMI and hip circumference, and breast cancer risk was only found among non-HRT users, while an inverse but nonsignificantly association was found among HRT users. Obese postmenopausal women (BMI > 30 kg/m^2) who never used HRT before had a 31% excess risk compared with women with BMI <25 kg/m^2 (p for trend ≤ 0.002) (Lahmann et al., 2004b). According to a large nested case-control study within the EPIC cohort with 613 postmenopausal breast cancer cases and 1139 matched controls, the RR for developing postmenopausal breast cancer per 5 kg/m^2 increase in BMI was 1.11 (95% CI, 0.99–1.25) (Rinaldi et al., 2006a).

Recent evidence also indicated that adult height was positively associated with breast cancer risk. For premenopausal breast cancer, a large Norwegian cohort showed a positive effect in women taller than 167 cm compared with women less than 159 cm (RR = 2.63, 95% CI, 1.48–4.68) (Vatten and Kvinnsland, 1990a). A large case-control study found that risk was increased about twofold among women who were tall and thin compared with women who were heavy and short (Swanson et al., 1996). An increasing risk for premenopausal breast cancer development was also reported from nine countries, data from EPIC study (RR = 1.05, 95% CI, 1.00–1.16 for height increment per 5 cm) (Lahmann et al., 2004b). A Swedish cohort showed a statistically significant 30% reduced risk among premenopausal women shorter than 160 cm compared with taller ones (Weiderpass et al., 2004). For postmenopausal women, a positive association between adult height and breast cancer was consistently reported. A significantly increasing risk was reported in the large prospective mortality study in United States (CPS-II) for women taller than 66 inches versus shorter (RR = 1.64, 95% CI, 1.23–2.18) (Petrelli et al., 2002). As noted in subgroup studies (Lahmann et al., 2003; Tehard et al., 2004), the pooled nine EPIC countries data showed a slightly but significantly increasing risk by height increment per 5cm (RR = 1.10, 95% CI, 1.05–1.16) in postmenopausal women (Lahmann et al., 2004b). Result from the NHS study suggested that the adult height was positively associated with postmenopausal breast cancer incidence (RR = 1.57, 95% CI, 1.23–2.01; p for trend < 0.0001) for participants taller than 175 cm compared with those shorter than 160 cm, and each 5 cm increment corresponded to an 11% increase (95% CI, 6–17%) in risk of postmenopausal breast cancer development (Baer et al., 2006).

Central Adiposity

In 2003, Harvie et al. (2003) systematically reviewed the relationship between central obesity, in terms of waist circumference or WHR, and the risk of breast cancer in pre- and postmenopausal women, based on eight eligible identified publications of cohort and case-control data (Mannisto et al., 1996; Ng et al., 1997; Kaaks et al., 1998; Huang et al., 1999; Sonnenschein et al., 1999; Folsom et al., 2000; Muti et al., 2000; Morimoto et al., 2002). Pooled results from cohort studies suggested a 39% lower risk of breast cancer in postmenopausal women with the smallest waist (compared with the largest) and a 24% lower risk in women with the smallest WHR, while little effect was found in premenopausal women. After adjusted for BMI, the associations between waist circumference or WHR and breast cancer risk were no longer significant in postmenopausal women, but became negatively associated with risk among premenopausal women (Harvie et al., 2003). A meta-analysis of the published literature on WHR and breast cancer risk reported that the overall risk for developing breast cancer in women with high

WHR was 1.62 (95% CI, 1.28–2.04). The summary risks were 1.79 (95% CI, 1.22–2.62) for premenopausal women and 1.50 (95% CI, 1.10–2.04) for postmenopausal women (Connolly et al., 2002).

Inconsistent results, however, have been shown among individual studies on central adiposity and premenopausal breast cancer risk. Some studies suggested that neither waist/hip circumference nor WHR was related to premenopausal breast cancer risk (Petrek et al., 1993; Franceschi et al., 1996; Swanson et al., 1996; Kaaks et al., 1998; Huang et al., 1999; Hall et al., 2000; Friedenreich et al., 2002; Borugian et al., 2003; Lahmann et al., 2004b) while others showed increasing risks (Schapira et al., 1990; Mannisto et al., 1996; Ng et al., 1997; Sonnenschein et al., 1999; Hall et al., 2000), and one French prospective study even found a protective effect (Tehard and Clavel-Chapelon, 2006).

For postmenopausal women, high central adiposity has been consistently reported to be associated with higher breast cancer risk in epidemiological studies (Ballard-Barbash et al., 1990; Folsom et al., 1990; Bruning et al., 1992; Sellers et al., 1992; Petrek et al., 1993; Franceschi et al., 1996; Mannisto et al., 1996; Ng et al., 1997; Kaaks et al., 1998; Huang et al., 1999; Hall et al., 2000; Friedenreich et al., 2002). The effect of high central adiposity for postmenopausal breast cancer development seems to be independent from BMI in the majority of the studies. A 10 year follow up of 603 postmenopausal breast cancer case cohort study in Canada showed that WHR was directly related to breast cancer mortality (for highest quartile vs. lowest, RR = 3.3, 95% CI, 1.1–10.4) (Borugian et al., 2003). In the nested case-control EPIC study, postmenopausal breast cancer risk was positively related to waist circumference (RR = 1.12, 95% CI, 1.02–1.24) and hip circumferences (RR = 1.14, 95% CI, 1.02–1.27), per 10 cm increase, respectively (Rinaldi et al., 2006a).

Birth Weight and Birth Size

Michels and Xue (2006) have recently reviewed the available evidence based on 26 studies on the association between birth weight and the risk of breast cancer. Many, but not all, studies suggested a consistent positive association between birth weight and breast cancer risk in younger or premenopausal women but with either null or a reduced association among postmenopausal women (Le Marchand et al., 1988; Michels et al., 1996; Sanderson et al., 1996; Ekbom et al., 1997; Sanderson et al., 1998; Mogren et al., 1999; Innes et al., 2000; Stavola et al., 2000; Andersson et al., 2001; Hilakivi-Clarke et al., 2001; Hubinette et al., 2001; Kaijser et al., 2001; Sanderson et al., 2002; Titus-Ernstoff et al., 2002; Vatten et al., 2002; Ahlgren et al., 2003; Kaijser et al., 2003; McCormack et al., 2003; Mellemkjaer et al., 2003; Ahlgren et al., 2004; dos Santos Silva et al., 2004; Hodgson et al., 2004; Lahmann et al., 2004a; McCormack et al., 2005; Vatten et al., 2005). Through combining published results, comparing women with high birth weight to those with low birth weight, the RR for breast cancer development was 1.20 (95% CI, 1.07–1.35) for premenopausal women and 1.04 (95% CI, 0.91–1.19) for postmenopausal breast cancer women among the cohort studies, and 1.36 (95% CI, 1.15–1.61) and 1.04 (95% CI, 0.66–1.64), respectively, among case-control studies (Michels and Xue, 2006).

Several individual studies have indicated that birth weights above 4 kg increases premenopausal breast cancer risk (Ekbom et al., 1992, 1997; Andersson et al., 2001; Hilakivi-Clarke et al., 2001; Hubinette et al., 2001; Vatten et al., 2002; Ahlgren et al., 2003; dos Santos Silva et al., 2004). A British cohort found that women who weighed $\geq$4 kg at birth were five times (RR = 5.03, 95% CI, 1.13–22.5) more likely to develop premenopausal breast cancer than those who weighed <3 kg (p for trend = 0.03); and the RR per 1 kg increase in birth weight in this study was 2.31 (95% CI, 0.95–5.64) (dos Santos Silva et al., 2004). On the basis of a large Danish cohort of 106,504 women, a RR of 1.17 (95% CI, 1.02–1.33) for women with birth weight >4 kg versus >2.5 kg was reported (Ahlgren et al., 2004), and the attributable risk of birth weight was 7% (Ahlgren et al., 2006). The role for low birth weight on breast cancer risk is less worked out, although several recent large-scale case-control or cohort studies, mainly conducted in Scandinavia or North America, have presented supporting data for a protective role for low birth weight for premenopausal breast cancer (Barba et al., 2006; Michels et al., 2006; Park et al., 2006; Troisi et al., 2006; Lof et al., 2007). In the NHS and NHS-II studies, a low birth weight (birth weight < 5.5 lb vs. >8.5 lb) was associated with a decreased incidence of breast cancer among premenopausal women (RR = 0.66, 95% CI, 0.47–0.93) (Michels et al., 2006). The protective effect of low birth weight for premenopausal breast cancer was also found in a Swedish cohort study with RR of 0.65 (95% CI, 0.43–0.99), comparing women with low birth weight ($\leq$2.5 kg) to women with the highest birth weight (>3 kg) (Lof et al., 2007). Birth weight is highly correlated to birth length. In a Swedish cohort study, the positive association between birth weight and premenopausal breast cancer risk disappeared when adjusted for birth length and head circumference (McCormack et al., 2003). However, the numbers of cases were low in that study. A number of studies have examined the effect from birth length itself (Ekbom et al., 1992, 1997; Andersson et al., 2001; Hilakivi-Clarke et al., 2001; Hubinette et al., 2001; Vatten et al., 2002; Ahlgren et al., 2003; dos Santos Silva et al., 2004). All studies found a positive association, though most not statistically significant.

Some individual studies have reported a positive association between birth weight and postmenopausal breast cancer risk. A Danish cohort study found a significant positive association (risk increase 9% per kg) between birth weight and breast cancer risk (Ahlgren et al., 2004). The increasing risk was also observed in a nested case-control study in Sweden [odds ratio (OR) = 1.06, 95% CI, 1.00–1.12, per 0.1 kg) and persisted after adjustment for other perinatal and adult risk factors (Lahmann et al., 2004a). A weak J-shaped pattern was observed in U.S. women aged between 50 and 79 years with the highest risk in the birth weight category >4.5 kg (OR = 1.18, 95% CI, 0.92–1.51) (Titus-Ernstoff et al., 2002). Findings from two recent studies suggested that the positive association between birth weight and breast cancer risk was present irrespective of age at breast cancer diagnosis (Kaijser et al., 2003; Ahlgren et al., 2004). However, nonsignificant positive (Le Marchand et al., 1988; Michels et al., 1996; Ekbom et al., 1997; Michels et al., 2006) or inverse (Sanderson et al., 1996; McCormack et al., 2005) trends for postmenopausal breast cancer were observed in some other studies.

Young Adult Body Size and Weight Change During the Lifetime and Breast Cancer Risk

The evidence for the association between young adult body size, weight changes (gain or loss) and breast cancer risk is rather limited and inconsistent. An earlier review estimated that weight gain throughout adult life was associated with a risk ranging from 0.5 to 1.2 in premenopausal women and from 1.4 to 2.5 in postmenopausal women. Weight loss, on the other hand, was associated with a risk of 0.7 to 0.9 in premenopausal women and 0.8 to 1.5 in postmenopausal women (Ballard-Barbash, 1994).

Among premenopausal women, some studies indicated that heavier weight or BMI during their young adulthood, generally reported for ages between 18 and 20 years, was associated with a 25% to 40% decreased risk for breast cancer (Paffenbarger et al., 1980; Le Marchand et al., 1988; London et al., 1989; Chu et al., 1991; Brinton and Swanson, 1992; Sellers et al., 1992; Huang et al., 1997; Coates et al., 1999; Peacock et al., 1999). The U.S. NHS study gave a risk estimate of 0.74 (95% CI, 0.54–1.00) for the top sextile of weight gain (>25 kg) from age 18 years (Huang et al., 1997). In the NHS-II cohort, the body fatness at each age was reported to be inversely associated with premenopausal breast cancer incidence and RR were 0.48 (95% CI, 0.35–0.55) and 0.57 (95% CI, 0.39–0.83) for the most overweight compared with the most lean in childhood and adolescence, respectively, and the results were independent of adult BMI and menstrual cycle characteristics (Baer et al., 2005). A large prospective cohort study in Norway and Sweden reported associations between perceived body shape at age 7 and BMI at age 18, with heavier builds at both ages reducing risk. However, changes in body size from age 7 or 18 to adulthood did not affect breast cancer risk (Weiderpass et al., 2004). A German case-control study found that larger body build at menarche had a protective effect against premenopausal breast cancer, compared with smaller build (OR = 0.69, 95% CI, 0.49–0.96), and suggested that this effect may be more pronounced for women who were lean in adolescence and early adulthood (Verla-Tebit and Chang-Claude, 2005). However, some data reported that adult weight gain and central obesity increase the risk of premenopausal breast cancer (Willett et al., 1985; Schapira et al., 1990, 1991a; Peacock et al., 1999). A Danish cohort study showed that high stature at 14 years of age, low BMI at 14 years of age, and peak growth at an early age were independent risk factors for breast cancer, with attributable risks of 15%, 15%, and 9%, respectively (Ahlgren et al., 2006). Null effect from young body size and weight change for premenopausal breast cancer risk was observed in some studies (Friedenreich et al., 2002; Lahmann et al., 2005; Whiteman et al., 2005).

For the risk of postmenopausal breast cancer, a positive association was shown consistently in retrospective and prospective studies from young adult body size and weight changes through adult life (Paffenbarger et al., 1980; Le Marchand et al., 1988; Ingram et al., 1989; London et al., 1989; Ballard-Barbash et al., 1990; Folsom et al., 1990; Chu et al., 1991; Brinton and Swanson, 1992; Harris et al., 1992; Franceschi et al., 1996; Mannisto et al., 1996; Ziegler et al., 1996; Huang et al., 1997; Magnusson et al., 1998; Enger et al., 2000; Friedenreich et al., 2002; Radimer et al., 2004). RR between 1.2 and 2.3 for the highest versus lowest categories for weight gained between age 18 or 20 and the reference age were reported (Friedenreich, 2001b; IARC, 2002). In a Swedish case-control study, women who had gained 30 kg or more since age 18 had an OR of 2.04 (95% CI, 1.20–3.48) compared with those who had maintained their weight unchanged (Magnusson et al., 1998). A Finnish prospective study indicated that tallness in childhood was associated with increased risk of developing breast cancer ($p = 0.01$ at age 7 years). The relative risk for breast cancer was 1.27 (95% CI, 0.97–1.78) for every 1 kg increase in birth weight and 1.21 (95% CI, 1.06–1.38) for every 1 kg/m^2 decrease in BMI at age 7 (Hilakivi-Clarke et al., 2001). In a U.S. case-control study, the increasing association between breast cancer and weight change from age 18 to usual adult weight was only found among Hispanics but not in non-Hispanic white women and largely restricted to women who were lean at age 18 and those with hormone receptor–positive tumors (Wenten et al., 2002). A large Swedish cohort study showed that women with weight gain >21 kg had a RR of 1.75 (95% CI, 1.11–2.77) compared with women with lower weight gains (Lahmann et al., 2003), and for every 5 kg gain in weight, the risk was increased by 1.08 (95% CI, 1.04–1.12) (Lahmann et al., 2004c). In a pooled data from six EPIC countries, a positive association between weight gain and postmenopausal breast cancer risk was found only among noncurrent HRT users (RR = 1.50, 95% CI, 1.06–2.13) for women who gained 15 to 20 kg versus women who kept a stable weight ($\pm$2 kg) (p for trend $\leq$0.0002). A pooled RR per weight gain increment of 5 kg of 1.08 (95% CI, 1.04–1.12) was reported among non-HRT-users postmenopausal women (Lahmann et al., 2005). Result from NHS study suggested that 15.0% (95% CI, 12.8–17.4%) of breast cancer cases be attributable to weight gain over 2 kg since age 18 and 4.4% (95% CI, 3.6–5.5%) to weight gain over 2 kg since menopause. Among those who did not use postmenopausal hormones, the population attributable risks were 24.2% (95% CI, 19.8–29.1%) for a weight gained since age 18 and 7.6% (95% CI, 5.9–9.7%) for weight gained since menopause (Eliassen et al., 2006).

Data on an association between weight loss and breast cancer risk is sparse and mainly reported a nonsignificant slightly reduced risk (Ballard-Barbash et al., 1990; Brinton and Swanson, 1992; Ziegler et al., 1996; Huang et al., 1997; Parker and Folsom, 2003; Harvie et al., 2005; Eliassen et al., 2006). One study in premenopausal women found a statistically significant decreasing risk from weight loss between age 20 and enrolment, which, however, only appeared among low-grade of breast cancer cases (Coates et al., 1999). Nevertheless, unintentional weight loss was not found to decrease cancer risk in a US prospective study of 21,707 postmenopausal women (RR = 0.81, 95% CI, 0.66–1.00 for women who experienced weight loss over 20 lb compared with women who had not lost such an amount of weight) (Parker and Folsom, 2003).

Modification of the Association Between Body Size and Risk of Breast Cancer

Adiposity affects circulating hormonal levels, particularly in postmenopausal women. Endogenous hormones levels and use of exogenous estrogens and progestins may be strong modifiable risk factors for breast cancer. Obesity is associated with early age of menarche and late age of menopause, which maximize the number of ovulatory cycles and therefore increases breast cancer risk. It is also suggested that obesity associated with decreased fertility or infertility, which increases the lifetime cumulative exposure of mammary epithelium to estrogen, might increase the risk of breast cancer (IARC, 2002; Carmichael and Bates, 2004). It has been proposed that the association of birth weight and body size throughout life with premenopausal breast cancer risk may be due, in part, to relationships with sex hormones. HRT may particularly affect the association between body size and postmenopausal breast cancer (Magnusson et al., 1998).

A recent study from the NHS-II cohort suggested that the effects of adiposity on premenopausal sex hormone levels may be one mechanism through which adult adiposity, but not birth weight or childhood body size, affects premenopausal breast cancer risk (Tworoger et al., 2006). As some results shown above, the effect modification by HRT on the association between obesity and postmenopausal breast cancer risk has been addressed by several studies (Willett et al., 1985; Swanson et al., 1989; Harris et al., 1992; Collaborative Group on Hormonal Factors in Breast Cancer, 1997; Huang et al., 1997; Magnusson et al., 1998; van den Brandt et al., 2000; Morimoto et al., 2002; Lahmann et al., 2003; Feigelson et al., 2004; Modugno et al., 2006), and the effect of weight gain has been found unequivocal among non-HRT-users but not among HRT users (Magnusson et al., 1998). On the basis of an Oxford Pooling Project, which combined 51 cohorts data, the RR associated with duration of current or recent HRT use for five years or longer decreased progressively with increasing BMI (1.73, 1.29, and 1.02, for BMIs of <22.5, 22.5–24.9, and >25.0 kg/m^2, respectively) (Collaborative Group on Hormonal Factors in Breast Cancer, 1997). The NHS study showed that the risk increased from 1.2 among all women to 1.9 among non-HRT-users (Huang et al., 1999). In another large case-control study, the association between weight gain and postmenopausal breast cancer risk was reduced among current HRT users, although the test for interaction was not statistically significant (Trentham-Dietz et al., 2000). The nine EPIC countries data showed that the positive association between hip circumference and postmenopausal breast cancer was restricted to obese women who had never used HRT (Lahmann et al., 2004b), which was also confirmed in EPIC subpopulation studies (Huang et al., 1997; Lahmann et al., 2003, 2004a). The increase in breast cancer risk associated with adiposity was substantially reduced after adjustment for any exogenous estrogens use (Rinaldi et al., 2006a). Stratification according to tumor estrogen receptor (ER) status in a Canadian cohort study showed that the increased breast cancer mortality was restricted to ER-positive postmenopausal women (Borugian et al., 2003). One case-control study showed a risk of 2.45 (95% CI, 1.73–3.47) for women in the highest versus the lowest BMI among women with ER- and progesterone receptor (PgR)-positive tumors and was not increased among those with ER-negative or PgR-negative tumors or with ER-positive but PgR-negative tumors. However, this modified association did not appear among premenopausal women (Enger et al., 2000). The stronger association among non-HRT-users provides strong support for the hypothesis that the mechanism for increased risk is largely due to increases in endogenous estrogen production among heavier women.

Family history of breast and ovarian cancer may also modify the associations between body size and breast cancer risk in postmenopausal women. In a cohort of postmenopausal women, among women with elevated WHR, only those with a positive family history of breast cancer were at increased risk. The combination of high WHR with a family history of breast and ovarian cancer was associated with more than fourfold increases in risk of breast cancer (Sellers et al., 1992). In another large U.S. cohort risk associated with waist circumference and WHR appeared to vary slightly according to the family history of breast cancer (Huang et al., 1999). Among women having a family history of breast cancer, risk estimates for the highest compared to the lowest quintile were 1.23 for waist and 0.73 for WHR. Conversely, among women without a family history, risk estimates were 1.45 for waist and 1.40 for WHR (Huang et al., 1999).

Non-insulin-dependent diabetes mellitus (type 2) and postmenopausal breast cancer share a number of risk factors, including obesity, increased WHR, and a positive family history. A prospective cohort study in Iowa indicated a complex interrelation between these factors. Diabetes was not found to be associated with breast cancer risk (RR = 0.97) while family history of breast cancer and breast cancer incidence was slightly modified by individual history of diabetes. Conversely, a family history of breast cancer was associated with a RR of five-year diabetes mortality of 1.94 (95% CI, 1.17–3.24), which persisted after stratification by WHR (Sellers et al., 1994). Other studies also noted that a high BMI is significantly associated with an increased risk of inflammatory breast cancer (IBC), which is the most lethal form of breast cancer in both premenopausal and postmenopausal women (Chang et al., 1998). In a study of 68 women with IBC treated in United States, a significantly increased risk of IBC versus non–breast cancer (OR = 4.52, 95% CI, 1.85–11.04), comparing women in the highest with lowest BMI tertile was found, and the risk was not significantly modified by menopausal status (Chang et al., 1998).

Physical activity may reduce lifetime exposure to sex steroid hormones, and exposure to insulin and insulin-like growth factors thus prevent overweight or obesity and may protect against breast cancer. Numerous observational studies have assessed the association between physical activity and breast cancer risk. Although most studies reported that high physical activity is associated with decreased risk, inconsistent results have been also reported in some studies. Nevertheless, systematic reviews done by International Agency for Research on Cancer (IARC) or individual researchers found a fairly consistent inverse association between physical activities and the occurrence or mortality of breast cancer (Friedenreich and Rohan, 1995; Gammon et al., 1998; Friedenreich, 2001a; IARC, 2002; Vainio et al., 2002; Monninkhof et al., 2007). The decreased risk was observed for both occupational and recreational activities, among pre- and postmenopausal women, for activity measured at different time periods in life and for different levels of intensity and dose-response relationship of activity. It was indicated in a most recent meta-analysis, which included 19 cohort studies and 29 case-control studies that for pre- and postmenopausal breast cancer combined, physical activity was associated with a modest (15–20%) decreased risk. Stronger evidence appeared for postmenopausal breast cancer (ranging from 20–80%), while a much weaker evidence for premenopausal breast cancer. A trend analysis indicated a 6% (95% CI, 3–8%) decrease in breast cancer risk for each additional hour of physical activity per week assuming sustained level of activity (Monninkhof et al., 2007).

An increase in body weight is generally accounted for by excess energy intake relative to energy expenditure. Efforts to control weight gain usually involve either reducing energy intake via dietary energy restriction, or increasing energy expenditure via physical activity, or both. However, it is not clear whether preventing weight gain by dietary energy restriction, physical activity, or their combination has comparable effects on the risk for cancer (Thompson et al., 2004).

MECHANISM-BASED HYPOTHESIS BETWEEN BODY SIZE AND BREAST CANCER

The biological mechanisms explaining why obesity increases breast cancer risk in postmenopausal women but reduces the risk in premenopausal women have not been fully elucidated (Velie et al., 2005). The following hypotheses of biomechanism have been proposed to explain the relation between body size and breast cancer risk.

Proposed Biological Cancer-Promoting Mechanisms

Chronic Hyperinsulinemia

Abdominal fatness is associated with chronically elevated levels of insulin (hyperinsulinemia) and insulin resistance. Chronic hyperinsulinemia may increase breast cancer risk by carcinogenic effects mediated directly by insulin receptors in neoplastic target cells or by secondary carcinogenic effects due to changes in circulating insulin-like growth factor-I (IGF-I) or endogenous sex steroids caused by the hyperinsulinemia (Calle and Kaaks, 2004). Nevertheless, a recent analysis within the EPIC cohort did not find support for the hypothesis that chronic hyperinsulinemia generally was associated with an increased breast cancer risk irrespective of age, although the analysis could not rule that increased levels of insulin might contribute to an increased breast cancer risk after menopause (Verheus et al., 2006).

Elevated Circulating IGF-I and IGFBP-3

IGF-I might contribute to carcinogenesis since IGF-I promote cellular proliferation and inhibit apoptosis in many types of tissue, including both normal and neoplastic breast cells (Sachdev and Yee, 2001). The major binding protein of IGF-I, insulin growth factor–binding protein-3 (IGFBP-3), not only regulates IGF-I but it has also been shown to inhibit cell growth itself (Yu and Rohan, 2000). Indeed, in many studies increased serum levels of IGF-I and IGFBP-3 have been associated with increased risk of breast cancer, primarily among premenopausal women (Renehan et al., 2004), but also in older women (Rinaldi et al., 2006b). However, there is no clear linear relationship between circulating levels of IGF-I and the degree of obesity (Calle and Kaaks, 2004; Gram et al., 2006).

Elevated Circulating Estrogens

Obesity influences the synthesis and bioavailability of endogenous sex steroids by several mechanisms (Calle and Kaaks, 2004). For instance, adipose tissue expresses various enzyme systems that catalyze the production of estrogens from its precursors. In postmenopausal women, BMI is positively associated with increased levels of the estrogens, estrone and estradiol. Furthermore, adipose tissue increase circulating levels of insulin and IGF-I, which results in lower levels of sex hormone globulin (SHBG) and an increase in bioavailability of circulating estradiol. A pooled cohort study indicated that the association between BMI and breast cancer risk could almost entirely be attributed to increasing levels of endogenous estrogen levels caused by obesity (Key et al., 2003). This effect may address the stronger positive association among non-HRT-users compared with HRT-users between BMI and postmenopausal breast cancer risk.

Adipokines

In addition to the obesity-related changes in hormones (insulin and sex steroids), and IGF-I described above, proteins secreted by the adipocytes, so-called adipokines have been suggested to play a role in the link between obesity and breast cancer (Calle and Kaaks, 2004). In this context obesity-associated dysfunction of, e.g., leptin, TNF-α, and adiopenectin are interesting, although more research is needed to elucidate this most recent hypothesis.

Reversal Association Between Obesity and Breast Cancer Risk in Premenopausal Women

It has been suggested that the reduced breast cancer risk observed in obese premenopausal women is due to the increased frequency of anovalutory cycles, resulting in decreased levels of estradiol (Velie et al., 2005). Indeed, this hypothesis have been supported by several studies which have reported decreased serum levels of estradiol and increased serum levels of SHBG in obese premenopausal women, while increased levels of estradiol and decreased levels of SHBG have been found in obese postmenopausal women (Velie et al., 2005).

Proposed Mechanisms for the Link Between Size at Birth and Subsequent Breast Cancer Risk

The biological mechanisms underlying the association between birth weight and breast cancer risk are not fully clear. In utero exposures to elevated levels of hormones (estrogens or androgens) or insulin growth factors have been suggested as possible biological mechanisms (Velie et al., 2005). Growth factors have been suggested to influence breast cancer risk by increasing the number of susceptible stem cells in the mammary gland or by initiating tumors through DNA mutations (Michels and Xue, 2006).

BODY SIZE AND THE DIAGNOSIS OF BREAST CANCER

Most studies show that overweight is associated with a more advanced stage of breast cancer at diagnosis, especially when considering tumor size as a marker for breast cancer stage (Carmichael and Bates, 2004). In a population based case-control study, risk of late-stage disease (defined as tumor > 2 cm) was increased with higher BMI (OR = 1.46, 95% CI, 1.10–1.93 for the highest vs. the lowest tertile) (Hall et al., 1999). In a large Norwegian cohort study, RR estimates for stage I breast cancer for women in the top BMI quintile compared with the lowest were 0.80, 0.54, 0.54 and 0.63 for women aged 30 to 34, 35 to 39, 40 to 44 and 45 to 49 years. RR estimates for stage I–IV breast cancer were 1.2, 1.2, 0.97, and 1.4, respectively, for the same five-year age groups. However, the only statistically significant RR were those for stage I breast cancer among women 35 to 49 years (Tretli, 1989). Another study showed that obese women (BMI $\geq$ 27.3 kg/m^2) had an increased risk to have a more advanced breast cancer (tumor > 2 cm) at diagnosis compared to women who were not obese (OR = 1.57, 95% CI, 1.15–2.14). The association was stronger in women younger than 50 years (OR = 2.34, 95% CI, 1.34–4.08) compared with women older than 50 years (OR = 1.30, 95% CI, 0.89–1.91) (Cui et al., 2002). Furthermore, a recent Canadian study of 519 breast cancer patients reported that obese women had larger tumor sizes at diagnosis compared with normal- and overweight women (Porter et al., 2006). The evidence of studies about the risk from node status was less consistent than studies for tumor size. Some authors have reported that obese women were more likely to have lymph node metastases (Schapira et al., 1991b; Daniell et al., 1993; Porter et al., 2006), while others have not (Cui et al., 2002).

It is not clear why obesity appears to be associated with more advanced breast cancer at diagnosis. One explanation may be that obese patients are more likely to have a delayed diagnosis. Obese women often have larger breasts which might make it more difficult to identify breast abnormalities. Obesity is also more common in lower socioeconomic classes, which is associated with later presentation to a health professional. Delayed diagnosis of breast cancer has been suggested in obese women (Arndt et al., 2002), although this was not confirmed by a recent study (Porter et al., 2006). Secondly, the association between obesity and advanced tumor stage at diagnosis may actually due to some physiological features that are associated with both obesity and tumor progression. For instance, obesity influences the levels of hormones (e.g., estrogens or cortisol) and insulin growth factors, and these levels are also thought to play role for tumor progression (Porter et al., 2006).

BODY SIZE AND THE TREATMENT OF BREAST CANCER

The common treatments for breast cancer are surgery, radiotherapy, chemotherapy, and hormonal treatment. Obesity may influence all these treatments (Carmichael, 2006).

Surgery

Several recent reports suggest that obese women are more likely to have complications like infections of the surgical site when undergoing surgery for breast cancer (Nieto et al., 2002; Vilar-Compte et al., 2004). Furthermore, obesity is also associated with the need for more extensive surgery since having a high BMI increases the risk for a failed procedure when using the less invasive procedure sentinel node biopsy. In a review of 2495 sentinel lymph node biopsy (2.48% failure rate) BMI was statistically significantly higher in the failure group, and the success of the sentinel lymph node biopsy was inversely related to BMI ($r = 0.98$, $p = 0.002$) (Derossis et al., 2003).

Radiotherapy

Obesity is associated with increased incidence of complications of radiotherapy such as lymphoedema of the arm and breast (Meek, 1998; Kocak and Overgaard, 2000; Goffman et al., 2004). Furthermore, obese women often have larger breasts, which make it more difficult to provide an optimal dose. A recent report suggested that women with very large breasts may undergo reduction mammoplasty to allow optimal benefit from adjuvant radiotherapy (Newman et al., 2001).

Chemotherapy

Oncologists often give reduced doses of adjuvant chemotherapy to obese breast cancer patients (Carmichael, 2006). This is done in order to avoid overdosing resulting from an assumed altered drug distribution in obese women. Doses are reduced empirically (i.e., reducing the dose after the final dose calculation) or by using ideal instead of actual body weight when calculating the dose. However, several recent reports have argued that there is few data to support such a "dose-reduction policy" in obese women (Madarnas et al., 2001; Poikonen et al., 2001; Colleoni et al., 2005; Griggs et al., 2005). In a retrospective cohort of 9672 women treated with doxorubicin hydrochloride and cyclophosphamide, febrile neutropenia, the most common form of adverse effect of this treatment, was not more common among overweight and obese women receiving full weight-based doses than among normal- and underweight women. Furthermore, severely obese women were less likely to be hospitalized for febrile neutropenia when they received full doses (Griggs et al., 2005). There is also some indirect evidence that chemotherapy is less efficient in obese women. Poikonen et al. (2001) reported that when blood leukocyte nadir was used as a surrogate marker for the drug effect, obese patients had somewhat higher leukocyte nadir values. Empiric dose reductions for patients with high BMI have also been suggested to result in shortened disease-free survival (Rosner et al., 1996). There is a recently published review from four randomized trials of the International Breast Cancer Study Group assessing adjuvant CMF (cyclophosphamide, methotrexate, and 5-fluoroouracil) conducted between 1978 and 1993 in several countries in premenopausal women with node-positive breast cancer (Colleoni et al., 2005). The results confirmed that obese patients were more likely to receive a reduced dose of chemotherapy than nonobese patients (39% vs. 16%). Furthermore, for obese patients as well as for the total population, a reduction of the chemotherapy dose ($<85\%$ compared with $\geq 85\%$) was associated with a worse outcome for the ER-negative cohort (RR = 0.68, 95% CI, 0.54–0.86 for disease-free survival and RR = 0.72, 95% CI, 0.56–0.94 for overall survival). The corresponding associations for the ER-positive cohort were not statistically significant. These findings indicated that for patients with ER-absent tumors and ER-low tumors reductions in chemotherapy should be avoided.

Endocrine Treatment

Antiestrogen treatment has been suggested to be less efficient in obese women since they have larger amounts of body fat, which promotes an increased aromatization of peripheral androgens to estrogens (which takes place in fat cells). This suggestion was supported by the higher incidence of amenorrhea in nonobese women than in obese women. In a recent study, women with lymph node-negative and ER-positive cancer, obesity was not associated with any change in tamoxifen efficacy (Dignam et al., 2003).

BODY SIZE AND THE PROGNOSIS OF BREAST CANCER

As consistently shown in the systematic reviews and most individual observational studies, heavier women experienced poorer survival and increased likelihood of recurrence, irrespective of menopausal status, and the effect consisted after adjustment for stage and treatment (Greenberg et al., 1985; McNee et al., 1987; Hebert et al., 1988; Mohle-Boetani et al., 1988; Lees et al., 1989; Verreault et al., 1989; Coates et al., 1990; Kyogoku et al., 1990; Tretli et al., 1990; Vatten et al., 1991; Giuffrida et al., 1992; Senie et al., 1992; Demark-Wahnefried et al., 1993; Bastarrachea et al., 1994; den Tonkelaar et al., 1995; Zhang et al., 1995; Ballard-Barbash and Swanson, 1996; Maehle and Tretli, 1996; Chlebowski et al., 2002; IARC, 2002; Carmichael and Bates, 2004; Loi et al., 2005; Carmichael, 2006; Tao et al., 2006). A meta-analysis which reviewed 8029 cases of breast cancer estimated that the overall adverse effect of obesity on the prognosis of breast cancer was 1.56 (95% CI, 1.22–2.00) (Ryu et al., 2001). Weight gain is reported in the majority of women undergoing adjuvant therapy for breast cancer (Heasman et al., 1985; Goodwin et al., 1988; Camoriano et al., 1990; Demark-Wahnefried et al., 1993; Demark-Wahnefried et al., 1997). A study of 391 premenopausal women found that women who gained more than 5.9 kg were 1.5 times more likely to recurrence and 1.8 times more likely to die than women who gained less weight (Camoriano et al., 1990). A 10 year follow-up cohort of 166 breast cancer patients reported that the android body fat distribution (indicated by a higher suprailiac-thigh ratio) (RR = 2.6, 95% CI, 1.63–4.17) and adult weight gain (RR = 1.2, 95% CI, 1.0–1.3) were statistically significant prognostic indicators for survival (Kumar et al., 2000). An U.S. study reported that body weight loss (BWL) is a major prognostic factor in breast cancer, with a significant ($p < 0.001$) correlation with recurrence (Marinho et al., 2001). Nevertheless, null or adverse prognostic effects from obesity were also appeared in some studies (Sohrabi et al., 1980; Greenberg et al., 1985; Jain and Miller, 1994; Katoh et al., 1994; den Tonkelaar et al., 1995; Obermair et al., 1995; Menon et al., 1999; Marret et al., 2001; Carmichael et al., 2004). Neither WHR nor waist circumference was independently associated with poorer overall survival and disease-free survival in a Chinese study (Tao et al., 2006).

As indicated above, higher BMI is associated with a more advanced stage of breast cancer at diagnosis in terms of tumor size, but data on lymph node status is not so consistent. In several studies, the association between obese women with breast cancer prognosis was limited to or more pronounced among women with stage I and II disease (Verreault et al., 1989; Tretli et al., 1990; Enger et al., 2004), ER- and PgR-positive status (Coates et al., 1990; Giuffrida et al., 1992; Maehle and Tretli, 1996) and negative nodes (Mohle-Boetani et al., 1988; Newman et al., 1997). In some epidemiological studies, the excess incidence of breast cancer among lean young women was limited to tumors that were less than 2.0 cm in diameter, not associated with metastases to lymph nodes, and well differentiated (Willett et al., 1985). There was a 70% increased risk in the upper quintile of BMI among women with stage I disease and a 40% increased risk for stage II disease, while no association was found for late stage III and stage IV disease (Tretli et al., 1990). In a cohort of 1238 women with unilateral breast cancer treated with modified radical mastectomy and followed for 15 years, the risk of dying from breast cancer relative to BMI varied markedly by hormone receptor status (Maehle and Tretli, 1996). Further study of that cohort showed that obese patients had a 1.53 higher risk of lymph node metastases compared to slim patients ($p = 0.02$). In the PgR-negative group, obesity gave a 3.08 times higher risk of lymph node metastases ($p = 0.03$). BMI did not show a statistically significant relationship with prognosis if only hormone receptor status was considered. However, if lymph node status and hormone receptor status were taken together, the association was strong and reversed in the lymph node-positive group with ER-negative tumors (Maehle et al., 2004). It was indicated that among women with hormone receptor–positive tumors, obese women had a risk of death three times higher than thin women, while among women with hormone receptor–negative tumors, thin women had a risk of death six times higher than obese women, even after adjustment for lymph node status, tumor diameter, and mean nuclear area. Based on a clinical trial of women with node-negative, ER-breast cancer, obesity did not increase recurrence risk, but was associated with greater risk for second cancers (RR = 1.5, 95% CI, 1.1–2.1), contra lateral breast cancer (CBC) (RR = 2.1, 95% CI, 1.2–3.6 in postmenopausal women), and mortality, particularly non–breast cancer deaths (Dignam et al., 2006).

Furthermore, the differences in reported survival in breast cancer patients with anthropometrical characteristics may also partly be explained by the use of differing definitions of body size by various studies. However, the possibility of publication bias against negative studies should not be dismissed, and certain modified risk factors need to be noted. There is indirect evidence that poor survival in women with breast cancer in lower socioeconomic classes may be partly explained by the greater incidence of obesity in lower socioeconomic classes (Stoll, 1996; Haybittle et al., 1997). The host factors such as cellular immunity and nutrition that may determine metastases and recurrence of breast cancer may be unfavorable in deprived obese patients of lower socioeconomic status. It is also suggested that women from lower socioeconomic classes tend to have poor access and utilization of the diagnostic and therapeutic support for breast cancer (Carmichael and Bates, 2004). All treatment modalities for breast cancer such as surgery, radiotherapy, chemotherapy, and hormonal treatment may be adversely affected by the presence of obesity (Carmichael and Bates, 2004). In NHS study, the positive associations between weight before diagnosis and breast cancer recurrence and death were most apparent in women who never smoked (Kroenke et al., 2005). Obesity is also associated with significantly worse outcome in women with IBC (Chang et al., 2000). Recent published papers showed that type 2 diabetes mellitus was associated with negative prognostic factors at breast cancer presentation, as the mean BMI and tumor stage and size were higher among diabetic patients and the differences remained significant after adjustment for BMI. Moreover, after adjustment for BMI, breast cancer among diabetic patients was more often hormone receptor negative (Wolf et al., 2006).

BODY SIZE AND THE PREVENTION OF BREAST CANCER

The prevalence of overweight and obesity in adult and children has increased rapidly over the last two decades in most countries. In United States, it is estimated from the CPS-II that up to 50% of postmenopausal breast cancer deaths can be attributed to obesity (Petrelli et al., 2002). It is feared that increasing obesity in women will manifest its effect of increased incidence of breast cancer in women in the coming years.

Obesity contributes toward development and poor prognosis of breast cancer and also influences the diagnosis and treatment of the disease. Overweight and obesity are among the few risk factors for breast cancer that can be modified throughout life. Therefore, maintaining a relatively low weight, especially for women approaching menopause should be an integral part of any strategy to prevent breast cancer and improve breast cancer outcome (Carmichael, 2006). Epidemiological studies, animal experiments, and mechanistic investigation all support a beneficial effect of weight control in the prevention of cancer. The available evidence on the avoidance of weight gain suggested lack of a cancer preventive effect for premenopausal women, and inadequate evidence for preventive effect of intentional weight loss for breast cancer. However, sufficient evidence exists for a postmenopausal breast cancer preventive effect of avoidance of weight gain. It was estimated that up to 18,000 deaths in U.S. women older than 50 years may be avoided if women could maintain a BMI of less than 25 kg/m^2 throughout their adult life (Petrelli et al., 2002), and a 10% breast cancer incidence decrease and a consequent reduction in mortality would be reached through reduction of obesity in Europe (Carmichael et al., 2004). Furthermore, as reviewed above, there is evidence that higher weight at birth also increases the breast cancer risk in adult (Michels and Xue, 2006). Overweight or obese pregnant women usually will give birth to larger-sized babies (Kramer et al., 2002; Surkan et al., 2004), and therefore weight control in these women are strongly encouraged for the benefit of both women themselves and their female offsprings.

CONCLUSION

The evidence that obesity, measured as BMI, WHR, or weight gain during lifetime, adversely affects women's health is overwhelming and indisputable. An inverse association between obesity and premenopausal breast cancer risk has been found in countries with high incidence rates of breast cancer, among heavier women with poorer survival and increased risk of recurrence comparing with women having normal weight. Overweight and obesity clearly increase postmenopausal breast cancer risk and affect negatively the outcomes of breast cancer treatments and therefore overall breast cancer survival. Adult weight gain has been shown to be a strong and consistent predictor of postmenopausal breast cancer risk and to be associated with adverse prognosis of breast cancer. Weight loss among overweight or obese women possibly also reduces the risk of postmenopausal breast cancer, but so far no firm conclusion can be drawn. A consistent positive association is shown between birth weight and breast cancer risk in younger or premenopausal women, while the effect on postmenopausal women is less evident.

Most epidemiological studies based on tumor size suggest that obesity is associated with a more advanced stage of breast cancer at diagnosis, although data based on lymph node status is less consistent. Obesity influences breast cancer treatments in several ways. Obese breast cancer patients often have more complications when treated by surgery or radiotherapy. Majority of the literature has reported that obesity is associated with poor prognosis of breast cancer in both pre- and postmenopausal women.

The biological mechanism explaining the association between obesity and breast cancer are only partially understood. Elevated circulating estrogens, chronic hyperinsulinemia, increased levels of IGF-I and its binding protein IGFBP-3, or the involvement of adipokines may all play a role. Recent data indicates that the effects of obesity on breast cancer risk are largely mediated by increased estrogen levels.

RECOMMENDATION

Controlling of the obesity epidemic worldwide will require the participation of all segments of society and substantial investments, particularly in public education and community environments that promote working and other physical activities. It has been suggested that work site and school programs including at least one hour of physical activity on most days, and transportation systems encouraging walking and using of bicycles should be widely implemented. Certain strategies for breast cancer research related to body size and recommendations for public health action have been proposed by the IARC (2002).

Recommendations for Research

1. Critically evaluate methods for assessing body size and develop standardized and validated measuring indicators.
2. Develop, maintain, or enhance national surveillance programs for monitoring prevalence and trends in body size and studying environmental factors.
3. Conduct more observational epidemiological studies in diverse population to assess the association between body size and breast cancer risk; study the effect of voluntary weight reduction on cancer risk in overweight and obese individuals in different subpopulations.
4. Conduct experimental and mechanistic studies to clarify the mechanisms of body size and weight gain influencing breast cancer development and prognosis in animal models.
5. Conduct long-term clinical intervention studies in subgroups of age and ethnicity to alter behavioral patterns (regarding dietary intake and physical activity) which may influence weight change; carry out community intervention studies to prevent weight gain.

Recommendations for Public Health

Obesity cannot be prevented or managed solely at the level of the individual. Governments, the food industry, international agencies, media, communities, and individuals all need to work together to modify the environment. Though a number of recommendations assuming a certain level of infrastructure may not existing in developing countries, the underlying targets to improve dietary quality and ensure appropriate levels of physical activity for healthy weight are relevant and should be incorporated into strategies (IARC, 2002).

1. Governmental and non-governmental organizations: A public health policy, plan, and health education campaign are urgently required to address the rising problems of obesity and breast cancer. Public education should provide timely and accurate information on the epidemic of obesity. Governments at local and national levels, as well as non-governmental organizations should provide adequate funding for healthy lifestyle education and proper access for physical programs in schools and in public. In developing countries, there are dietary traditions, behavioral patterns, and infrastructures that potentially could aid programs for prevention of weight gain.
2. Health professionals: Health professionals should counsel individuals about a healthy range of body weight. For persons currently within the healthy range, it is recommended that weight gain during adult life should not exceed 5 kg.
3. Families and individuals: Prevention of overweight and obesity should begin early in life, based on a healthy lifestyle. However, it is never too late to benefit from starting to be more active. Parents and individuals should limit the purchase and the availability at home of high-energy foods and beverages with low nutritional value, such as soda beverages and baked snacks, and instead provide healthy foods, in particular an abundant supply of fruits and vegetables and whole grain products.

REFERENCES

Ahlgren M, Melbye M, Wohlfahrt J, Sorensen TI. Growth patterns and the risk of breast cancer in women. N Engl J Med 2004; 351(16):1619–1626.

Ahlgren M, Melbye M, Wohlfahrt J, Sorensen TI. Growth patterns and the risk of breast cancer in women. Int J Gynecol Cancer 2006; 16(suppl 2):569–575.

Ahlgren M, Sorensen T, Wohlfahrt J, Haflidadottir A, Holst C, Melbye M. Birth weight and risk of breast cancer in a cohort of 106,504 women. Int J Cancer 2003; 107(6): 997–1000.

Andersson SW, Bengtsson C, Hallberg L, Lapidus L, Niklasson A, Wallgren A, Hulthen L. Cancer risk in Swedish women: the relation to size at birth. Br J Cancer 2001; 84(9): 1193–1198.

Andersson SW, Niklasson A, Lapidus L, Hallberg L, Bengtsson C, Hulthen L. Poor agreement between self-reported birth weight and birth weight from original records in adult women. Am J Epidemiol 2000; 152(7):609–616.

Arndt V, Sturmer T, Stegmaier C, Ziegler H, Dhom G, Brenner H. Patient delay and stage of diagnosis among breast cancer patients in Germany—a population based study. Br J Cancer 2002; 86(7):1034–1040.

Baer HJ, Colditz GA, Rosner B, Michels KB, Rich-Edwards JW, Hunter DJ, Willett WC. Body fatness during childhood and adolescence and incidence of breast cancer in premenopausal women: a prospective cohort study. Breast Cancer Res 2005; 7(3):R314–R325.

Baer HJ, Rich-Edwards JW, Colditz GA, Hunter DJ, Willett WC, Michels KB. Adult height, age at attained height, and incidence of breast cancer in premenopausal women. Int J Cancer 2006; 119(9):2231–2235.

Ballard-Barbash R. Anthropometry and breast cancer. Body size—a moving target. Cancer 1994; 74(suppl 3):1090–1100.

Ballard-Barbash R, Schatzkin A, Taylor PR, Kahle LL. Association of change in body mass with breast cancer. Cancer Res 1990; 50(7):2152–2155.

Ballard-Barbash R, Swanson CA. Body weight: estimation of risk for breast and endometrial cancers. Am J Clin Nutr 1996; 63(suppl 3):437S–441S.

Barba M, McCann SE, Nie J, Vito D, Stranges S, Fuhrman B, Trevisan M, Muti P, Freudenheim JL. Perinatal exposures and breast cancer risk in the Western New York Exposures and Breast Cancer (WEB) Study. Cancer Causes Control 2006; 17(4):395–401.

Bastarrachea J, Hortobagyi GN, Smith TL, Kau SW, Buzdar AU. Obesity as an adverse prognostic factor for patients receiving adjuvant chemotherapy for breast cancer. Ann Intern Med 1994; 120(1):18–25.

Berclaz G, Li S, Price KN, Coates AS. Body mass index as a prognostic feature in operable breast cancer: the International Breast Cancer Study Group experience. Ann Oncol 2004; 15(6):875–884.

Bergstrom A, Pisani P, Tenet V, Wolk A, Adami HO. Overweight as an avoidable cause of cancer in Europe. Int J Cancer 2001; 91(3):421–430.

Borugian MJ, Sheps SB, Kim-Sing C, Olivotto IA, Van Patten C, Dunn BP, Coldman AJ, Potter JD, Gallagher RP, Hislop TG. Waist-to-hip ratio and breast cancer mortality. Am J Epidemiol 2003; 158(10):963–968.

Bouchardy C, Le MG, Hill C. Risk factors for breast cancer according to age at diagnosis in a French case-control study. J Clin Epidemiol 1990; 43(3):267–275.

Brinton LA, Swanson CA. Height and weight at various ages and risk of breast cancer. Ann Epidemiol 1992; 2(5):597–609.

Bruning PF, Bonfrer JM, Hart AA, van Noord PA, van der Hoeven H, Collette HJ, Battermann JJ, de Jong-Bakker M, Nooijen WJ, de Waard F. Body measurements, estrogen availability and the risk of human breast cancer: a case-control study. Int J Cancer 1992; 51(1):14–19.

Calle EE, Kaaks R. Overweight, obesity and cancer: epidemiological evidence and proposed mechanisms. Nat Rev Cancer 2004; 4(8):579–591.

Camoriano JK, Loprinzi CL, Ingle JN, Therneau TM, Krook JE, Veeder MH. Weight change in women treated with adjuvant therapy or observed following mastectomy for node-positive breast cancer. J Clin Oncol 1990; 8(8):1327–1334.

Carmichael AR. Obesity as a risk factor for development and poor prognosis of breast cancer. BJOG 2006; 113(10): 1160–1166.

Carmichael AR, Bates T. Obesity and breast cancer: a review of the literature. Breast 2004; 13(2):85–92.

Carmichael AR, Bendall S, Lockerbie L, Prescott RJ, Bates T. Does obesity compromise survival in women with breast cancer? Breast 2004; 13(2):93–96.

Chang S, Alderfer JR, Asmar L, Buzdar AU. Inflammatory breast cancer survival: the role of obesity and menopausal status at diagnosis. Breast Cancer Res Treat 2000; 64(2): 157–163.

Chang S, Buzdar AU, Hursting SD. Inflammatory breast cancer and body mass index. J Clin Oncol 1998; 16(12): 3731–3735.

Chie WC, Li CY, Huang CS, Chang KJ, Lin RS. Body size as a factor in different ages and breast cancer risk in Taiwan. Anticancer Res 1998; 18(1B):565–570.

Chlebowski RT, Aiello E, McTiernan A. Weight loss in breast cancer patient management. J Clin Oncol 2002; 20(4): 1128–1143.

Chu SY, Lee NC, Wingo PA, Senie RT, Greenberg RS, Peterson HB. The relationship between body mass and breast cancer among women enrolled in the Cancer and Steroid Hormone Study. J Clin Epidemiol 1991; 44(11):1197–1206.

Coates RJ, Clark WS, Eley JW, Greenberg RS, Huguley CM Jr., Brown RL. Race, nutritional status, and survival from breast cancer. J Natl Cancer Inst 1990; 82(21):1684–1692.

Coates RJ, Uhler RJ, Hall HI, Potischman N, Brinton LA, Ballard-Barbash R, Gammon MD, Brogan DR, Daling JR, Malone KE, Schoenberg JB, Swanson CA. Risk of breast cancer in young women in relation to body size and weight gain in adolescence and early adulthood. Br J Cancer 1999; 81(1):167–174.

Collaborative Group on Hormonal Factors in Breast Cancer. Breast cancer and hormone replacement therapy: collaborative reanalysis of data from 51 epidemiological studies of 52,705 women with breast cancer and 108,411 women without breast cancer. Lancet 1997; 350(9084):1047–1059.

Colleoni M, Li S, Gelber RD, Price KN, Coates AS, Castiglione-Gertsch M, Goldhirsch A. Relation between chemotherapy dose, oestrogen receptor expression, and body-mass index. Lancet 2005; 366(9491):1108–1110.

Connolly BS, Barnett C, Vogt KN, Li T, Stone J, Boyd NF. A meta-analysis of published literature on waist-to-hip ratio and risk of breast cancer. Nutr Cancer 2002; 44(2):127–138.

Cui Y, Whiteman MK, Flaws JA, Langenberg P, Tkaczuk KH, Bush TL. Body mass and stage of breast cancer at diagnosis. Int J Cancer 2002; 98(2):279–283.

Daling JR, Malone KE, Doody DR, Johnson LG, Gralow JR, Porter PL. Relation of body mass index to tumor markers and survival among young women with invasive ductal breast carcinoma. Cancer 2001; 92(4):720–729.

Daniell HW, Tam E, Filice A. Larger axillary metastases in obese women and smokers with breast cancer—an influence by host factors on early tumor behavior. Breast Cancer Res Treat 1993; 25(3):193–201.

de Waard F. Breast cancer incidence and nutritional status with particular reference to body weight and height. Cancer Res 1975; 35(11 pt 2):3351–3356.

Demark-Wahnefried W, Rimer BK, Winer EP. Weight gain in women diagnosed with breast cancer. J Am Diet Assoc 1997, 97(5):519–526, 529 (quiz 527–528).

Demark-Wahnefried W, Winer EP, Rimer BK. Why women gain weight with adjuvant chemotherapy for breast cancer. J Clin Oncol 1993; 11(7):1418–1429.

den Tonkelaar I, de Waard F, Seidell JC, Fracheboud J. Obesity and subcutaneous fat patterning in relation to survival of postmenopausal breast cancer patients participating in the DOM-project. Breast Cancer Res Treat 1995; 34(2): 129–137.

Derossis AM, Fey JV, Cody HS, Borgen PI III. Obesity influences outcome of sentinel lymph node biopsy in early-stage breast cancer. J Am Coll Surg 2003; 197(6):896–901.

Dignam JJ, Wieand K, Johnson KA, Fisher B, Xu L, Mamounas EP. Obesity, tamoxifen use, and outcomes in women with estrogen receptor-positive early-stage breast cancer. J Natl Cancer Inst 2003; 95(19):1467–1476.

Dignam JJ, Wieand K, Johnson KA, Raich P, Anderson SJ, Somkin C, Wickerham DL. Effects of obesity and race on prognosis in lymph node-negative, estrogen receptor-negative breast cancer. Breast Cancer Res Treat 2006; 97(3):245–254.

dos Santos Silva I, De Stavola BL, Hardy RJ, Kuh DJ, McCormack VA, Wadsworth ME. Is the association of birth weight with premenopausal breast cancer risk mediated through childhood growth? Br J Cancer 2004; 91(3): 519–524.

Ekbom A, Hsieh CC, Lipworth L, Trichopoulos D, Adami HO. Intrauterine environment and breast cancer risk in women: a population-based study. J Natl Cancer Inst 1997; 89: 71–76.

Ekbom A, Trichopoulos D, Adami HO, Hsieh CC, Lan SJ. Evidence of prenatal influences on breast cancer risk. Lancet 1992; 340(8826):1015–1018.

Eliassen AH, Colditz GA, Rosner B, Willett WC, Hankinson SE. Adult weight change and risk of postmenopausal breast cancer. JAMA 2006; 296(2):193–201.

Enger SM, Greif JM, Polikoff J, Press M. Body weight correlates with mortality in early-stage breast cancer. Arch Surg 2004; 139(9):954–58 (discussion 958–960).

Enger SM, Ross RK, Paganini-Hill A, Carpenter CL, Bernstein L. Body size, physical activity, and breast cancer hormone receptor status: results from two case-control studies. Cancer Epidemiol Biomarkers Prev 2000; 9(7):681–687.

Feigelson HS, Jonas CR, Teras LR, Thun MJ, Calle EE. Weight gain, body mass index, hormone replacement therapy, and postmenopausal breast cancer in a large prospective study. Cancer Epidemiol Biomarkers Prev 2004; 13(2):220–224.

Folsom AR, Kaye SA, Prineas RJ, Potter JD, Gapstur SM, Wallace RB. Increased incidence of carcinoma of the breast associated with abdominal adiposity in postmenopausal women. Am J Epidemiol 1990; 131(5):794–803.

Folsom AR, Kushi LH, Anderson KE, Mink PJ, Olson JE, Hong CP, Sellers TA, Lazovich D, Prineas RJ. Associations of general and abdominal obesity with multiple health outcomes in older women: the Iowa Women's Health Study. Arch Intern Med 2000; 160(14):2117–2128.

Franceschi S, Favero A, La Vecchia C, Baron AE, Negri E, Dal Maso L, Giacosa A, Montella M, Conti E, Amadori D. Body size indices and breast cancer risk before and after menopause. Int J Cancer 1996; 67(2):181–186.

Friedenreich CM. Physical activity and cancer prevention: from observational to intervention research. Cancer Epidemiol Biomarkers Prev 2001a; 10(4):287–301.

Friedenreich CM. Review of anthropometric factors and breast cancer risk. Eur J Cancer Prev 2001b; 10(1):15–32.

Friedenreich CM, Courneya KS, Bryant HE. Case-control study of anthropometric measures and breast cancer risk. Int J Cancer 2002; 99(3):445–452.

Friedenreich CM, Rohan TE. A review of physical activity and breast cancer. Epidemiology 1995; 6(3):311–317.

Galanis DJ, Kolonel LN, Lee J, Le Marchand L. Anthropometric predictors of breast cancer incidence and survival in a multi-ethnic cohort of female residents of Hawaii, United States. Cancer Causes Control 1998; 9(2):217–224.

Gammon MD, John EM, Britton JA. Recreational and occupational physical activities and risk of breast cancer. J Natl Cancer Inst 1998; 90(2):100–117.

Gibson R. Principles of nutritional assessment. New York: Oxford University Press, 2005.

Giuffrida D, Lupo L, La Porta GA, La Rosa GL, Padova G, Foti E, Marchese V, Belfiore A. Relation between steroid receptor status and body weight in breast cancer patients. Eur J Cancer 1992; 28(1):112–115.

Goffman TE, Laronga C, Wilson L, Elkins D. Lymphedema of the arm and breast in irradiated breast cancer patients: risks in an era of dramatically changing axillary surgery. Breast J 2004; 10(5):405–411.

Goodwin PJ, Boyd NF. Body size and breast cancer prognosis: a critical review of the evidence. Breast Cancer Res Treat 1990; 16(3):205–214.

Goodwin PJ, Panzarella T, Boyd NF. Weight gain in women with localized breast cancer—a descriptive study. Breast Cancer Res Treat 1988; 11(1):59–66.

Gram IT, Norat T, Rinaldi S, Dossus L, Lukanova A, Tehard B, Clavel-Chapelon F, van Gils CH, van Noord PA, Peeters PH, Bueno-de-Mesquita HB, Nagel G, Linseisen J, Lahmann PH, Boeing H, Palli D, Sacerdote C, Panico S, Tumino R, Sieri S, Dorronsoro M, Quiros JR, Navarro CA, Barricarte A, Tormo MJ, Gonzalez CA, Overvad K, Paaske Johnsen S, Olsen A, Tjonneland A, Travis R, Allen N, Bingham S, Khaw KT, Stattin P, Trichopoulou A, Kalapothaki V, Psaltopoulou T, Casagrande C, Riboli E,

Kaaks R. Body mass index, waist circumference and waist-hip ratio and serum levels of IGF-I and IGFBP-3 in European women. Int J Obes (Lond) 2006; 30(11): 1623–1631; [Epub Mar 21, 2006].

Greenberg ER, Vessey MP, McPherson K, Doll R, Yeates D. Body size and survival in premenopausal breast cancer. Br J Cancer 1985; 51(5):691–697.

Griggs JJ, Sorbero ME, Lyman GH. Undertreatment of obese women receiving breast cancer chemotherapy. Arch Intern Med 2005; 165(11):1267–1273.

Hall HI, Coates RJ, Uhler RJ, Brinton LA, Gammon MD, Brogan D, Potischman N, Malone KE, Swanson CA. Stage of breast cancer in relation to body mass index and bra cup size. Int J Cancer 1999; 82(1):23–27.

Hall IJ, Newman B, Millikan RC, Moorman PG. Body size and breast cancer risk in black women and white women: the Carolina Breast Cancer Study. Am J Epidemiol 2000; 151(8):754–764.

Harris RE, Namboodiri KK, Wynder EL. Breast cancer risk: effects of estrogen replacement therapy and body mass. J Natl Cancer Inst 1992; 84(20):1575–1582.

Harvie M, Hooper L, Howell AH. Central obesity and breast cancer risk: a systematic review. Obes Rev 2003; 4(3): 157–173.

Harvie M, Howell A, Vierkant RA, Kumar N, Cerhan JR, Kelemen LE, Folsom AR, Sellers TA. Association of gain and loss of weight before and after menopause with risk of postmenopausal breast cancer in the Iowa women's health study. Cancer Epidemiol Biomarkers Prev 2005; 14(3): 656–661.

Haybittle J, Houghton J, Baum M. Social class and weight as prognostic factors in early breast cancer. Br J Cancer 1997; 75(5):729–733.

Heasman KZ, Sutherland HJ, Campbell JA, Elhakim T, Boyd NF. Weight gain during adjuvant chemotherapy for breast cancer. Breast Cancer Res Treat 1985; 5(2):195–200.

Hebert JR, Augustine A, Barone J, Kabat GC, Kinne DW, Wynder EL. Weight, height and body mass index in the prognosis of breast cancer: early results of a prospective study. Int J Cancer 1988; 42(3):315–318.

Heymsfield S, Baumgartner R, Ross R. Evaluation of total and regional body composition. In: Bray G, Bouchard C, James W, eds. Handbook of Obesity. New York: Marcel Dekker, 1998.

Hilakivi-Clarke L, Forsen T, Eriksson JG, Luoto R, Tuomilehto J, Osmond C, Barker DJ. Tallness and overweight during childhood have opposing effects on breast cancer risk. Br J Cancer 2001; 85(11):1680–1684.

Hislop TG, Coldman AJ, Elwood JM, Brauer G, Kan L. Childhood and recent eating patterns and risk of breast cancer. Cancer Detect Prev 1986; 9(1–2):47–58.

Hjartaker A, Adami HO, Lund E, Weiderpass E. Body mass index and mortality in a prospectively studied cohort of Scandinavian women: the women's lifestyle and health cohort study. Eur J Epidemiol 2005; 20(9):747–754.

Hodgson ME, Newman B, Millikan RC. Birthweight, parental age, birth order and breast cancer risk in African-American and white women: a population-based case-control study. Breast Cancer Res 2004; 6(6):R656–R667.

Hsieh CC, Trichopoulos D, Katsouyanni K, Yuasa S. Age at menarche, age at menopause, height and obesity as risk factors for breast cancer: associations and interactions in an international case-control study. Int J Cancer 1990; 46(5): 796–800.

Huang Z, Hankinson SE, Colditz GA, Stampfer MJ, Hunter DJ, Manson JE, Hennekens CH, Rosner B, Speizer FE, Willett WC. Dual effects of weight and weight gain on breast cancer risk. JAMA 1997; 278(17):1407–1411.

Huang Z, Willett WC, Colditz GA, Hunter DJ, Manson JE, Rosner B, Speizer FE, Hankinson SE. Waist circumference, waist:hip ratio, and risk of breast cancer in the Nurses' Health Study. Am J Epidemiol 1999; 150(12):1316–1324.

Hubinette A, Lichtenstein P, Ekbom A, Cnattingius S. Birth characteristics and breast cancer risk: a study among like-sexed twins. Int J Cancer 2001; 91(2):248–251.

IARC. IARC Handbooks of Cancer Prevention: Weight Control and Physical Activity. Lyon: IARC Press, 2002.

Ingram D, Nottage E, Ng S, Sparrow L, Roberts A, Willcox D. Obesity and breast disease. The role of the female sex hormones. Cancer 1989; 64(5):1049–1053.

Innes K, Byers T, Schymura M. Birth characteristics and subsequent risk for breast cancer in very young women. Am J Epidemiol 2000; 152(12):1121–1128.

Jain M, Miller AB. Pre-morbid body size and the prognosis of women with breast cancer. Int J Cancer 1994; 59(3): 363–368.

Kaaks R, Van Noord PA, Den Tonkelaar I, Peeters PH, Riboli E, Grobbee DE. Breast-cancer incidence in relation to height, weight and body-fat distribution in the Dutch "DOM" cohort. Int J Cancer 1998; 76(5):647–651.

Kaijser M, Akre O, Cnattingius S, Ekbom A. Preterm birth, birth weight, and subsequent risk of female breast cancer. Br J Cancer 2003; 89(9):1664–1666.

Kaijser M, Lichtenstein P, Granath F, Erlandsson G, Cnattingius S, Ekbom A. In utero exposures and breast cancer: a study of opposite-sexed twins. J Natl Cancer Inst 2001; 93(1): 60–62.

Katoh A, Watzlaf VJ, D'Amico F. An examination of obesity and breast cancer survival in post-menopausal women. Br J Cancer 1994; 70(5):928–933.

Key TJ, Appleby PN, Reeves GK, Roddam A, Dorgan JF, Longcope C, Stanczyk FZ, Stephenson HE Jr., Falk RT, Miller R, Schatzkin A, Allen DS, Fentiman IS, Wang DY, Dowsett M, Thomas HV, Hankinson SE, Toniolo P, Akhmedkhanov A, Koenig K, Shore RE, Zeleniuch-Jacquotte A, Berrino F, Muti P, Micheli A, Krogh V, Sieri S, Pala V, Venturelli E, Secreto G, Barrett-Connor E, Laughlin GA, Kabuto M, Akiba S, Stevens RG, Neriishi K, Land CE, Cauley JA, Kuller LH, Cummings SR, Helzlsouer KJ, Alberg AJ, Bush TL, Comstock GW, Gordon GB, Miller SR. Body mass index, serum sex hormones, and breast cancer risk in postmenopausal women. J Natl Cancer Inst 2003; 95(16):1218–1226.

Kocak Z, Overgaard J. Risk factors of arm lymphedema in breast cancer patients. Acta Oncol 2000; 39(3):389–392.

Kolonel LN, Nomura AM, Lee J, Hirohata T. Anthropometric indicators of breast cancer risk in postmenopausal women in Hawaii. Nutr Cancer 1986; 8(4):247–256.

Kramer MS, Morin I, Yang H, Platt RW, Usher R, McNamara H, Joseph KS, Wen SW. Why are babies getting bigger? Temporal trends in fetal growth and its determinants. J Pediatr 2002; 141(4):538–542.

Kroenke CH, Chen WY, Rosner B, Holmes MD. Weight, weight gain, and survival after breast cancer diagnosis. J Clin Oncol 2005; 23(7):1370–1378.

Kumar NB, Cantor A, Allen K, Cox CE. Android obesity at diagnosis and breast carcinoma survival: Evaluation of the effects of anthropometric variables at diagnosis, including body composition and body fat distribution and weight gain during life span, and survival from breast carcinoma. Cancer 2000; 88(12):2751–2757.

Kyogoku S, Hirohata T, Takeshita S, Nomura Y, Shigematsu T, Horie A. Survival of breast-cancer patients and body size indicators. Int J Cancer 1990; 46(5):824–831.

La Vecchia C, Negri E, Franceschi S, Talamini R, Bruzzi P, Palli D, Decarli A. Body mass index and post-menopausal breast cancer: an age-specific analysis. Br J Cancer 1997; 75(3): 441–444.

Lahmann PH, Gullberg B, Olsson H, Boeing H, Berglund G, Lissner L. Birth weight is associated with postmenopausal breast cancer risk in Swedish women. Br J Cancer 2004a; 91(9):1666–1668.

Lahmann PH, Hoffmann K, Allen N, van Gils CH, Khaw KT, Tehard B, Berrino F, Tjonneland A, Bigaard J, Olsen A, Overvad K, Clavel-Chapelon F, Nagel G, Boeing H, Trichopoulos D, Economou G, Bellos G, Palli D, Tumino R, Panico S, Sacerdote C, Krogh V, Peeters PH, Bueno-de-Mesquita HB, Lund E, Ardanaz E, Amiano P, Pera G, Quiros JR, Martinez C, Tormo MJ, Wirfalt E, Berglund G, Hallmans G, Key TJ, Reeves G, Bingham S, Norat T, Biessy C, Kaaks R, Riboli E. Body size and breast cancer risk: findings from the European Prospective Investigation into Cancer And Nutrition (EPIC). Int J Cancer 2004b; 111(5):762–771.

Lahmann PH, Lissner L, Berglund G. Breast cancer risk in overweight postmenopausal women. Cancer Epidemiol Biomarkers Prev 2004c; 13(8):1414.

Lahmann PH, Lissner L, Gullberg B, Olsson H, Berglund G. A prospective study of adiposity and postmenopausal breast cancer risk: the Malmo Diet and Cancer Study. Int J Cancer 2003; 103(2):246–252.

Lahmann PH, Schulz M, Hoffmann K, Boeing H, Tjonneland A, Olsen A, Overvad K, Key TJ, Allen NE, Khaw KT, Bingham S, Berglund G, Wirfalt E, Berrino F, Krogh V, Trichopoulou A, Lagiou P, Trichopoulos D, Kaaks R, Riboli E. Long-term weight change and breast cancer risk: the European prospective investigation into cancer and nutrition (EPIC). Br J Cancer 2005; 93(5):582–589.

Larsson I, Berteus Forslund H, Lindroos AK, Lissner L, Naslund I, Peltonen M, Sjostrom L. Body composition in the SOS (Swedish Obese Subjects) reference study. Int J Obes Relat Metab Disord 2004; 28(10):1317–1324.

Larsson I, Henning B, Lindroos AK, Naslund I, Sjostrom CD, Sjostrom L. Optimized predictions of absolute and relative amounts of body fat from weight, height, other anthropometric predictors, and age 1. Am J Clin Nutr 2006; 83(2):252–259.

Le Marchand L. Ethnic variation in breast cancer survival: a review. Breast Cancer Res Treat 1991; 18(suppl 1): S119–S126.

Le Marchand L, Kolonel LN, Earle ME, Mi MP. Body size at different periods of life and breast cancer risk. Am J Epidemiol 1988; 128(1):137–152.

Lees AW, Jenkins HJ, May CL, Cherian G, Lam EW, Hanson J. Risk factors and 10-year breast cancer survival in northern Alberta. Breast Cancer Res Treat 1989; 13(2):143–151.

Li CI, Stanford JL, Daling JR. Anthropometric variables in relation to risk of breast cancer in middle-aged women. Int J Epidemiol 2000; 29(2):208–213.

Lof M, Sandin S, Hilakivi-Clarke L, Weiderpass E. Birth weight in relation to endometrial and breast cancer risks in Swedish women. Br J Cancer 2007; 96(1):134–136.

Loi S, Milne RL, Friedlander ML, McCredie MR, Giles GG, Hopper JL, Phillips KA. Obesity and outcomes in premenopausal and postmenopausal breast cancer. Cancer Epidemiol Biomarkers Prev 2005; 14(7):1686–1691.

London SJ, Colditz GA, Stampfer MJ, Willett WC, Rosner B, Speizer FE. Prospective study of relative weight, height, and risk of breast cancer. JAMA 1989; 262(20):2853–2858.

Lubin F, Ruder AM, Wax Y, Modan B. Overweight and changes in weight throughout adult life in breast cancer etiology. A case-control study. Am J Epidemiol 1985; 122(4):579–588.

Lukanova A, Bjor O, Kaaks R, Lenner P, Lindahl B, Hallmans G, Stattin P. Body mass index and cancer: results from the Northern Sweden Health and Disease Cohort. Int J Cancer 2006; 118(2):458–466.

Madarnas Y, Sawka CA, Franssen E, Bjarnason GA. Are medical oncologists biased in their treatment of the large woman with breast cancer? Breast Cancer Res Treat 2001; 66(2):123–133.

Maehle BO, Tretli S. Pre-morbid body-mass-index in breast cancer: reversed effect on survival in hormone receptor negative patients. Breast Cancer Res Treat 1996; 41(2): 123–130.

Maehle BO, Tretli S, Thorsen T. The associations of obesity, lymph node status and prognosis in breast cancer patients: dependence on estrogen and progesterone receptor status. Apmis 2004; 112(6):349–357.

Magnusson C, Baron J, Persson I, Wolk A, Bergstrom R, Trichopoulos D, Adami HO. Body size in different periods of life and breast cancer risk in post-menopausal women. Int J Cancer 1998; 76(1):29–34.

Magnusson CM, Roddam AW, Pike MC, Chilvers C, Crossley B, Hermon C, McPherson K, Peto J, Vessey M Beral V. Body fatness and physical activity at young ages and the risk of breast cancer in premenopausal women. Br J Cancer 2005; 93(7):817–824.

Mannisto S, Pietinen P, Pyy M, Palmgren J, Eskelinen M, Uusitupa M. Body-size indicators and risk of breast cancer according to menopause and estrogen-receptor status. Int J Cancer 1996; 68(1):8–13.

Marinho LA, Rettori O, Vieira-Matos AN. Body weight loss as an indicator of breast cancer recurrence. Acta Oncol 2001; 40(7):832–837.

Marret H, Perrotin F, Bougnoux P, Descamps P, Hubert B, Lefranc T, Le Floch O, Lansac J, Body G. Low body mass index is an independent predictive factor of local recurrence after conservative treatment for breast cancer. Breast Cancer Res Treat 2001; 66(1):17–23.

McCormack VA, dos Santos Silva I, De Stavola BL, Mohsen R, Leon DA, Lithell HO. Fetal growth and subsequent risk of breast cancer: results from long term follow up of Swedish cohort. BMJ 2003; 326(7383):248.

McCormack VA, dos Santos Silva I, Koupil I, Leon DA, Lithell HO. Birth characteristics and adult cancer incidence: Swedish cohort of over 11,000 men and women. Int J Cancer 2005; 115(4):611–617.

McNee RK, Mason BH, Neave LM, Kay RG. Influence of height, weight, and obesity on breast cancer incidence and recurrence in Auckland, New Zealand. Breast Cancer Res Treat 1987; 9(2):145–150.

Meek AG. Breast radiotherapy and lymphedema. Cancer 1998; 83(suppl 12 American):2788–2797.

Mellemkjaer L, Olsen ML, Sorensen HT, Thulstrup AM, Olsen J, Olsen JH. Birth weight and risk of early-onset breast cancer (Denmark). Cancer Causes Control 2003; 14(1): 61–64.

Menon KV, Hodge A, Houghton J, Bates T. Body mass index, height and cumulative menstrual cycles at the time of diagnosis are not risk factors for poor outcome in breast cancer. Breast 1999; 8(6):328–333.

Michels KB, Trichopoulos D, Robins JM, Rosner BA, Manson JE, Hunter DJ, Colditz GA, Hankinson SE, Speizer FE, Willett WC. Birthweight as a risk factor for breast cancer. Lancet 1996; 348(9041):1542–1546.

Michels KB, Xue F. Role of birthweight in the etiology of breast cancer. Int J Cancer 2006; 119(9):2007–2025.

Michels KB, Xue F, Terry KL, Willett WC. Longitudinal study of birthweight and the incidence of breast cancer in adulthood. Carcinogenesis 2006; 27(12):2464–2468.

Modugno F, Kip KE, Cochrane B, Kuller L, Klug TL, Rohan TE, Chlebowski RT, Lasser N, Stefanick ML. Obesity, hormone therapy, estrogen metabolism and risk of postmenopausal breast cancer. Int J Cancer 2006; 118(5):1292–1301.

Mogren I, Damber L, Tavelin B, Hogberg U. Characteristics of pregnancy and birth and malignancy in the offspring (Sweden). Cancer Causes Control 1999; 10(1):85–94.

Mohle-Boetani JC, Grosser S, Whittemore AS, Malec M, Kampert JB, Paffenbarger RS Jr. Body size, reproductive factors, and breast cancer survival. Prev Med 1988; 17(5): 634–642.

Monninkhof EM, Elias SG, Vlems FA, van der Tweel I, Schuit AJ, Voskuil DW, van Leeuwen FE. Physical activity and breast cancer: a systematic review. Epidemiology 2007; 18(1):137–157.

Morimoto LM, White E, Chen Z, Chlebowski RT, Hays J, Kuller L, Lopez AM, Manson J, Margolis KL, Muti PC, Stefanick ML, McTiernan A. Obesity, body size, and risk of postmenopausal breast cancer: the Women's Health Initiative (United States). Cancer Causes Control 2002; 13(8):741–751.

Muti P, Stanulla M, Micheli A, Krogh V, Freudenheim JL, Yang J, Schunemann HJ, Trevisan M, Berrino F. Markers of insulin resistance and sex steroid hormone activity in relation to breast cancer risk: a prospective analysis of abdominal adiposity, sebum production, and hirsutism (Italy). Cancer Causes Control 2000; 11(8):721–730.

Newman LA, Kuerer HM, McNeese MD, Hunt KK, Gurtner GC, Vlastos GS, Robb G, Singletary SE. Reduction mammoplasty improves breast conservation therapy in patients with macromastia. Am J Surg 2001; 181(3): 215–220.

Newman SC, Lees AW, Jenkins HJ. The effect of body mass index and oestrogen receptor level on survival of breast cancer patients. Int J Epidemiol 1997; 26(3):484–490.

Ng EH, Gao F, Ji CY, Ho GH, Soo KC. Risk factors for breast carcinoma in Singaporean Chinese women: the role of central obesity. Cancer 1997; 80(4):725–731.

Nieto A, Lozano M, Moro MT, Keller J, Carralafuente C. Determinants of wound infections after surgery for breast cancer. Zentralbl Gynakol 2002; 124(8–9):429–433.

Obermair A, Kurz C, Hanzal E, Bancher-Todesca D, Thoma M, Bodisch A, Kubista E, Kyral E, Kaider A, Sevelda P, et al. The influence of obesity on the disease-free survival in primary breast cancer. Anticancer Res 1995; 15(5B): 2265–2269.

Okasha M, McCarron P, McEwen J, Smith GD. Body mass index in young adulthood and cancer mortality: a retrospective cohort study. J Epidemiol Community Health 2002; 56(10): 780–784.

Paffenbarger RS Jr., Kampert JB, Chang HG. Characteristics that predict risk of breast cancer before and after the menopause. Am J Epidemiol 1980; 112(2):258–268.

Park SK, Garcia-Closas M, Lissowska J, Sherman ME, McGlynn KA, Peponska B, Bardin-Mikoajczak A, Zatonski W, Szeszenia-Dabrowska N, Brinton LA. Intrauterine environment and breast cancer risk in a population-based case-control study in Poland. Int J Cancer 2006; 119(9): 2136–2141.

Parker ED, Folsom AR. Intentional weight loss and incidence of obesity-related cancers: the Iowa Women's Health Study. Int J Obes Relat Metab Disord 2003; 27(12): 1447–1452.

Pathak DR, Whittemore AS. Combined effects of body size, parity, and menstrual events on breast cancer incidence in seven countries. Am J Epidemiol 1992; 135(2):153–168.

Peacock SL, White E, Daling JR, Voigt LF, Malone KE. Relation between obesity and breast cancer in young women. Am J Epidemiol 1999; 149(4):339–346.

Petrek JA, Peters M, Cirrincione C, Rhodes D, Bajorunas D. Is body fat topography a risk factor for breast cancer? Ann Intern Med 1993; 118(5):356–362.

Petrelli JM, Calle EE, Rodriguez C, Thun MJ. Body mass index, height, and postmenopausal breast cancer mortality in a prospective cohort of US women. Cancer Causes Control 2002; 13(4):325–332.

Poikonen P, Blomqvist C, Joensuu H. Effect of obesity on the leukocyte nadir in women treated with adjuvant cyclophosphamide, methotrexate, and fluorouracil dosed according to body surface area. Acta Oncol 2001; 40(1): 67–71.

Porter GA, Inglis KM, Wood LA, Veugelers PJ. Effect of obesity on presentation of breast cancer. Ann Surg Oncol 2006; 13(3):327–332; [Epub Jan 30, 2006].

Radimer KL, Ballard-Barbash R, Miller JS, Fay MP, Schatzkin A, Troiano R, Kreger BE, Splansky GL. Weight change and the risk of late-onset breast cancer in the original Framingham cohort. Nutr Cancer 2004; 49(1):7–13.

Rapp K, Schroeder J, Klenk J, Stoehr S, Ulmer H, Concin H, Diem G, Oberaigner W, Weiland SK. Obesity and incidence of cancer: a large cohort study of over 145,000 adults in Austria. Br J Cancer 2005; 93(9):1062–1067.

Renehan A, Zwahlen M, Minder C, O'Dwyer S, Shalet S, Egger M. Insulin-growth factor (IGF)-I, IGF binding protein-3, and cancer risk; systematic review and meta-regression analysis. Lancet 2004; 363:1346–1353.

Rinaldi S, Key TJ, Peeters PH, Lahmann PH, Lukanova A, Dossus L, Biessy C, Vineis P, Sacerdote C, Berrino F, Panico S, Tumino R, Palli D, Nagel G, Linseisen J, Boeing H, Roddam A, Bingham S, Khaw KT, Chloptios J, Trichopoulou A, Trichopoulos D, Tehard B, Clavel-Chapelon F, Gonzalez CA, Larranaga N, Barricarte A, Quiros JR, Chirlaque MD, Martinez C, Monninkhof E, Grobbee DE, Bueno-de-Mesquita HB, Ferrari P, Slimani N, Riboli E, Kaaks R. Anthropometric measures, endogenous sex steroids and breast cancer risk in postmenopausal women: a study within the EPIC cohort. Int J Cancer 2006a; 118(11):2832–2839.

Rinaldi S, Peeters PH, Berrino F, Dossus L, Biessy C, Olsen A, Tjonneland A, Overvad K, Clavel-Chapelon F, Boutron-Ruault MC, Tehard B, Nagel G, Linseisen J, Boeing H, Lahmann PH, Trichopoulou A, Trichopoulos D, Koliva M, Palli D, Panico S, Tumino R, Sacerdote C, van Gils CH, van Noord P, Grobbee DE, Bueno-de-Mesquita HB, Gonzalez CA, Agudo A, Chirlaque MD, Barricarte A, Larranaga N, Quiros JR, Bingham S, Khaw KT, Key T, Allen NE, Lukanova A, Slimani N, Saracci R, Riboli E, Kaaks R. IGF-I, IGFBP-3 and breast cancer risk in women: The European Prospective Investigation into Cancer and Nutrition (EPIC). Endocr Relat Cancer 2006b; 13(2): 593–605.

Roberts S. Can self-reported data accurately describe the prevalence of overweight? Public Health 1995; 109: 275–284.

Rosner GL, Hargis JB, Hollis DR, Budman DR, Weiss RB, Henderson IC, Schilsky RL. Relationship between toxicity and obesity in women receiving adjuvant chemotherapy for breast cancer: results from cancer and leukemia group B study 8541. J Clin Oncol 1996; 14(11):3000–3008.

Rowland M. Self-reported weight and height. Am J Clin Nutr 1990; 52:1125–1133.

Ryu SY, Kim CB, Nam CM, Park JK, Kim KS, Park J, Yoo SY, Cho KS. Is body mass index the prognostic factor in breast cancer?: a meta-analysis. J Korean Med Sci 2001; 16(5): 610–614.

Sachdev D, Yee D. The IGF system and breast cancer. Endocr Relat Cancer 2001; 8:197–209.

Sanderson M, Shu XO, Jin F, Dai Q, Ruan Z, Gao YT, Zheng W. Weight at birth and adolescence and premenopausal breast cancer risk in a low-risk population. Br J Cancer 2002; 86(1):84–88.

Sanderson M, Williams MA, Daling JR, Holt VL, Malone KE, Self SG, Moore DE. Maternal factors and breast cancer risk among young women. Paediatr Perinat Epidemiol 1998; 12(4):397–407.

Sanderson M, Williams MA, Malone KE, Stanford JL, Emanuel I, White E, Daling JR. Perinatal factors and risk of breast cancer. Epidemiology 1996; 7(1):34–37.

Schapira DV, Kumar NB, Lyman GH, Cox CE. Abdominal obesity and breast cancer risk. Ann Intern Med 1990; 112(3):182–186.

Schapira DV, Kumar NB, Lyman GH, Cox CE. Obesity and body fat distribution and breast cancer prognosis. Cancer 1991a; 67(2):523–528.

Schapira DV, Kumar NB, Lyman GH, Cox CE. Obesity and body fat distribution and breast cancer prognosis. Cancer 1991b; 67(2):523–528.

Sellers TA, Kushi LH, Potter JD, Kaye SA, Nelson CL, McGovern PG, Folsom AR. Effect of family history, body-fat distribution, and reproductive factors on the risk of postmenopausal breast cancer. N Engl J Med 1992; 326(20):1323–1329.

Sellers TA, Sprafka JM, Gapstur SM, Rich SS, Potter JD, Ross JA, McGovern PG, Nelson CL, Folsom AR. Does body fat distribution promote familial aggregation of adult onset diabetes mellitus and postmenopausal breast cancer? Epidemiology 1994; 5(1):102–108.

Senie RT, Rosen PP, Rhodes P, Lesser ML, Kinne DW. Obesity at diagnosis of breast carcinoma influences duration of disease-free survival. Ann Intern Med 1992; 116(1):26–32.

Sohrabi A, Sandoz J, Spratt JS, Polk HC Jr. Recurrence of breast cancer. Obesity, tumor size, and axillary lymph node metastases. JAMA 1980; 244(3):264–265.

Sonnenschein E, Toniolo P, Terry MB, Bruning PF, Kato I, Koenig KL, Shore RE. Body fat distribution and obesity in pre- and postmenopausal breast cancer. Int J Epidemiol 1999; 28(6):1026–1031.

Stavola BL, Hardy R, Kuh D, Silva IS, Wadsworth M, Swerdlow AJ. Birthweight, childhood growth and risk of breast cancer in a British cohort. Br J Cancer 2000; 83(7):964–968.

Stoll BA. Obesity and breast cancer. Int J Obes Relat Metab Disord 1996; 20(5):389–392.

Surkan PJ, Hsieh CC, Johansson AL, Dickman PW, Cnattingius S. Reasons for increasing trends in large for gestational age births. Obstet Gynecol 2004; 104(4):720–726.

Swanson CA, Brinton LA, Taylor PR, Licitra LM, Ziegler RG, Schairer C. Body size and breast cancer risk assessed in women participating in the Breast Cancer Detection Demonstration Project. Am J Epidemiol 1989; 130(6): 1133–1141.

Swanson CA, Coates RJ, Schoenberg JB, Malone KE, Gammon MD, Stanford JL, Shorr IJ, Potischman NA, Brinton LA. Body size and breast cancer risk among women under age 45 years. Am J Epidemiol 1996; 143(7):698–706.

Tao MH, Shu XO, Ruan ZX, Gao YT, Zheng W. Association of overweight with breast cancer survival. Am J Epidemiol 2006; 163(2):101–107.

Tehard B, Clavel-Chapelon F. Several anthropometric measurements and breast cancer risk: results of the E3N cohort study. Int J Obes (Lond) 2006; 30(1):156–163.

Tehard B, Lahmann PH, Riboli E, Clavel-Chapelon F. Anthropometry, breast cancer and menopausal status: use of repeated measurements over 10 years of follow-up-results of the French E3N women's cohort study. Int J Cancer 2004; 111(2):264–269.

Thompson HJ, Zhu Z, Jiang W. Weight control and breast cancer prevention: are the effects of reduced energy intake equivalent to those of increased energy expenditure? J Nutr 2004; 134(suppl 12):3407S–3411S.

Titus-Ernstoff L, Egan KM, Newcomb PA, Ding J, Trentham-Dietz A, Greenberg ER, Baron JA, Trichopoulos D, Willett WC. Early life factors in relation to breast cancer risk in postmenopausal women. Cancer Epidemiol Biomarkers Prev 2002; 11(2):207–210.

Tornberg SA, Carstensen JM. Relationship between Quetelet's index and cancer of breast and female genital tract in 47,000 women followed for 25 years. Br J Cancer 1994; 69(2): 358–361.

Trentham-Dietz A, Newcomb PA, Egan KM, Titus-Ernstoff L, Baron JA, Storer BE, Stampfer M, Willett WC. Weight change and risk of postmenopausal breast cancer (United States). Cancer Causes Control 2000; 11(6): 533–542.

Tretli S. Height and weight in relation to breast cancer morbidity and mortality. A prospective study of 570,000 women in Norway. Int J Cancer 1989; 44(1):23–30.

Tretli S, Haldorsen T, Ottestad L. The effect of pre-morbid height and weight on the survival of breast cancer patients. Br J Cancer 1990; 62(2):299–303.

Troisi R, Hatch EE, Titus-Ernstoff L, Palmer JR, Hyer M, Strohsnitter WC, Robboy SJ, Kaufman R, Herbst A, Adam E, Hoover RN. Birth weight and breast cancer risk. Br J Cancer 2006; 94(11):1734–1737.

Troy L, Michels K, Hunter D, Spiegelman D, Manson JE, Colditz GA, Stampfer MJ, Willett WC. Self-reported birthweight and history of having been breastfeed among younger women: an assessment of validity. Int J Epidemiol 1996; 25:122–127.

Tworoger SS, Eliassen AH, Missmer SA, Baer H, Rich-Edwards J, Michels KB, Barbieri RL, Dowsett M, Hankinson SE. Birthweight and body size throughout life in relation to sex hormones and prolactin concentrations in premenopausal women. Cancer Epidemiol Biomarkers Prev 2006; 15(12): 2494–2501.

Ursin G, Longnecker MP, Haile RW, Greenland S. A meta-analysis of body mass index and risk of premenopausal breast cancer. Epidemiology 1995; 6(2):137–141.

Vainio H, Kaaks R, Bianchini F. Weight control and physical activity in cancer prevention: international evaluation of the evidence. Eur J Cancer Prev 2002; 11(suppl 2):S94–S100.

van den Brandt PA, Spiegelman D, Yaun SS, Adami HO, Beeson L, Folsom AR, Fraser G, Goldbohm RA, Graham S, Kushi L, Marshall JR, Miller AB, Rohan T, Smith-Warner SA, Speizer FE, Willett WC, Wolk A, Hunter DJ. Pooled analysis of prospective cohort studies on height, weight, and breast cancer risk. Am J Epidemiol 2000; 152(6):514–527.

Vatten LJ, Foss OP, Kvinnsland S. Overall survival of breast cancer patients in relation to preclinically determined total serum cholesterol, body mass index, height and cigarette smoking: a population-based study. Eur J Cancer 1991; 27(5):641–646.

Vatten LJ, Kvinnsland S. Body height and risk of breast cancer. A prospective study of 23,831 Norwegian women. Br J Cancer 1990a; 61(6):881–885.

Vatten LJ, Kvinnsland S. Body mass index and risk of breast cancer. A prospective study of 23,826 Norwegian women. Int J Cancer 1990b; 45(3):440–444.

Vatten LJ, Kvinnsland S. Prospective study of height, body mass index and risk of breast cancer. Acta Oncol 1992; 31(2): 195–200.

Vatten LJ, Maehle BO, Lund Nilsen TI, Tretli S, Hsieh CC, Trichopoulos D, Stuver SO. Birth weight as a predictor of breast cancer: a case-control study in Norway. Br J Cancer 2002; 86(1):89–91.

Vatten LJ, Nilsen TI, Tretli S, Trichopoulos D, Romundstad PR. Size at birth and risk of breast cancer: prospective population-based study. Int J Cancer 2005; 114(3):461–464.

Velie EM, Nechuta S, Osuch JR. Lifetime reproductive and anthropometric risk factors for breast cancer in postmenopausal women. Breast Dis 2005; 24:17–35.

Verheus M, Peeters PH, Rinaldi S, Dossus L, Biessy C, Olsen A, Tjonneland A, Overvad K, Jeppesen M, Clavel-Chapelon F, Tehard B, Nagel G, Linseisen J, Boeing H, Lahmann PH, Arvaniti A, Psaltopoulou T, Trichopoulou A, Palli D, Tumino R, Panico S, Sacerdote C, Sieri S, van Gils CH, Bueno-de-Mesquita BH, Gonzalez CA, Ardanaz E, Larranaga N, Garcia CM, Navarro C, Quiros JR, Key T, Allen N, Bingham S, Khaw KT, Slimani N, Riboli E, Kaaks R. Serum C-peptide levels and breast cancer risk: results from the European Prospective Investigation into Cancer and Nutrition (EPIC). Int J Cancer 2006; 119(3):659–667.

Verla-Tebit E, Chang-Claude J. Anthropometric factors and the risk of premenopausal breast cancer in Germany. Eur J Cancer Prev 2005; 14(4):419–426.

Verreault R, Brisson J, Deschenes L, Naud F. Body weight and prognostic indicators in breast cancer. Modifying effect of estrogen receptors. Am J Epidemiol 1989; 129(2):260–268.

Vilar-Compte D, Jacquemin B, Robles-Vidal C, Volkow P. Surgical site infections in breast surgery: case-control study. World J Surg 2004; 28(3):242–246; [Epub Feb 17, 2004].

Weiderpass E, Braaten T, Magnusson C, Kumle M, Vainio H, Lund E, Adami HO. A prospective study of body size in different periods of life and risk of premenopausal breast cancer. Cancer Epidemiol Biomarkers Prev 2004; 13 (7):1121–1127.

Wenten M, Gilliland FD, Baumgartner K, Samet JM. Associations of weight, weight change, and body mass with breast cancer risk in Hispanic and non-Hispanic white women. Ann Epidemiol 2002; 12(6):435–444.

Whiteman MK, Hillis SD, Curtis KM, McDonald JA, Wingo PA, Marchbanks PA. Body mass and mortality after breast cancer diagnosis. Cancer Epidemiol Biomarkers Prev 2005; 14(8):2009–2014.

WHO. Obesity: preventing and managing the global epidemic. Report of a WHO consultation. World Health Organ Tech Rep Ser 2000; 894:1–253.

Willett WC. Browne ML, Bain C, Lipnick RJ, Stampfer MJ, Rosner B, Colditz GA, Hennekens CH, Speizer FE. Relative weight and risk of breast cancer among premenopausal women. Am J Epidemiol 1985; 122(5):731–740.

Wolf I, Sadetzki S, Gluck I, Oberman B, Ben-David M, Papa MZ, Catane R, Kaufman B. Association between diabetes mellitus and adverse characteristics of breast cancer at presentation. Eur J Cancer 2006; 42(8):1077–1082.

Yong LC, Brown CC, Schatzkin A, Schairer C. Prospective study of relative weight and risk of breast cancer: the Breast Cancer Detection Demonstration Project follow-up study, 1979 to 1987–1989. Am J Epidemiol 1996; 143(10):985–995.

Yu H, Rohan T. Role of insulin-growth factor family in cancer development and progression. Int J Cancer 2000; 88:828–832.

Zhang S, Folsom AR, Sellers TA, Kushi LH, Potter JD. Better breast cancer survival for postmenopausal women who are less overweight and eat less fat. The Iowa Women's Health Study. Cancer 1995; 76(2): 275–283.

Ziegler RG, Hoover RN, Nomura AM, West DW, Wu AH, Pike MC, Lake AJ, Horn-Ross PL, Kolonel LN, Siiteri PK, Fraumeni JF Jr. Relative weight, weight change, height, and breast cancer risk in Asian-American women. J Natl Cancer Inst 1996; 88(10):650–660.

22

Antiangiogenic Therapy of Breast Cancer: Rationale and Clinical Results

RAFFAELE LONGO, FRANCESCO TORINO, ROBERTA SARMIENTO, FRANCESCA CACCIAMANI, and GIAMPIETRO GASPARINI

Division of Medical Oncology, S. Filippo Neri Hospital, Rome, Italy

INTRODUCTION

Angiogenesis, the process of new blood vessel formation, plays a central role in breast cancer (BC) development, invasion, and metastasis (Folkman, 1971). Hyperplastic murine breast papillomas (Brem et al., 1993, 1977) and histologically normal lobules adjacent to cancerous breast tissue (Jensen et al., 1982) support angiogenesis in preclinical models, suggesting that angiogenesis is one of the early events involved in the transformation of mammary hyperplasia to malignancy.

Hypoxia has a key role in promoting angiogenesis. The hypoxia-inducible factors HIF-1 and HIF-2 are heterodimeric transcription factors consisting of α and β subunits. The β subunit is constitutively expressed while the α subunit is under hypoxic condition protected from degradation (Salceda and Caro, 1997; Wang et al., 1995). HIF-1α expression progressively increases from normal breast tissue to ductal hyperplasia to ductal carcinoma in situ (DCIS) up to invasive ductal carcinoma (IDC). HIF-1α is overexpressed in poorly differentiated tumors and it is associated to increased proliferation index and expression of the vascular endothelial growth factor (VEGF) (Bos et al., 2001).

VEGF is the most powerful proangiogenic factor (Kim et al., 1993). The biologic effects of VEGF are mediated by specific endothelial surface cell receptors: VEGF-R_1 (flt-1), VEGF-R_2 (flk-1/kdr), and VEGF-R_3. VEGF-R_1 is a "decoy" receptor involved in the recruitment of endothelial progenitor cells and vascular maintenance, VEGF-R_2 induces endothelial cell proliferation and migration and regulates vascular permeability, while VEGF-R_3 stimulates lymphangiogenesis (Kim et al., 1993). *VEGF* gene expression is upregulated by a number of stimuli, including hypoxia, nitric oxide, various growth factors, estrogens, progestins, loss of *p53*, activation of *ras*, v-*src*, and HER-2/*neu* (Sledge, 2002).

In BC, the switch to the angiogenic phenotype is associated to the progression from DCIS to IC (Hanahan and Folkman, 1996). In C3(1)/Tag mice, VEGF levels increase eightfold in invasive tumors compared with preneoplastic lesions. Also angiopoietin-2 is upregulated in IC compared with premalignant tumors. Treatment of nude mice with endostatin, an endogenous angiogenesis inhibitor, significantly downregulates VEGF, VEGF-Rs, and angiopoietin-2, blocking tumor growth and delaying the conversion of neoplastic lesions to IC (Calvo et al., 2002).

Clinicopathologic correlations confirm the central role of angiogenesis in BC progression. The fibrocystic lesions with high vascular density are associated with greater risk of BC transformation (Guinebretiere et al., 1994).

Microvessel density (MVD) is higher in histopathologically aggressive DCIS lesions (Guidi et al., 1994) and it is associated with VEGF overexpression (Guidi et al., 1997).

Intratumor MVD is surrogate marker of a measure of the extent of new blood vessel growth and of the degree of angiogenesis in human tumors. Increased MVD in primary tumors adversely affects disease-free survival and overall survival in patients with BC. A study from Guidi et al. compared intratumoral MVD in primary BC tissue and axillary lymph node metastases and evaluated the relationship of primary- and metastatic-tumor MVD with disease-free survival and overall survival in women treated with adjuvant chemotherapy. Tissue sections from 47 primary tumors and 91 axillary metastatic lymph nodes were examined for the presence or absence of focal areas of intense neovascularization (vascular "hot spots"). The authors reported that the presence of elevated vascularization in axillary lymph node mtastasis, but not in primary BC, was associated to statistically significantly worse disease-free survival and overall survival by univariate analysis. This study suggests that the assessment of neovascularization in axillary lymph node metastases may provide clinically useful prognostic information.

Several studies have found an inverse correlation of VEGF overexpression with overall survival in both node-positive and node-negative BC (Gasparini, 1996; Gasparini et al., 1997). Increased VEGF expression is also associated with impaired response to tamoxifen or chemotherapy in patients with advanced BC (Foekens et al., 2001). Recently, VEGF expression has been successfully quantified by immunohistochemistry in BC tumor specimens (Ragaz et al., 2004). The expression and intensity of expression were found to correlate with a significantly worse clinical outcome.

Angiogenesis is involved in all the phases of tumor growth, and its inhibition induces a control of tumor growth and metastasis. Anticancer chemotherapy is known to have a direct cytotoxicity effect on tumor cells. The changes in circulating VEGF and endostatin levels during chemotherapy in patients with BC were analyzed and their correlations with efficacy of chemotherapy were studied by Tang et al., as presented at the 29th Annual San Antonio Breast Cancer Symposium. One hundred and twenty serum samples were collected from 40 patients with metastatic BC at three times: before chemotherapy and at the end of the first and of the fifth to sixth cycles of chemotherapy, and analyzed for VEGF and endostatin levels using enzyme-linked immunosorbent assay (ELISA). Tumor angiogenesis activity was evaluated using the serum soluble vascular cell adhesion molecule (VCAM-1) measured by ELISA. Systemic chemotherapy for BC resulted in a significant decrease of serum VEGF levels. The authors suggest that chemotherapy combined with antiangiogenic agents is helpful for accelerating the death of tumor cells and elevating the efficacy of treatment (Tang et al., 2006).

ANTIANGIOGENIC AGENTS

Bevacizumab

A number of antiangiogenic agents entered in clinical trials in oncology, either alone or in combination with other therapies. Up to now the most promising agent is bevacizumab (bev), a humanized monoclonal antibody directed against VEGF-A (Table 1).

A phase II study of bev monotherapy at escalating doses conducted in 75 patients with heavely pretreated metastatic BC (MBC) reported a 9.3% objective response rate (RR) with 17% of patients responding or stable at 22 weeks; four (7%) patients continued therapy without progression for more than 12 months (Cobleigh et al., 2003). Another phase II trial in 55 metastatic pretreated BC patients evaluated the safety and activity of bev (10 mg/kg every two weeks) combined with vinorelbine (25 mg/m^2/wk), showing an RR of 31% with one complete response. Treatment was well tolerated, with moderate grade of hypertension, proteinuria, and epistaxis. No major bleedings or thrombotic events were registered (Rugo, 2004).

A phase III trial randomly assigned 462 patients with anthracycline- and taxane-refractory disease to receive capecitabine with or without bev. As expected, hypertension requiring treatment (17.9% vs. 0.5%), proteinuria (22.3% vs. 7.4%), and thromboembolic events (7.4% vs. 5.6%) were more frequent in the combined arm. In each

Table 1 Antiangiogenic Compounds Tested in Human Breast Cancer

Naturally occurring inhibitors	Clinical study
Endostatin	Phase I
Matrix metalloproteinase inhibitors	
Marimastat	Phase II
BAY 12-9566	Phase I–II
CGS27023A	Phase I–II
Antiendothelial growth factors	
Bevacizumab	Phase III
SU5416	Phase I
Angiozyme	Phase I
Suramin	Phase I–II
Inhibitors of endothelial cell proliferation and migration	
Antiintegrin avb3 Mab	Phase I
TNP-470	Phase I
Agents with various mechanism of action	
Thalidomide	Phase I–II
ZD1839	Phase I–II
PNU-145156	Phase I
COX-2 inhibitors	Phase II
Antiestrogens	Phase II–III

group 12% of patients discontinued therapy because of toxicity. The combined therapy significantly increased RR (9.1% vs. 19.8%; $p = 0.001$), but because many of the responses in the combination group were relatively short-lived, progression-free survival (PFS) and overall survival (OS) were similar in both groups (4.17 vs. 4.86 months and 14.5 vs. 15.1 months, respectively) (Miller, 2003). Although attempts to correlate VEGF RNA overexpression (by in situ hybridization) and response in this study were unsuccessful, the sample size was too small for a definitive conclusion.

A large international phase III trial (E2100) evaluated paclitaxel (90 mg/m^2 weekly for three of four weeks) with or without bev (10 mg/kg every two weeks) in chemotherapy-naive patients. This trial completed the accrual in late May of 2004 and enrolled over 700 women. The interim analysis showed a better RR and PFS in the experimental group (28.2% vs. 14.2%, and 10.9 vs. 6.11 months, both statistically significant). The combined treatment was well tolerated, with hypertension, proteinuria, and sensory peripheral neuropathy being the most frequently observed side effects (Miller, 2003).

An ongoing trial coordinated by the North Central Cancer Treatment Group (NCCTG) is testing the combination of docetaxel, capecitabine, and bevacizumab as first-line chemotherapy.

Bev has also been tested in the neoadjuvant setting. One study compared docetaxel alone or combined with bev. The responsive patients underwent definitive surgery followed by four cycles of doxorubicin/cyclophosphamide and tamoxifen (if hormone receptor positive). There were five complete clinical responses and 24 partial responses, and therapy was generally well tolerated (Overmoyer et al., 2004).

In the study by Wedam et al. (2006), 21 patients with inflammatory and locally advanced BC were treated with bev for cycle 1 at 15 mg/kg on day one, followed by six cycles of bev with doxorubicin and docetaxel every three weeks. After locoregional therapy, patients received eight cycles of bev alone and hormonal therapy when indicated. Tumor biopsies and dynamic contrast-enhanced magnetic resonance imaging (DCE-MRI) were obtained at baseline, and after cycles 1, 4, and 7 of therapy. After completion of chemotherapy, 8 of the 13 patients experienced a confirmed partial response. There was also the evidence of a decrease in vascular permeability assessed by DCE-MRI after the first cycle of bev monotherapy.

The phosphorylation of VEGFR-2, at tyrosine sites 951 and 996, was evaluated by immunohistochemistry (IHC) and compared to baseline. The phosphorylation status decreased after the first infusion of bev and persisted during chemotherapy. In addition, there were no significant changes in MVD, VEGF-A, or VEGFR-2 expression (Wedam et al., 2006).

The Eastern Cooperative Oncology Group (ECOG) adjuvant feasibility trial evaluating bev (10 mg/kg every 2 weeks) in combination with dose-dense doxorubicin and cyclophosphamide followed by paclitaxel in node-positive BC (E 2104 trial) is ongoing.

Preclinical models of the combination of bev and docetaxel demonstrate synergistic suppression of capillary vessel formation. On the basis of this evidence, Silverman et al. have presented the vascular and antitumor effects of the combination bev/docetaxel versus docetaxel alone for treatment of locally advanced disease at the 29th Annual San Antonio Breast Cancer Symposium. Circulating VEGF, basic fibroblastic growth factor (bFGF), serum markers intracellular adhesion molecule (ICAM), VCAM-1 and E-selectin, tumor MVD, and DCE-MRI were serially assessed during and after treatment. In a randomized phase II trial 49 patients with locally unresectable BC were randomized to receive neoadjuvant therapy with bev (10 mg/kg weekly × 8) and docetaxel (two 8-week cycles of 35 mg/mq weekly × 6 with a 2-week break) or docetaxel alone. Like in other studies, an increase in plasma VEGF levels was seen with the combination schedules. DCE-MRI findings support greater effect of the combination schedule than docetaxel alone on tumor blood flow (Silverman et al., 2006).

There is preclinical and clinical rationale supporting the combination of bev with trastuzumab. HER-2 appears to play a role in the regulation of VEGF (Koukourakis et al., 1999). An in vitro study demonstrated increased HIF-1α and VEGF mRNA expression in HER-2-overexpressing BC cell lines (Laughner et al., 2001). In another experimental study, exposure to trastuzumab significantly decreased VEGF in HER-2-overexpressing cells (Epstein et al., 2002). In vivo experiments have shown a better reduction in tumor xenograft volume using the combination of trastuzumab and bev compared with single-agent control (Koukourakis et al., 1999). In a cohort of 611 patients with primary BC and a median follow-up of greater than 50 months, there was a significant coexpression of HER-2 and VEGF (Konecny et al., 2004). A recent phase I trial evaluating the tolerability of trastuzumab and bev showed no negative pharmacokinetic interaction. Clinical responses were observed in five of nine patients, including one patient with prior disease progression on chemotherapy plus trastuzumab (Pegram et al., 2004). A phase II trial evaluating the clinical efficacy and safety of trastuzumab and bev combination as first-line treatment of Her2-amplified BC documented 13 out of 28 clinical responses and 9 out of 28 stable disease at week 8. Most common grade I/II adverse events were: fever, chills, headache, infusion reaction, fatigue, epistaxis, and aspartate aminotransferase/alanine aminotransferase (AST/ALT) increase. Six cardiac adverse events were reported: 2 grade 1, 3 grade 2 and 1 grade 4 (Pegram et al., 2006).

There is also a rationale supporting the simultaneous blockade of VEGF and EGFR pathways. Also EGFR regulates VEGF (Maity et al., 2000; Clarke et al., 2001) and several studies have demonstrated that the blockade of EGFR has also antiangiogenic effects (Bruns et al., 2000; Petit et al., 1997). Furthermore, increased production of VEGF is one possible mechanism by which tumor cells escape to anti-EGFR therapy (Rugo, 2004). One study has tested the strategy of combining bev and erlotinib. This combination demonstrated activity and the authors found that changes in circulating endothelial cells and circulating tumor cells correlate with clinical response (Abrams et al., 2003).

Tyrosine Kinase Inhibitors

SU011248 (Sunitinib Malate) is a multitarget tyrosine kinase inhibitor (VEGF-R_1, VEGF-R_2), platelet-derived growth factor receptor (PDGF-R), c-kit receptor, and Flt-3 (Gasparini et al., 2005a,b). SU011248 demonstrated preclinical activity in BC models (Abrams et al., 2003; Murray et al., 2003). Physiologic imaging during treatment with SU011248 revealed that [^{11}C] carbon monoxide and [^{18}F] fluoromethane imaging might be a useful surrogate of response (Miller et al., 2003). A phase II study of SU011248 in MBC resistant to anthracycline and taxane is ongoing. Preliminary toxicity data are available in 22 patients and the most frequently reported drug-related adverse events of any grade include diarrhea (32%), nausea (27%), fatigue (23%), and hypertension (14%). Preliminary efficacy data are available in 23 patients and four partial responses and five stable diseases were observed (Schneider and Miller, 2005). In a recent phase II study evaluating SU11248 monotherapy in 51 patients with refractory MBC, seven patients (14%) showed a partial response and one patient had prolonged stable disease (11 months). Toxicity, albeit manageable, required dose adjustments and includes fatigue, diarrhea, mucositis, anorexia, hypertension, neutropenia, and thrombocytopenia (Miller, 2003).

PTK787/ZK (Vatalanib) is a pan-VEGF, PDGF-R, c-kit, and c-Fms receptor tyrosine kinase inhibitor (Gasparini et al., 2005). Patients with a variety of advanced cancers received this agent and it was generally well tolerated. The Hoosier Oncology Group activated a phase I/II study of PTK787 in combination with trastuzumab in patients with newly diagnosed HER-2-overexpressing, locally recurrent, or metastatic BC.

Our oncology group is conducting a dose finding study with PTK787/ZK in combination with vinorelbine and trastuzumab in patients with metastatic BC HER-2/*neu* positive progressed after anthracyclines- and/or taxanes-based chemotherapy for metastatic disease. Four dose levels are planned: the primary objective of the present study is to determine the maximum tolerated dose (MTD) and the pharmacokinetics interactions of vinorelbine and PTK787/ZK in combination with fixed standard dosage of weekly trastuzumab.

ZD6474 is an inhibitor of VEGF-R_2 and the EGF-R tyrosine kinases (Gasparini et al., 2005). In a cohort of 7,12-dimethylbenz[a]anthracene-treated rats, there was the inhibition of the formation of atypical ductal hyperplasia and carcinoma in situ by more than 95% and no invasive disease occurred (Heffelfinger et al., 2004). A phase II trial in previously treated MBC was recently reported. The drug is well tolerated, with 26% of patients experiencing cutaneous rash (but none worse than grade 2). There were no objective responses and one patient had stable disease (Miller et al., 2004). This was, however, a heavily pretreated population with a median of four prior chemotherapeutic regimens.

Our center participated in an international phase I/II trial investigating the role of AG-013736, a VEGF-R tyrosine kinase inhibitor, combined with docetaxel versus docetaxel and placebo, as first-line treatment. The analysis of the phase I study showed that this combination was safe and efficacious. The phase II is ongoing and has currently enrolled 57 patients (Rugo, 2004).

On the basis of experimental data indicating that estrogens stimulate VEGF expression (Nakamura et al., 1996). Traina et al. performed a phase II study with the combination of letrozole and bev in hormone receptor-positive tumors. The preliminary analysis documented promising results in terms of tolerability and efficacy (Traina et al., 2005).

VEGF expression is not a predictive factor for bev or other anti-VEGF compounds and many prospective trials are examining also other biomarkers. The identification of effective predictive indicators may further improve the selection of patients for antiangiogenic therapy, so enhancing the therapeutic benefit in more rationally selected patients (Hurwitz et al., 2004; Gasparini et al., 2005; Moses et al., 2004).

In a mouse model, Yoshiji et al. demonstrated that VEGF is essential for early but not late growth of human BC (Yoshiji et al., 1997). In another in vivo model, VEGF levels significantly decrease after the angiogenic switch, and bFGF maintains the vascular phenotype of tumor cells until late stages of tumor progression; then both the angiogenic factors are operative (Toi et al., 1995). Relf et al. confirmed that VEGF acts as mitogen in the earliest stages of primary BC, but as the cancer progressed, angiogenesis was supported by more proangiogenic factors: bFGF, transforming growth factor beta-1 (TGFβ-1), placenta growth factor (PLGF), platelet-derived endothelial cell growth factor, and pleiotrophin inclusive (Relf et al., 1997). Overall, these studies suggest that the optimal setting of administration of anti-VEGF agents could be the adjuvant therapy.

Ribozymes

Angiozyme (Ribozyme) is a chemically stabilized ribozyme targeting the VEGFR-1 mRNA. A phase I/II study was undertaken in patients with refractory solid tumors (Weng et al., 2001). A phase II trial in pretreated MBC patients has been performed. Although there was evidence of biologic activity with a decrease in serum VEGFR-1 levels (in patients that had detectable baseline levels), there were no objective responses (Hortobagyi et al., 2002).

Cyclooxygenase-2

Cyclooxygenase-2 (COX-2) expression in BC is variable but it is associated with parameters of biological aggressiveness, such as large tumor size, axillary node metastasis, hormonal receptor-negative disease, and HER-2/*neu* amplification (Arun and Goss, 2004). In addition, moderate to high COX-2 expression is found in a significant proportion of preinvasive and invasive BCs (Heffelfinger et al., 2004). Several experimental studies in animal models showed a pivotal role of COX-2 in various tumor processes, including apoptosis, angiogenesis, invasiveness, inflammation, and induction of aromatase, a cytochrome P450 enzyme that catalyses estrogen production (Gasparini et al., 2003).

Selective and nonselective COX-2 inhibitors significantly reduced carcinogen-induced rat mammary tumors and may have a role in the prevention and treatment of BC (Dannenberg and Howe, 2003). A meta-analysis of clinical studies indicates that the use of aspirin or nonsteroidal anti-inflammatory drugs reduce the risk of BC by approximately 20% (Khuder and Mutgi, 2001).

Celecoxib was tested in combination with trastuzumab in a phase II study in HER-2-positive MBC with a good tolerability but negative results (Dang et al., 2002). In another phase II trial, the combination of celecoxib and exemestane showed promising activity without relevant side effects (Canney, 2000). In the neoadjuvant setting, celecoxib in combination with 5-fluorouracil, epirubicin, cyclophosphamide (FEC) regimen or exemestane was superior to chemotherapy or hormone therapy alone, respectively (Chow et al., 2003; Chow and Toi, 2005).

A number of trials are planned to test the combination of celecoxib with other hormonal and/or cytotoxic agents in metastatic and adjuvant/neoadjuvant setting or coxibs alone as chemopreventive agents.

The above results should be reconsidered taking into account the emerged important cardiovascular and thromboembolic toxicity correlated to the prolonged use of such agents (Bresalier et al., 2005; Solomon et al., 2005; Nussmeier et al., 2005). Several mechanisms can explain this unexpected toxicity. Coxibs reduce the levels of COX-2-mediated prostacyclin that inhibits aggregation of platelets and proliferation of vascular smooth-muscle cells and induces vasodilatation, without affecting the levels of thromboxane A_2, the chief COX-1 mediated product of platelets that causes platelets' aggregation, vasoconstriction, and vascular proliferation. In addition, coxibs increase blood pressure, decrease angiogenesis, and destabilize aterosclerotic plaques (Gasparini et al., 2003; Bresalier et al., 2005; Nussmeier et al., 2005).

MMPIs

Marimastat is an oral MMP inhibitor. A pilot feasibility study of this drug evaluated patients with high-risk BC (Table 2). Marimastat was given either as single agent following completion of adjuvant chemotherapy or concurrently with tamoxifen. Arthralgia and arthritis were the most commonly reported toxicities. Six patients (19%) who received the 5-mg (twice daily) dose and 11 patients (35%) who received the 10-mg (twice daily) dose discontinued therapy because of toxicity, although plasma drug levels were rarely within the target range for biologic

Table 2 Mechanisms of Action of Inhibitors of Angiogenesis

Drug	Mechanism of action
Endostatin	Naturally occurring inhibitor: • Interference with VEGF and FGF-2 • Induction of endothelial cell apoptosis • Inhibition of matrix metalloproteinases
Marimastat BAY 12-9566 CGS27023A	Matrix metalloproteinases inhibitors
Ribozyme	Inhibition of mRNA of Flt-1 (VEGFR)
SU5416	Inhibition of Flk-1 (VEGFR)
Bevacizumab	RhuMab VEGF antibody
Vitaxin	Inhibition of integrin avb3
TNP-470	Inhibition of methione aminopeptidase-2 expressed in endothelial/ nonendothelial cells
Suramin	Antagonism of angiogenesis growth factor
Thalidomide	Downregulation of VEGF
ZD1839	Inhibition of EGF receptor
PNU-1451565	Inhibition of FGF
Celecoxib	Inhibition of COX-2
2-Methoxyestradiol	

activity (40 to 200 ng/mL). These findings were discouraging, as the toxicity prohibited the maintenance of plasma biologically active concentrations (Miller et al., 2003). In a phase III trial (E2196), 190 patients with MBC, responsive or stable after a first-line chemotherapy, were randomly assigned to receive marimastat or placebo. There was no significant difference in progression-free survival (4.7 vs. 3.1 months; $p = 0.16$) or overall survival (26.6 vs. 24.7 months; $p = 0.86$). Musculoskeletal toxicity was the most important toxicity. In that study, high plasma marimastat levels, at month 1 or 3, were associated with a greater risk of progression and death (Sparano et al., 2004).

METRONOMIC CHEMOTHERAPY

Several cytotoxic agents routinely used in chemotherapy have moderate antiangiogenic activity (Sweeney and Sledge, 1999). The enhancement of antiangiogenic activity typically requires prolonged exposure to low drug concentrations (Slaton et al., 1999). Several reports confirm the antiangiogenic activity of metronomic dose and schedule in preclinical models. The combination of low, frequent dose chemotherapy plus an agent that selectively targets the endothelial cell compartment (TNP-470 and anti-VEGF-2) controlled tumor growth much more effectively than the cytotoxic agent alone (Browder et al., 2000; Klement et al., 2000; Wild et al., 2004).

Thus far, few clinical trials have tested antiangiogenic schedules of chemotherapy, so-called metronomic therapy (Hanahan et al., 2000). Preclinical data suggests that the mechanism responsible for the antiangiogenic effect is the induction of increased plasma levels of thrombospondin-1 (a potent and endothelial specific inhibitor of angiogenesis) (Bocci et al., 2003). A phase II study of low-dose methotrexate (2.5 mg twice daily for 2 days each week) and cyclophosphamide (50 mg daily) in patients with previously treated MBC found an overall RR of 19% (an additional 13% of patients were stable for six months or more). Serum VEGF levels decreased in all patients remaining on therapy for at least 2 months but did not correlate with response (Colleoni et al., 2002). These studies suggest that activated endothelial cells may be more sensitive, or even selectively sensitive, to protracted low-dose chemotherapy compared with other types of normal cells, thus creating a potential therapeutic window. Such selective sensitivity has been confirmed in in vitro studies (Bocci et al., 2002). The Dana-Farber/Harvard Cancer Center (Boston, Massachusetts, U.S.) is enrolling patients in a phase II randomized study of metronomic low-dose cyclophosphamide and methotrexate with or without bevacizumab in women with MBC. Twenty-six patients have been enrolled thus far with no grade 3 or 4 toxicity to date (Harold J. Burstein, personal communication).

CONCLUSIONS

BC is a heterogeneous disease characterized by tumor-specific mutations and dysregulated cellular pathways. Targeting these pathways with novel agents may be the key to fighting cancer in the future. Understanding the specific genetic mutations and molecular pathways driving breast tumorigenesis will make targeted therapy possible. Trastuzumab provides the proof of principle that anticancer agents can be targeted based on the molecular biology of each individual tumor.

As documented with the combined use of trastuzumab and bev, the multitarget therapy, is at its infancy, but anyway it looks as one of the more promising new therapeutic strategies to improve clinical outcome of BC patients. Several other double or triplet combined therapies are under clinical evaluation based on antiangiogenic, anti-COX-2, or anti-EGFR compounds, supported by translational evaluation of laboratory biomarkers with the aim to select in each single patient the most relevant growth factors in play that may be the suitable target for tailored treatments.

In addition, it is important to understand the potential mechanisms of antiangiogenic resistance in order to ameliorate or bypass such clinical problems.

Extensive preclinical data support a combined approach with multiple antiangiogenic and chemotherapeutic agents having additive or synergistic combinatorial activity (Browder et al., 2000; Klement et al., 2000; Sweeney and Sledge, 1999; Teicher et al., 1992). The mechanistic rationale for many of these combinations is poorly understood, and not intuitive, as both radiotherapy and chemotherapy depend on an effective blood supply for therapeutic efficacy. A potential explanation may lie in the inherent inefficiency of the tumor vasculature. Antiangiogenic therapy normalizes the intratumoral vascular network resulting in improved tissue oxygenation and decreased interstitial pressure and ultimately favoring the delivery of cytotoxic agents (Jain, 2001).

Another strategy is based on the combination of multiple antiangiogenic agents. As tumor progression is associated with expression of an increased number of proangiogenic factors, the use of multiple antiangiogenic agents to simultaneously inhibit this redundant process may bypass the acquired resistance to each single agent. This approach is, of course, not unique to antiangiogenic therapy, having previously been used to limit resistance to cytotoxic, antimicrobial, and antiviral therapies. The combination of antiangiogenic agents has been tested in preclinical models with promising results (Brem et al., 1993; Scappaticci et al., 2001).

Also the blockades of VEGF and EGFR (Rugo, 2004) pathways as well as VEGF and HER-2 pathways (Pegram et al., 2004) are under evaluation.

Another important topic is the identification of the optimal clinical setting. It is rare that a treatment is more effective in large rather than in small tumors. The adjuvant setting is the logical place to accomplish this goal. The use of antiangiogenics as adjuvant therapy has its own potential barriers. The toxicity of chronic antiangiogenic therapy remains largely unexplored, as is the toxicity of combinations of chemotherapy with antiangiogenic therapy. Although intuitively, the impact of angiogenesis inhibition is expected to be greatest in patients with micrometastatic disease, proof of this concept will require commitment of substantial human and financial resources to randomized adjuvant trial.

Finally, the selection of patients to be treated is critical by the use of predictive surrogate markers of activity. Antiangiogenic therapy has been applied as a general therapy given on a population basis rather than as a targeted therapy. This is because the response to antiangiogenic agents is not related to the target impression. If a patient's tumor does not express VEGF and therefore fails to respond to an anti-VEGF therapy, is the tumor resistant or is the therapy merely misguided? As insensitivity due to lack of therapeutic target results in resistance at the patient level, proper targeting is a means of overcoming such resistance. So we need to optimize the strategies to overcome the mechanisms of resistance. In addition, we must become more astute at recognizing the correlations between the biology and clinical outcomes. This will require a comprehensive effort to perform tissue collection for testing as part of the development of antiangiogenic agents. The design of new generation trials (such as E2100) testing the efficacy of these therapies in a less refractory setting, as well as trials which are targeting multiple pathways, will also hopefully shed light on the true potentials of these agents.

REFERENCES

Abrams TJ, Murray LJ, Pesenti E, Holway VW, Colombo T, Lee LB, Cherrington JM, Pryer NK. Preclinical evaluation of the tyrosine kinase inhibitor SU11248 as a single agent and in combination with "standard of care" therapeutic agents for the treatment of breast cancer. Mol Cancer Ther 2003; 2:1011–1021.

Arun B, Goss P. The role of COX-2 inhibition in breast cancer treatment and prevention. Semin Oncol 2004; 31(suppl 7): 22–29.

Bocci G, Francia G, Man S, Lawler J, Kerbel RS. Thrombospondin 1, a mediator of the antiangiogenic effects of low-dose metronomic chemotherapy. Proc Natl Acad Sci U S A 2003; 100:12917–12922.

Bocci G, Nicolaou KC, Kerbel RS. Protracted low-dose effects on human endothelial cell proliferation and survival in vitro reveal a selective antiangiogenic window for various chemotherapeutic drugs. Cancer Res 2002; 62:6938–6943.

Bos R, Zhong H, Hanrahan CF, Mommers EC, Semenza GL, Pinedo HM, Abeloff MD, Simons JW, van Diest PJ, van der Wall E. Levels of hypoxia-inducible factor-1 alpha during breast carcinogenesis. J Natl Cancer Inst 2001; 93:309–314.

Brem H, Gresser I, Grosfeld J, Folkman J. The combination of antiangiogenic agents to inhibit primary tumor growth and metastasis. J Pediatr Surg 1993; 28:1253–1257.

Brem SS, Gullino PM, Medina D. Angiogenesis: a marker for neoplastic transformation of mammary papillary hyperplasia. Science 1977; 195:880–882.

Bresalier RS, Sandler RS, Quan H, Bolognese JA, Oxenius B, Horgan K, Lines C, Riddell R, Morton D, Lanas A, Konstam MA, Baron JA. Adenomatous polyp Prevention on Vioxx (APPROVe) Trial Investigators. Cardiovascular events associated with rofecoxib in a colorectal adenoma chemoprevention trial. N Engl J Med 2005; 352:1092–1102.

Browder T, Butterfield CE, Kraling BM, Shi B, Marshall B, O'Reilly MS, Folkman J. Antiangiogenic scheduling of chemotherapy improves efficacy against experimental drug-resistant cancer. Cancer Res 2000; 60:1878–1886.

Bruns CJ, Solorzano CC, Harbison MT, Ozawa S, Tsan R, Fan D, Abbruzzese J, Traxler P, Buchdunger E, Radinsky R, Fidler IJ. Blockade of the epidermal growth factor receptor signaling by a novel tyrosine kinase inhibitor leads to apoptosis of endothelial cells and therapy of human pancreatic carcinoma. Cancer Res 2000; 60:2926–2935.

Calvo A, Yokoyama Y, Smith LE, Ali I, Shih SC, Feldman AL, Libutti SK, Sundaram R, Green JE. Inhibition of the mammary carcinoma angiogenic switch in C3(1)/SV40 transgenic mice by a mutated form of human endostatin. Int J Cancer 2002; 101:224–234.

Canney PA. A phase II study of the efficacy and tolerability of the combination of exemestane with the cylooxigenase-2 inhibitor celecoxib in postmenopausal women with advanced breast cancer. Proc Am Soc Clin Oncol 2000; 22:158 (abstr).

Chow LW, Toi M. Celecoxib antiaromatase neoadjuvant (CAAN) Trial for locally advanced breast cancer. Breast Cancer Res Treat 2005; 94:S240 (abstr 5095).

Chow LW, Toi M, Takebayashi Y. Neoadjuvant celecoxib and 5-fluorouracil/epirubicin/cyclophosphamide (FEC) for the treatment of locally advanced breast cancer (LABC). Proc Am Soc Clin Oncol 2003; 22:327 (abstr).

Clarke K, Smith K, Gullick WJ, Harris AL. Mutant epidermal growth factor receptor enhances induction of vascular endothelial growth factor by hypoxia and insulin-like growth factor-1 via a PI3 kinase dependent pathway. Br J Cancer 2001; 84:1322–1329.

Cobleigh MA, Langmuir VK, Sledge GW, Miller KD, Haney L, Novotny WF, Reimann JD, Vassel A. A phase I/II dose-escalation trial of bevacizumab in previously treated metastatic breast cancer. Semin Oncol 2003; 30(5 suppl 16): 117–124.

Colleoni M, Rocca A, Sandri MT, Zorzino L, Masci G, Nole F, Peruzzotti G, Robertson C, Orlando L, Cinieri S, de BF, Viale G, Goldhirsch A. Low-dose oral methotrexate and cyclophosphamide in metastatic breast cancer: antitumor activity and correlation with vascular endothelial growth factor levels. Ann Oncol 2002; 13:73–80.

Dang CT, Dickler MN, Moasser MM, Theodoulou M, Seidman A, Norton L, Hudis CA. Celecoxib © and trastuzumab (herceptin) (H) is feasible after H for HER-2/neu overexpressing (H2+) metastatic breast cancer (MBC) patients (pts). Proc Am Soc Clin Oncol 2002; 21:2003 (abstr).

Dannenberg AJ, Howe LR. The role of COX-2 in breast and cervical cancer. Prog Exp Tumor Res 2003; 37:90–106.

Epstein M, Ayala R, Tchekmedyian N, Borgstrom P, Pegram M, Slamon D. HER2/neu-overexpressing human breast cancer xenografts exhibit increased angiogenic potential mediated by vascular endothelial growth factor (VEGF). Breast Cancer Res Treat 2002; 76:S143 (abstr 570).

Foekens JA, Peters HA, Grebenchtchikov N, Look MP, Meijer-van Gelder ME, Geurts-Moespost A, van der Kwast TH, Sweep CG, Klijn JG. High tumor levels of vascular endothelial growth factor predict poor response to systemic therapy in advanced breast cancer. Cancer Res 2001; 61:5407–5414.

Folkman J. Tumor angiogenesis: therapeutic implications. N Engl J Med 1971; 285:1182–1186.

Gasparini G, Fox SB, Verderio P, Bevilacqua P, Boracchi P, Dante S, Marubini E, Harris AL. Determination of angiogenesis adds information to estrogen receptor status in predicting the efficacy of adjuvant tamoxifen in node-positive breast cancer patients. Clin Cancer Res 1996; 2(7):1191–1198.

Gasparini G, Longo R, Fanelli M, Teicher BA. Combination of antiangiogenic therapy with other anticancer therapies: results, challenges, and open questions. J Clin Oncol 2005a; 23(8):1295–1311.

Gasparini G, Longo R, Sarmiento R, Morabito A. COX-2 inhibitors (Coxibs): a new class of anticancer agents? Lancet Oncol 2003; 4:605–615.

Gasparini G, Longo R, Toi M, Ferrara N. Angiogenic inhibitors: a new therapeutic strategy in oncology. Nat Clin Pract Oncol 2005b; 2(11):562–77.

Gasparini G, Toi M, Gion M, Verderio P, Dittadi R, Hanatani M, Matsubara I, Vinante O, Bonoldi E, Boracchi P, Gatti C, Suzuki H, Tominaga T. Prognostic significance of vascular endothelial growth factor protein in node-negative breast carcinoma. J Natl Cancer Inst 1997; 89:139–147.

Guidi AJ, Fischer L, Harris JR, Schnitt SJ. Microvessel density and distribution in ductal carcinoma in situ of the breast. J Natl Cancer Inst 1994; 86:614–619.

Guidi AJ, Schnitt SJ, Fischer L, Tognazzi K, Harris JR, Dvorak HF, Brown LF. Vascular permeability factor (vascular endothelial growth factor) expression and angiogenesis in patients with ductal carcinoma in situ of the breast. Cancer 1997; 80:1945–1953.

Guinebretiere JM, Le Monique G, Gavoille A, Bahi J, Contesso G. Angiogenesis and risk of breast cancer in women with fibrocystic disease. J Natl Cancer Inst 1994; 86:635–636.

Hanahan D, Bergers G, Bergsland E. Less is more, regularly: metronomic dosing of cytotoxic drugs can target tumor angiogenesis in mice. J Clin Invest 2000; 105:1045–1047.

Hanahan D, Folkman J. Patterns and emerging mechanisms of the angiogenic switch during tumorigenesis. Cell 1996; 86:353–364.

Heffelfinger SC, Yan M, Gear RB, Schneider J, LaDow K, Warshawsky D. Inhibition of VEGFR2 prevents DMBA-induced mammary tumor formation. Lab Invest 2004; 84:989–998.

Hortobagyi G, Weng D, Elias A, et al. ANGIOZYME treatment of stage IV metastatic breast cancer patients: assessment of serum markers of angiogenesis. Breast Cancer Res Treat 2002; 76:S97 (abstr 362).

Hurwitz H, Fehrenbacher L, Novotny W, Cartwright T, Hainsworth J, Heim W, Berlin J, Baron A, Griffing S, Holmgren E, Ferrara N, Fyfe G, Rogers B, Ross R, Kabbinavar F. Bevacizumab plus irinotecan, fluorouracil, and leucovorin for metastatic colorectal cancer. N Engl J Med 2004; 350:2335–2342.

Jain RK. Normalizing tumor vasculature with anti-angiogenic therapy: a new paradigm for combination therapy. Nat Med 2001; 7:987–989.

Jensen HM, Chen I, DeVault MR, Lewis AE. Angiogenesis induced by "normal" human breast tissue: a probable marker for precancer. Science 1982; 218:293–295.

Khuder SA, Mutgi AB. Breast cancer and NSAID use: a meta-analysis. Br J Cancer 2001; 84:1188–1192.

Kim KJ, Li B, Winer J, Armanini M, Gillet N, Phillips HS, Ferrara N. Inhibition of vascular endothelial growth factor-induced angiogenesis suppresses tumour growth in vivo. Nature 1993; 362:841–844.

Klement G, Baruchel S, Rak J, Man S, Clark K, Hicklin DJ, Bohlen P, Kerbel RS. Continuous low-dose therapy with vinblastine and VEGF receptor-2 antibody induces sustained tumor regression without overt toxicity. J Clin Invest 2000; 105:R15–R24.

Konecny GE, Meng YG, Untch M, Wang HJ, Bauerfeind I, Epstein M, Stieber P, Vernes JM, Gutierrez J, Hong K, Beryt M, Hepp H, Slamon DJ, Pegram MD. Association between HER-2/neu and vascular endothelial growth factor expression predicts clinical outcome in primary breast cancer patients. Clin Cancer Res 2004; 10: 1706–1716.

Koukourakis MI, Giatromanolaki A, O'Byrne KJ, Cox J, Krammer B, Gatter KC, Harris AL. bcl-2 and c-erbB-2 proteins are involved in the regulation of VEGF and of thymidine phosphorylase angiogenic activity in non-small-cell lung cancer. Clin Exp Metastasis 1999; 17:545–554.

Laughner E, Taghavi P, Chiles K, Mahon PC, Semenza GL. HER2 (neu) signaling increases the rate of hypoxia-inducible factor 1alpha (HIF-1alpha) synthesis: novel mechanism for HIF-1-mediated vascular endothelial growth factor expression. Mol Cell Biol 2001; 21:3995–4004.

Maity A, Pore N, Lee J, Solomon D, O'Rourke DM. Epidermal growth factor receptor transcriptionally up-regulates vascular endothelial growth factor expression in human glioblastoma cells via a pathway involving phosphatidylinositol 3′-kinase and distinct from that induced by hypoxia. Cancer Res 2000; 60:5879–5886.

Miller KD. E2100: a phase III trial of paclitaxel versus paclitaxel/bevacizumab for metastatic breast cancer. Clin Breast Cancer 2003; 3(6):421–422.

Miller KD, Burstein HJ, Elias AD, Rugo HS, Cobleigh MA, Wolff AC, Eisenberg PD, Collier M, Adams BJ, Baum CM. Phase II study of SU11248, a multitargeted tyrosine kinase inhibitor (TKI) in patients (pts) with previously treated metastatic breast cancer (MBC). Breast Cancer Res Treat 2005a; 94:S61 (abstr 1066).

Miller KD, Chap LI, Holmes FA, Cobleigh MA, Marcom PK, Fehrenbacher L, Dickler M, Overmoyer BA, Reimann JD, Sing AP, Langmuir V, Rugo HS. Randomized phase III trial of capecitabine compared with bevacizumab plus capecitabine in patients with previously treated metastatic breast cancer. J Clin Oncol 2005b; 23:792–799.

Miller K, Miller M, Mehrotra S, et al. The search for surrogates—physiologic imaging in a breast cancer xenograft model during treatment with SU11248. Breast Cancer Res Treat 2003; 82:S18 (abstr 38).

Miller K, Trigo J, Stone A, Wheeler C, Barge A, Sledge GW, Baselga J. A phase II trial of ZD6474, a vascular endothelial growth factor receptor-2 (VEGFR-2) and epidermal growth factor receptor (EGFR) tyrosine kinase inhibitor, in patients with previously treated metastatic breast cancer (MBC). Breast Cancer Res Treat 2004; 88:S240 (abstr 6060).

Moses MA, Harper J, Fernández CA. A role for antiangiogenic therapy in breast cancer. Curr Oncol Rep 2004; 6:42–48.

Murray LJ, Abrams TJ, Long KR, Ngai TJ, Olson LM, Hong W, Keast PK, Brassard JA, O'farrell AM, Cherrington JM, Pryer NK. SU11248 inhibits tumor growth and CSF-1R-dependent osteolysis in an experimental breast cancer bone metastasis model. Clin Exp Metastasis 2003; 20:757–766.

Nakamura J, Savinov A, Lu Q, Brodie A. Estrogen regulates vascular endothelial growth/permeability factor expression in 7,12-dimethylbenz(a)anthracene-induced rat mammary tumors. Endocrinology 1996; 137:5589–5596.

Nussmeier NA, Whelton AA, Brown MT, Langford RM, Hoeft A, Parlow JL, Boyce SW, Verburg KM. Complications of the COX-2 inhibitors parecoxib and valdecoxib after cardiac surgery. N Engl J Med 2005; 352:1081–1091.

Overmoyer B, Silverman P, Leeming R, Shenk R, Lyons J, Ziats N, Jesberger J, Dumadag L, Remick S, Chen H. Phase II trial of neoadjuvant docetaxel with or without bevacizumab in patients with locally advanced breast cancer. Breast Cancer Res Treat 2004; 88:S106 (abstr 2088).

Pegram M, Chan D, Dichmann RA, Tan-Chiu E, Yeon C, Durna L, Lin SL, Slamon D. Phase II combined biological therapy targeting the HER2 proto-oncogene and the vascular endothelial growth factor using trastuzumab (T) and bevacizumab (B) as first line treatment of HER2-amplified breast cancer. 29th Symposium Of San Antonio Breast Cancer 2006 (abstr 301).

Pegram MD, Yeon C, Ku NC, Gaudreault J, Slamon DJ. Phase I combined biological therapy of breast cancer using two humanized monoclonal antibodies directed against HER2 proto-oncogene and vascular endothelial growth factor (VEGF). Breast Cancer Res Treat 2004; 88:S124 (abstr 3039).

Petit AM, Rak J, Hung MC, Rockwell P, Goldstein N, Fendly B, Kerbel RS. Neutralizing antibodies against epidermal growth factor and ErbB-2/neu receptor tyrosine kinases down-regulate vascular endothelial growth factor production by tumor cells in vitro and in vivo: angiogenic implications for signal transduction therapy of solid tumors. Am J Pathol 1997; 151:1523–1530.

Ragaz J, Miller K, Badve S, Dayachko Y, Dunn S, Nielsen T, Brodie A, Huntsman D, Bajdik C, George S. Adverse association of expressed vascular endothelial growth factor (VEGF), Her2, Cox2, uPA and EMSY with long-term outcome of stage I-III breast cancer (BrCa). Results from the British Columbia Tissue Microarray Project. Proc Am Soc Clin Oncol 2004; 23:8 (abstr 524).

Relf M, LeJeune S, Scott PA, Fox S, Smith K, Leek R, Moghaddam A, Whitehouse R, Bicknell R, Harris AL. Expression of the angiogenic factors vascular endothelial cell growth factor, acidic and basic fibroblast growth factor, tumor growth factor beta-1, platelet-derived endothelial cell growth factor, placenta growth factor, and pleiotrophin in human primary breast cancer and its relation to angiogenesis. Cancer Res 1997; 57(5):963–969.

Rugo HS. Bevacizumab in the treatment of breast cancer: rationale and current data. The Oncologist 2004; 9(suppl 1): 43–49.

Salceda S, Caro J. Hypoxia-inducible factor 1alpha (HIF-1alpha) protein is rapidly degraded by the ubiquitin-proteasome system under normoxic conditions. Its stabilization by hypoxia depends on redox-induced changes. J Biol Chem 1997; 272:22642–22647.

Scappaticci FA, Smith R, Pathak A, Schloss D, Lum B, Cao Y, Johnson F, Engleman EG, Nolan GP. Combination angiostatin and endostatin gene transfer induces synergistic antiangiogenic activity in vitro and antitumor efficacy in leukemia and solid tumors in mice. Mol Ther 2001; 3:186–196.

Schneider BP, Miller KD. Angiogenesis of breast cancer. J Clin Oncol 2005; 23:1782–1790.

Silverman P, Lyons J, Fu P, Remick S, Chen H, Ziats N, Wasman J, Hartman P, Jesberger J, Leeming R, Shenk R, Dumadag L, Overmoyer B. Randomized phase II study of docetaxel +/− bevacizumab for locally advanced unresectable breast cancer: impact on biomarkers of angiogenesis. 29th Symposium of San Antonio Breast Cancer 2006 (abstr 5086).

Slaton JW, Perrotte P, Inoue K, Dinney CP, Fidler IJ. Interferon-alpha-mediated down-regulation of angiogenesis-related genes and therapy of bladder cancer are dependent on optimization of biological dose and schedule. Clin Cancer Res 1999; 5:2726–2734.

Sledge GW Jr. Vascular endothelial growth fact in breast cancer: biologic and therapeutic aspects. Semin Oncol 2002; 29(suppl 11):104–110.

Solomon SD, McMurray JJ, Pfeffer MA, Wittes J, Fowler R, Finn P, Anderson WF, Zauber A, Hawk E, Bertagnolli M. Adenoma Prevention with Celecoxib (APC) Study Investigators. Cardiovascular risk associated with celecoxib in a clinical trial for colorectal adenoma prevention. N Engl J Med 2005; 352:1071–1080.

Sparano JA, Bernardo P, Stephenson P, Gradishar WJ, Ingle JN, Zucker S, Davidson NE. Randomized phase III trial of marimastat versus placebo in patients with metastatic breast cancer who have responding or stable disease after first-line chemotherapy: Eastern Cooperative Oncology Group Trial E2196. J Clin Oncol 2004; 22:4631–4638.

Sweeney C, Sledge G. Chemotherapy agents as antiangiogenic therapy. Cancer Conference Highlights 1999; 3:2–4.

Tang J, Zhao J, Pan L, Xu Z. Effects of systemic chemotherapy on circulating angiogenic factors levels in patients with breast cancer. 29th Symposium of San Antonio Breast Cancer, 2006 (abstr 5090).

Teicher BA, Sotomayor EA, Huang ZD. Antiangiogenic agents potentiate cytotoxic cancer therapies against primary and metastatic disease. Cancer Res 1992; 52:6702–6704.

Toi M, Inada K, Hoshina S, Suzuki H, Kondo S, Tominaga T. Vascular endothelial growth factor and platelet-derived endothelial cell growth factor are frequently coexpressed in highly vascularized human breast cancer. Clin Cancer Res 1995; 1(9):961–964.

Traina TA, Dickler MN, Caravelli JF, Yeh BM, Brogi E, Panageas K, Flores SA, Norton L, Park J, Hudis C, Rugo H. A phase II trial of letrozole in combination with Bevacizumab, an anti-VEGF antibody, in patients with hormone receptor-positive metastatic breast cancer. Breast Cancer Res Treat 2005; 94:S93 (abstr 2030).

Wang GL, Jiang BH, Rue EA, Semenza GL. Hypoxia-inducible factor 1 is a basic-helix-loop-helix-PAS heterodimer regulated by cellular O2 tension. Proc Natl Acad Sci U S A 1995; 92:5510–5514.

Wedam S, Low J, Yang SX, Chow CK, Choyke P, Danforth D, Hewitt SM, Berman A, Steinberg SM, Liewehr DJ, Plehn J, Doshi A, Thomasson D, McCarthy N, Koeppen H, Sherman M, Zujewski J, Camphausen K, Chen H, Swain SM. Antiangiogenic and antitumor effects of bevacizumab in patients with inflammatory and locally advanced breast cancer. J Clin Oncol 2006; 24:769–777.

Weng DE, Weiss P, Kellackey C, Ganapathi R, Parker VP, Usman N, Cowens JW, Smith JA, Jackson TE, Radka SF, Di Francesco A, Kim JA, Borden EC. Angiozyme pharmacokinetic and safety results: a phase I/II study in patients with refractory solid tumors. Proc Am Soc Clin Oncol 2001; 20:99a (abstr 393).

Wild R, Dings R, Subramanian I, Ramakrishnan S. Carboplatin selectively induces the VEGF stress response in endothelial cells: potentiation of antitumor activity by combination treatment with antibody to VEGF. Int J Cancer 2004; 110:343–351.

Yoshiji H, Harris SR, Thorgeirsson UP. Vascular endothelial growth factor is essential for initial but not continued in vivo growth of human breast carcinoma cells. Cancer Res 1997; 57(18):3924–3928.

23

Cytotoxic Therapy and Other Non-Hormonal Approaches for the Treatment of Metastatic Breast Cancer

CHRISTINE M. PELLEGRINO and JOSEPH A. SPARANO

Department of Oncology, Montefiore Medical Center, Albert Einstein College of Medicine, Bronx, New York, U.S.A.

INTRODUCTION

Approximately one-third of patients relapse after primary therapy for operable disease, or initially present with metastatic breast cancer. Although metastatic breast cancer is treatable, it is an incurable condition that is typically associated with a median survival of approximately 18 to 24 months. The goals of systemic therapy include palliation of symptoms, preventing or delaying the development of disease-associated symptoms, and prolongation of survival. Although regarded as incurable, recent declines in breast cancer mortality have been in part attributed to improved therapies for early and advanced stage disease (Berry et al., 2005, 2006). Current options for systemic therapy include hormonal therapy for those with estrogen receptor (ER)- and/or progesterone receptor (PR)-positive disease, trastuzumab for those with disease that overexpresses Her2/neu, and cytotoxic chemotherapy. Cytotoxic therapy is generally reserved for patients with hormone receptor (HR)-positive disease who have failed one or more hormonal regimens, patients with HR-negative disease where there is no role for hormonal therapy, or those with who have symptomatic disease that requires prompt symptom relief. This chapter will focus on the efficacy of cytotoxic therapy and other nonhormonal approaches for the treatment of patients with metastatic breast cancer. The emphasis will be on clinical trials that are either randomized phase III trials, or selected phase II trials that have had a substantial impact on the field. End points that will be reviewed for selected studies include response rate, median time to disease progression (or treatment failure), median survival, and the incidence of severe (grade 3) and life threatening (grade 4) toxicities.

CLINICAL BENEFITS OF SYSTEMIC THERAPY

Effect of Cytotoxic Therapy on Survival and Symptom Palliation

Factors associated with shortened survival included HR-negative disease, visceral dominant disease, three or more disease sites, a disease-free interval of less than 24 months, and a history of prior systemic treatment (Clark et al., 1987). Population-based and hospital-based studies evaluating survival during the pre and postchemotherapy era suggests that cytotoxic chemotherapy prolongs survival by an average of about 9 to 12 months (Ross et al., 1985; Brincker, 1988). Numerous studies have demonstrated that objective response to therapy is associated with improved survival. The correlation between response rate and survival was evaluated by reviewing 79 comparisons between arms with unequal response rates in 50 published trials that included chemotherapy for metastatic breast cancer (A'Hern et al., 1988). In 73% of comparisons, the group with the higher response rate also demonstrated a significantly longer median survival, and weighted linear regression showed a statistically significant relationship between relative response and survival. A review of experience at the MD Anderson Cancer Center illustrates this point (Rahman et al., 1999). This retrospective report included 1581 patients treated between 1973 and 1982 with doxorubicin-based therapy. Complete response occurred in 17% and partial response occurred in 48%. Median progression-free survival (PFS) and overall survival (OS) were 22.4 months and 41.8 months, respectively, for complete responders, and 14 months and 24.6 months for partial responders. For those who had progressive disease during therapy, the median OS was only 3.8 months. The median time to achieve an objective response was about five months. These results illustrate the importance of achieving a response to cytoxic therapy as a surrogate for improved survival.

The correlation between survival and response in patients treated with cytotoxic therapy supports using response rate as an end point in clinical trials. On the other hand, others have pointed out that patients who survive a sufficient duration of time to have the opportunity to exhibit response will have a predictably longer survival than other patients, even if the therapy has no effect on survival (Buyse and Piedbois, 1996). The United States Food and Drug Administration (FDA) uses clinical benefit as its criterion for approving new agents. In an analysis of FDA approvals over a 13 year period between 1990 and 2002, the FDA granted marketing approval to 71 oncology drug applications, including three new hormonal agents (anastozole, letrozole, fulvestant), two new cytotoxic agents (paclitaxel, docetaxel), and other agents (trastuzumab, pamidronate, and zoledronate) for breast cancer (Johnson et al., 2003). Regular approvals were granted based on end points demonstrating that the drug provided a longer life, a better life, or a favorable effect on an established surrogate for a longer or better life. Accelerated approval was granted based on surrogate end points that were less well established but reasonably likely to predict a longer or a better life. Tumor response was the approval basis in 26 of 57 regular approvals, supported by relief of tumor-specific symptoms in nine of these 26 regular approvals. Relief of tumor-specific symptoms provided critical support for approval in 13 of 57 regular approvals. Approval was based on tumor response in 12 of 14 of the accelerated approvals.

Although virtually all trials focus on response rate and survival, few provide information regarding the impact of therapy on symptom relief. One group reported that symptom relief in breast cancer usually correlates with objective response (Geels et al., 2000). In their study of 300 patients with metastatic breast cancer who were participating in a clinical trial that evaluated a doxorubicin-containing regimen, the investigators asked patients and their caretakers about symptoms (Table 1). Some symptoms were disease related (e.g., pain), whereas others were related to measures aimed at symptom relief (e.g., constipation associated with narcotics). Physician-reported symptoms (as assessed by chart review by nurses or data managers) underestimated the extent of symptomatology compared with patient-reported symptoms, consistent with previous reports (Macquart-Moulin et al., 1997). Most importantly, however, the authors demonstrated a strong correlation between objective tumor response and both physician- and patient-reported symptom relief (Fig. 1), thereby validating the use of response as a surrogate for evaluating new treatment modalities. A meta-analysis evaluating 21 clinical trials including several tumor types and breast cancer demonstrated similar findings (Victorson et al., 2006).

Table 1 Incidence of Cancer-Related Symptoms in Patients with Metastatic Breast Cancer

Symptoms	Case-report form[a]	Patient reported
Cancer pain	38%	81%
Constipation	27%	46%
Lethargy	26%	89%
Shortness of breath	24%	62%
Cough	20%	51%
Nausea	16%	44%
Mood	15%	71%
Anorexia	13%	55%
Insomnia	9%	68%

[a]As recorded in the case report form by nurse or other research associate, based on review of physician notes and other medical records.

Definition of Response and Other Endpoints

Response is often loosely defined in clinical practice but is rigidly defined in clinical trials. Clinical indicators of response include relief of pain, decreased narcotic requirements, less dyspnea or cough, diminished fatigue, and improved performance status and sense of well being. In general, response criteria have relied on at least 50% reduction in the sum of the products of bidimensionally measurable lesions (Oken et al., 1982). Many lesions are often difficult to measure bidimensionally due to lack of a discrete lesion (e.g., bone metastases, effusions, lymphangitic metastases), small lesions, or confluence of more than one lesion. The United States National Cancer Institute (NCI) and the European Organization for Research and Treatment of Cancer (EORTC) developed a set of standardized response criteria for solid tumors (RECIST) that relies on unidimensional measurement of indicator lesions demonstrating at least 30% reduction in the sum of unidimensional measurements (Therasse et al., 2000). This system has shown to correlate well with bidimensional

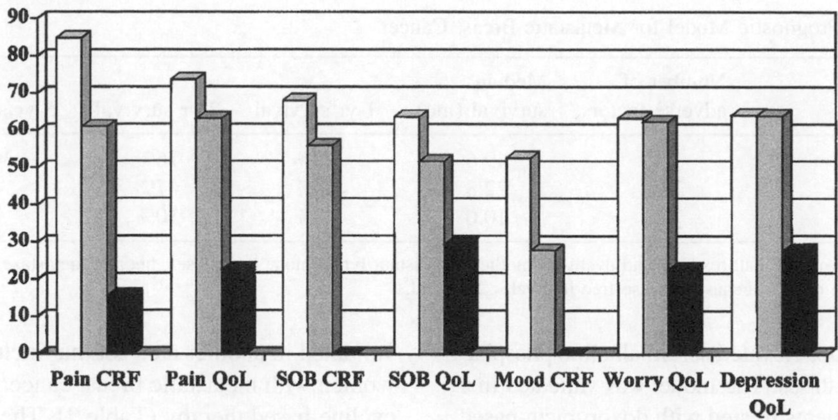

Figure 1 Proportion of patients with symptom response according to each objective response category: significant results with both CRF and QoL data. *Abbreviations*: CRF, case report form; QoL, quality of life; □, complete or partial response; ▒, stable disease; ■, progressive disease. *Source*: From Geels et al. (2000).

measurements, has fairly consistent inter- and intra-observer reproducibility, and is generally less time consuming than performing bidimensional measurements.

Other end points that are commonly used include time to disease progression (TTP), PFS, and time to treatment failure (TTF). TTP is generally defined as the time from treatment initiation until disease progression (with deaths from other causes censored), and may be influenced by the proportion demonstrating response, the durability of those responses, and by the proportion and durability of those experiencing stable disease. The definition of PFS is similar, but also includes deaths not due to breast cancer. TTF includes not only disease progression as an event, but also includes serious adverse events or other events that prompt discontinuation of treatment, and deaths from any cause, thereby reflecting both treatment- and disease-associated morbidity.

Patterns and Timing of Recurrence

Although breast cancer may recur decades after initial presentation, the majority of patients relapse within ten years, with the greatest risk occurring during the first five years. Patterns of relapse in 3585 patients with operable breast cancer who were followed for a median of 8.1 years were evaluated in one study; 45% of the study population recurred (Saphner et al., 1996). The annual hazard rate for recurrence was greatest at between one and three years after presentation (about 12–13 recurrences/100 patients/yr), then progressively decreased each year before plateauing at about 4% to 5% annually between 5 and 10 years, then decreasing further to about 2% annually thereafter (there was no information beyond 12 years). The hazard rate for recurrence was about twofold higher during only the first two years for ER-negative compared with ER-positive tumors, whereas it was approximately equivalent beyond two years. In contrast, the annual hazard rate for axillary node positive disease was increased relative to patients with negative axillary nodes for up to 10 years.

The patterns of recurrence in 1015 patients with metastatic breast cancer were evaluated by the San Antonio group (Clark et al., 1987). The most common initial sites of metastases include soft tissue (45%), bone (40%), lung (20%), liver (10–15%), other visceral sites (9%), contralateral breast (9%), and brain (6%). ER-negative disease was more likely than ER-positive disease to be associated with liver metastases (17% vs. 10%), lung metastases (28% vs. 15%), and soft tissue metastases (51% vs. 41%), and to have multiple sites of metastases (44% vs. 31%). Features that were associated with a significantly worse outcome in multivariate analysis of 901 patients included brain, liver, lung, or bone metastases, increasing number of positive lymph nodes at the time of initial surgery, short disease-free interval, and ER-negative disease. In contrast to ductal carcinoma, lobular carcinoma has a greater propensity for recurrence in serosal surfaces (i.e., meninges, pleura, and peritoneum) as well as the ovaries and endometrium (Harris et al., 1984).

Prognostic Factor Models

Several groups have proposed models that may be useful in predicting response or survival in patients with metastatic breast cancer. Such models may be useful in selecting patients for a more conservative treatment approach or for stratification in randomized clinical trials.

The MD Anderson group studied 546 patients with metastatic breast cancer treated with doxorubicin-based chemotherapy and developed a model predictive for response and survival (Hortobagyi et al., 1983). Adverse prognostic variables included elevated serum lactate dehydrogenase, poor performance status, lung metastases,

Table 2 Prognostic Model for Metastatic Breast Cancer

Risk group	Number of adverse factors	Median survival (mo)	1-yr survival	2-yr survival	5-yr survival
Low	≤1	49.6	96%	76%	36%
Intermediate	2–3	22.8	80%	47%	14%
High	≥4	10.0	41%	10%	0%

Adverse prognostic features: prior adjuvant chemotherapy, distant lymph node metastases, hepatic metastases, elevated serum lactate dehydrogenase, disease-free interval <24 months.

extensive prior irradiation, elevated serum alkaline phosphatase, and extent of metastases. The model was validated in a second group of 200 patients treated with doxorubicin-based therapy. The model accurately estimates survival based upon a mathematical formula, which may not be practical for routine clinical use.

Yamamoto reported a prognostic model based upon a prognostic factor analysis that was performed in 233 Japanese women with metastatic breast cancer (Yamamoto et al., 1998). This model employed simple dichotomous variables, with assignment of risk group based upon the number of adverse prognostic features. In multivariate analysis, features associated with a worse outcome included history of prior adjuvant chemotherapy, distant lymph node metastases, hepatic metastases, elevated serum lactate dehydrogenase, and short disease-free interval (<24 months). The authors developed a model that was validated in another data set that included 315 consecutive women with metastatic breast cancer that received anthracycline-based therapy (Table 2). The median survival was best for patients with zero to one factors (49.6 months), intermediate for those with two to three factors (22.8 months), and poorest for those with four to five factors (10.0 months). Such a model may be more practical and useful in the clinical setting.

CYTOTOXIC THERAPY

Cytotoxic Agents with Single-Agent Activity

The cytotoxic agents that are most commonly used for the treatment of metastatic breast cancer and have substantial single-agent activity are shown in Table 3. These include the alkylating agents (i.e., cyclophosphamide, melphalan,

Table 3 Cytotoxic Agents that have Single Agent Activity as First-line Therapy in Breast Cancer

Drug class	Mechanisms of action	Agents	Single-agent response rate	Reference
Alkylating agents	DNA adduct formation	Cyclophosphamide	36%	Henderson, 1991
		Melphalan	25%	
		Thiotepa	25%	
Anthracyclines	DNA intercalation, Inhibits topoisomerase-II	Doxorubicin	43%	Henderson, 1991
		Epirubicin	38%	Bastholt et al., 1996
Antimetabolites	Inhibits DHFR and TS	Methotrexate	26%	Henderson, 1991
		5-Fluorouracil	28%	Henderson, 1991
		Capecitabine	25%	O'Shaughnessy et al., 1998
Anthracenediones	DNA intercalation, Inhibits topoisomerase-II	Mitoxantrone	27%	Henderson, 1991
Nucleoside analogs	Inhibits DNA synthesis	Gemcitabine	37%	Blackstein et al., 2002
Platinum analogs	DNA adduct formation	Cisplatin	45%	Sledge et al., 1988
		Carboplatin	35%	Martin, 1992
Taxanes and Epothilones	Inhibits microtubule depolymerization	Paclitaxel	25%	Paridaens et al., 2000
		Docetaxel	48%[a]	Chan et al., 1999
		Ixabepilone	42%	Roche et al., 2007
Vinca alkaloids	Inhibit microtubule formation	Vinblastine	21%[b]	Henderson, 1991
		Vinorelbine	41%	Fumoleau et al., 1993
Other agents	DNA intercalation	Mitomycin-C	22%[b]	Henderson, 1991

[a]Includes some patients who received docetaxel as second-line therapy.
[b]Response rate when used as second-line therapy.
Abbreviations: DHFR, dihydrofolate reductase; TS, thymidylate synthase.

thiotepa), antimetabolites (i.e., methotrexate, pemetrexed, 5-fluorouracil, capecitabine) (Henderson, 1991; Oshaughnessy et al., 2001; Llombart-Cussac et al., 2007), anthracyclines [doxorubicin, epirubicin (Henderson, 1991; Bastholt et al., 1996)], anthracenediones (mitoxantrone) (Henderson, 1991), nucleoside analogues (gemcitabine) (Blackstein et al., 2002), platinum salts (cisplatin, carboplatin) (Sledge et al., 1988; Martin et al., 1992), antitubulin agents (paclitaxel, docetaxel, vinorelbine) (Fumoleau et al., 1993; Chan et al., 1999; Paridaens et al., 2000; Roche et al., 2007), and other agents (mitomycin-C) (Henderson, 1991).

Combination Regimens

The relatively low objective response rates, differing mechanisms of action, and partially nonoverlapping toxicities created interest in using these agents in combination. The dose and schedules of commonly used agents and/or combinations are shown in Table 4. The most commonly used combinations have included alkylators and antimetabolites in the 1970s (e.g., CMF), anthracycline-based combinations in the 1980s and 1990s (e.g., FAC, FEC), and taxane-containing combinations more recently. Because anthracycline- and taxane-based therapy is now more commonly used in the adjuvant setting, many relapsed patients who have had prior adjuvant anthracyclines are not able to receive anthracycline-based therapy (due to the cumulative lifetime maximum dose), and may also have disease that is resistant to taxane therapy (if there is a short disease-free interval). This has fostered the increased use of single-agent taxane therapy or taxane-based combinations for metastatic disease, particularly for those who have not had adjuvant taxane therapy.

Table 4 Commonly Used Chemotherapy Agents/Regimens for Metastatic Disease

Drug	Dose/Route	Schedule
CMF regimens		
Classical CMF		
Cyclophosphamide	100 mg/m^2 PO	Days 1–14 every 28 days
Methotrexate	40 mg/m^2 IV	Days 1, 8 every 28 days
5-fluoruracil	600 mg/m^2 IV	Days 1, 8 every 28 days
Intravenous CMF		
Cyclophosphamide	600 mg/m^2 IV	
Methotrexate	40 mg/m^2 IV	Every 21 days
5-fluorouracil	600 mg/m^2 IV	
Doxorubicin-based regimens		
AC		
Doxorubicin (Adriamycin)	600 mg/m^2	Every 21 days
Cyclophosphamide	60 mg/m^2	
FAC		
5-fluorouracil	500 mg/m^2 IV	Every 21 days
Doxorubicin (Adriamycin)	50 mg/m^2 IV	
Cyclophosphamide	500 mg/m^2 IV	
CAF		
Cyclophosphamide	100 mg/m^2 PO	Days 1–14 every 28 days
Doxorubicin (Adriamycin)	30 mg/m^2 IV	Days 1, 8 every 28 days
5-fluorouracil	500 mg/m^2 IV	Days 1, 8 every 28 days
Epirubicin-based regimen (FEC)		
5-fluorouracil	500 mg/m^2 IV	Every 21 days
Epirubicin	50, 75, or 100 mg/m^2 IV	
Cyclophosphamide	500 mg/m^2 IV	
Antimicrotubule Agents		
Paclitaxel	175 mg/m^2 IV	Every 21 days
	80 mg/m^2 IV	Weekly
Nab-paclitaxel	260 mg/m^2 IV	Every 21 days
	100–150 mg/m^2 IV	Weekly for 3 or 4 wk
Docetaxel	60–100 mg/m^2 IV	Every 21 days
Vinorelbine	25–30 mg/m^2	Weekly
Ixabepilone	40 mg/m^2	Every 21 days

In the early days of cytotoxic therapy for metastatic breast cancer, the only agents available included alkylators and antimetabolites. These agents generally produced response rates of 15% to 25% when used as single agents, prompting their use in combination with the expectation that they would have additive antitumor effects. Of the various combination tested, CMF and variations of the CMF regimen were the most commonly used in clinical practice. Two trials that evaluated CMF were particularly noteworthy. One trial compared "classical" CMF (that included oral cyclophosphamide) with IV CMF (Table 4) in 232 eligible patients with metastatic breast cancer (Engelsman, 1991). Classical CMF resulted in a superior response rate (48% vs. 29%), similar response duration (11 months), and a superior survival (17 vs. 12 months), and was associated with less nausea and vomiting but more mucositis and alopecia. These findings suggested that the classical CMF regimen is the preferable regimen for metastatic breast cancer. Another trial compared IV CMF given at its standard dose or 50% of its usual dose in 133 patients with metastatic breast cancer (Tannock, 1988). The conventional dose therapy was associated with a significantly better response rate (30% vs. 11%) in patients with measurable disease and improved survival (median 15.6 vs. 12.8 months). Taken together, these results would favor the use of classical CMF when feasible; when IV CMF must be used, it should be used at its full dose.

CYTOTOXIC AGENTS COMMONLY USED FOR METASTATIC BREAST CANCER

Doxorubicin

Mechanism of Action and Metabolism

Doxorubicin and other anthracyclines exert their cytotoxic effects by inducing the formation of covalent topoisomerase-DNA complexes, and by intercalating between adjacent DNA base pairs. The effects on topoisomerase inhibit the religation portion of the ligation-religation reaction in replicating DNA, and the intercalation results in single-and double-strand DNA breaks. Doxorubicin undergoes hepatic metabolism, and it is generally recommended that its dose be reduced in patients with hepatic dysfunction (Donelli et al., 1998).

Phase III Trials of Doxorubicin

Since the 1970s, doxorubicin-based combinations have been commonly used for the initial treatment of patients with metastatic disease. This was based largely on the results of several randomized trials demonstrating a response and in some cases survival advantage for patients treated with anthracycline-based therapy. For example, the Cancer and Acute Leukemia Group B (CALGB) compared CMF with CAF and CAF plus vincristine and prednisone (CAFVP) in 395 patients with metastatic breast cancer (Aisner et al., 1987). The objective response rate was significantly higher for CAF or CAFVP compared with CMF (55% vs. 58% vs. 37%); the CAF regimen was also associated with a significantly better median survival than CMF (24.7 vs. 14.9 months). A pooled analysis of five randomized trials previously cited that included a total of 1088 patients with metastatic breast cancer indicated that doxorubicin-based regimens were associated with a significantly lower hazard rate for treatment failure [HR 0.69; 95% confidence intervals (CI) 0.59–0.81] and death (HR 0.78; 95% CI 0.67–0.90), but were also associated with more nausea and vomiting, alopecia, leukopenia, and cardiac toxicity (A'Hern et al., 1993).

Cardiac Toxicity of Doxorubicin

Cardiac dysfunction is a well-described toxicity of anthracycline therapy that limits the cumulative amount of drug that can be administered. The anthracyclines mediate their cardiac effects via reactive free-radical intermediates (e.g., superoxide, hydrogen peroxide, and hydroxyl radical) that are produced by chemical reduction via iron-catalyzed pathways (Myers, 1998). The resulting damage to myocardial cells leads to the release of toxic cellular metabolites, generation of inflammatory cytokines, calcium overload, and adrenergic dysfunction, all resulting in a cascade of events culminating in further myocardial cell damage. The myocardial injury produces typical histological changes characterized by myofibril loss, vacuolar swelling of the sarcoplasmic reticulum, loss of contractile elements and organelles, and mitochondrial and nuclear degeneration (Billingham, 1978; Billingham et al., 1978; Friedman et al., 1978). The toxic hydrogen peroxide molecule is inactivated by catalase (which converts it to water and oxygen) and glutathione peroxidase (which uses glutathione to reduce hydrogen peroxide to water and oxidized glutathione) (Doroshow et al., 1980). Cardiac tissue is prone to doxorubicin-induced injury because it is relatively lacking in catalase, and because doxorubicin produces rapid destruction of glutathione peroxidase. Factors associated with an increased risk of anthracycline-induced cardiac toxicity included advanced age ($\geq$70 years), previous mediastinal irradiation, history of atherosclerotic heart disease or hypertension, and liver dysfunction (Von Hoff et al., 1979).

Phase III Trials of Doxorubicin and Dexrazoxane

Dexrazoxane is a *bis*-dioxopiperazine compound that has been shown to have a protective effect against doxorubicin-induced cardiomyopathy. It is hydrolyzed to form a chelating agent that is similar in structure to EDTA, chelates with iron intracellularly, and inhibits the generation of free

Table 5 Phase III Trials of Doxorubicin with and without Dexrazoxane

Reference	Number	Treatment arms	Response rate	Median TTP (mo)	Median survival (mo)
Speyer and Wasserheit, 1998	92	FAC	45%	9.3	NS
		FAC plus Dex	48%	10.3	NS
Speyer et al., 1992	150	FAC	37%	9.4	16.7
		FAC plus Dex	41%	10.1	18.3
Swain et al., 1997	349	FAC	61%[a]	8.7	18.4
		FAC plus Dex	48%	8.5	19.9
Swain et al., 1997	185	FAC	49%	8.3	18.4
		FAC plus Dex	54%	7.8	15.3
Marty et al., 2006	164	ABT	35%	7.0	16.0
		ABT-Dex	35%	7.8	13.5

[a]Statistically significant difference.
Abbreviations: FAC, 5-fluorouracil, Adriamycin (doxorubicin), and cyclophosphamide (see Table 4 for doses); Dex, dexrazoxane; NS, not stated; ABT, anthracyclines-based therapy.

radicals that are responsible for the cardiotoxic effects of doxorubicin. The role of dexrazoxane was evaluated in four phase III trials that compared 5-fluorouracil (500 mg/m^2), doxorubicin (50 mg/m^2), and cyclophosphamide (500 mg/m^2) used alone (FAC) or in combination with dexrazoxane (given at a 20:1 or 10:1 ratio to the doxorubicin dose) (Table 5). Dexrazoxane reduced the risk of doxorubicin-associated congestive heart failure (CHF) by about one-half (Speyer et al., 1992; Swain et al., 1997a, b; Speyer and Wasserheit, 1998; Swain, 1998), and allowed about one-third of patients to receive at least 700 mg/m^2 of doxorubicin, a cumulative dose at which about 20% of patients would be expected to develop CHF if dexrazoxane were not used. In a combined analysis of two trials, the addition of dexrazoxane (10:1 ratio) was associated with significantly more grade 3 to 4 leukopenia (78% vs. 68%), a finding consistent with the mildly myelosuppressive effect of dexrazoxane when given as a single agent (Liesmann et al., 1981). The objective response rate was significantly lower for patients treated with dexrazoxane in one trial, although this effect was not observed in the other trials. In addition, there was no significant difference in median time to progression and survival in any of the trials. A retrospective analysis was performed in a subset of 201 patients (of a total of 534 patients enrolled in two trials) who were randomized to receive either FAC plus a placebo for six courses followed by continued FAC with open label dexrazoxane beginning at course 7, or FAC plus placebo for at least seven courses (Swain et al., 1997). This select group of the study population consisted of patients who had not had disease progression or prohibitive toxicity after six cycles of therapy. The incidence of cardiac toxicity was significantly reduced by the delayed administration of dexrazoxane (25% vs. 60%). These studies formed the basis for the approval of dexrazoxane for patients with metastatic breast cancer who have received at least 300 mg/m^2 of doxorubicin (for the treatment of metastatic disease) and who are judged by their physician to benefit from continued doxorubicin-based therapy. Dexrazoxane is not recommended for use as initial therapy with doxorubicin for metastatic disease.

In contrast to the previously described trials that evaluated dexrazoxane in patients who had no prior adjuvant anthracyclines, another phase III trial included 164 women with metastatic breast cancer previously treated with anthracyclines who were randomized to receive anthracycline-based chemotherapy with ($N = 85$) or without ($N = 79$) dexrazoxane for a maximum of six cycles. Patients treated with dexrazoxane had significantly less cardiac toxicity (39% vs. 13%, $p < 0.001$) and a reduced incidence of CHF (11% vs. 1%, $p < 0.05$), without a significant difference in response rate or other toxicities (Marty et al., 2006).

Liposomal Doxorubicin

Liposomal Preparations

Liposomes are closed vesicular structures capable of enveloping water-soluble molecules that were initially described in the 1960s (Bangham and Horne, 1964). They may serve as a vehicle for delivering cytotoxic agents more specifically to tumor and by limiting exposure of normal tissues to the drug. Current preparations of liposomes fall into two broad classes based on their recognition by the mononuclear phagocyte system (MPS). One class of liposomes are readily recognized and phagocytized by the MPS. This is due to binding of plasma proteins to the liposome surface, thereby inducing uptake by macrophages in the liver, spleen, lungs, and bone marrow. It has been shown in animal models that most of the injected cytotoxic agent is rapidly taken up by the MPS, minimizing exposure of normal tissues, and thus diminishing some acute and chronic toxicities (Kanter et al., 1993a, 1993b). D-99 is an example of such a preparation. Its liposomes are about 150 to 250 nm in size and include cholesterol and the acidic lipid egg phosphatidylcholine. Patients with a history of hypersensitivity to eggs or egg products should therefore not receive this agent. The drug is prepared in the pharmacy immediately prior to use by admixing doxorubicin with the liposome preparation and a buffer solution. The negatively charged membrane-associated lipids serve to form "ion pairs" with doxorubicin (which is positively charged at physiological pH), which favors entry of doxorubicin into the liposome. A second class of agents include liposomes that are designed to avoid detection by the MPS system. This results in prolonged residence time of the drug in the plasma. There is also evidence that some of these preparations may result in greater tumor penetration by the anthracycline. One such example of this class is liposomal daunorubicin. The liposome consists of a lipid bilayer of distearoylphosphatidylcholine and cholesterol in a 2:1 molar ratio, and has a mean diameter of 45 nm. A second example is pegylated liposomal doxorubicin (PLD). The liposomal carrier for this product includes cholesterol, HSPC (fully hydrogenated soy phosphatidylcholine), and the polyethylene glycol preparation MPEG-DSPE (*N*-[carbamoyl]-methoxypolyethylene glycol 2000]-1,2-dis-tearoylsn-glycero-3-phosphoethanolamine sodium salt). Its size is approximately 85 nm. Both liposomal daunorubicin and PLD circulate in the plasma for a relatively long period compared with D-99 or conventional doxorubicin. Relative to conventional doxorubicin, PLD has a very limited volume of distribution (2.5–3.0 L/m^2 vs. 240–690 L/m^2) due to its confinement to the vascular space, slower clearance from the circulation (0.04 L/hr/m^2 vs. 27.5–59.6 L/hr/m^2), prolonged beta half-life (55 vs. 0.43–2.0 hours), and approximately threefold greater area under the curve (AUC) (Gabizon et al., 2003). The rationale for their development and use in breast cancer has been extensively reviewed (Robert et al., 2004).

Tumor Penetration of Liposomal Anthracyclines

Several lines of evidence suggest that some liposomal anthracyclines may preferentially localize to tumorous tissue in a variety of animal models, including a mouse mammary carcinoma (Vaage et al., 1992; Symon et al., 1999). Some clinical studies in humans have shown better tumor localization and penetration. For example, tumor uptake was demonstrated in 12 of 17 patients (71%) treated with In^{111} labeled pegylated liposomes (Gabizon et al., 1991). Doxorubicin levels were also found to be 4- to 16-fold higher in malignant pleural effusions after equivalent IV dose of PLD compared with doxorubicin (Gabizon et al., 1994). Finally, tumor tissue uptake of doxorubicin was evaluated in two patients with metastatic breast cancer who underwent palliative resection of a bone metastasis (Symon et al., 1999). One patient received 50 mg/m^2 of PLD six days prior to resection, and the second received 35 mg/m^2 12 days prior to resection. Patient one had a plasma drug level of 7 μg/mL, a tumor level of 6.5 μg/g, and a level in normal muscle of 0.6 μg/g. Patient two had a plasma level of 0.94 μg/mL, a tumor level of 1.4 μg/g, and a muscle level of 0.15 μg/g. These studies demonstrated a preferential distribution of PLD in tumorous tissue relative to normal muscle.

Comparison of D-99 with Doxorubicin and Epirubicin

D-99 has been the most extensively studied liposomal anthracycline in breast cancer (Table 6). A phase III trial in 216 patients with metastatic breast cancer compared conventional D-99 (75 mg/m^2) given as a 60 minute IV infusion every 3 weeks with conventional doxorubicin given at the same dose and schedule (Harris et al., 2002). Treatment was continued until progressive disease or prohibitive cardiac toxicity. Cardiac toxicity was defined as clinical CHF or a decrease in the left ventricular ejection fraction (LVEF) by at least 20% and within the normal range, or by at least 10% to below the normal range. There was no significant difference in the response rate between the two agents (33% vs. 29%). D-99 caused less grade 3 to 4 toxicity, including vomiting (10% vs. 25%), stomatitis (9% vs. 16%), fever/infection (6% vs. 11%), CHF (0% vs. 4%), and fewer protocol defined declines in ejection fraction. Two phase III trials that compared D-99 with conventional anthracyclines when used in conjunction with cyclophosphamide were also reported. One study compared D-99 (60 mg/m^2) and cyclophosphamide (600 mg/m^2) with an identical dose of doxorubicin and cyclophosphamide every three weeks in 297 women with metastatic breast cancer (Batist et al., 2001). Treatment was continued until progressive disease or prohibitive cardiac toxicity. There was no significant difference in response rate (43% vs. 43%) or median PFS (5.2 vs. 5.5 months.). Patients treated with D-99 experienced less grade 4 neutropenia (62% vs. 75%), stomatitis (4% vs. 16%), diarrhea (2% vs. 7%), CHF (0% vs. 4), and other cardiotoxic events (6% vs. 22%). A similar trial was performed in 160 women with metastatic breast cancer that compared D-99 (75 mg/m^2) and cyclophosphamide (600 mg/m^2) with epirubicin (75 mg/m^2) and

Table 6 Phase III Trials of Liposomal Doxorubicin Vs. Doxorubicin or Epirubicin

Reference	Number	Treatment arms	Response rate	Median TTP (mo)	Median survival (mo)
Harris et al., 2002	216	D-99 (75 mg/m^2)	28%	NS	NS
		Doxorubicin (75 mg/m^2)	25%	NS	NS
Batist et al., 2001	297	Cyclophosphamide plus D-99 (60 mg/m^2)	43%	5.2	NR
		Cyclophosphamide plus Doxorubicin (60 mg/m^2)	43%	5.5	NR
Chan et al., 2004	160	Cyclophosphamide plus D-99 (75 mg/m^2)	46%	7.6[a]	18.5
		Cyclophosphamide plus Epirubicin (75 mg/m^2)	39%	6.0	16.0
Keller et al., 2004	301	PLD 50 mg/m^2 every 4 wk	10%	2.9	11.0
		Vinorelbine or mitomycin/vinblastine	12%	2.5	9.0
O'Brien et al., 2004	509	PLD 50 mg/m^2 every 4 wk	33%	6.9	21.0
		Doxorubicin 60 mg/m^2 every 3 wk	38%	7.8	22.0

[a]Statistically significant difference.
Abbreviations: NR, not reached; NS, not stated; PLD, pegylated liposomal doxorubicin.

cyclophosphamide every three weeks (Chan et al., 2004). There was no significant difference in response rate (46% vs. 39%), although median PFS was improved with D-99 (7.6 vs. 6.0 months). There was significantly more stomatitis with D-99 (33% vs. 9%), but there was no difference in the incidence of CHF (4% vs. 4%) or grade 3 to 4 neutropenia (47% vs. 36%). Due to clinical evidence of a dose-response relationship for doxorubicin (Jones et al., 1987) and a lesser toxicity associated with D-99, a phase II trial of dose-escalated D-99 (135 mg/m^2) plus G-CSF was performed, but demonstrated an equivalent objective response (46%) with substantially more toxicity, suggesting no advantage for dose-escalated liposomal anthracyclines (Shapiro et al., 1999; Mrozek et al., 2005).

Phase III Trials of PLD

Two phase III trials have also evaluated PLD (Table 6). Kelller et al. randomly assigned 301 patients who had disease progression following first- or second-line taxane-containing regimen for metastatic disease to either PLD (50 mg/m^2 every four weeks); or comparator-vinorelbine (30 mg/m^2 weekly) or mitomycin C (10 mg/m^2 day 1 and every 4 weeks) plus vinblastine (5 mg/m^2 day 1, day 14, day 28, and day 42) every six to eight weeks (Keller et al., 2004). PFS and OS were similar for PLD and comparator [PFS: hazard ratio, 1.26; 95% CI 0.98–1.62; $p = 0.11$; median, 2.9 months (PLD) and 2.5 months (comparator); OS: HR, 1.05; 95% CI 0.82–1.33; $p = 0.71$; median, 11.0 months (PLD) and 9.0 months (comparator)]. Most frequently reported adverse events were nausea (23% to 31%), vomiting (17% to 20%), and fatigue (9% to 20%) and were similar among treatment groups. PLD-treated patients experienced more palmar-plantar erythrodysesthesia (37%; 18% grade 3, one patient grade 4) and stomatitis (22%, 5% grades 3/4). Neuropathy (11%), constipation (16%), and neutropenia (14%) were more common with vinorelbine. Alopecia was low in both the PLD and vinorelbine groups (3% and 5%).

O'Brien et al. randomized 509 patients with metastatic breast cancer and normal cardiac function to receive either PLD 50 mg/m^2 (every 4 weeks) or doxorubicin 60 mg/m^2 (every 3 weeks). PLD and doxorubicin were comparable with respect to PFS (6.9 vs. 7.8 months, respectively; hazard ratio = 1.00; 95% CI 0.82–1.22). Subgroup results were consistent. Overall risk of cardiotoxicity was significantly higher with doxorubicin than PLD (HR = 3.16; 95%CI 1.58–6.31; $p < 0.001$). OS was similar (21 and 22 months for PLD and doxorubicin, respectively; HR = 0.94; 95% CI 0.74–1.19). Alopecia (overall, 66% vs. 20%; pronounced, 54% vs. 7%), nausea (53% vs. 37%), vomiting (31% vs. 19%) and neutropenia (10% vs. 4%) were more often associated with doxorubicin than PLD. Palmar-plantar erythrodysesthesia (48% vs. 2%), stomatitis (22% vs. 15%) and mucositis (23% vs. 13%) were more often associated with PLD than doxorubicin (O'Brien et al., 2004).

Epirubicin

Mechanism of Action and Pharmacology

Epirubicin (4′-epi-doxorubicin) is a semisynthetic stereoisomer of doxorubicin that differs by a reorientation (epimerization) of the hydroxyl group in the 4′ position of the daunosamine ring. It has comparable antitumor activity but is significantly less cardiotoxic than the parent compound in animal models (Casazza, 1979). Relative to doxorubicin, it is more lipophilic, is more rapidly cleared from the plasma, and has a shorter plasma half-life (30 vs. 45 hours). Like doxorubicin, epirubicin is also metabolized by the liver and its dose must be modified in patients with hepatic dysfunction (Coukell and Faulds, 1997).

Comparison of Epirubicin with Doxorubicin

In clinical trials comparing equimolar doses of doxorubicin in humans, epirubicin has less hematologic, nonhematologic (nausea and vomiting, alopecia, mucositis), and cardiac toxicity. The ratio of epirubicin: doxorubicin that produces equivalent hematologic toxicity is 1:1.2, nonhematologic toxicity is 1:1.5, and cardiac toxicity 1:1.8. The maximum cumulative recommended dose in order to prevent cardiomyopathy, therefore, is between 950 to 1000 mg/m^2. There have been seven randomized trials that have compared epirubicin with doxorubicin, including four trials that compared single-agent therapy and three that compared combination therapy (Italian Epirubicin Study Group, 1988; Hortobagyi et al., 1989; Gundersen et al., 1990; Gasparini et al., 1991; French Epiribuicin Study Group, 1991; Findlay and Walker-Dilks, 1998). The power of many of these studies was limited due to their small sample size. A meta-analysis of these trials reveals no significant difference in overall response rate, complete response rate, or one-year mortality when the drugs were used at equimolar doses (Findlay and Walker-Dilks, 1998). Epirubicin was associated with significantly less toxicity, however, including CHF (hazard ratio 0.38), other cardiotoxic effects (HR 0.43), grade 3 to 4 nausea or vomiting (HR 0.76), and grade 3 to 4 neutropenia (HR 0.52).

Evaluation of the Optimal Dose of Epirubicin

Several trials have also evaluated escalated doses of epirubicin (Table 7). One randomized trial evaluated 209 patients with metastatic breast cancer who were randomized to receive either 100 mg/m^2 or 50 mg/m^2 of epirubicin plus prednisolone every three weeks, with the high dose given for eight courses and the low dose given for 16 courses (Habeshaw et al., 1991). High-dose epirubicin resulted in a higher objective response rate (41% vs. 23%), but there was no significant difference in progression free interval or OS. High-dose epirubicin was associated with significantly more alopecia and grade 3 to 4 myelosuppression (10% vs. 3%), mucositis (9% vs. 1%), and nausea and vomiting (35% vs. 15%). Another trial compared epirubicin 50 mg/m^2 every three weeks with 50 mg/m^2 given on days 1 and 8 every 3 weeks in 164 patients with locally advanced or metastatic breast cancer (Focan et al., 1993). The more intensive schedule resulted in a significantly improved objective response rate (69% vs. 41%), median response duration (22 vs. 14 months), and median time to progression (19.2 vs. 8 months), although there was no difference in survival. High-dose epirubicin was associated with significantly more grade 3 to 4 neutropenia (incidence by treatment course 12% vs. 6%). Another report evaluated epirubicin at one of four different dose levels (40, 60, 90, or 135 mg/m^2 every three weeks) in 287 women with metastatic breast cancer (Bastholt et al., 1996). The 90 mg/m^2 dose level was associated with the best therapeutic index because of a higher response (38% vs. 20%) and improved median time to progression (8.4 vs. 4.6 months) compared with the lower dose levels, and equivalent efficacy with less grade 3 to 4 toxicity compared with the higher dose level.

Evaluation of the Optimal Schedule of Epirubicin

In one report, epirubicin (50 mg/m^2), cyclophosphamide (500 mg/m^2), and 5-fluorouracil (500 mg/m^2) was given either every four weeks or in divided doses on a weekly basis in 148 evaluable patients (Blomqvist et al., 1993). There was a significantly better outcome for the every four-week schedule with regard to response rate (47% vs. 30%),

Table 7 Phase III Trials Evaluating Escalating Doses of Epirubicin

Reference	Number	Treatment arms	Response rate	Median TTP (mo)	Median survival (mo)
Habeshaw et al., 1991	209	E-50	23%	4.0	10.6
		E-100	41%[a]	7.0	10.1
Focan et al., 1993	164	FEC-50	41%	8.0	23.6
		FEC-100	69%[a]	19.2[a]	27.1
Bastholt et al., 1996	287	E-40	20%	4.4	13.6
		E-60	20%	4.7	14.0
		E-90	38%[a]	8.4[b]	14.6
		E-135	36%[a]	8.4[b]	11.3

[a]Statistically significant difference.
[b]Trend toward significant difference favoring doses $\geq$ 90 mg/m^2.
Abbreviations: FAC, 5-fluorouracil, Adriamycin (doxorubicin), and cyclophosphamide; FEC, 5-fluorouracil, epirubicin, and cyclophosphamide; A, Adriamycin (doxorubicin); E, epirubicin, number adjacent to regimen refers to dose of anthracycline in mg/m^2.

median time to progression (9.2 vs. 5.4 months), and median survival (21.2 vs. 11.8 months). There was significantly more leukopenia, nausea, and alopecia in the every four week group. Other studies found no difference in response rate when epirubicin was compared with doxorubicin given by either a weekly schedule (Gasparini et al., 1991) or by continuous infusion (Hortobagyi et al., 1989).

Comparison of Single-Agent Epirubicin with Combination Therapy

The French Epirubicin Study Group (1991) compared singe agent epirubicin (75 mg/m^2) with two FEC regimens which contained the same dose of cyclophosphamide (500 mg/m^2) and 5-fluorouracil (500 mg/m^2) but two differing doses of epirubicin (50 mg/m^2 and 75 mg/m^2) in 391 patients. The response rate favored the FEC regimens compared with single-agent epirubicin (45% vs. 31%), but there was no significant difference in median response duration, time to progression, or survival. The FEC regimen produced more neutropenia, nausea and vomiting, and alopecia.

Mitoxantrone

Mechanism of Action of Metabolism

Mitoxantrone is an anthraquinone that is structurally related to doxorubicin. It lacks the aminosugar moiety of doxorubicin, but retains the planar polycyclic aromatic ring structure that permits intercalation in DNA. Mitoxantrone does not produce the quinone type free radicals that are responsible for anthracycline cardiotoxicity. The metabolism and elimination of mitoxantrone are not well characterized (Faulds et al., 1991).

Comparison of Mitoxantrone with Doxorubicin

In general, mitoxantrone seems to be less effective than doxorubicin. It is associated with less alopecia, mucositis, nausea, vomiting, and cardiomyopathy than doxorubicin. However, some evidence suggests that mitoxantrone may be more leukemogenic when used in the adjuvant setting (Chaplain et al., 2000), and cases of myelodysplasia and leukemia have also been reported in patients with metastatic disease (Sparano et al., 1996; Melillo et al., 1997).

There have been several trials evaluating mitoxantrone used as first-line therapy for patients with metastatic breast cancer (Table 8). One trial compared mitoxantrone (12 mg/m^2) with doxorubicin (50 mg/m^2) when used in combination with vincristine and prednisolone in 115 patients with metastatic breast cancer (Leonard et al., 1987). There was a significantly higher response rate associated with vincristine, Novantrone (mitoxantrone), prednisolone (VNP) (61% vs. 35%), although there was no significant difference in median time to progression or survival. There was no significant difference in the incidence of severe toxicities between the two arms, although VNP produced less alopecia. Another trial compared CNF with CAF as first-line therapy in 331 patients with metastatic breast cancer (Bennett et al., 1988). There was trend toward higher response rate (37% vs. 29%) and median response duration (eight vs. six months) for doxorubicin, although there was no difference in median survival. CNF was associated with significantly less severe adverse events (34% vs. 62%), including severe alopecia (39% vs. 4%) and cardiac toxicity. In another report, CNF was compared with CAF in 100 patients (Alonso et al., 1995).

Table 8 Phase III Trials Comparing Mitoxantrone with Doxorubicin as First-Line or Second-Line Therapy

Reference	Number	First- or second-line therapy	Treatment arms	Response rate	Median TTP (mo)	Median survival (mo)
Leonard et al., 1987	115	First line	VNP-14	35%	6.2[b]	11
			VAP-50	61%[a]	7.9[b]	11
Bennett et al., 1988	331	First line	CNF-10	29%	6.0	12.6
			CAF-50	37%	8.0	12.8
Alonso et al., 1995	100	First line	CNF-12	68%	NS	19
			CAF-50	68%	NS	18
Henderson et al., 1989	325	Second line	Mitoxantrone 14 mg/m^2	21%	2.3	9.1
			Doxorubicin 75 mg/m^2	29%	3.5	8.9
Cowan et al., 1991	411	Second line	Mitoxantrone 14 mg/m^2	14%	2.2	5.9[a]
			Doxorubicin 60 mg/m^2	28%	4.4	10.5
			Bisantrene 320 mg/m^2	13%	2.2	9.7

Number adjacent to regimen refers to dose of anthracycline/anthracenedione in mg/m^2.
[a]Significantly different difference.
[b]Median TTP reported in responders only, not significantly different.
Abbreviations: VNP, vincristine, Novantrone (mitoxantrone), prednisolone; VAP, vincristine, Adriamycin (doxorubicin), prednisolone; CAF, cyclophosphamide, Adriamycin (doxorubicin), and 5-fluorouracil; CNF, cyclophosphamide, Novantrone (mitoxantrone), 5-fluorouracil; NS, not stated.

There was no significant difference in response rate, median time to progression, or survival. There was significantly more severe alopecia associated with CAF, although CNF produced more grade 1 to 2 myelosuppression and treatment delays. Classical CMF has also been compared with mitoxantrone (6.5 mg/m^2) and methotrexate (30 mg/m^2) given every three weeks in 116 patients with locally advanced or metastatic breast cancer (Harper-Wynne et al., 1999). There was a trend toward a higher response rate for CMF (29% vs.15%), although there was no significant difference in median time to treatment failure, survival, or quality of life between the two groups. The mitoxantrone-containing arm was associated with less myelosuppression and fewer dose reductions and treatment delays.

Several studies have also evaluated mitoxantrone as second-line therapy (Table 8). One trial compared single-agent mitoxantrone (14 mg/m^2) with doxorubicin (75 mg/m^2) in 325 women who had failed one prior nonanthracycline-containing regimen for metastatic breast cancer (Henderson et al., 1989). There was no significant difference in response rate (21% vs. 29%), median time to progression (2.3 vs. 3.5 months), or median survival (9.1 vs. 8.9 months). Mitoxantrone produced less severe toxicity, including nausea or vomiting (10% vs. 25%), stomatitis (1% vs. 8%), alopecia (5% vs. 61%), and less cardiac toxicity. Another study compared mitoxantrone with doxorubicin and bisantrene in 201 patients who had failed prior chemotherapy, demonstrating a significantly higher response rate for doxorubicin (28%) compared with mitoxantrone (14%) or bisantrene (13%) (Cowan et al., 1991). Doxorubicin was also associated with improved median TTF (4.4 vs. 2.2 vs. 2.2 months) and median survival (10.5 vs. 5.9 vs. 9.7 months). Likewise, another trial compared mitoxantrone (12 mg/m^2) with doxorubicin (60 mg/m^2) in 90 patients with metastatic breast cancer who had failed CMF for metastatic disease (Neidhart et al., 1986). There was a trend toward a higher response rate for doxorubicin (30% vs. 17%), although it was not significantly different. There was less nausea, vomiting, alopecia, and fatigue with mitoxantrone.

Taxanes

Mechanism of Action and Metabolism

The taxanes paclitaxel and docetaxel inhibit mitosis by binding to tubulin, promoting assembly of microtubules, and inhibiting their depolymerization (Schiff et al., 1979). In addition to their microtubule effects, the taxanes have other effects on various biological processes that may contribute to their antineoplastic activity, such as induction of apoptosis, inhibition of angiogenesis, cell motility, invasiveness, and metalloproteinase production (Sparano, 2000). Both drugs undergo hepatic metabolism, and their dose must be modified in patients with hepatic dysfunction (Bruno et al., 1998; Venook et al., 1998). Both paclitaxel and docetaxel are insoluble in water, requiring that they be solubilized in polyoxyethanol (for paclitaxel) or polysorbate 80 (for docetaxel). As these solvents have been associated with toxicity, this has led to development of solvent-free taxane preparations such as ABI-007, an albumin-stabilized nanoparticle formulation of paclitaxel, which may be administered over a shorter period of time and does not require steroid premedication to prevent hypersensitivity (Spencer and Faulds, 1994; Fulton and Spencer, 1996; Wagstaff et al., 2003; Robinson and Keating, 2006). Other formulations of paclitaxel and docetaxel are being developed.

Single-Agent Paclitaxel: Duration of Infusion

A number of trials have evaluated the optimal dose and schedule of paclitaxel for metastatic breast cancer (Table 9). One study compared paclitaxel (250 mg/m^2) given as a 3-hour or a 24-hour IV infusion in 563 patients with stage IV (84%) or stage IIIB breast cancer (16%) (Smith et al., 1999). Filgrastim was used only if there was infection or febrile neutropenia. All patients had no prior therapy for metastatic or locally advanced disease. The primary objective of the trial was tumor response after four cycles of therapy. The 24-hour infusion produced a significantly higher response rate after four cycles (51% vs. 41%) and overall (54% vs. 44%), although there was no significant difference in median PFS (7.2 vs. 6.3 months) or median OS (21.9 vs. 21.1 months). The overall incidence of grade 3 to 4 toxicity was equivalent in the two arms (58% vs. 59%), although grade 4 toxicity was more common in the 24-hour group (23% vs. 12%). The 24-hour infusion was associated with more grade 3 to 4 granulocytopenia (81% vs. 73%), infection (12% vs. 7%), febrile neutropenia (18% vs. 5%), vomiting (8% vs. 3%), and diarrhea (4% vs. 1%). On the other hand, the three-hour infusion was associated with more grade 3 to 4 neurosensory (22% vs. 13%) and neuromotor (17% vs. 12%) toxicity.

Another study also compared paclitaxel (175 mg/m^2) given as either a 24-hour or 3-hour infusion in 521 patients with metastatic breast cancer (Peretz, 1995). The protocol called for escalation of the paclitaxel dose in each arm until dose-limiting toxicity occurred. There was no difference in response rate ($\sim$30%), although the 24-hour arm was associated with significantly better median TTP (4.6 vs. 3.8 months) and survival (13.4 vs. 9.8 months). If adjusted for baseline prognostic factors, the difference favoring TTP ($p = 0.099$) and survival ($p = 0.081$) no longer retained statistical significance, although this was not a planned analysis. The 24-hour infusion was associated with significantly more grade 4 neutropenia (79% vs. 30%), febrile neutropenia (17% vs. 1%), mucositis (any grade 45% vs. 22%), and diarrhea (any grade, 41% vs. 25%). On the other

Table 9 Phase III Trials Evaluating the Dose Schedule or Preparation of Paclitaxel

Reference	Number	First-line	Treatment arms	Response rate	Median TTP (mo)	Median survival (mo)
Smith et al., 1999	563[a]	100%	250 mg/m^2 3 hr infusion 24 hr infusion	44% 54%[b]	6.3 7.1	21.1 21.9
Peretz et al., 1995	521	44%	175 mg/m^2 3-hr infusion 24-hr infusion	29% 31%	3.8 4.6[b]	9.8 13.4[b]
Holmes et al., 1998	179	NS	250 mg/m^2, 3-hr infusion 140 m/m^2, 96-hr infusion	23% 29%	NS NS	11 10
Nabholtz et al., 1996	471	30%	3-hr infusion 175 mg/m^2 135 mg/m^2	29% 22%	4.2 3.0[b]	11.7 10.5
Winer et al., 2004	474	24%	3-hr infusion 175 mg/m^2 210 mg/m^2 250 mg/m^2	22% 26% 21%	3.9 4.2 5.4[b]	10.7 11.7 12.7
Seidman et al., 2004	735	69%	175 mg/m^2 every 3 wk 90 m/mg^2 weekly	28% 40%[b]	5.0 9.0[b]	20.0 24.0
Gradishar et al., 2005	454	42%	Every 3 wk Paclitaxel 175 mg/m^2 ABI-007 260 mg/m^2	19% 33%[b]	4.0 5.4[b]	24.0 23.6

[a]Includes 16% of patients who had stage IIIB disease.
[b]Statistically significant difference.
Abbreviation: NS, not stated.

hand, neuropathy was more common with the three-hour infusion (any grade, 78% vs. 65%).

Another study compared paclitaxel given at its maximum tolerable dose via either a 3-hour infusion (250 mg/m^2) or a 96-hour infusion (140 mg/m^2) in 179 patients with metastatic breast cancer (Holmes, 1998). There was no significant difference in the response rate (23% vs. 29%) or median survival (11 vs. 10 months), although there was a trend toward a longer response duration with the 96 hour infusion (4.5 vs. 7.5 months).

Single-Agent Paclitaxel: Evaluating the Optimal Dose Every Three Weeks

Several trials have evaluated the optimal dose of paclitaxel given as a three-hour IV infusion. One study compared 175 mg/m^2 versus 135 mg/m^2 dose of paclitaxel given as a three-hour infusion every three weeks in 471 patients with metastatic breast cancer (Nabholtz et al., 1996). About 70% of patients had failed one prior therapy for metastatic disease, 67% had prior exposure to anthracyclines, and 18% were considered anthracycline resistant (progression was best response to anthracyclines, or relapsed with six months of adjuvant anthracycline). There was no significant difference in overall response rate (29% vs. 22%) or median survival (11.7 vs. 10.5 months), although the higher dose was associated with a significant improvement in median TTP (4.2 vs. 3.0 months). The response rate was similar in patients who had been previously exposed to anthracyclines, and those who were considered to have anthracycline-resistant disease. The high-dose arm was associated with more grade 3 to 4 leukopenia (34% vs. 24%), neuropathy (7% vs. 3%), febrile neutropenia (4% vs. 2%), and grade 3 myalgia/arthralgia (16% vs. 9%). A quality of life adjusted time to progression analysis that was corrected for baseline prognostic factors revealed an advantage for the higher dose of paclitaxel. The CALBG compared three different doses of paclitaxel every three weeks in 474 patients with metastatic breast cancer, of whom 76% had prior chemotherapy for metastatic disease (Winer et al., 2004). There was no significant difference in the response rate among the three arms (22% vs. 26% vs. 21%). There was a borderline significant correlation between paclitaxel dose and median TTP that favored the highest dose (3.9 vs. 4.2 vs. 5.4 months), although there was no significant difference in median survival (10.7 vs. 11.7 vs. 12.7 months). The standard-dose arm (175 mg/m^2) was associated with significantly less grade 4 granulocytopenia (35% vs. 44% vs. 52%), grade 3 sensory neuropathy (8% vs. 18% vs.

31%), grade 3 motor neuropathy (7% vs. 12% vs. 12%), and grade 3 myalgias (3% vs. 6% vs. 11%).

Single-Agent Paclitaxel: Weekly Schedules

Preclinical data suggest that more prolonged drug exposure is associated with a greater antineoplastic effect in vitro, and that low taxane concentrations are cytotoxic (Jordan et al., 1996). Based on these principles, a number of studies have .evaluated weekly taxane therapy. Paclitaxel given as a weekly one- hour infusion (80–100 mg/m^2) in 30 patients with metastatic breast cancer produced an objective response rate of 53% (Seidman et al., 1998). A multicenter trial of the weekly paclitaxel (80 mg/m^2) resulted in a 21% objective response rate in 130 patients, although most patients (82%) had failed at least one prior regimen (Perez et al., 2001). The CALGB subsequently compared paclitaxel given every three weeks (175 mg/m^2) versus weekly (90 mg/m^2) in 735 women with metastatic breast cancer, some of whom also received trastuzumab (all if Her2/neu positive, and one half of those who were Her2/neu negative), and 158 of whom were treated in prior trial evaluating every three-week paclitaxel. The weekly arm demonstrated an improved response rate (40% vs. 28%, $p = 0.0017$) and median TTP (nine months vs. five months; $p = 0.0008$) for the weekly schedule, with no significant difference in survival (24 vs. 20 months) (Seidman, 2004). The weekly schedule produced more grade 3 sensory/motor neuropathy (23/8% vs. 12/4%, $p = 0.001/0.04$), but less grade 3 to 4 neutropenia (8% vs. 15%, $p = 0.013$).

Albumin-Bound Paclitaxel

ABI-007 is a nanometer-sized albumin-bound paclitaxel particle initially developed to avoid the toxicities associated with polyethylated castor oil. It is administered as a colloidal suspension of 130 nanometer particles, and allows the safe infusion of significantly higher doses and shorter infusion schedules (30 minutes) without steroid premedication (Robinson and Keating, 2006). In addition, the albumin-bound nanoparticle was designed to preferentially deliver paclitaxel to tumors by biologically interacting with albumin receptors that mediate drug transport; in vitro studies have demonstrated a 4.5-fold increase in paclitaxel transport across endothelial cells for ABI-007 compared with standard paclitaxel. Gradishar et al. reported a phase III study comparing albumin-bound paclitaxel (260 mg/m^2) with standard paclitaxel (175 mg/m^2) in 454 patients with metastatic breast cancer (Gradishar et al., 2005). Albumin-bound paclitaxel demonstrated significantly higher response rates (33% vs. 19%, $p = 0.001$) and time to progression (5.4 vs. 4.0 months, $p = 0.006$), less grade 4 neutropenia (9% vs. 22%, $p < 0.001$), but more grade 3 sensory neuropathy (10% vs. 2%, $p < 0.001$). A randomized phase II study has demonstrated the efficacy and safety of weekly administration of ABI-007 (Gradishar, 2007).

Single-Agent Paclitaxel Compared with Other Agents or Combinations

The results of several trials that compared single-agent paclitaxel with other agents or combinations are outlined in Table 10. An Australian group compared paclitaxel (200 mg/m^2, three-hour infusion) for eight cycles with CMFP for six cycles in 209 eligible patients with metastatic breast cancer (Bishop et al., 1999). When comparing paclitaxel with CMF, there was no significant difference in response rate (29% vs. 35%) or median TTP (5.3 vs. 6.4 months). There was a trend toward improved survival with paclitaxel (17.3 vs. 13.9 months) and the proportion surviving at two years (39% vs. 20%). Although approximately 40% of patients in both arms were crossed over to epirubicin as specified by the protocol, the interpretation of the survival advantage is confounded by a lack of crossover to paclitaxel for patients initially assigned to CMF. Paclitaxel produced significantly less grade 3 to 4 leukopenia (29% vs. 66%), thrombocytopenia (1% vs. 12%), mucositis (3% vs. 6%), nausea or vomiting (1% vs. 8%), infection (1% vs. 7%), and febrile neutropenia (1% vs. 9%). On the other hand, paclitaxel produced more alopecia (76% vs. 24%), grade 3 to 4 neuropathy (10% vs. 0%) and myalgia/arthralgia (20% vs. 1%). There was no difference in the overall quality of life score as assessed by the patient (visual analog scale) or physician (Spitzer index).

The EORTC compared paclitaxel (200 mg/m^2, three-hour infusion) with doxorubicin (75 mg/m^2) every three weeks for up to seven cycles in 331 patients with metastatic breast cancer (Paridaens et al., 2000). Crossover was mandated if progression occurred during therapy, but was optional if progression occurred at a later time. Paclitaxel was associated with a significantly inferior response rate (25% vs. 41%) and median TTP (3.9 vs. 7.5 months), although there was no difference in median survival (15.6 vs. 18.3 months). The crossover response rate for paclitaxel (following progression on doxorubicin) was 16%, whereas the crossover response rate for doxorubicin (following progression on paclitaxel) was 30%. Paclitaxel was associated with less grade 4 neutropenia (40% vs. 85%) and febrile neutropenia (7% vs. 20%). It was also associated with less grade 3 to 4 mucositis (1% vs. 15%), nausea/vomiting (2% vs. 13%), and CHF (0% vs. 4%). Paclitaxel produced more grade 3 to 4 neuropathy (9% vs. 0%), and arthralgia/myalgia (4% vs. 0%). Quality of life analysis using the EORTC QLQ-C30 tool and the Rotterdam Symptoms Check List in 257 patients showed no overall difference in global function, although bone pain was better controlled with doxorubicin and side effects were less with paclitaxel.

Table 10 Phase III Trials Evaluating Paclitaxel or Docetaxel Monotherapy with Other Agents/Regimens as First or Second-line Therapy

Reference	Number	First- or second-line therapy	*Treatment arms*	Response rate	Median TTP (mo)	Median survival (mo)
Bishop et al., 1999	209	first line	Paclitaxel 200 mg/m^2 (3 hr)	29%	5.3	17.3
			CMFP	35%	6.4	13.9
Paridaens et al., 2000	331	first line	Paclitaxel 200 mg/m^2 (3 hr)	25%	4.1	15.4
			Doxorubicin 75 mg/m^2	41%[a]	7.3[a]	18.1
Sledge et al., 2003	732	first line	Paclitaxel 175 mg/m^2 (24 hr)	34%	6.0	22.2
			Doxorubicin 60 mg/m^2	36%	5.9	18.9
			Doxorubicin/paclitaxel (150/50 mg/m^2)	47%[a]	8.0[a,b]	22.0
Chan et al., 1999	326	first/second line	Docetaxel 100 mg/m^2	48%[a]	6.1	15.0
			Doxorubicin 75 mg/m^2	33%	4.9	14.0
Nabholtz et al., 1999	392	second line	Docetaxel 100 mg/m^2	30%[a]	4.4[a]	11.4[a]
			Mitomycin-C plus vinblastine	12%	2.6	8.7
Sjostrom et al., 1999	283	second line	Docetaxel 100 mg/m^2	42%[a]	6.3[a]	10.4
			Methotrexate plus 5-FU	21%	3.0	11.1
Bonneterre et al., 2002	175	second line	Docetaxel 100 mg/m^2	33%	6	13
			Vinorelbine plus 5-FU	36%	5	12

[a]Statistically significant difference ($p < 0.05$)
[b]Trial used time to treatment failure as end point, not time to progression.
Abbreviation: NR, not reached.

The Eastern Cooperative Oncology Group (ECOG) compared paclitaxel (175 mg/m^2, 24 hour infusion), doxorubicin (60 mg/m^2), and the combination (doxorubicin 50 mg/m^2 followed four hours later by paclitaxel 150 mg/m^2 via a 24 hour infusion plus filgrastim) every three weeks in 732 patients with metastatic breast cancer (Sledge et al., 2003). Patients initially assigned to doxorubicin received a maximum of eight cycles, followed by crossover to paclitaxel at progression. Those initially assigned to paclitaxel continued until disease progression. Patients initially assigned to the combination received the combination for a maximum of eight cycles, followed by single-agent paclitaxel (150 mg/m^2) until disease progression. The objective response rate favored the combination compared with paclitaxel or doxorubicin (47% vs. 34% vs. 36%), as did the median time to treatment failure (8.0 vs. 6.0 vs. 5.9 months). There was no significant difference in median survival (22.0 vs. 22.2 vs. 18.9 months). The crossover response rate for paclitaxel (following progression on doxorubicin) was 22%, whereas the crossover response rate for doxorubicin (following progression on paclitaxel) was 20%. There was no significant difference in the incidence of cardiac toxicity between the three arms. There was also no significant difference in quality of life between these three arms.

Single-Agent Docetaxel Compared with Other Agents or Combinations

The results of several trials that compared single-agent docetaxel with other agents or combinations regimens as first-line therapy are shown in Table 10. One trial compared docetaxel (100 mg/m^2) with doxorubicin (75 mg/m^2) every three weeks for seven cycles in 326 patients with metastatic breast cancer (Chan et al., 1999). Patients were required to have failed prior alkylator-based therapy either in the adjuvant setting (47%) or for the treatment of metastatic disease (53%). The objective response rate was significantly higher for docetaxel (48% vs. 33%), an advantage that was also observed in patients with visceral metastases (46% vs. 29%), liver metastases (54% vs. 26%), resistant disease (47% vs. 25%), or those who had relapsed within 12 months of completing adjuvant therapy (52% vs. 15%). There was no significant difference in median TTP (6.1 vs. 4.9 months) or median survival (15 vs. 14 months). Doxorubicin produced significantly more grade 3 to 4 vomiting (12% vs. 3%) and stomatitis (12% vs. 5%), febrile neutropenia (12% vs. 6%), need for red cell transfusions (21% vs. 7%), and CHF (4% vs. 0%). On the other hand, when considering all grades of toxicity, docetaxel produced more neurosensory toxicity (43% vs. 6%), neuromotor toxicity (18% vs. 3%), nail disorders (44% vs. 5%), skin toxicity (38% vs. 7%), diarrhea (50% vs. 17%), and allergic reactions (18% vs. 6%). There was no significant difference in overall quality of life scores using the EORTC C-30 instrument. A phase III trial compared docetaxel (100 mg/m^2) with paclitaxel (175 mg/m^2) given every three weeks in patients who progressed after an anthracycline-containing regimens, including 42% of patients who received the treatment as first-line chemotherapy (Jones, 2005). Docetaxel was associated with improved response

(32% vs. 25%, $p = 0.10$), TTF (5.7 vs. 3.6 months, $p < 0.0001$), and survival (15.4 vs. 12.7 months, $p = 0.03$). There was more hematologic and nonhematologic toxicities in the docetaxel arm, and no differences in global quality of life scores (Jones et al., 2005). Another trial compared docetaxel given every three weeks (100 mg/m^2) with a weekly schedule (35 mg/m^2/wk for 3 of 4 weeks) in 118 patients with metastatic breast cancer. There was a trend toward a higher response rater for the every three-week arm, with no difference in PFS (5.7 vs. 5.5 months) or OS (18.3 vs. 18.6 months).

Several trials evaluated single-agent docetaxel as second-line therapy (Table 10). One trial compared docetaxel (100 mg/m^2 every 3 weeks) with mitomycin (12 mg/m^2 every 6 weeks) plus vinblastine (6 mg/m^2 every 3 weeks) (MV) for a maximum of 10 three-week cycles in 392 patients with metastatic breast cancer (Nabholtz et al., 1999). All patients had progressive disease after prior anthracycline-containing therapy. Docetaxel resulted in a significantly higher response rate (30% vs. 12%), median TTP (4.4 vs. 2.6 months), and OS (11.4 vs. 8.7 months). Docetaxel produced more grade 3 to 4 neutropenia (93% vs. 63%), febrile neutropenia (9% vs. 0.5%), infection (11% vs. 1%), stomatitis (9% vs. 0.5%), diarrhea (7.5% vs. 0%), skin rash (4% vs. 0%), nail disorders (2.5% vs. 0%), asthenia (16% vs. 6.4%), and neurosensory toxicity (5% vs. 0%). MV produced more grade 3 to 4 thrombocytopenia (12% vs. 4%). With regard to quality of life, more patients treated with MV discontinued treatment (82% vs. 63%) due to disease progression, toxicity, or other factors, although longitudinal analysis showed no difference in the global health scores between the two treatments. Another study compared docetaxel (100 mg/m^2) with sequential methotrexate (200 mg/m^2 day 1, 8) and 5-FU (600 mg/m^2 day 1, 8) every three weeks in 283 patients with metastatic breast cancer (Sjostrom et al., 1999). All patients had anthracycline resistant breast cancer. Docetaxel produced a significantly better response rate (42% vs. 21%) and median TTP (6.3 vs. 3.0 months), although there was no significant difference in survival (10.4 vs. 11.1 months). Grade 3 to 4 toxicities that occurred more often with docetaxel included leukopenia (78% vs. 16%), febrile neutropenia (23% vs. 11%), infections (31% vs. 6%), asthenia (15% vs. 2%), neuropathy (5% vs. 0%), and nail toxicity (6% vs. 0%). Docetaxel also produced more grade 2 to 3 fluid retention (42% vs. 11%). Another group compared docetaxel (100 mg/m^2) with vinorelbine (25 mg/m^2 days 1, 5) and 5-FU (750 mg/m^2 for five days by continuous IV infusion) every three weeks in 175 patients with metastatic breast cancer (Bonneterre et al., 2002). All patients had failed prior anthracycline-based therapy, and had failed one prior therapy for metastatic disease. There was no significant difference in the treatment arms with regard to response rate (33% vs. 26%), median TTP (6 vs. 5 months), or survival (13 vs. 12 months).

Taxane-Anthracycline Combinations

Because the anthracyclines and taxanes are the most active cytotoxic agents for breast cancer, there have been many phase I and II or phase II trials evaluating anthracycline-taxane combinations in metastatic disease. These agents may exhibit clinical relevant pharmacokinetic interactions under certain circumstances. Paclitaxel has been shown to alter the plasma disposition of doxorubicin and its major metabolite (doxorubicinol), resulting in about a 30% increase in exposure to doxorubicin and its active metabolite (Gianni et al., 1997). This interaction is highly sequence and schedule dependent, and is observed if there is a relatively short (15 minute) interval between administration of the drugs, or with relatively short (3 hour) paclitaxel infusions (Sparano, 1998). Docetaxel, on the other hand, has been found to have no effect on the pharmacokinetics of doxorubicin when docetaxel is given as a one-hour infusion either one hour or 15 minutes after an injection of doxorubicin (D'Incalci et al., 1998). Paclitaxel also increases the plasma concentration time curves for the 7d-Aone and glucuronidated metabolites of epirubicin to a significantly greater extent than docetaxel (Esposito et al., 1999). These findings provide a potential explanation for the enhancement of cardiotoxicity when doxorubicin is used with paclitaxel. For example, several phase II studies have demonstrated a greater risk of CHF or subclinical cardiac dysfunction with doxorubicin-paclitaxel combinations (Gianni et al., 1995; Gehl et al., 1996; Sparano et al., 1999) but not with combinations of doxorubicin-docetaxel (Sparano et al., 2000) or epirubicin-paclitaxel (Conte et al., 1997).

Taxane-Based Combinations Compared with Other Combinations

Several phase III trials have evaluated anthracycline-taxane combinations (Table 11). One trial compared the combination of doxorubicin (50 mg/m^2) followed 24 hours later by paclitaxel (220 mg/m^2 three hour infusion) (AT) with FAC every three weeks for eight cycles in 267 patients with metastatic breast cancer (Jassem et al., 2001). The AT regimen produced a significantly better response rate (68% vs. 55%), median TTP (8.3 vs. 6.2 months), and median survival (23 vs. 18.3 months). Patients treated with FAC as initial therapy did not cross over to paclitaxel. AT produced more grade 3 to 4 toxicity, including neutropenia (89% vs. 65%), arthralgia/myalgia (10% vs. 0%), neuropathy (12% vs. 0%), and diarrhea (2% vs. 0%), whereas nausea or vomiting occurred more often with FAC (8% vs. 18%). There was

Table 11 Phase III Trials Evaluating Taxane Combinations with Other Regimens as First-line Therapy

Reference	Number	Treatment arms	Response rate	Median TTP (mo)	Median survival (mo)
Jassem et al., 2001	267	Paclitaxel (220 mg/m^2, 3 hr.) plus Doxorubicin 50 mg/m^2	68%[a]	8.3[a]	23.0[a]
		FAC	55%	6.2	18.3
Nabholtz et al., 2003	429	Docetaxel 75 mg/m^2 plus Doxorubicin 50 mg/m^2	59%[a]	8.7[a]	22.5
		Cyclophosphamide 600 mg/m^2 plus Doxorubicin 60 mg/m^2	47%	7.4	21.7
Langley et al., 2005	795	Epirubicin 75 mg/m^2 plus Paclitaxel 200 mg/m^2	65%	7.0	13.0
		Epirubicin 75 mg/m^2 plus Cyclophosphamide 600 mg/m^2	55%	7.1	14.0
Biganzoli et al., 2002	275	Doxorubicin 60 mg/m^2 plus Paclitaxel 175 mg/m^2	58%	5.9	NS
		Doxorubicin 60 mg/m^2 plus Cyclophosphamide 600 mg/m^2	54%	6.0	NS

[a]Statistically significant difference.
Abbreviations: NS, not stated; FAC, 5-fluorouracil, Adriamycin (doxorubicin), and cyclophosphamide.

no significant difference in the incidence of CHF, being less than 2% in both arms. The lack of an increase in cardiac toxicity is likely due to the long interval between administration of paclitaxel and doxorubicin.

The EORTC compared doxorubicin (60 mg/m^2) used with either paclitaxel [175 mg/m^2 three hour infusion, AT (adriamycin (doxorubicin) + taxol (paclitaxel))] or cyclophosphamide [600 mg/m^2, AC (adriamycin (doxorubicin) = cytoxan (cyclophosphamide))] in 275 patients with metastatic breast cancer (Biganzoli et al., 2002). Comparing AT with AC, there was no significant difference in response rate (58% vs. 54%), median TTP (5.9 vs. 6.0 months), or median survival.

Another group compared doxorubicin (50 mg/m^2) plus docetaxel (75 mg/m^2) AT (adriamycin (doxorubicin) + taxotere (docetaxel)) with doxorubicin (60 mg/m^2) plus cyclophosphamide (600 mg/m^2) every three weeks for up to eight cycles in 429 patients with metastatic breast cancer (Nabholtz et al., 2003). AT produced a significantly higher response rate (59% vs. 47%) and longer median TTP (8.7 vs. 7.4 months), but did not improve median survival. It produced significantly more febrile neutropenia (33% vs. 10%) and more grade 3 to 4 infection (7% vs. 2%), diarrhea (8% vs. 1%), and asthenia (8% vs. 3%). There was no significant difference in the incidence of CHF (2% for AT vs. 4% for AC), although patients treated with docetaxel received less doxorubicin (median cumulative dose of 378 mg/m^2 for AT vs. 420 mg/m^2 for AC).

Another trial compared epirubicin (60 mg/m^2) used with either paclitaxel [175 mg/m^2, three-hour infusion, ET (epirubicin + taxol (paclitaxel))] or cyclophosphamide [600 mg/m^2, EC (epirubicin + cytoxan (cyclophosphamide))] in 705 patients with metastatic breast cancer (Langley et al., 2005). Comparing ET with EC, there was no significant difference in response rate (65% vs. 55%) median PFS (7 vs. 7.1 months) or OS (13 vs. 14 months), with more toxicity in the ET arm.

Gemcitabine

Mechanism of Action and Metabolism

Gemcitabine is a nucleoside analog that mediates its cytotoxic effects by inhibiting DNA synthesis. It is metabolized intracellularly by nucleoside kinases to the active diphosphate (dFdCDP) and triphosphate (dFdCTP) nucleosides (Noble and Goa, 1997). The metabolite dFdCDP inhibits ribonucleotide reductase, thereby inhibiting generation of dexoynucleoside triphosphates such as dCTP that are necessary for DNA synthesis. The depletion of dCTP results in preferential incorporation of gemcitabine triphosphate into DNA, a process termed "self-potentiation." After incorporation of the gemcitabine nucleotides into DNA, only one additional nucleotide is added to the DNA strand before there is inhibition of DNA synthesis. DNA polymerase is then unable to remove the gemcitabine nucleotide and repair the growing DNA strands, a process called "masked chain termination." The clearance of gemcitabine is reduced in the elderly and in women. Elimination of the drug is dependent on renal excretion. The effects of renal and hepatic dysfunction on the disposition of the drug have not been assessed. Some evidence suggests that the drug may be more effective if given at a fixed infusion rate

Table 12 Phase III Trials of Gemcitabine as First or Second-line Therapy

Reference	Setting	Number	Treatment arms	Response rate	Median TTP (mo)	Median survival (mo)
Albain et al., 2004	first line	529	Paclitaxel 175 mg/m^2 every 3 wk	22%	3.9	15.8
			Paclitaxel plus gemcitabine 1250 mg/m^2 on days 1, 8	41%[a]	5.2[a]	18.6
Martin et al., 2007	second line or greater	252	Vinorelbine 30 mg/m^2 day 1, 8 every 21 days	26%	4.0	15.9
			Vinorelbine plus gemcitabine 1200 mg/m^2	36%	6.0[a]	16.4

[a]Statistically significant difference.

(10 mg/m^2/min) than the standard 30-minute infusion schedule because of saturation of intracellular phosphorylation enzymes that occurs with more rapid infusion rates.

Phase III Trials

There have been two phase III trials including gemcitabine as a variable in the randomization (Table 12). Albain et al. reported a phase III trial comparing paclitaxel versus paclitaxel plus gemcitabine as first-line therapy in anthracycline pretreated patients (Albain, 2004). The study compared standard paclitaxel (175 mg/m^2) every three weeks to a combination of paclitaxel dose plus gemcitabine (1250 mg/m^2 on days 1 and 8). The combination was associated with an improved response rate (41% vs. 22%, $p < 0.0001$), median TTP (5.2 vs. 3.9 months, $p < 0.0001$), and trend toward improved survival (18.6 vs. 15.8 months). There was more grade 3 to 4 hematologic toxicity associated with the combination arm, including febrile neutropenia (5% vs. 1%). Martin reported a phase III trial in 252 women with locally recurrent and metastatic breast cancer who had been pretreated with anthracyclines and taxanes were randomly assigned single-agent vinorelbine (30 mg/m^2, days 1 and 8) or gemcitabine plus vinorelbine (1200/30 mg/m^2, days 1 and 8) (Martin et al., 2007). Median PFS was 6.0 months (95% CI 4.8–7.1) for patients given gemcitabine plus vinorelbine and 4.0 months (2.9–5.1) for those assigned vinorelbine [hazard ratio 0.66 (0.50–0.88); $p = 0.0028$]. There was a numerically higher response rate for the combination arm (36% vs. 26%, $p = 0.093$), but no difference in OS (15.9 vs. 16.4 months). There was more grade 3 to 4 neutropenia (61% vs. 44%) and febrile neutropenia (11% vs. 6%) for the combination arm, but comparable nonhematologic toxicity.

Vinorelbine

Mechanism of Action and Metabolism

Vinorelbine is a semisynthetic vinca alkaloid that has a modification of the catharanthine moiety of vinblastine. It mediates its effect by binding to tubulin and inhibiting microtubule assembly. Vinorelbine may be more specific for mitotic microtubules than axonal microtubules compared with other vinca alkaloids such as vincristine and vinblastine. It undergoes hepatic elimination, and the dose should be modified in patients with hepatic dysfunction (Marty et al., 1992).

Phase II and Phase III Trials

Phase II trials in metastatic breast cancer have indicated clinical activity for vinorelbine when used as first- or second-line therapy (Lewis et al., 2002). There have been several phase III trials that evaluated vinorelbine as a component of therapy in metastatic breast cancer (Table 13). Two trials demonstrated no evidence for improved efficacy for the doxorubicin/vinorelbine regimen compared with doxorubicin alone (Norris et al., 2000) or CAF (Blajman et al., 1999) when used as first-line therapy for metastatic disease. Single-agent vinorelbine (30 mg/m^2 weekly) was compared with melphalan (25 mg/m^2 every four weeks) in 183 patients with anthracycline-refractory metastatic breast cancer (Jones et al., 1995). Although there was no significant difference in response rate (16% vs. 9%), vinorelbine was associated with a significant improvement in time to disease progression (2.8 vs. 1.9) and survival (8.2 vs. 7.2 months). Grade 3 to 4 toxicities included predominantly of granulocytopenia (75% vs. 71%), anemia (14% vs. 34%), and thrombocytopenia (0% vs. 59%), but febrile neutropenia was uncommon (10% vs. 8%). Another trial compared epirubicin (90 mg/m^2 ever three weeks) used alone or in combination with vinorelbine (25 mg/m^2 days 1 and 8) in 387 patients with metastatic breast cancer (Ejlertsen et al., 2004). The combination was associated with improved median PFS (10.1 vs. 8.2 months, $p = 0.019$), but not response (42% vs. 40%) or OS (19.1 vs. 18 months).

Capecitabine

Mechanism of Action and Metabolism

Capecitabine is an orally administered prodrug of 5-fluorouruacil. After absorption from the gastrointestinal

Table 13 Phase III Trials Evaluating Vinorelbine as First or Second-line Therapy

Reference	Number	First- or second-line therapy	Treatment arms	Response rate	Median TTP (mo)	Median survival (mo)
Jones et al., 1995	183	Second or greater	Vinorelbine 30 mg/m^2 weekly	16%	2.8[a]	8.2[a]
			Melphalan 25 mg/m^2 every 4 wk	9%	1.9	7.2
Blajman et al., 1999	177	First	Doxorubicin 50 mg/m^2 day 1 and Vinorelbine 25 mg/m^2 day 1, 8 q 3 wk	74%	7.5	17.8
			FAC	75%	9.0	17.31
Norris et al., 2000	303	First and second	Doxorubicin 50 mg/m^2 day 1 and Vinorelbine 25 mg/m^2 day 1, 8 q 3 wk	38%	6.2	13.8
			Doxorubicin 70 mg/m^2 day 1 q 3 wk	30%	6.1	14.4
Ejlertsen et al., 2004	387		Epirubicin 90 mg/m^2	42%	10.1[a]	19.1
			Epirubicin plus vinorelbine 25 mg/m^2 day 1, 8	40%	8.2	18.0

[a]Statistically significant difference.
Abbreviations: FAC, 5-fluorouracil, doxorubicin, cyclophosphamide (see Table 4 for doses).

tract, it is hydrolyzed in the liver by carboxylesterase to produce 5'-deoxy-5-fluorocytidine, which is converted by cytidine deaminase that is found principally in the liver and tumor tissue to 5'-deoxy-5-fluorouridine (Wagstaff et al., 2003). This metabolite is then converted to 5-fluorouracil by thymidine phosphorylase, an enzyme that is found in higher levels in most solid tumors compared with normal tissue, thereby resulting in relatively selective production of 5-fluorouracil in tumorous tissue (Ishikawa et al., 1998). The drug is well absorbed after oral administration, is rapidly converted to noncytotoxic intermediates, and results in significantly higher intratumoral levels of 5-flourouracil compared with plasma and normal tissue levels (Schuller et al., 1997). 5-fluorouracil exerts its antitumor effect principally by inhibiting thymidylate synthetase. The pharmacokinetics of the drug are not altered in patients with mild-to-moderate renal or hepatic dysfunction and thus require no modification in this setting.

Phase II Trials

A multicenter phase II trial of capecitabine was performed in 162 patients with paclitaxel-refractory breast cancer who had failed at least two (but not more than three) prior chemotherapy regimens (Blum et al., 1999). The initial dose was 2510 mg/m^2 per day given in two divided doses for 14 consecutive days, followed by a seven-day rest period, repeated in three week cycles. The response rate was 20%, the median response duration was 9.8 months, and median survival was 12.8 months. Common side effects included hand foot syndrome (56%), diarrhea (54%), nausea (52%), vomiting (37%), fatigue (36%), and dermatitis (15%), although these toxicities were grade 3 to 4, toxicities that occurred in more than 5% were diarrhea (14%) and hand foot syndrome (10%). Some have advocated the use of a lower daily dose (2000 mg/m^2/day) without compromise of activity (Hennessy et al., 2005).

Phase III Trials

O'Shaughenessy reported a comparision between capecitabine (2500 mg/m^2/day orally on days 1–14) plus docetaxel (75 mg/m^2) to single-agent docetaxel (100 mg/m^2 intravenously every 3 weeks) in 511 patients with anthracycline pretreated metastatic breast cancer (O'Shaughnessy et al., 2002) (Table 14). The combination arm was associated with improved response rate (42% vs. 30%; $p = 0.006$), median TTP (6.1 vs. 4.2 months, $p = 0.0001$), and OS (14.5 vs. 11.5 months, $p = 0.0126$). Gastrointestinal toxicity and hand-foot syndrome were higher in the combination, and myalgia, arthralgia, and neutropenic fever were all more common in single-agent docetaxel arm. There were more grade 3 adverse events in the combination arm (71% vs. 49%) and more grade 4 events in the docetaxel arm (31% vs. 25%).

Ixabepilone

Mechanism of Action and Metabolism

The epothilones are a novel class of antineoplastic agents that target microtubules. Naturally occurring epothilones, including epothilones A to D, are macrolides originally isolated from the bacterium *Sorangium cellulosum* (Watkins et al., 2005). Due to the promising antineoplastic activity of natural epothilones, numerous semisynthetic epothilone analogs have been synthesized. Epothilones

Table 14 Phase III Trials including Capecitabine Monotherapy or Combinations with Antitubulins

Reference	Number	Treatment arms	Response rate	Median TTP (mo)	Median survival (mo)
O'Shaughnessy et al., 2002	511	Docetaxel 100 mg/m^2 every 3 wk	30%	4.2	11.5
		Docetaxel plus capecitabine 2500 mg/m^2/day days 1–14	42%[a]	6.1[a]	14.5[a]
Vahdat et al., 2007	752	Capecitabine 2500 mg/m^2 days 1–14 every 3 wk	14%	4.2	TE
		Capecitabine 2000 mg/m^2 days 1–14 plus ixabepilone 40 mg/m^2 IV every 21 days	35%[a]	5.8[a]	TE

[a]Statistically significant difference.
Abbreviation: TE, too early.

promote cell death by stabilizing microtubules and inducing apoptosis. Ixabepilone is a semisynthetic analog of epothilone B, designed to optimize the antineoplastic characteristics of the natural product. Ixabepilone has demonstrated efficacy in cell lines and xenografts resistant to commonly used cytotoxic agents (Larkin and Kaye, 2006). It is metabolized by the liver, and the dose must be modified in patients with hepatic dysfunction.

Phase III Trial

A phase III trial that included 752 patients with metastatic breast cancer who had anthracycline and taxane pretreated and/or resistant disease were randomized to receive capecitabine alone (2500 mg/m^2/day on days 1–14 every 3 weeks) or capecitabine at a reduced dose (2000 mg/m^2/day on days 1–14) plus ixabepilone (40 mg/m^2 IV over 3 hours every 3 weeks) (Vahdat, 2007) (Table 14). The combination arm was associated with improved response rate (35% vs. 14%, $p < 0.0001$) and PFS (4.2 vs. 5.8 months, $p = 0.0003$), with follow-up insufficient at the time regarding survival. The combination with associated with more grade 3 to 4 neuropathy (23% vs. 0%), fatigue (9% vs. 3%), and hematologic toxicity such as neutropenia (68% vs. 11%), febrile neutropenia (4% vs. 1%), anemia (10% vs. 4%), and thrombocytopenia (8% vs. 4%), but comparable degrees of capecitabine-associated toxicities such as foot syndrome (18% vs. 17%), mucositis (6% vs. 9%), and diarrhea (2% vs. 3%). Patients with grade 2 baseline elevations in liver function were found to have a substantially increased risk of death to neutropenic infection (5 of 16, 31%), and were subsequently excluded from participation in the trial after this was identified. The risk of treatment-associated death was 2% in those with normal or baseline grade 1 liver function abnormalities (less than 2.5-fold elevation in transaminase level).

Platinum Analogs

Mechanism of Action and Metabolism

Cisplatin and carboplatin are platinum complexes with two ammonia groups in the *cis* position. Cisplatin undergoes an initial aquation reaction in which the chloride groups are replaced by water molecules. The aquated platinum complex binds preferentially to the N-7 position of guanine and adenine and produces DNA interstrand cross-links. Carboplatin has a similar mechanism of action, although it requires a higher drug concentration and longer incubation time in vitro to produce a comparable effect. Both drugs undergo renal elimination. Relative to cisplatin, carboplatin produces less nausea and vomiting, nephrotoxicity, and neuropathy, but more thrombocytopenia and neutropenia (Go and Adjei, 1999).

Phase II and III Trials

Cisplatin is inactive when used as second line therapy for metastatic breast cancer. Several studies have indicated, however, that both cisplatin and carboplatin have activity when used as first-line therapy. When used as first-line therapy, response has been reported in 45% of patients treated with cisplatin (Sledge et al., 1988; Sledge and Roth, 1989) and 25% to 35% for carboplatin (Martin et al., 1992; O'Brien et al., 1993). Response rates have been very low in patients with chemotherapy-refractory disease, but other studies evaluating taxane-platinum combinations have demonstrated considerable activity when used as first-line therapy (Loesch et al., 2002; Decatris et al., 2004). There has been one phase III trial including a platinum as a variable in Her2/neu positive disease that demonstrated improved response and median TTP when carboplatin was added to paclitaxel and trastuzumab (Robert et al., 2006) (Table 16).

Table 15 Phase III Trial of Maintenance Chemotherapy or with Other Agents

Reference	Number	Induction	Maintenance arms	Median TTP	Median survival
Coates et al., 1987	305	AC or CMF × 3	Continuous AC or CMF	6.0[a]	10.7
			Intermittent AC or CMF	4.0	9.4
Muss et al., 1991	250	FAC × 6	CMF	9.4	16.0
			No therapy	6.7	14.9
Cocconi et al., 1990	95	CMF × 6	CMF continuation	15.2	34.5
		CMF × 6 ⇒ AV × 2 ⇒ CMF × 6	No therapy	15.6	33.1
Falkson et al., 1998	141	CAF/CMF ⇒ CR	CMFPTH	18.7[a]	32.2
			No therapy	7.8	28.7
Ejlersten et al., 1993	318	CEF × 6 mos	CEF × 6 ⇒ CMF x 6	14[a]	23
			No therapy	10	18
French Epirubicin Study Group, 2000	392	FEC- 75 × 4	FEC-75 × 7	10.3[a]	17.9
		FEC-100 × 450 × 8	FEC-50 × 8	8.3[a]	18.9
		FEC-100 × 4	No therapy	6.2	16.3
Gennari et al., 2006	255	Epi or Dox plus paclitaxel	Paclitaxel 175 mg/m^2 every 3 wk × 8	8.0	28.0
			No therapy	9.0	29.0
Sparano et al., 2004	190	Dox or taxane-based therapy	Marimastat 10 mg BID	4.7	24.7
			Placebo	3.1	26.0
Mayordomo et al., 2004	1028	Induction chemotherapy	Theratope Vaccine	ND	ND
			Sham Vaccine		

[a]Statistically significant difference.
Abbreviation: ND, no difference.

DURATION OF CHEMOTHERAPY: MAINTENANCE THERAPY IN METASTATIC BREAST CANCER

Although there are clear benefits from administration of a short course of chemotherapy for four to six months, the benefits of more prolonged chemotherapy or other agents for responding patients is less certain. There have been several randomized trials that have addressed this issue (Table 15).

Less Than Four Months of Therapy

The Australian-New Zealand Breast Cancer Trials Group randomized 305 eligible women with metastatic breast cancer to receive doxorubicin (50 mg/m^2) and cyclophosphamide (750 mg/m^2) (AC) intravenously every three weeks or classical CMF every four weeks given either continuously until disease progression or intermittently (for 3 courses, followed by a 9–12 week rest period, then 3 additional courses, etc) (Coates et al., 1987). Although there was no significant difference in the efficacy of AC or CMF, the continuous regimen was associated with a significantly improved response rate (49% vs. 32%) and median time to disease progression (6.0 vs. 4.0 months). With regard to survival, there was trend toward an increased risk of death with intermittent therapy when adjusted for adverse prognostic factors (relative risk 1.26; 95% CI 0.99–1.62; $p = 0.07$). Quality of life was evaluated using a linear analogue patient self-assessment scale measuring physical well-being, mood, pain, appetite, and nausea or vomiting. Quality of life improved for all parameters after three months with the exception of nausea or vomiting, which worsened. Beyond the first course of therapy and before disease progression, quality of life was significantly better for those who received continuous therapy. Given that other groups have shown that the median time to response is approximately six to eight courses of therapy, the inferior outcome for the intermittent group may be attributable to premature termination of treatment in patients who might otherwise demonstrate response and symptom palliation had treatment continued. Although this study provides good evidence that administration of treatment until disease progression results in better palliation of symptoms than only three courses (9–12 weeks) of therapy, it does not address whether continuing treatment after achieving response is beneficial.

CMF Maintenance Beyond Four Months

The Piedmont Oncology Group studied 250 women with metastatic breast cancer treated with FAC for six courses (18 weeks) (Muss et al., 1991). Of the 233 patients evaluable for response, complete response occurred in 6%, partial response occurred in 24%, and stable disease occurred in 42%. Of the 169 patients who had stable or responding disease, 145 were randomized to either discontinue chemotherapy or to continue chemotherapy with classical CMF for a maximum of 12 cycles (or one year). The median TTP from the point of randomization favored continuous therapy (9.4 vs. 3.2 months). The median TTP did not significantly differ, however, if progression in the observation group was defined at the point where patients progressed after receiving reinduction (CMF) therapy (9.4 vs. 6.7 months; $p = 0.41$). There was no significant difference in OS. Maintenance treatment was associated with more toxicity than the no treatment group. The Italian Cooperative Group compared continuous classical CMF with classical CMF for six cycles followed by two cycles of doxorubicin-based therapy and no further therapy (Cocconi et al., 1990). There was no significant difference in response rate, median time to progression, or survival.

Epirubicin-Based Maintenance Therapy

A phase III trial was performed that included 318 evaluable women with metastatic breast cancer who were randomized to receive FEC (5-fluorouracil 600 mg/m^2, epirubicin 60 mg/m^2, cyclophosphamide 600 mg/m^2) every three weeks for a total of six months or until disease progression (for a maximum of 18 months) (Ejlertsen, 1993). Epirubicin was replaced by methotrexate (40 mg/m^2) when the cumulative epirubicin dose reached 1000 mg/m^2 (at about 12 months) or if cardiac toxicity developed. In addition, all patients received tamoxifen 30 mg daily until progression, and premenopausal women received ovarian irradiation. Considering all patients, maintenance therapy was associated with improved PFS (14 vs. 10 months) and survival (23 vs. 18 months). About 20% of patients requested discontinuation of maintenance therapy due to toxicity The French Epirubicin Study Group (2000) randomized 392 eligible patients to receive: (A) FEC-75 for 11 cycles (about eight months), (B) FEC-100 × four cycles followed by FEC-50 for eight cycles (also about eight months), and (C) FEC-100 for four cycles (about 3 months) followed by FEC-100 at the time of disease progression. The outcome favored the arms A and B (8 months of therapy) compared with arm C (3 months of therapy) in terms of response rate (61% vs. 48%) and median TTP (9.6 vs. 6.2 months), although there was no difference in survival (about 18.5 months vs. 16.3 months). This study confirmed the findings of the Australian-New Zealand study demonstrating that administration of three months of chemotherapy produces an inferior response rate and time to disease progression compared with a longer course.

Taxane-Based Maintenance Chemotherapy

The MANTA1 trial included 459 patients who received first-line combination chemotherapy with epirubicin or doxorubicin plus paclitaxel, of whom 255 who had a response or stable disease were randomly assigned to eight courses of maintenance paclitaxel versus no further chemotherapy (Gennari et al., 2006). A futility analysis performed including 215 of the randomly assigned patients revealed no difference in the median PFS between the two arms (8.0 vs. 9.0 months), nor in OS (28.0 vs. 29.0 months). When the Bayesian method for monitoring clinical trials was applied to these data there was only a 9% chance of observing a three-month improvement in median PFS in the group receivingmaintenance paclitaxel.

Maintenance Chemotherapy After Complete Remission

ECOG evaluated the role of maintenance chemohormonal therapy in 141 eligible patients who had a complete response to initial doxorubicin-containing chemotherapy (including some patients who had residual bone disease (Falkson et al., 1998). Patients were randomized to receive CMF plus prednisone, tamoxifen, and Halotestin [CMF(P)TH] or observation. Median TTP was improved with maintenance therapy (18.7 vs. 7.8 months), although median survival was not significantly impacted (32.2 vs. 28.7 months).

Other Approaches

ECOG compared the matrix metalloproteinase inhibitor marimastat (10 mg PO BID) with placebo in 190 patients with metastatic breast cancer who had responding or stable disease after first-line chemotherapy (Sparano et al., 2004). When comparing placebo with marimastat, there was no significant difference in median PFS (3.1 months vs. 4.7 months, $p = 0.16$) or OS (26.6 vs. 24.7 months). Patients treated with marimastat were more likely to develop grade 2 or 3 musculoskeletal toxicity, a known complication of the drug indicative of achieving a biological effect, compared with patients administered placebo (63% vs. 22%, $p < 0.0001$). A similar approach was employed evaluating Theratope, a cancer vaccine consisting of a synthetic form of the tumor-associated antigen Sialyl Tn (STn) conjugated to the carrier protein keyhole limpet hemocyanin (KLH). The trial included 1028 patients who were randomized to receive Theratope or a control injection consisting of the adjuvant plus KLH plus a single injection of cyclophosphamide prior to vaccination following a response or stable disease after induction chemotherapy. There was no difference in median TTP or OS, although there seemed to be a benefit for the vaccine in the subset of patients with HR-positive disease treated with concurrent endocrine therapy (Mayordomo, 2004).

Summary of Trials Evaluating Maintenance Therapy

Taken together, these studies suggest that treatment with at least six months of cytotoxic therapy is preferable to shorter courses, and that continued treatment beyond six months delays progression for an average of three to six months at the expense of treatment-associated toxicity. The decision regarding whether to continue treatment beyond six months should be individualized on the basis of factors such as response, symptom palliation, and treatment-associated toxicity. The literature suggests that patients can be reassured that treatment holidays do not adversely impact survival.

HIGH-DOSE THERAPY PLUS STEM CELL TRANSPLANTATION

Based upon preclinical and retrospective clinical data suggesting a dose-response curve for cytotoxic therapy, several studies have evaluated the role of high-dose chemotherapy plus stem cell transplantation for metastatic breast cancer. Initial findings from a number of phase II trials seemed promising, although some evidence suggests that these findings may be entirely attributed to selection bias (Rahman et al., 1997). The ECOG and Philadelphia Transplant Group reported the results of a phase III trial that evaluated high-dose therapy in 553 women with metastatic breast cancer who received standard CMF or CAF chemotherapy for metastatic disease (Stadtmauer et al., 2000). Of the 553 women initially registered, 199 had at least a partial response to therapy and were randomized to continued standard therapy with CMF for up to two years or high-dose cyclophosphamide, carboplatin, and thiotepa plus stem cell transplantation. In comparing the standard versus high-dose groups, there was no significant difference in the median time to disease progression (9.0 vs. 9.6 months) or OS at three years (38% vs. 32%). A previously reported phase III study had indicated an improvement in response and survival for tandem high-dose therapy, although the results of this trial are in question because of scientific misconduct by the study's lead investigator (Bezwoda et al., 1995). A systematic review which identified six randomized trials including high dose chemotherapy plus stem cell transplant concluded that there was insufficient evidence to recommend the procedure (Farquhar et al., 2005).

HER2 AS A THERAPEUTIC TARGET: TRASTUZUMAB AND LAPATINIB

The human epidermal growth factor receptors (HER) consist of a family of proteins that play an important role in cellular growth, differentiation, and survival (Slamon et al., 1989). There are currently four known members of this family, including epidermal growth factor receptor (also known as HER1, erbB1), HER2 (erbB2), HER3 (erbB3), and HER4 (erB4) (Hung, 1999). The receptors may become activated by forming homodimers or heterodimers, or by ligand binding. HER2 is the preferential dimerization partner of other members of the HER family. The *HER2* gene is a protooncogene located at the long arm of human chromosome 17(17q11.2-q12). It is also commonly referred to as HER2/*neu* because it is identical to the rat *neu* gene that was isolated from the rat neuroblastoma. Transfection of cell lines with HER2 enhances the metastatic potential of these cells in animal models by stimulating a variety of processes involved in the metastatic cascade, including proliferation, invasion, migration, seeding of distant sites, and growth. HER2 produces these effects by activating signal transduction pathways that induce downstream activation of cycle D1, a critical regulator of the cell cycle. Breast cancers that have HER2 gene amplification and protein overexpression exhibit greater metastatagenecity (are more likely to metastasize) and virulence (relapse sooner). Approximately 15% to 20% of newly diagnosed breast cancers exhibit amplification of the *HER2/neu* gene, usually associated with overexpression of Her2/neu protein.

Trastuzumab

Mechanism of Action

Trastuzumab (Herceptin®) is a humanized version of the murine monoclonal antibody 4D5 that was formulated by inserting the complementarity-determining regions of 4D5 into the framework of a consensus human IgG. The biological basis for the activity of trastuzumab is unknown, but may involve multiple mechanisms including but not limited to modulation of signal transduction pathways that favor apoptosis, perturbation of the cell cycle, antibody-dependent cellular cytotoxicity, complement-dependent cytotoxicity, and inhibition of nuclear excision repair mechanisms that confer alkylator agent resistance (Hudis, 2007).

Phase III Trials

Several trials have evaluated trastuzumab for metastatic breast cancer (Table 16). The pivotal trial that led to the approval of trastuzumab included 469 women with metastatic breast cancer, all of whom had received no prior chemotherapy for metastatic disease and who had disease

Table 16 Phase III Trials of Anti-Her2/neu Directed Therapy

Reference	Treatment	Number	Setting	Response rate	Median TTP (mo)	Median survival (mo)
Slamon et al., 1998	AC[a]	291	first line	38%	5.7	24.5
	AC plus trastuzumab	178	first line	50%	7.6[a]	33.4[a]
	Paclitaxel			15%	2.5	18.4
	Paclitaxel plus trastuzumab			38%[a]	6.5[a]	22.1[a]
Marty et al., 2006	Docetaxel	186	first line	34%	6.1	22.7
	Docetaxel plus trastuzumab		first line	61%[a]	11.7[a]	31.2[a]
Robert et al., 2006	Paclitaxel-trastuzumab	196	first line	36%	7.1	32.2
	Paclitaxel-trastuzumab plus carboplatin AUC 6 every 3 wk		first line	52%[a]	10.7[a]	35.7
Geyer et al., 2006	Capecitabine 2500 mg/m^2/day days 1–14 every 21 days	321	progressive disease after prior anthracyclines, taxane, and trastuzumab	14%	4.6	TE
	Capecitabine 2000 mg/m^2/day, days 1–14 every 21 days plus lapatinib 1250 mg daily			23%	8.6[a]	TE

[a]Statistically significant difference. Dosing: Trastuzumab dosing—4 mg/kg loading dose, then 2 mg/kg weekly; AC—doxorubicin (Adriamycin) 60 mg/m^2, cyclophosphamide 600 mg/m2 every 3 weeks; Paclitaxel—175 mg/m2 every 3 weeks; docetaxel 100 mg/m2 every 3 weeks.
Abbreviation: TE, too early.

that was demonstrated to exhibit HER2 protein overexpression (Slamon et al., 2001). Patients with no prior history of adjuvant anthracycline therapy ($N = 291$) received doxorubicin (60 mg/m^2) or epirubicin (75 mg/m^2) plus cyclophosphamide (600 mg/m^2) (AC) for six cycles. Patients who had a previous history of anthracycline exposure ($N = 178$) received paclitaxel (175 mg/m^2 three hour infusion) for six cycles. Patients were randomized to receive trastuzumab (4 mg/kg loading dose, followed by 2 mg/kg IV weekly) or no trastuzumab. For all patients, the addition of trastuzumab to chemotherapy was associated with significantly improved response (50% vs. 32 percent, $p < 0.001$), median TTP (7.4 vs. 4.6 months; $p < 0.001$), response duration (9.1 vs. 6.1 months, $p < 0.001$), and survival (25.1 vs. 20.3 months, $p = 0.01$). There was a benefit in survival for the trastuzumab group despite a high crossover for patients assigned to receive chemotherapy only as initial therapy. Similar trends were observed for patients treated with AC or paclitaxel (Table 16). There was prohibitive cardiotoxicity when trastuzumab was combined with AC (described below). For patients treated with paclitaxel, when considering all grades of toxicity, the addition of trastuzumab resulted in a significantly greater incidence of fever (49% vs. 23%), chills (41% vs. 4%), abdominal pain (34% vs. 22%), infection (47% vs. 27%), nausea (51% vs. 9%), diarrhea (45% vs. 29%), cough (41% vs. 22%), rhinitis (22% vs. 5%), sinusitis (21% vs. 7%), and rash (38% vs. 18%). The response rate with trastuzumab is approximately 15% when used as a single agent for second-line therapy, and 23% when used as first-line therapy as a single agent (Shak, 1999; Vogel et al., 2002). This suggests that the optimal use of this agent may be in combination with conventional cytotoxic therapy rather than as a single agent.

A second phase III trial compared chemotherapy alone or in combination with trastuzumab as first-line therapy in 186 patients with Her2/neu positive metastatic breast cancer (Marty et al., 2005). Patients were randomly assigned to six cycles of docetaxel (100 mg/m^2 every three weeks) alone or in combination with trastuzumab (4 mg/kg loading dose followed by 2 mg/kg weekly until disease progression). The addition of trastuzumab was associated with an improved response rate (61% vs. 34%, $p = 0.0002$), TTP (11.7 vs. 6.1 months, $p = 0.0001$), TTF (9.8 vs. 5.3 months, $p = 0.0001$), response duration (11.7 vs. 5.7 months, $p = 0.009$), and OS (31.2 vs. 22.7 months, $p = 0.0325$). The addition of trastuzumab was associated with more grade 3 to 4 neutropenia (32% vs. 22%) and febrile neutropenia (23% vs. 17%).

Another phase III trial evaluated the efficacy and safety of trastuzumab and paclitaxel with or without carboplatin as first-line therapy in 196 patients women with Her2/neu positive metastatic breast cancer (Robert et al., 2006). All patients received trastuzumab (4 mg/kg loading dose plus 2 mg/kg weekly thereafter until disease progresses ion) plus either paclitaxel (175 mg/m^2 every three weeks) or paclitaxel plus carboplatin (AUC 6) for six cycles. The addition of carboplatin was associated with an improved response rate (52% vs. 36%, $p = 0.040$), PFS (10.7 vs. 7.1 months, $p = 0.03$), but no significant difference in OS (35.7 vs. 32.2 months). Improved clinical outcomes for the carboplatin arm were most evident in HER-2/neu 3+

disease with regard to response (57% vs. 36%) and median PFS (13.8 vs. 7.6 months). There was more myelosuppression and neuropathy in the carboplatin arm. A subsequent randomized phase II trial demonstrated better tolerability and comparable or greater efficacy when carboplatin and paclitaxel were given on a weekly schedule (Perez et al., 2005).

Cardiac Toxicity of Trastuzumab

An unexpected side effect of trastuzumab that was noted during the course of the pivotal trial was cardiac dysfunction. The incidence of cardiac dysfunction was significantly greater for patients treated with trastuzumab plus AC (28% vs. 7%) or trastuzumab plus paclitaxel (11% vs. 1%) compared with chemotherapy alone. Cardiac dysfunction was defined as (*i*) cardiomyopathy, characterized by a decrease in cardiac ejection fraction associated with abnormal myocardial wall motion that was either global or more severe in the septum, (*ii*) symptoms of CHF (including dyspnea, increased cough, and paroxysmal nocturnal dyspnea), (*iii*) signs of CHF (including peripheral edema, S3 gallop, and tachycardia), or (*iv*) a decline in cardiac ejection fraction from baseline of at least 5% to below 55% with signs and symptoms or a decrease in cardiac ejection fraction of at least 10 points to below 55% without signs or symptoms. The incidence of CHF was also increased for patients treated with trastuzumab plus AC (19% vs. 3%) or trastuzumab plus paclitaxel (4% vs. 1%) compared with chemotherapy alone. The majority of patients with CHF improved with medical therapy. The cumulative doses of doxorubicin administered in the AC arm ($\sim$350 mg/m^2) and in the paclitaxel arm ($\sim$250 mg/m^2) were well below the level typically associated with cardiac toxicity. Cardiac dysfunction has also been noted with single-agent trastuzumab. It is noteworthy that the incidence of cardiac dysfunction was higher in patients receiving trastuzumab as second-line therapy (7%), most of whom had received prior anthracycline for the treatment of early stage and/or advanced disease (Cobleigh et al., 1999). In contrast, the incidence of cardiac dysfunction was only about 1% in patients who received trastuzumab as first therapy for metastatic disease, of whom only about one-half had received prior adjuvant doxorubicin.(Vogel et al., 2001) A retrospective analysis of the clinical trial database that included 1024 patients treated with trastuzumab was reported; an analysis of several clinical factors including age, weight, history of hypertension, cumulative doxorubicin dose, HER2 expression level, and treatment revealed only advanced age (>60 years) and concurrent doxorubicin therapy to be significantly associated with cardiac dysfunction (Seidman et al., 2002).

Lapatinib

Mechanism of Action and Metabolism

Lapatinib is an orally administered small molecule inhibitor of HER2/neu and erbB1tyrosine kinases, leading to inhibition of mitogen-activated protein kinase (MAPK) and phosphatidylinositol-3-kinase (PI3K) signaling in erbB1-expressing and erbB2-overexpressing tumor cell lines, including cell lines that are trastuzumab resistant. It extensively metabolized by the hepatic CYP3A4/5 pathway, its metabolism may be significantly altered by inhibitors (e.g., clarithromycin, ketoconazole, grapefruit juice, antiretroviral protease inhibitors) or inducers (e.g., rifampin, anticonvulsants, dexamethasone) of the CYP3A4/5 system. There is no pharmacokinetic interaction with capecitabine. Its bioavalailability is improved if taken with food; there is high inter- and intrapatient variability when taken after a meal. Although less bioavailable, when taken on an empty stomach, this is recommended because of more consistent absorption. The dose should be reduced in patients with severe hepatic dysfunction, and should be used only in patients with normal cardiac function (Moy et al., 2007).

Phase III Trials

A phase III, open-label trial was performed in 321 patients with HER2/neu positive metastatic breast cancer who had progressive disease after trastuzumab plus taxane therapy which compared capecitabine (2500 mg/m^2/day on days 1–14 every 21 days) to capecitabine (at 2000 mg/m^2/day on days 1–14) plus lapatinib (1250 mg continuously) (Geyer et al., 2006) (Table 16). The addition of lapatinib resulted in a significant improvement in median TTP (36.9 vs. 19.7 weeks, $p = 0.00016$), and PFS (36.9 vs. 17.9 weeks, $p = 0.000045$), with a trend toward improved response rate (22.5% vs. 14.3%, $p = 0.113$). There were also fewer relapses within the central nervous system in the lapatinib group ((11 vs. 4 events). There was no significant difference in events requiring discontinuation of therapy ((14% vs. 11%). Diarrhea was more common on the combination arm (58%) compared with capecitabine alone (39%), as were hand-foot syndrome (43% vs. 34%) and rash (35% vs. 30%).

ANGIOGENESIS AS A THERAPEUTIC TARGET: BEVACIZUMAB

Mechanism of Action

Clinical studies have suggested a correlation between microvessel density and/or vascular endothelial growth factor (VEGF) expression and poor clinical outcome, and the inhibition of microvascular growth is believed to retard the growth of all tissues, including metastatic tissue. Bevacizumab is a recombinant, humanized monoclonal

Table 17 Phase III Trials of Anti-VEGF Directed Therapy with Bevacizumab

Reference	Treatment	Number	Setting	Response rate	Median TTP (mo)	Median Survival (mo.)
Miller et al., 2005	Capecitabine 2500 mg/m^2/day, days 1–14 every 21 days	462	Progressive disease after prior anthracyclines,	9%	4.2	14.1
	Capecitabine plus bevacizumab 15 mg/kg IV every 3 wk		taxane, and trastuzumab	20%	4.9	15.5
Miller et al., 2007	Paclitaxel 90 mg/m2 day 1, 8, 15 every 28 days	722	first-line chemotherapy	14%	6.1	TE
	Paclitaxel plus bevacizumab 10 mg/kg IV every 2 wk			30%	11.4	

Abbreviation: TE, too early.

antibody, which binds to, and neutralizes, VEGF preventing its association with endothelial receptors. VEGF binding initiates angiogenesis (endothelial proliferation and the formation of new blood vessels), leading to growth and progression of many types of human cancer (Schneider and Miller, 2005).

Phase III Trials

Bevacizumab has modest activity as a single agent in metastatic breast cancer. In a phase two trial, the response rate in 75 patients with refractory disease was only 9.3% (Cobleigh et al., 2003). There have been two phase III trials evaluating bevacizumab in metastatic breast cancer (Table 17). Miller reported a phase III trial that compared capecitabine (2500 mg/m^2/day for 14 of 21 days) alone or in combination with bevacizumab (15 mg/kg every 3 weeks) in 462 patients with metastatic breast cancer who had progressive disease after prior anthracycline and taxane therapy (Miller et al., 2005). Although the addition of bevacizumab was associated with a significantly increased response (20% vs. 9%; $p = 0.001$); there was no improvement in the primary end point of PFS (4.9 vs. 4.2 months) or OS (15.1 vs. 14.5 months).

Grade 3 to 4 hypertension requiring treatment occurred significantly more often with bevacizumab (17.9% vs. 0.5%). A second phase III trial performed by the ECOG compared weekly paclitaxel (90 mg/m^2 days 1, 8, 15 every 28 days) alone or in combination with bevacizumab (10 mg/kg every two weeks) in 722 patients with metastatic breast cancer who had no prior chemotherapy for metastatic disease. The addition of bevacizumab was associated with a significantly increased response (30% vs. 14%; $p < 0.0001$) and TTP p (11.4 vs. 6.1 months, HR 0.51, 95% CI 0.43–0.62, $p < 0.0001$). The median number of events had not yet been reached to permit an OS analysis at the time of the report. Forest plot analysis for time to progression revealed an advantage of bevacizumab in all subgroups, including ER-positive and ER-negative disease, visceral disease, short disease-free interval (<24 months), more than three disease sites, and prior adjuvant taxane therapy. As in the study conduced in patients with more advanced disease, grade 3 to 4 toxicities that were more prevalent in the bevacizumab arm included grade 3 to 4 hypertension (15% vs. 2%), bleeding (2% vs. 0%), proteinuria (2% vs. 0%), but no cardiac toxicity or thromboembolic events (Miller, 2007).

BONE STROMA AS A THERAPEUTIC TARGET: BISPHOSPHONATES

Bone metastases are a common complication of metastatic breast cancer, occurring in about 50% of patients with metastases, of whom it is the sole site of disease in about 25% (Nielsen et al., 1991). The most common sites of metastases include the ribs, spine, pelvis, and proximal long bones. Complications of skeletal metastases include pain, vertebral compression fracture, pathological fracture, spinal cord compression, and hypercalcemia. These complications are due not only to tumor-associated bone invasion and destruction, but also due to osteolysis that is mediated by tumor-associated osteoclast activating factors. The bisphosphonates are potent group osteoclast inhibitors that inhibit bone resorption without inhibiting bone mineralization. A phase III trial was performed that compared the bisphosphonate pamidronate (90 mg given as a 2-hour IV infusion every 3–4 weeks for up to 2 years) with a placebo infusion in 380 patients with metastatic breast cancer who were receiving standard chemotherapy and who had at least one lytic bone metastasis that measured at least 1 cm (Hortobagyi et al., 1996, 1998). It is noteworthy that about 60% of patients enrolled on the study had bone as their only site of metastases. The median time to a first skeletal-related event (i.e., need for radiation, nonvertebral pathological fracture, hypercalcemia, bone surgery, and spinal cord compression) was significantly longer for patients treated with pamidronate (13.1 vs. 7.0 months), and fewer patients developed skeletal related complications (43% vs. 56%), worsening bone pain or worsening performance status. The difference favoring pamidronate persisted at 15, 18, 21, and 24 months. A similar benefit was also noted for pamidronate in patients receiving hormonal therapy (Theriault et al., 1999). An American Society of Clinical Oncology (ASCO) expert panel concluded that IV bisphosphonates are indicated in patients with osteolytic bone metastases, particularly if they are symptomatic, and that treatment should continue (even if a skeletal-related event has occurred) until there is evidence of a substantial decline in the general performance status (Hillner et al., 2000, 2003). A subsequent randomized phase III trial compared zolendronic acid (4 mg or 8 mg intravenously as a 15 minute IV infusion) with pamidronate in 1130 patients with breast cancer and lytic bone metastases, showing comparable efficacy and safety for the 4 mg dose; the 8 mg dose proved to be no more effective and was associated with renal dysfunction (Berenson et al., 2001; Rosen et al., 2001). A subsequent update of the ASCO guidelines recommended that there was insufficient evidence supporting the efficacy of one bisphosphonate over the other. The panel also concluded that starting bisphosphonates in women who demonstrate bone destruction through imaging but have normal plain radiographs was reasonable (irrespective of skeletal pain), but that beginning bisphosphonates based on an abnormal bone scan but without evidence of bone destruction was not recommended (Hillner et al., 2003). Renal function must be monitored in patients receiving parental bisphosphonate therapy, and doses withheld or modified in accordance with labeled instructions.

SYSTEMATIC REVIEWS OF CYTOTOXIC THERAPY

Several systematic reviews have been reported evaluating a variety of questions regarding which agents to use, whether they should be used concurrently or sequentially, and other issues.

Systematic Review of Chemotherapy

Fossati reported a systematic review of randomized clinical trials performed in metastatic breast cancer reported between 1975 and 1997 that were identified by a MEDLINE and EMBASE search (Fossati et al., 1998). The data extracted from each report included tumor response, the hazard ratio for mortality, and proportion with severe side effects. A total of 189 randomized trials were identified, of which all provided response data and 133 (70%) provided data or Kaplan–Meier curves necessary for calculation of the hazard ratios. One hundred sixty five were two arm trials, and 24 studies included three or more arms. The trials were categorized into twelve separate groups by their primary comparison, including six groups that included chemotherapy as a component of therapy (Table 18):

- Polychemotherapy versus single-agent therapy: Polychemotherapy was associated with a higher objective response rate (48% vs. 34%) and a significant reduction in the hazard rate for death whether the comparison was anthracycline combinations versus single-agent anthracyclines (HR 0.87; 95% CI 0.76–0.97), or nonanthracycline combinations versus single-agents (HR 0.70; 95% CI 0.59–0.84).
- Anthracycline versus nonanthracycline chemotherapy: Anthracyclines were associated with a significantly higher response rate (51% vs. 45%) but had no significant effect on survival. Anthracyclines produced more nausea and vomiting, leukopenia, alopecia, and neurological and cardiac toxicity. There was a modest reduction rate in the hazard rate for death (HR 0.89; 95% CI 0.82–0.97) if the comparison regimen did not contain prednisone, whereas there was a disadvantage for anthracyclines (HR 1.16; 95% CI 1.02–1.32) when compared with a regimen that contained prednisone.
- Other chemotherapy versus CMF: There was a slightly higher response rate for the non-CMF regimens (49% vs. 44%), but the non-CMF regimens produced significantly more nausea and vomiting, leukopenia, alopecia, and neurological toxicity. There was no significant difference in the hazard rate for death.

Table 18 Systematic Review of Chemotherapy for Metastatic Breast Cancer

Comparison	Number of trials	Number of patients	Response rate	Hazard rate for death
PolyCHT vs. single agent	15	2442	48% vs. 34%[a]	0.82[a]
Anthracycline vs. nonanthracycline CHT	30	5241	51% vs. 45%[a]	No difference
Other CHT vs. CMF	17	3041	49% vs. 44%[a]	No difference
Epirubicin vs. doxorubicin	10	1512	44% vs. 47%	No difference
High vs. low-intensity CHT	19	3193	44% vs. 33%[a]	0.90[a]
Chemohormonal therapy vs. CHT alone	25	3606	56% vs. 46%	No difference

[a]Statistically significant difference.
Abbreviation: CHT, chemotherapy.

- Epirubicin versus doxorubicin: There was no significant difference in response rate (44% vs. 47%). Epirubicin produced less leukopenia and cardiac toxicity. Epirubicin was associated with a trend toward a higher risk for death (HR 1.13; 95% CI 1.00–1.27), although this was not statistically significant.
- Standard-dose versus low-dose chemotherapy: Standard-dose chemotherapy was associated with a significantly higher response rate (44% vs. 33%), but was associated with more nausea and vomiting, leukopenia, mucositis, and alopecia. Standard-dose therapy was associated with a significant reduction in the hazard rate for death (HR 0.90; 95% CI 0.83–0.97).
- Chemotherapy versus chemohormonal therapy: Hormonal therapy consisted of tamoxifen, medroxyprogesterone acetate, estrogen, oophorectomy, and other hormones. There was a higher response rate for chemohormonal therapy (56% vs. 46%), but there was a higher risk of cardiac toxicity, hot flashes, and edema. There was no significant effect on the hazard rate for death.

Single-Agent Vs. Combination Chemotherapy

Carrick evaluated the results of randomized trials comparing single-agent versus combination chemotherapy (Carrick et al., 2005). Of the 37 eligible trials, 28 included time-to-event data. Based on an estimated 4220 deaths in 5707 women, there was a modest advantage for combination chemotherapy regimens compared with single agents with a hazard ratio for OS of 0.88 (95% CI 0.83–0.94, $p < 0.0001$) and no evident heterogeneity. Results are similar if the analysis was limited to trials for those receiving first-line chemotherapy. Combination regimens were also associated with improved TTP [overall HR of 0.78 (95% CI 0.73–0.83, $p < 0.00001$] and response rates [odds ratio (OR) 1.28, CI 1.15–1.42, $p < 0.00001$] although significant heterogeneity was observed ($p = 0.002$ and $p < 0.00001$, respectively), likely reflecting the varying efficacy of the comparator regimens used in the trials. Combination regimens were associated with more toxicity. The authors concluded that combination regimens were associated with improved response rate and TTP, and modestly improved survival with more toxicity.

Systematic Review of Anthracycline-Containing Therapy

Lord reported a systematic review of studies including antitumor antibiotics, and identified 33 trials, including 29 trials with anthracyclines, and 26 that included time-to-event data for OS (Lord et al., 2004). The observed 4084 deaths in 5284 randomized women did not demonstrate a statistically significant difference in survival between regimens that contained antitumor antibiotics and those that did not (HR 0.97, 95% CI 0.91–1.03, $p = 0.35$) and no significant heterogeneity. Antitumor antibiotic regimens were associated with improved TTP (HR 0.84, 95% CI 0.77–0.91) and tumor response rates (OR 1.34, 95% CI 1.21–1.48), although significant heterogeneity was observed for these outcomes, and the associations were consistent when the analysis was restricted to the 29 trials that reported on anthracyclines. Patients receiving anthracycline-containing regimens were also more likely to experience toxic events compared to patients receiving non-antitumor antibiotic regimens. No statistically significant difference was observed in any outcome between mitoxantrone-containing and non-antitumor antibiotic-containing regimens. The authors concluded that compared to regimens without antitumor antibiotics, regimens that contained these agents showed a statistically significant advantage for tumor response and TTP, were associated with more toxicity, and were not associated with improved survival.

Systematic Review of Taxane-Containing Therapy

Ghersi evaluated the results of randomized trials comparing taxane-containing chemotherapy regimens with regimens not containing a taxane in women with metastatic breast cancer (Ghersi et al., 2005). Of 21 eligible trials, 16 had published some results and 12 data on OS. An estimated 2621 deaths among 3643 women suggest a significant difference in OS in favor of taxane-containing regimens (HR 0.93, 95% CI 0.86–1.00, $p = 0.05$). The treatment effect on survival was similar if only trials of first-line chemotherapy were included, although not statistically significant. There was also an advantage for taxanes in TTP (HR 0.92, 95% CI 0.85–0.99, $p = 0.02$) and overall response (OR 1.34, 95% CI 1.18–1.52, $p < 0.001$). There was significant heterogeneity across the trials ($p < 0.001$), partly because of the varying efficacy of the comparator regimens. The authors concluded that taxane-containing regimens improved OS in women with metastatic breast cancer. Taxane-containing regimens are more effective than some, but not all, nontaxane-containing regimens.

Three-Drug Vs. Two-Drug Chemotherapy Regimens

Jones evaluated randomized trials that evaluated a first-line regimen of at least two chemotherapy drugs, and compared it to that same regimen plus the addition of one or more chemotherapy drugs (Jones et al., 2006). The analysis identified 17 trials (2674 patients), including 15 trials that included response data and 11 that included time-to-event data for OS. There was no difference in OS (HR 0.96; 95% CI 0.87–1.07, $p = 0.47$) or in TTP (HR 0.93; 95% CI 0.81–1.07, $p = 0.31$), and no significant heterogeneity. Addition of a drug to the regimen was associated with improved response rates (OR 1.21, 95% CI 1.01–1.44, $p = 0.04$), although there was significant heterogeneity for this outcome across the trials. Where measured, acute toxicities such as alopecia, nausea and vomiting, and leukopenia were more common with the addition of a drug. The authors concluded that the addition of one or more drugs to the regimen shows a statistically significant advantage for response, but was associated with more toxicity and did not improve time to progression or survival.

GENERAL APPROACH TO TREATMENT

The selection of treatment is influenced by several factors, including disease-specific and patient-specific factors. Disease-specific factors include biological features (such as ER and/or PR expression and Her2/neu expression), the extent of the disease (number of disease sites, presence of visceral metastases and/or bone metastases), and the disease-related symptoms. Patient-specific factors include comorbid illnesses (e.g., heart disease may preclude anthracyclines), organ function (neuropathy or liver dysfunction may preclude taxanes), age, and performance status. Impaired performance status may be due to advanced age, comorbid illness, advanced breast cancer, or all of these factors. A suggested algorithm for the management of metastatic breast cancer is shown in Figure 2.

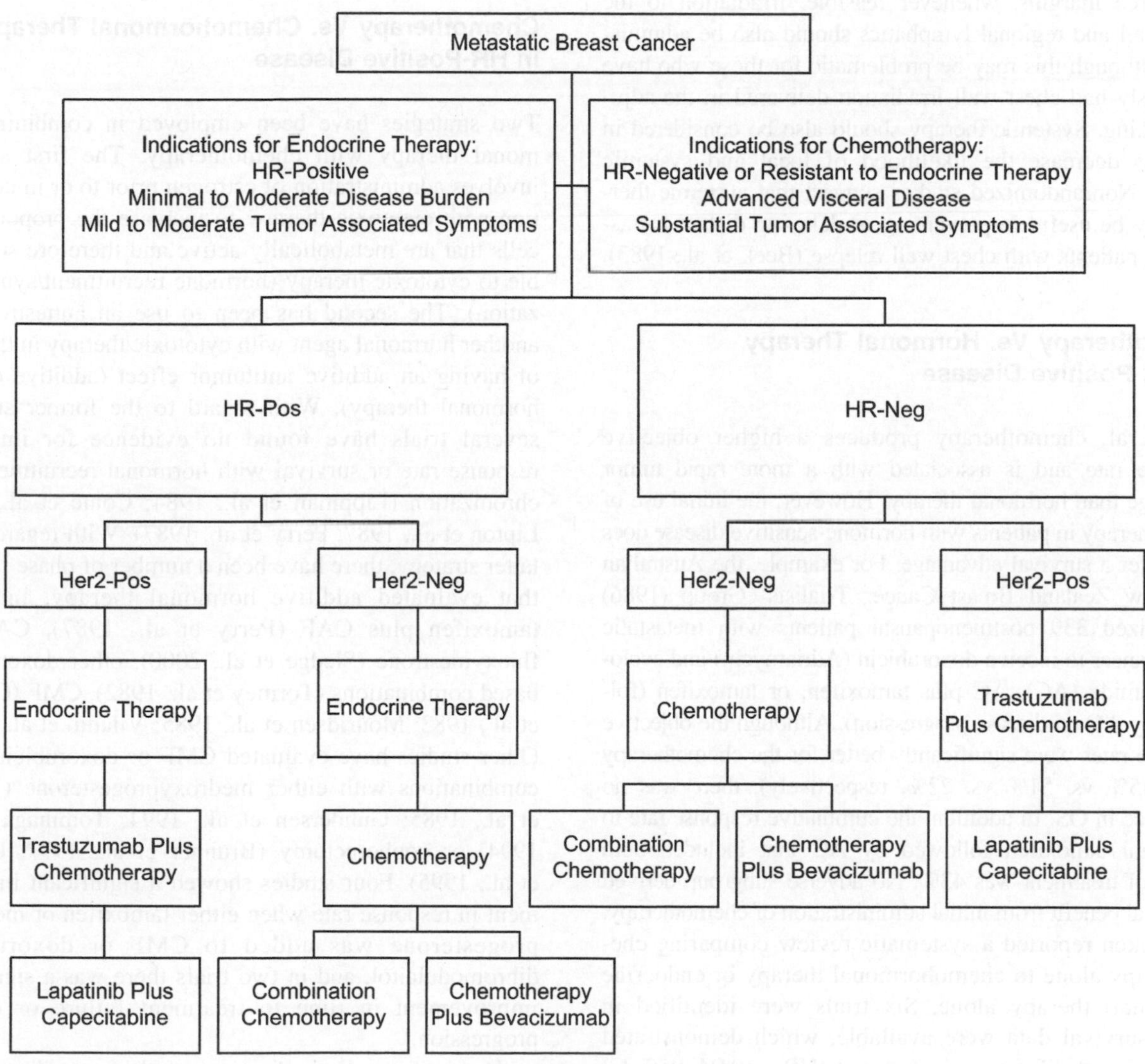

Figure 2 Algorithm for the use of cytotoxic therapy in the management of breast cancer.

One Site of Disease

Selected patients may be cured with surgical resection. With solitary lung metastases, one group reported a 50% five-year disease-free survival (Lanza et al., 1992). Resection of hepatic lesions has also resulted in treatment-free survival is some selected patients (Pocard et al., 2000). Patients with single cerebral metastases may benefit from surgical resection, even if there are other sites of systemic metastases. Resection of bone metastases is generally reserved for patients with or high risk for pathological fracture, and is generally followed by local irradiation. Patients with chest wall recurrence should undergo a thorough evaluation for metastatic disease, including a careful history and physical examination, bone scan, and computerized tomography of the chest and abdomen, as clinically unsuspected metastases are not uncommon (Rosenmann et al., 1988). The tumor should be resected with an attempt to establish adequate tumor-free margins, whenever feasible. Irradiation to the chest wall and regional lymphatics should also be administered, although this may be problematic for those who have previously had chest wall irradiation delivered in the adjuvant setting. Systemic therapy should also be considered in order to decrease the likelihood of local and systemic relapse. Nonrandomized studies suggest that systemic therapy may be useful in preventing or delaying distant metastases in patients with chest wall relapse (Beck et al., 1983).

Chemotherapy Vs. Hormonal Therapy for HR-Positive Disease

In general, chemotherapy produces a higher objective response rate and is associated with a more rapid tumor shrinkage than hormonal therapy. However, the initial use of chemotherapy in patients with hormone-sensitive disease does not confer a survival advantage. For example, the Australian and New Zealand Breast Cancer Trialists' Group (1986) randomized 339 postmenopausal patients with metastatic breast cancer to receive doxorubicin (Adriamycin) and cyclophosphamide (AC), AC plus tamoxifen, or tamoxifen (followed by AC on disease progression). Although the objective response rates were significantly better for the chemotherapy arms (45% vs. 51% vs. 22%, respectively), there was no difference in OS. In addition, the cumulative response rate to sequential tamoxifen followed by AC that included both phases of treatment was 43%. No adverse subgroup derived a survival benefit from initial administration of chemotherapy.

Wilcken reported a systematic review comparing chemotherapy alone to chemohormonal therapy or endocrine (hormonal) therapy alone. Six trials were identified in which survival data were available, which demonstrated no significant difference in survival (HR = 0.94, 95% CI 0.79–1.12, $p = 0.5$), and no significant heterogeneity (Wilcken et al., 2003). A pooled estimate of reported response rates in eight trials involving 817 women showed a significant advantage for chemotherapy over endocrine therapy with RR = 1.25 (1.01–1.54, $p = 0.04$), although the two largest trials showed trends in opposite directions (test for heterogeneity was $p = 0.0018$). There was little information available on toxicity and quality of life. Six of the seven fully published trials commented on increased toxicity with chemotherapy, mentioning nausea, vomiting, and alopecia. Three of the seven mentioned aspects of quality of life, with differing results. Only one trial formally measured quality of life, concluding that it was better with chemotherapy. The authors concluded that in women with metastatic breast cancer and where HR are present, a policy of treating first with endocrine therapy rather than chemotherapy is recommended except in the presence of rapidly progressive disease.

Chemotherapy Vs. Chemohormonal Therapy in HR-Positive Disease

Two strategies have been employed in combining hormonal therapy with chemotherapy. The first strategy involves administration of estrogen prior to or in conjunction with cytotoxic therapy to increase the proportion of cells that are metabolically active and therefore susceptible to cytotoxic therapy (hormone recruitment/synchronization). The second has been to use an antiestrogen or another hormonal agent with cytotoxic therapy in the hope of having an additive antitumor effect (additive chemohormonal therapy). With regard to the former strategy, several trials have found no evidence for improved response rate or survival with hormonal recruitment/synchronization (Lippman et al., 1984; Conte et al., 1986; Lipton et al., 1987; Perry et al., 1987). With regard to the latter strategy, there have been a number of phase III trials that evaluated additive hormonal therapy, including tamoxifen plus CAF (Perry et al., 1987), CAF and fluoxymestrone (Sledge et al., 2000), other doxorubicin-based combinations (Tormey et al., 1982), CMF (Cocconi et al., 1983; Mouridsen et al., 1985; Viladiu et al., 1985). Other studies have evaluated CMF or doxorubicin-based combinations with either medroxyprogesterone (Viladiu et al., 1985; Gundersen et al., 1994; Tominaga et al., 1994) or oophorectomy (Brunner et al., 1977; Falkson et al., 1995). Four studies showed a significant improvement in response rate when either tamoxifen or medroxyprogesterone was added to CMF or doxorubicin-dibromodulcitol, and in two trials there was a significant improvement in time to treatment failure or disease progression.

The interpretation of many of these studies is confounded by the inclusion of patients with ER-negative or unknown disease, or failure of prior hormonal therapy. Nevertheless, these studies demonstrate no convincing evidence that hormonal therapy should be given concurrently with systemic chemotherapy, a finding that is reinforced by the systematic analysis reported by Fossati. This suggests that these treatment modalities are best used sequentially rather than concurrently.

Non-Localized (Disseminated) Disease

The majority of patients with metastatic breast cancer have multiple sites within an organ involved, or multiple organs involved. Patients with hormone-sensitive disease and no symptoms or mild-to-moderate symptoms should receive hormonal therapy. Local irradiation should be considered for patients with a localized site of disease, especially bony disease, that is symptomatic or that is at risk for producing a catastrophic complication (e.g., spinal cord compression, pathological fracture). Systemic chemotherapy should be reserved for patients with hormone-insensitive disease, or patients with symptomatic hormone-sensitive disease who have failed all hormonal therapy options or who are moderately severely symptomatic and in urgent need for symptom palliation. The options available for cytotoxic-containing chemotherapy include single-agent therapy or combination-cytotoxicity therapy. For patients with Her2/neu positive disease, first-line cytoxic therapy should always be used in combination with trastuzumab. The benefit of continued trastuzumab after disease progression on trastuzumab plus cytotoxic therapy is uncertain (Tripathy et al., 2004). For patients with Her2/neu negative disease, options included single-agent cytotoxic therapy, single-agent cytotoxic therapy plus bevacizumab, or combination-cytotoxic therapy. Bevacizumab seems to be effective only when used in combination with chemotherapy, and when used as first-line therapy. Several professional organizations have provided evidence based recommendations or guidelines for selecting cytotoxic therapy (Carlson et al., 2006; Beslija et al., 2007).

Clinical Trials

Since metastatic breast cancer is an incurable disease associated with a short survival, it is not unreasonable to consider every individual with the disease a candidate for a clinical trial. For phase III trials, the goals are generally to improve response rate, symptom palliation, and/or survival, or to diminish toxicity when compared with standard therapy. For phase II trials, the goal is to identify an effective new agent or combination. Clinical trials performed in patients with metastatic disease may also be useful for identifying new treatment strategies to be employed in the adjuvant setting. The CALGB performed a randomized phase III trial that compared standard CAF chemotherapy ($N = 144$ patients) as initial therapy for metastatic disease with one of four other cytotoxic agents ($N = 178$ patients) that proved to be less effective, including trimetrexate, melphalan, amonafide, carboplatin, or elsamitrucin (Costanza et al., 1999). Patients assigned to initially receive the phase II agent received no more than four cycles, and then went on immediately to CAF either after a maximum of four cycles of therapy or if disease progression occurred before the fourth cycle. Comparing the initial versus delayed CAF arm, there was no significant difference in the cumulative response rate after completing CAF (52% vs. 44%), median response duration (21.4 vs. 15.0; $p = 0.069$), or median survival (19.6 vs. 16.6 months; $p = 0.074$), although there was a trend favoring initial CAF. In multivariate analysis, the only factors that adversely affected response included prior adjuvant chemotherapy and visceral disease, and the only factors that adversely affected survival were poor performance status (1 vs. 0), visceral metastases, and the more prior treatment modalities. These findings suggest that it may be reasonable and ethical to offer selected patients with metastatic breast cancer, an investigational agent as first-line therapy, particularly if such a patient lacks visceral disease, has an excellent performance status, and has had limited prior therapy, and particularly if the agent being tested has demonstrated activity in phase I trials.

CONCLUSION

There are many active cytotoxic agents that are available for the treatment of metastatic breast cancer. Although cytotoxic therapy relieves tumor-associated symptoms and prolongs survival, these benefits must be weighed against its inherent toxicity. No firm conclusions can be reached regarding a standard of care that should be administered to all patients. One exception may be the use of trastuzumab, which should be administered to all patients with Her2/neu overexpressing disease selected to receive chemotherapy. The choice of when to initiate cytotoxic therapy and which agent(s) to administer is dependent on the biology of the disease (e.g., ER or Her2/neu expression), the extent of the disease, the prior treatment history, the presence of other medical conditions, and the goals of therapy in that particular individual.

REFERENCES

A'Hern RP, Ebbs SR, Baum MB. Does chemotherapy improve survival in advanced breast cancer? A statistical overview. Br J Cancer 1988; 57(6):615–618.

A'Hern RP, Smith IE, Ebbs SR. Chemotherapy and survival in advanced breast cancer: the inclusion of doxorubicin in Cooper type regimens. Br J Cancer 1993; 67(4):801–805.

Aisner J, Weinberg V, Perloff M, Weiss R, Perry M, Korzun A, Ginsberg S, Holland JF. Chemotherapy versus chemoimmunotherapy (CAF v CAFVP v CMF each +/− MER) for metastatic carcinoma of the breast: a CALGB study. Cancer and Leukemia Group B. J Clin Oncol 1987; 5(10): 1523–1533.

Albain KS, Nag S, Calderillo-Ruiz G, Jordaan JP, Llombart A, Pluzanska A, Pawlicki M, Melemed AS, O'Shaughnessy J, Reyes JM. Global Phase III study of gemcitabine plus paclitaxel (GT) vs. paclitaxel (T) as frontline therapy for metastatic breast cancer (MBC): First report of overall survival. Proc Am Soc Clin Oncol 2004 18:510 (abstr).

Alonso MC, Tabernero JM, Ojeda B, Llanos M, Sola C, Climent MA, Segui MA, Lopez JJ. A phase III randomized trial of cyclophosphamide, mitoxantrone, and 5-fluorouracil (CNF) versus cyclophosphamide, adriamycin, and 5-fluorouracil (CAF) in patients with metastatic breast cancer. Breast Cancer Res Treat 1995; 34(1):15–24.

Australian and New Zealand Clinical Trials Group. A randomized trial in postmenopausal patients with advanced breast cancer comparing endocrine and cytotoxic therapy given sequentially or in combination. The Australian and New Zealand Breast Cancer Trials Group, Clinical Oncological Society of Australia. J Clin Oncol 1986; 4(2):186–193.

Bangham AD, Horne RW. Negative staining of phospholipids and their structural modification by surface-active agents as observed in the electron microscope. J Mol Biol 1964; 8:660–668.

Bastholt L, Dalmark M, Gjedde SB, Pfeiffer P, Pedersen D, Sandberg E, Kjaer M, Mouridsen HT, Rose C, Nielsen OS, Jakobsen P, Bentzen SM. Dose-response relationship of epirubicin in the treatment of postmenopausal patients with metastatic breast cancer: a randomized study of epirubicin at four different dose levels performed by the Danish Breast Cancer Cooperative Group. J Clin Oncol 1996; 14(4):1146–1155.

Batist G, Ramakrishnan G, Rao CS, Chandrasekharan A, Gutheil J, Guthrie T, Shah P, Khojasteh A, Nair MK, Hoelzer K, Tkaczuk K, Park YC, Lee LW. Reduced cardiotoxicity and preserved antitumor efficacy of liposome-encapsulated doxorubicin and cyclophosphamide compared with conventional doxorubicin and cyclophosphamide in a randomized, multicenter trial of metastatic breast cancer. J Clin Oncol 2001; 19(5):1444–1454.

Beck TM, Hart NE, Woodard DA, Smith CE. Local or regionally recurrent carcinoma of the breast: results of therapy in 121 patients. J Clin Oncol 1983; 1(6):400–405.

Bennett JM, Muss HB, Doroshow JH, Wolff S, Krementz ET, Cartwright K, Dukart G, Reisman A, Schoch I. A randomized multicenter trial comparing mitoxantrone, cyclophosphamide, and fluorouracil with doxorubicin, cyclophosphamide, and fluorouracil in the therapy of metastatic breast carcinoma. J Clin Oncol 1988; 6(10): 1611–1620.

Berenson JR, Rosen LS, Howell A, Porter L, Coleman RE, Morley W, Dreicer R, Kuross SA, Lipton A, Seaman JJ. Zoledronic acid reduces skeletal-related events in patients with osteolytic metastases. Cancer 2001; 91(7): 1191–1200.

Berry DA, Cronin KA, Plevritis SK, Fryback DG, Clarke L, Zelen M, Mandelblatt JS, Yakovlev AY, Habbema JD, Feuer EJ. Effect of screening and adjuvant therapy on mortality from breast cancer. N Engl J Med 2005; 353(17):1784–1792.

Berry DA, Inoue L, Shen Y, Venier J, Cohen D, Bondy M, Theriault R, Munsell MF. Modeling the impact of treatment and screening on U.S. breast cancer mortality: a Bayesian approach. J Natl Cancer Inst Monogr 2006; (36):30–36.

Beslija S, Bonneterre J, Burstein H, Cocquyt V, Gnant M, Goodwin P, Heinemann V, Jassem J, Kostler WJ, Krainer M, Menard S, Petit T, Petruzelka L, Possinger K, Schmid P, Stadtmauer E, Stockler M, Van Belle S, Vogel C, Wilcken N, Wiltschke C, Zielinski CC, Zwierzina H. Second consensus on medical treatment of metastatic breast cancer. Ann Oncol 2007; 18(2):215–225.

Bezwoda WR, Seymour L, Dansey RD. High-dose chemotherapy with hematopoietic rescue as primary treatment for metastatic breast cancer: a randomized trial. J Clin Oncol 1995; 13(10):2483–2489.

Biganzoli L, Cufer T, Bruning P, Coleman R, Duchateau L, Calvert AH, Gamucci T, Twelves C, Fargeot P, Epelbaum R, Lohrisch C, Piccart MJ. Doxorubicin and paclitaxel versus doxorubicin and cyclophosphamide as first-line chemotherapy in metastatic breast cancer: The European Organization for Research and Treatment of Cancer 10961 Multicenter Phase III Trial. J Clin Oncol 2002; 20(14): 3114–3121.

Billingham M. Use of the myocardial biopsy to monitor cardiotoxicity. Cancer Treat Rep 1978; 62(10):1607.

Billingham ME, Mason JW, Bristow MR, Daniels JR. Anthracycline cardiomyopathy monitored by morphologic changes. Cancer Treat Rep 1978; 62(6):865–872.

Bishop JF, Dewar J, Toner GC, Smith J, Tattersall MH, Olver IN, Ackland S, Kennedy I, Goldstein D, Gurney H, Walpole E, Levi J, Stephenson J, Canetta R. Initial paclitaxel improves outcome compared with CMFP combination chemotherapy as front-line therapy in untreated metastatic breast cancer. J Clin Oncol 1999; 17(8):2355–2364.

Blackstein M, Vogel CL, Ambinder R, Cowan J, Iglesias J, Melemed A. Gemcitabine as first-line therapy in patients with metastatic breast cancer: a phase II trial. Oncology 2002; 62(1):2–8.

Blajman C, Balbiani L, Block J, Coppola F, Chacon R, Fein L, Bonicatto S, Alvarez A, Schmilovich A, Delgado FM. A prospective, randomized Phase III trial comparing combination chemotherapy with cyclophosphamide, doxorubicin, and 5-fluorouracil with vinorelbine plus doxorubicin in the treatment of advanced breast carcinoma. Cancer 1999; 85(5):1091–1097.

Blomqvist C, Elomaa I, Rissanen P, Hietanen P, Nevasaari K, Helle L. Influence of treatment schedule on toxicity and efficacy of cyclophosphamide, epirubicin, and fluorouracil in metastatic breast cancer: a randomized trial comparing weekly and every-4-week administration. J Clin Oncol 1993; 11(3):467–473.

Blum JL, Jones SE, Buzdar AU, LoRusso PM, Kuter I, Vogel C, Osterwalder B, Burger HU, Brown CS, Griffin T. Multicenter phase II study of capecitabine in paclitaxel-refractory metastatic breast cancer. J Clin Oncol 1999; 17(2):485–493.

Bonneterre J, Roche H, Monnier A, Guastalla JP, Namer M, Fargeot P, Assadourian S. Docetaxel vs 5-fluorouracil plus vinorelbine in metastatic breast cancer after anthracycline therapy failure. Br J Cancer 2002; 87(11):1210–1215.

Brincker H. Distant recurrence in breast cancer. Survival expectations and first choice of chemotherapy regimen. Acta Oncol 1988; 27(6A):729–732.

Brunner KW, Sonntag RW, Alberto P, Senn HJ, Martz G, Obrecht P, Maurice P. Combined chemo- and hormonal therapy in advanced breast cancer. Cancer 1977; 39(suppl 6):2923–2933.

Bruno R, Hille D, Riva A, Vivier N, ten Bokkel Huinnink WW, van Oosterom AT, Kaye SB, Verweij J, Fossella FV, Valero V, Rigas JR, Seidman AD, Chevallier B, Fumoleau P, Burris HA, Ravdin PM, Sheiner LB. Population pharmacokinetics/pharmacodynamics of docetaxel in phase II studies in patients with cancer. J Clin Oncol 1998; 16(1):187–196.

Buyse M, Piedbois P. On the relationship between response to treatment and survival time. Stat Med 1996; 15 (24):2797–2812.

Carlson RW, Brown E, Burstein HJ, Gradishar WJ, Hudis CA, Loprinzi C, Mamounas EP, Perez EA, Pritchard K, Ravdin P, Recht A, Somlo G, Theriault RL, Winer EP, Wolff AC. NCCN Task Force Report: adjuvant therapy for breast cancer. J Natl Compr Canc Netw 2006; 4(suppl 1): S1–S26.

Carrick S, Parker S, Wilcken N, Ghersi D, Marzo M, Simes J. Single agent versus combination chemotherapy for metastatic breast cancer. Cochrane Database Syst Rev 2005; (2): CD003372.

Casazza AM. Experimental evaluation of anthracycline analogs. Cancer Treat Rep 1979; 63(5):835–844.

Chan S, Davidson N, Juozaityte E, Erdkamp F, Pluzanska A, Azarnia N, Lee LW. Phase III trial of liposomal doxorubicin and cyclophosphamide compared with epirubicin and cyclophosphamide as first-line therapy for metastatic breast cancer. Ann Oncol 2004; 15(10):1527–1534.

Chan S, Friedrichs K, Noel D, Pinter T, Van Belle S, Vorobiof D, Duarte R, Gil Gil M, Bodrogi I, Murray E, Yelle L, von Minckwitz G, Korec S, Simmonds P, Buzzi F, Gonzalez Mancha R, Richardson G, Walpole E, Ronzoni M, Murawsky M, Alakl M, Riva A, Crown J. Prospective randomized trial of docetaxel versus doxorubicin in patients with metastatic breast cancer. J Clin Oncol 1999; 17(8): 2341–2354.

Chaplain G, Milan C, Sgro C, Carli PM, Bonithon-Kopp C. Increased risk of acute leukemia after adjuvant chemotherapy for breast cancer: a population-based study. J Clin Oncol 2000; 18(15):2836–2842.

Clark GM, Sledge GW, Jr., Osborne CK, McGuire WL. Survival from first recurrence: relative importance of prognostic factors in 1,015 breast cancer patients. J Clin Oncol 1987; 5(1):55–61.

Coates A, Gebski V, Bishop JF, Jeal PN, Woods RL, Snyder R, Tattersall MH, Byrne M, Harvey V, Gill G. Improving the quality of life during chemotherapy for advanced breast cancer. A comparison of intermittent and continuous treatment strategies. N Engl J Med 1987; 317(24): 1490–1495.

Cobleigh MA, Langmuir VK, Sledge GW, Miller KD, Haney L, Novotny WF, Reimann JD, Vassel A. A phase I/II dose-escalation trial of bevacizumab in previously treated metastatic breast cancer. Semin Oncol 2003; 30(5 suppl 16): 117–124.

Cobleigh MA, Vogel CL, Tripathy D, Robert NJ, Scholl S, Fehrenbacher L, Wolter JM, Paton V, Shak S, Lieberman G, Slamon DJ. Multinational study of the efficacy and safety of humanized anti-HER2 monoclonal antibody in women who have HER2-overexpressing metastatic breast cancer that has progressed after chemotherapy for metastatic disease. J Clin Oncol 1999; 17(9):2639–2648.

Cocconi G, Bisagni G, Bacchi M, Buzzi F, Canaletti R, Carpi A, Ceci G, Colozza A, De Lisi V, Lottici R, Passalacqua R, Peracchia G. A comparison of continuation versus late intensification followed by discontinuation of chemotherapy in advanced breast cancer. A prospective randomized trial of the Italian Oncology Group for Clinical Research (G.O.I.R.C.). Ann Oncol 1990; 1(1):36–44.

Cocconi G, De Lisi V, Boni C, Mori P, Malacarne P, Amadori D, Giovanelli E. Chemotherapy versus combination of chemotherapy and endocrine therapy in advanced breast cancer. A prospective randomized study. Cancer 1983; 51(4):581–588.

Conte PF, Alama A, Di Marco E, Canavese G, Rosso R, Nicolin A. Cytokinetic parameters of locally advanced human breast cancer treated with diethylstilbestrol and chemotherapy. Basic Appl Histochem 1986; 30(2):227–231.

Conte PF, Baldini E, Gennari A, Michelotti A, Salvadori B, Tibaldi C, Danesi R, Innocenti F, Gentile A, Dell'Anna R, Biadi O, Mariani M, Del Tacca M. Dose-finding study and pharmacokinetics of epirubicin and paclitaxel over 3 hours: a regimen with high activity and low cardiotoxicity in advanced breast cancer. J Clin Oncol 1997; 15(7): 2510–2517.

Costanza ME, Weiss RB, Henderson IC, Norton L, Berry DA, Cirrincione C, Winer E, Wood WC, Frei E, 3rd, McIntyre OR, Schilsky RL. Safety and efficacy of using a single agent or a phase II agent before instituting standard combination chemotherapy in previously untreated metastatic breast cancer patients: report of a randomized study—Cancer and Leukemia Group B 8642. J Clin Oncol 1999; 17(5):1397–1406.

Coukell AJ, Faulds D. Epirubicin. An updated review of its pharmacodynamic and pharmacokinetic properties and therapeutic efficacy in the management of breast cancer. Drugs 1997; 53(3):453–482.

Cowan JD, Neidhart J, McClure S, Coltman CA, Jr., Gumbart C, Martino S, Hutchins LF, Stephens RL, Vaughan CB, Osborne CK. Randomized trial of doxorubicin, bisantrene, and mitoxantrone in advanced breast cancer: a Southwest Oncology Group study. J Natl Cancer Inst 1991; 83(15): 1077–1084.

D'Incalci M, Schuller J, Colombo T, Zucchetti M, Riva A. Taxoids in combination with anthracyclines and other agents: pharmacokinetic considerations. Semin Oncol 1998; 25(6 suppl 13):16–20.

Decatris MP, Sundar S, O'Byrne KJ. Platinum-based chemotherapy in metastatic breast cancer: current status. Cancer Treat Rev 2004; 30(1):53–81.

Donelli MG, Zucchetti M, Munzone E, D'Incalci M, Crosignani A. Pharmacokinetics of anticancer agents in patients with impaired liver function. Eur J Cancer 1998; 34(1):33–46.

Doroshow JH, Locker GY, Myers CE. Enzymatic defenses of the mouse heart against reactive oxygen metabolites: alterations produced by doxorubicin. J Clin Invest 1980; 65(1):128–135.

Ejlertsen B, Mouridsen HT, Langkjer ST, Andersen J, Sjostrom J, Kjaer M. Phase III study of intravenous vinorelbine in combination with epirubicin versus epirubicin alone in patients with advanced breast cancer: a Scandinavian Breast Group Trial (SBG9403). J Clin Oncol 2004; 22(12): 2313–2320.

Ejlertsen B, Pfeiffer P, Pedersen D, Mouridsen HT, Rose C, Overgaard M, Sandberg E, Kristensen B. Decreased efficacy of cyclophosphamide, epirubicin, and 5-fluorouracil in metastatic breast cancer when reducing treatment duration from 18 to 6 months. Eur J Cancer 1993; 29A:527–531.

Engelsman E, Klijn JC, Rubens RD, Wildiers J, Beex LV, Nooij MA, Rotmensz N, Sylvester R. Classical CMF versus a 3-weekly intravenous CMF schedule in postmenopausal patients with advanced breast cancer. An EORTC Breast Cancer Co-operative Group Phase III Trial (10808). Eur J Cancer 1991; 27(8):966–970.

Esposito M, Venturini M, Vannozzi MO, Tolino G, Lunardi G, Garrone O, Angiolini C, Viale M, Bergaglio M, Del Mastro L, Rosso R. Comparative effects of paclitaxel and docetaxel on the metabolism and pharmacokinetics of epirubicin in breast cancer patients. J Clin Oncol 1999; 17(4):1132.

Falkson G, Gelman RS, Pandya KJ, Osborne CK, Tormey D, Cummings FJ, Sledge GW, Abeloff MD. Eastern Cooperative Oncology Group randomized trials of observation versus maintenance therapy for patients with metastatic breast cancer in complete remission following induction treatment. J Clin Oncol 1998; 16(5):1669–1676.

Falkson G, Holcroft C, Gelman RS, Tormey DC, Wolter JM, Cummings FJ. Ten-year follow-up study of premenopausal women with metastatic breast cancer: an Eastern Cooperative Oncology Group study. J Clin Oncol 1995; 13(6): 1453–1458.

Farquhar C, Marjoribanks J, Basser R, Hetrick S, Lethaby A. High dose chemotherapy and autologous bone marrow or stem cell transplantation versus conventional chemotherapy for women with metastatic breast cancer. Cochrane Database Syst Rev 2005; (3):CD003142.

Faulds D, Balfour JA, Chrisp P, Langtry HD. Mitoxantrone. A review of its pharmacodynamic and pharmacokinetic properties, and therapeutic potential in the chemotherapy of cancer. Drugs 1991; 41(3):400–449.

Findlay BP, Walker-Dilks C. Epirubicin, alone or in combination chemotherapy, for metastatic breast cancer. Provincial Breast Cancer Disease Site Group and the Provincial Systemic Treatment Disease Site Group. Cancer Prev Control 1998; 2(3):140–146.

Focan C, Andrien JM, Closon MT, Dicato M, Driesschaert P, Focan-Henrard D, Lemaire M, Lobelle JP, Longree L, Ries F. Dose-response relationship of epirubicin-based first-line chemotherapy for advanced breast cancer: a prospective randomized trial. J Clin Oncol 1993; 11(7):1253–1263.

Fossati R, Confalonieri C, Torri V, Ghislandi E, Penna A, Pistotti V, Tinazzi A, Liberati A. Cytotoxic and hormonal treatment for metastatic breast cancer: a systematic review of published randomized trials involving 31,510 women. J Clin Oncol 1998; 16(10):3439–3460.

French Epirubicin Study Group. A prospective randomized trial comparing epirubicin monochemotherapy to two fluorouracil, cyclophosphamide, and epirubicin regimens differing in epirubicin dose in advanced breast cancer patients. The French Epirubicin Study Group. J Clin Oncol 1991; 9(2): 305–312.

French Epirubicin Study Group. Epirubicin-based chemotherapy in metastatic breast cancer patients: role of dose-intensity and duration of treatment. J Clin Oncol 2000; 18(17): 3115–3124.

Friedman MA, Bozdech MJ, Billingham ME, Rider AK. Doxorubicin cardiotoxicity. Serial endomyocardial biopsies and systolic time intervals. JAMA 1978; 240(15): 1603–1606.

Fulton B, Spencer CM. Docetaxel. A review of its pharmacodynamic and pharmacokinetic properties and therapeutic efficacy in the management of metastatic breast cancer. Drugs 1996; 51(6):1075–1092.

Fumoleau P, Delgado FM, Delozier T, Monnier A, Gil Delgado MA, Kerbrat P, Garcia-Giralt E, Keiling R, Namer M, Closon MT. Phase II trial of weekly intravenous vinorelbine in first-line advanced breast cancer chemotherapy. J Clin Oncol 1993; 11(7):1245–1252.

Gabizon A, Catane R, Uziely B, Kaufman B, Safra T, Cohen R, Martin F, Huang A, Barenholz Y. Prolonged circulation time and enhanced accumulation in malignant exudates of doxorubicin encapsulated in polyethylene-glycol coated liposomes. Cancer Res 1994; 54(4):987–992.

Gabizon A, Chisin R, Amselem S, Druckmann S, Cohen R, Goren D, Fromer I, Peretz T, Sulkes A, Barenholz Y. Pharmacokinetic and imaging studies in patients receiving a formulation of liposome-associated adriamycin. Br J Cancer 1991; 64(6):1125–1132.

Gabizon A, Shmeeda H, Barenholz Y. Pharmacokinetics of pegylated liposomal Doxorubicin: review of animal and human studies. Clin Pharmacokinet 2003; 42(5):419–436.

Gasparini G, Dal Fior S, Panizzoni GA, Favretto S, Pozza F. Weekly epirubicin versus doxorubicin as second line therapy in advanced breast cancer. A randomized clinical trial. Am J Clin Oncol 1991; 14(1):38–44.

Geels P, Eisenhauer E, Bezjak A, Zee B, Day A. Palliative effect of chemotherapy: objective tumor response is associated with symptom improvement in patients with metastatic breast cancer. J Clin Oncol 2000; 18(12):2395–2405.

Gehl J, Boesgaard M, Paaske T, Vittrup Jensen B, Dombernowsky P. Combined doxorubicin and paclitaxel in advanced breast cancer: effective and cardiotoxic. Ann Oncol 1996; 7(7):687–693.

Gennari A, Amadori D, De Lena M, Nanni O, Bruzzi P, Lorusso V, Manzione L, Conte PF. Lack of benefit of maintenance paclitaxel in first-line chemotherapy in metastatic breast cancer. J Clin Oncol 2006; 24(24):3912–3918.

Geyer CE, Forster J, Lindquist D, Chan S, Romieu CG, Pienkowski T, Jagiello-Gruszfeld A, Crown J, Chan A, Kaufman B, Skarlos D, Campone M, Davidson N, Berger M, Oliva C, Rubin SD, Stein S, Cameron D. Lapatinib plus capecitabine for HER2-positive advanced breast cancer. N Engl J Med 2006; 355(26):2733–2743.

Ghersi D, Wilcken N, Simes J, Donoghue E. Taxane containing regimens for metastatic breast cancer. Cochrane Database Syst Rev 2005; (2):CD003366.

Gianni L, Munzone E, Capri G, Fulfaro F, Tarenzi E, Villani F, Spreafico C, Laffranchi A, Caraceni A, Martini C. Paclitaxel by 3-hour infusion in combination with bolus doxorubicin in women with untreated metastatic breast cancer: high antitumor efficacy and cardiac effects in a dose-finding and sequence-finding study. J Clin Oncol 1995; 13(11):2688–2699.

Gianni L, Vigano L, Locatelli A, Capri G, Giani A, Tarenzi E, Bonadonna G. Human pharmacokinetic characterization and in vitro study of the interaction between doxorubicin and paclitaxel in patients with breast cancer. J Clin Oncol 1997; 15(5):1906–1915.

Go RS, Adjei AA. Review of the comparative pharmacology and clinical activity of cisplatin and carboplatin. J Clin Oncol 1999; 17(1):409–422.

Gradishar W, Krasnojon D, Cheporov S, Makhson A, Manikhas G, Clawson A, Hawkins MJ. Randomized comparison of weekly or every-3-week (q3w) nab-paclitaxel compared to q3w docetaxel as first-line therapy in patients (pts) with metastatic breast cancer (MBC). ASCO Annual Meeting Proceedings (Post-Meeting Edition). J Clin Oncol 2007; 25 (18S):1032 (abstr).

Gradishar WJ, Tjulandin S, Davidson N, Shaw H, Desai N, Bhar P, Hawkins M, O'Shaughnessy J. Phase III trial of nanoparticle albumin-bound paclitaxel compared with polyethylated castor oil-based paclitaxel in women with breast cancer. J Clin Oncol 2005; 23(31):7794–7803.

Gundersen S, Hannisdal E, Lundgren S, Wist E. Weekly doxorubicin with or without high-dose medroxyprogesterone acetate in hormone-resistant advanced breast cancer. A randomised study. The Norwegian Breast Cancer Group. Eur J Cancer 1994; 30A(12):1775–1778.

Gundersen S, Kvinnsland S, Klepp O, Lund E, Host H. Weekly Adriamycin vs. 4-epidoxorubicin every second week in advanced breast cancer. A randomized trial. The Norwegian Breast Cancer Group. Eur J Cancer 1990; 26(1):45–48.

Habeshaw T, Paul J, Jones R, Stallard S, Stewart M, Kaye SB, Soukop M, Symonds RP, Reed NS, Rankin EM. Epirubicin at two dose levels with prednisolone as treatment for advanced breast cancer: the results of a randomized trial. J Clin Oncol 1991; 9(2):295–304.

Harper-Wynne C, English J, Meyer L, Bower M, Archer C, Sinnett HD, Lowdell C, Coombes RC. Randomized trial to compare the efficacy and toxicity of cyclophosphamide, methotrexate and 5-fluorouracil (CMF) with methotrexate mitoxantrone (MM) in advanced carcinoma of the breast. Br J Cancer 1999; 81(2):316–322.

Harris L, Batist G, Belt R, Rovira D, Navari R, Azarnia N, Welles L, Winer E. Liposome-encapsulated doxorubicin compared with conventional doxorubicin in a randomized multicenter trial as first-line therapy of metastatic breast carcinoma. Cancer 2002; 94(1):25–36.

Harris M, Howell A, Chrissohou M, Swindell RI, Hudson M, Sellwood RA. A comparison of the metastatic pattern of infiltrating lobular carcinoma and infiltrating duct carcinoma of the breast. Br J Cancer 1984; 50(1):23–30.

Henderson IC. Chemotherapy for metastatic disease. In: Harris JR, Hellman S, Henderson IC, et al (eds). Breast Diseases. 2nd ed. Philadelphia, PA: J.B. Lippincott Company, 1991:604–665

Henderson IC, Allegra JC, Woodcock T, Wolff S, Bryan S, Cartwright K, Dukart G, Henry D. Randomized clinical trial comparing mitoxantrone with doxorubicin in previously treated patients with metastatic breast cancer. J Clin Oncol 1989; 7(5):560–571.

Hennessy BT, Gauthier AM, Michaud LB, Hortobagyi G, Valero V. Lower dose capecitabine has a more favorable therapeutic index in metastatic breast cancer: retrospective analysis of patients treated at M. D. Anderson Cancer Center and a review of capecitabine toxicity in the literature. Ann Oncol 2005; 16(8):1289–1296.

Hillner BE, Ingle JN, Berenson JR, Janjan NA, Albain KS, Lipton A, Yee G, Biermann JS, Chlebowski RT, Pfister DG. American Society of Clinical Oncology guideline on the role of bisphosphonates in breast cancer. American Society of Clinical Oncology Bisphosphonates Expert Panel. J Clin Oncol 2000; 18(6):1378–1391.

Hillner BE, Ingle JN, Chlebowski RT, Gralow J, Yee GC, Janjan NA, Cauley JA, Blumenstein BA, Albain KS, Lipton A, Brown S. American Society of Clinical Oncology 2003 update on the role of bisphosphonates and bone health issues in women with breast cancer. J Clin Oncol 2003; 21(21):4042–4057.

Holmes FA, Valero V, Buzdar A, Booser DJ, Winn R, Tolcher A, Seidman A, Goodwin W, Bearden J, Baysinger L, Hortobagyi GN, Arbuck SA. Final results: randomized phase III trials of paclitaxel by 3-hr versus 96-hr infusion in patients with metastatic breast cancer; the long & short of it. Proc Am Soc Clin Oncol 1998; 17:110a.

Hortobagyi GN, Smith TL, Legha SS, Swenerton KD, Gehan EA, Yap HY, Buzdar AU, Blumenschein GR. Multivariate analysis of prognostic factors in metastatic breast cancer. J Clin Oncol 1983; 1(12):776–786.

Hortobagyi GN, Theriault RL, Porter L, Blayney D, Lipton A, Sinoff C, Wheeler H, Simeone JF, Seaman J, Knight RD. Efficacy of pamidronate in reducing skeletal complications in patients with breast cancer and lytic bone metastases. Protocol 19 Aredia Breast Cancer Study Group. N Engl J Med 1996; 335(24):1785–1791.

Hortobagyi GN, Theriault RL, Lipton A, Porter L, Blayney D, Sinoff C, Wheeler H, Simeone JF, Seaman JJ, Knight RD, Heffernan M, Mellars K, Reitsma DJ. Long-term prevention of skeletal complications of metastatic breast cancer with pamidronate. Protocol 19 Aredia Breast Cancer Study Group. J Clin Oncol 1998; 16(6):2038–2044.

Hortobagyi GN, Yap HY, Kau SW, Fraschini G, Ewer MS, Chawla SP, Benjamin RS. A comparative study of doxorubicin and epirubicin in patients with metastatic breast cancer. Am J Clin Oncol 1989; 12(1):57–62.

Hudis CA. Trastuzumab–mechanism of action and use in clinical practice. N Engl J Med 2007; 357(1):39–51.

Italian Epirubicin Study Group. Phase III randomized study of fluorouracil, epirubicin, and cyclophosphamide v fluorouracil, doxorubicin, and cyclophosphamide in advanced breast cancer: an Italian multicoated trial. Italian Multicentre Breast Study with Epirubicin. J Clin Oncol 1988; 6(6):976–982.

Ishikawa T, Sekiguchi F, Fukase Y, Sawada N, Ishitsuka H. Positive correlation between the efficacy of capecitabine and doxifluridine and the ratio of thymidine phosphorylase to dihydropyrimidine dehydrogenase activities in tumors in human cancer xenografts. Cancer Res 1998; 58:685–690.

Jassem J, Pienkowski T, Pluzanska A, Jelic S, Gorbunova V, Mrsic-Krmpotic Z, Berzins J, Nagykalnai T, Wigler N, Renard J, Munier S, Weil C. Doxorubicin and paclitaxel versus fluorouracil, doxorubicin, and cyclophosphamide as first-line therapy for women with metastatic breast cancer: final results of a randomized phase III multicenter trial. J Clin Oncol 2001; 19(6):1707–1715.

Johnson JR, Williams G, Pazdur R. End points and United States Food and Drug Administration approval of oncology drugs. J Clin Oncol 2003; 21(7):1404–1411.

Jones SE, Erban J, Overmoyer B, Budd GT, Hutchins L, Lower E, Laufman L, Sundaram S, Urba WJ, Pritchard KI, Mennel R, Richards D, Olsen S, Meyers ML, Ravdin PM. Randomized phase III study of docetaxel compared with paclitaxel in metastatic breast cancer. J Clin Oncol 2005; 23(24):5542–5551.

Jones D, Ghersi D, Wilcken N. Addition of drug/s to a chemotherapy regimen for metastatic breast cancer. Cochrane Database Syst Rev 2006; 3:CD003368.

Jones RB, Holland JF, Bhardwaj S, Norton L, Wilfinger C, Strashun A. A phase I–II study of intensive-dose adriamycin for advanced breast cancer. J Clin Oncol 1987; 5:172–178.

Jones S, Winer E, Vogel C, Laufman L, Hutchins L, O'Rourke M, Lembersky B, Budman D, Bigley J, Hohneker J. Randomized comparison of vinorelbine and melphalan in anthracycline-refractory advanced breast cancer. J Clin Oncol 1995; 13(10):2567–2574.

Jordan MA, Wendell K, Gardiner S, Derry WB, Copp H, Wilson L. Mitotic block induced in HeLa cells by low concentrations of paclitaxel (Taxol) results in abnormal mitotic exit and apoptotic cell death. Cancer Res 1996; 56(4): 816–825.

Kanter PM, Bullard GA, Ginsberg RA, Pilkiewicz FG, Mayer LD, Cullis PR, Pavelic ZP. Comparison of the cardiotoxic effects of liposomal doxorubicin (TLC D-99) versus free doxorubicin in beagle dogs. In Vivo 1993a; 7(1):17–26.

Kanter PM, Bullard GA, Pilkiewicz FG, Mayer LD, Cullis PR, Pavelic ZP. Preclinical toxicology study of liposome encapsulated doxorubicin (TLC D-99): comparison with doxorubicin and empty liposomes in mice and dogs. In Vivo 1993b; 7(1):85–95.

Keller AM, Mennel RG, Georgoulias VA, Nabholtz JM, Erazo A, Lluch A, Vogel CL, Kaufmann M, von Minckwitz G, Henderson IC, Mellars L, Alland L, Tendler C. Randomized phase III trial of pegylated liposomal doxorubicin versus vinorelbine or mitomycin C plus vinblastine in women with taxane-refractory advanced breast cancer. J Clin Oncol 2004; 22(19):3893–3901.

Langley RE, Carmichael J, Jones AL, Cameron DA, Qian W, Uscinska B, Howell A, Parmar M. Phase III trial of epirubicin plus paclitaxel compared with epirubicin plus cyclophosphamide as first-line chemotherapy for metastatic breast cancer: United Kingdom National Cancer Research Institute trial AB01. J Clin Oncol 2005; 23 (33):8322–8330.

Lanza LA, Natarajan G, Roth JA, Putnam JB, Jr. Long-term survival after resection of pulmonary metastases from carcinoma of the breast. Ann Thorac Surg 1992; 54(2): 244–247; discussion 248.

Larkin JM, Kaye SB. Epothilones in the treatment of cancer. Expert Opin Investig Drugs 2006; 15(6):691–702.

Leonard RC, Cornbleet MA, Kaye SB, Soukop M, White G, Hutcheon AW, Robinson S, Kerr ME, Smyth JF. Mitoxantrone versus doxorubicin in combination chemotherapy for advanced carcinoma of the breast. J Clin Oncol 1987; 5(7):1056–1063.

Leonard R, O'Shaughnessy J, Vukelja S, Gorbounova V, Chan-Navarro CA, Maraninchi D, Barak-Wigler N, McKendrick JJ, Harker WG, Bexon AS, Twelves C. Detailed analysis of a randomized phase III trial: can the tolerability of capecitabine plus docetaxel be improved without compromising its survival advantage? Ann Oncol 2006; 17(9):1379–1385.

Lewis R, Bagnall AM, King S, Woolacott N, Forbes C, Shirran L, Duffy S, Kleijnen J, ter Riet G, Riemsma R. The clinical effectiveness and cost-effectiveness of vinorelbine for breast cancer: a systematic review and economic evaluation. Health Technol Assess 2002; 6(14):1–269.

Liesmann J, Belt R, Haas C, Hoogstraten B. Phase I evaluation of ICRF-187 (NSC-169780) in patients with advanced malignancy. Cancer 1981; 47(8):1959–1962.

Lippman ME, Cassidy J, Wesley M, Young RC. A randomized attempt to increase the efficacy of cytotoxic chemotherapy in metastatic breast cancer by hormonal synchronization. J Clin Oncol 1984; 2(1):28–36.

Lipton A, Santen RJ, Harvey HA, Manni A, Simmonds MA, White-Hershey D, Bartholomew MJ, Walker BK, Dixon RH, Valdevia DE. A randomized trial of aminoglutethimide +/− estrogen before chemotherapy in advanced breast cancer. Am J Clin Oncol 1987; 10(1):65–70.

Llombart-Cussac A, Martin M, Harbeck N, Anghel RM, Eniu AE, Verrill MW, Neven P, De Greve J, Melemed AS, Clark R, Simms L, Kaiser CJ, Ma D. A randomized, double-blind, phase II study of two doses of pemetrexed as first-line chemotherapy for advanced breast cancer. Clin Cancer Res 2007; 13(12):3652–3659.

Loesch D, Robert N, Asmar L, Gregurich MA, O'Rourke M, Dakhil S, Cox E. Phase II multicenter trial of a weekly paclitaxel and carboplatin regimen in patients with advanced breast cancer. J Clin Oncol 2002; 20(18):3857–3864.

Lord S, Ghersi D, Gattellari M, Wortley S, Wilcken N, Simes J. Antitumour antibiotic containing regimens for metastatic breast cancer. Cochrane Database Syst Rev 2004; (4):CD003367.

Macquart-Moulin G, Viens P, Bouscary ML, Genre D, Resbeut M, Gravis G, Camerlo J, Maraninchi D, Moatti JP. Discordance between physicians' estimations and breast cancer patients' self-assessment of side-effects of chemotherapy: an issue for quality of care. Br J Cancer 1997; 76(12): 1640–1645.

Martin M, Diaz-Rubio E, Casado A, Santabarbara P, Lopez Vega JM, Adrover E, Lenaz L. Carboplatin: an active drug in metastatic breast cancer. J Clin Oncol 1992; 10(3):433–437.

Martin M, Ruiz A, Munoz M, Balil A, Garcia-Mata J, Calvo L, Carrasco E, Mahillo E, Casado A, Garcia-Saenz JA, Escudero MJ, Guillem V, Jara C, Ribelles N, Salas F, Soto C, Morales-Vasquez F, Rodriguez CA, Adrover E, Mel JR. Gemcitabine plus vinorelbine versus vinorelbine monotherapy in patients with metastatic breast cancer previously treated with anthracyclines and taxanes: final results of the phase III Spanish Breast Cancer Research Group (GEICAM) trial. Lancet Oncol 2007; 8(3):219–225.

Marty M, Cognetti F, Maraninchi D, Snyder R, Mauriac L, Tubiana-Hulin M, Chan S, Grimes D, Anton A, Lluch A, Kennedy J, O'Byrne K, Conte P, Green M, Ward C, Mayne K, Extra JM. Randomized phase II trial of the efficacy and safety of trastuzumab combined with docetaxel in patients with human epidermal growth factor receptor 2-positive metastatic breast cancer administered as first-line treatment: the M77001 study group. J Clin Oncol 2005; 23(19):4265–4274.

Marty M, Espie M, Llombart A, Monnier A, Rapoport BL, Stahalova V. Multicenter randomized phase III study of the cardioprotective effect of dexrazoxane (Cardioxane) in advanced/metastatic breast cancer patients treated with anthracycline-based chemotherapy. Ann Oncol 2006; 17 (4):614–622.

Marty M, Extra JM, Dieras V, Giacchetti S, Ohana S, Espie M. A review of the antitumour activity of vinorelbine in breast cancer. Drugs 1992; 44(suppl 4):29–35; discussion 66–69.

Mayordomo J, Tres A, Miles D, Finke L, Jenkins H. Long-term follow-up of patients concomitantly treated with hormone therapy in a prospective controlled randomized multicenter clinical study comparing STn-KLH vaccine with KLH control in stage IV breast cancer following first-line chemotherapy. J Clin Oncol 2004; 22:2603 (abstr).

Melillo LM, Sajeva MR, Musto P, Perla G, Cascavilla N, Minervini MM, D'Arena G, Carotenuto M. Acute myeloid leukemia following 3M (mitoxantrone, mitomycin and methotrexate) chemotherapy for advanced breast cancer. Leukemia 1997; 11(12):2211–2213.

Miller KD, Chap LI, Holmes FA, Cobleigh MA, Marcom PK, Fehrenbacher L, Dickler M, Overmoyer BA, Reimann JD, Sing AP, Langmuir V, Rugo HS. Randomized phase III trial of capecitabine compared with bevacizumab plus capecitabine in patients with previously treated metastatic breast cancer. J Clin Oncol 2005; 23(4):792–799.

Miller K, Wang M, Gralow J, Dickler M, Cobleigh M, Perez EA, Shenkier T, Cella D, Davidson NE. Paclitaxel plus bevacizumab versus paclitaxel alone for metastatic breast cancer. N Engl J Med 2007; 57(26):2666–2676.

Mouridsen HT, Rose C, Engelsman E, Sylvester R, Rotmensz N. Combined cytotoxic and endocrine therapy in postmenopausal patients with advanced breast cancer. A randomized study of CMF vs CMF plus tamoxifen. Eur J Cancer Clin Oncol 1985; 21(3):291–299.

Moy B, Kirkpatrick P, Kar S, Goss P. Lapatinib. Nat Rev Drug Discov 2007; 6(6):431–432.

Mrozek E, Rhoades CA, Allen J, Hade EM, Shapiro CL. Phase I trial of liposomal encapsulated doxorubicin (Myocet; D-99) and weekly docetaxel in advanced breast cancer patients. Ann Oncol 2005; 16(7):1087–1093.

Muss HB, Case LD, Richards F, 2nd, White DR, Cooper MR, Cruz JM, Powell BL, Spurr CL, Capizzi RL. Interrupted versus continuous chemotherapy in patients with metastatic breast cancer. The Piedmont Oncology Association. N Engl J Med 1991; 325(19):1342–1348.

Myers C. The role of iron in doxorubicin-induced cardiomyopathy. Semin Oncol 1998; 25(4 suppl 10):10–14.

Nabholtz JM, Falkson C, Campos D, Szanto J, Martin M, Chan S, Pienkowski T, Zaluski J, Pinter T, Krzakowski M, Vorobiof D, Leonard R, Kennedy I, Azli N, Murawsky M, Riva A, Pouillart P. Docetaxel and doxorubicin compared with doxorubicin and cyclophosphamide as first-line chemotherapy for metastatic breast cancer: results of a randomized, multicenter, phase III trial. J Clin Oncol 2003; 21(6):968–975.

Nabholtz JM, Gelmon K, Bontenbal M, Spielmann M, Catimel G, Conte P, Klaassen U, Namer M, Bonneterre J, Fumoleau P, Winograd B. Multicenter, randomized comparative study of two doses of paclitaxel in patients with metastatic breast cancer. J Clin Oncol 1996; 14(6):1858–1867.

Nabholtz JM, Senn HJ, Bezwoda WR, Melnychuk D, Deschenes L, Douma J, Vandenberg TA, Rapoport B, Rosso R, Trillet-Lenoir V, Drbal J, Molino A, Nortier JW, Richel DJ, Nagykalnai T, Siedlecki P, Wilking N, Genot JY, Hupperets PS, Pannuti F, Skarlos D, Tomiak EM, Murawsky M, Alakl M, Aapro M. Prospective randomized trial of docetaxel versus mitomycin plus vinblastine in patients with metastatic breast cancer progressing despite previous anthracycline-containing chemotherapy. 304 Study Group. J Clin Oncol 1999; 17(5):1413–1424.

Neidhart JA, Gochnour D, Roach R, Hoth D, Young D. A comparison of mitoxantrone and doxorubicin in breast cancer. J Clin Oncol 1986; 4(5):672–677.

Nielsen OS, Munro AJ, Tannock IF. Bone metastases: pathophysiology and management policy. J Clin Oncol 1991; 9(3):509–524.

Noble S, Goa KL. Gemcitabine. A review of its pharmacology and clinical potential in non-small cell lung cancer and pancreatic cancer. Drugs 1997; 54(3):447–472.

Norris B, Pritchard KI, James K, Myles J, Bennett K, Marlin S, Skillings J, Findlay B, Vandenberg T, Goss P, Latreille J, Rudinskas L, Lofters W, Trudeau M, Osoba D, Rodgers A. Phase III comparative study of vinorelbine combined with doxorubicin versus doxorubicin alone in disseminated metastatic/recurrent breast cancer: National Cancer Institute of Canada Clinical Trials Group Study MA8. J Clin Oncol 2000; 18(12):2385–2394.

O'Brien ME, Talbot DC, Smith IE. Carboplatin in the treatment of advanced breast cancer: a phase II study using a pharmacokinetically guided dose schedule. J Clin Oncol 1993; 11(11):2112–2117.

O'Brien ME, Wigler N, Inbar M, Rosso R, Grischke E, Santoro A, Catane R, Kieback DG, Tomczak P, Ackland SP, Orlandi F, Mellars L, Alland L, Tendler C. Reduced cardiotoxicity and comparable efficacy in a phase III trial of pegylated liposomal doxorubicin HCl (CAELYX/Doxil) versus conventional doxorubicin for first-line treatment of metastatic breast cancer. Ann Oncol 2004; 15(3):440–449.

Oken MM, Creech RH, Tormey DC, Horton J, Davis TE, McFadden ET, Carbone PP. Toxicity and response criteria of the Eastern Cooperative Oncology Group. Am J Clin Oncol 1982; 5(6):649–655.

O'Shaughnessy JA, Blum J, Moiseyenko V, Jones SE, Miles D, Bell D, Rosso R, Mauriac L, Osterwalder B, Burger HU, Laws S. Randomized, open-label, phase II trial of oral capecitabine (Xeloda) vs. a reference arm of intravenous CMF (cyclophosphamide, methotrexate and 5-fluorouracil) as first-line therapy for advanced/metastatic breast cancer. Ann Oncol 2001; 12(9):1247–1254.

O'Shaughnessy J, Miles D, Vukelja S, Moiseyenko V, Ayoub JP, Cervantes G, Fumoleau P, Jones S, Lui WY, Mauriac L, Twelves C, Van Hazel G, Verma S, Leonard R. Superior survival with capecitabine plus docetaxel combination therapy in anthracycline-pretreated patients with advanced breast cancer: phase III trial results. J Clin Oncol 2002; 20(12):2812–2823.

O'Shaughnessy J, Moiseyenko J, Bell D, Nabholtz JM, Miles D, Gorbunova V, Laws S, Griffin T, Osterwalder B. A randomized phase II study of Xeloda™ (capecitabine) vs. CMF as first-line chemotherapy of breast cancer in women > 55 years. Proc Am Soc Clin Oncol 1998; 17:(abstr 398).

Paridaens R, Biganzoli L, Bruning P, Klijn JG, Gamucci T, Houston S, Coleman R, Schachter J, Van Vreckem A, Sylvester R, Awada A, Wildiers J, Piccart M. Paclitaxel versus doxorubicin as first-line single-agent chemotherapy for metastatic breast cancer: a European Organization for Research and Treatment of Cancer Randomized Study with cross-over. J Clin Oncol 2000; 18(4):724–733.

Peretz T, Sulkes A, Chollet P, Gelmon K, Paridaens R, Gorbonuva V, Catimel G, Kuhnle H, ten Bokkel Huinink W, Khayat D, Ditrich C, Klaassen U, Bergh J, Wilking N, Nabholtz JM, Calabresi F, Tubiana-Hulin M, Chazard M, Gallant G, Diergarten K, Westberg R, Bogaert J, Renard J, Weil C. A multicenter, randomized study of two schedules of paclitaxel in patients with advanced breast cancer. Proc Eur J Cancer 1995; 31(s75):345 (abstr).

Perez EA, Suman VJ, Rowland KM, Ingle JN, Salim M, Loprinzi CL, Flynn PJ, Mailliard JA, Kardinal CG, Krook JE, Thrower AR, Visscher DW, Jenkins RB. Two concurrent phase II trials of paclitaxel/carboplatin/trastuzumab (weekly or every-3-week schedule) as first-line therapy in women with HER2-overexpressing metastatic breast cancer: NCCTG study 983252. Clin Breast Cancer 2005; 6(5):425–432.

Perez EA, Vogel CL, Irwin DH, Kirshner JJ, Patel R. Multicenter phase II trial of weekly paclitaxel in women with metastatic breast cancer. J Clin Oncol 2001; 19(22):4216–4223.

Perry MC, Kardinal CG, Korzun AH, Ginsberg SJ, Raich PC, Holland JF, Ellison RR, Kopel S, Schilling A, Aisner J. Chemohormonal therapy in advanced carcinoma of the breast: Cancer and Leukemia Group B protocol 8081. J Clin Oncol 1987; 5(10):1534–1545.

Pocard M, Pouillart P, Asselain B, Salmon R. Hepatic resection in metastatic breast cancer: results and prognostic factors. Eur J Surg Oncol 2000; 26(2):155–159.

Rahman ZU, Frye DK, Buzdar AU, Smith TL, Asmar L, Champlin RE, Hortobagyi GN. Impact of selection process on response rate and long-term survival of potential high-dose chemotherapy candidates treated with standard-dose doxorubicin-containing chemotherapy in patients with metastatic breast cancer. J Clin Oncol 1997; 15(10):3171–3177.

Rahman ZU, Frye DK, Smith TL, Asmar L, Theriault RL, Buzdar AU, Hortobagyi GN. Results and long term follow-up for 1581 patients with metastatic breast carcinoma treated with standard dose doxorubicin-containing chemotherapy: a reference. Cancer 1999; 85(1):104–111.

Robert N, Leyland-Jones B, Asmar L, Belt R, Ilegbodu D, Loesch D, Raju R, Valentine E, Sayre R, Cobleigh M, Albain K, McCullough C, Fuchs L, Slamon D. Randomized phase III study of trastuzumab, paclitaxel, and carboplatin compared with trastuzumab and paclitaxel in women with HER-2-overexpressing metastatic breast cancer. J Clin Oncol 2006; 24(18):2786–2792.

Robert N J, Vogel CL, Henderson IC, Sparano JA, Moore MR, Silverman P, Overmoyer BA, Shapiro CL, Park JW, Colbern GT, Winer EP, Gabizon AA. The role of the liposomal anthracyclines and other systemic therapies in the management of advanced breast cancer. Semin Oncol 2004; 31 (6 suppl 13):106–146.

Robinson DM, Keating GM. Albumin-bound Paclitaxel: in metastatic breast cancer. Drugs 2006; 66(7):941–948.

Roche H, Yelle L, Cognetti F, Mauriac L, Bunnell C, Sparano J, Kerbrat P, Delord JP, Vahdat L, Peck R, Lebwohl D, Ezzeddine R, Cure H. Phase II clinical trial of ixabepilone (BMS-247550), an epothilone b analog, as first-line therapy in patients with metastatic breast cancer previously treated with anthracycline chemotherapy. J Clin Oncol 2007; 25 (23):3415–3420.

Rosen LS, Gordon D, Kaminski M, Howell A, Belch A, Mackey J, Apffelstaedt J, Hussein M, Coleman RE, Reitsma DJ, Seaman JJ, Chen BL, Ambros Y. Zoledronic acid versus pamidronate in the treatment of skeletal metastases in patients with breast cancer or osteolytic lesions of multiple myeloma: a phase III, double-blind, comparative trial. Cancer J 2001; 7(5):377–387.

Rosenman J, Churchill CA, Mauro MA, Parker LA, Newsome J. The role of computed tomography in the evaluation of post-mastectomy locally recurrent breast cancer. Int J Radiat Oncol Biol Phys 1988; 14:57–62.

Ross MB, Buzdar AU, Smith TL, Eckles N, Hortobagyi GN, Blumenschein GR, Freireich EJ, Gehan EA. Improved survival of patients with metastatic breast cancer receiving combination chemotherapy. Cancer 1985; 55(2):341–346.

Saphner T, Tormey DC, Gray R. Annual hazard rates of recurrence for breast cancer after primary therapy. J Clin Oncol 1996; 14(10):2738–2746.

Schiff PB, Fant J, Horwitz SB. Promotion of microtubule assembly in vitro by taxol. Nature 1979; 277(5698):665–667.

Schneider BP, Miller KD. Angiogenesis of breast cancer. J Clin Oncol 2005; 23(8):1782–1790.

Schuller J, Cassady J, Reigner BG, Durston S, Roos B, Ishitsuka H, Utoh M, Dumont E. Tumor selectivity of Xeloda in colorectal cancer patients. Proc Am Soc Clin Oncol 1997; 16(227a) (abstr).

Seidman AD, Berry D, Cirrincione C, Harris L, Dressler L, Muss H, Norton L, Winer E, Hudis C. CALGB 9840:Phase III study of weekly (W) paclitaxel (P) via 1-hour infusion versus standard (S) 3 hour infusion every third week in the treatment of metastatic breast cancer (MBC), with trastuzumab(T) for HER2 positive MBC and randomized for T in HER2 normal MBC. Proc Am Soc Clin Oncol 2004; 22:512 (abstr).

Seidman AD, Hudis CA, Albanell J, Tong W, Tepler I, Currie V, Moynahan ME, Theodoulou M, Gollub M, Baselga J, Norton L. Dose-dense therapy with weekly 1-hour paclitaxel infusions in the treatment of metastatic breast cancer. J Clin Oncol 1998; 16(10):3353–3361.

Seidman A, Hudis C, Pierri MK, Shak S, Paton V, Ashby M, Murphy M, Stewart SJ, Keefe D. Cardiac dysfunction in the trastuzumab clinical trials experience. J Clin Oncol 2002; 20(5):1215–1221.

Shak S. Overview of the trastuzumab (Herceptin) anti-HER2 monoclonal antibody clinical program in HER2-overexpressing metastatic breast cancer. Herceptin Multinational Investigator Study Group. Semin Oncol 1999; 26(4 suppl 12):71–77.

Shapiro CL, Ervin T, Welles L, Azarnia N, Keating J, Hayes DF. Phase II trial of high-dose liposome-encapsulated doxorubicin with granulocyte colony-stimulating factor in metastatic breast cancer. TLC D-99 Study Group. J Clin Oncol 1999; 17(5):1435–1441.

Sjostrom J, Blomqvist C, Mouridsen H, Pluzanska A, Ottosson-Lonn S, Bengtsson NO, Ostenstad B, Mjaaland I, Palm-Sjovall M, Wist E, Valvere V, Anderson H, Bergh J. Docetaxel compared with sequential methotrexate and 5-fluorouracil in patients with advanced breast cancer after anthracycline failure: a randomised phase III study with crossover on progression by the Scandinavian Breast Group. Eur J Cancer 1999; 35(8):1194–1201.

Slamon DJ, Godolphin W, Jones LA, Holt JA, Wong SG, Keith DE, Levin WJ, Stuart SG, Udove J, Ullrich A. Studies of the HER-2/neu proto-oncogene in human breast and ovarian cancer. Science 1989; 244(4905):707–712.

Slamon DJ, Leyland-Jones B, Shak S, Fuchs H, Paton V, Bajamonde A, Fleming T, Eiermann W, Wolter J, Pegram M, Baselga J, Norton L. Use of chemotherapy plus a monoclonal antibody against HER2 for metastatic breast cancer that overexpresses HER2. N Engl J Med 2001; 344(11):783–792.

Slamon D, Leyland-Jones B, Shak S, Paton V, Bajamonde A, Fleming T, Eiermann W, Wolter J, Baselga J, Norton L. Addition of Herceptin™ (humanized anti-her2 antibody) to first line chemotherapy for her2 overexpressing metastatic breast cancer markedly increased anticancer activity: a randomized, multinational controlled phase III trial. Proc Am Soc Clin Oncol 1998; 17(98a) (abstr 377).

Sledge GW Jr., Hu P, Falkson G, Tormey D, Abeloff M. Comparison of chemotherapy with chemohormonal therapy as first-line therapy for metastatic, hormone-sensitive breast cancer: An Eastern Cooperative Oncology Group study. J Clin Oncol 2000; 18(2):262–266.

Sledge GW Jr., Loehrer PJ Sr., Roth BJ, Einhorn LH. Cisplatin as first-line therapy for metastatic breast cancer. J Clin Oncol 1988; 6(12):1811–1814.

Sledge GW Jr., Roth BJ. Cisplatin in the management of breast cancer. Semin Oncol 1989; 16(4 suppl 6):110–115.

Sledge GW, Neuberg D, Bernardo P, Ingle JN, Martino S, Rowinsky EK, Wood WC. Phase III trial of doxorubicin, paclitaxel, and the combination of doxorubicin and paclitaxel as front-line chemotherapy for metastatic breast cancer: an intergroup trial (E1193). J Clin Oncol 2003; 21(4):588–592.

Smith RE, Brown AM, Mamounas EP, Anderson SJ, Lembersky BC, Atkins JH, Shibata HR, Baez L, DeFusco PA, Davila E, Tipping SJ, Bearden JD, Thirlwell MP. Randomized trial of 3-hour versus 24-hour infusion of high-dose paclitaxel in patients with metastatic or locally advanced breast cancer: National Surgical Adjuvant Breast and Bowel Project Protocol B-26. J Clin Oncol 1999; 17(11):3403–3411.

Sparano JA. Compilation of phase I and II trial data of docetaxel and doxorubicin in the treatment of advanced breast cancer and other malignancies. Semin Oncol 1998; 25(6 suppl 13):10–15.

Sparano JA. Taxanes for breast cancer: an evidence-based review of randomized phase II and phase III trials. Clin Breast Cancer 2000; 1(1):32–40; discussion 41–42.

Sparano JA, Bernardo P, Stephenson P, Gradishar WJ, Ingle JN, Zucker S, Davidson NE. Randomized phase III trial of marimastat versus placebo in patients with metastatic breast cancer who have responding or stable disease after first-line chemotherapy: Eastern Cooperative Oncology Group trial E2196. J Clin Oncol 2004; 22(23):4683–4690.

Sparano JA, Hu P, Rao RM, Falkson CI, Wolff AC, Wood WC. Phase II trial of doxorubicin and paclitaxel plus granulocyte colony-stimulating factor in metastatic breast cancer: an Eastern Cooperative Oncology Group Study. J Clin Oncol 1999; 17(12):3828–3834.

Sparano JA, O'Neill A, Schaefer PL, Falkson CI, Wood WC. Phase II trial of doxorubicin and docetaxel plus granulocyte colony-stimulating factor in metastatic breast cancer: Eastern Cooperative Oncology Group Study E1196. J Clin Oncol 2000; 18(12):2369–2377.

Sparano JA, Robert N, Silverman P, Lazarus H, Malik U, Venkatraj U, Sarta C. Phase I trial of high-dose mitoxantrone plus cyclophosphamide and filgrastim in patients with advanced breast carcinoma. J Clin Oncol 1996; 14 (9):2576–2583.

Spencer CM, Faulds D. Paclitaxel. A review of its pharmacodynamic and pharmacokinetic properties and therapeutic potential in the treatment of cancer. Drugs 1994; 48(5):794–847.

Speyer JL, Green MD, Zeleniuch-Jacquotte A, Wernz JC, Rey M, Sanger J, Kramer E, Ferrans V, Hochster H, Meyers M. ICRF-187 permits longer treatment with doxorubicin in women with breast cancer. J Clin Oncol 1992; 10(1):117–127.

Speyer J, Wasserheit C. Strategies for reduction of anthracycline cardiac toxicity. Semin Oncol 1998; 25(5):525–537.

Stadtmauer EA, O'Neill A, Goldstein LJ, Crilley PA, Mangan KF, Ingle JN, Brodsky I, Martino S, Lazarus HM, Erban JK, Sickles C, Glick JH. Conventional-dose chemotherapy compared with high-dose chemotherapy plus autologous hematopoietic stem-cell transplantation for metastatic breast cancer. Philadelphia Bone Marrow Transplant Group. N Engl J Med 2000; 342(15):1069–1076.

Swain SM. Adult multicenter trials using dexrazoxane to protect against cardiac toxicity. Semin Oncol 1998; 25(4 suppl 10):43–47.

Swain SM, Whaley FS, Gerber MC, Ewer MS, Bianchine JR, Gams RA. Delayed administration of dexrazoxane provides cardioprotection for patients with advanced breast cancer treated with doxorubicin-containing therapy. J Clin Oncol 1997a; 15(4):1333–1340.

Swain SM, Whaley FS, Gerber MC, Weisberg S, York M, Spicer D, Jones SE, Wadler S, Desai A, Vogel C, Speyer J, Mittelman A, Reddy S, Pendergrass K, Velez-Garcia E, Ewer MS, Bianchine JR, Gams RA. Cardioprotection with dexrazoxane for doxorubicin-containing therapy in advanced breast cancer. J Clin Oncol 1997b; 15(4):1318–1332.

Symon Z, Peyser A, Tzemach D, Lyass O, Sucher E, Shezen E, Gabizon A. Selective delivery of doxorubicin to patients with breast carcinoma metastases by stealth liposomes. Cancer 1999; 86(1):72–78.

Tannock IF, Boyd NF, DeBoer G, Erlichman C, Fine S, Larocque G, Mayers C, Perrault D, Sutherland H. A randomized trial of two dose levels of cyclophosphamide, methotrexate, and fluorouracil chemotherapy for patients with metastatic breast cancer. J Clin Oncol 1988; 6: 1377–1387.

Therasse P, Arbuck SG, Eisenhauer EA, Wanders J, Kaplan RS, Rubinstein L, Verweij J, Van Glabbeke M, van Oosterom AT, Christian MC, Gwyther SG. New guidelines to evaluate the response to treatment in solid tumors. European Organization for Research and Treatment of Cancer, National Cancer Institute of the United States, National Cancer Institute of Canada. J Natl Cancer Inst 2000; 92(3):205–216.

Theriault RL, Lipton A, Hortobagyi GN, Leff R, Gluck S, Stewart JF, Costello S, Kennedy I, Simeone J, Seaman JJ, Knight RD, Mellars K, Heffernan M, Reitsma DJ. Pamidronate reduces skeletal morbidity in women with advanced breast cancer and lytic bone lesions: a randomized, placebo-controlled trial. Protocol 18 Aredia Breast Cancer Study Group. J Clin Oncol 1999; 17(3):846–854.

Tominaga T, Abe O, Ohshima A, Hayasaka H, Uchino J, Abe R, Enomoto K, Izuo M, Watanabe H, Takatani O. Comparison of chemotherapy with or without medroxyprogesterone acetate for advanced or recurrent breast cancer. Eur J Cancer 1994; 30A(7):959–964.

Tormey DC, Falkson G, Crowley J, Falkson HC, Voelkel J, Davis TE. Dibromodulcitol and adriamycin +/− tamoxifen in advanced breast cancer. Am J Clin Oncol 1982; 5(1):33–39.

Tripathy D, Slamon DJ, Cobleigh M, Arnold A, Saleh M, Mortimer JE, Murphy M, Stewart SJ. Safety of treatment of metastatic breast cancer with trastuzumab beyond disease progression. J Clin Oncol 2004; 22(6):1063–1070.

Vaage J, Mayhew E, Lasic D, Martin F. Therapy of primary and metastatic mouse mammary carcinomas with doxorubicin encapsulated in long circulating liposomes. Int J Cancer 1992; 51(6):942–948.

Vahdat LT, Thomas E, Li R, Jassem J, Gomez H, Chung H, Peck R, Mukhopadhyay P, Klimovsky J, Roché H. Phase III trial of ixabepilone plus capecitabine compared to capecitabine alone in patients with metastatic breast cancer (MBC) previously treated or resistant to an anthracycline and resistant to taxanes. ASCO Annual Meeting Proceedings (Post-Meeting Edition), June 20 Supplement. J Clin Oncol, 2007; 25(18S):1006 (abstr).

Venook AP, Egorin MJ, Rosner GL, Brown TD, Jahan TM, Batist G, Hohl R, Budman D, Ratain MJ, Kearns CM, Schilsky RL. Phase I and pharmacokinetic trial of paclitaxel in patients with hepatic dysfunction: Cancer and Leukemia Group B 9264. J Clin Oncol 1998; 16(5): 1811–1819.

Victorson D, Soni M, Cella D. Metaanalysis of the correlation between radiographic tumor response and patient-reported outcomes. Cancer 2006; 106(3):494–504.

Viladiu P, Alonso MC, Avella A, Beltran M, Borras J, Ojeda B, Bosch FX. Chemotherapy versus chemotherapy plus hormonotherapy in postmenopausal advanced breast cancer patients. A randomized trial. Cancer 1985; 56(12): 2745–2750.

Vogel C, Cobleigh MA, Tripathy D, Gutheil JC, Harris LN, Fehrenbacher L, Slamon DJ, Murphy M, Novotny WF, Burchmore M, Shak S, Stewart SJ. First-line, single-agent Herceptin(trastuzumab) in metastatic breast cancer: a preliminary report. Eur J Cancer 2001; 37(suppl 1):S25–S29.

Vogel CL, Cobleigh MA, Tripathy D, Gutheil JC, Harris LN, Fehrenbacher L, Slamon DJ, Murphy M, Novotny WF, Burchmore M, Shak S, Stewart SJ, Press M. Efficacy and safety of trastuzumab as a single agent in first-line treatment of HER2-overexpressing metastatic breast cancer. J Clin Oncol 2002; 20(3):719–726.

Von Hoff DD, Layard MW, Basa P, Davis HL, Jr., Von Hoff AL, Rozencweig M, Muggia FM. Risk factors for doxorubicin-induced congestive heart failure. Ann Intern Med 1979; 91 (5):710–717.

Wagstaff AJ, Ibbotson T, Goa KL. Capecitabine: a review of its pharmacology and therapeutic efficacy in the management of advanced breast cancer. Drugs 2003; 63(2):217–236.

Watkins EB, Chittiboyina AG, Jung JC, Avery MA. The epothilones and related analogues—a review of their syntheses and anti-cancer activities. Curr Pharm Des 2005; 11 (13):1615–1653.

Wilcken N, Hornbuckle J, Ghersi D. Chemotherapy alone versus endocrine therapy alone for metastatic breast cancer. Cochrane Database Syst Rev 2003; (2):CD002747.

Winer EP, Berry DA, Woolf S, Duggan D, Kornblith A, Harris LN, Michaelson RA, Kirshner JA, Fleming GF, Perry MC, Graham ML, Sharp SA, Keresztes R, Henderson IC, Hudis C, Muss H, Norton L. Failure of higher-dose paclitaxel to improve outcome in patients with metastatic breast cancer: cancer and leukemia group B trial 9342. J Clin Oncol 2004; 22(11):2061–2068.

Yamamoto N, Watanabe T, Katsumata N, Omuro Y, Ando M, Fukuda H, Takue Y, Narabayashi M, Adachi I, Takashima S. Construction and validation of a practical prognostic index for patients with metastatic breast cancer. J Clin Oncol 1998; 16(7):2401–2408.

24

Adjuvant and Neoadjuvant Systemic Chemotherapy and Biologic Therapy for Operable and Locally Advanced Breast Cancer

JOSEPH A. SPARANO

Department of Oncology, Montefiore Medical Center, Albert Einstein College of Medicine, Bronx, New York, U.S.A.

INTRODUCTION

Relapse in local and distant sites is common after primary surgical treatment of breast cancer. It has been more than 30 years since it was shown that administration of cytotoxic chemotherapy after surgery reduces the risk of local and systemic relapse (Fisher et al., 1975; Bonadonna et al., 1976). Adjuvant regimens initially consisted of alkylating agents used alone (e.g., L-phenylalanine mustard) or in combination with antimetabolites (e.g., cyclophosphamide, methotrexate, and 5-fluorouracil) but have subsequently evolved to include additional agents (e.g., doxorubicin, taxanes) used in combination or sequentially, typically given for four to eight treatment cycles lasting two to six months (Carlson et al., 2006).

In addition to common short-term acute toxicities such as nausea, vomiting, alopecia, and myelosuppression, long-term toxicities include infertility, premature menopause, cardiomyopathy, acute leukemia, and neuropathy (Shapiro and Recht, 2001).

Prognostic factors associated with an increased risk of local and systemic recurrence include the number of axillary lymph nodes harboring metastases, the extent of axillary lymph node involvement, primary tumor size, nuclear and/or histological grade, expression of the estrogen receptor (ER), progesterone receptor (PR), and Her2/neu protein, and other factors (Goldhirsch et al., 2003). Some prognostic factors also serve as predictive factors since their expression predicts benefit from specific therapies such as adjuvant hormonal therapy (e.g., ER and PR expression) or adjuvant trastuzumab (e.g., Her2/neu expression). Indications for adjuvant chemotherapy have expanded from including only premenopausal women with positive axillary lymph nodes in the 1970s to currently include even those at relatively low risk of recurrence, such as women up to 60 or 70 years of age with ER-positive axillary lymph node–negative tumors measuring at least 1 cm, or even smaller tumors that have unfavorable histological features or are ER-negative (Carlson et al., 2006; Goldhirsch et al., 2003). In addition, more recent studies have evaluated the potential advantages and disadvantages of administering chemotherapy before surgery (Kaufmann et al., 2006). In this chapter, the evidence supporting the use of chemotherapy given either preoperatively or postoperatively in patients with operable non-locally advanced, operable locally advanced, and inoperable locally advanced disease is reviewed. Chemotherapy given preoperatively is often referred to as "primary systemic therapy" (PST) and given postoperatively is referred to as

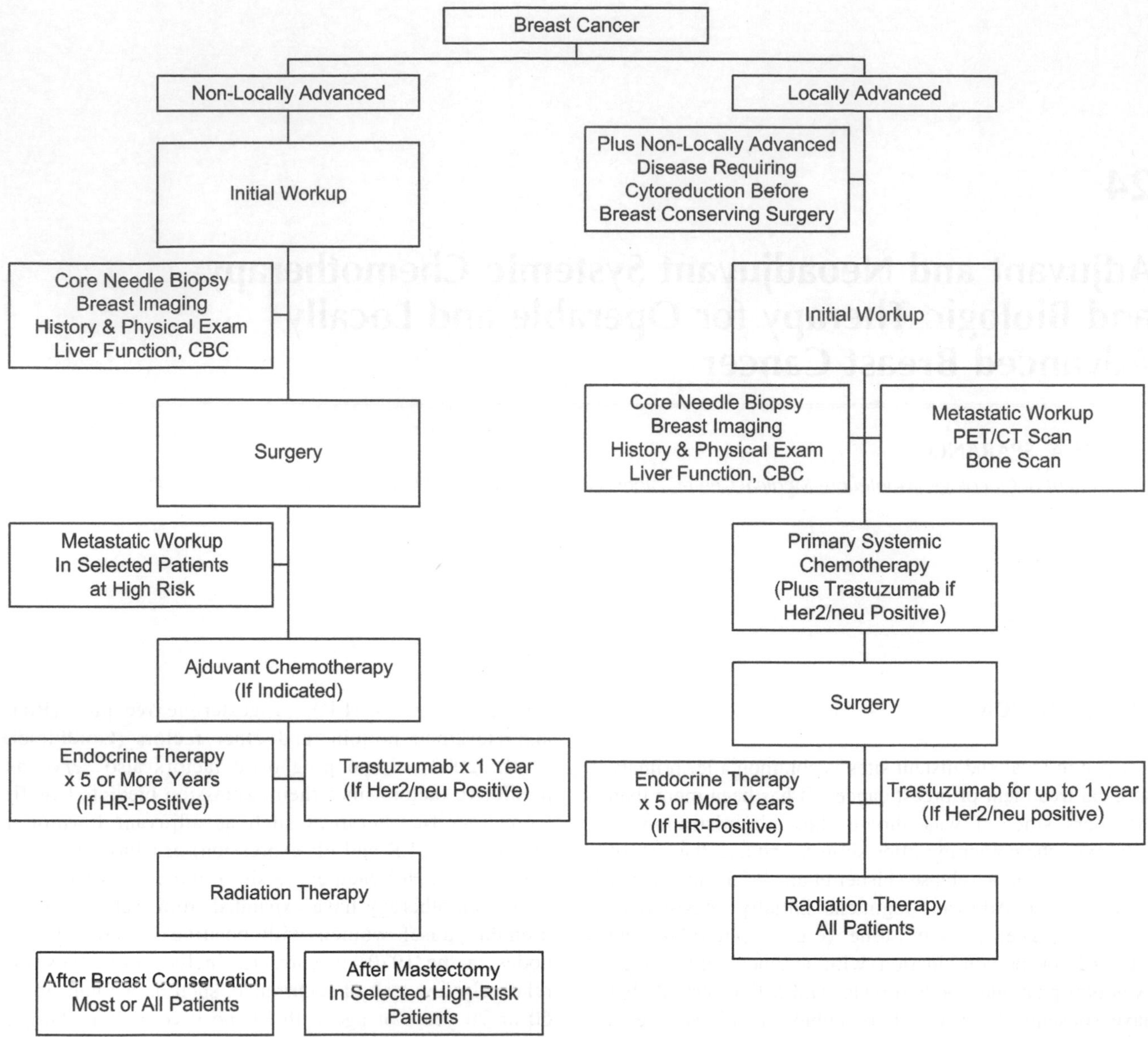

Figure 1 Management of operable and locally advanced breast cancer.

"adjuvant" therapy, which will be the terms used in this chapter.

APPROACH TO THE PATIENT WITH BREAST CANCER

An approach to the initial management of locally advanced breast cancer (LABC) and nonlocally advanced breast cancer (non-LABC) includes the following essential elements and is shown schematically in Figure 1.

- Diagnostic core biopsy, including evaluation for nuclear and/or histological grade, and ER, PR, Her2/neu receptor expression
- Imaging of the ipsilateral and contralateral breast with mammography, plus sonography and/or magnetic resonance imaging (MRI) in selected cases
- A workup to exclude the presence of occult systemic metastases before surgery for all patients with LABC, and selected patients with non-LABC after surgery
- Image-guided clip placement for selected patients with operable breast cancer (usually when diagnosis is made by stereotactic core biopsy), and all patients with LABC who are potential candidates for breast conserving surgery
- Surgical treatment of the primary tumor and axilla, including axillary dissection or sentinel lymph node biopsy (SNB) in selected patients

- Systemic chemotherapy after surgery in selected cases of non-LABC based on risk of recurrence (prognostic factors), or before surgery in LABC and selected patients with non-LABC who require tumor cytoreduction to facilitate breast conservation. Surgery should consist of mastectomy (in all patients with inflammatory carcinoma and most cases of LABC) or breast conservation surgery (in most cases of non-LABC and selected patients with non-inflammatory LABC)
- Irradiation to the breast (in all patients with prior breast-conserving surgery) or chest wall and regional lymphatics (in selected high-risk patients following mastectomy)
- Adjuvant hormonal therapy for five years or longer in all patients who have a tumor that is hormone receptor (HR)-positive
- Adjuvant trastuzumab for one year in patients with Her2/neu-positive disease who have a sufficiently elevated risk of recurrence that warrants adjuvant chemotherapy (and combined with preoperative chemotherapy in patients with LABC); for patients treated with preoperative trastuzumab, the total duration of preoperative and postoperative trastuzumab should be one year.

Diagnosis

All patients should have histological confirmation of the diagnosis prior to definitive surgery or initiating systemic therapy. For patients with nonpalpable lesions, image-guided core biopsy (usually with 3–5 or more cores) or needle localization biopsy may be required in order to establish a tissue diagnosis; the latter may be both diagnostic and therapeutic if adequate surgical margins have been achieved, and if the axilla was adequately evaluated. Histological confirmation by core needle biopsy is preferable to cytological confirmation for several reasons. First, it provides sufficient amount of tissue to accurately determine histological grade, ER, PR, and Her2/neu expression. Second, for patients enrolled on clinical trials, it affords the ability to archive tissue for evaluation of biomarkers predictive of chemotherapy, endocrine therapy, trastuzumab, or novel therapies.

Breast Imaging

All patients must have bilateral mammography, and in selected cases sonography and/or MRI. The American College of Radiology has recommended MRI for the following indications in patients with known or suspected breast cancer: (1) lesion characterization when other modalities are inconclusive, (2) before, during, and/or after primary systemic chemotherapy (PST) to evaluate chemotherapeutic response and the extent of residual disease prior to surgical treatment, with consideration of placement of MRI-compatible localization tissue markers prior to PST, (3) infiltrating lobular carcinoma, (4) infiltrating ductal carcinoma when breast conservation is considered, (5) suspected invasion deep to fascia, and (6) evaluation of the contralateral breast, which may detect unsuspected contralateral disease in about 3% of patients (American College of Radiology, 2007).

Excluding Metastatic Disease

In addition to breast imaging, all patients should have a complete history and physical examination, complete blood count, liver function tests, serum creatinine, and chest X ray. Noninvasive cardiac assessment of left ventricular ejection fraction (LVEF) is indicated for patients who will receive anthracycline-based therapy. Bone scan and computerized tomography (CT) of the chest and abdomen are recommended to rule out occult metastatic disease in patients with LABC who are considered for preoperative chemotherapy or for patients who have already had surgery and are at high risk for having occult metastases (e.g., 4 or more positive axillary lymph nodes). For patients with 10 or more positive axillary lymph nodes, occult metastases may be present in up to 25% of patients who undergo computerized tomography, bone scan, and bone marrow biopsy (Crump et al., 1996). Newer imaging modalities such as positron emission tomography (PET) after injection of fluorine-18 fluorodeoxyglucose (FDG) used in combination with computerized tomography (PET-CT) may be more sensitive in detecting local-regional spread or in excluding metastatic disease (Quon and Gambhir, 2005).

Evaluation of the Axilla

SNB and/or axillary lymph node dissection (ALND) are indicated in patients with non-LABC in order to adequately stage or treat the axilla. The false-negative rate for SNB is approximately 10% and is highly dependent on surgical skill and experience (Mabry and Giuliano, 2007). An expert panel convened by the American Society of Clinical Oncology performed an evidence-based literature review, which identified one published prospective randomized controlled trial in which SNB was compared with ALND, four limited meta-analyses, and 69 published single-institution and multicenter trials in which the test performance of SNB in patients who subsequently had ALND was evaluated. The panel concluded that the available evidence demonstrated that SNB, when performed by experienced clinicians, was a safe and acceptably accurate

Table 1 Treatment Effect of Adjuvant Anthracycline-Based Chemotherapy at 15 Years: Early Breast Cancer Trialists' Overview

		Recurrence		Death	
	Comparison	<50 yr	50–69 yr	<50 yr	50–50 yr
ER status					
Positive	Chemotherapy + tam vs. tam alone	0.64 (+0.08)	0.85 (+0.04)	0.65(+0.10)	0.89 (+0.04)
Negative	Chemotherapy vs. none	0.61 (+0.07)	0.67 (+0.07)	0.68 (+0.08)	0.74 (+0.08)
Nodal status					
Positive	Chemotherapy vs. none (±tam)	0.63 (+0.05)	0.83 (+0.03)	0.70 (+0.05)	0.90 (+0.03)
Negative	Chemotherapy vs. none (±tam)	0.64 (+0.05)	0.90 (+0.03)	0.72 (+0.06)	0.77 (+0.06)

Odds ratio for recurrence or death shown (with standard error in parenthesis).

method for identifying early-stage breast cancer without involvement of the axillary lymph nodes, and is associated with less morbidity; however, the comparative effects on tumor recurrence or patient survival are unknown. The panel also concluded that completion ALND remains standard treatment for patients with axillary metastases identified on SNB (Lyman et al., 2005).

There is insufficient information regarding the role of SNB in patients with LABC who have nonpalpable lymph nodes, or after PST. For patients with clinically enlarged nodes, confirmation of involved lymph nodes prior to PST may be accomplished by fine needle aspiration cytology, sometimes sonographically guided. For patients with a clinically negative or equivocal axillary exam, sonography may be useful in identifying enlarged and/or suspicious lymph nodes and facilitating sonographically directed aspiration cytology prior to PST. For patients enrolled on clinical trials evaluating PST in which the axillary lymph node status is a trial end point, evaluation of the axilla may be necessary. Some experts have recommended performing SNB prior to PST because it permits accurate information about axillary lymph node involvement without the confounding effect of prior PST (Sabel et al., 2003). Other experts have favored the use of SNB after PST because it takes advantage of the downstaging effect, thereby sparing axillary dissection in those who have been downstaged, and at the time of definitive surgery (Mamounas et al., 2005a).

OPERABLE/NONLABC

Treatment Effect of Adjuvant Chemotherapy

Evidence from multiple studies, including the Early Breast Cancer Trialists' meta-analysis, indicates that adjuvant chemotherapy substantially reduces the risk of recurrence, although the treatment effect varies with age and tumor biology (Early Breast Cancer Trialists, 2005). The last published analysis included 194 randomized trials of adjuvant chemotherapy or hormonal therapy that began by 1995. Many trials involved chemotherapy regimens including CMF (cyclophosphamide, methotrexate, 5-fluorouracil), anthracycline-based combinations such as FAC (5-fluorouracil, doxorubicin, cyclophosphamide) or FEC (5-fluorouracil, epirubicin, cyclophosphamide), and endocrine therapies such as tamoxifen or ovarian suppression. There were no studies in the analysis that included taxanes, trastuzumab, or aromatase inhibitors. Treatment with up to six months of anthracycline-based polychemotherapy (e.g., with FAC or FEC) reduced the annual breast cancer death rate by about 38% (±5%) for women younger than 50 years, and by about 20% (±4%) for those aged 50 to 69 years, largely irrespective of the use of tamoxifen and of ER status, nodal status, or other tumor characteristics (Table 1). Anthracycline-based regimens were significantly more effective than CMF chemotherapy in reducing the risk of recurrence ($2p = 0.0001$) and breast cancer mortality ($2p < 0.00001$). There was little information regarding women age 70 years or older.

Incremental Benefit from Adjuvant Taxane Therapy

Several trials have now demonstrated that taxanes, whether given concurrently with or sequentially following anthracycline-based therapy, produce an incremental reduction in the risk of recurrence (Table 2). This has been confirmed in a recent meta-analysis of adjuvant and neoadjuvant (i.e., preoperative) taxane trials (Nowak et al., 2004). The clinical questions addressed by these trials may be classified into three categories including evaluation of (1) sequential use of anthracycline and taxanes compared with non-taxane regimens, (2) the optimal taxane schedule, and (3) substituting taxanes for other agents.

Sequential Anthracycline-Taxane Regimens

Several trials demonstrated that adding four cycles of paclitaxel or docetaxel given every three weeks sequentially

Table 2 Randomized Trials of Adjuvant Taxane Therapy

References	No.	Patient selection	Follow-up	Arms	DFS	Hazard ratio	OS	Hazard ratio	Comment
Sequential taxane use									
Henderson et al., 2003	3121	Positive axillary nodes	69 mo	AC × 4	65%	Referent arm	77%	Referent arm	DFS and OS at 5 yr shown
				AC × 4 → P × 4	70%	0.83 ($p = 0.0023$)	80%	0.82 ($p = 0.0011$)	2 × 2 factorial design evaluating dose escalation showed no difference between 60 vs. 75 vs. 90 mg/m^2
Mamounas et al., 2005b	3060	Positive axillary node	65 mo	AC × 4	72%	Referent arm	85%	Referent arm	DFS and OS at 5 yr shown
				AC × 4 → P × 4	76%	0.83 ($p = 0.006$)	85%	0.93 ($p = 0.46$)	All patients 50 or older and younger patients with ER-positive tumors received concurrent tamoxifen
Taxane schedule and type									
Citron et al., 2003	2005	Positive axillary nodes	36 mo	AC → P or A → P → C at 3 weeks vs.	75%	Referent arm	NR	Referent arm	DFS and OS at 4 yr shown
				AC → P or A → P → C at 2 weeks	82%	0.74 ($p = 0.01$)	NR	0.69 ($p = 0.013$)	
Sparano et al., 2007	4988	Positive axillary nodes or (88%) high-risk node negative (12%)	60 mo	AC × 4 → P × 4	81%	Referent arm	89%	Referent arm	DFS and OS at 5 yr shown
				AC × 4 → P × 12	84%	0.70 ($p = 0.02$)	92%	No difference	
				AC × 4 → D × 4	83%	0.76 ($p = 0.02$)	89%	No difference	
				AC × 4 → D × 12	81%	0.91 ($p =$ NS)	89%	No difference	
Substituting taxanes for other agents									
Martin et al., 2005	1491	Positive axillary nodes	55 mo	FAC × 6	68%	Referent arm	81%	Referent arm	DFS and OS at 5 yr shown
				TAC × 6	75%	0.72 ($p = 0.001$)	87%	0.70 ($p = 0.008$)	
Jones et al., 2006	1016	0–3 positive axillary nodes	66 mo	AC × 4	80%	Referent arm	87%	Referent arm	DFS and OS at 5 yr shown
				TC × 4	86%	0.67 ($p = 0.0.15$)	90%	0.76 ($p = 0.13$)	
Goldstein et al., 2005	2885	0–3 positive axillary nodes	48 mo	AC × 4	87%	Referent arm	94%	Referent arm	DFS and OS at 4 yr
				AD × 4	97%	No difference	93%	No difference	
Roche et al., 2006	1999	Positive axillary nodes	60 mo	FEC × 6	73%	Referent arm	87%	Referent arm	DFS and OS at 5 yr shown
				FEC × 3 → D × 3	78%	0.82 ($p = 0.034$)	91%	0.73 ($p < 0.05$)	
Martin et al., 2005	1298	Positive axillary nodes	46 mo	FEC × 6	79%	Referent arm	92%	Referent arm	DFS and OS at 4 yr shown
				FEC × 4 → P × 8	85%	0.63 ($p = 0.0008$)	94%	0.74 ($p = 0.1391$)	

Abbreviations: DFS, disease-free survival; OS, overall survival.

Chemotherapy regimens: AC—doxorubicin 60 mg/m^2, cyclophosphamide 600 mg/m^2 every three weeks; FAC—5-fluorouracial 500 mg/m^2, doxorubicin 50 mg/m^2, cyclophosphamide 500 mg/m^2 every three weeks; TAC—docetaxel 75 mg/m^2, doxorubicin 50 mg/m^2, cyclophosphamide 500 mg/m^2 every three weeks; TC—docetaxel 75 mg/m^2, cyclophosphamide mg/m^2 every three weeks; P × 5—paclitaxel 175 mg/m^2 (Henderson et al., 2003; Sparano, 2007) or 225 mg/m^2 (Mamounas et al., 2005a) every three weeks; P × 12—paclitaxel 80 mg/m^2 weekly × 12 weeks; D × 4—docetaxel 100 mg/m^2 every three weeks (Sparano, 2007); D × 12—docetaxel 35 mg/m^2 weekly × 12 (Sparano, 2007); AD—doxorubicin 60 mg/m^2, docetaxel 60 mg/m^2 (Goldstein et al., 2005); FEC—5-fluorouracial 500 mg/m^2, epirubicin 90 mg/m^2 (Martin et al., 2005) or 100 mg/m^2 (Roche et al., 2006; followed by paclitaxel 100 mg/m^2 weekly × 8), cyclophosphamide 500 mg/m^2 every three weeks.

following anthracycline-based adjuvant therapy reduced the risk of recurrence. For example, trials C9344 and B28 both demonstrated that administration of four cycles of paclitaxel following four cycles of doxorubicin-cyclophosphamide given every three weeks reduced the risk of recurrence by about 17% (Mamounas et al., 2005b; Henderson et al., 2003). However, the disparity in the number of cycles of therapy in the taxane arms (8) compared with the non-taxane arms (4) raised the question as to whether the benefit observed for the taxane arms was attributable to a longer duration of cytotoxic therapy or due specifically to the sequential addition of taxanes. The Early Breast Cancer Trialist's overview demonstrated no advantage for chemotherapy treatment duration of more than six months. However, other trials have shown that shorter durations of therapy may be less effective. For example, six cycles of adjuvant FEC given every three weeks (18 weeks) was found to be more effective than three cycles of adjuvant FEC (9 weeks) (Fumoleau et al., 2003). However, other trials found the sequential use of an anthracycline-based combination followed by a taxane to be more effective than administration of an equivalent number of anthracycline-containing combination without taxanes, whether given preoperatively (Smith et al., 2002) or postoperatively (Roche et al., 2006).

Taxane Schedule and Type

Several trials evaluated the optimal taxane schedule. In C9741, 3001 patients with axillary lymph node–positive breast cancer were randomly assigned to receive four cycles of doxorubicin-cyclophosphamide (AC) followed sequentially by four cycles of paclitaxel either every three weeks or every two weeks with granulocyte colony–stimulating factor support (Table 2). There was a clear advantage for the every two-week regimen, although the benefit seemed to be driven largely by the effect in HR-negative disease (Citron et al., 2003). Another study comparing an every three- versus every two-week schedule of FEC demonstrated no advantage for the two-week schedule, suggesting that scheduling may be an important issue for taxane but not non-taxane regimens (Venturini et al., 2005). In E1199, 4950 eligible patients with axillary lymph node–positive and high-risk node-negative disease were randomly assigned to receive four cycles of doxorubicin-cyclophosphamide chemotherapy every 3 weeks followed by either four cycles of paclitaxel every 3 weeks, four cycles of docetaxel every 3 weeks, 12 doses of paclitaxel given weekly for 12 weeks, or 12 doses of docetaxel given weekly for 12 weeks (Sparano et al., 2007). Compared with the standard every three-week AC-paclitaxel arm, there was an improvement in disease-free survival (DFS) for both the weekly paclitaxel arm and every three-week docetaxel arm, but not the weekly docetaxel arm. Weekly paclitaxel was also associated with improvement in overall survival.

Substituting Taxanes for Other Agents

Some, but not all, trials have demonstrated benefit for substituting a taxane for other agents in combination regimens. In BCIRG001, the combination of docetaxel, doxorubicin, and cyclophosphamide (TAC) resulted in a 30% reduction in the risk of recurrence when compared with 5-flourouracil, doxorubicin, and cyclophosphamide (FAC), both given every three weeks for six cycles, in patients with positive axillary lymph nodes; comparable benefit was seen in both HR-positive and HR-negative diseases (Table 2) (Martin et al., 2005). A particular strength of this trial was the centralized testing for HR and Her/neu expression in a single-reference laboratory, and a prespecified analysis plan for comparing the treatment arms independently in HR-positive and HR-negative populations. Likewise, the docetaxel-cyclophosphamide (TC) combination was associated with about a 30% reduction in the risk of recurrence when compared with doxorubicin-cyclophosphamide (AC) combination, both given every three weeks for four cycles, in patients with zero to three positive axillary lymph nodes (Jones et al., 2006). On the other hand, the doxorubicin-docetaxel (AT) combination was no more effective than the AC combination, both given every three weeks for four cycles, in patients with zero to three positive axillary lymph nodes in trial E2197 (Goldstein et al., 2005).

Two other trials compared a strategy of substituting taxane therapy for anthracycline-based therapy after an initial period of anthracycline therapy. In the PACS 01 trial, 1999 patients with operable node-positive breast cancer were randomized to receive FEC for six cycles or for three cycles followed by three cycles of docetaxel given every three weeks (Roche et al., 2006). After a median follow-up of five years, there was improved DFS and overall survival for the docetaxel-containing arm. In the GEICAM 9906 trial, 1348 women with operable node-positive breast cancer were randomized to receive FEC for six cycles or for three cycles every three weeks followed by eight doses of weekly paclitaxel (Rodríguez-Lescure et al., 2007). There was an improvement in DFS for the weekly paclitaxel arm.

SELECTION FOR ADJUVANT CHEMOTHERAPY AND ESTIMATING BENEFIT

Although adding chemotherapy reduces the risk of recurrence on average by about 30%, the absolute benefit for an individual patient may range from up to 30% or more for high-risk women with 10 or more positive axillary lymph nodes to as little as 1% for women with low-risk ER-positive, axillary lymph node-negative disease (Fisher et al., 2001). Although selection of both adjuvant endocrine therapy and trastuzumab relies largely on predictive factors, treatment recommendations for chemotherapy are based on the recurrence risk as estimated by prognostic factors. If the residual risk of recurrence exceeds approximately 5% to 10% despite adjuvant hormonal therapy in ER-positive disease, or in any patient with an ER-negative tumor, chemotherapy is generally recommended for individuals who are medically fit and less than 60 to 70 years of age (Carlson et al., 2006). Decision aids such as Adjuvant!(Olivotto et al., 2005), decision boards (Whelan et al., 2004), and other tools are often useful to assist patients and caregivers with information regarding absolute benefits that might be expected from chemotherapy (Whelan and Loprinzi, 2005). Although such aids may assist some patients in making a more informed decision regarding whether to accept adjuvant chemotherapy, when faced with a choice, many patients and their clinicians err on the side of overtreatment because of the imprecise nature of predicting treatment benefit (Simes and Coates, 2001).

The Adjuvant! decision aid (www.adjuvantonline.com) has emerged as a particularly practical and useful tool that is widely used and has been validated in a large population-based study. The model estimates 10-year outcomes of relapse-free survival (RFS) and overall survival after the user inputs standard clinical features, such as age, tumor grade, ER status, nodal status, comorbidities, and therapeutic options (such as type of chemotherapy and endocrine therapy). In an external validation model using 4083 women with T1-2, N0-1, M0 breast cancer diagnosed in British Columbia between 1989 and 1993, 10-year predicted and observed outcomes were within 1% for overall survival, breast cancer–specific survival, and event-free survival. Predicted and observed outcomes were within 2% for most demographic, pathological, and treatment-defined subgroups (Olivotto et al., 2005). However Adjuvant! overestimated certain outcomes in women younger than 35 years of age with lymphatic or vascular invasion.

Several multigene molecular markers have been shown to predict outcome more reliably than standard clinical features (van 't Veer et al., 2002; Paik et al., 2004; Foekens et al., 2006) and may be comparable in their ability to predict clinical outcomes (Fan et al., 2006) (discussed in chapter 2). Some have also been shown to predict benefit from adjuvant chemotherapy (Paik et al., 2006). These markers may be used to assist in making more informed treatment decisions regarding chemotherapy, particularly in low-risk patients with ER-positive disease (Sparano et al., 2005). Clinical trials now ongoing will further refine the role of these markers in clinical practice (Sparano, 2006).

INCREMENTAL BENEFIT FROM THE ADDITION OF ENDOCRINE THERAPY TO CHEMOTHERAPY

Endocrine therapy may produce substantial incremental benefit when added to adjuvant chemotherapy in patients with HR-positive disease, which accounts for approximately 65% of all breast cancer. The Early Breast Cancer Trialists' meta-analysis indicated that for ER-positive disease, use of up to five years of adjuvant tamoxifen reduced the annual breast cancer death rate by 31% (±3%), irrespective of chemotherapy use and age, PR status, or other tumor characteristics (Table 1) (Early Breast Cancer Trialists, 2005). Several trials have now demonstrated that aromatase inhibitors reduce the risk of relapse by approximately 20% when compared with tamoxifen in postmenopausal women and are now recommended as standard option either alone or sequentially following a two- to five-year course of tamoxifen (reviewed in chapter 10) (Baum, 2005; Coates et al., 2007; Goss et al., 2005; Coombes et al., 2004, 2007).

INCREMENTAL BENEFIT FROM THE ADDITION OF TRASTUZUMAB TO CHEMOTHERAPY

Approximately 15% of all breast cancers overexpress Her2/neu protein, which is known to be associated with an increased risk of relapse (Slamon et al., 1989). It was subsequently shown that the humanized anti-Her2/neu monoclonal antibody trastuzumab was effective for the management of metastatic breast cancer (as discussed in chapter 24) (Cobleigh et al., 1999; Slamon et al., 2001). Subsequent studies demonstrated that trastuzumab also reduced the risk of recurrence by approximately 50% when given either following completion of adjuvant chemotherapy or concurrently with and after taxane therapy in women with Her2/neu-positive disease, a finding that was demonstrated consistently in five different trials (Table 3). All trials required confirmation of Her2/neu protein overexpression by immunohistochemistry or gene amplification by fluorescent in situ hybridization (FISH) in local or central laboratories by standard methodologies (Wolff et al., 2007).

A combined analysis of two trials (NSABP B31 and North American Breast Intergroup trial N9831) included 3676 women with positive axillary lymph nodes (94%) or high-risk node-negative (6%) disease, all of whom received standard AC chemotherapy every three weeks for 4 cycles, followed by paclitaxel given every three weeks for 4 cycles (B31) or weekly for 12 cycles (N9831). In both studies, patients were randomly assigned to receive chemotherapy only or chemotherapy plus trastuzumab given concurrently with and following paclitaxel (4 mg/kg loading dose week 1, followed by 2 mg/kg

Table 3 Randomized Trials of Adjuvant Trastuzumab Therapy in Her2/neu-Positive Breast Cancer

References	No.	Patient selection	Follow-up	Chemotherapy regimen	DFS	Hazard ratio	OS	Hazard ratio	Comment
Romond et al., 2005	3676	Positive axillary nodes	24 mo	AC × 4 → P × 4 or P × 12					
				• Without trastuzumab	67%	Referent arm	77%	Referent Arm	DFS and OS at 4 yr shown
				• With trastuzumab for 52 weeks (concurrent with paclitaxel × 12 weeks)	85%	0.48 ($p < 0.0001$)	80%	0.82 ($p = 0.0011$)	
Piccart-Gebhart et al., 2005 Smith et al., 2007	3387	Positive axillary nodes (57%), high-risk node negative (32%)	24 mo	Adjuvant chemotherapy followed by					
				• No trastuzumab	74%	Referent arm	90%	Referent arm	DFS and OS at 3 yr shown
				• Trastuzumab for 52 weeks after chemotherapy	81%	0.64 ($p < 0.001$)	92%	0.66 ($p = 0.0115$)	
Joenssu et al., 2006	232	Positive axillary nodes (90%) or high-risk node negative (10%)	36 mo	V or D × 3 cycles → FEC × 3					
				• No trastuzumab	79%	Referent arm	86%	Referent arm	RFS (not DFS) and OS shown at 3 yr
				• Trastuzumab weekly × nine weeks concurrent with V or D	89%	0.42 ($p = 0.01$)	94%	0.41 ($p = 0.07$)	
Slamon et al., 2006	3222	Positive axillary nodes (71%) or high-risk node negative (29%)	23 mo	AC × 4 → D × 4	81%	Referent arm	93%	Referent arm	Results for DFS and OS at 3 yr from 2nd interim analysis
				AC × 4 → D × 4 + trastuzumab for 52 wk (weekly concurrent with docetaxel × 12 weeks then every 3 wk)	87%	0.61 ($p < 0.0001$)	97%	0.59 ($p < 0.004$)	
				DC × 6 cycles + trastuzumab for 52 weeks, (weekly concurrent with chemotherapy × 18 weeks, then every 3 wk)	86%	0.67 ($p = 0.003$)	95%	0.066 ($p = 0.017$)	

Abbreviations: NR, not reported in abstract; ND, not different, data not shown; NS, not stated; DFS, disease-free survival; OS, overall survival.
Chemotherapy regimens: AC—doxorubicin 60 mg/m^2, cyclophosphamide 600 mg/m^2 every tjree weeks; P—paclitaxel 80 mg/m^2 weekly × 12 or 175 mg/m^2 every three weeks × 4; V—vinorelbine 25 mg/m^2 weekly × nine weeks; D—docetaxel 100 mg/m^2 every three weeks × 3; FEC—5-fluorouracial 600 mg/m^2, epirubicin 60 mg/m^2, cyclophosphamide 600 mg/m^2 every three weeks; DC—docetaxel 75 mg/m^2, carboplatin AUC 6 every three weeks × 16 cycles.

weekly for 51 weeks); the N9831 trial included a third arm that evaluated sequential administration of paclitaxel followed by trastuzumab that was not included in the combined analysis (Romond et al., 2005). After a median follow-up of two years at the first planned interim analysis, the hazard ratio favored trastuzumab for DFS (0.48; $p < 0.0001$) and overall survival (0.67; $p = 0.015$).

A third trial (HERA) performed by the Breast International Group included 5081 women with axillary lymph node–positive (57%), node-negative (32%), or unknown axillary status (11% due to neoadjuvant chemotherapy) who had received at least four cycles of adjuvant or neoadjuvant chemotherapy (and surgery); patients were randomized to receive no adjuvant trastuzumab or adjuvant trastuzumab (8 mg/kg loading dose followed by 6 mg/kg every 3 weeks) for either one year or two years (Piccart-Gebhart et al., 2005). After a median follow-up of one year at the first planned interim analysis comparing the one year trastuzumab arm with no trastuzumab, the hazard ratio likewise favored trastuzumab for DFS (0.54; $p < 0.0001$). A subsequent report after a median follow-up of two years revealed a significant reduction in the risk of death with one year of adjuvant trastuzumab (0.66; $p = 0.0115$) (Smith et al., 2007).

A fourth trial performed by the Finnish Herceptin Study Group (FinHer) randomized 232 women with axillary node–positive or high-risk node-negative disease to receive nine weekly trastuzumab doses (4 mg/kg, then 2 mg/kg weekly) concurrently with an antitubulin agent (weekly vinorelbine for 9 doses or docetaxel every 3 weeks for 3 doses) followed by three cycles of FEC. Trastuzumab was associated with a significantly lower risk of recurrence (0.42; $p = 0.01$) (Joensuu et al., 2006).

A fifth study performed by the Breast Cancer International Research Group (BCIRG006) evaluated 3222 women with either axillary lymph node-positive (68%) or high-risk node-negative (32%) breast cancer to four cycles of adjuvant AC followed by four cycles of docetaxel every three weeks (AC-T), the same regimen plus trastuzumab for one year (AC-TH) starting concurrently with docetaxel, or six cycles of carboplatin and docetaxel every three weeks plus trastuzumab given for one year (TCH) (Slamon et al., 2006). At the second planned interim analysis after a median follow-up of 23 months, both the AC-TH and TCH arms were associated with an improved DFS (0.061; $p < 0.0001$ and 0.67, $p = 0.0003$, respectively) and overall survival (0.59; $p = 0.004$ and 0.66, $p = 0.017$) compared with the non-trastuzumab-containing arm.

Taken together, these trials demonstrate a very clear and consistent benefit for adjuvant trastuzumab in reducing the risk of relapse and death for Her2/neu-positive disease. The optimal dose rate is 2 mg/kg/wk, plus the equivalent of a 4 mg/kg loading dose in order to rapidly achieve blood levels that are believed to be therapeutic. All studies utilized weekly trastuzumab given concurrently with chemotherapy, and most used an every three-week schedule after chemotherapy was completed. The optimal duration of therapy appears to be one year, although continued follow-up of the HERA study will be required to determine whether two years of therapy is more effective than one year. Results of the FinHer study suggest that a short course of adjuvant trastuzumab given concurrently with chemotherapy may be equally effective as longer durations, although experience with the short schedule is limited. Another trial (E2198) found comparable outcomes with short and long durations of adjuvant trastuzumab; it included 234 patients who were randomized either to adjuvant paclitaxel every 3 weeks with trastuzumab (4 mg/kg loading dose followed by 2 mg/kg weekly for 9 weeks) followed by standard AC for four cycles (without trastuzumab) or to the same regimen followed by trastuzumab weekly for 52 weeks. DFS at five years was 76% for the short duration and 73% for the long duration of trastuzumab ($p = 0.55$), and overall survival rates at five years (88% vs. 83%; $p = 0.29$) and rates of cardiac toxicity (1.7% vs. 2.4%; $p =$ NS) were also similar (Sledge et al., 2006). Although the study was adequately powered as a safety trial, it was insufficiently powered to permit definitive efficacy comparison of the two treatment arms. Nevertheless, these studies raise the question as to whether shorter durations of adjuvant trastuzumab may be equally effective as one year of adjuvant therapy.

Adjuvant trastuzumab was associated with an increased risk of cardiac toxicity in all of the studies reported. All studies excluded patients with known cardiac disease, and all required a normal LVEF at baseline confirmed by either nuclear scan or echocardiography. Cardiac monitoring with either nuclear scan or echocardiography was performed in both trials at baseline, after AC chemotherapy (3 months), after paclitaxel chemotherapy (6 months), and again at 9 and 18 months after initiation of chemotherapy. In the B31-N9831 combined analysis, New York Heart Associated class III or IV congestive heart failure or death from cardiac causes at three years was 0.8% in the control group and 4.1% in the trastuzumab group (Romond et al., 2005). An independent analysis of cardiac events in the B31 found that among patients with normal post-AC LVEF who began post-AC treatment, 5 of 814 control patients (0.6%) subsequently had confirmed cardiac events compared with 31 of 850 (3.6%) trastuzumab-treated patients; 27 patients treated with trastuzumab who developed cardiac dysfunction have been followed for at least six months after the cardiac event, of whom 26 were asymptomatic at last assessment and 18 remained on cardiac medication (Tan-Chiu et al., 2005). Trastuzumab was discontinued in 4% of patients because of symptomatic cardiotoxicity and in 14% because of asymptomatic decreases in LVEF (of at least 16% if the LVEF remained above normal or between 11% and 15% if the LVEF decreased below normal). In the HERA trial, symptomatic cardiac toxicity occurred in 0.1% in the observation arm and 2.3% in the one year trastuzumab arm ($p < 0.001$), and 10% or greater decline in LVEF (or decline to below normal) occurred in 2.2% in the observation arm compared with 7.1% in the one year trastuzumab arm ($p < 0.001$). In BCIRG 006, symptomatic cardiac toxicity occurred in 0.4% in the AC-T control arm, 1.9% in the AC-TH arm, and 0.4% in the TC-H arm (Slamon et al., 2006).

RATIONALE FOR PRIMARY SYSTEMIC (NEOADJUVANT) CHEMOTHERAPY

Administration of chemotherapy prior to surgery, called "primary systemic chemotherapy" or "neoadjuvant chemotherapy," offers several potential advantages to postoperative therapy for both practical and theoretical reasons (Wolff and Davidson, 2000). Practical advantages include the high clinical response rate, the correlation between short-term response and long-term outcomes, and facilitation of breast conservation surgery in patients with large tumor–breast ratio who may not be optimal candidates for breast conservation otherwise. Theoretical advantages that have not yet been proven include selection of patients for additional therapy based on the extent of residual disease, or the use of non-cross-resistant therapy before or after surgery if there was an inadequate response to initial therapy. Potential disadvantages include the small but definite risk of disease progression during therapy, and the possibility that this strategy may represent overtreatment for some patients with favorable disease characteristics. Theoretical concerns include the potential for alteration of the biological characteristics of the primary tumor, although some reports and preclinical data suggest that PST does not influence the grade or ER and/or PR expression (Frierson and Fechner, 1994; Seno et al., 1998). Such concerns may be obviated by obtaining core needle biopsy rather than fine needle aspiration at diagnosis before PST. Preclinical data also suggests that removal of the primary tumor may induce cytokinetic effects on distant metastases that favor postoperative chemotherapy administration (Fisher, 1980; Fisher et al., 1989), although this has not been borne out in randomized clinical trials. For patients with LABC, the advantages of PST outweigh any disadvantages, particularly for those individuals who may be candidates for breast conservation after sufficient cytoreduction.

Randomized Trials Comparing Primary Systemic with Adjuvant Chemotherapy

There have been nine randomized trials comparing preoperative versus postoperative chemotherapy in patients with operable breast cancer. Some of these studies included a relatively small proportion of patients who had noninflammatory LABC and also included patients who would have been appropriate candidates for breast conservation without preoperative therapy. The studies were primarily designed to evaluate whether preoperative chemotherapy was more effective than postoperative chemotherapy in reducing the risk of relapse. In general, they showed no difference in DFS or overall survival between the two approaches, although a higher proportion of patients treated with PST had breast conservation and were less likely to have positive axillary nodes at surgery, due to the downstaging effect of preoperative therapy.

Mauri et al. (2005) performed a meta-analysis of nine randomized studies, including a total of 3946 patients, which compared PST with adjuvant chemotherapy (Fig. 2). No statistically or clinically significant difference was found in relapse [summary risk ratio (RR) = 0.99, 95% confidence intervals (CI) = 0.91–1.07], distant relapse (summary RR = 0.94, 95% CI = 0.83–1.06), or survival (summary RR = 1.00, 95% CI = 0.90–1.12). Neoadjuvant therapy was associated with an increased risk of locoregional disease recurrence (RR = 1.22, 95% CI = 1.04–1.43), especially in trials where more patients in the neoadjuvant arm received radiation therapy without surgery (RR = 1.53, 95% CI = 1.11–2.10). There was substantial heterogeneity across trials in the rates of complete clinical response (range = 7–65%; p for heterogeneity of <0.001), pathological response (range = 4–29%; p for heterogeneity of <0.001), and breast conservation (range = 28–89% in neoadjuvant arms, p for heterogeneity of <0.001).

Several individual trials merit additional discussion, including the B18 trial, the EORTC trial, and the ECTO trial. The National Surgical Adjuvant Breast and Bowel Project (NSABP) reported the largest and most cleanly designed study (B18) that compared four cycles of doxorubicin (60 mg/m^2) and cyclophosphamide (600 mg/m^2) given every three weeks either preoperatively or postoperatively in 1523 patients (Fisher et al., 1997, 1998). Objective response in the neoadjuvant group occurred in 79%, including a 35% clinical complete response (cCR) and 9% pathological CR rate (pCR). Response was dependent on tumor size; clinical CR occurred in 35% of those with T2 lesions compared with only 17% of those with T3 lesions. There was no difference between the two arms at five years in DFS (67%), distant disease–free survival (DDFS) (73%), or overall survival (80%). Patients treated with PST were more likely to be treated with lumpectomy than mastectomy (67% vs. 60%) and were less likely to

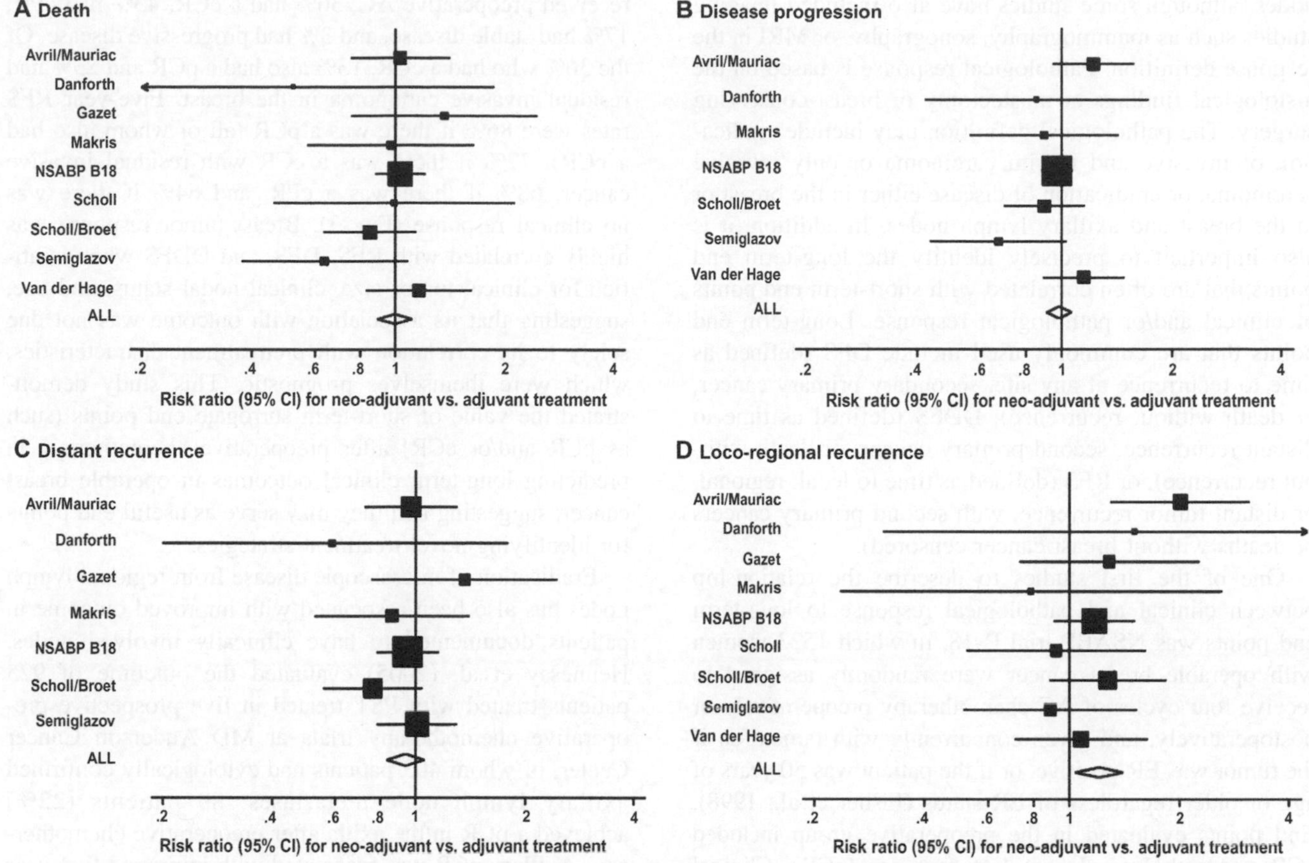

Figure 2 Meta-analysis for primary outcomes with neoadjuvant therapy compared with adjuvant therapy for breast cancer.

have positive axillary lymph nodes at axillary dissection (41% vs. 57%).

Likewise, van Der Hage et al. (2001) reported on behalf of the European Organization for the Research and Treatment of Cancer (EORTC) a phase III trial in which 698 patients with operable stage I–IIIB disease were randomized to receive four cycles of FEC given preoperatively versus the same regimen given postoperatively (the first cycle administered within 36 hours after surgery). At a median follow-up of 56 months, there was no significant difference in overall survival [hazard ratio (HR) 1.16; $p = 0.38$), progression-free survival (HR 1.15; $p = 0.27$), and time to local-regional recurrence (LRR) (HR 1.13; $p = 0.61$). Fifty-seven patients (23%) were downstaged by the preoperative chemotherapy, although breast conservation rates were similar in the two treatment arms.

Finally, Gianni et al. (2005a,b) reported the results of the only phase III trial that compared preoperative versus postoperative administration of concurrent anthracycline-taxane therapy [referred to as the European Cooperative Trial in Operable breast cancer (ECTO)]. The trial included 1355 women with operable breast cancer who had primary tumor measuring more than 2 cm. Patients were randomized to adjuvant doxorubicin (75 mg/m^2 every 3 weeks $\times$ 4) followed by IV CMF (day 1 and 8 every 28 days for 4 cycles), adjuvant doxorubicin (60 mg/m^2), and paclitaxel (200 mg/m^2 over 3 hours every 21 days for 4 cycles) followed by CMF (AT-CMF), or sequential AT-CMF given before surgery. After a median follow-up of 43 months, freedom from progression was significantly improved for women receiving adjuvant AT-CMF than A-CMF (HR 0.65, range 0.48–0.90; $p = 0.01$). There was no difference in the freedom from progression rates between those who received AT-CMF given as adjuvant or preoperative therapy (HR 0.83, range 0.59–1.16; $p = 0.27$). There were also no significant differences with regard to breast conservation, local relapse, DFS, or overall survival between the pre- and postoperative arms.

Prognostic Significance of Clinical and Pathological Response to PST

The importance of achieving a complete clinical and especially pathological response has been noted in several studies. In reviewing trials using clinical and/or pathological response as an end point, it is important to consider the definitions used, especially when performing cross trial comparisons. In general, clinical response is based on physical examination of the breast and regional lymph nodes, although some studies have also included imaging studies such as mammography, sonography, or MRI in the response definition. Pathological response is based on the histological findings at mastectomy or breast-conserving surgery. The pathological definition may include eradication of invasive and in situ carcinoma or only invasive carcinoma, or eradication of disease either in the breast or in the breast and axillary lymph nodes. In addition, it is also important to precisely identify the long-term end points that are often correlated with short-term end points of clinical and/or pathological response. Long-term end points that are commonly used include DFS (defined as time to recurrence at any site, secondary primary cancer, or death without recurrence), DDFS (defined as time to distant recurrence, second primary cancer, or death without recurrence), or RFS (defined as time to local, regional, or distant tumor recurrence, with second primary cancers or deaths without breast cancer censored).

One of the first studies to describe the relationship between clinical and pathological response to long-term end points was NSABP trial B-18, in which 1523 women with operable breast cancer were randomly assigned to receive four cycles of AC chemotherapy preoperatively or postoperatively, and given concurrently with tamoxifen if the tumor was ER-positive, or if the patient was 50 years of age or older regardless of ER status (Fisher et al., 1998). End points evaluated in the preoperative group included cCR and pathological complete response (pCR). Clinical response was based on physical examination alone. cCR was defined as complete disappearance of all palpable tumor and nodal masses, whereas clinical partial response (cPR) was defined as a 50% or greater reduction in the product of the two greatest perpendicular diameters of the palpable tumor (or sum of the products if there was more than one palpable tumor). pCR was defined as no histological evidence of residual invasive cancer cells in the breast at the time of surgery. Of the 683 women who received preoperative AC, 36% had a cCR, 43% had cPR, 17% had stable disease, and 3% had progressive disease. Of the 36% who had a cCR, 13% also had a pCR and 23% had residual invasive carcinoma in the breast. Five-year RFS rates were 86% if there was a pCR (all of whom also had a cCR), 77% if there was a cCR with residual invasive cancer, 68% if there was a cPR, and 64% if there was no clinical response (Fig. 3). Breast tumor response was highly correlated with RFS, DFS, and DDFS when stratified for clinical tumor size, clinical nodal status, and age, suggesting that its association with outcome was not due solely to its correlation with pretreatment characteristics, which were themselves prognostic. This study demonstrated the value of short-term surrogate end points (such as pCR and/or cCR) after preoperative chemotherapy in predicting long-term clinical outcomes in operable breast cancer, suggesting that they may serve as useful end points for identifying novel treatment strategies.

Eradication of microscopic disease from regional lymph nodes has also been associated with improved outcome in patients documented to have clinically involved nodes. Hennessy et al. (2005) evaluated the outcome of 925 patients treated with PST treated in five prospective preoperative chemotherapy trials at MD Anderson Cancer Center, of whom 403 patients had cytologically confirmed axillary lymph node metastases; 89 patients (22%) achieved a pCR in the axilla after preoperative chemotherapy. Axillary pCR was associated with improved five-year RFS (87% vs. 60%) and overall survival (93% vs. 72%; $p < 0.0001$). Residual primary tumor in the breast did not affect outcome of those with an axillary pCR.

Carey et al. (2005) evaluated the outcome of 132 patients with stage IIA–IIIB breast cancer who received preoperative chemotherapy based on the posttreatment stage. A higher pathological stage of residual tumor after preoperative chemotherapy was associated with a significantly lower rate of distant DFS and was reported to be 95% for stage 0 (i.e.,

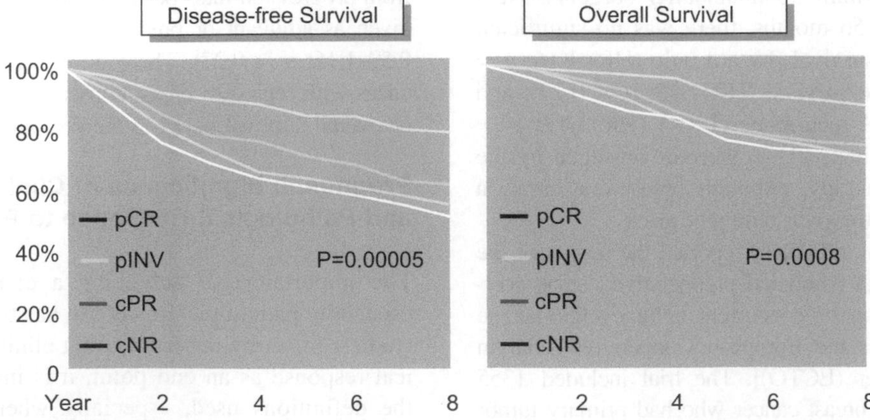

Figure 3 Relationship between clinical and pathological response in the breast to long-term outcomes after treatment with doxorubicin-cyclophosphamide in NSABP B18.

pCR), 84% for stage I, 72% for stage II, and 47% for stage III, and 18% for stage IIIC (p trend < 0.001).

Several other classifications of pathological response have been proposed but have not been shown to more accurately predict long-term clinical outcomes (Chevallier et al., 1993; Sataloff et al., 1995). A limitation of relying purely on complete pathological or clinical response as an end point is that it fails to identify patients with residual invasive carcinoma who may have derived benefit from therapy. In an effort to address this problem, Symmans et al. (2006) retrospectively reviewed posttreatment surgical specimens from 432 patients in two completed neoadjuvant trials evaluating FAC alone ($N = 189$) or paclitaxel followed by FAC (T/FAC) ($N = 243$). Specimens were systematically evaluated for (1) the largest two dimensions (in millimeters) of the residual tumor bed in the breast (largest tumor bed if multicentric disease), (2) the percentage of the tumor bed area that contained in situ and/or invasive carcinoma (estimated as 0%, 1%, 5%, 10%, 20%, 30%, 40%, 50%, 60%, 70%, 80%, or 90%), (3) the histological estimate of the percentage of the carcinoma in the tumor bed that was in situ (estimated as 0%, 1%, 5%, 10%, 20%, 30%, 40%, 50%, 60%, 70%, 80%, or 90%), (4) the number of positive metastatic lymph nodes, and (5) the largest diameter (in millimeters) of the largest nodal metastases. This information was modeled into an index called the "residual cancer burden" (RCB) (http://www3.mdanderson.org/app/medcalc/index.cfm?pagename=jsconvert3). RCB was a continuous predictor of distant relapse–free survival after T/FAC (HR 1.86, 95% CI 1.51–2.30) or FAC (HR 1.67, 95% CI 1.38–2.01) with median follow-up of five and eight years, respectively. The resistant category RCB-3 predicted relapse more strongly than stage III disease and identified a larger group of high-risk patients. These findings suggest that the posttreatment RCB algorithm may provide more accurate prognostic information than provided by pretreatment clinical stage, and may be used to identify individuals who have less than a complete pathological response who derive substantive benefit from PST.

Molecular Profiling to Predict Response to Preoperative Chemotherapy

Several studies have also evaluated whether gene expression profiling might identify tumors more likely to respond to preoperative chemotherapy and to specific cytotoxic agents. Cleator et al. (2006) evaluated gene expression patterns using Affymetrix U133A chips (which comprise ~22,000 genes) in 40 patients treated with preoperative AC for six cycles, of whom 22 (55%) had complete and 7 (18%) had partial clinical response. When evaluating gene expression profile of those who had a cCR versus others (using a false discovery rate of 5%), 253 genes were differently expressed, including genes responsible for upregulation of cell cycle, survival, stress response, and estrogen-related pathways in the sensitive tumors, and transcription, signal transduction, and amino acid metabolism pathways in the resistant tumors. Gianni et al. evaluated a panel of 384 genes in 89 patients with LABC treated with three cycles of preoperative doxorubicin and cyclophosphamide, followed by 12 weekly paclitaxel doses, all of whom had pretreatment core biopsies obtained. Eighty-six genes correlated with pCR (unadjusted $p < 0.05$); pCR was more likely with higher expression of proliferation-related genes and immune-related genes, and with lower expression of ER-related genes (Gianni et al., 2005b). In 82 independent patients treated with neoadjuvant paclitaxel and doxorubicin, DNA microarray data were available for 79 of the 86 genes. In univariate analysis, 24 genes correlated with pCR with $p < 0.05$ (false discovery, four genes) and 32 genes showed correlation with $p < 0.1$ (false discovery, eight genes). The Recurrence Score was positively associated with the likelihood of pCR ($p = 0.005$), suggesting that the patients who are at greatest recurrence risk are more likely to have benefit from chemotherapy. Hess et al. (2006) developed a multigene predictor of pCR to preoperative weekly paclitaxel and FAC in a training set of 82 patients with stage I–III breast cancer using oligonucleotide microarrays on fine-needle aspiration specimens and validated it in 51 similar patients. The pCR rate was 26% in both the training and validation cohorts. A total of 56 probes were identified as differentially expressed between pCR versus residual disease, at a false discovery rate of 1%, and 780 distinct classifiers were evaluated in cross validation. Although many predictors performed equally well, a nominally best 30-probe classifier selected for validation demonstrated significantly higher sensitivity (92% vs. 61%) than a clinical predictor including age, grade, and ER status. The negative predictive value (96% vs. 86%) and area under the curve (0.877 vs. 0.811) were nominally better but not statistically significant. The combination of genomic and clinical information yielded a predictor not significantly different from the genomic predictor alone. There was also good reproducibility of the predictive signature in 31 samples that were evaluated in replicate.

Taken together, these data suggest that although genomic classifiers hold promise for predicting benefit from specific therapies given preoperatively or postoperatively, there is insufficient evidence to support their use to predict benefit from specific chemotherapy regimens given preoperatively at this time.

Randomized Trials Comparing Different Chemotherapy Regimens for PST

Several randomized phase II or III trials have evaluated different regimens as PST for operable breast cancer and/or LABC (Table 4). These studies may be broadly

Table 4 Randomized Trials Comparing Different Taxane-Based Regimens for Primary Systemic Therapy

References	No.	Patient selection	T3 tumor	T4 tumor	Clinically palpable nodes	Treatment arms	Clinical response rate	Clinical CR rate	Breast path CR	Pathologically negative nodes	Breast conservation
Treatment duration											
Bear et al., 2006	2411	T1c-T3, N01	45% > 4 cm	0%	30%	AC × 4 → surgery OR AC × 4 → surgery → D × 4 (combined results)	85%	40%	14%	51%	62%
						AC × 4 → D × 4 → surgery	91%	64%	26%	58%	64%
							($p < 0.001$)	($p < 0.001$)	($p < 0.001$)	($p < 0.001$)	($p =$ NS)
von Minckwitz et al., 2005	913	T2-3, N0-2	8%	0%	40%	AD × 4 → surgery	75%	31%	7%	55%	66%
						AC × 4 → D × 4 → surgery	85%	56%	14%	61%	75%
							($p < 0.001$)			($p = 0.13$)	($p < 0.005$)
Substituting taxanes for other agents											
Buzdar et al., 1999	174	T1-3, N0-1	28%	0%	61%	FAC × 4 → surgery	79%	24%	23%	44%	35%
						P × 4 → surgery	80%	27%	14%	37%	46%
Dieras et al., 2004	200	T2-3, N0-1	38%	0%	58%	AC × 4 → surgery	70%	7%	10%	39%	45%
						AP × 4 → surgery	89%	15%	16%	41%	56%
Evans et al., 2005	363	T > 3 cm	NR	14%	NR	AC × 4 → surgery	61%	17%	21%	39%	20%
						AD × 4 → surgery	70%	20%	24%	34%	20%
							($p = 0.06$)				
Smith et al., 2002	102		44%	16%	20%	CVAP × 4 → CVAP × 4 → surgery	64%	56%	15%	56%	NR
						CVAP × 4 → D × 4 → surgery	85%	33%	31%	60%	NR

Drug scheduling											
Therasse et al., 2003	448	Locally advanced	NR	86%	>40%	CEF × 6 4 → surgery	54%	31%	14%	NR	NR
						Dose escalated EC × 6 4 → surgery	56%	27%	10%.	NR	NR
Green et al., 2005	258	T1-3, N0-1	11%	1%	44%	P × 4 → FAC × 4 → surgery	83%	39%	16%	NR	38%
						P × 12 → FAC × 4 → surgery	85%	56%	28% ($p = 0.02$)	NR	47% ($p = 0.05$)
Ellis et al., 2006	265	Locally advanced	NR	~30%	NR	Weekly AC 4 → paclitaxel→ surgery	NR	NR	27%	NR	NR
						Standard AC → paclitaxel → surgery	NR	NR	17% ($p = 0.06$)	NR	NR

Note: Breast pCR defined as no invasive carcinoma (includes patients with residual in situ disease): Breast pCR in some studies includes pCR in breast and lymph nodes (von Minckwitz et al., 2005; Dieras et al., 2004; Green et al., 2005); clinical response includes physical exam only, or physical exam plus imaging in selected studies (Buzdar et al., 1999).

Abbreviation: NR, not reported.

Chemotherapy regimens: AC—doxorubicin 60 mg/m^2, cyclophosphamide 600 mg/m^2 IV every three weeks (all studies); D—docetaxel 100 mg/m^2 every three weeks (Bear et al., 2006); AD—doxorubicin 50 mg/m^2, docetaxel 175 mg/m^2 every three weeks plus filgrastim; AC every three weeks × 4, then D every three weeks × 4 (von Minckwitz et al., 2005); CVAP—cyclophosphamide 1000 mg/m^2, vincristine 1.5 mg/m^2, doxorubicin 50 mg/m^2, prednisone 50 mg daily × 5 days; D—docetaxel 100 mg/m^2 (Smith et al., 2002); FAC—5-fluorouracil 500 mg/m^2 day 1 and 4, doxorubicin 50 mg/m^2 via 72-hour IV infusion, cyclophosphamide 500 mg/m^2 day 1 and 4 every three weeks; P—paclitaxel 50 mg/m^2 via 24-hour infusion (Buzdar et al., 1999); AP—doxorubicin 60 mg/m^2, paclitaxel 200 mg/m^2 every three weeks (Dieras et al., 2004); AD—doxorubicin 60 mg/m^2 and docetaxel 75 mg/m^2 every three weeks (Evans et al., 2005); CEF—cyclophosphamide 75 mtg/m^2/day orally days 1 to 14, epirubicin 60 mg/m^2 days 1, 8, 5-flourouracil 500 mg/m^2 days 1, 8, or EC—epirubicin 120 mg/m^2 and cyclophosphamide 830 mg/m^2 IV plus G-CSF (Therasse et al., 2003); P × 4—paclitaxel 225 mg/m^2 via 24-hour infusion every three weeks or weekly for 12 consecutive doses (at 80 mg/m^2) in clinically node negative patients or given for three of four weeks for a total of 12 doses (at 150 mg/m^2) in node-positive patients, all followed by FEC every three weeks (5-fluorouracil 500 mg/m^2, doxorubicin 50 mg/m^2 as a 72-hour IV infusion, and cyclophosphamide 500 mg/m^2) (Green et al., 2005); Weekly AC—doxorubicin 24 mg/m^2/wk plus oral cyclophosphamide (60 mg/m^2/day) for 15 weeks plus G-CSF, or standard AC every 3 weeks for 5 doses, both followed by weekly paclitaxel 80 mg/m^2 for 12 weeks (Ellis, 2006).

classified into several categories: (1) treatment duration, (2) substituting taxanes for other agents, (3) drug scheduling, and (4) drug sequencing.

Treatment Duration

Bear et al. (2006) reported the results of NSABP B27, in which 2411 women with stage I–IIIA breast cancer were randomly assigned to four cycles of preoperative AC (as in the B18 trial), followed by four additional preoperative cycles of docetaxel (100 mg/m^2 every 3 weeks), or AC followed by surgery, followed by docetaxel. Tamoxifen was also given concurrently with chemotherapy in all patients. Patients treated with preoperative docetaxel had a significantly improved cCR rate (64% vs. 40%; $p < 0.001$) and breast pCR rate (26% vs. 14%; $p < 0.001$), but similar breast conservation rates (62% vs. 64%). An unexpected and somewhat disappointing aspect of this trial was that although there was a nearly twofold increase in the pCR rate for the preoperative docetaxel arm, it did not transplant into improved DFS for the docetaxel-containing arms. Potential explanations include inadequate statistical power to detect such improvements, and concurrent administration of tamoxifen, which may have attenuated the benefit of chemotherapy.

The German Breast Group performed a phase III trial in 913 patients with stage IIA–IIIB breast cancer, which compared the combination of concurrent dose-dense doxorubicin (50 mg/m^2) and docetaxel (75 mg/m^2) and filgrastim every two weeks for four cycles with standard sequential doxorubicin (60 m/m^2) and cyclophosphamide (600 mg/m^2) for four cycles followed by docetaxel (100 mg/m^2) for four cycles given every three weeks (von Minckwitz et al., 2005). All patients also received tamoxifen 20 mg daily concurrently with chemotherapy. There was a significantly higher breast and nodal pCR rate for the sequential arm (14% vs. 7%, $p < 0.001$), which was the primary study end point. Response was also higher for the sequential arm when assessed by clinical exam (75% vs. 63%; $p < 0.001$) and imaging including mammography and sonography (75% vs. 69%; $p < 0.001$). The breast conservation rate also favored the sequential arm (63% vs. 58%; $p = 0.05$). The results of this trial provide additional support for the use of at least eight cycles of preoperative chemotherapy and suggest that an abbreviated course of a dose-dense anthracycline-taxane combination may be insufficient.

Substituting Taxanes for Other Agents

Buzdar et al. (1999) compared paclitaxel (250 mg/m^2) versus FAC every three weeks for four cycles in 174 patients with stage II–IIIA breast cancer prior to mastectomy or lumpectomy and axillary dissection. Comparing paclitaxel with FAC, there was no significant difference in the clinical response rate (80% vs. 79%) or cCR rate (27% vs. 24%), although the pCR rate was higher with FAC (1% vs. 12%). The estimated two-year DFS was not significantly different for the two arms (94% vs. 89%).

Dieras et al. (2004) compared doxorubicin plus either cyclophosphamide (AC) or paclitaxel (AP) for four cycles in 247 patients with clinical stage II–IIIA breast cancer in a multicenter randomized phase II trial (Dieras et al., 2004). About 60% of patients on both arms had clinically enlarged axillary lymph nodes, and 38% had primary tumors measuring at least 5 cm. All patients subsequently underwent surgery and local irradiation. Patients were randomized to receive AP in a 2:1 fashion. The AP arm was associated with a higher overall clinical response rate (89% vs. 70%), cCR rate (16% vs. 7%), and pCR rate (16% vs. 10%). In addition, more AP patients were able to have breast-conserving therapy (58% vs. 45%). After a median follow-up of approximately 31 months, there was no significant difference in disease-free or overall survival.

Evans et al. (2005) compared doxorubicin plus either cyclophosphamide (AC) or docetaxel (AD) for four cycles in 363 patients with LABC or tumors more than 3 cm in size in a multicenter randomized phase III trial. All patients subsequently underwent surgery and local irradiation. The AD arm was associated with a higher overall clinical response rate (70% vs. 61%; $p = 0.06$), but a comparable cCR rate (20% vs. 17%), breast pCR rate (21% vs. 24%), and breast conservation rate (20% for both arms).

Smith et al. (2002) performed a randomized trial in patients with LABC or large primary tumors (at least 3 cm). All patients received cyclophosphamide, doxorubicin, vincristine, and prednisone (CAVP) as primary therapy. Of the 163 patients treated with CVAP, 63% had an objective response and were randomized to receive either four additional cycles of CAVP ($N = 47$) or four cycles of docetaxel ($N = 50$). There was an improvement in clinical response rate (85% vs. 64%; $p = 0.03$) and pCR rate (31% vs. 15%; $p = 0.06$) for patients randomized to receive docetaxel. Of the 58 patients (37%) who had no response to the initial course of CAVP and were crossed over to docetaxel, objective response occurred in 46%, including 11% who had a clinical CR and 2% who had a pCR.

Drug Scheduling

Therasse et al. (2003) compared FEC with dose-escalated epirubicin and cyclophosphamide (EC) in 448 patients with LABC, of whom 207 had inflammatory and 241 had noninflammatory disease. There was no significant difference in the clinical CR rate (31% vs. 27%). Pathological response could not be accurately determined because of differences in the local therapy permitted. After a median follow-up of 5.5 years, there was no significant difference in progression-free survival or overall survival.

Green et al. (2005) evaluated 258 patients with clinical stage I–IIIA breast cancer treated with preoperative paclitaxel given either every three weeks for four cycles ($N = 131$) or weekly for 12 doses given by one of several weekly schedules depending upon the clinical lymph nodes status ($N = 127$), followed by four cycles of FAC given every three weeks for four cycles. Although clinical response was similar in two arms, the weekly taxane schedule was associated with a higher pCR rate (28% vs. 16%; $p = 0.02$) and higher breast conservation rate (49% vs. 41%).

Ellis et al. (2006) reported the results of Southwest Oncology Group (SWOG) trial 0012, a phase III trial in 372 patients with LABC who were randomized to preoperative chemotherapy consisting of standard AC every three weeks for five cycles, or weekly doxorubicin (24 mg/m^2) and daily oral cyclophosphamide (60 mg/m^2/day) for 15 weeks plus granulocyte colony–stimulating factor (5 μg/kg/day × 6/7 weekly). Both groups then received weekly paclitaxel (80 mg/m^2) for 12 weeks. Of the 265 patients who were evaluable at the time of the report, there was a higher breast pCR in the weekly doxorubicin arm (27% vs. 17%; $p = 0.06$). When adjusted for HR status and the presence of inflammatory carcinoma, there was significantly higher pCR rate in the weekly doxorubicin arm (odds ratio 1.98; 95% CI 1.05–3.74; $p = 0.034$). The weekly doxorubicin arm was associated with more hand-foot syndrome, stomatitis, and less neutropenia.

Drug Sequencing

No trials have compared the clinical impact of different drug sequences of cytotoxic agents on clinical outcomes. However, some evidence suggests that administration of taxanes prior to other agents may be preferable. Antiangiogenic therapy may initially improve blood flow in tumors that exhibit disordered vascular beds, thereby improving drug delivery of cytotoxic agents that are given after it (Hansen-Algenstaedt et al., 2000). Taxanes are known to have potent angiogenic effects (Hotchkiss et al., 2002) and may also improve tumor blood flow by reduction in tumor-associated vascular compression (Padera et al., 2004). A study providing proof of principle indicated that preoperative paclitaxel more effectively reduced interstitial fluid pressure (IFP) in primary breast cancer than doxorubicin-cyclophosphamide (Taghian et al., 2005). In this study, 54 patients with breast cancers measuring at least 3 cm were randomly assigned to receive neoadjuvant dose-dense doxorubicin at 60 mg/m^2 every two weeks for four cycles followed by nine cycles of weekly paclitaxel at 80 mg/m^2 (group 1) or vice versa (group 2). IFP measured by wick-in-needle technique and pO_2 (Eppendorf) were measured in tumors at baseline and after completing the administration of the first and second regimens. Paclitaxel, when administered first, decreased the mean IFP by 36% ($p = 0.02$) and improved the tumor pO_2 by almost 100% ($p = 0.003$). In contrast, doxorubicin did not have a significant effect on either parameter, and this difference was independent of the tumor size or response measured by ultrasound. Although no phase III trials have directly compared the pCR rate after neoadjuvant sequential AC-taxane therapy by using differing sequences (AC → taxane vs. taxane → AC), studies evaluating the taxane first sequence have demonstrated pCR rates that are comparable or higher to the usual AC → taxane sequence (Green et al., 2005).

Trials Evaluating Combination of Targeted Agents with Cytotoxic Therapy

Several trials have evaluated combining agents targeting specific biological pathways with standard cytotoxic therapy. These have generally been single-arm phase II or randomized phase II trials and have largely consisted of trials evaluating the trastuzumab plus cytotoxic therapy in Her2/neu-positive disease (Table 5).

Trastuzumab Plus Chemotherapy

Several trials have also evaluated the role of neoadjuvant trastuzumab, usually in patients with locally advanced disease, including combinations with paclitaxel (Burstein et al., 2003; Mohsin et al., 2005), docetaxel (Mohsin et al., 2005; Hurley et al., 2006), docetaxel and cisplatin (Hurley et al., 2006), and sequential paclitaxel followed by FEC (Buzdar et al., 2005, 2007). The trials varied with regard to patient selection, duration of preoperative trastuzumab, and the type and schedule of concurrent chemotherapy administered. Nevertheless, these studies have demonstrated the safety and efficacy of preoperative trastuzumab combined with several chemotherapy regimen.

Buzdar et al. (2005) reported the results of a randomized phase II trial, which demonstrated that the addition of trastuzumab to standard chemotherapy significantly improved the pCR rate in the breast and lymph nodes. Forty-two patients with Her2/neu-positive disease were randomly assigned to either four cycles of paclitaxel (225 mg/m^2 given by 24-hour infusion every 3 weeks) followed by four cycles of FEC every 3 weeks given either alone or in combination with weekly trastuzumab

Table 5 Phase II Trials Evaluating Preoperative Targeted Agents Plus Chemotherapy

References	Chemotherapy	Target	Agent	Schedule	No.	Breast pCR
Burstein et al., 2003	Pac 175 mg/m^2 q 3 wk × 4	Her2/neu	Trastuzumab	Weekly × 12	40	18%
Hurley et al., 2006	Doc 75 mg/m^2 + CDDP 70 mg/m^2 q 3 wk × 4	Her2/neu	Trastuzumab	Weekly × 12	48	23%
Buzdar et al., 2005	Pac 225 mg/m^2 q 3 wk × 4 → FEC75 × 4	Her2/neu	Trastuzumab	Weekly × 24 vs. none	23 vs. 19	65% vs. 26% ($p = 0.02$)
Wedam et al., 2006	Dox 50 mg/m^2 + Doc 75 mg/m^2 q 3 wk × 6	VEGF	Bevacizumab	15 mg/kg q 3 wk × 6	21	0%
Sparano, 2006	Dox 60 mg/m^2 + Cyclophosphamide 600 mg/m^2 q 2 wk × 4	Ras	Tipifarnib	200 mg PO BID days 2–7 each cycle	21	33%

Abbreviations: Pac, paclitaxel; Doc, docetaxel; CDDP, cisplatin; VEGF, vascular endothelial growth factor; trastuzumab dose 4 mg/kg loading dose, followed by 2 mg/kg.

for 24 weeks. The primary objective was to demonstrate a 20% improvement in pCR (assumed 21–41%) with the addition of trastuzumab to chemotherapy. The planned sample size was 164 patients. After 34 patients had completed therapy, the Data Monitoring Committee stopped the trial because of superiority of trastuzumab plus chemotherapy: pCR rates were 25% and 68% for chemotherapy ($N = 16$) and trastuzumab plus chemotherapy ($N = 18$), respectively ($p = 0.02$). The decision was based on the calculation that if the study continued to 164 patients, there was a 95% probability that trastuzumab plus chemotherapy would be superior. No clinical congestive heart failure was observed; 10% or grater decrease in the cardiac ejection fraction was observed in five patients (26%) in the chemotherapy arm alone and seven patients (30%) in the chemotherapy plus trastuzumab arm. Although the study was small, it clearly demonstrated that adding trastuzumab to preoperative chemotherapy significantly improved the pCR rate. It also raises the question as to whether additional trastuzumab would be necessary after surgery, especially since one adjuvant trial demonstrated comparable benefit for a shortened nine-week trastuzumab course (Joensuu et al., 2006). Given the substantial body of evidence favoring a one year course of trastuzumab, it would seem prudent to administer trastuzumab postoperatively to patients who have received a short course of preoperative trastuzumab so that the total duration of trastuzumab therapy given pre- and postoperatively is approximately one year.

One trial evaluated the biological and clinical effects of a short course of preoperative trastuzumab given as a single agent (Mohsin et al., 2005). Weekly trastuzumab was given for the first three weeks, followed by a combination of trastuzumab and docetaxel for 12 weeks before surgery. Sequential core biopsies were taken at baseline and within weeks 1 and 3 after the first dose of trastuzumab. Core biopsies were assessed by immunohistochemistry for cell cycle and proliferation (Ki67, p27, phosphorylated [p]-MAPK), apoptosis and survival (apoptotic index, p-Akt), epidermal growth factor receptor, and total and p-HER-2. There was early clinical tumor regression with a median decrease of –20% (range 0–60.4%) after only three weeks of trastuzumab, with eight patients (23%) meeting clinical criteria for partial response. Apoptosis was significantly induced (median increase from 3.5% to 4.7%; $p = 0.006$) within week 1, a 35% increase above baseline. No significant change in epidermal growth factor receptor score was observed after one week, and total or p-HER-2 expression was unchanged. Tumors with high baseline Ki67 were less likely to respond ($p = 0.02$). Pathological response in the breast was not seen. Nevertheless, this trial demonstrated that trastuzumab alone induces significant increase in apoptosis after a single dose.

Angiogenesis Inhibitors Plus Chemotherapy

Angiogenesis has been validated as an important therapeutic target, and several trials have demonstrated substantial clinical benefit by targeting angiogenesis in colorectal, lung, and breast carcinoma. Vascular endothelial growth factor (VEGF) mediates tumor angiogenesis primarily via VEGF receptor 2 (VEGFR2), and its biological effects may be inhibited by the recombinant humanized monoclonal antibody bevacizumab (Schneider and Miller, 2005). Several trials have evaluated bevacizumab in combination with cytotoxic therapy in patients with LABC. Wedam et al. (2006) treated 21 patients with inflammatory and LABC with bevacizumab for cycle 1 (15 mg/kg on day 1) followed by six cycles of bevacizumab with doxorubicin and docetaxel every three weeks. Tumor biopsies and dynamic contrast-enhanced magnetic resonance imaging (DCE-MRI) were obtained at baseline and after cycles 1, 4, and 7. Bevacizumab induced significant decreases in phosphorylated VEGFR2 in tumor cells (median decrease 67%; $p = 0.004$) and increased tumor apoptosis (median increase 129%; $p = 0.0008$), and the changes persisted after the addition of chemotherapy. DCE-MRI indicated a median decrease of 34% in the inflow transfer rate constant ($p = 0.003$), 15% in the backflow extravascular-extracellular rate constant ($p = 0.0007$), and 14% in extravascular-extracellular volume fraction ($p = 0.002$) after bevacizumab alone, indicating evidence of reduced blood flow in vivo. With regard to clinical response, 14 patients had a cPR and there were no pCRs. Lyons et al. treated 49 patients who were randomized to preoperative docetaxel alone (35 mg/m^2 weekly for 6 of 8 weeks, given for 2 cycles) or docetaxel plus bevacizumab (10 mg/kg every 2 weeks). There was a reduction in tumor blood flow measured by DCE-MRI and a reduction of tumor microvessel density, but no pCRs were noted. This study demonstrated that bevacizumab induces biological effects in vivo, but further studies will be required to determine whether bevacizumab or other agents targeting angiogenesis will be useful for operable or LABC.

Farnesyl Transferase Inhibitors Plus Chemotherapy

Ras proteins belong to the low molecular weight guanosine nucleotide–binding GTPases (G protein) superfamily that play a critical role in cell growth; oncogenic mutations of the three known human *ras* genes are found in 30% of all human cancers (Li and Sparano, 2003). Although oncogenic *ras* mutations are uncommon in breast cancer, hyperactivation of Ras protein and its downstream effectors is very common due to either overexpression of upstream components, such as EGFR and HER-2/neu (Smith et al., 2000). Upstream events may lead to activation of the pathway without Ras protein overexpression or due to and estrogen-dependent aberrant pathway in breast cancer models. Ras protein overexpression in breast cancer (not associated with *ras* mutations) has been associated with poor prognosis, and RhoC overexpression (a downstream effector of Ras) is associated with regional and/or distant metastases and with inflammatory carcinoma (Kleer et al., 2005). Posttranslational modification at the carboxyl terminus of Ras mediated by farnesyl transferase (FTase) is essential for mediation of its downstream effects, and FTase inhibitors (FTIs) have been shown to potentiate the cytotoxic effect of chemotherapy in preclinical modes and have single-agent activity in metastatic breast cancer (Kelland et al., 2001; Johnston et al., 2003). On the basis of these considerations, the FTI tipifarnib was combined with dose-dense AC given for four cycles in 21 patients with LABC (Sparano et al., 2006). Tipifarnib significantly inhibited FTase in primary breast cancer in all five patients evaluated, and the breast pCR occurred in seven patients (33%), including five of 12 (42%) with ER-positive disease. Additional studies will be required to confirm these preliminary findings, but they do provide an example of how other targeted agents may be combined with standard therapy.

LOCALLY ADVANCED BREAST CANCER

LABC includes several clinical presentations of breast cancer that are associated with a high rate of local and systemic recurrence when treated with local therapy alone. This includes tumors that are very large but resectable, tumors in which it is technically difficult to establish tumor-free margins due to skin or chest wall involvement, and tumors of any size associated with extensive axillary adenopathy or regional nonaxillary lymph nodes. For patients treated with surgery alone, fewer than 30% survive disease-free beyond five years and approximately 30% to 50% develop local recurrence (Fracchia et al., 1980). For irradiation, approximately 20% survive disease-free (Zucali et al., 1976).

The definition of LABC generally includes the following clinical presentations and their corresponding stages by the sixth edition (2002) of the American Joint Committee on Cancer in the absence of distant metastases (Singletary et al., 2003).

- Large primary tumors (>5 cm, T3) occurring without axillary lymph node metastases (stage IIB) or with ipsilateral moveable (N1) or fixed or matted (N2) axillary lymph node metastases (stage IIIA)
- Tumors of any size that are associated with axillary lymph node metastases that are fixed to one another or to other structures (stage IIIA)
- Tumors of any size that show extension to the chest wall (T4a) or skin, including edema, ulceration, or satellite skin nodules (T4b), or both extension to chest wall and skin changes (T4c) (stage IIIB)
- Inflammatory (T4d) carcinoma with or without axillary nodal metastases (stage IIIB)
- Tumors of any size associated with axillary nodes and ipsilateral infraclavicular nodes (N3a) or internal mammary nodes (N3b), or ipsilateral supraclavicular nodes (N3c) (stage IIIC)

Historical Perspectives on Prognostic Features in LABC

Haagensen and Stout (1943) first described the features of LABC more than 50 years ago when they reported that several "grave signs" were associated with a low cure rate with radical mastectomy. The "grave signs" included edema or ulceration of the skin, fixation of the tumor to the chest wall, and axillary lymph nodes that were either larger than 2.5 cm in diameter or fixed to each other or other structures. Patients with two or more features were considered "categorically inoperable," as only two percent survived disease-free beyond five years. By today's criteria, these findings would generally be indicative of T4 lesions or N2 adenopathy. Large primary tumor size is associated with a worse prognosis even in the absence of "grave signs." This is due in large part to the direct correlation between tumor size and the incidence and number of lymph node metastases, although there also seems to be an effect that is independent of axillary metastases. Another important adverse prognostic feature is inflammatory carcinoma, which typically presents with erythema, edema, and increased warmth of the skin of the involved breast. The resultant brawny induration of the skin may result in an orange peel (or so called "peau d'orange") appearance. Biopsy of the skin typically reveals infiltration of tumor cells into the dermal lymphatics, although the diagnosis may be made even in the absence of this histopathological finding. Inflammatory carcinoma is associated with a distinctly worse prognosis compared with noninflammatory presentations of LABC (Buzdar et al., 1995).

Several other factors are known to be associated with a higher risk of recurrence, including increasing number of axillary lymph node metastases, extranodal extension of tumor cells outside of the lymph node, medial location of the tumor, poor nuclear or histological grade, ER and PR-negative disease, and overexpression of the Her2/neu (Gasparini et al., 1993).

Although knowledge of prognostic and/or predictive factors may be useful for stratifying patients in randomized clinical trials, or selecting specific therapies such as endocrine therapy or trastuzumab, it is difficult to predict outcome because of the multiple prognostic factors that have been identified. Rouzier et al. (2006) sought to address this problem by developing a nomogram to predict expected pCR rate and distant metastasis–free survival (DMFS) after preoperative chemotherapy. After evaluating baseline clinical variables and outcome in 496 patients treated with preoperative anthracycline-based chemotherapy, a nomogram was developed that was tested in two independent cohorts of patients, including 337 treated with preoperative anthracycline-based therapy and 237 patients who received preoperative paclitaxel and anthracycline. The pCR nomogram based on clinical stage, ER status, histological grade, and number of preoperative chemotherapy cycles had good discrimination and calibration in the training and the anthracycline-treated validation sets (concordance indices, 0.77, 0.79). Clinical information may be entered into a web-based algorithm (http://www.mdanderson.org/care_centers/breastcenter/dIndex.cfm?pn=448442B2-3EA5-4BAC-98310076A9553E63), with the information required including type of therapy, age, T stage, initial tumor size, histological type, histological grade, ER expression, and presence or absence of multifocality. The model provides a predicted probability of achieving a pCR, of having residual tumor less than 3 cm, and of being able to have breast-conserving surgery. The model also provides a predictive probability of being without recurrence at 5 and 10 years for patients treated with three to four cycles of doxorubicin-based chemotherapy based on pretreatment factors (histological type, grade, and ER expression) and residual disease at surgery (pathological tumor size and number of positive axillary nodes). Adjuvant! should not be employed in patients treated with preoperative therapy because treatment results in downstaging, which impacts tumor stage and nodal status variables that are entered in the model.

Diagnosis, Pretreatment Evaluation, and Multimodality Management

An algorithm for the management of patients with operable or LABC treated with PST is shown in Figure 1. PST is indicated for the majority of patents with LABC and for patients with large tumor–breast ratio for whom cytoreduction may facilitate breast conservation. There are several important issues that must be carefully considered in patients treated with PST, including (1) establishing the diagnosis, (2) excluding metastatic disease, (3) breast imaging, (4) evaluation of the axilla, (5) pre- and post-chemotherapy surgical planning, and (6) postoperative local irradiation and systemic therapy, if indicated.

Surgical Issues After PST

Several important surgical issues need to be considered in managing patients who have received PST, including assuring appropriate breast conservation surgery in patients whose tumor may or may not complete regress after therapy and management of the axilla.

All patients with operable or LABC who are candidates for PST should be evaluated by a multidisciplinary team including a surgeon, medical oncologist, radiologist, and radiation oncologist, and the local treatment goals planned prior to initiating PST. The location and characteristics of the primary tumor and regional lymph nodes need to be accurately recorded in the medical record. For patients who may be considering breast conservation, sonographically or mammographcally directed radiopaque clip placement in the center of the tumor, and/or multiple clip placements bracketing the tumor bed, should be performed to facilitate accurate tumor localization at surgery. Patients should be consistently evaluated after each chemotherapy cycle in order to determine clinical response. Posttreatment imaging with mammography, sonography, and/or MRI is indicated for those being considered for breast conservation in order to facilitate achieving tumor-free margins.

Some studies have demonstrated the feasibility of performing SNB after PST. Mamounas et al. reported the feasibility and accuracy of SNB in 428 patients enrolled in NSABP B-27. Lymphatic mapping was performed with radioactive colloid (15%), with lymphazurin blue dye alone (30%), or with both (55%). Success rate for the identification and removal of a sentinel node was 85% and increased significantly with the use of radioisotope compared with lymphazurin alone (88% vs. 78%; $p = 0.03$). There were no significant differences in success rate according to clinical tumor size, clinical nodal status, age, or calendar year of random assignment. Of 343 patients who had SNB and axillary dissection, the sentinel nodes were positive in 125 patients and were the only positive nodes in 70 patients (56%). Of the 218 patients with negative sentinel nodes, nonsentinel nodes were positive in 15 (false-negative rate, 11%; 15 of 140 patients). There were no significant differences in false-negative rate according to clinical patient and tumor characteristics, method of lymphatic mapping, or breast tumor response to chemotherapy. These results are comparable to those obtained from multicenter studies evaluating SNB before systemic therapy and suggest that the sentinel node concept is applicable following PST.

Locoregional failure is a concern for patients with LABC treated with breast-conserving surgery (BCS), as it is known to be associated with increased risk of distant disease and death. Among 2669 patients with operable breast cancer and positive axillary nodes treated initially with surgery in five NSABP trials, 424 patients (16%) experienced locoregional failure, including 259 (10%) with ipsilateral breast tumor recurrence (IBTR) and 165 (6%) with other local-regional recurrence (oLRR) (Wapnir et al., 2006). The 10-year cumulative incidence of IBTR and oLRR was 9% and 6%, respectively. Most locoregional failures occurred within five years (62% for IBTR and 81% for oLRR). The five-year DDFS rates after IBTR and oLRR were 51% and 19%, respectively, and five-year overall survival rates were 60% and 24%, respectively. Hazard ratios for mortality associated with IBTR and oLRR were 2.6 and 5.9, respectively. Chen et al. (2004) reviewed the experience with BCS in patients managed at MD Anderson Cancer Center after PST. The analysis included 340 patients treated with PST followed by BCS and radiation therapy between 1987 and 2000. Clinical stage at diagnosis (according to the 2003 American Joint Committee on Cancer system) was I in 4%, II in 58%, and III in 38% of patients. Only 4% had positive surgical margins. At a median follow-up period of 60 months, 29 patients (9%) had developed LRR, 16 of which were IBTRs. Five-year actuarial rates of IBTR-free and LRR-free survival were 95% and 91%, respectively. Variables that positively correlated with IBTR and LRR were clinical N2 or N3 disease, pathological residual tumor larger than 2 cm, a multifocal pattern of residual disease, and lymphovascular space invasion in the specimen. The presence of any one of these factors was associated with five-year actuarial IBTR-free and LRR-free survival rates of 87% to 91% and 77% to 84%, respectively. Initial T category (T1–2 vs. T3–4) correlated with LRR but did not correlate with IBTR (5-year IBTR-free rates of 96% vs. 92%, respectively; $p = 0.19$). This report provides reassurance that BCS may be performed in patients following PST, resulting in acceptably low rates of LRR and IBTR in appropriately selected patients, even in those with T3 or T4 disease. This same group has proposed a scoring system that may assist in estimating the risk of LRR after BCS or mastectomy (Huang et al., 2006).

Nonrandomized Trials of PST in LABC and Non-LABC

A number of trials have evaluated the role of PST in LABC and non-LABC given either before surgery, irradiation, or both. In general, these studies have demonstrated PST to be a feasible approach, resulting in an objective response rate of approximately 70% to 80%, cCR rate of 20% to 30%, and pathological complete response rate of 5% to 10%. Rapid progression to inoperable disease was uncommon. Most studies included doxorubicin as a component of therapy.

The largest experience evaluating PST in LABC at a single institution has been reported by the MD Anderson group. Patients were treated on seven successive trials conducted over 20-year period that evaluated doxorubicin-based regimens (Buzdar et al., 1995; Hortobagyi et al., 1988). The group included 752 patients with inflammatory ($N = 178$) and noninflammatory ($N = 598$) LABC, including some patients who had regional lymph node metastases that involved the supraclavicular and/or internal mammary nodes. In the initial study that included 174 evaluable patients, response was evaluated after three cycles of FAC: 88% of patients had at least a partial response, including 17% who had a cCR. Additional therapy consisted of continued adjuvant FAC (administered until a cumulative doxorubicin dose of 450 mg/m^2), "maintenance CMF" for one to two years, and local irradiation given before or after adjuvant therapy. At

15 years, the estimated survival was 54% for stage IIIA disease and 24% for stage IIIB disease. The same group has also reported a 32% 10-year survival for patients with ipsilateral supraclavicular lymph node metastases treated with a similar combined modality approach (and have therefore been reclassified from stage IV to stage IIIC disease in the sixth edition of the AJCC staging) (Brito et al., 2001).

RANDOMIZED TRIALS OF IRRADIATION FOLLOWING MASTECTOMY

Factors associated with a high rate of local recurrence after mastectomy include having a large (>5 cm) primary tumor, at least four positive axillary lymph nodes, extension of tumor beyond the lymph node capsule, or a positive surgical margin. In one large retrospective analysis of patients treated with mastectomy without irradiation in four clinical trials, 55% of 2016 patients had a disease recurrence, including 13% who had an isolated locoregional failure and 8% who had a locoregional failure and distant failure as the first site of failure (Cuzick et al., 1994; Recht et al., 1999).

Cuzick et al. (1994) performed a meta-analysis of eight randomized trials initiated before 1975 in which radiotherapy was the randomized option and surgery was the same for both treatment arms. An increase in all-cause mortality in 10-year survivors that was apparent in the first analysis of this data was no longer significant, although a numerical difference in favor of nonirradiated patients persisted. Irradiation resulted in an excess of cardiac deaths, although this was offset by a reduced number of deaths due to breast cancer. This analysis demonstrated that irradiation administered by relatively primitive techniques by today's standards reduced breast cancer mortality, an effect that was offset by delayed toxicity of the treatment. Whelan et al. (2000) reported the results of a more recent meta-analysis that included 18 trials that were reported between 1967 and 1999, which found that locoregional irradiation given after mastectomy reduced the risk of local recurrence by 75%, any recurrence by 31%, and mortality by 17%.

The results of four studies are noteworthy in that they were first to unequivocally demonstrate a benefit for irradiation or included patients with LABC (Table 6). The Danish Breast Cancer Cooperative Group randomized 1708 women treated between 1982 and 1987, all of whom were premenopausal and had either positive axillary nodes, a tumor size of more than 5 cm, and/or invasion of the cancer to skin or pectoralis fascia (Overgaard et al., 1997). All patients underwent a modified radical mastectomy and a level I ALND. Some level II nodes were also removed, although a complete level II dissection was not routinely performed. The median number of axillary lymph nodes removed was seven. All patients received CMF for nine cycles. About one-half of all patients were randomly assigned to also receive radiation therapy. The radiation began within one week of the first cycle of CMF and was completed prior to starting the second cycle. Those assigned to receive radiation received eight rather than nine cycles of CMF. The radiation field included the chest wall, supraclavicular nodes, infraclavicular nodes, axillary nodes, and the internal mammary nodes in the four upper intercostal spaces. The dose of radiation for most patients was 50 Gy given in 25 fractions over a period of five weeks. The recommended field arrangement involved the use of an anterior photon field against the supraclavicular, infraclavicular, and axillary nodes, and an anterior electron field against the internal mammary nodes and the chest wall. The use of electrons to the chest wall and internal mammary nodes was intended to reduce exposure of the heart to radiation. Most patients were treated at one of six departments that used a linear accelerator. At 10 years, DFS was 48% in the radiation group compared with 34% in the control group. Likewise,

Table 6 Randomized Trials of Postmastectomy Chest Wall Irradiation

References	Follow-up (yr)	Arms	T3/T4	No.	LRR	DFS	OS
Overgaard et al., 1997	9.5	RT	28%/0%	852	9%[a]	48%[a]	54%[a]
		No RT	25%/0%	856	32%	34%	45%
Overgaard et al., 1999	9.9	RT	35%/0%	686	8%[a]	36%[a]	45%[a]
		No RT	35%/0%	689	35%	24%	35%
Ragaz et al., 1997	12.5	RT	NR	164	13%[a]	56%[a]	64%[a]
		No RT	NR	154	25%	41%	54%
Olson et al., 1997	9.1	RT	45%/34%	164	15%[a]	60%	46%
		No RT	47%/13%	146	24%	56%	47%

Abbreviations: NR, not reported; LRR, local-regional recurrence; DFS, disease-free survival; OS, overall survival; a, not significant.

overall survival was improved, being 54% at 10 years in those assigned to receive radiation compared with 45% in the control group. Radiotherapy reduced the risk of local recurrence from 32% to 9%. There was no effect of radiotherapy on the proportion of patients that presented with distant metastases without local recurrence. Using a statistical model that adjusted for a variety of prognostic variables, the authors reported that radiotherapy reduced the risk of death by about 30%, and reduced the risk of any type of recurrence or death by about 40%. A study performed by the same group in postmenopausal women treated with tamoxifen revealed that irradiation reduced the risk of local recurrence (35% vs. 8%) and resulted in an improvement in DFS (36% vs. 24%) and overall survival (45% vs. 36%) (Overgaard et al., 1999).

The British Columbia Cancer Agency reported a similar trial that included 318 Canadian women treated between 1978 and 1986, all of whom were premenopausal and were required to have at least one positive axillary node (Ragaz et al., 1997). All patients underwent a modified radical mastectomy and a level I ALND. Unlike the Danish study, all patients also had a complete level II node dissection. This resulted in a higher median number of axillary lymph nodes removed in the Canadian study (11) compared with the Danish premenopausal study (7). All patients received CMF for 6 to 12 months. Irradiation began between the fourth and fifth cycles of CMF. The radiation field included the chest wall, supraclavicular nodes, infraclavicular nodes, axillary nodes, and the internal mammary nodes, a field that was similar to the Danish study. The dose of radiation was about 25% lower, being 37.5 Gy given in 16 fractions over a period of three to four weeks. All fields were treated with a cobalt 60 unit. At 10 years, DFS was 56% in the radiation group compared with 41% in the control group. Likewise, overall survival was improved, being 64% at 10 years in those assigned to receive radiation compared with 54% in the control group. The DFS in both groups was about 7% to 8% better in the Canadian study compared with the Danish premenopausal study, probably because the Canadian trial included fewer patients with large tumors. About one-fourth of patients in the Danish trial had tumor larger than five centimeters, compared with less than 4% in the Canadian trial. The benefits for radiotherapy were seen in patients with one to three positive nodes and in those with four or more positive nodes.

Olson et al. evaluated postmastectomy irradiation in 332 patients with noninflammatory LABC that was technically resectable, of whom 46% had T3 lesions and 38% had T4 lesions. Patients underwent mastectomy followed by six cycles of doxorubicin-based adjuvant therapy. The median number of positive axillary lymph nodes was 8, compared with 1 to 3 in the Danish and Canadian trials. Although the risk of local recurrence was reduced from 24% to 15%, there was no significant difference in DFS or overall survival (Olson et al., 1997).

The American Society of Clinical Oncology has issued guidelines for postmastectomy irradiation (Recht et al., 2001). The panel recommended radiation for patients with four or more positive axillary nodes, or T3 tumors with any number of positive axillary nodes. The panel recommended that the radiation field always include the chest wall and the supraclavicular region if there were four or more positive nodes, and that full axillary irradiation not be given in patients who have undergone level I and II axillary dissection due to the risk of lymphedema.

INFLAMMATORY BREAST CANCER

Inflammatory breast cancer (IBC) is associated with a worse prognosis than noninflammatory LABC (Jaiyesimi et al., 1992). It is characterized clinically by erythema (often with an erysipeloid edge), edema, and brawny induration of the skin that produces the so-called "peau d'orange" (orange peel) appearance. It may be confused with cellulitis or mastitis. It is associated with a palpable mass in about one-half of cases. It has been recognized for more than a century that this appearance is due to infiltration of tumor cells in the dermal lymphatics that produces capillary congestion, thereby resulting in edema and erythema of the skin. IBC accounts for approximately 6% of all breast cancer in the United States and occurs more commonly in younger and African American women (Levine et al., 1985). It is a very common presentation of breast cancer in Tunisia, where it accounts for about one-half of all cases (Tabbane et al., 1977; Mourali et al., 1978, 1980; Costa et al., 1982; Attia-Sobol et al., 1993). It usually presents with a relatively short interval between symptoms or signs and clinical presentation, whereas in other cases it may occur as a consequence of a neglected slowly growing tumor. One retrospective analysis of 109 patients who had either IBC ($N = 62$) or a neglected LABC with secondary evidence of clinical inflammatory signs ($N = 47$) suggested a similar prognosis when treated with combined modality therapy (Attia-Sobol et al., 1993). Up to one-third of patients with IBC may have distant metastases at the time of presentation, compared with only about 5% for patients with noninflammatory LABC (Levine et al., 1985). The tumor is often high grade and is ER/PR negative. Molecular alterations that have been associated with IBC include Her2/neu overexpression, p53 mutations (Sawaki et al., 2006), overexpression of caveolin 1 and 2 (Van den Eynden et al., 2006), and overexpression of RhoC in conjunction with loss of WNT-1-induced secreted protein 3 (WISP3) (Kleer et al., 2004). Several studies have used molecular profiling techniques. Bieche et al. (2004) reported that 27 of the 538 genes were significantly upregulated in IBC compared with non-IBC, including genes encoding transcription factors, growth factors, and growth factor receptors. Others have reported a signature that appears to be distinct for inflammatory disease (Bertucci et al., 2004; Van Laere et al., 2005; Charafe-Jauffret et al., 2004).

There is some controversy if the presence of dermal lymphatic invasion is mandatory for the diagnosis, and regarding its prognostic significance. Ellis reported that patients who had clinical manifestations of IBC but lacked dermal lymphatic invasion histologically had a better prognosis, although this conclusion was based on a retrospective analysis of eight cases (Ellis and Teitelbaum, 1974). Saltzstein (1974) proposed that patients with "clinically occult inflammatory carcinoma," characterized by dermal lymphatic invasion by tumor cells without clinical signs of IBC, had a poor prognosis consistent with IBC; however, this observation was likewise based on a small number of cases. Levine et al. (1985) reported a three-year survival rate of 34% in 153 patients with both clinical and histological evidence of dermal lymphatic involvement ($N = 153$), 60% for those with clinical signs alone ($N = 2937$), and 52% in those with dermal lymphatic involvement without clinical signs ($N = 81$).

Management of IBC

Treatment with surgery, irradiation, or the combination is inadequate for IBC (Singletary et al., 1994). With surgery alone, median survival is generally less than two years, and the local recurrence rate is high (Bozzetti et al., 1981). Following the report by Haagensen about the ineffectiveness of surgery for the treatment of breast cancer associated with "grave signs," many groups investigated irradiation as the primary therapy; median survival ranged between 9 and 28 months, and few patients survived beyond five years (Barker et al., 1976; Chu et al., 1980; Bozzetti et al., 1981; Perez and Fields, 1987). Local and systemic control is also poor when surgery and irradiation are used in combination (Zucali et al., 1976).

Nonrandomized Studies of Chemotherapy Plus Local Therapy for Inflammatory Carcinoma

The observation that local treatment modalities did little to improve survival due to the rapid development of metastatic disease prompted investigators to evaluate the role of chemotherapy in conjunction with local therapy, and generally indicated a more favorable outcome (De Lena et al., 1978; Israel et al. 1986; Swain and Lippman 1989; Low et al., 2004). Several nonrandomized studies suggested a role for systemic chemotherapy.

Rouesse et al. (1986) reported three consecutive studies conducted at the Institut Gustave-Roussy. The first trial consisted of 60 patients treated before 1975 with irradiation alone. Subsequent studies utilized different induction chemotherapy regimens followed by identical postirradiation maintenance chemotherapy. Induction chemotherapy consisted of doxorubicin, vincristine, methotrexate (AVM) for three cycles in the second study, and AVM plus cyclophosphamide and 5-fluorouracil (AVCMF) for three cycles in the third study. There was a significant improvement in four-year DFS for patients treated with AVCMF (46%) compared with AVM (28%) and irradiation alone (16%). Likewise, there was also significantly better survival for patients treated with AVCMF (66%) compared with AVM (44%) and irradiation alone (28%). A statistically significant improvement in four-year DFS and overall survival was demonstrated for patients receiving induction chemotherapy with AVCMF (46% and 66%, respectively) compared with patients receiving induction chemotherapy with AVM (28% and 44%, respectively). The four-year DFS and overall survival of historical controls treated with radiotherapy alone were 16% and 28%, respectively.

Perez et al. (1994) treated 179 patients with IBC with irradiation alone ($N = 33$), irradiation and chemotherapy ($N = 35$), irradiation and surgery ($N = 25$), or chemotherapy, irradiation, and surgery ($N = 96$). The 10-year DFS was significantly better for those treated with all three modalities (35%) compared with irradiation and surgery (24%) or irradiation alone or in combination with chemotherapy (0%). Although this was a nonrandomized study, it suggested that combined modality therapy could provide survival benefit in IBC compared with single modality treatment.

Chevallier et al. (1993) reported three studies of combined modality therapy in 178 patients with IBC. In the first study, 64 patients received CMF or doxorubicin, vincristine, cyclophosphamide, and 5-fluorouracil (ACVF) plus irradiation. In the second study, 83 patients received either doxorubicin-based chemotherapy followed by surgery ($N = 38$) or irradiation (N = 22) if there was a complete or partial response, or irradiation ($N = 23$) if there was supraclavicular adenopathy or progressive disease after chemotherapy. In the third study, 31 patients received estrogen priming plus FEC followed by surgery or irradiation. The objective response rates were 56%, 74%, and 94% for the first, second, and third studies, respectively, suggesting an advantage for hormonal synchronization. There was no significant difference in the three arms, however, in the median DFS (17, 19, and 22 months, respectively). Subsequent studies in metastatic breast cancer revealed no benefit for estrogen synchronization (Lippman et al., 1984; Lipton et al., 1987; Paridaens et al., 1993). Likewise, a phase III trial evaluating estrogen priming as adjuvant therapy in patients with stage II–IIIA breast cancer demonstrated no benefit (Bontenbal et al., 2000).

Buzdar et al. (1995) reported the results of 178 patients treated at the MD Anderson Cancer Center in four consecutive studies all of whom received three cycles of FAC prior to local therapy. The four studies also included: (1) radiotherapy to the primary tumor followed by maintenance chemotherapy for 24 months ($N = 40$), (2) mastectomy followed by adjuvant FAC and irradiation ($N = 23$), (3) the same regimen as the second study plus the addition of vincristine and prednisone ($N = 43$), (4) the same treatment as the previous studies with doxorubicin given as a 48-hour IV infusion ($N = 72$). There was no significant difference in DFS or OS between the groups. The local control rate was 82%, and about one-third of patients survived 10 years, with some relapses seen after 10 years.

CONCLUSIONS

Chemotherapy, hormonal therapy, and immunotherapy with trastuzumab have all been shown to significantly reduce the risk of recurrence when used postoperatively in appropriately selected patients with operable breast cancer who have received primary surgical therapy. For patients with LABC who are not optimal surgical candidates, preoperative chemotherapy produces clinical response in most patients, clinical downstaging in the majority of patients, and facilitates breast conservation in some patients. Management of both operable and locally advanced disease requires a multimodality treatment approach including surgeons, radiologists, medical oncologists, radiation oncologists, and pathologists.

REFERENCES

ACR practice guideline for the performance of magnetic resonance imaging (MRI) of the breast. Reston, VA: American College of Radiology, 2007. Available at: http://www.acr.org/s_acr/bin.asp?CID=549&DID=17775&DOC=FILE.PDF. Accessed March 8, 2007.

Attia-Sobol J, Ferriere JP, Cure H, Kwiatkowski F, Achard JL, Verrelle P, Feillel V, de Latour M, Lafaye C, Deloche C, et al. Treatment results, survival and prognostic factors in 109 inflammatory breast cancers: univariate and multivariate analysis. Eur J Cancer 1993; 29A(8):1081–1088.

Barker JL, Nelson AJ, Montague E. Inflammatory carcinoma of the breast. Radiology 1976; 121(1):173–176.

Baum M. Adjuvant endocrine therapy in postmenopausal women with early breast cancer: where are we now? Eur J Cancer 2005; 41(12):1667–1677.

Bear HD, Anderson S, Smith RE, Geyer CE Jr., Mamounas EP, Fisher B, Brown AM, Robidoux A, Margolese R, Kahlenberg MS, Paik S, Soran A, Wickerham DL, Wolmark N. Sequential preoperative or postoperative docetaxel added to preoperative doxorubicin plus cyclophosphamide for operable breast cancer: National Surgical Adjuvant Breast and Bowel Project Protocol B-27. J Clin Oncol 2006; 24(13):2019–2027.

Bertucci F, Finetti P, Rougemont J, Charafe-Jauffret E, Nasser V, Loriod B, Camerlo J, Tagett R, Tarpin C, Houvenaeghel G, Nguyen C, Maraninchi D, Jacquemier J, Houlgatte R, Birnbaum D, Viens P. Gene expression profiling for molecular characterization of inflammatory breast cancer and prediction of response to chemotherapy. Cancer Res 2004; 64(23):8558–8565.

Bieche I, Lerebours F, Tozlu S, Espie M, Marty M, Lidereau R. Molecular profiling of inflammatory breast cancer: identification of a poor-prognosis gene expression signature. Clin Cancer Res 2004; 10(20):6789–6795.

Bonadonna G, Brusamolino E, Valagussa P, Rossi A, Brugnatelli L, Brambilla C, de Lena M, Tancini G, Bajetta E, Musumeci R, Veronesi U. Combination chemotherapy as an adjuvant treatment in operable breast cancer. N Engl J Med 1976; 294(8):405–410.

Bontenbal M, van Putten WL, Burghouts JT, Baggen MG, Ras GJ, Stiegelis WF, Beudeker M, Janssen JT, Braun JJ, van der Linden GH, van der Velden PC, van Geel AN, Helle P, Leisink M, Foekens JA, Klijn JG. Value of estrogenic recruitment before chemotherapy: first randomized trial in primary breast cancer. J Clin Oncol 2000; 18(4):734–742.

Bozzetti F, Saccozzi R, de Lena M, Salvadori B. Inflammatory cancer of the breast: analysis of 114 cases. J Surg Oncol 1981; 18(4):355–361.

Brito RA, Valero V, Buzdar AU, Booser DJ, Ames F, Strom E, Ross M, Theriault RL, Frye D, Kau SW, Asmar L, McNeese M, Singletary SE, Hortobagyi GN. Long-term results of combined-modality therapy for locally advanced breast cancer with ipsilateral supraclavicular metastases: The University of Texas M.D. Anderson Cancer Center experience. J Clin Oncol 2001; 19(3):628–633.

Burstein HJ, Harris LN, Gelman R, Lester SC, Nunes RA, Kaelin CM, Parker LM, Ellisen LW, Kuter I, Gadd MA, Christian RL, Kennedy PR, Borges VF, Bunnell CA, Younger J, Smith BL, Winer EP. Preoperative therapy with trastuzumab and paclitaxel followed by sequential adjuvant doxorubicin/cyclophosphamide for HER2 overexpressing stage II or III breast cancer: a pilot study. J Clin Oncol 2003; 21(1):46–53.

Buzdar AU, Singletary SE, Booser DJ, Frye DK, Wasaff B, Hortobagyi GN. Combined modality treatment of stage III and inflammatory breast cancer. M.D. Anderson Cancer Center experience. Surg Oncol Clin N Am 1995; 4(4): 715–734.

Buzdar AU, Singletary SE, Theriault RL, Booser DJ, Valero V, Ibrahim N, Smith TL, Asmar L, Frye D, Manuel N, Kau SW, McNeese M, Strom E, Hunt K, Ames F, Hortobagyi GN. Prospective evaluation of paclitaxel versus combination chemotherapy with fluorouracil, doxorubicin, and cyclophosphamide as neoadjuvant therapy in patients with operable breast cancer. J Clin Oncol 1999; 17(11): 3412–3417.

Buzdar AU, Valero V, Ibrahim NK, Francis D, Broglio KR, Theriault RL, Pusztai L, Green MC, Singletary SE, Hunt KK, Sahin AA, Esteva F, Symmans WF, Ewer MS, Buchholz TA, Hortobagyi GN. Neoadjuvant therapy with paclitaxel followed by 5-fluorouracil, epirubicin, and cyclophosphamide chemotherapy and concurrent trastuzumab in human epidermal growth factor receptor 2-positive operable breast cancer: an update of the initial randomized study population and data of additional patients treated with the same regimen. Clin Cancer Res 2007; 13(1):228–233.

Buzdar AU, Ibrahim NK, Francis D, Booser DJ, Thomas ES, Theriault RL, Pusztai L, Green MC, Arun BK, Giordano SH, Cristofanilli M, Frye DK, Smith TL, Hunt KK, Singletary SE, Sahin AA, Ewer MS, Buchholz TA, Berry D, Hortobagyi GN. Significantly higher pathologic complete remission rate after neoadjuvant therapy with trastuzumab, paclitaxel, and epirubicin chemotherapy: results of a randomized trial in human epidermal growth factor receptor 2-positive operable breast cancer. J Clin Oncol 2005; 23 (16):3676–3685.

Carey LA, Metzger R, Dees EC, Collichio F, Sartor CI, Ollila DW, Klauber-DeMore N, Halle J, Sawyer L, Moore DT, Graham ML. American Joint Committee on Cancer tumor-node-metastasis stage after neoadjuvant chemotherapy and breast cancer outcome. J Natl Cancer Inst 2005; 97 (15):1137–1142.

Carlson RW, Brown E, Burstein HJ, Gradishar WJ, Hudis CA, Loprinzi C, Mamounas EP, Perez EA, Pritchard K, Ravdin P, Recht A, Somlo G, Theriault RL, Winer EP, Wolff AC. NCCN Task Force report: adjuvant therapy for breast cancer. J Natl Compr Canc Netw 2006; 4(suppl 1):S1–S26.

Charafe-Jauffret E, Tarpin C, Bardou VJ, Bertucci F, Ginestier C, Braud AC, Puig B, Geneix J, Hassoun J, Birnbaum D, Jacquemier J, Viens P. Immunophenotypic analysis of inflammatory breast cancers: identification of an 'inflammatory signature'. J Pathol 2004; 202(3):265–273.

Chen AM, Meric-Bernstam F, Hunt KK, Thames HD, Oswald MJ, Outlaw ED, Strom EA, McNeese MD, Kuerer HM, Ross MI, Singletary SE, Ames FC, Feig BW, Sahin AA, Perkins GH, Schechter NR, Hortobagyi GN, Buchholz TA. Breast conservation after neoadjuvant chemotherapy: the MD Anderson Cancer Center experience. J Clin Oncol 2004; 22(12):2303–2312.

Chevallier B, Bastit P, Graic Y, Menard JF, Dauce JP, Julien JP, Clavier B, Kunlin A, D'Anjou J. The Centre H. Becquerel studies in inflammatory non metastatic breast cancer. Combined modality approach in 178 patients. Br J Cancer 1993; 67(3):594–601.

Chu AM, Wood WC, Doucette JA. Inflammatory breast carcinoma treated by radical radiotherapy. Cancer 1980; 45(11): 2730–2737.

Citron ML, Berry DA, Cirrincione C, Hudis C, Winer EP, Gradishar WJ, Davidson NE, Martino S, Livingston R, Ingle JN, Perez EA, Carpenter J, Hurd D, Holland JF, Smith BL, Sartor CI, Leung EH, Abrams J, Schilsky RL, Muss HB, Norton L. Randomized trial of dose-dense versus conventionally scheduled and sequential versus concurrent combination chemotherapy as postoperative adjuvant treatment of node-positive primary breast cancer: first report of Intergroup Trial C9741/Cancer and Leukemia Group B Trial 9741. J Clin Oncol 2003; 21(8): 1431–1439.

Cleator S, Tsimelzon A, Ashworth A, Dowsett M, Dexter T, Powles T, Hilsenbeck S, Wong H, Osborne CK, O'Connell P, Chang JC. Gene expression patterns for doxorubicin (Adriamycin) and cyclophosphamide (cytoxan) (AC) response and resistance. Breast Cancer Res Treat 2006; 95(3):229–233.

Coates AS, Keshaviah A, Thurlimann B, Mouridsen H, Mauriac L, Forbes JF, Paridaens R, Castiglione-Gertsch M, Gelber RD, Colleoni M, Lang I, Del Mastro L, Smith I, Chirgwin J, Nogaret JM, Pienkowski T, Wardley A, Jakobsen EH, Price KN, Goldhirsch A. Five years of letrozole compared with tamoxifen as initial adjuvant therapy for postmenopausal women with endocrine-responsive early breast cancer: update of study BIG 1-98. J Clin Oncol 2007; 25(5): 486–492.

Cobleigh MA, Vogel CL, Tripathy D, Robert NJ, Scholl S, Fehrenbacher L, Wolter JM, Paton V, Shak S, Lieberman G, Slamon DJ. Multinational study of the efficacy and safety of humanized anti-HER2 monoclonal antibody in women who have HER2-overexpressing metastatic breast cancer that has progressed after chemotherapy for metastatic disease. J Clin Oncol 1999; 17(9):2639–2648.

Coombes RC, Hall E, Gibson LJ, Paridaens R, Jassem J, Delozier T, Jones SE, Alvarez I, Bertelli G, Ortmann O, Coates AS, Bajetta E, Dodwell D, Coleman RE, Fallowfield LJ, Mickiewicz E, Andersen J, Lonning PE, Cocconi G, Stewart A, Stuart N, Snowdon CF, Carpentieri M, Massimini G, Bliss JM van de Velde C. A randomized trial of exemestane after two to three years of tamoxifen therapy in postmenopausal women with primary breast cancer. N Engl J Med 2004; 350(11):1081–1092.

Coombes RC, Kilburn LS, Snowdon CF, Paridaens R, Coleman RE, Jones SE, Jassem J, Van de Velde CJ, Delozier T, Alvarez I, Del Mastro L, Ortmann O, Diedrich K, Coates AS, Bajetta E, Holmberg SB, Dodwell D, Mickiewicz E, Andersen J, Lonning PE, Cocconi G, Forbes J, Castiglione M, Stuart N, Stewart A, Fallowfield LJ, Bertelli G, Hall E, Bogle RG, Carpentieri M, Colajori E, Subar M, Ireland E, Bliss JM. Survival and safety of exemestane versus tamoxifen after 2–3 years' tamoxifen treatment (Intergroup Exemestane Study): a randomised controlled trial. Lancet 2007; 369(9561):559–570.

Costa J, Webber BL, Levine PH, Muenz L, O'Conor GT, Tabbane F, Belhassen S, Kamaraju LS, Mourali N. Histopathological features of rapidly progressing breast carcinoma in Tunisia: a study of 94 cases. Int J Cancer 1982; 30(1):35–37.

Crump M, Goss PE, Prince M, Girouard C. Outcome of extensive evaluation before adjuvant therapy in women with breast cancer and 10 or more positive axillary lymph nodes. J Clin Oncol 1996; 14(1):66–69.

Cuzick J, Stewart H, Rutqvist L, Houghton J, Edwards R, Redmond C, Peto R, Baum M, Fisher B, Host H, et al. Cause-specific mortality in long-term survivors of breast cancer who participated in trials of radiotherapy. J Clin Oncol 1994; 12(3):447–453.

De Lena M, Zucali R, Viganotti G, Valagussa P, Bonadonna G. Combined chemotherapy-radiotherapy approach in locally advanced (T3b-T4) breast cancer. Cancer Chemother Pharmacol 1978; 1(1):53–59.

Dieras V, Fumoleau P, Romieu G, Tubiana-Hulin M, Namer M, Mauriac L, Guastalla JP, Pujade-Lauraine E, Kerbrat P, Maillart P, Penault-Llorca F, Buyse M, Pouillart P. Randomized parallel study of doxorubicin plus paclitaxel and doxorubicin plus cyclophosphamide as neoadjuvant treatment of patients with breast cancer. J Clin Oncol 2004; 22(24):4958–4965.

Early Breast Cancer Trialists' Collaborative Group (EBCTCG). Effects of chemotherapy and hormonal therapy for early breast cancer on recurrence and 15-year survival: an overview of the randomised trials. Lancet 2005; 365 (9472):1687–1717.

Ellis DL, Teitelbaum SL. Inflammatory carcinoma of the breast. A pathologic definition Cancer 1974; 33(4):1045–1047.

Ellis GK, Barlow WE, Russell CA, Royce ME, Perez EA, Livingston RB. SWOG 0012, a randomized phase III comparison of standard doxorubicin (A) and cyclophosphamide (C) followed by weekly paclitaxel (T) versus weekly doxorubicin and daily oral cyclophosphamide plus G-CSF (G) followed by weekly paclitaxel as neoadjuvant therapy for inflammatory and locally advanced breast cancer. Proc Am Soc Clin Oncol 2006; 24(18S):LBA537.

Evans TR, Yellowlees A, Foster E, Earl H, Cameron DA, Hutcheon AW, Coleman RE, Perren T, Gallagher CJ, Quigley M, Crown J, Jones AL, Highley M, Leonard RC, Mansi JL. Phase III randomized trial of doxorubicin and docetaxel versus doxorubicin and cyclophosphamide as primary medical therapy in women with breast cancer: an anglo-celtic cooperative oncology group study. J Clin Oncol 2005; 23(13):2988–2995.

Fan C, Oh DS, Wessels L, Weigelt B, Nuyten DS, Nobel AB, van't Veer LJ, Perou CM. Concordance among gene-expression-based predictors for breast cancer. N Engl J Med 2006; 355(6):560–569.

Fisher B. Laboratory and clinical research in breast cancer—a personal adventure: the David A. Karnofsky memorial lecture. Cancer Res 1980; 40(11):3863–3874.

Fisher B, Carbone P, Economou SG, Frelick R, Glass A, Lerner H, Redmond C, Zelen M, Band P, Katrych DL, Wolmark N, Fisher ER. 1-Phenylalanine mustard (L-PAM) in the management of primary breast cancer. A report of early findings. N Engl J Med 1975; 292(3):117–122.

Fisher B, Saffer E, Rudock C, Coyle J, Gunduz N. Effect of local or systemic treatment prior to primary tumor removal on the production and response to a serum growth-stimulating factor in mice. Cancer Res 1989; 49(8):2002–2004.

Fisher B, Brown A, Mamounas E, Wieand S, Robidoux A, Margolese RG, Cruz AB Jr., Fisher ER, Wickerham DL, Wolmark N, DeCillis A, Hoehn JL, Lees AW, Dimitrov NV. Effect of preoperative chemotherapy on local-regional disease in women with operable breast cancer: findings from National Surgical Adjuvant Breast and Bowel Project B-18. J Clin Oncol 1997; 15(7):2483–2493.

Fisher B, Bryant J, Wolmark N, Mamounas E, Brown A, Fisher ER, Wickerham DL, Begovic M, DeCillis A, Robidoux A, Margolese RG, Cruz AB Jr., Hoehn JL, Lees AW, Dimitrov NV, Bear HD. Effect of preoperative chemotherapy on the outcome of women with operable breast cancer. J Clin Oncol 1998; 16(8):2672–2685.

Fisher B, Jeong JH, Dignam J, Anderson S, Mamounas E, Wickerham DL, Wolmark N. Findings from recent National Surgical Adjuvant Breast and Bowel Project adjuvant studies in stage I breast cancer. J Natl Cancer Inst Monogr 2001; (30):62–66.

Foekens JA, Atkins D, Zhang Y, Sweep FC, Harbeck N, Paradiso A, Cufer T, Sieuwerts AM, Talantov D, Span PN, Tjan-Heijnen VC, Zito AF, Specht K, Hoefler H, Golouh R, Schittulli F, Schmitt M, Beex LV, Klijn JG, Wang Y. Multicenter validation of a gene expression-based prognostic signature in lymph node-negative primary breast cancer. J Clin Oncol 2006; 24(11):1665–1671.

Fracchia AA, Evans JF, Eisenberg BL. Stage III carcinoma of the breast. A detailed analysis. Ann Surg 1980; 192(6): 705–710.

Frierson HF Jr., Fechner RE. Histologic grade of locally advanced infiltrating ductal carcinoma after treatment with induction chemotherapy. Am J Clin Pathol 1994; 102(2): 154–157.

Fumoleau P, Kerbrat P, Romestaing P, Fargeot P, Bremond A, Namer M, Schraub S, Goudier MJ, Mihura J, Monnier A, Clavere P, Serin D, Seffert P, Pourny C, Facchini T, Jacquin JP, Sztermer JF, Datchary J, Ramos R, Luporsi E. Randomized trial comparing six versus three cycles of epirubicin-based adjuvant chemotherapy in premenopausal, node-positive breast cancer patients: 10-year follow-up results of the French Adjuvant Study Group 01 trial. J Clin Oncol 2003; 21(2):298–305.

Gasparini G, Pozza F, Harris AL. Evaluating the potential usefulness of new prognostic and predictive indicators in node-negative breast cancer patients. J Natl Cancer Inst 1993; 85(15):1206–1219.

Gianni L, Baselga J, Eiermann W, Guillem Porta V, Semiglazov V, Lluch A, Zambetti M, Sabadell D, Raab G, Llombart Cussac A, Bozhok A, Martinez-Agullo A, Greco M, Byakhov M, Lopez Lopez JJ, Mansutti M, Valagussa P, Bonadonna G. Feasibility and tolerability of sequential doxorubicin/paclitaxel followed by cyclophosphamide, methotrexate, and fluorouracil and its effects on tumor response as preoperative therapy. Clin Cancer Res 2005a; 11(24 pt 1):8715–8721.

Gianni L, Zambetti M, Clark K, Baker J, Cronin M, Wu J, Mariani G, Rodriguez J, Carcangiu M, Watson D, Valagussa P, Rouzier R, Symmans WF, Ross JS, Hortobagyi GN, Pusztai L, Shak S. Gene expression profiles in paraffin-embedded core biopsy tissue predict response to chemotherapy in women with locally advanced breast cancer. J Clin Oncol2005b; 23(29):7265–7277.

Goldhirsch A, Wood WC, Gelber RD, Coates AS, Thurlimann B, Senn HJ. Meeting highlights: updated international expert consensus on the primary therapy of early breast cancer. J Clin Oncol 2003; 21(17):3357–3365.

Goldstein LJ, O'Neill A, Sparano J, Perez E, Shulman L, Martino S, Davidson N. E2197: Phase III AT (doxorubicin/ docetaxel) vs AC (doxorubicin/cyclophosphamide) in the adjuvant treatment of node positive and high risk node negative breast cance. Proc Am Soc Clin Oncol 2005; 23 (16S, suppl 1): abstr 512.

Goss PE, Ingle JN, Martino S, Robert NJ, Muss HB, Piccart MJ, Castiglione M, Tu D, Shepherd LE, Pritchard KI, Livingston RB, Davidson NE, Norton L, Perez EA, Abrams JS, Cameron DA, Palmer MJ, Pater JL. Randomized trial of letrozole following tamoxifen as extended adjuvant therapy in receptor-positive breast cancer: updated findings from NCIC CTG MA.17. J Natl Cancer Inst 2005; 97(17): 1262–1271.

Green MC, Buzdar AU, Smith T, Ibrahim NK, Valero V, Rosales MF, Cristofanilli M, Booser DJ, Pusztai L, Rivera E, Theriault RL, Carter C, Frye D, Hunt KK, Symmans WF, Strom EA, Sahin AA, Sikov W, Hortobagyi GN. Weekly paclitaxel improves pathologic complete remission in operable breast cancer when compared with paclitaxel once every 3 weeks. J Clin Oncol 2005; 23(25):5983–5992.

Haagensen CD, Stout AP. Carcinoma of the breast. II: criteria of operability. Ann Surg 1943; 118:859–870.

Hansen-Algenstaedt N, Stoll BR, Padera TP, Dolmans DE, Hicklin DJ, Fukumura D Jain RK. Tumor oxygenation in hormone-dependent tumors during vascular endothelial growth factor receptor-2 blockade, hormone ablation, and chemotherapy. Cancer Res 2000; 60(16):4556–4560.

Henderson IC, Berry DA, Demetri GD, Cirrincione CT, Goldstein LJ, Martino S, Ingle JN, Cooper MR, Hayes DF, Tkaczuk KH, Fleming G, Holland JF, Duggan DB, Carpenter JT, Frei E III, Schilsky RL, Wood WC, Muss HB, Norton L. Improved outcomes from adding sequential paclitaxel but not from escalating doxorubicin dose in an adjuvant chemotherapy regimen for patients with node-positive primary breast cancer. J Clin Oncol 2003; 21(6): 976–983.

Hennessy BT, Hortobagyi GN, Rouzier R, Kuerer H, Sneige N, Buzdar AU, Kau SW, Fornage B, Sahin A, Broglio K, Singletary SE, Valero V. Outcome after pathologic complete eradication of cytologically proven breast cancer axillary node metastases following primary chemotherapy. J Clin Oncol 2005; 23(36):9304–9311.

Hess KR, Anderson K, Symmans WF, Valero V, Ibrahim N, Mejia JA, Booser D, Theriault RL, Buzdar AU, Dempsey PJ, Rouzier R, Sneige N, Ross JS, Vidaurre T, Gomez HL, Hortobagyi GN, Pusztai L. Pharmacogenomic predictor of sensitivity to preoperative chemotherapy with paclitaxel and fluorouracil, doxorubicin, and cyclophosphamide in breast cancer. J Clin Oncol 2006; 24(26):4236–4244.

Hortobagyi GN, Ames FC, Buzdar AU, Kau SW, McNeese MD, Paulus D, Hug V, Holmes FA, Romsdahl MM, Fraschini G, et al. Management of stage III primary breast cancer with primary chemotherapy, surgery, and radiation therapy. Cancer 1988; 62(12):2507–2516.

Hotchkiss KA, Ashton AW, Mahmood R, Russell RG, Sparano JA, Schwartz EL. Inhibition of endothelial cell function in vitro and angiogenesis in vivo by docetaxel (Taxotere): association with impaired repositioning of the microtubule organizing center. Mol Cancer Ther 2002; 1(13):191–200.

Huang EH, Strom EA, Perkins GH, Oh JL, Chen A M, Meric-Bernstam F, Hunt KK, Sahin AA, Hortobagyi GN, Buchholz TA. Comparison of risk of local-regional recurrence after mastectomy or breast conservation therapy for patients treated with neoadjuvant chemotherapy and radiation stratified according to a prognostic index score. Int J Radiat Oncol Biol Phys 2006; 66(2):352–357.

Hurley J, Doliny P, Reis I, Silva O, Gomez-Fernandez C, Velez P, Pauletti G, Powell JE, Pegram MD, Slamon DJ. Docetaxel, cisplatin, and trastuzumab as primary systemic therapy for human epidermal growth factor receptor 2-positive locally advanced breast cancer. J Clin Oncol 2006; 24(12):1831–1838.

Israel L, Breau JL, Morere JF. Two years of high-dose cyclophosphamide and 5-fluorouracil followed by surgery after 3 months for acute inflammatory breast carcinomas. A phase II study of 25 cases with a median follow-up of 35 months. Cancer 1986; 57(1):24–28.

Jaiyesimi IA, Buzdar AU, Hortobagyi G. Inflammatory breast cancer: a review. J Clin Oncol 1992; 10(6):1014–1024.

Joensuu H, Kellokumpu-Lehtinen PL, Bono P, Alanko T, Kataja V, Asola R, Utriainen T, Kokko R, Hemminki A, Tarkkanen M, Turpeenniemi-Hujanen T, Jyrkkio S, Flander M, Helle L, Ingalsuo S, Johansson K, Jaaskelainen AS, Pajunen M, Rauhala M, Kaleva-Kerola J, Salminen T, Leinonen M, Elomaa I, Isola J. Adjuvant docetaxel or vinorelbine with or without trastuzumab for breast cancer. N Engl J Med 2006; 354(8): 809–820.

Johnston SR, Hickish T, Ellis P, Houston S, Kelland L, Dowsett M, Salter J, Michiels B, Perez-Ruixo JJ, Palmer P, Howes A. Phase II study of the efficacy and tolerability of two dosing regimens of the farnesyl transferase inhibitor, R115777, in advanced breast cancer. J Clin Oncol 2003; 21(13):2492–2499.

Jones SE, Savin MA, Holmes FA, O'Shaughnessy JA, Blum JL, Vukelja S, McIntyre KJ, Pippen JE, Bordelon JH, Kirby R, Sandbach J, Hyman WJ, Khandelwal P, Negron AG, Richards DA, Anthony SP, Mennel RG, Boehm KA, Meyer WG, Asmar L. Phase III trial comparing doxorubicin plus cyclophosphamide with docetaxel plus cyclophosphamide as adjuvant therapy for operable breast cancer. J Clin Oncol 2006; 24(34):5381–5387.

Kaufmann M, Hortobagyi GN, Goldhirsch A, Scholl S, Makris A, Valagussa P, Blohmer JU, Eiermann W, Jackesz R, Jonat W, Lebeau A, Loibl S, Miller W, Seeber S, Semiglazov V, Smith R, Souchon R, Stearns V, Untch M, von Minckwitz G. Recommendations from an international expert panel on the use of neoadjuvant (primary) systemic treatment of operable breast cancer: an update. J Clin Oncol 2006; 24(12):1940–1949.

Kelland LR, Smith V, Valenti M, Patterson L, Clarke PA, Detre S, End D, Howes AJ, Dowsett M, Workman P, Johnston SR. Preclinical antitumor activity and pharmacodynamic studies with the farnesyl protein transferase inhibitor R115777 in human breast cancer. Clin Cancer Res 2001; 7(11):3544–3550.

Kleer CG, Zhang Y, Pan Q, Gallagher G, Wu M, Wu ZF, Merajver SD. WISP3 and RhoC guanosine triphosphatase cooperate in the development of inflammatory breast cancer. Breast Cancer Res 2004; 6(2):R110–R115.

Kleer CG, Griffith KA, Sabel MS, Gallagher G, van Golen KL, Wu ZF, Merajver SD. RhoC-GTPase is a novel tissue biomarker associated with biologically aggressive carcinomas of the breast. Breast Cancer Res Treat 2005; 93(2): 101–110.

Levine PH, Steinhorn SC, Ries LG, Aron JL. Inflammatory breast cancer: the experience of the surveillance, epidemiology, and end results (SEER) program. J Natl Cancer Inst 1985; 74(2):291–297.

Li T, Sparano JA. Inhibiting ras signaling in the therapy of breast cancer. Clin Breast Cancer 2003; 3(6):405–416.

Lippman ME, Cassidy J, Wesley M, Young RC. A randomized attempt to increase the efficacy of cytotoxic chemotherapy in metastatic breast cancer by hormonal synchronization. J Clin Oncol 1984; 2(1):28–36.

Lipton A, Santen RJ, Harvey HA, Manni A, Simmonds MA, White-Hershey D, Bartholomew MJ, Walker BK, Dixon RH, Valdevia DE, et al. A randomized trial of aminoglutethimide +/- estrogen before chemotherapy in advanced breast cancer. 1987; 10(1):65–70.

Low JA, Berman AW, Steinberg SM, Danforth DN, Lippman ME, Swain SM. Long-term follow-up for locally advanced and inflammatory breast cancer patients treated with multimodality therapy. J Clin Oncol 2004; 22(20):4067–4074.

Lyman GH, Giuliano AE, Somerfield MR, Benson AB III, Bodurka DC, Burstein HJ, Cochran AJ, Cody HS III, Edge SB, Galper S, Hayman JA, Kim TY, Perkins CL, Podoloff DA, Sivasubramaniam VH, Turner RR, Wahl R, Weaver DL, Wolff AC, Winer EP. American Society of Clinical Oncology guideline recommendations for sentinel lymph node biopsy in early-stage breast cancer. J Clin Oncol 2005; 23(30):7703–7720.

Mabry H, Giuliano AE. Sentinel node mapping for breast cancer: progress to date and prospects for the future. Surg Oncol Clin N Am 2007; 16(1):55–70.

Mamounas EP, Brown A, Anderson S, Smith R, Julian T, Miller B, Bear HD, Caldwell CB, Walker AP, Mikkelson W M, Stauffer JS, Robidoux A, Theoret H, Soran A, Fisher B, Wickerham DL, Wolmark N. Sentinel node biopsy after neoadjuvant chemotherapy in breast cancer: results from National Surgical Adjuvant Breast and Bowel Project Protocol B-27. J Clin Oncol 2005a; 23(12):2694–2702.

Mamounas EP, Bryant J, Lembersky B, Fehrenbacher L, Sedlacek SM, Fisher B, Wickerham DL, Yothers G, Soran A Wolmark N. Paclitaxel after doxorubicin plus cyclophosphamide as adjuvant chemotherapy for node-positive breast cancer: results from NSABP B-28. J Clin Oncol 2005b; 23(16):3686–3696.

Martin M, Pienkowski T, Mackey J, Pawlicki M, Guastalla JP, Weaver C, Tomiak E, Al-Tweigeri T, Chap L, Juhos E, Guevin R, Howell A, Fornander T, Hainsworth J, Coleman R, Vinholes J, Modiano M, Pinter T, Tang SC, Colwell B, Prady C, Provencher L, Walde D, Rodriguez-Lescure A, Hugh J, Loret C, Rupin M, Blitz S, Jacobs P, Murawsky M, Riva A, Vogel C. Adjuvant docetaxel for node-positive breast cancer. N Engl J Med 2005; 352(22):2302–2313.

Mauri D, Pavlidis N, Ioannidis JP. Neoadjuvant versus adjuvant systemic treatment in breast cancer: a meta-analysis. J Natl Cancer Inst 1978; 97(3):188–194.

Mohsin SK, Weiss HL, Gutierrez MC, Chamness GC, Schiff R, Digiovanna MP, Wang CX, Hilsenbeck SG, Osborne CK, Allred DC, Elledge R, Chang JC. Neoadjuvant trastuzumab induces apoptosis in primary breast cancers. J Clin Oncol 2005; 23(11):2460–2468.

Mourali N, Levine PH, Tabanne F, Belhassen S, Bahi J, Bennaceur M, Herberman RB. Rapidly progressing breast cancer (poussee evolutive) in Tunisia: studies on delayed hypersensitivity. Int J Cancer 1978; 22(1):1–3.

Mourali N, Muenz LR, Tabbane F, Belhassen S, Bahi J, Levine PH. Epidemiologic features of rapidly progressing breast cancer in Tunisia. Cancer 1980; 46(12):2741–2746.

Nowak AK, Wilcken NR, Stockler MR, Hamilton A, Ghersi D. Systematic review of taxane-containing versus non-taxane-containing regimens for adjuvant and neoadjuvant treatment of early breast cancer. Lancet Oncol 2004; 5(6):372–380.

Olivotto IA, Bajdik CD, Ravdin PM, Speers CH, Coldman AJ, Norris BD, Davis GJ, Chia SK, Gelmon KA. Population-based validation of the prognostic model ADJUVANT! for early breast cancer. J Clin Oncol 2005; 23(12):2716–2725.

Olson JE, Neuberg D, Pandya KJ, Richter MP, Solin LJ, Gilchrist KW, Tormey DC, Veeder M, Falkson G. The role of radiotherapy in the management of operable locally advanced breast carcinoma: results of a randomized trial by the Eastern Cooperative Oncology Group. Cancer 1997; 79(6):1138–1149.

Overgaard M, Hansen PS, Overgaard J, Rose C, Andersson M, Bach F, Kjaer M, Gadeberg CC, Mouridsen HT, Jensen MB, Zedeler K. Postoperative radiotherapy in high-risk premenopausal women with breast cancer who receive adjuvant chemotherapy. Danish Breast Cancer Cooperative Group 82b Trial. N Engl J Med 1997; 337(14):949–955.

Overgaard M, Jensen MB, Overgaard J, Hansen PS, Rose C, Andersson M, Kamby C, Kjaer M, Gadeberg CC, Rasmussen BB, Blichert-Toft M, Mouridsen HT. Postoperative radiotherapy in high-risk postmenopausal breast-cancer patients given adjuvant tamoxifen: Danish Breast Cancer Cooperative Group DBCG 82c randomised trial. Lancet 1999; 353(9165):1641–1648.

Padera TP, Stoll BR, Tooredman JB, Capen D, Di Tomaso E, Jain RK. Pathology: cancer cells compress intratumour vessels. Nature 2004; 427(6976):695.

Paik S, Shak S, Tang G, Kim C, Baker J, Cronin M, Baehner FL, Walker MG, Watson D, Park T, Hiller W, Fisher ER, Wickerham DL, Bryant J, Wolmark N. A multigene assay to predict recurrence of tamoxifen-treated, node-negative breast cancer. N Engl J Med 2004; 351(27):2817–2826.

Paik S, Tang G, Shak S, Kim C, Baker J, Kim W, Cronin M, Baehner FL, Watson D, Bryant J, Costantino JP, Geyer CEJr., Wickerham DL, Wolmark N. Gene expression and benefit of chemotherapy in women with node-negative, estrogen receptor-positive breast cancer. J Clin Oncol 2006; 24(23):3726–3734.

Paridaens R, Heuson JC, Julien JP, Veyret C, van Zyl J, Klijn JG, Sylvester R, Mignolet F. Assessment of estrogenic recruitment before chemotherapy in advanced breast cancer: a double-blind randomized study. European Organization for Research and Treatment of Cancer Breast Cancer Cooperative Group. J Clin Oncol 1993; 11(9):1723–1728.

Perez CA, Fields JN. Role of radiation therapy for locally advanced and inflammatory carcinoma of the breast. Oncology (Williston Park) 1987; 1(1):81–94.

Perez CA, Fields JN, Fracasso PM, Philpott G, Soares RL Jr., Taylor ME, Lockett MA, Rush C. Management of locally advanced carcinoma of the breast. II. Inflammatory carcinoma. Cancer 1994; 74(suppl 1):466–476.

Piccart-Gebhart MJ, Procter M, Leyland-Jones B, Goldhirsch A, Untch M, Smith I, Gianni L, Baselga J, Bell R, Jackisch C, Cameron D, Dowsett M, Barrios CH, Steger G, Huang CS, Andersson M, Inbar M, Lichinitser M, Lang I, Nitz U, Iwata H, Thomssen C, Lohrisch C, Suter TM, Ruschoff J, Suto T, Greatorex V, Ward C, Straehle C, McFadden E, Dolci MS, Gelber RD. Trastuzumab after adjuvant chemotherapy in HER2-positive breast cancer. N Engl J Med 2005; 353(16): 1659–1672.

Quon A, Gambhir SS. FDG-PET and beyond: molecular breast cancer imaging. J Clin Oncol 2005; 23(8):1664–1673.

Ragaz J, Jackson SM, Le N, Plenderleith IH, Spinelli JJ, Basco VE, Wilson KS, Knowling MA, Coppin CM, Paradis M, Coldman AJ, Olivotto IA Adjuvant radiotherapy and chemotherapy in node-positive premenopausal women with breast cancer. N Engl J Med 1997; 337(14):956–962.

Recht A, Gray R, Davidson NE, Fowble BL, Solin LJ, Cummings FJ, Falkson G, Falkson HC, Taylor SG IV, Tormey DC. Locoregional failure 10 years after mastectomy and adjuvant chemotherapy with or without tamoxifen without irradiation: experience of the Eastern Cooperative Oncology Group. J Clin Oncol 1999; 17(6):1689–1700.

Recht A, Edge SB, Solin LJ, Robinson DS, Estabrook A, Fine RE, Fleming GF, Formenti S,Hudis C, Kirshner JJ, Krause DA, Kuske RR, Langer AS, Sledge GWJr., Whelan TJ, Pfister DG. Postmastectomy radiotherapy: clinical practice guidelines of the American Society of Clinical Oncology. J Clin Oncol 2001; 19(5):1539–1569.

Roche H, Fumoleau P, Spielmann M, Canon JL, Delozier T, Serin D, Symann M, Kerbrat P, Soulie P, Eichler F, Viens P, Monnier A, Vindevoghel A, Campone M, Goudier MJ, Bonneterre J, Ferrero JM, Martin AL, Geneve J, Asselain B. Sequential adjuvant epirubicin-based and docetaxel chemotherapy for node-positive breast cancer patients: the FNCLCC PACS 01 Trial. J Clin Oncol 2006; 24(36): 5664–5671.

Rodríguez-Lescure Á, Martin M, Ruiz A, Alba E, Calvo L, García-Asenjo JL, Guitian M, de la Cruz A, Aranda I, de Álava E. Subgroup analysis of GEICAM 9906 trial comparing six cycles of $FE_{90}C$ (FEC) to four cycles of $FE_{90}C$ followed by 8 weekly paclitaxel administrations (FECP): Relevance of HER2 and hormonal status (HR). Proc Asco 2007:185, abstr 10598.

Romond EH, Perez EA, Bryant J, Suman VJ, Geyer CE Jr., Davidson NE, Tan-Chiu E, Martino S, Paik S, Kaufman PA, Swain SM, Pisansky TM, Fehrenbacher L, Kutteh LA, Vogel VG, Visscher DW, Yothers G, Jenkins RB, Brown AM, Dakhil SR, Mamounas EP, Lingle WL, Klein PM, Ingle JN, Wolmark N. Trastuzumab plus adjuvant chemotherapy for operable HER2-positive breast cancer. N Engl J Med 2005; 353(16):1673–1684.

Rouesse J, Friedman S, Sarrazin D, Mouriesse H, Le Chevalier T, Arriagada R, Spielmann M, Papacharalambous A, May-Levin F. Primary chemotherapy in the treatment of inflammatory breast carcinoma: a study of 230 cases from the Institut Gustave-Roussy. J Clin Oncol 1986; 4(12): 1765–1771.

Rouzier R, Pusztai L, Garbay JR, Delaloge S, Hunt KK, Hortobagyi GN, Berry D, Kuerer HM. Development and validation of nomograms for predicting residual tumor size and the probability of successful conservative surgery with neoadjuvant chemotherapy for breast cancer. Cancer 2006; 107(7):1459–1466.

Sabel MS, Schott AF, Kleer CG, Merajver S, Cimmino VM, Diehl KM, Hayes DF, Chang AE, Pierce LJ. Sentinel node biopsy prior to neoadjuvant chemotherapy. Am J Surg 2003; 186(2):102–105.

Saltzstein SL. Clinically occult inflammatory carcinoma of the breast. Cancer 1974; 34(2):382–328.

Sataloff DM, Mason BA, Prestipino AJ, Seinige UL, Lieber CP, Baloch Z. Pathologic response to induction chemotherapy in locally advanced carcinoma of the breast: a determinant of outcome. J Am Coll Surg 1995; 180(3):297–306.

Sawaki M, Ito Y, Akiyama F, Tokudome N, Horii R, Mizunuma N, Takahashi S, Horikoshi N, Imai T, Nakao A, Kasumi F, Sakamoto G, Hatake K. High prevalence of HER-2/neu and p53 overexpression in inflammatory breast cancer. Breast Cancer 2006; 13(2):172–178.

Schneider BP, Miller KD. Angiogenesis of breast cancer. J Clin Oncol 2005; 23(8):1782–1790.

Seno R, Sparano JA, Fineberg SA. Gross and histologic features of locally advanced breast cancer after neoadjuvant chemotherapy. Anat Pathol 1998; 3:169–180.

Shapiro CL, Recht A. Side effects of adjuvant treatment of breast cancer. N Engl J Med 2001; 344(26):1997–2008.

Simes RJ, Coates AS. Patient preferences for adjuvant chemotherapy of early breast cancer: how much benefit is needed? J Natl Cancer Inst Monogr 2001; (30):146–152.

Singletary SE, Ames FC, Buzdar AU. Management of inflammatory breast cancer. World J Surg 1994; 18(1):87–92.

Singletary SE, Allred C, Ashley P, Bassett LW, Berry D, Bland KI, Borgen PI, Clark GM, Edge SB, Hayes DF, Hughes LL, Hutter RV, Morrow M, Page DL, Recht A, Theriault RL, Thor A, Weaver DL, Wieand HS, Greene FL. Staging system for breast cancer: revisions for the 6th edition of the AJCC Cancer Staging Manual. Surg Clin North Am 2003; 83(4):803–819.

Slamon DJ, Godolphin W, Jones LA, Holt JA, Wong SG, Keith DE, Levin WJ, Stuart SG, Udove J, Ullrich A, et al. Studies of the HER-2/neu proto-oncogene in human breast and ovarian cancer. Science 1989; 244(4905):707–712.

Slamon DJ, Leyland-Jones B, Shak S, Fuchs H, Paton V, Bajamonde A, Fleming T, Eiermann W, Wolter J, Pegram M, Baselga J, Norton L. Use of chemotherapy plus a monoclonal antibody against HER2 for metastatic breast cancer that overexpresses HER2. N Engl J Med 2001; 344(11):783–792.

Slamon DJ, Romond EH, Perez EA. Advances in adjuvant therapy for breast cancer. Clin Adv Hematol Oncol 2006;

4(3): suppl 1, 4–9; discussion suppl 10; quiz 2 p following suppl 10.

Sledge GW, O'Neill A, Thor A, Kahanic SP, Zander PJ, Davidson N. Adjuvant trastuzumab: long-term results of E2198. Breast Cancer Res Treat2006; 95(suppl 1): abstr 2075.

Smith CA, Pollice AA, Gu LP, Brown KA, Singh SG, Janocko LE, Johnson R, Julian T, Hyams D, Wolmark N, Sweeney L, Silverman JF, Shackney SE. Correlations among p53, Her-2/neu, and ras overexpression and aneuploidy by multiparameter flow cytometry in human breast cancer: evidence for a common phenotypic evolutionary pattern in infiltrating ductal carcinomas. Clin Cancer Res 2000; 6(1): 112–126.

Smith IC, Heys SD, Hutcheon AW, Miller ID, Payne S, Gilbert FJ, Ah-See AK, Eremin O, Walker LG, Sarkar TK, Eggleton SP, Ogston KN. Neoadjuvant hemotherapy in breast cancer: significantly enhanced response with docetaxel. J Clin Oncol 2002; 20(6):1456–1466.

Smith I, Procter M, Gelber RD, Guillaume S, Feyereislova A, Dowsett M, Goldhirsch A, Untch M, Mariani G, Baselga J, Kaufmann M, Cameron D, Bell R, Bergh J, Coleman R, Wardley A, Harbeck N, Lopez RI, Mallmann P, Gelmon K, Wilcken N, Wist E, Sanchez Rovira P, Piccart-Gebhart MJ. 2-year follow-up of trastuzumab after adjuvant chemotherapy in HER2-positive breast cancer: a randomised controlled trial. Lancet 2007; 369(9555):29–36.

Sparano JA. TAILORx: trial assigning individualized options for treatment (Rx). Clin Breast Cancer 2006; 7(4):347–350.

Sparano JA, Fazzari MJ, Childs G. Clinical application of molecular profiling in breast cancer. Future Oncol 2005; 1(4):485–496.

Sparano JA, Moulder S, Kazi A, Vahdat L, Li T, Pellegrino C, Munster P, Malafa M, Lee D, Hoschander S, Hopkins U, Hershman D, Wright JJ, Sebti SM. Targeted inhibition of farnesyltransferase in locally advanced breast cancer: a phase I and II trial of tipifarnib plus dose-dense doxorubicin and cyclophosphamide. J Clin Oncol 2006; 24(19): 3013–3018.

Sparano JA, Wang M, Martino S, et al. Phase III study of doxorubicin-cyclophosphamide followed by paclitaxel or docetaxel given every 3 weeks or weekly in patients with axillary node-positive or high-risk node-negative breast cancer: results of North American Breast Cancer Intergroup Trial E1199. Proc Asco 2007; 25(185), (abstr 516).

Swain SM, Lippman ME. Treatment of patients with inflammatory breast cancer. Important Adv Oncol 1989; 129–150.

Symmans W, Peintinger F, Hatzis C, et al. A new measurement of residual cancer burden to predict survival after neoadjuvant chemotherapy. J Clin Oncol 2007; 25: 4412–4422.

Tabbane F, Muenz L, Jaziri M, Cammoun M, Belhassen S, Mourali N. Clinical and prognostic features of a rapidly progressing breast cancer in Tunisia. Cancer 1977; 40(1): 376–382.

Taghian AG, Abi-Raad R, Assaad SI, Casty A, Ancukiewicz M, Yeh E, Molokhia P, Attia K, Sullivan T, Kuter I, Boucher Y, Powell SN. Paclitaxel decreases the interstitial fluid pressure and improves oxygenation in breast cancers in patients treated with neoadjuvant chemotherapy: clinical implications. J Clin Oncol 2005; 23(9):1951–1961.

Tan-Chiu E, Yothers G, Romond E, Geyer CEJr., Ewer M, Keefe D, Shannon RP, Swain SM, Brown A, Fehrenbacher L, Vogel VG, Seay TE, Rastogi P, Mamounas EP, Wolmark N, Bryant J. Assessment of cardiac dysfunction in a randomized trial comparing doxorubicin and cyclophosphamide followed by paclitaxel, with or without trastuzumab as adjuvant therapy in node-positive, human epidermal growth factor receptor 2-overexpressing breast cancer: NSABP B-31. J Clin Oncol 2005; 23(31): 7811–7819.

Therasse P, Mauriac L, Welnicka-Jaskiewicz M, Bruning P, Cufer T, Bonnefoi H, Tomiak E, Pritchard KI, Hamilton A, Piccart MJ. Final results of a randomized phase III trial comparing cyclophosphamide, epirubicin, and fluorouracil with a dose-intensified epirubicin and cyclophosphamide + filgrastim as neoadjuvant treatment in locally advanced breast cancer: an EORTC-NCIC-SAKK multicenter study. J Clin Oncol 2003; 21(5):843–850.

van der Hage JA, van de Velde CJ, Julien JP, Tubiana-Hulin M, Vandervelden C, Duchateau L. Preoperative chemotherapy in primary operable breast cancer: results from the European Organization for Research and Treatment of Cancer trial 10902. J Clin Oncol 2001; 19(22):4224–4237.

van 't Veer LJ, Dai H, van de Vijver MJ, He YD, Hart AA, Mao M, Peterse HL, van der Kooy K, Marton MJ, Witteveen AT, Schreiber GJ, Kerkhoven RM, Roberts C, Linsley PS, Bernards R, Friend SH. Gene expression profiling predicts clinical outcome of breast cancer. Nature 2002; 415(6871): 530–536.

van den Eynden GG, van Laere SJ, van der Auwera I, Merajver SD, van Marck EA, van Dam P, Vermeulen PB, Dirix LY, van Golen KL. Overexpression of caveolin-1 and -2 in cell lines and in human samples of inflammatory breast cancer. Breast Cancer Res Treat 2006; 95(3):219–228.

van Laere S, van der Auwera I, van den Eynden GG, Fox SB, Bianchi F, Harris AL, van Dam P, van Marck EA, Vermeulen PB, Dirix LY. Distinct molecular signature of inflammatory breast cancer by cDNA microarray analysis. Breast Cancer Res Treat 2005; 93(3):237–246.

Venturini M, Del Mastro L, Aitini E, Baldini E, Caroti C, Contu A, Testore F, Brema F, Pronzato P, Cavazzini G, Sertoli MR, Canavese G, Rosso R, Bruzzi P. Dose-dense adjuvant chemotherapy in early breast cancer patients: results from a randomized trial. J Natl Cancer Inst 2005; 97(23): 1724–1733.

von Minckwitz G, Raab G, Caputo A, Schutte M, Hilfrich J, Blohmer JU, Gerber B, Costa SD, Merkle E, Eidtmann H, Lampe D, Jackisch C, du Bois A, Kaufmann M. Doxorubicin with cyclophosphamide followed by docetaxel every 21 days compared with doxorubicin and docetaxel every 14 days as preoperative treatment in operable breast cancer: the GEPARDUO study of the German Breast Group. J Clin Oncol 2005; 23(12):2676–2685.

Wapnir IL, Anderson SJ, Mamounas EP, Geyer CE Jr., Jeong JH, Tan-Chiu E, Fisher B, Wolmark N. Prognosis after ipsilateral breast tumor recurrence and locoregional recurrences in five National Surgical Adjuvant Breast and Bowel Project node-positive adjuvant breast cancer trials. J Clin Oncol 2006; 24(13):2028–2037.

Wedam SB, Low JA, Yang SX, Chow CK, Choyke P, Danforth D, Hewitt SM, Berman A, Steinberg SM, Liewehr DJ, Plehn J, Doshi A, Thomasson D, McCarthy N, Koeppen H, Sherman M, Zujewski J, Camphausen K, Chen H, Swain SM. Antiangiogenic and antitumor effects of bevacizumab in patients with inflammatory and locally advanced breast cancer. J Clin Oncol 2006; 24(5):769–777.

Whelan TJ, Julian J, Wright J, Jadad AR, Levine ML. Does locoregional radiation therapy improve survival in breast cancer? A meta-analysis. J Clin Oncol 2000; 18(6):1220–1229.

Whelan T, Levine M, Willan A, Gafni A, Sanders K, Mirsky D, Chambers S, O'Brien MA, Reid S, Dubois S. Effect of a decision aid on knowledge and treatment decision making for breast cancer surgery: a randomized trial. JAMA 2004; 292(4):435–441.

Whelan TJ, Loprinzi C. Physician/patient decision aids for adjuvant therapy. J Clin Oncol 2005; 23(8):1627–1630.

Wolff AC, Davidson NE. Primary systemic therapy in operable breast cancer. J Clin Oncol 2000; 18 (7):1558–1569.

Wolff AC, Hammond ME, Schwartz JN, Hagerty KL, Allred DC, Cote RJ, Dowsett M, Fitzgibbons PL, Hanna WM, Langer A, McShane LM, Paik S, Pegram MD, Perez EA, Press MF, Rhodes A, Sturgeon C, Taube SE, Tubbs R, Vance GH, van de Vijver M, Wheeler TM, Hayes DF. American Society of Clinical Oncology/College of American Pathologists guideline recommendations for human epidermal growth factor receptor 2 testing in breast cancer. J Clin Oncol 2007; 25(1):118–145.

Zucali R, Uslenghi C, Kenda R, Bonadonna G. Natural history and survival of inoperable breast cancer treated with radiotherapy and radiotherapy followed by radical mastectomy. Cancer 1976; 37(3):1422–1431.

25

BRCA1, *BRCA2*, and Hereditary Breast Cancer

BETSY A. BOVE

Clinical Molecular Genetics, Department of Pathology, Fox Chase Cancer Center, Philadelphia, Pennsylvania, U.S.A.

INTRODUCTION

Mutations in the *BRCA1* and *BRCA2* genes account for the largest percentage of hereditary breast cancers. Since their discovery in the mid-1990s, much has been learned regarding their structure and function, their mutational spectrum, the clinical implications of their mutations, and the management of their mutation carriers. While a large proportion of hereditary breast cancers remain unassociated with mutation in the breast cancer–susceptibility genes, it is thought that alternate types of mutations will be discovered outside the technical limitations of the generally accepted polymerase chain reaction (PCR)-based methods for mutation detection. Large insertions and deletions already account for more than 60 of the over 1200 known *BRCA* alterations. Changes in methylation patterns and in gene regulatory regions will likely contribute to an additional percentage of heritable breast cancer predisposition. As well, other genes have been identified that modify the affects of *BRCA* mutations and likely more are just on the horizon in the molecular research laboratory. The use of functional assays will help identify carriers and is a more effective approach than the current methods of carrier risk prediction. The *BRCA* genes have been determined and suggested to be involved in DNA repair, transcription regulation, mitotic progression, viral response, and ubiquitination. The identification of their roles in these molecular pathways will help determine and realize molecular targeted therapies that will specifically inhibit the viability of cancer cells without destroying normal healthy ones. While other genes that contribute to a much lesser extent to the epidemiology of hereditary cancers have been named, data from recent experiments indicate it is unlikely that another gene that will have a major contribution to the cause of hereditary breast disease will be identified. Time will tell.

MOLECULAR GENETICS OF HEREDITARY BREAST CANCER

Much has been published over the past 10 years since the discovery of the first breast cancer–susceptibility genes regarding the causes of hereditary and familial breast and ovarian cancers. Family history is still the strongest known epidemiological risk factor (Bowcock, 1997) while approximately 70% to 90% of all breast cancers occur sporadically. The remaining breast cancer cases are inheritable and caused by *BRCA1*, *BRCA2*, (Brody and Biesecker, 1998) and other identified (Sakorafas and Tsiotou, 2000) and unidentified tumor suppressor genes. In this chapter, we discuss these genes.

Breast Cancer Susceptibility Genes

Hall and colleagues (Hall et al., 1990) identified a link between a locus on chromosome 17q and site-specific breast cancer in 1990 by gene linkage, and this same locus was reportedly associated with the hereditary breast-ovarian cancer syndrome (Narod et al., 1991). *BRCA1* was isolated in 1994 (Miki et al., 1994) and less than two years later, *BRCA2* was identified (Wooster et al., 1994; Wooster et al., 1995; Tavitigian et al., 1996). The mode of transmission, autosomal dominant, implies a mode of genetic transmission where a single mutant allele is sufficient to initiate and/or promote breast cancer. Whole branches of a family may be unaffected, while other branches contain multiple breast cancers.

BRCA1

BRCA1, located on the long arm of chromosome 17 at q21, is composed of 24 exons, 22 that are coding, distributed over roughly 100 kilobase pairs (kbp) of genomic DNA (Miki et al., 1994; Lane et al., 1995). The 7.8-kb transcript is detected in numerous tissues, including the breast and ovary, and encodes an 1863–amino acid protein (Miki et al., 1994). *BRCA1* also encodes for at least two more protein products of smaller size because of alternative splicing (Thakur et al., 1997; Wilson et al., 1997; Xu et al., 1999; ElShamy and Livingston, 2004). One of the variants, BRCA1-delta11, is identical to the full-length form except for the absence of exon 11 (Xu et al., 1999). The other is BRCA1-IRIS, which is a 1399–residue polypeptide encoded by an uninterrupted open reading frame that extends from codon 1 of the known *BRCA1* open reading frame to a termination point 34 triplets into intron 11 (ElShamy and Livingston, 2004). An alternative splice variant of *BRCA1* containing an additional in-frame exon (insertion of 66 nucleotides between exons 13 and 14 called exon 13A-containing transcript) has also been identified (Fortin et al., 2005). *BRCA1* full-length form contains multiple functional domains, including a highly conserved N-terminal RING (really interesting new gene) finger, two nuclear localization signals (NLS) that are located in the exon 11, an 'SQ' cluster between amino acids 1280–1524, and C-terminal BRCT domains (Paterson, 1998).

BRCA2

BRCA2, located on the long arm of chromosome 13 at band q12–13, is composed of 27 exons, 26 that are coding, distributed over about 70 kbp of genomic DNA. The approximately 12,000-base transcript is ubiquitously expressed and encodes for a 3418–amino acid protein. BRC repeats spanning the ovarian cancer cluster region (OCCR) and the nuclear localization region are putative functional domains. The human *BRCA1* or *BRCA2* gene has only approximately 60% level of homology with its murine counterparts, perhaps suggesting the rapid evolution of these genes and proteins (Lane et al., 1995).

Fanconi Anemia Genes

Fanconi anemia (FA) is an inherited disorder associated with progressive aplastic anemia, multiple congenital abnormalities, and predisposition to malignancies including leukemia and solid tumors (Fanconi, 1967). FA is inherited as an autosomal recessive trait, but is genetically heterogeneous with multiple complementation groups that include an x-linked form (Meetei et al., 2004). Twelve groups have been described, named FA-1, B, C, D1, D2, E, F, G, I, J, L, and M (Mathew, 2006). The FA proteins form nuclear multi protein complexes referred to collectively as the FA pathway (Taniguchi and D'Andrea, 2006). FA proteins include a ubiquitin ligase (*FANCL*), a monoubiquitinated protein (*FANCD2*), and a helicase (*FANCJ/BACH1/BRIP1*) (Taniguchi and D'Andrea, 2006). The association of the FA genes with breast cancer arose when *FANCD1* was found to be the *BRCA2* gene (Howlett et al., 2002) and provided the first direct link between FA proteins and DNA repair (Mathew, 2006), as both *BRCA1* and *BRCA2* have been associated with proteins having a function in DNA repair systems.

Research indicates that FA proteins work together with *BRCA2/RAD51*-mediated homologous recombination in double-strand break (DSB) repair through the C-terminal domain (CTD), whereas the FA pathway plays a role that is independent of the CTD of *BRCA2* in interstrand cross-link repair (Kitao et al., 2006). *FANCG*, shown to interact with recombination proteins *XRCC3* and *BRCA2*, may have a role in building multiprotein complexes that facilitate homologous recombination repair (Hussain et al., 2006). FA gene products have been shown to functionally or physically interact with *BRCA1*, *RAD51*, and the *MRE11/RAD50/NBS1* complex, suggesting that the FA complex may be involved in the repair of DNA DSBs (Yang et al., 2005). Both *ATR* and *BRCA1* are required to activate the FA pathway (Zhu and Dutta, 2006). The defined roles of these protein complexes have not been identified. Germline mutations of the *NBS1* gene have been documented to have a significantly, though moderately increased, age-related risk of breast cancer in the Polish population (Steffen et al., 2006) and the Northern Finnish population (Heikkinen et al., 2006). Monoallelic mutations in *BRCA2* cause susceptibility to breast and other cancers, while biallelic mutations cause FA (Mathew, 2006) (Table 1). Seal et al. (2003) concluded that FA gene mutations, other than in *BRCA2*, may be low-penetrant alleles, but are unlikely to make a significant contribution to the risk of familial breast cancer (Seal et al., 2003). Low penetrant or significant yet to be determined in breast cancer risk, the following data has accumulated regarding FA mutated alleles.

Two new studies show that the FA complementation group N results from biallelic mutations in *PALB2* (for

Table 1 Other Genetic Conditions Associated with Increased Breast Cancer Risk

Syndrome	Mutant Gene
Li-Fraumeni	*TP53/CHK2*
Cowden	*PTEN*
Fanconi Anemia	*BACH1(FANCJ,BRIP1)/PALB2*
Peutz-Jeghers	*STK11(LKB1)*
Ataxia telangiectasia	*ATM*

"partner and localizer of *BRCA2*") (Xia et al., 2007; Reid et al., 2007), which encodes a recently identified interaction partner of the breast cancer–susceptibility protein *BRCA2* (Xia et al., 2006). A third study shows that monallelic *PALB2* mutations are associated with breast cancer susceptibility (Rahman et al., 2007), providing yet more links between Fanconi anemia, homologous recombination repair, and cancer predisposition (Patel, 2007). The *BRCA2-PALB2* interaction is crucial for certain key *BRCA2* DNA damage-response functions as well as its tumor suppression activity (Xia et al., 2006). Erkko et al. showed by screening for *PALB2* mutations in Finland that a frameshift mutation, 1592delT, is present at significantly elevated frequency in familial breast cancer cases compared with ancestry-matched population controls (Erkko et al., 2007). The truncated PALB2 protein caused by this mutation retained little *BRCA2*-binding capacity and was deficient in homologous recombination and cross-link repair. Further screening of 1592delT in unselected breast cancer individuals revealed a roughly fourfold enrichment of this mutation in patients compared with controls. The authors suggest that *PALB2* is a breast cancer–susceptibility gene (Erkko et al., 2007).

The *BACH1* helicase was originally identified as a protein that binds to the BRCT repeats of *BRCA1* (Cantor et al., 2001). Also known as *BRIP* or *FANCJ* of the FA gene group, the gene has been screened for breast cancer susceptibility. While two missense mutations were found in the gene in early-onset familial breast cancer cases (Cantor et al., 2001), it was concluded that germline pathogenic mutations are extremely rare or absent in familial breast cancer (Luo et al., 2002; Karppinen et al., 2003; Rutter et al., 2003b; Vahteristo et al., 2006; Lewis et al., 2005). Recent evidence may indicate truncating mutations in *BACH1* to be low-penetrant breast cancer–susceptibility alleles (Seal et al., 2006). It is predicted that *BRCA1* regulates the *BACH1* helicase activity to coordinate the timely displacement of *RAD51* from nucleofilaments, promoting error-free repair and ultimately maintaining chromosomal integrity (Cantor and Andreassen, 2006).

In other gynecological cancers, lack of ubiquitinated *FANCD2* was found in 2 of 25 ovarian cancer cell lines (Taniguchi et al., 2003). *FANCF* methylation was observed in 4 of 19 primary ovarian tumors (*FANCF* is silenced by hypermethylation) (Taniguchi et al., 2003), in 27 of 91 primary cervical cancers, in 3 of 9 cervical cancer cell lines, and in 0 of 20 normal cervical epithelial (Narayan et al., 2004). A variant detected in the putative promoter region of *FANCD2* with consensus binding sites for some transcriptional factors indicate that a relationship between *FANCD2* and sporadic breast cancer risk may exist (Barroso et al., 2006).

CHK2

Human *CHK2* is the homologue of the yeast genes, *Csd1* and *Rad53*G_2, which are kinases activated after DNA damage (Shieh et al., 2000). One consequence of the inactivation is the arrest of cells at the G_2 checkpoint thus preventing damaged cells from entering into mitosis. Studies in yeast show that alterations in these genes result in the loss of checkpoint function, an important step in the genesis of many cancers. In addition, recent studies suggest that *CHK2* acts not only at the G_2 checkpoint but also at G_1 as well, apparently by stabilizing the *p53* protein that leads to arrest of the cell cycle in G_1 (Tominaga et al., 1999; Chehab et al., 2000). These important biological findings raise the possibility that *CHK2* might be involved in familial aggregation of breast and other cancers.

The *CHK2* gene was first indicated in cancer susceptibility in 1999 when Bell et al. (1999) discovered three *CHK2* germline mutations among four classical Li-Fraumeni and 18 Li-Fraumeni-like families, suggesting that *CHK2* could be a new predisposition gene to Li-Fraumeni syndrome (LFS). Two of the alterations found (1100delC in the kinase domain in exon 10 and the 470T>C I157T missense mutation in the FHA domain in exon3) have been widely studied for inherited susceptibility to breast cancer (Nevanlinna and Bartek, 2006). These two alterations have since been identified in breast cancer patients and rarely in Li-Fraumeni families (Allinen et al., 2001; Vahteristo et al., 2001; Bougeard et al., 2001; Lee et al., 2001; Sodha et al., 2002; Siddiqui et al., 2005. Overall, lower risks have been documented for I157T than 1100delC and negligible risk had been seen originally for both among familial non-*BRCA1/2* breast cancer patients in the United Kingdom, North America, and the Netherlands (Schutte et al., 2003).

However, the data now seem to be consistent, showing an increased risk of breast cancer in carriers of *CHK2* mutation, which is roughly twofold compared with non-carriers (Narod and Lynch, 2007). It is evident, however, that the contribution of *CHK2* mutations to the burden of breast cancer varies by ethnic group. The *CHK2* 1100delC mutation appears to be most prevalent in the Netherlands (4%), despite earlier findings, and is high in Finland (2.5%) (Kilpivaara et al., 2005) and Germany (2.3%) as well (Rashid et al., 2005). The 1100delC mutation is rare in Australia (Jekimovs et al., 2005), Spain (Osorio et al., 2004), and among Ashkenazi Jews (Offit et al., 2003).

The IVS2+1G>A splicing mutation has been associated possibly with a two- to fourfold elevated risk for breast cancer (Cybulski et al., 2004; Bogdanova et al., 2005). As this allele is rare, very large patient cohorts will be needed to evaluate the associated risk reliably (Dufault et al., 2004). Two other alleles suggested to be founder alleles specific to the Ashkenazi population are S428F in the kinase domain in exon 11 and P85L in the N-terminal region of exon 1 (Shaag et al., 2005). The former had a 1.37% frequency among 1673 controls and 2.88% among 1632 breast caner patients and was associated with two-fold elevated risk. The latter did not differ between cases and controls. Walsh et al. (2006) searched for large genomic rearrangements in *CHK2* is a series of 300 high-risk breast cancer families with four or more cases of breast or ovarian cancer and discovered a novel 5.6-kb genomic deletion in two Czechoslovakian families. The deleterious mutation CHEK2del5567 has been identified in other populations (Walsh et al., 2006; Cybulski et al., 2007). Other populations may as well carry *CHK2* large rearrangements.

Arguably, *CHK2* is the most important breast cancer–susceptibility gene to be identified since *BRCA2* was found in 1995 (Narod and Lynch, 2007). However, it will be an enormous challenge to evaluate a specific chemo-preventive agent or clinical trial drug in such a small subgroup, and few patients will consider prophylactic surgery at a lifetime risk level of 15% to 20%. However, all familial breast cancer-predisposing genes identified to date are components of the genome maintenance machinery that responds to DNA damage, of which *CHK2* is a member. The cellular response capabilities of DNA damaging therapies should be considered. Subsequent studies will be necessary to determine the extent of *CHK2* mutations in hereditary breast cancer-prone families.

Ataxia-Telangiectasia Mutated

Ataxia-telangiectasia mutated (*ATM*), the gene for ataxia-telangiectasia was mapped by genetic linkage analysis in 1988 and was identified by positional cloning in 1995 (Gatti et al., 1988; Savitsky et al., 1995). Over 300 distinct *ATM* mutations have been reported (see www.benaroya-research.org), and the prevalence of such *ATM* mutations has been shown to be 0.5% to 1% in Western populations (Swift et al., 1986; Renwick et al., 2006). Missense mutation account for only about 10% of ataxia patients, and like *BRCA1* and *BRCA2*, it is difficult to identify missense mutations that are causative for disease. Carriers of deleterious mutations have a 100-fold increased risk of cancer, including childhood lymphoid cancers and epithelial cancers in adults, including breast cancer (Morrell et al., 1986). Swift first proposed that relatives of ataxia-telangiectasia might be at increased risk of breast cancer nearly 20 years ago (Swift et al., 1987). He found the relative risk (RR) of cancer for men to be 2.3, while for women it was 3.1 with breast cancer being the most strongly associated cancer. Recent studies of a large ataxia population estimated the overall RR of breast cancer in carriers to be 2.23, and it was higher in women younger than 50 years at 4.9 (Thompson et al., 2005). Since prevalence had been estimated in the general population to be up to 1%, even a relatively modest increase in breast cancer risk in carriers could be appreciable.

Renwick et al. (2006) recently conducted an analysis to confirm the role of *ATM* alterations in predisposition to breast cancer. Conflicting evidence existed because of a small sample size and the fact that few studies had data from full-screen analysis of *ATM* in both cases and controls. It had also been suggested that those alterations that cause ataxia may be different from those that cause predisposition to breast cancer (Gatti et al., 1999). The Renwick study used 443 *BRCA1/2* negative familial breast cancer cases and 521 controls, all full screened for *ATM*. They identified two *ATM* mutations that cause ataxia in controls and 12 in familial breast cancer cases; of the 37 nonsynonymous missense variants identified, 12 were present in both cases and controls, 15 were present exclusively in cases, and 10 were present exclusively in controls. These data confirm the difficulty in identifying the phenotypic consequences of alterations that do not cause truncation (Renwick et al., 2006). Renwick's data suggest that the majority of missense variants are not associated with increased risks of breast cancer (Renwick et al., 2006). The RR of breast cancer associated with *ATM* mutations was estimated to be 2.37, which is very similar to the risks estimated from epidemiological analyses (Thompson et al., 2005). Broadly, the analyses demonstrate that, at least in the U.K. population, the combined *ATM* mutation prevalence is similar to that of *CHK2*1100delC, that *ATM* mutations are associated with similar risks of breast cancer, and that they make a contribution to breast cancer incidence that is similar to *CHK2*1100delC—that of low-penetrance susceptibility alleles (Renwick et al., 2006; Nevanlinna and Bartek, 2006; Ahmed and Rahman, 2006). The age-and mutation-specific risks should be further investigated in larger studies. Of keen interest is the developing role of DNA repair genes in the etiology of breast cancer: *BRCA1*, *BRCA2*, *TP53*, *CHK2*, and now *ATM* (Table 2).

Table 2 Human Instability Syndromes

Syndrome	Gene	Repair deficiency	Cancer predisposition
Ataxia telangiectasia, AT	*ATM*	response to DSBs	lymphoma leukemia
AT-like syndrome	*AT-LD MRE11*	response to DSBs	not described
Nijmegen breakage, NBS	*NSB1*	HR, NHEJ	Lymphoma
Familial breast/ovarian cancer	*BRCA1*	HR, NER, MMR	breast, ovarian
Familial breast cancer	*BRCA2*	HR, repair of cross links	breast, male breast, ovarian, prostate
Fanconi anemia, FA	*FANC A-G, D1*[a]	HR, repair of cross links	Leukemia
D2, L Blooms, BS	*BLM*	HR, recQ-related helicase	all

[a]Biallelic mutations in *BRCA2* are found in *FANCD1* patients.
Source: Adapted from Eyfjord and Bodvarsdottir (2005).

TP53

The *p53* exists at low levels in virtually all normal cells. Wild-type *p53* functions as a suppressor of neoplastic growth, and mutation or deletion, or both, of the normal gene eliminates this suppression. (Chen et al., 1990; Bartek et al., 1990).

The human *TP53* gene codes for a protein product (referred to as *p53*) that has an important biological function as a cell cycle checkpoint. Wild-type *p53* acts as a negative regulator of cell growth and is induced following DNA damage and mediates cell cycle arrest in late G_1. In some contexts, wild-type *p53* can induce apoptosis (programmed cell death), and in the absence of the wild-type protein leads to resistance to ionizing radiation and chemotherapeutic agents. For example, in normal cells with DNA damaged by ultraviolet or γ irradiation, progression through the cell cycle is blocked at G_1 coincident with a sharp rise in the levels of the *p53*. During the subsequent arrest of growth, repair of DNA is completed before the cells proceed into S-phase. If, however, genomic damage is excessive the cell undergoes apoptosis, which requires normally functioning *p53*. Cells can escape apoptosis in the absence of a functional *p53* protein, thus allowing the cell to survive and replicate its damaged DNA, which in turn leads to the propagation of the mutation. The *p53* has therefore been described as the "guardian of the genome" as it prevents entry into S-phase unless, or until, the genome has been cleared of potentially damaging mutations. In addition, because many chemotherapeutic drugs are believed to kill tumor cells by inducing apoptosis, loss of the *p53* function may also directly decrease the sensitivity of the cells to such cytotoxic agents, enhancing the emergence of drug-resistant populations of cancer cells.

The biochemical mechanisms by which the *p53* acts in regulating cell proliferation are not fully understood; however, the *p53* appears to mediate growth suppression in part through its specific DNA-binding and transcriptional regulatory abilities (El-Deiry et al., 1994; Ko and Prives, 1996). In particular, wild-type *p53* can enhance the expression of a number of genes, including *p21/WAF-1/CIP1*. *p21*, encodes a protein capable of inhibiting cyclin-dependent kinases and arresting cell division. In contrast, mutant forms of the *p53* no longer possess the ability to arrest cell growth and induce apoptosis. This phenomenon is likely because the mutant *p53* are unable to bind to specific DNA response sequences and to activate the transcription of genes with an adjacent *p53* recognition sequence.

To date the *TP53* gene is the most commonly altered gene yet identified in human tumors (e.g., sporadic osteosarcomas, soft tissue sarcomas, brain tumors, leukemias, and carcinomas of the breast, colon, lung, and ovary) occurring in a large fraction (perhaps even half) of the total cancers in the United States and United Kingdom. In contrast to the retinoblastoma gene, *RB*, where the hereditary syndrome served as the basis for identification of the causal gene, *TP53* was discovered and subsequently found to have a role in hereditary cancer. In 1990, Li and colleagues identified germline *TP53* mutations in a series of families with LFS that features diverse childhood cancers as well as early-onset breast cancers (Malkin et al., 1990).

LFS is a rare autosomal dominant cancer syndrome that in its classic form is defined by the existence of both a proband with a sarcoma and two other first-degree relatives with a cancer by age 45 years (Li et al., 1988; Birch et al., 1994). Families with LFS have a high risk of many cancer types (50% risk of cancer by age 30; >90% by age 70) (Tonin, 2000). The tumor types that arise in these families are quite variable, with breast cancer, soft tissue sarcomas, brain tumors, osteosarcomas, and leukemias being the most frequently observed cancers and adrenocortical carcinomas, melanomas, gonadal germ cell tumors, and carcinomas of the lung, pancreas, and prostate appearing to lesser extents (Frebourg et al., 1995).

Breast cancer appears to be the most frequent cancer diagnosed in adults with LFS. It accounts for approximately 27% of all tumors in individuals with germline

TP53 mutations (Kleihues et al., 1997; Varley et al., 1997). The absolute risk of breast cancer in a female mutation carrier has not been estimated precisely, but appears to be approximately 50% by age 50 years (Li et al., 1988). Functional analyses of mutant proteins derived from the germline of patients with LFS have shown that germline *TP53* mutations can inactivate the transcriptional regulatory activity and tumor suppressor function of the wild-type protein. Many of the germline mutations detected in LFS are identical to those that occur somatically in spontaneous tumors. Outside the LFS, in population-based studies of breast cancer, *TP53* germline mutations are found in less than 1% of cases diagnosed under the age of 35 (Malkin et al., 1990; Borressen et al., 1992; Sidransky et al., 1992; Walsh et al., 2006).

In a recent study by Olivier et al., *TP53* mutations within exons 5 to 8 conferred an elevated risk of breast cancer–specific death of 2,27 compared with patients with no such mutation among 1794 breast cancer patients. Specific missense mutations (codon 179 and R248W) seem to be associated with an even worse prognosis (Olivier et al., 2006). Previous studies have emphasized that missense mutations in the DNA binding motifs have a worse prognosis. A common Arg/Pro polymorphism at codon 72 of the *TP53* gene has been investigated as a risk factor for cancer in different populations. So far, the results have been controversial. Damin et al. (2006) have recently suggested that it might be implicated in breast carcinogenesis in their evaluation of 118 women with primary breast carcinoma. Kyndi et al. (2006) found the polymorphism to be a possible prognostic value only related to LOH in their study of 204 Danish women.

Mary Claire King and colleagues have conducted a study of 300 probands from families with four or more cases of breast or ovarian cancer and screened them with multiple DNA-based and RNA-based methods to detect genomic rearrangements in *BRCA1* and *BRCA2* and germline mutations of all classes in *CHK2, TP53,* and *PTEN.* They predict from these results that among patients with breast cancer and severe family histories of cancer who test negative for *BRCA1* and *BRCA2*, approximately 12% can be expected to carry a large genomic deletion or duplication in one of these genes, and approximately 5% can be expected to carry a mutation in *CHK2* or *TP53* (1%) (Walsh et al., 2006).

PTEN

An additional autosomal dominant cancer syndrome associated with hereditary forms of breast cancer is Cowden disease or Cowden syndrome. Cowden disease is associated with germline mutations in the *PTEN/MMAC1* gene at chromosome 10q22–23 (Li et al., 1997; Nelen et al., 1997; Steck et al., 1997). It is a rare autosomal dominant syndrome in which affected members tend to develop bilateral breast cancer along with other malignancies, including thyroid and uterine cancer (Hanssen and Fryns, 1995). The risk of breast cancer in women with Cowden disease is significant and is estimated to be 30% to 50% by the age of 50 years (Radford and Zehnbauer, 1996; Sabate et al., 2006). To date, mutations in *PTEN* do not appear to account for hereditary breast cancer susceptibility outside families that are affected by Cowden disease (Rhei et al., 1997); however, additional studies are ongoing to determine the true extent of *PTEN* mutations in familial and sporadic forms of breast cancer. In a recent study among Cowden individuals, *PTEN* mutations were found in all patients presenting with benign or malignant breast pathology (Sabate et al., 2006). In sporadic disease, no strong association with any common haplotype has been found (Haiman et al., 2006).

The level of *PTEN* expression, however, has been associated with breast cancer outside the Cowden disease syndrome. Engin et al. (2006) evaluated 85 primary breast cancer patients and found the loss of *PTEN* protein expression in 32.5% of the cases. Lymph node metastases (Tsutsui et al., 2005a; Piekarski and Biernat, 2006), disease progression (Bose et al., 2006), and aggressive phenotype (Tsutsui et al., 2005b) have all been associated with breast carcinoma. Agrawal and Eng (2006) have observed recently that differential expression of *PTEN* could play a role in the pathogenesis of sporadic breast cancers and the Cowden syndrome and may lend a novel way of making a rapid molecular diagnosis of the syndrome without mutation analysis.

STK11

The *STK11/LKB1* gene was mapped to 19p13.3 following the demonstration of chromosome 19p allele loss in intestinal hamartomas and linkage analysis from Peutz–Jeghers syndrome (PJS) patients (Godard et al., 1971; Hemminki et al., 1998). PJS is a rare autosomal dominant disorder characterized by melanocytic macules of the lips, multiple gastrointestinal hamartomatous polyps, and an increased risk for various neoplasms, including breast and gastrointestinal cancers (Godard et al., 1971; Tomlinson and Houlston, 1997). A fivefold increased risk of early-onset breast cancer appears to be associated with PJS (Tomlinson and Houlston, 1997), suggesting that *STK11/LKB1* may be a candidate breast cancer–susceptibility gene.

However recent data involving 419 individuals with PJS, 297 having documented *STK11/LKB1* mutations, evaluated by the Kaplan–Meier method showed that cancer risks were similar in PJS patients with identified *STK11/LKB1* mutations and those with no detectable mutation (Hearle et al., 2006). There are data that suggest that mutations in exon 6 of *LKB1* are associated with a higher cancer risk than mutations within other regions of the gene (Mehenni et al., 2006). Like *BRCA1* and *BRCA2*, it appears that *STK11/LKB1* mutations can cause ovarian tumors when present in the germline, but occur rarely in the soma (Wang et al., 1999). Its involvement in breast cancer appears to be only in patients with the syndrome (Hemminki et al., 1998; Jenne et al., 1998; de Jong et al., 2002).

Approximately 30% of sporadic breast cancer samples express low levels of *LKB1*. Low levels correlate with shorter relapse-free survival (Fenton et al., 2006). Overexpression of the *LKB1* protein in breast cancer cells has been found to result in significant inhibition of in vitro invasion. In vivo, *LKB1* expression reduced tumor growth in the mammary fat pad, microvessel density, and lung metastasis of mice. Overexpression of the *LKB1* protein in human breast cancer is significantly associated with a decrease in microvessel density, suggesting a negative regulatory role in human breast cancer (Zhuang et al., 2006b). In light of this evidence regarding prognosis and expression levels, it has been suggested that *LKB1* immunohistochemistry (IHC) merits evaluation as a potential prognostic marker for breast carcinoma (Fenton et al., 2006).

Other Genes?

Despite the above dozen or so genes discussed that contribute to the cause of hereditary breast cancer, that still leaves approximately 54% of familial breast cancers without a known genetic component. A recent genome-wide linkage search for breast cancer–susceptibility genes by Smith et al. of 149 multiple case breast cancer families suggested regions that may harbor novel breast cancer–susceptibility genes, including regions on chromosome 4 close to marker D4S392 and on chromosome arm 2p (Smith et al., 2006). They also indicate, however, that no single gene is likely to account for a large fraction of the familial aggregation of breast cancer that is not due to mutations in *BRCA1* or *BRCA2* (Smith et al., 2006). Other cancer genes, such as *Myc*, *c-ERBB2*, *cyclin D1*, *MDGI* and *TSG101*, have been shown to be involved in the tumorigenesis of breast cancers although they do not give rise to familial breast cancer syndromes (Sakorafas and Tsiotou, 2000). Recently, *RAD50* and *NBS1* (a member of one of the Fanconi gene pathway complexes) have been suggested to be breast cancer–susceptibility genes associated with genomic instability (Heikkinen et al., 2006). It is possible that each plays a role in cancer development (Tonin et al., 1996); however, further studies are necessary. A list of literature cited genes involved in causing breast cancer are included in Table 3.

Table 3 Causes of Hereditary Susceptibility to Breast Cancer

Gene	Contribution to hereditary breast cancer
BRCA1	20%
BRCA2/FANCD1	20%
TP53	<1%
PTEN	<1%
CHK2	5%
ATM	<1%
NBS1	<1%
STK11/LKB1	<1%
PALB2	<1%
RAD50	<1%
BRIP1BACH1/FANCJ	<1%
Undiscovered genes	54%

Source: Adapted from Wooster and Weber (2003).

Epidemiology

BRCA-Related Breast Cancer

Early linkage studies estimated that 90% of breast-ovarian cancer families, those with four or more cases of early-onset breast cancer and at least one case of ovarian cancer, were linked to *BRCA1* (FitzGerald et al., 1996; Langston et al., 1996; Couch et al., 1997). However, data derived from linkage studies tend to overestimate the fraction of hereditary breast cancer from mutations in *BRCA1* and *BRCA2*, as has been shown by more recent studies performed on families who may not be suitable for linkage analysis but who are more typical of the spectrum of breast cancer families seen by practicing physicians. Two of these later studies have estimated that the proportion of the familial risk of breast cancer that is accounted for by *BRCA1* and *BRCA2* is approximately 15% (Peto et al., 1999; Peto and Mack, 2000). More recently, in light of better detection methods, *BRCA1* and *BRCA2* have been estimated to account for about 40% of the familial risk with much of the remaining risk likely explained by combinations of more common, lower-penetrant variants (Wooster and Weber, 2003; Walsh and King, 2007). The fact that the proportion of families without linkage is much larger among families with fewer than six cases is consistent with the hypothesis that susceptibility alleles in other breast cancer genes confer risks lower than those conferred by *BRCA1* or *BRCA2* but are, correspondingly, more common in the population. This scenario might also be the case with regard to early-onset breast cancers. Multiple studies that have evaluated early-onset breast cancer patients have found that mutations in *BRCA1* and *BRCA2* account for a small proportion of these cancers (Struewing et al., 1996; Malone et al., 2000; Shen et al., 2000).

Search Strategies for Other High Penetrance Genes

The likelihood that other breast cancer–susceptibility genes exist has been evaluated by "twin studies" as well as mathematical models. The largest twin study was conducted by Lichtenstein et al. (2000) where it was estimated that genetic factors account for approximately 27% of breast cancer phenotypic variance (Hopper and Carlin, 1992, 2000a; Lichtenstein et al., 2000; Antoniou and Easton, 2006). Another by Peto and Mack (2000) lead them to hypothesize that genetic susceptibility to breast cancer may be the result of multiple low-penetrance alleles which may coexist in high penetrant combinations, that is, a type of polygenic model (Peto and Mack, 2000; Mack et al., 2002). They also propose that the high constant risk could reflect a model in which women reach a high risk of breast cancer at a genetically determined age.

Cui et al. (2001) used data on families ascertained through a "population-based" series of breast cancer patients and found that the familial clustering was a mixed model of inheritance, including both a recessive and a polygenic component (Cui et al., 2001). Antoniou et al. (2002) attempted an alternative approach using a model that took into account the reduced sensitivity of mutation testing. This analysis found that familial segregation of breast cancer is best explained by a model that includes the effects of *BRCA1*, *BRCA2*, and a polygenic component representing the effects of a large number of genes, each conferring a small effect on risk and combining multiplicatively (Antoniou et al., 2002). There was no significant evidence for another major gene. In a recent reanalysis of some of this same data, there was evidence that the polygenic variance decreased with age (Antoniou et al., 2006; Antoniou and Easton, 2006). This model provides explanation to the observation of age-specific familial RRs of breast cancer, and is the basis for the breast and ovarian analysis of disease incidence and carrier estimation algorithm (BOADICEA) model, which can be used for genetic counseling purposes (Antoniou et al., 2004). An alternative model to BOADICEA was developed by Tyrer et al. (2004), which assumes the effects of *BRCA1, BRCA2*, and of a third, dominantly inherited hypothetical gene. In reality, the progress in finding other genes has not proven successful. Two genome-wide linkage screens have been published, one finding linkage on 2q32 (a study of 14 multiple case families from Finland) and the other larger study of 149 families found linkage on 4q (Tyrer et al., 2004; Smith et al., 2006) each with less than impressive LOD scores (<1). Other studies have suggested linkage to chromosomes 8p and 13q12–13 (Kerangueven et al., 1995; Seitz et al., 1997), neither confirmed by the first two studies. These data lend support to the idea, as the twin studies did, that no one gene will be responsible for a significant fraction of breast cancer susceptibility.

"Case control" association studies to identify breast cancer genes have also been unsuccessful. Association studies have researched candidate genes on the basis of their potential roles in carcinogenesis, DNA repair pathway genes among the most popular for study. Several positive associations have been reported but none of these has been convincingly replicated (Pharoah et al., 2004). Very stringent significant levels ($p < 0.0001$ or better) are required to avoid a high false-positive rate (Antoniou and Easton, 2006). To support this end, the Breast Cancer Association Consortium (BCAC) has been established, a group of over 20 institutions working as a collaborative effort to combine data. A recent report by the group detailed results of the evaluation of 16 single-nucleotide polymorphisms (SNPs) (Breast Cancer Association, 2006). Only two alleles were found to be associated with an increased risk of breast cancer: *PGR* V660L and *TGFB1* L10P. These data continue to be evaluated in follow-up studies.

So in comparison with the *BRCA* genes, germline mutations in *TP53*, *PTEN*, *CHK2*, *ATM*, and the other genes discussed above combined account for only a fraction (no more that 10%) of the familial aggregation of breast cancer, indicating that additional culprit genes remain to be identified. Simulation studies have shown that, even with complete correlation among relatives in the exposure to the environmental factor, such risk factors need to confer at least a 10-fold increase in risk to lead to even modest increase to the familial RR (Hopper and Carlin, 1992). Among the known risk factors for breast cancer, none confers such high risks (Antoniou and Easton, 2006).

Male Breast Cancer

Linkage to both *BRCA1* (Pich et al., 2000; Bernard-Gallon et al., 2003; Struewing et al., 1995b) and *BRCA2* (Wooster et al., 1994; Thorlacius et al., 1995) genes occur in cancer families with male breast cancer. It has been published that 14% of male breast cancers are attributed to *BRCA2* mutations; almost all of these patients have a family history of male and/or female breast cancer (Couch et al., 1996; Roa et al., 1996). Furthermore, *BRCA2* (not *BRCA1*) gene rearrangements have been reported in male breast cancer families (Tournier et al., 2004; Woodward et al., 2005). Noteworthy, however, is that these risk estimates are derived from families that are studied for research purposes, who are characterized by early onset of cancer, multiple tumors, or both, and have met stringent criteria for autosomal dominant inheritance of cancer predisposition. They are likely to represent a sample biased toward increased risk and may overestimate the cancer risk associated with *BRCA1* and *BRCA2* mutations (Burke et al., 1997). Male *BRCA2* mutation carriers have an approximate 6% lifetime risk for breast cancer, a dramatic 100- to 200-fold increased risk as compared with the general population by age 70 (Weber, 1996; Wolpert et al., 2000).

Other *BRCA* Cancers

BRCA1 mutation carriers have been estimated in the past to have a risk for *colon* cancer which is approximately fourfold greater than that of the general population and a risk for prostate cancer, which is approximately threefold greater (Ford et al., 1994; Thompson and Easton, 2002). However, the evidence to date is against a major genetic basis for combined breast and colorectal cancer susceptibility (Brinkman et al., 2006). Weber and colleagues have suggested from data regarding breast cancer in families with multiple primary cancers that the presence of multiple primary cancers of any kind may predict for an increased likelihood of finding a *BRCA1* or *BRCA2* mutation (Shih et al., 2000).

In some studies, Ashkenazi Jewish men were examined for the association between founder mutations in *BRCA1* and *prostate* cancer risk, but no association has been detected between *BRCA1* mutation and prostate cancer risk (Kirchhoff et al., 2004). The role of *BRCA1* mutation in prostate cancer is quite limited (Dong, 2006). The *BRCA2* gene has on the other hand been consistently shown to play a role in prostate cancer. The common Ashkenazi founder mutation is significantly associated with prostate cancer risk (Kirchhoff et al., 2004). A founder mutation of *BRCA2*, 5bp deletion, has been identified in the Icelandic population, and an association of this mutation with prostate cancer has also been detected. It has been estimated that germline mutations in *BRCA2* may account for about 5% of prostate cancer in familial clusters, particularly significant in prostate cancers diagnosed at a younger age (Edwards et al., 2003). Outside the men with *BRCA2* mutations, data suggest that most of the increased risk of breast cancer following prostate cancer can be explained by estrogen treatment (Karlsson et al., 2006).

In addition to cancers of the breast, ovary, and prostate, *BRCA2* mutations may be associated with increased risk for other cancers. Risks for all cancers in addition to breast and ovary have been shown elevated; with some population subgroups differing with regard to how frequently elevated risks are found at individual sites (Friedenson, 2005). Statistically significant increases in risks have been observed for pancreatic cancer (Greer and Whitcomb, 2006), gall bladder and bile duct cancer, stomach cancer, and malignant melanoma (Hall et al., 2006; BCLC, 2000). It has been noted, however, that in pancreatic cancer the inactivation of the wild-type allele in the tumor may not always be the first somatic event during the molecular evolution of a cancer. It may be necessary for earlier genetic alterations before biallelic inactivation of a recessive tumor susceptibility gene such as *BRCA2* (Goggins et al., 2000). At present the identification of individuals at increased risk for ocular melanoma (OM) due to mutations in *BRCA2* is small (Houlston and Damato, 1999), leading to the assumption that there may be additional loci that contribute to familial aggregation of OM and to the familial association between OM and breast cancer (Sinilnikova et al., 1999). A novel ocular and cutaneous malignant melanoma susceptibility locus has been mapped to chromosome 9q21.32 (Jonsson et al., 2005). Further elucidation of excess risks for extra-breast cancers in *BRCA1* and *BRCA2* mutation carriers is the subject of continuing research.

Mutations in Both *BRCA* Genes

When considering the high prevalence of carcinoma of the breast and ovary in the general population, one should expect to encounter families where both mutations are segregating. Results of family studies and segregation analyses have indicated that a general or mixed western population frequency for mutations in both genes combined is between 0.06% and 0.26% (Ford et al., 1995; Whittemore et al., 1997; Antoniou et al., 2002; Whittemore et al., 2004b), with most estimates toward the lower end of this range. Such was the case reported by Ramus et al. (1997) (Gayther et al., 1997), who described a patient from a Hungarian family who manifested both breast and ovarian cancer and was found to have truncating mutations in both the *BRCA1* and *BRCA2* genes. This patient carried the 185delAG mutation in *BRCA1* as well as the 6174delT mutation in *BRCA2*. Both of these mutations are common in Ashkenazi Jewish breast cancer patients (Tonin et al., 1995a; Couch et al., 1996; Neuhausen et al., 1996; Berman et al., 1996a; Ramus et al., 1997), and each mutation has been shown to occur in approximately 1% of the Ashkenazi population (Struewing et al., 1995a; Oddoux et al., 1996; Roa et al., 1996) (discussed in further detail below). Given the frequencies of these mutations, it is interesting to note that no one has yet reported a Jewish individual who has inherited, both maternally and paternally, either two *BRCA1* or two *BRCA2* mutations. Several groups have evaluated the functional requirements for *BRCA1* and *BRCA2* in embryogenesis using mouse "knockout" models. In all studies, *BRCA1*- and *BRCA2*-deficient mouse embryos show developmental arrest after days 5 to 6 and 6.5 to 9.5 of gestation, respectively. Thus, in addition to their importance in tumor development (at least in humans), these genes are also required for embryonic development to proceed to completion (at least in mice). On the basis of mouse studies, one would predict that human embryos that are homozygous for mutant *BRCA1* or for mutant *BRCA2* might also fail to develop to completion.

MUTATION

Mutation Spectrum

Germline mutations in *BRCA1* were initially detected in five of eight families that demonstrated linkage to *BRCA1* and in four of 44 randomly selected breast and ovarian tumors (Futreal et al., 1994; Miki et al., 1994). The mutations detected in these randomly selected tumors were also present in the germline, indicating that the mutations were indeed inherited. Since this initial report, hundreds of studies have continued to evaluate high-risk cancer families for disease-associated mutations in both *BRCA1* and *BRCA2*. *BRCA1* and *BRCA2* have been estimated to account for about 40% of the familial risk with much of the remaining risk likely explained by combinations of more common, lower-penetrant variants (Wooster and Weber, 2003; Walsh and King, 2007).

The mutations detected are scattered over the entire coding sequence (5,592 bp and 10,254 bp, respectively) as well as the surrounding intervening sequences and fall into several categories. The majority of the mutations reported in *BRCA1* and *BRCA2* are either point mutations or small insertions and deletions. Well over 1000 different mutations (deleterious mutations, naturally occurring polymorphisms, and unclassified variants) have been identified in *BRCA1* and *BRCA2*, and genetic testing for mutations in these genes in high-risk families is now well established (Walsh et al., 2006). To aid in these studies, a centralized mutation database was established that serves as a warehouse to store the *BRCA1* and *BRCA2* sequence variants detected in cancer-prone families being studied throughout the world (BIC).

Frameshift/Nonsense

Testing for mutations in these genes has become one of the most widely used hereditary cancer tests, with over 70,000 patients tested to date (Tavtigian et al., 2006). Of the mutations that have clearly been associated with the disease, approximately 80% to 85% are frameshift or nonsense mutations. These alterations span the length of the large genes, and result in considerable heterogeneity in the size of the mutant protein as they cause premature termination of protein translation. They are considered to be deleterious. Frameshift mutations result primarily from the deletions or insertions of a few nucleotides (e.g., 1, 2, 4) within a coding region or exon (e.g., CAG GTT AGT to CAG GTT TAG T) or from sequence changes affecting the splice donor (e.g., CTAgt to CTAtt) or splice acceptor sites (e.g., cagGTA to catGTA) (splice site mutation). Single base insertions or deletions occur most frequently at adenine (A), and with decreasing frequencies at thymine (T), and guanine (G) or cytosine (C). While G>A base substitutions are the most common in both *BRCA1* and *BRCA2*, G>T substitutions occur more frequently in *BRCA1* (BIC).

Nonsense mutations result from the substitution of a single nucleotide within a codon, which codes for an amino acid. This substitution results in converting the coding codon to a stop codon (e.g., AAG to TAG). All of these mutations are predicted to results in the expression of a truncated or severely defective protein. Although 13.5% of patients tested through full sequence analyses of both *BRCA1* And *BRCA2* at the nation's major testing site are found to carry a deleterious mutation (frameshift or nonsense), 12% of patients who do not carry a clearly deleterious variant are found to carry an uncertain variant (Frank et al., 2002). A second group of single-nucleotide substitution sequence variants are referred to as missense mutations. Unlike nonsense mutations, the substitution results in a functional codon, but encodes for a different amino acid at that position (e.g., CAG to CAC, Gln to His). The problem with missense changes, in the *BRCA* genes and others, is that it is not always simple to determine if the amino acid substitution will adversely affect the protein's function and thereby contribute to the disease phenotype (discussed further under "Clinical Implications"). If the missense change is commonly found in control populations (ethnically matched disease-free individuals with no family history of breast and/or ovarian cancer), it is deemed to be a naturally occurring polymorphism. However, many of these variants are found in only a limited number of families and are referred to as Variants of Unknown Significance.

Variants of Unknown Significance

Some controversy exists regarding classifying sequence variants as disease-associated (i.e., deleterious mutations) or benign (i.e., polymorphisms). The frequent discovery of Variants of Unknown Significance is a major problem from a clinical standpoint since many patients who undergo genetic testing are left to interpret these ambiguous results while trying to make important health care decisions. Recently, Goldgar et al. developed a method for analysis of unclassified missense substitutions in *BRCA1* and *BRCA2* that integrates four types of data: segregation of sequence variants of interest in pedigrees; pooled family histories of index cases who carry the variant versus all index cases tested; co-occurrence of the variant with clearly deleterious variants in the same gene; and cross-species protein multiple sequence alignment, followed by the comparison of the physiochemical characteristics of the amino acids observed at the point of the mutation. Each of these data types has its own strengths and weaknesses. One strength of the integrated method is that each of the four types of data analysis that it has integrated was developed as an independent estimator of the likelihood that a sequence variant confers a high cancer risk versus being neutral or of little clinical significance (Goldgar et al., 2004).

In a study performed by the BCLC, it was reported that among the *BRCA1*-linked families tested, mutations were detected in only 63% of the affected probands (Ford et al., 1995). These limitations brought into question the validity and accuracy of most diagnostic testing. Commercial companies that test for a fee tend to focus solely on sequencing the coding exons and the immediate adjacent intronic sequences. However, later studies have shown that not all *BRCA1* or *BRCA2* mutations are detected by PCR-based methods that focus primarily on coding sequence, since there are a number of families found strongly linked to *BRCA1* and *BRCA2* for which no mutations have been detected (Ford et al., 1995; Swensen et al., 1997; Puget et al., 1999). Furthermore, studies suggest that a substantial fraction of *BRCA1* (and potentially *BRCA2*) mutations may be large deletions or rearrangements that are not detected by standard screening methods.

Large Rearrangements

More than 60 different large genomic rearrangements involving one or more exons of the *BRCA1* gene have been described (Armaou et al., 2007) since the first reported *BRCA1* rearrangement in 1997 (Puget et al., 1997). Fifty-four arc deletions, eight are duplications, one is a triplication, and three combine both deletion and insertion events (Armaou et al., 2007). Most of them are caused by recombination between *Alu* repeats, whereas four rearrangements have been generated through unequal homologous recombination events that do not involve *Alu* repeats; they are the result of recombination between the *BRCA1* gene and the *BRCA1* pseudogene (Smith et al., 1996; Puget et al., 2002; Preisler-Adams et al., 2006). Six rearrangements have shown a founder effect and at least one genomic rearrangement has been detected in each of the *BRCA1* exons (Armaou et al., 2007; *BRCA1* Exon 13 Duplication Screening Group 2000b). The proportion of the *BRCA1* mutations due to genomic rearrangements varies in different countries from the highest of 27% in the Netherlands (Hogervorst et al., 2003) to 19% in Italy (Agata et al., 2006), 15% in American families (Puget et al., 1999), 12 % in French families (Gad et al., 2002), 8.2% in Spain (de la Hoya et al., 2006) and 8% in German families (Hofmann et al., 2003). The prevalence of five previously reported, frequently tested, and recurrent *BRCA1* genetic rearrangements in more than 20,000 patients from hereditary breast/ovarian cancer families has recently been determined in a large North American patient population. The results showed a 6-kb duplication of exon 13 identified in 2.01%, a 26-kb deletion encompassing exons 14–20 identified in 0.27%, a 510-bp deletion of exon 22 identified in 0.19%, and a 3.4-kb deletion of exon 13 identified in 0.04% (Hendrickson et al., 2005). A previously reported 7.1kb deletion of exons 8–9 was not found. The prevalence of the five in this population is then 2.51%. Some alterations in the panel likely remain culture-specific and will not prove useful in screening a mixed population. Full gene screen for large insertions/deletions in *BRCA1* will help determine the frequency of this type of alteration in the general population.

While screening for *BRCA1* rearrangements has become part of the routine molecular diagnosis of predisposition to breast/ovarian cancer, relatively few *BRCA2* germline rearrangements have been reported (Casilli et al., 2006). A recent follow-up study found that 7.7% of *BRCA2* mutations arc germline rearrangements (Casilli et al., 2006). These data are in agreement with another recent study of 121 selected breast and breast-ovarian cancer families from Italy, where three deletions were found and their contribution to the *BRCA2* spectrum was estimated to be 11% (Mazoyer, 2005). Conversely, a study in Finland found no large genomic *BRCA2* rearrangements among 36 male breast cancer patients (Karhu et al., 2006). These data suggest that the contribution of rearrangements to the mutation spectrum of *BRCA2* may in fact be comparable to that of rearrangements in the mutation spectrum of *BRCA1*, currently estimated at about 15% (Mazoyer, 2005) but that statistics are likely to be population specific. Additionally, while the prevalence of *BRCA* rearrangements appears low (Ellis et al., 2006; Frolov et al., 2002), *BRCA2* rearrangements have been identified in sporadic breast tumors (van der Looij et al., 2000; Armaou et al., 2007). There is published data that *BRCA2* germline rearrangements are present in a significant number of male breast cancer families (Tournier et al., 2004).

Regulatory Mutations

In addition to large rearrangements that contribute to the frequency of *BRCA* mutations, inferred regulatory mutations have been suspected to occur in the *BRCA* genes that lead to the absence of a stable transcript from the mutant allele (Ford et al., 1995; Feunteun and Lenoir, 1996). The presence of these regulatory mutations that prevent transcription from the mutated allele has been inferred on the basis of the observation that at least one carrier was heterozygous for a *BRCA1* polymorphism at the genomic level but apparently homozygous at the cDNA level (Miki et al., 1994; Gayther et al., 1995; Xu et al., 1997). These types of mutations are much more difficult to detect and are routinely ignored by those performing diagnostic tests, but are being investigated in the research environment. Large deletions (hundreds to thousands of base pairs) may be responsible for other reported inferred regulatory mutations in *BRCA1* (and likely *BRCA2*) as well as mutations in the promoter, in potential regulatory elements in the 5′ and 3′ untranslated regions (UTRs), or in the polyadenylation signal (Puget et al., 1999). Neuhausen and colleagues were the first to report a 14-kb *Alu*-mediated deletion in *BRCA1* that eliminates transcription by removing both known transcription start sites (Swensen et al., 1997). A report of a possible transposon-like element (Presneau et al., 1999) represents a new type of *BRCA1/BRCA2* gene alteration that may effect gene expression or control of expression. More recently by a combination of comparative genomics and functional analysis a successful strategy has been used to identify two novel regulatory elements in intron 2 of *BRCA1* and provide the first direct evidence that conserved noncoding sequences in *BRCA1* regulate gene expression (Wardrop and Brown, 2005).

A reduction in expression of the *BRCA1* is thought to be a key event in development of some sporadic breast and ovarian cancers (Sobczak and Krzyzosiak, 2002; Pietschmann et al., 2005; Hughes, 2006). The vast majority of breast cancer-related *BRCA1* and *BRCA2* mutations identified to date are germline mutations, whereas, somatic mutations are found but rarely (<10%) in sporadic ovarian cancers (Hosking et al., 1995; Merajver et al., 1995) and even less in sporadic breast tumors (Khoo et al., 1999; van der Looij et al., 2000). Increasing evidence suggests that the *BRCA* and FA pathways may be inactivated by multiple mechanisms in a substantial proportion of sporadic cancers, and that these cancers could display "BRCA-ness" (Turner et al., 2004). So, the decrease in expression in some sporadic disease will be attributed to a mechanism other than mutation.

BRCA1 contains two separate promoters that induce transcription of messenger ribonucleic acid mRNAs with different 5′UTRs. In certain breast cancers, *BRCA1* expression is downregulated by a switch from expression of a shorter 5′UTR, which enables efficient translation, to expression of a different longer 5′UTR, which contains secondary structure and upstream open reading frames (uORFs) that strongly inhibit translation (Sobczak and Krzyzosiak, 2002; Pietschmann et al., 2005; Hughes, 2006). A stable secondary structure formed by a truncated *Alu* element and upstream AUG codons are responsible for reduced translation of mRNA. Changes in the 3′UTR have the potential also to affect the rate or amount of translation to functional protein. A novel insertion/deletion in the 3′UTR of *BRCA1* was identified in the Iranian hereditary breast/ovarian cancer kindred (Pietschmann et al., 2005). The alteration was absent in age-matched Iranian control groups.

Methylated-Mediated Suppression

Methlyation-mediated suppression of detoxification, DNA repair, and tumor suppressor genes has been implicated in cancer development and progression. Hypermethylation of CpG-island promoters is known to be strongly associated with gene silencing. Once established, methylation is passed on to daughter cells during DNA replication by the activity of DNA methyltransferases, thereby conserving the overall pattern of methylated CpG-islands (Herman and Baylin, 2003). The methylation patterns of virtually all types of cancer, including breast carcinoma, have been found to differ extensively from that of the corresponding normal tissue. An alternative mechanism for *BRCA1* inactivation, other than by mutation or regulatory mechanisms, has been suggested to be gene silencing by these epigenetic mechanisms (Birgisdottir et al., 2006). *BRCA1* methylation has only been found in breast and ovarian tumors and has been associated with allelic imbalance at the *BRCA1* locus and reduced *BRCA1* gene expression (Esteller et al., 2001; Esteller, 2000). *BRCA2* promoter hypermethylation has not been found in breast tumors, although it has been reported in ovarian tumors (Collins et al., 1997; Hilton et al., 2002). Gene expression profiling has revealed similarities between *BRCA1* methylated and familial *BRCA1* tumors (Hedenfalk et al., 2001; van 't Veer et al., 2002). This lends support to the idea that epigenetic silencing of the *BRCA1* gene might channel tumor progression, similar to an underlying *BRCA1* germline mutation resulting in a *BRCA*-like phenotype. A recent report, however, shows high levels of *BRCA1* expression and a low frequency of *BRCA1* promoter methylation in basal-like sporadic tumors suggesting a more complex situation (Matros et al., 2005). Bean et al. have recently found as well that *BRCA1* promoter hypermethylation is not associated with breast cancer risk as measured by mathematical risk models (Bean et al., 2007). Continued research will help define the role of methylation, if any, in *BRCA1/2* related breast cancer.

Founder or Recurrent Mutations in *BRCA1* and *BRCA2*

Although there has been no clustering of mutations along the *BRCA1* gene, surveys of large numbers of linked families and high-risk women have revealed a few mutations that are seen recurrently (Shattuck-Eidens et al., 1995; Couch et al., 1996). The same has transpired with

Table 4 *BRCA1* and *BRCA2* Founder Mutations

Ashkenazi Jewish	185delAG, *BRCA1*	1/40
	5382insC, *BRCA1*	
	6174delT, *BRCA2*	
Icelandic	999del5, *BRCA2*	1/170
Dutch	IVS12-1643del3835, *BRCA1*	1/333
	IVS21-36del510, *BRCA1*	

Recurrent mutations: Spanish, Belgian, Swedish, German, and Polish.
Source: From Breast Cancer Information Core (BIC), NHGRI.

our experience with *BRCA2*. Present data have supported that the type and frequency of the mutations have different geographic and ethnic distributions. First realized for example were that certain groups of women of Eastern European decent have a higher than expected rate of mutation of *BRCA1* (Egan et al., 1996). Additionally, certain mutations in *BRCA1* were found to account for a significant proportion of hereditary breast cancer in the Dutch population (Petrij-Bosch et al., 1997). The following is a brief review of the known *BRCA1* or *BRCA2* founder mutations, primarily focusing on the individuals of Ashkenazi Jewish decent (Table 4).

Ashkenazi Jews

Breast cancer risk

Ashkenazi Jews represent more than 90% of the 6 million Jews in the United States and Canada. The risk of breast cancer is greater for Jews than for non-Jews (Newill, 1961; Salber et al., 1969), particularly for early-onset cancer, and was documented well before the discovery of *BRCA1* and *BRCA2*. In a large case-control study (Egan et al., 1996), the RR for breast cancer associated with Jewish ethnicity was 1.10 (95% confidence interval [CI] = 0.84–1.44); the effect of family history was about twofold higher for Jewish women. While this statistically significant increase may be because of genetic and nongenetic factors, one possible explanation is a higher frequency of mutations in the breast cancer–susceptibility gene *BRCA1* and *BRCA2*.

Carrier risk

Multivariate analysis identified three strong, significant predictors of *BRCA1* mutation status in Jewish cases, diagnosis at ages 35 to 44 years in the cases, early diagnosis age in a relative, and family history of ovarian cancer. While the carrier rate in non-Jewish populations is too low to consider genetic screening, the carrier rate in Ashkenazi Jews is high and genetic screening poses fewer technical barriers. Jewish ancestry has repeatedly emerged as a significant predictor of a positive *BRCA* gene test result (Couch et al., 1997; Shattuck-Eidens et al., 1997; Frank et al., 1998) and genetic risk analysis without assessment of Jewish ancestry in incomplete (Rubinstein et al., 2002). The high genetic cancer risks of Ashkenazi *BRCA* founder mutations, the aggressive nature of ovarian and early-onset breast cancers, and the increasing effectiveness of medical interventions make crucial further dialogue and research to keep guidelines for genetic screening appropriate (Rubinstein, 2004). There is emerging evidence for other genetic factors in the Ashkenazim such as the HER2 1655V polymorphism, which conveys a modest effect on lifetime breast cancer risk that is stronger at younger ages and in women with a family history of breast cancer (Rutter et al., 2003a).

The *BRCA* mutation carrier rate in the general population has been estimated at about 1 in 345 to 1 in 1000, far lower than in Ashkenazi Jews (Ford et al., 1995; Andersen, 1996; Whittemore et al., 1997; Peto et al., 1999). Other studies produced data in agreement with earlier reports (Struewing et al., 1997; Warner et al., 1999; Hartge et al., 1999) of 10.2% carrier rate for *BRCA1* mutations and 1.1% carrier rate for *BRCA2* mutations among Jewish women. The incidence of alterations is as high as 1/40 to 1/50, accounting for approximately 50% of early-onset breast cancer in Ashkenazi Jewish women (Collins, 1996; Bowcock, 1997). Thus, 38% of Jewish women with breast cancer under the age of 30 years would be expected to have germline *BRCA1* or *BRCA2* mutations (Ford et al., 1995; Struewing et al., 1995a). The proportion of breast cancer cases in the general population because of *BRCA1* is estimated to be 5.3% in women younger than 40 years, 2.2% between 40 and 49 years old, and 1.1% between 50 and 70 years (Ford et al., 1995). The proportion of carriers of *BRCA2* mutations in the general population is equally low. Thus, further analysis is merited in high-risk, founder mutation-negative families to identify the nonfounder mutations and provide accurate counseling (Roa et al., 1996; Frank et al., 2002; Kauff et al., 2002a). Only 78% to 96% of Ashkenazi Jews with detectable mutations using DNA sequence analysis carry one of the founder mutations.

But Jewish women are disproportionately impacted by *BRCA* mutations throughout life, with a 10% carrier rate for breast cancer diagnosed at any age and a 21% to 31% carrier rate for breast cancer diagnosed by the age of 40 years (Hartge et al., 1999). In an Israeli study, 30% of breast cancers diagnosed in Jewish women younger than 40 years had one of the three founder mutations and 10% of Jewish women diagnosed older than 40 years were carriers (Abeliovich et al., 1997). Comparable rates in non-Jewish population are 6.1% for breast cancer diagnosed before the age of 50 years, and only 1.2% of women diagnosed who are 50 years or older are carriers (Peto et al., 1999).

Founder mutations

Ashkenazi Jewish women have been found to have high incidence of three founder mutations: 185delAG and

5382insC in *BRCA1*, and 6174delT in *BRCA2* (Struewing et al., 1995a; Tonin et al., 1996; Berman et al., 1996a). The cumulative incidence of these three mutations in Ashkenazi Jews is approximately 2.5% (Struewing et al., 1995a; Tonin et al., 1996; Devilee, 1999). The frequency of these three mutations is approximately five times higher than the frequency of *BRCA1* and *BRCA2* mutations in the general population (Struewing et al., 1995a; Oddoux et al., 1996; Roa et al., 1996; Struewing et al., 1997). In the Ashkenazi general population, the carrier frequencies of these founder mutations are approximately 1% for 185delAG (Struewing et al., 1996), 0.13% for 5382insC, and 1.35% for 6174delT (Oddoux et al., 1996; Roa et al., 1996). The carrier frequency of the 185delAG alteration has been estimated to account for 16% and 39%, respectively, of the breast and ovarian cancer diagnosed before the age of 50 years in this ethnic subgroup (Struewing et al., 1995a). These studies were supported by a study that found that 21% of Jewish women with diagnosed breast cancer at 40 years or younger were *BRCA1* 185delAG mutation carriers (FitzGerald et al., 1996). Six of eighty Ashkenazi Jewish women (8%) diagnosed with breast cancer before the age of 42 years were carriers of the 6174delT alteration (Struewing et al., 1995a). Studies of all three founder mutation in Jewish women with prevalent breast cancer, unselected for family history, have found mutation rates of 7% (Fodor et al., 1998) and 12% (Warner et al., 1999) suggesting a significant contribution of founder mutations across the age spectrum.

BRCA *penetrance*

Lifetime penetrance estimates based on genotyping of probands have ranged widely in Jewish and non-Jewish populations, and the RRs of breast cancer of the three founder mutations in Ashkenazi Jewish families not selected for either the number of affected members or age at onset of breast cancer are uncertain. Penetrance, the lifetime risk of cancer, was estimated from the original linkage studies as being especially high, about 85% for breast cancer, and 40% to 65% for ovarian cancers in *BRCA1* carriers and 20% for *BRCA2* carriers (Easton et al., 1995; Ford et al., 1998). Since then, many but not all studies have found much lower penetrance estimates (Rubinstein, 2004). Unlike the original linkage analysis, the later studies have included incident breast cancer cases in the general population unselected for family history, unselected ovarian cancer cases in Jewish women, cases from breast cancer risk evaluation clinics, and pooled pedigree data from multiple studies.

Breast cancer penetrance for non-Jewish population ranged from 40% to 73% (age 70 years) for *BRCA1* and 37 (age 70 years) to 74% (age 80 years) for *BRCA2*. Lifetime penetrance of breast cancer (to age 70 years) for Jewish population ranged from 36% to 60% for *BRCA1* and from 21% to 56% for *BRCA2*. Several studies in Jewish populations fall well within range of the results in non-Jewish populations. Interestingly, several studies have shown a birth cohort effect, whereby *BRCA* carriers born after 1930 or 1940 have higher lifetime cancer risks that women born earlier (Narod et al., 1995; Chang-Claude et al., 1997; Antoniou et al., 2003; King et al., 2003).

Male breast cancer

About 0.8% of breast cancers occur in men. Risk factors include age, testicular disease, benign breast conditions, gynecomastia, previous liver diseases, never being married, Jewish ancestry, African ancestry, family history of female breast cancer, Klinefelter syndrome, androgen insensitivity syndrome caused by mutations in the androgen receptor gene, and mutations in *BRCA1* and *BRCA2* (Steinitz et al., 1981; Sasco et al., 1993; Lynch et al., 1999; Brenner et al., 2002; Giordano et al., 2002). Studies show generally low *BRCA2* mutation rates for unselected male breast cancer cases or when family history is negative (Lynch et al., 1999; Giordano et al., 2002). About 4% to 8% of non-Jewish male breast cancer cases versus 19% of Jewish male breast cancer cases carry germline *BRCA* mutations (Struewing et al., 1999). Although *BRCA2* is the gene best known for its association with male breast cancer (Wooster et al., 1995; Ford et al., 1998), over a third of mutations in men having testing for the two genes were found in the *BRCA1* gene (Frank et al., 2002). The highest genetic attributable risk for male breast cancer, 40%, was found in the Icelandic population, because of the *BRCA2* founder mutation 999del5 (Thorlacius et al., 1997). The penetrance to age 70 for male breast cancer has been estimated as 6% for *BRCA2* and is presumably less for male *BRCA1* carriers (Easton et al., 1997; Liede et al., 2004). Men who choose to have genetic testing do so primarily in order to clarify risks to their daughters. Closer follow-up is warranted, but the needs of male carriers have not been addressed fully (Liede et al., 2000b).

Other cancers

The Ashkenazi founder mutations, like other mutations in *BRCA1* and *BRCA2*, may predispose an individual to other cancers. Ovarian cancer is a component of the autosomal dominant hereditary breast-ovarian cancer syndrome and may be due to a mutation in either of the *BRCA* genes. The lifetime risk of ovarian cancer conferred by a *BRCA1* mutation was originally estimated to be 60% (Ford et al., 1994; Easton et al., 1995), and the risk for carriers of a *BRCA2* mutation was originally estimated to be 27% (Ford et al., 1998). It is noteworthy that a risk estimate made on the basis of a sample of mostly unaffected Jewish individuals was much lower (Struewing et al., 1997). In a more recent study, ovarian cancer penetrance for *BRCA1* and *BRCA2* combined was 22% (6–65%) by 80 years (ABCSG, 2000) (30–45% for *BRCA1* and 10–20% for *BRCA2*). The rate of ovarian cancer among Israeli Jews born in Europe or North America is among the highest reported (Parkin and Iscovich, 1997). This excessive risk may be due to the high frequency of founder mutations in this population.

While breast and ovarian carcinomas are predominant in Ashkenazi families carrying these mutations, there is evidence in the literature supporting a higher incidence of prostate (Ford et al., 1994), pancreatic (Simard et al., 1994; Tulinius et al., 1994; Tonin et al., 1995b; Johannsson et al., 1996; Phelan et al., 1996), and colorectal cancers (Berman et al., 1996b). Recent studies lend support to the association of colorectal cancer with *BRCA* mutation carriers (Drucker et al., 2000), while data regarding an association with pancreatic and prostate cancers are still contradictory (Lehrer et al., 1998; Hubert et al., 1999; Lal et al., 2000). Kadouri et al. found recently a 2.5-fold increase in any other cancer and a fourfold of colon cancer risk among *BRCA1* founder carriers. Corresponding hazard ratios in *BRCA2* founder carriers were nonsignificant, except for markedly elevated lymphoma risk (Kadouri et al., 2007).

Population-Specific Mutations

As described above for the Ashkenazi Jews where an ethnic increase in cancer incidence arises from founder effects, clear ethnic differences have been observed for other populations. A part of the observed ethnic differences in cancer susceptibility may be explained by genetic factors. Recurring mutations in *BRCA1* and *BRCA2* are identified and further evaluated to determine if they are founder mutations (having a shared haplotype) or if they have arisen two or more times by chance. Founder or recurrent mutations for *BRCA1* and *BRCA2* have been described in French Canadians (Simard et al., 1994), Swedes (Johannsson et al., 1996), Icelanders (Thorlacius et al., 1996), Norwegians (Andersen et al., 1996), Finns (Huusko et al., 1998), Dutch (Peelen et al., 1997; Petrij-Bosch et al., 1997), Russians (Gayther et al., 1997), Japanese (Inoue et al., 1995), and African Americans (Gao et al., 1997b) in early testing and in most populations tested more recently. A high frequency of novel *BRCA1* germline mutations have been reported to be present in families from Tuscany, Italy, as well (Caligo et al., 1996). Common mutations have been found in British (Gayther et al., 1995; Markoff et al., 1997, 2000b), Sardinian (Pisano et al., 2000), Scottish (Liede et al., 2000a), Belgian (Claes et al., 1999), and Polish populations (Gorski et al., 2000).

Minorities

African Americans

The proportion of breast cancer attributed to mutations in *BRCA1* or *BRCA2* has varied widely among different studies and different ethnic groups. It is not known if the proportions vary among blacks, whites, Asians, or Hispanics, and if the spectrum of mutations reflects those of founder ancestors. Only recently has information about genetic testing begun to appear in the literature regarding these other ethnic minorities. One of the largest ethnic minorities in the United States, the African American population, remains understudied, despite having a proportionately high incidence of early-onset breast cancer. African American women make up a significant proportion of women who are diagnosed with early-onset disease, have tumors that are larger in size, and have greater involvement of lymph nodes (Aziz et al., 1999; Gapstur et al., 1996; Ries et al., 1996; Elmore et al., 1998). From 1973 to 1993, the incidence rate of breast cancer in African Americans and whites increased 36.9% and 24.0%, respectively, and during the same time, the mortality rate decreased 4.3% in white patients with breast cancer, but increased 18.0% for African American women. The mortality rate of breast cancer in young whites decreased by 21.5%, this rate remained almost the same (–0.7%) in young African Americans (Ries et al., 1996).

Two recent studies conferred that early-onset age and larger number of affected relatives to be predictive of carrying a mutation on one of the two *BRCA* genes in African American families (Nanda et al., 2005; Malone et al., 2006). Both studies found ovarian cancer to be less common in black versus white families, but that ovarian cancer was predictive of carrier status. The Malone et al. study is the largest study to date of *BRCA1/BRCA2* in black women with breast cancer, and is the first to present multivariate analyses of predictors of mutation status in a population-based setting.

Early studies found that the prevalence of *BRCA1* mutations was low in African American women enrolled in a population-based case-control study (Newman et al., 1998). In this study, no protein-truncating *BRCA1* mutations were found in 88 cases and 79 controls. In 2000, Gao and colleagues reported that the prevalence of *BRCA1/2* mutations ranged from 12% to 21% in a clinic-based series of African American women who had a personal and family history of breast and/or ovarian cancer, finding one novel *BRCA1* and three novel *BRCA2* mutations; no recurrent mutations were identified. Frank and colleagues (2002) reported that the prevalence of mutations was 19% and 16% in African American and non-Ashkenazi European individuals, respectively (Frank et al., 2002). However, recent work has shown that the prevalence of

BRCA1/2 mutations is similar among African Americans and other ethnic groups who have a personal and family history of breast and/or ovarian cancer (Halbert et al., 2005).

The vast majority of African Americans originated from western Africa, where breast cancer is considered a rare aggressive disease predominantly affecting young women (Parkin and Iscovich, 1997). In 1993, one of the two families with evidence of linkage between breast cancer and genetic markers flanking *BRCA1* was a family of African American descent (Chamberlain et al., 1993). Since then, a number of unique mutations in the *BRCA1* and *BRCA2* genes have been reported in this population. In one study three novel *BRCA1* mutations were identified in five of nine (56%) African American families screened for mutations (Gao et al., 1997b). A recent review on hereditary breast cancer in African Americans reported that 26 different *BRCA1* mutations and 18 distinct *BRCA2* mutations have been identified in Africans or African American individuals. Most of these are unique mutations, but a few recurrent mutations have been identified (Frank et al., 2002; Olopade et al., 2003; Gao et al., 1997a; Mefford et al., 1999). A significantly higher frequency of variants of uncertain significance has been identified in African Americans (Haffty et al., 2006). Taken together, African Americans have a unique mutation spectrum in the *BRCA1* and *BRCA2* genes, but recurrent mutations are likely to be more widely dispersed and therefore not readily identifiable in this population.

Hispanics

Breast cancer is the most commonly diagnosed cancer in Hispanic women, and is the leading cancer cause of death, exceeding even lung cancer (Weitzel et al., 2005). The prevalence of *BRCA* mutations among high-risk Hispanic families is unknown. The Hispanic population is not evenly distributed across the United States, and consists of a range of individuals from different countries of origin (Rumbaut, 1995). This variability in geographic concentration and diversity or origin of Hispanics has contributed to the difficulty in studying these populations. For these reasons and others, it is not surprising that large racial disparities exist between white and minority populations in the use of genetic counseling and *BRCA1* and *BRCA2* mutation detection testing (Armstrong et al., 2005; Hall and Olopade, 2005).

The largest published study of the prevalence of *BRCA* mutations in a largely immigrant Hispanic population residing in an urban center in the United States has been only recently published by (Weitzel et al., 2005). Six recurrent mutations accounted for 47% (16 of 34) of the deleterious mutations in this cohort. The *BRCA1* 185delAG mutation was prevalent (3.6%) in this clinic-based cohort of predominantly Mexican descent, and shared the Ashkenazi Jewish founder haplotype. Torres et al., 2006 found a high proportion of founder mutations in breast/ovarian cancer families from Colombia. Germline mutations were identified in 24.5% of 53 families. Two recurrent *BRCA1* mutations accounted for 100% of all *BRCA1* mutations and the recurrent *BRCA2* mutation for 40% of all *BRCA2* mutations. Haplotype analysis suggested that each had arisen from a common ancestor. The prevalence of *BRCA1* or *BRCA2* mutations was 50% in multiple-case breast cancer families, and was 33% for the breast-ovarian cancer families. These data suggest a substantial proportion of hereditary breast/ovarian cancer in Colombia that differed completely to that previously reported in the above California study. This information reinforces that specific genetic risk assessment strategies for the different Hispanic population in South America and in the United States need to be developed.

Mutation Detection

By consistently finding fewer mutation carriers than expected, it is possible to assess that the mutation detection system does not detect all DNA changes in a gene. For a time the most widely used screening method because of its simplicity and low cost was single-stranded conformation polymorphism (SSCP), though this method still reaches a variable sensitivity of only 70 to 80% and requires optimization of conditions for each amplicon tested (Glavac and Dean, 1993). Direct nucleotide sequencing is considered the gold standard technique for mutation detection for genes such as *BRCA1* and *BRCA2*. Variations of this standard, such as digital detection sequencing (Ruparel et al., 2004), have been developed to reduce cost and for ease of high throughput.

Other common techniques for the identification of base pair substitutions are denaturing gradient gel electrophoresis (DGGE) (Fodde and Losekoot, 1994), conformation sensitive gel electrophoresis (CSGE) (Markoff et al., 1998), and allele specific oligonucleotide hybridization (ASO) (Richter and Seth, 1998). Each of these methods has its limitations and is either low in sensitivity and reproducibility or high in costs and difficult to perform (Cotton, 1993; Ravnik-Glavac and Dean, 1994). Array-based technologies have been applied to these original concepts that have solved some but not all technical and budgetary problems (Yim et al., 2005; Kuperstein et al., 2006). Use of heteroduplex analysis, which relies on the heteroduplexes formed after the hybridization of mutant and wild-type DNA possessing differing mobilities in nondenaturing gels, has previously been limited to detection of insertion/deletions (Cotton, 1997). High-throughput and array-based adaptations of this method has broadened its mutation detection capabilities to single-nucleotide substitutions

(Esteban-Cardenosa et al., 2004; Weber et al., 2004; Velasco et al., 2005).

Another disadvantage of the above-mentioned techniques is the lack of selectivity with respect to the position of a sequence variation. Techniques relying on conformational changes in DNA also detect neutral polymorphism alterations that are of little, if any, significance. The *BRCA1* gene possesses a large number of harmless polymorphisms scattered over the whole gene. If these sequence variations cannot be rapidly distinguished from clinically relevant mutations, every alteration that is found by prescreening has to be sequenced. Advances in mutation detection involve the use of enzyme mutation detection (Del Tito et al., 1998; Oleykowski et al., 1998; Kulinski et al., 2000). These enzymes cleave DNA duplexes at sites containing mispaired DNA bases. DNA fragments resulting from cleavage can be detected by conventional analytical methods such as gel electrophoresis. Enzyme detection is a single-tube assay that requires PCR amplification of the DNA of interest, formation of heteroduplex DNA, enzymatic mismatch cleavage, and analysis by gel electrophoresis. Unlike previous mutation techniques, the enzyme mutation detection technique uses a single protocol to identify point mutations, deletion, and insertions for all DNA fragments. Mutations have been shown to be identified in mixed samples containing up to a 20-fold excess of normal DNA (Del Tito et al., 1998). Sensitivity and specificity have been determined to be 100% and 94% respectively (Del Tito et al., 1998).

Oefner and coworkers have reported yet another technique for the identification of single-base substitutions and small deletions/insertions (Oefner and Underhill, 1995; Underhill et al., 1997). Heteroduplex DNAs are separated from homoduplex strands by ion-pairing reversed phase liquid chromatography via a special high performance liquid chromatography (HPLC) column. Partial heat denaturation decreases the retention time of mismatched DNA molecules compared with their intact double-stranded counterparts. While the DHPLC technique is highly sensitive, efficient (as it can be automated), and economical, preparation for mutation analysis requires standardization for each amplicon tested. Additionally, in that *BRCA1* and *BRCA2* are highly polymorphic there will be occasion that a unique alteration is detected within a polymorphism cluster so that direct sequencing will be required to determine the specific unique variation.

Methods based on hybridization of test DNA or RNA with multiple, defined oligonucleotides or cDNA probes attached to a solid glass or nylon matrix have been developed and are referred to as "oligonucleotide microassays" or "DNA microarrays" or "gene chips." By analyzing different hybridization patterns or levels between control and test DNA or RNA, oligonucleotide microarrays have been used for the analysis of many large genes, *de novo* DNA sequencing, comparative sequence analysis, and gene expression studies (Southern, 1996; Wallace, 1997; Lipshutz et al., 1999). However, relatively little is published about the sensitivity and specificity of microarray methods to detect sequence alteration compared with gel-based DNA sequence analysis. The possibilities suggest that microarray methods can be improved.

Although sequencing the entire coding region of a large gene is a sensitive technique for overall detection of mutations, it is more time consuming and labor intensive than analysis by DNA microarray technology (Wen et al., 2000). Universal DNA array technology has been used for detection of small insertions and deletions in *BRCA1* and *BRCA2* by Favis and colleagues, who portend that rapid identification of these specific types of alterations is permitted in the context of both clinical diagnosis and population studies (Favis et al., 2000). This study made use of a multiplex assay using a modified PCR to evenly amplify each amplicon (PCR/PCR) (Belgrader et al., 1996), followed by a ligase detection reaction (LDR) (Khanna et al., 1999). Frolov et al. (2002) used a DNA array-based method for detection of large rearrangements in the *BRCA1* gene. The authors suggest the potential to screen clinical tumor samples for genomic rearrangements simultaneously in a large number of cancer-associated genes. Mutations, the three Ashkenazi founder mutations in this case, were identified by screening reaction products with a universal DNA microarray (Gerry et al., 1999) which uncouples mutation detection from array hybridization and provides for high sensitivity.

Mutation detection technologies for *BRCA1* and *BRCA2* have been designed to detect germline genomic alterations in the coding regions and splice site regions of these two large genes. As mentioned in the discussion of mutation spectrum, it seems possible and likely that regulatory changes may play an equally important role in determining *BRCA* gene expression and control. Alterations in the 5′ and 3′ regions of the gene, alterations in other noncoding regions with possible regulatory roles, and changes in methylation patterns are all viable research candidates to pursue to identify the pathways for controlling *BRCA1* and *BRCA2* expression. Molecular methods that can be used routinely to identify these changes may enable us to realize a greater portion of hereditary breast cancer being attributable to these genes, as have the methods developed for identifying large genomic rearrangements.

The ability to conduct large-scale population-based studies to search for mutations in *BRCA1* and *BRCA2* is constrained by the lack of an inexpensive method with high throughput and sensitivity for mutation detection. While the search for a sensitive and specific method is necessary, cost will continue to present an obstacle to individuals who decide to pay for their own testing in order to avoid any prejudicial loss of health and life insurance or for those growing in number who are uninsured. As well, those insurance companies who will cover the cost of testing will search for a cost competitive method for evaluation that is comprehensive, sensitive, and specific.

CLINICAL IMPLICATIONS

Risk Estimation for Determining *BRCA1/2* Mutation Carriers

Early detection of breast cancer is critical for the success of treatment. Women with mutations in either *BRCA1* or *BRCA2* have been documented to have a lifetime risk of breast cancer of 65% and 45% and a lifetime risk of ovarian cancer of 39% and 11% respectively (Antoniou et al., 2003), though estimates vary within an accepted range (Table 5). This lifetime risk is 10 times greater than that of the general population. These two genes are responsible for approximately 40% of all hereditary breast cancers (Wooster and Weber, 2003). So the development of genetic tests for the two critically important breast cancer genes, *BRCA1* and *BRCA2*, which enable accurate risk assessment for individuals in high-risk families has been predicted to have substantial medical benefits.

None of the cancer susceptibility tests currently available is appropriate for screening of asymptomatic individuals in the general population. Only between 5% and 10% of breast cancer cases are considered to result from hereditary predisposition (Deng and Scott, 2000). Low gene frequency (estimated prevalence of approximately 1 in 800 to 1 in 1000) (Ford et al., 1995) and the absence of any undisputed cancer prevention option initially made widespread population screening for these mutations not only unfeasible, but also undesirable. Now, however, identification of these *BRCA* carriers before they present with cancer is important since prophylactic surgery can reduce morbidity and mortality in these individuals (Struewing et al., 1995a; Hartmann et al., 1999; Rebbeck et al., 1999b; Hartmann et al., 2001; Meijers-Heijboer et al., 2001; Kauff et al., 2002b; Rebbeck et al., 2004). Many advisory bodies, including the American Society of Clinical Oncologists (ASCO), have now recommended that testing be restricted to but freely offered to women at high-risk of developing breast or ovarian cancer as indicated by family history, as prevention and treatment options have expanded (Table 6).

Table 5 *BRCA1* and *BRCA2* Carrier Cancer Risk

	Breast cancer	Ovarian cancer	Male breast cancer
BRCA1	60–80%	30–45%	1–5%
BRCA2	60–80%	10–20%	5–10%

Table 6 Features that Indicate Increased Likelihood of Having *BRCA1* or *BRCA2* Mutation

1. Multiple cases of early onset breast cancer
2. Ovarian cancer (with family history of breast or ovarian cancer)
3. Breast and ovarian cancer in the same woman
4. Bilateral breast cancer
5. Ashkenazi Jewish heritage
6. Male breast cancer

The prevalence of germline *BRCA* mutations in such high-risk families is estimated at 3.4 to 15.5% (Frank et al., 2002; Huang et al., 2002; Antoniou et al., 2003; Myriad, 2004; Nelson et al., 2005). These low figures have led to the development of models that can more accurately assess the pretest probability of identifying a *BRCA1/2* gernline mutation (Couch et al., 1997; Parmigiani et al., 1998; Berry et al., 2002; Frank et al., 2002; Evans et al., 2004). The Claus model (Claus et al., 1994) was one of the first, offering the most comprehensive assessment of family history at the time. It was supplemented by the Gail model (Gail et al., 1989) for the purposes of making decisions about preventive cancer drugs.

Mendelian models like BRCAPRO (Parmigiani et al., 1998) evaluate the probability that an individual is a gene mutation carrier, while other models such as Penn (Couch et al., 1997), Manchester (Evans et al., 2004), and Frank–Myriad (Frank et al., 2002) determine the likelihood of identifying a mutation on the basis of known family history. Although the performance of some of these models has been previously examined, no single model has been universally adopted (Berry et al., 2002; Euhus et al., 2002; de la Hoya et al., 2003; Marroni et al., 2004; Barcenas et al., 2006; James et al., 2006). Previous model validation studies have considered only a subset of the available models, have not compared the results with germline testing, and have not considered the barriers of the use of models in clinical practice (Kang et al., 2006). Kang and colleagues evaluated all four models with the shortcomings of other studies in mind; their findings suggest that routine use of Penn, Manchester, BRCAPRO, or Myriad for predicting *BRCA* mutation status in clinical practice is not currently justified.

Risk models are developed and applied on the basis of pedigrees constructed from clinical histories, themselves often inaccurate. *BRCA* germline mutation testing represents a further source of significant error. The true prevalence of *BRCA* mutations is often underestimated because of the limitations of molecular testing (sensitivity of molecular techniques 70%) (Eng et al., 2001). Performance of the models was not due to type of mutation testing. Furthermore, models are often derived on the basis of mutation testing results from one uncharacterized individual in a high-risk family. Exclusion of a *BRCA* mutation in one individual does not necessarily indicate that the family is mutation negative. As uncontrollable factors such as cost, death and unavailability often dictate the choice of individual within a family for mutation testing, it is clear that *BRCA* mutational status is not a "gold standard test." Models are not currently available to adjust predictions of breast cancer risk for a negative *BRCA* test. Given these limitations in developing and applying risk models, Kang et al., advocate the development of risk prediction models that are less reliant on clinical history.

The second approach for risk estimation involves the several geographic or cultural populations, notably among the Ashkenazi and among Icelanders, in which a few mutations are "common" particularly among cases but also in the general geographic or cultural population. These populations have such mutations because of some facet of their genetic history rather than any specific feature of *BRCA1* or *BRCA2*. Low cost, rapid mutation detection techniques can be developed for such mutations compared with full gene analysis. Such studies examine the risk of cancer in relatives whose mutation carrier status is estimated from that of their relative who provided a DNA sample. Early studies were published for the Ashkenazi (Struewing et al., 1997) and for the Icelandic population (Thorlacius et al., 1998). However, in recent studies fewer mutations were found in the Ashkenazi Jewish population than predicted. This exposes a controversial issue within the breast cancer genetics research community. It is expected that the mutational spectra of *BRCA1* and *BRCA2*, as well as the influence of environmental and genetic modifiers, will be more diverse among the families studied in a breast cancer linkage consortium (BCLC) than among a single ethnic group. Hence, the same mutation could cause different cancer risk in different families through modifying effects. Population-based estimates will then represent the average of considerable risk heterogeneity. Until there is more information available regarding the effect of genetic and environmental modifier, individual risk assessment will remain difficult.

The third approach is to attempt to look for mutations in a large set of systematically identified persons and to examine the risk of cancer in relatives who also carry mutations; the only difference form the second approach is the mutation testing of relatives.

Studies of families, segregation analyses, and other indirect analytic method have produced estimate for general or western populations of 0.056% (Antoniou et al., 2002) and 0.24% (Whittemore et al., 2004b) for *BRCA1*, 0.072% for *BRCA2* (Antoniou et al., 2002), and 0.06% (Ford et al., 1995) and 0.14% (Whittemore et al., 1997) for the two genes combined. Risch et al. (2006) found estimates greater at 0.32% and 0.69% for the two genes, and because they are based on empirical ovarian cancer mutation frequencies and RRs that lie within the ranges of published values, they are likely to be substantially correct.

Penetrance—How Likely a *BRCA1/2* Mutation Carrier Will Develop Cancer

Deleterious Risk

Information on risks for cancer associated with mutation in *BRCA1* and *BRCA2* is important for genetic screening and counseling of patients with cancer and of women with family histories of cancer. Cancer risks associated with carrying a mutation may extend beyond ovarian and breast cancer, may differ among the various mutations within the genes, and may also apply to males (Risch et al., 2006). A large and recent study to investigate penetrance was conducted by Risch and colleagues investigating *BRCA* mutations among 1171 unselected patients with newly incident ovarian cancer in Ontario, Canada, with respect to cancers reported among their relatives. Despite study, limitations of low overall participation, personal histories were not confirmed, the patient population was multiethnic with a preponderance from the British Isles or other European countries, and only slightly more than 10% were mutation positive, there were clear advantages. The population-based case sampling was representative of all incident ovarian cancers arising in a defined geographic area of North America. Additionally, a strength of the study was the use of Ontario-population cancer incidence and mortality rates to estimate cumulative incidence of cancer to those aged 80 years.

The study found the hereditary proportion of invasive ovarian tumors was approximately 13%. The cumulative risk of breast cancer among *BRCA1* mutation carriers to those aged 80 years was 90%, somewhat greater than the previously reported values of 45% to 87%, whereas that of ovarian cancer (24%) was slightly below the previously reported values of 28% to 66%. For *BRCA2* mutation carriers, the cumulative risk of breast cancer to those aged 80 years was 41%, in the range of previously reported values (36–75%). That of ovarian cancer for *BRCA2* (8.4%) was lower than previously reported (11–32%). The validation of mutation carriage frequencies for Ashkenazi Jews indicates that the population RRs are likely to be accurate.

The position of the *BRCA* mutation within the coding region of the gene may influence the risk of breast or ovarian cancer (Narod, 2006). Risch and colleagues found a trend on increasing risk of breast cancer associated with increasingly downstream location of mutations in the *BRCA1* coding sequence and a peak on ovarian cancer risk associated with mutations in the middle of the coding sequence. They had previously noted the finding for breast cancer (Risch et al., 2001), and similar results for both breast and ovarian cancers have been reported in a meta-analysis of 22 studies (Antoniou et al., 2003). An analysis of *BRCA1* mutations in 356 families of the BCLC also confirmed that ovarian cancer risk may peak in the central section of the gene (Thompson and Easton, 2002).

In contrast to a previous report (Risch et al., 2001), the authors found overall an increased risk of breast cancer associated with carriage of *BRCA2* mutations. The association appeared to be restricted to non-OCCR mutations, particularly those in the region 3' of the OCCR. Mutations in the OCCR (defined by nucleotides 4075–6503) were not associated with breast cancer. A similar pattern of lower risks for breast cancer associated with *BRCA2* mutations in the OCCR than with those outside of the OCCR was noted in the meta-analysis (Antoniou et al., 2003) and in a study of 164 families of the BCLC (Thompson and Easton, 2001). A previous study (Thompson and Easton, 2002) also found a lower risk of ovarian cancer associated with 3′ *BRCA1* mutations than with 5′ and central *BRCA1* mutations confirming original observations (Gayther et al., 1995). For *BRCA2*, Lubinski et al. (2004) found a mildly increased number of ovarian cancers associated with mutations in nucleotides 3500–7400 and beyond nucleotide 9300, compared with a uniform mutation location distribution. This encompasses the OCCR defined in 1995 by an increased ovarian cancer risk by 1.9 times with mutation contained in this region (Thompson and Easton, 2001).

As the authors previously reported (Risch et al., 2001), elevated risks of stomach cancer and of leukemias and lymphomas were associated with *BRCA1* mutations. Also, increased risks were observed for liver and gallbladder cancer associated with both *BRCA1* and *BRCA2* mutations reported by the BCLC (Ford et al., 1994; BCLC, 1999). Testicular cancers have been reported in families of *BRCA1* mutation carriers (Tonin et al., 1998). The increased risk of male breast cancer associated with *BRCA2* mutation has also been reported (Liede et al., 2002; Syrjakoski et al., 2004), as has the lack of association between *BRCA2* mutation and increased risk of prostate cancer (Anton-Culver et al., 2000; Lehrer et al., 1998; Sinclair et al., 2000). Positive prostate cancer associations for non-OCCR mutations were found in the BCLC analysis of 173 *BRCA2* mutation-positive families (BCLC, 1999) and in a study in Iceland, in which the founder mutation 999del5 is located on the 5' side of the OCCR (Tulinius et al., 2002). The latter also found the increased risk of prostate cancer associated only with non-OCCR *BRCA2* mutations. Until such findings can be convincingly corroborated, they should not be used in genetic counseling.

Missense Risk

While deleterious mutation testing results are associated with a penetrance range, a significant portion of those receiving *BRCA* genetic testing results (13%) are left with a often inconclusive report—that of the identification of a variant of uncertain significance (Frank et al., 2002). This class of alterations includes missense mutation, mutation in regulator regions, and mutations in splicing enhancer regions for which the effect on protein function has not been determined. Unclassified variants now account for 40% of all sequence alterations excluding common polymorphisms that are identified by mutation screening of *BRCA1* and *BRCA2* (Monteiro and Couch, 2006). Unclassified variants, which can also be found in other cancer-predisposing genes such as *MLH1*, *MSH2*, and *ATM*, represent a major clinical issue as the inability to tell a carrier of an unclassified variant whether the mutation is cancer predisposing or not constitutes a significant problem for risk assessment, genetic counseling, and informed decision making about cancer prevention and therapeutics.

Widely recognized as a problem in *BRCA* risk assessment, several data sources have been used in an attempt to evaluate missense mutations: the Bayesian method to analyze pedigrees (Thompson et al., 2003), methods using of information from interspecies sequence variation (Fleming et al., 2003; Abkevich et al., 2004), integrated methods to combine information from different sources in a comprehensive framework (Goldgar et al., 2004; Chenevix-Trench et al., 2006), functional assays to assess the effect of amino acid changes on protein function (Humphrey et al., 1997; Vallon-Christersson et al., 2001; Coyne et al., 2004; Phelan et al., 2005; Morris et al., 2006), methods based on co-occurrence with a deleterious mutations (Judkins et al., 2005), and structure-based analysis to generate computation prediction models (Mirkovic et al., 2004; Monteiro and Couch, 2006). Although still far from clinical application, these methods have provided important information (Carvalho et al., 2007).

A series of recent approaches based on sequence analysis have been used to predict the possible effect of unclassified variants on protein function (Fleming et al., 2003; Abkevich et al., 2004; Kashuk et al., 2005). Lacking in these studies is the knowledge gleamed from three-dimensional architecture of the protein. Several different domains of *BRCA1* and *BRCA2* have been characterized by crystal three-dimensional structures (Williams et al., 2001; Williams and Glover, 2003; Ekblad et al., 2002; Williams et al., 2004; Glover et al., 2004; Baer, 2001;

Gaiser et al., 2004; Shiozaki et al., 2004; Botuyan et al., 2004; Joo et al., 2002; Clapperton et al., 2004; Yang et al., 2002; Brzovic et al., 2001). Through a detailed understanding of structure-function relationships, we should be able to generate reliable computation prediction methods for assessment of risk at the atomic level for unclassified variants (Monteiro and Couch, 2006). There are still significant hurdles to overcome that will take a close collaboration of structural and molecular biologists, epidemiologist, computer scientists, geneticists, and genetic counselors (Monteiro and Couch, 2006). It seems clear that in the case of most rare variants, no single data source is informative enough to unambiguously classify them into neutral or deleterious (Goldgar et al., 2004; Monteiro and Couch, 2006).

The most recent study to employ the advised multisource approach by Carvalho et al., used a transcription-based assay to assess the effect of 22 variants in light of all available clinical, genetic, and structural information. The method has shown previously an excellent agreement with existing genetic data (Vallon-Christersson et al., 2001; Phelan et al., 2005). They found the following missense mutations to be compatible with a deleterious classification: T1700A, V1713A, G1788D, S1655F, G1706E, V1736A, G1738R, G1738E, R1753T, L1764P, and I1766S (Carvalho et al., 2007). The authors used a threshold level of transcription activity to determine deleterious mutations, so they advised caution in the classification until further evidence for these threshold is obtained. There have been only a rare few missense mutations in *BRCA1* that have been accepted as deleterious. M1775R (Phelan et al., 2005), C61G (Brzovic et al., 1998), P1749R (Jin et al., 2000) have been frequently cited.

These findings, along with a few other missense alterations that have been proven clinically relevant, suggest that a certain proportion of uncharacterized variants may affect *BRCA1* function and increase breast and ovarian cancer risk. Any physician who offers genetic testing should be aware, and able to communicate through the procedure of informed consent, the benefits and limits of current testing procedures.

Modifiers of Breast Cancer Risk in *BRCA1/BRCA2* Mutation Carriers

Another area for study in genetic predisposition to breast cancer is to determine whether there are modifiers of risk to *BRCA1/2* mutation carriers. Penetrance estimates based on mutation-positive families ascertained through population-based series of breast cancer patients have generally been lower than estimates based on families with multiple-affected individuals (Ford et al., 1998; Antoniou et al., 2003). Risks vary with age at diagnosis and the type of cancer, indicating that the carrier's risk is modified by genetic factors.

Rare, high-penetrance germline mutations in genes such as *BRCA1* or *BRCA2* account for less than 25% of the familial risk of breast cancer, and much of the remaining variation in genetic risk is likely to be explained by combinations of more common, lower-penetrance variants (Pharoah et al., 2002). Collaborative studies are needed to achieve the sample sizes necessary to detect a more modest effect. The Breast Cancer Association Consortium (BCAC) was established in 2005 to facilitate such collaborative studies in breast cancer. The consortium currently comprises over 20 international collaborating research groups, with a potential combined sample size of up to 30,000 cases and 30,000 controls. The first combined data analysis involved 16 SNPs that had been investigated in at least three independent studies with at least 10,000 genotyped subjects in total (BCAC, 2006). After subsequent study, two SNPs evaluated showed significant associations with invasive breast cancer: *CASP8* D302H and *TGFb1* L10P (Cox et al., 2007) in the *Caspase 8* gene. It is suggested that these two variants may account for approximately 0.3% and 0.2% of the excess familial risk of breast cancer, respectively, in populations of European ancestry (Cox et al., 2007). *Caspase 8* is an important initiator of apoptosis and is activated by external death signals and in response to DNA damage (Hengartner, 2000). Smaller studies have been conducted involving candidate polymorphic genes that encode for enzymes implicated in the metabolism of estrogen, detoxification of reactive oxygen species, alcohol and one-carbon metabolism pathways, or proteins that play a role in DNA repair or cell signaling processes.

CYP1A1 encodes aryl hydrocarbon hydroxylase (AHH) which catalyses the 2-hyroxylation of estradiaol in several tissues, including the breast (Hellmold et al., 1998). The polymorphism m1 (Msp1) is associated with a modest increase of breast cancer risk in the white population, and m2 (codon 462, isoleucine/valine) is associated with a moderately increased breast cancer risk only in postmenopausal women (de Jong et al., 2002). A specific polymorphism (17.5-kb region deletion) in *CYP2D6*, another member of the cytochrome P450 family that codes for debrisoquine hydroxylase, has been associated with an increased breast cancer susceptibility (de Jong et al., 2002).

Polymorphisms leading to the absence of different *GST* (glutathione S-transferase) isoenzymes affect the tolerance of the organism to chemical challenges and may influence cancer susceptibility (Dumitrescu and Cotarla, 2005). A pooled analysis of studies on *GSTM1* null genotype has found a small and only marginally significant association with increased breast cancer risk (de Jong et al., 2002). A meta-analysis study fount that an isoleucine to valine substitution at codon 105 in *GSTP1* has been associated with a moderately increased breast cancer risk in homozygous carriers (de Jong et al., 2002). Polymorphisms in the rate-limiting enzyme involved in alcohol oxidation, alcohol dehydrogenase (*ADH*) may modulate breast cancer risk, as alcohol is a well-documented risk factor. Premenopausal women with the *ADH1C*1,1* genotype have been found to be a 1.8 times higher risk for breast cancer than women with the other two genotypes (Coutelle et al., 2004; Freudenheim et al., 1999).

MTHFR (5,10-methylenetetrahydrofolate reductase) encodes an enzyme crucial for DNA synthesis and maintenance of DNA methylation patterns, dependent on folate intake. Two functional polymorphisms in *MTHFR* gene, C677T and A1298C, which result in a decreased enzyme activity in the variant carriers, are associated with an increased risk of developing breast cancer (Campbell et al., 2002; Ergul et al., 2003).

As discussed previously, all high-penetrant breast cancer alleles known are DNA repair genes. Low-penetrant alleles have also been found from the genes involved in the many DNA repair pathways. One *XRCC1* 399Q variant allele (a gene involved in base excision repair) has been shown to be sufficient to confer an increased risk of breast cancer in African American carriers (Duell et al., 2001). Having any combination of three or more variant alleles for *XRCC1* Arg194Trp, *XRCC3* Thr241Met (implicated in homologous recombination repair), or *ERCC4*/XPF Arg415Gln (implicated in nucleotide excision repair) results in an increased risk of breast cancer (Smith et al., 2003). The *RAD51* gene, which participates in homologous recombination DSB repair in the same pathway as the *BRCA1* and *BRCA2* gene products, is a candidate for modifying effect. An SNP *RAD51*-135G>C in the 5′UTR of the gene has been found to elevate breast cancer risk among *BRCA2* carriers (Kadouri et al., 2004), but had no effect (Kadouri et al., 2004) or a reduction in risk for *BRCA1* carriers (Jakubowska et al., 2003). The homozygote *BRCA2* Asn372His polymorphism has been associated with an increased risk of breast cancer in different European populations, as well as a large Australian population (Goode et al., 2002). Other polymorphisms in genes, such as estrogen receptor (*ER*), heat shock protein 70 (*HSP70*) or tumor necrosis factor α (*TNF*α), integrin beta 3 (*ITGB3*) (Jakubowska et al., 2007), and *E2F6 (Yang et al., 2006)* may also influence the risk of developing breast cancer (de Jong et al., 2002) and have all been considered candidates for "modifier genes" in breast cancer.

Lastly is assessing risk, there is insufficient data to make a recommendation concerning environmental and lifestyle factors that potentially modify the genetic influence of mutations in *BRCA1* and *BRCA2* in the development of breast or ovarian cancer. The use of chemopreventive agents (Fisher et al., 1998; Gronwald et al., 2006), hormone replacement therapy (HRT) (Rebbeck et al., 2005), the use of oral contraceptives (Narod et al., 1998; Narod et al., 2002), smoking (Brunet et al., 1998 Colilla et al., 2006), reproductive factors (Rebbeck et al., 2001; Narod, 2006), dietary fat intake, alcohol intake, low-antioxidant vitamin intake, antioxidants (Kowalska et al., 2005; Nkondjock et al., 2006), radiation exposure, and decreased physical activity may each affect an individual's estimated risk for the cancer predisposition (Table 7).

Table 7 Modifiers of *BRCA* Mutation Penetrance

Mutation location
Genes at other loci
Exposures

Pathology of *BRCA1*- AND *BRCA2*-Associated Breast Tumors

Vast amounts of data have emerged showing that breast tumors from patients with germline mutation in the *BRCA1* and *BRCA2* genes are morphologically and genetically different from each other, as well as from hereditary tumors not associated with *BRCA1* and *BRCA2* mutations and sporadic cases and from age-matched controls (Lakhani et al., 1997; Lakhani et al., 1998; Lakhani et al., 1999; Honrado et al., 2006; Armes et al., 1998). This suggests that *BRCA* mutations lead to different further genetic alterations that are specifically involved in the development of each of these types of breast tumor. Identifying these molecular differences will help to identify tumor markers that can predict the presence of gene alterations.

BRCA1 tumors are more often of medullary carcinoma (11%) than has been reported in *BRCA2* cases (2%) or in sporadic cases (1%) (Lakhani et al., 2000). *BRCA1* tumors are of higher grade and are scarce or absent ductal in situ components (Lakhani et al., 1997) and lack a positive correlation between tumor size and lymph node involvement (Foulkes et al., 2003). These latter two aspects have been associated with the fast growth of these tumors (Brekelmans et al., 2001). *BRCA2* tumors are not specifically associated with a subtype and are intermediate in grade between *BRCA1* and sporadic (Lakhani et al., 2000; Palacios et al., 2003; Eerola et al., 2005a).

BRCA1 tumors are better characterized for immunohistochemical markers because they have a much more specific immunohistochemical phenotype than *BRCA2* tumors, sharing characteristics of sporadic (Honrado et al., 2006). Most noteworthy is that between 63 and 90% of *BRCA1* carcinomas have been reported to be *ER* negative (Palacios et al., 2003; Robson et al., 2004; Foulkes et al., 2004a; Eerola et al., 2005a; Oldenburg et al., 2006). Similarly, PR is more frequently negative in *BRCA1* than in *BRCA2* or sporadic tumors. For *BRCA2* tumors, 60% to 90% have been reported to be *ER* positive and 40% to 80% PR positive (Palacios et al., 2003; Robson et al., 2004; Eerola et al., 2005a; Oldenburg et al., 2006). These differences in grade, *ER*, and PR have been shown age specific as well (Eerola et al., 2005b). The number of tumors with HER2 expression of 3+ in the DAKO score system is very low or nonexistent for both *BRCA1* and *BRCA2* (Lakhani et al., 2002; Palacios et al., 2003). On the other hand, *BRCA1* tumors underexpress proteins related to the inhibition of the cyclin-CDK complexes, such as p16, *p27*, and *p21* (Foulkes et al., 2004a; Palacios et al., 2005).

BRCA1 tumors have a higher proliferative index than sporadic tumors (Armes et al., 1999; Palacios et al., 2003). It follows then that *BRCA1* tumors overexpress proteins that promote cell cycle progression such as cyclin E, A or B1 (Foulkes et al., 2004a; Chappuis et al., 2005; Palacios et al., 2005). In *BRCA2* tumors, the expression of proteins related to cell cycle is similar to that observed in sporadic tumors with respect to both cyclins promoting cell cycle progression (cyclins D, E, A, and B1) and cyclin-CDK complex inhibitors (p16, *p27*, and *p21*) (Palacios et al., 2005), which are overexpressed compared with *BRCA1* tumors.

In *BRCA1* and *BRCA2* tumors, expression of *p53* has been reported to be positive more frequently than in sporadic tumors (Palacios et al., 2003; Eerola et al., 2005a). This is in accordance with the hypothesis that down regulation of *p53* is an important event to overcome cell cycle arrest and promote tumorigenesis in *BRCA1*- and *BRCA2*-deficient tumors (Xu et al., 2001b; Ongusaha et al., 2003; Cheung et al., 2004). *BRCA1* tumors are more likely to exhibit low levels of the antiapoptotic protein BCL2 and the proapoptotic protein BAX than sporadic tumors (Freneaux et al., 2000; Palacios et al., 2003) and at the same time overexpress the proapoptotic protein *Caspase 3* and the antiapoptotic protein surviving (Palacios et al., 2005). The overexpression of numerous markers related with protecting cells from undergoing apoptosis such as BCL2 and NFKB, and expression of the proapoptotic marker BAX has been reported in *BRCA2* tumors (Armes et al., 1999; Freneaux et al., 2000; Palacios et al., 2003; Palacios et al., 2005). BCL2 in sporadic tumors has been associated with *ER* and PR positivity, and a low Ki-67 proliferation index (Linke et al., 2006; Ruiz et al., 2006), which are all typical characteristics of *BRCA2* tumors.

BRCA1 tumors overexpress *CHK2* and PCNA and underexpress *RAD50* with respect to sporadic tumors, and do not show differences in the expression of other proteins such as *RAD51*, *ATM* or *XRCC3* (Honrado et al., 2005). In *BRCA2* tumors overexpression of *CHK2* has been observed as well but in contrast to *BRCA1* tumors, there is no reduction of *RAD50* expression compared with sporadic tumors. Also, the nuclear expression of *RAD51* in *BRCA2* tumors is very low compared with *BRCA1* and sporadic tumors while cytoplasmic *RAD51* staining is observed more frequently in *BRCA2* tumors with respect to *BRCA1* and sporadic tumors (Honrado et al., 2005). *BRCA2* integrity is necessary to transport *RAD51* to the nucleus. It is noteworthy that this is one of the few markers that help to distinguish *BRCA2* positive from sporadic tumors.

Recently, numerous reports have been published about the basal-like phenotype and its association with *BRCA1* tumors (Perou et al., 2000; Sorlie et al., 2001; Sorlie et al., 2003; Sotiriou et al., 2003; Foulkes et al., 2003, 2004b, 2004a; Arnes et al., 2005; Jacquemier et al., 2005; Turner and Reis-Filho, 2006). The basal-like phenotype is characterized by the expression of markers typical of the normal basal/myoepithelium such as cytokeratins 5/6, 14, 17, epidermal growth factor receptor (*EGFR*), p-cadherin, osteonectin, fascin, caveolin-1, which are more frequently positive in *BRCA1* tumors (Palacios et al., 2003; van der Groep et al., 2004; Arnes et al., 2005; Lakhani et al., 2005; Pinilla et al., 2006; Rodriguez-Pinilla et al., 2006). Recently, it has been reported that two proteins, nerve growth factor receptor *NGFR*/p75ntr (Reis-Filho et al., 2006) and the small heat-shock protein a-basic-crystallin (ab-crystallin) (Moyano et al., 2006) that were commonly expressed in basal-like tumors are predictors of good prognosis and poor survival, respectively, in breast cancer patients independent of other prognostic markers. Lastly, there is a group of other markers more frequently expressed in *BRCA1* tumors that are not basal/myoepithelial markers but have been proposed as markers associated with the basal-like phenotype: cyclin E, p53, Skp2, and negativity for *p27* (Signoretti et al., 2002; Nielsen et al., 2004; Palacios et al., 2004; Foulkes et al., 2004a; Lakhani et al., 2005) (Table 8).

The importance of this association between *BRCA1* and the basal-like phenotype is the correlation with poor prognostics and the possibility of specific treatment like anti-epidermal *EGFR* agents (Honrado et al., 2006). A higher frequency of *EGFR* mutation in *BRCA1* and *BRCA2* tumors (45%) than in sporadic ones (15%) has been published, although the mutations are located in exon 20 in contrast to those reported in gefitinib-sensitive nonsmall-cell lung carcinoma that are located in exons 18–21 (Weber et al., 2005). The effect of *EGFR* mutation in *BRCA1/2* tumors, in anti-*EGFR* cancer therapy, is still unknown.

Gene expression profiling of cancer tumors has been advanced by the introduction of microarray technology. Thousands of genes can be analyzed in a single experiment

Table 8 Immunophenotype of *BRCA1*, *BRCA2*, and Sporadic Tumors

Antibodies	*BRCA1*	*BRCA2*	Sporadic
ER, PR	−	+	+
BCL-2, BAX	−	+	+
Cyclin D1	−	+	+
P16, *p27*, *p21*	−	+	+
RAD50	−	+	+
RAD51 (cytoplasm)	−	+	−
HER-2	−	−	+
CHK2	+	+	−
RAD51 (nucleus)	+	−	+
P53, Ki-67	+	−	−
Cyclins (E, A, B1)	+	−	−
Skp2	+	−	−
CK5/6, 14, 17	+	−	−
EGFR, P-cadherin	+	−	−

Source: From Honrado et al. (2006).

for expression levels in a specific tumor, or for reaction to a specific therapeutic drug. Several key publication in this field have focused on sporadic breast cancer (Perou et al., 2000; van 't Veer et al., 2002; van de Vijver et al., 2002; Chang et al., 2003; Sorlie et al., 2003) and show how molecular signatures are able to subclassify tumors in previously unknown classes. Much less is known about hereditary breast tumors. The study by Hedenfalk et al., 2001 is the only one focused specifically on *BRCA1* and *BRCA2* breast tumors (Hedenfalk et al., 2001). The study evaluated seven *BRCA1* tumors, seven *BRCA2* tumors, and seven sporadic tumors. They found 176 genes that significantly differed in their expression levels between *BRCA1* and *BRCA2* associated tumors, and identified 51 genes whose differences were able to best distinguish between the three types of tumors analyzed. Confirming immunohistochemical data cyclin D1 was over expressed in *BRCA2* with respect to *BRCA1* tumors. The same confirmation of IHC results were found with *ER* and PR. Genes involved in DNA repair, such as *MSH2* and *PDCD5*, were over expressed in *BRCA1* tumors. This could indicate a mechanism to overcome *BRCA1* deficiency (Honrado et al., 2006).

The array study was able to classify *BRCA1* and *BRCA2* tumors by 9 and 11 genes, respectively. The study was able to classify all *BRCA1* positive tumors and all except one *BRCA1* negative tumors; the only sporadic tumor that was incorrectly classified as *BRCA1* showed somatic hypermethylation of the *BRCA1* promoter and a consequent lack of expression of the gene, which now is known to mimic the behavior of a read *BRCA1* tumor (Wei et al., 2005). As predicted, the *BRCA2* tumors were not accurately classified in that they are not as accurately characterized as are *BRCA1* tumors.

A second study analyzed the expression profiling of a set of 98 breast tumors, including 18 from patients with *BRCA1* germline mutations (van 't Veer et al., 2002). The authors found a signature of 100 genes that was able to distinguish *BRCA1* tumors from the other *ER*-negative sporadic cases (van 't Veer et al., 2002). The same set of 18 *BRCA1* tumors was included together with 97 sporadic tumors in the gene expression analysis performed by Sorlie et al. (2003) who defined five subgroups of breast tumors: *ER* positive subdivided into luminal A and B, and *ER* negative subdivided into basal-like, ERBB2+ and normal-like tumors (Sorlie et al., 2003). All *BRCA1* tumors fell within the basal-like subgroup confirming the histopathological data (Foulkes et al., 2003; Palacios et al., 2004; Lakhani et al., 2005; Rodriguez-Pinilla et al., 2006).

These studies represent the potential for identifying the biological pathways specifically altered when a germline mutation in *BRCA1* or *BRCA2* exists. It is difficult to amass large numbers of *BRCA* tumors, so validation of these profiling data will take much time. It has been suggested that because of their involvement in DNA repair, heterozygosity for *BRCA1* and *BRCA2* mutations can already be associated with some level of genetic instability (Arnold et al., 2006; Warren et al., 2003; Kote-Jarai et al., 2004). In the case of *BRCA1*, more cellular processes may be affected by haploinsufficiency, given that the gene is known to be involved in a wide variety of pathways such as chromatin remodeling, transcription regulation, cell cycle checkpoint control, or maintenance of the inactive X chromosome (Scully and Livingston, 2000; Venkitaraman, 2002).

In a recent study by Kote-Jarai et al. (2004) the authors were able to differentiate breast fibroblasts from *BRCA1* mutation carriers from those derived from reduction mammoplasties, after inducing DNA damage by radiation (Kote-Jarai et al., 2004). By using a cDNA microarray, they identified 79 clones that could distinguish between both classes with 85% accuracy; some of the clones found to be downregulated in *BRCA1* carriers corresponded to DNA repair genes such as *RAD51* and *RAD 23*, suggesting that heterozygous mutations are already affecting this process. The *p27* gene was also downregulated suggesting that this must be a very early event. The possibility of detecting gene expression alterations in normal tissues open interesting perspectives in terms of directing genetic testing and improving risk assessment (Honrado et al., 2006).

Management of Unaffected Mutation Carriers

Ovarian Cancer Risk

The lifetime risk of ovarian cancer for women with *BRCA1* mutations is estimated at 40 to 50% (Ford et al., 1994; Antoniou et al., 2003; King et al., 2003) and in those with *BRCA2* mutations at 10% to 20% (Antoniou et al., 2003; King et al., 2003), though estimates vary. It has been consistently shown that prophylactic oophorectomy (PO) in women with *BRCA1/2* mutations reduces the risk of ovarian cancer by approximately 90% (Kauff et al., 2002b; Rebbeck et al., 2002; Rutter et al., 2003b). In addition to this reduction in the risk of ovarian cancer, an approximately 50% breast cancer risk reduction after PO has also been observed (Rebbeck et al., 2002). This reduction may be one of the several reasons for the variability in penetrance estimates for breast cancer across studies. Data with short-term follow-up also suggest that oophorectomy is associated with an improvement in breast cancer–specific survival, ovarian cancer–specific survival, and overall survival (Domchek et al., 2006). Data are accumulating as well to specify benefit of bilateral prophylactic oophorectomy according to mutations present in either *BRCA1* or *BRCA2* (Kauff et al., 2006). Randomized clinical trials are unlikely in light of the current knowledge regarding risk reduction. Recruiting women to an arm of a trial without the option of PO would be not acceptable to most nor ethical given the absence of effective screening for ovarian cancer.

Despite the large magnitude of ovarian cancer risk reduction with PO, other cancer risks remain. Primary peritoneal cancers have been reported in women with *BRCA1/2* mutations following PO with an estimated frequency of 2%to 4%, and occur more frequently in *BRCA1* compared to *BRCA2* carriers (Piver et al., 1993; Kauff et al., 2002b; Rebbeck et al., 2002; Casey et al., 2005). Occult ovarian and fallopian tube carcinomas have been found at the time of PO in 2% to 10% of *BRCA1/2* mutation carriers (Salazar et al., 1996; Lu et al., 2000; Colgan et al., 2001; McEwen et al., 2004; Powell et al., 2005). Cancers of the fallopian tube also represent a part of the hereditary breast/ovarian cancer syndrome associated with *BRCA1/2* mutations (Aziz et al., 2001; Carcangiu et al., 2004) with a lifetime risk or 3% (Brose et al., 2002). These observations support the recommendation that a thorough pathologic examination with serial sectioning of the ovaries and fallopian tubes removed by PO should be undertaken to confirm the absence of tumor at the time of surgery (Domchek and Weber, 2006).

The use of oral contraceptive pills (OCP) appears to decrease the risk of ovarian cancer by up to 50% in *BRCA1* and *BRCA2* carriers, although one report did not find this effect (Narod et al., 1998; Modan et al., 2001; Whittemore et al., 2004a). Data are inconsistent regarding the effect of OCP on breast cancer risk (Narod et al., 2002; Milne et al., 2005). Given the excess mortality associated with ovarian cancer compared with breast cancer, a reasonable risk reduction strategy is OCP use before child bearing, and oophorectomy once child bearing is complete (Domchek and Weber, 2006).

Women who carry *BRCA1/2* mutations should weigh the risks and benefits of total abdominal hysterectomy (TAH) at the time of PO on the basis of their personal medical history and with the following four consideration: (1) impact on HRT; (2) uterine and cervical cancer risk; (3) impact on decisions regarding tamoxifen; (4) fallopian tube carcinoma risk (Domchek and Weber, 2006). Women who are likely to benefit most from having a TAH at the time of PO are unaffected premenopausal women who will also be faced with decisions on HRT and future tamoxifen use (Domchek and Weber, 2006).

Breast Cancer Risk

Breast cancer risk estimates for *BRCA1* and *BRCA2* mutation carriers vary, and there is no simple relationship between carrier status and cancer risk. But cumulative evidence suggests that lifetime risk of breast cancer is 60% to 80% (Ford et al., 1994; Antoniou et al., 2003; King et al., 2003), although the risk may be slightly lower in women with *BRCA2* mutations. Cohort effects have been reported with an increase in breast cancer risk seen in younger cohorts (King et al., 2003); and as noted above, rates of oophorectomy are likely to influence penetrance data (Kramer et al., 2005). Several groups have confirmed that prophylactic mastectomy (PM) reduces breast cancer risk in mutation carriers by 90% (Hartmann et al., 2001; Meijers-Heijboer et al., 2001; Rebbeck et al., 2004). As opposed to ovarian cancer however, chemoprevention and enhanced screen as alternative strategies for treatment are supported (Domchek and Weber, 2006).

Limited data are available on the use of tamoxifen for chemoprevention of breast cancer in *BRCA1/2* mutation carriers, but an initial study showed 50% reduction in contralateral disease following at least 2 years of tamoxifen (Narod et al., 2000). This observation was confirmed more recently in two studies by Gronward and Pierce (Gronwald et al., 2006; Pierce et al., 2006). However, data from a recent prevention trial did not yield statistically significant conclusions regarding the use of tamoxifen as primary prevention in *BRCA1/2* mutation carriers (King et al., 2001). Until further information is available, it is generally believed that carriers should be offered tamoxifen, raloxifene, or enrollment on chemoprevention trials (Domchek and Weber, 2006). Raloxifene reduces the risk of invasive breast cancer by 76% in postmenopausal women during three years of treatment (Cummings et al., 1999).

For cancer surveillance, multiple studies have demonstrated that yearly magnetic resonance imaging (MRI) has improved sensitivity for the detection of malignancy in *BRCA1/2* mutation carriers as well as other high-risk women, and detects earlier stage cancers than mammography alone (Kriege et al., 2004; Warner et al., 2004;

Table 9 Modifying *BRCA* Carrier Cancer Risk

Chemoprevention	SERMS, oral contraceptives
Screening	mammography, MRI, CA-125, vaginal ultrasound
Surgery	tubal ligation, bilateral oophorectomy, prophylactic mastectomy

Leach et al., 2005). The sensitivity for MRI (77%) was significantly greater than for mammography (36%), ultrasound (US) (33%) and clinical breast exam (CBE) (9%), whereas MRI had a decreased specificity (95.4%) compared with mammography (99.8%), US (96%) and CBE (99.3%). The combination of MRI, mammography, and US had a sensitivity of 95%. The role of US in screening *BRCA1/2* mutation carriers is not clear at the current time. Warner et al., 2004 demonstrated that adding US to mammography modestly increased sensitivity, however, its inclusion triggered more biopsies than microsatellite instability (MSI) after the first year of screening. As for the concern for radiation risk with routine mammography, a multicenter case-control study with 3200 *BRCA1/2* mutation carriers has demonstrated no increased risk in breast cancer associated with mammography (Narod et al., 2006). It has been recommended staggering the MRI and mammogram every six months (Domchek and Weber, 2006) (Table 9).

It is generally thought that the impact of lifestyle risks are relatively modest, however breastfeeding, exercise, and maintenance of a stable weight have all been demonstrated to decrease breast cancer risk in *BRCA1/2* mutation carriers (King et al., 2003; Jernstrom et al., 2004). In contrast, spontaneous and therapeutic abortion is not associated with an increased risk of breast cancer in this population (Andrieu et al., 2006).

Several studies have addressed the question of whether *BRCA1/2* mutation carriers can be safely treated with local breast-conserving therapy as opposed to mastectomy. Data suggest that breast-conserving therapy is not associated with excess radiation toxicity (Pierce et al., 2000; Haffty et al., 2002; Pierce et al., 2006). The choice between breast conservation versus mastectomy for treatment of breast cancer in *BRCA1/2* mutation carriers who are otherwise good candidates for breast conservation should center on the excess risk of a second primary breast cancer (Domchek and Weber, 2006).

Systemic therapy for breast cancer in *BRCA1/2* mutation carriers remains dictated by standard prognostic features. *BRCA1*-associated tumors are more frequently of the basal phenotype (estrogen receptor, progesterone receptor, and HER2/new negative) (Lakhani et al., 1998, 2002). Since *BRCA* proteins are now known to be important for error-free DNA DSB repair by homologous recombination (Venkitaraman, 2002), it is believed they may have enhanced sensitivity to chemotherapy that induces DNA interstrand cross-links, such as platinum agents (Kennedy et al., 2004). In contrast, other preclinical models suggest that intact *BRCA1* is necessary for chemotherapeutic effects of paclitaxel and therefore *BRCA1*-null tumors may be relatively chemoresistant (Domchek and Weber, 2006). Interestingly, Lakhani et al. (2005) have recently demonstrated that 67% of *BRCA1*-related breast cancers express *EGFR* as compared with 21% of sporadic breast cancer controls. Therefore, *EGFR*-targeted therapy, used successfully in the treatment of non-small cell lung cancer, may be of potential benefit in breast cancer patients. Ashworth and colleagues have demonstrated that poly(ADP-ribose) polymerase (PARP) inhibitors cause marked chromosomal instability and apoptosis in *BRCA1* and *BRCA2* null cells (Farmer et al., 2005) and the concept has received increasing attention as potential DNA repair pathway inhibitors. Weber et al., have identified the tumor stroma as a potential landscape for neoplastic initiation (Weber et al., 2006). They consider that normalization of an impaired stroma can alter and potentially reverse preneoplastic or maybe even neoplastic breast epithelium. These new discoveries could alter the standard treatment of *BRCA* carrier cancers in the future, tailoring a more molecular targeted and tumor specific therapy.

STRUCTURE AND FUNCTION OF *BRCA1* AND *BRCA2*

The breast cancer genes *BRCA1* and *BRCA2* are very large genes with multiple functions. The exact functions of *BRCA1* have not been fully described but it now seems apparent that it has roles in DNA damage repair, transcriptional regulation, cell cycle control, and most recently in ubiquitylation. The main role of *BRCA2* appears to involve regulating the function of *RAD 51* in the repair by homologous recombination.

BRCA1/2 and DNA Repair

DSB Repair

BRCA1 was first discovered to be involved in DNA repair with the observation that it associates and colocalizes with *RAD51* in nuclear foci in mitotic cells (Scully et al., 1997c). These foci were also observed to contain *BRCA2* and the *BRCA1*-binding protein BRCA1-associated ring domain 1 (BARD1), both before and after DNA damage (Jin et al., 1997; Scully et al., 1997b; Chen et al., 1998). While *BRCA2* is directly involved in *RAD51*-mediated repair, affecting the choice between gene conversion (GC) and single-strand annealing (SSA), *BRCA1* acts upstream of these pathways (Stark et al., 2004). The involvement of *BRCA1* in the repair of DSBs by GC is consistent with its association and colocalization with *RAD51* in nuclear foci, and *BRCA1* is required for their formation (Bhattacharyya et al., 2000). Nonhomologous end-joining (NHEJ) has been reported to be unaffected in *BRCA1*-deficient cells, although data concerning the role of *BRCA1* within this repair pathway have been conflicting (Moynahan et al., 1999; Baldeyron et al., 2002; Zhong et al., 2002; Stark et al., 2004). *BRCA1* has been shown recently to be important in promoting precise NHEJ, while inhibiting more error-prone microhomology-mediated NHEJ (Wang et al., 2006; Zhuang et al., 2006a). Therefore, in addition to promoting error-free repair of DSBs by HR, *BRCA1* also reduces the mutagenic potential of NHEJ contributing to genomic stability (Gudmundsdottir and Ashworth, 2006).

Complexes

BRCA1 has been associated with many proteins involved in the DNA repair process. *BRCA2* and *RAD51* have been observed to coexist in a complex with *BRCA1* named BRCC (*BRCA1-BRCA2*-Containing Complex) that also contains BARD1 and other components (Dong et al., 2003). This complex displays an E3 ubiquitin ligase activity, which has been implicated in the regulation of factors involved in DNA repair. Another *BRCA1* containing complex is named BASC (*BRCA1* Associated Genome Surveillance Complex) (Wang et al., 2000). This complex includes tumor suppressors, DNA damage sensors and signal transducers (including the MRN complex), the mismatch repair proteins MSH2, MSH6 and MLH1, the Bloom syndrome helicase BLM, the *ATM* kinase, DNA replication factor C (RFC) and PCNA. The MRN complex is thought to be involved in the end-processing of DSBs in GC, SSA, and microhomology-mediated NHEJ. *BRCA1* colocalizes with the MRN complex in foci upon DNA damage and it also inhibits the nucleolytic activity of *MRE11* in vitro, thereby potentially influencing the choice of repair pathway after a DSB (Zhong et al., 1999; Wang et al., 2000; Paull et al., 2001). The association of *BRCA1* with MSH2 and MSH6 in the BASC complex also links *BRCA1* to a subpathway of nucleotide excision repair (NER) that preferentially repairs base lesions from the transcribed strand, as these two MSH proteins are know to be involved in this process (Wang et al., 2000). *BRCA1* is required for the repair of oxidative 8-oxoguanine lesions by transcription-coupled DNA repair (Gowen et al., 1998) and to enhance the global genomic repair (GGR) subpathway of NER by inducing the expression of the NER genes XPC, DDB2, and GADD45 (Harkin et al., 1999; Hartman and Ford, 2002). Cell lines from women with *BRCA1* mutations have been shown to be deficient in the repair of oxidative lesions by NER (Rodriguez et al., 2007). An association of *BRCA1* with a complex that contains the proteins SW1 and SNF links *BRCA1* to chromatin remodeling which is important to facilitate access of proteins involved in DNA processing, such as transcription and repair, to DNA (Bochar et al., 2000).

Damage Response

BRCA1 participates in the signaling cascade involved in the response to DNA damage. *ATM* and *ATR* phosphorylate *BRCA1* in response to different stimuli and they appear to have both distinct and overlapping phosphorylation sites, only some of which have been characterized (Gudmundsdottir and Ashworth, 2006). *ATM* phosphorylates *BRCA1* on several different residues (Ser1423, Ser1524, Ser1387) in response to IR (Cortez et al., 1999; Gatei et al., 2000). *ATR*, which is activated by UV-damage and hydroxyurea-induced replication arrest, also phosphorylates *BRCA1* on several residues, including Ser1423 during the G2-M phase (Tibbetts, 2000; Gatei et al., 2001; Okada and Ouchi, 2003) and colocalize at stalled replication forks (Tibbetts, 2000; Gatei et al., 2001). In response to IR, *ATM* phosphorylates and activates another checkpoint kinase, *CHK2*, which in turn can phosphorylate *BRCA1* on Ser988 (Lee et al., 2000). Recently, *CHK2* phosphorylation of the Ser988 of *BRCA1* was also shown to be important for the role of *BRCA1* in the repair of DSBs by promoting error-free HR and by inhibiting the error-prone microhomology-mediated subpathway of NHEJ (Zhang et al., 2004; Wang et al., 2006; Zhuang et al., 2006a). The DNA damage-response kinases *ATM*, *ATR*, and *CHK2*, therefore, modulate the function of *BRCA1* through prosphorylation, affecting cell cycle regulation and fidelity of DNA repair (Gudmundsdottir and Ashworth, 2006).

Cell Cycle Control

The role of *BRCA1* in cell cycle checkpoint has recently been reviewed (Kennedy et al., 2004; Deng, 2006). *BRCA1* has been reported to stimulate the transcription of the *p21* gene which results in cell cycle arrest at the G1-S phase boundary and is a coactivator for *p53*, indicating a complex mechanism of control (Somasundaram et al., 1997; Ouchi et al., 1998; Zhang et al., 1998). *BRCA1* has also been shown to be required for the *ATM/ATR*-mediated phosphorylation of several proteins following DNA damage, including *CHK2* and *p53* at Ser15, which is necessary for G1-S arrest via transcriptional induction of *p21* (Foray et al., 2003; Fabbro et al., 2004). *BRCA1* regulates the G2-M phase checkpoint at multiple levels (Gudmundsdottir and Ashworth, 2006). Establishment of the G2-M checkpoint requires phosphorylation of the CDC2 kinase, while removal of this phosphorylation by

CDC25C activates the CDC2/cyclinB complex to initiate mitosis. DNA damage leads to inhibition of CDC25C activity through phosphorylation by the CHK1 kinase and nuclear exclusion of CDC25C through binding to 14-3-3a, leading to cell cycle arrest at the G2-M checkpoint. *BRCA1* is essential for activating the CHK1 kinase and it also induces the expression of the 14-3-3 proteins and the WEE1 kinase, which is another inhibitor of CDEC2 activity (Yarden et al., 2002). In addition, *BRCA1* has been demonstrated to induce the expression of GADD45, which activates the G2-M checkpoint by inhibiting the activity of the CDC2-cyclinB complex (Mullan et al., 2001; Xu et al., 2001a).

BARD1/*BRCA1*

BRCA1 exists as a heterodimeric complex with BARD1, a structurally related protein that, like *BRCA1* contains a N-terminal RING-finger domain and two C-terminal BRCT motifs (Wu et al., 1996). Together they exhibit E3 ubiquitin ligase activity, which can be disrupted by cancer-predisposing mutations within the RING domain of *BRCA1* (Hashizume et al., 2001; Ruffner et al., 2001). The ubiquitin ligase activity is important for *BRCA1* to execute its role within the DNA damage-response pathway (Ruffner et al., 2001). BARD1 has also been shown to participate with *BRCA1* in the homology-directed repair of DSBs (Westermark et al., 2003; Fabbro et al., 2004). Recently, the *BRCA1*-BARD1 complex has been demonstrated to ubiquitinate RNA polymerase II following DNA damage resulting in its degradation and subsequent inhibition of transcription and RNA processing (Kleiman et al., 2005; Starita et al., 2005). This process could help in eliminating prematurely terminated transcripts that could produce truncated proteins and also to clear the damaged DNA region, creating access, and possibly acting as a recruiting factor for DNA repair proteins (Gudmundsdottir and Ashworth, 2006).

BRCA2 and *RAD51*-Mediated Recombination

The direct interaction between *BRCA2* and *RAD51* and their colocalization in nuclear foci after DNA damage was the first evidence for a role for *BRCA2* within the repair of DSBs by HR (Sharan et al., 1997; Chen et al., 1998; Moynahan et al., 2001; Tutt et al., 2001). *BRCA2* appears to regulate the function of *RAD51* in error-free repair of DSBs through HR by GC and in the last few years, much data have been published regarding the interaction between these two proteins and how it affects the repair of DSBs (Gudmundsdottir and Ashworth, 2006).

A decrease in GC causes deletion events predominantly through the use of the SSA pathway. NHEJ, however, is apparently unaffected in *BRCA2*-deficient cells (Patel et al., 1998; Yu et al., 2000). Loss of *BRCA2*, therefore, results in the repair of DSBs by a more error-prone mechanism possibly explaining the apparent chromosome instability associated with *BRCA2* deficiency. *BRCA2* has also been implicated in the response to stalled replication and in preserving the stability of stalled replication forks (Lomonosov et al., 2003).

BRCA2 binds directly to *RAD51* through its C-terminus and the BRC repeats located in the middle of the protein. Of the eight BRC repeats in the *BRCA2* protein, *RAD51* has been shown to bind to BRC1-4, BRC7, and BRC8, which are the more highly conserved repeats (Bignell et al., 1997; Wong et al., 1997). *BRCA2* is thought to be required for the transport of *RAD51* into the nucleus and to sites of DNA damage, where *RAD51* would be released to form the nucleoprotein filament required for recombination to take place. While *BRCA2* has NLS, these have not been identified in *RAD51*, prompting the idea that *BRCA2* facilitated the transport of *RAD51* into the nucleus (Spain et al., 1999; Davies et al., 2001). There is some evidence that the formation of *RAD51* foci in undamaged S phase cells may be *BRCA2* independent (Tarsounas et al., 2003) and occur in smaller numbers at stalled or broken replication forks. A model has been proposed that *BRCA2* is involved in both sequestering and mobilizing *RAD51* and holds *RAD51* in a state of readiness until DA damage or replication arrest, when the complex becomes localized to sites of DSBs (Gudmundsdottir and Ashworth, 2006).

For HR to take place, *RAD51* must be released from *BRCA2* to form a nucleoprotein filament on ssDNA, which then invades and pairs with a homologous DNA duplex, initiating strand exchange between the paired DNA molecules. The *BRCA2* BRC repeats along with the DNA/DSS1-binding domain (DBD) are important in this role (Galkin et al., 2005; Saeki et al., 2006) and studies imply that the key role of *BRCA2* is to deliver *RAD51* to sites of DNA damage. *BRCA2* might facilitate *RAD51*-mediated recombination and might have a role at the dsDNA-ssDNA junction of the resected DSB (Yang et al., 2002). The DBD-binding protein, DSS1, has also been shown to be important for properly controlled recombination (Kojic et al., 2005). The C-terminus of *BRCA2* is phosphorylated at S3291 by cyclin-dependent kinases in a cell cycle-dependent manner (Esashi et al., 2005) to modulate another interaction with *RAD51* and possibly provides a mechanism for the regulation of recombinational repair. The exact mechanism of how the two *BRCA2* binding regions, the BRC repeats and the C-Terminus, work together to control *RAD51* function is not yet known. It has been published recently that the BRC repeats mediate homologous recombination independent of the *BRCA2* C-terminal DNA-binding domain through a previously unrecognized role in control of *RAD51* activity (Shivji et al., 2006).

BRCA2 and Cell Cycle Regulation

BRCA2 associates with the DNA-binding protein BRAF35 (*BRCA2* associated factor 35) through a region contained within BRC6, 7, and 8 of *BRCA2* (Marmorstein et al., 2001). BRAF was observed to bind to branched DNA structures, such as those formed during recombinational repair, implicating BRAF35 in the DNA damage response. BUBR1, which is important for the correct attachment of chromosomes to the mitotic spindle, was found to interact with and phosphorylate the C-terminus of *BRCA2* (Futamura et al., 2000), but the significance of this remains to be elucidated. A role for *BRCA2* in cytokinesis has also been proposed as the cell cycle is extended from anaphase onset to the completion of cell division in *BRCA2*-deficient cells compared with wild-type cells (Daniels et al., 2004). *BRCA2* has also been reported to be phosphorylated in a cell cycle-dependent manner by Polo-like kinase 1 (Plk1) (Lin et al., 2003; Lee et al., 2004).

BRCA2/DSS1 and DNA Repair

The *BRCA2*-binding protein DSS1 is a highly-conserved 70 amino acid protein that interacts with the C-terminal DNA binding domain (DBD) of *BRCA2* (Crackower et al., 1996; Marston et al., 1999). It binds to *BRCA2* in an extended conformation, interacting with numerous residues within the helical domain, OB1 and OB2 of *BRCA2*, most of which are highly conserved (Yang et al., 2002). In both mouse and human cells, silencing of DSS1 using RNA interference (RNAi) compromised the ability of these cells to form colonies. Importantly DSS1 was shown to be required for the formation of DNA damage-induced *RAD51* foci, suggesting a role for DSS1 in *BRCA2*- and *RAD51*-dependent repair by HR (Gudmundsdottir et al., 2004; Li et al., 2006). DSS1 has been shown to be dispensable for the interaction between *BRCA2* and *RAD51*, but conflicting views exist as to whether DSS1 is required for the stability of *BRCA2* (Gudmundsdottir et al., 2004; Kojic et al., 2005; Li et al., 2006). *BRCA2* has proven to be largely insoluble in the absence of DSS1, potentially implicating DSS1 in maintaining the correct conformation of *BRCA2* (Yang et al., 2002; Kojic et al., 2003). The mechanism of how DSS1 depletion induces degradation of *BRCA2* remains to be elucidated.

DSS1: Proteasome and DNA Repair

A possible role for the proteasome in the repair of DSBs has emerged with the discovery that DSS1 is involved both in DSB repair and is a subunit of the proteasome. A functional link to the proteasome is provided by the demonstration that DSS1 is required for efficient ubiquitin-dependent protein degradation (Funakoshi et al., 2004; Sone et al., 2004; Josse et al., 2006). Using ChIP (chromatin immunoprecipitation) analysis, DSS1 was shown to bind to DNA at the site of a specific DSB along with components of the 19S and the 20S proteasome complexes, linking proteolysis to the repair of DSBs. In support of that, DSS1 was shown to be important for the repair of DSBs by both HR and NHEJ (Krogan et al., 2004).

Transcriptional Regulation

The functions of *BRCA1* and *BRCA2* are likely interdependent, so the above discussions on the roles of *BRCA1* and *BRCA2* in DNA repair will likely overlap with roles in transcription. *BRCA1* has three main features thought to be important for function: an amino-terminal RING finger domain, a pair of NLS in the central region of the molecule, and a pair of *BRCA1* C-terminal (BRCT) domains. The RING finger domain is thought to be important for its association with a number of proteins, in particular BARD1, and *BRCA1*-BARD1 heterodimers have been shown to act as ubiquitin ligases (Wu et al., 1996; Hashizume et al., 2001). The NLS are consistent with *BRCA1* being a predominantly nuclear protein. The BRCT domains (aa 1653–1736 and 1760–1855) were first identified in *BRCA1* but have now been shown to be present in an ever expanding group of proteins whose common functions are in DNA damage repair and cell cycle control (Bork et al., 1997). The *BRCA1* protein has been show to tolerate truncations of up to eight aa from its carboxy-terminus, but further deletion results in drastic BRCT folding defects as shown by proteolytic methods and computational predictive methods (Williams and Glover, 2003). BRCT domains have now been postulated to be phosphopeptide-binding motifs with high affinity for phosphoserine and phosphothreonine residues (Manke et al., 2003).

Experiments using the C-terminus of *BRCA1* (aa1560–1863) fused to a GAL4 DNA binding domain showed that *BRCA1* could activate transcription in both yeast and mammalian cells (Monteiro et al., 1996). Furthermore, germline point mutations of this C-terminal region found in patients with early-onset breast or ovarian cancer were deficient in transcriptional activation, suggesting that the ability of *BRCA1* to regulate transcription was key to its tumor suppressor activity (Monteiro et al., 1996). *BRCA1* has been found to copurify with the RNA polymerase II (RNA pol II) holoenzyme complex through an association with RNA helicase A (Anderson et al., 1998), suggesting that *BRCA1* is a component of the core transcriptional machinery (Scully et al., 1997a). RNA helicase A is known to interact with the transcriptional coactivator p300/CBP (Anderson et al., 1998) and *BRCA1* also interacts with p300/CBP but these associations appear to involve different regions of the p300/CBP molecule (Pao et al., 2000). *BRCA1* has been shown to modulate the phosphorylation status of the CTD of RNA polII, negatively regulating phosphorylation by the Cdk-activating kinase (CAK) (Moisan et al., 2004). This suggests that *BRCA1* through regulation of CAK may control cell cycle or enhance NER/TCR at the sites of DNA damage (Moisan et al., 2004).

RNA polII may also be a target for *BRCA1*/BARD1 ubiquitin ligase activity following DNA damage (Hashizume et al., 2001). RNA polII and the coupled 3′-RNA processing machinery stalled at the sites of DNA damage may be targeted by *BRCA1*/BARD1 for degradation, permitting access for repair machinery (Kleiman et al., 2005). *BRCA1* is thought to specifically target Rpb1 (the largest subunit of RNA polII) for ubiquitylation, an event that was dependent on phosphorylation of Rpb1 on a specific serine (serine 5 of the C-terminal heptad repeat YSPTSPS) (Starita et al., 2005). There are 52 repeats of this heptad in RNA polII CTD and multiple phosphorylations are required to generate the hyperphosphorylated RNA polII form associated with elongation. The association of hypophosphorylated *BRCA1* with preferentially the hyperphosphorylated form of RNA polII suggests that *BRCA1* does not affect direct promoter activation but plays roles in transcription related to chromatin remodeling as well as transcription-couples repair (Krum et al., 2003). *BRCA1* was also shown by yeast two-hybrid to associate with the zinc-finger containing nuclear protein NUFIP (Cabart et al., 2004). NUFIP stimulates activator-independent transcription by RNA polII both in vitro and in vivo and associates with preinitiation, open transcription and elongation complexes and facilitates the ATP-dependent dissociation of hyperphosphorylated RNA polII from open transcription complexes (Cabart et al., 2004). NUFIP also interacts with the positive elongation factor pTEFb, placing *BRCA1* in a complex with other proteins involved in mRNA elongation (Cabart et al., 2004). *BRCA1* may therefore utilize its association with RNA polII to stimulate mRNA transcription while simultaneously monitoring the fidelity of DNA removing RNA polII from actively transcribing genes upon encountering damaged DNA (Mullan et al., 2006). It has been published as well that the *BRCA1* COOH-terminal region acts as an RNA polymerase II carboxyl-terminal domain kinase inhibitor that modulates *p21*(WAF1/CIP1) expression (Moisan and Gaudreau, 2006).

The retinoblastoma suppressor (Rb-) associated protein (RbAp46) (Chen et al., 2001), which is also a growth suppressor, was identified to interact with and alter the transcriptional activity of *BRCA1*. The function of this interaction is unknown but it is disrupted by DNA damage so RbAp46 may act to sequester *BRCA1* in the absence of DNA damage. The BRCT domain was also found to interact with another Rb-associated protein, RbAp48, as well as Rb itself (Yarden and Brody, 1999). The ability of *BRCA1* to act as either a coactivator or corepressor of transcription may involve its ability to recruit both the basal transcription machinery (through RNA polII interaction), proteins implicated in chromatin remodeling, such as the histone deacetylases HDAC1 and HDAC2 (Yarden and Brody, 1999) or components of the SWI/SNF-related chromatin-remodeling complex (Bochar et al., 2000). *BRCA1* interacts directly with the BRG1 subunit of the SWI/SNF complex (Bochar et al., 2000). Remodeling can be achieved with only the BRG1-BAF155 minimal complex, whereas transcription requires the presence of an activation domain (Kadam et al., 2000). This activation function may be *BRCA1*'s role in collaboration with sequence-specific transcription factors (Mullan et al., 2006).

There are a number of other reports linking *BRCA1* to chromatin remodeling. Targeting *BRCA1* to an amplified region of a chromosome has been shown to cause localized chromatin decondensation (Ye et al., 2001). *BRCA1* has been shown to interact with hGCN5 and TRRAP in a histone acetyltransferase (HAT) complex (Oishi et al., 2006). HATs are important for the optimal transcriptional activity of many transcription factors since they acetylate the amino-terminal lysine residues of core histones to reduce their positive charge and thus reducing their binding affinity for DNA (Mullan et al., 2006).

ER

BRCA1 is known to mediate ligand-independent transcriptional repression by *ER*-α (Zheng et al., 2001). *BRCA1* acts as a buffer in this case to quench *ER*-α transcriptional activity in the absence of estrogen stimulation. A number of reports show that *BRCA1* also inhibits estrogen-dependent transcription (Fan et al., 1999). Overexpression of *BRCA1* inhibited the induction of over 90% of estrogen-inducible genes (Xu et al., 2005). *BRCA1* may regulate the activity of VEGF through its ability to modulate *ER*-α function (Kawai et al., 2002). Signaling to extracellular signal-related kinase (ERK) in response to estradiol is also stunted in the presence of wild type but not mutant *BRCA1* (Razandi et al., 2004). The transcriptional repression activity of *BRCA1* for *ER*-α is postulated to occur by the association of the amino-terminus of *BRCA1* (aa 1-300) with the C-terminal activation function (AF-2) of *ER*-α (Fan et al., 1999) and is thought to involve histone deacetylase activity (Zheng et al., 2001). *BRCA1* down-regulates the expression of p300, which also interacts with AF-2 (Fan et al., 2002a). Cyclin D1 has also been reported to compete with *BRCA1* for *ER*-α binding through a common hinge domain (Wang et al., 2005). The cofactor of *BRCA1*, COBRA1 is a subunit of the human-negative elongation factor (NELF), binds to *ER*-α and negatively regulated *ER*-α activity (Aiyar et al., 2004). Another coregulator of *BRCA1* transcription is MED1/TRAP220, which was shown to interact with the BRCT region of *BRCA1* (Wada et al., 2004). MED1/TRAP220 is a key coactivator for many transcription factors most notably nuclear receptors (Zhang et al., 2005).

p53

BRCA1 (aa 224–500) was shown to interact with the C-terminus of *p53* and in doing so alters the transcriptional activity of *p53* (Zhang et al., 1998). The second BRCT domain (aa 1760–1863) was also shown capable of interaction with *p53* in vitro and was sufficient to stimulate *p53*-dependent transcription from the *p21*cip1/WAF1 promoter (Chai et al., 1999). BRCA1-stabilized *p53* was found to specifically regulate the transcription of genes involved in DNA repair and growth arrest rather than proapoptotic genes (MacLachlan et al., 2002). The *p53* in turn acts to downregulate *BRCA1* levels in a negative feedback loop (MacLachlan et al., 2000). It may also effect *BRCA1* subcellular localization since *BRCA1* is exported from the nucleus via a CRM1- and *p53*-dependent mechanism (Feng et al., 2004). *BRCA1* may promote the accumulation of *p53* through its ability to regulate the levels of p14ARF since *BRCA1* cannot stabilize *p53* in p14ARF-deficient cells (Somasundaram et al., 1999). Another mode of *BRCA1* stabilization of *p53* may occur through its role in facilitating *p53* phosphorylation in response to DNA damage. It is required for the *ATM* and *ATR* to phosphorylate *p53* at Ser15 (Fabbro et al., 2004). This phosphorylation event is critical for G1/S arrest in response to gamma-irradiation through induction of *p21*cip1/WAF1.

STAT1

BRCA1 (aa 502–802) has been reported to interact with the C-terminus of the transcription factor STAT1 (Ouchi et al., 2000). Other transcription target include IRF7, MxA, 2,5 OAS and ISG54, accompanied by apoptosis (Andrews et al., 2002). One of these transcriptional targets, interferon regulatory factor 7 (IRF7), is a key molecule in the amplification of the interferon cascade in response to viral infection suggesting that *BRCA1* may play a transcriptional role in the innate immune response to viral infection (Marie et al., 1998). Another downstream target of *BRCA1* was 2,5 oligoadenylate synthase (2,5 OAS) which was shown to act as a mediator of apoptosis in a *BRCA1* and IFNδ-dependent manner (Mullan et al., 2005).

c-Myc

In yeast, two-hybrid screen c-Myc was identified as a *BRCA1*-interacting partner, an interaction that required the helix-loop-helix region of c-Myc, a region that is also involved in Myc-Max dimerization (Wang et al., 1998). Two amino-terminal regions of *BRCA1* (aa 175–303 and aa 443–511) were required for interaction with c-Myc (Wang et al., 1998). *BRCA1* was found to inhibit Myc-mediated transcription and reversed the transforming activity of c-Myc in association with other oncogenes such as Ras (Wang et al., 1998). *BRCA1* (aa 298–693) and (aa 1301–1863) was also found to interact with another Myc-interacting protein, Nmi (N-Myc-interacting protein) (Li et al., 2002). Nmi is thought to function as an adaptor molecule, facilitating the formation of an Nmi-Myc-*BRCA1* complex. Nmi cotransfected with *BRCA1* was shown to significantly inhibit c-Myc induced transcription of the human telomerase reverse transcriptase gene, human telomerase reverse transcriptase (HTERT) promoter (Li et al., 2002). Data suggest that both the *BRCA1* amino-terminus and an intact RING domain are required for effective suppression of c-Myc transcription and subsequently TERT activity (Xiong et al., 2003). Recently, data have shown that *BRCA1*, through its interaction with Myc, leads to the downregulation of a number of other transcriptional targets including psoriasin (S100A7) (Kennedy et al., 2005).

CtIP

An association of *BRCA1* with CtIP is abrogated following DNA damage indicating that *BRCA1* and/or CtIP phosphorylation may disrupt this interaction (Li et al., 1999). A potential model was proposed suggesting that *ATM* phosphorylation of *BRCA1* and its associated corepressor CtIP following DNA damage led to the dissociation of *BRCA1* and CtIP, resulting in the BRCA1-mediated up regulation of GADD45 (Li et al., 2000). In contrast, it was also reported that CtIP was found in a complex associating with *BRCA1* and BARD1 and that this complex was stable following DNA damage (Yu and Baer, 2000; Wu-Baer and Baer, 2001). These discrepancies will eventually be resolved, with the agreement that the *BRCA1*-CtIP interaction plays an important role in the DNA damage-dependent induction of genes such as GADD45.

ZBRK1

ZBRK1 is a transcriptional corepressor and was shown to bind to a specific sequence within GADD45 intron 3 after complexing with *BRCA1* (Zheng et al., 2000). ZBRK1 appeared to repress GADD45 transcription in a *BRCA1*-dependent manner, and the GADD45 promoter is possibly derepressed following *BRCA1* activation by stress or damage stimuli (Zheng et al., 2000). XBRK1 has two repression domains with the CTD acting in a *BRCA1*-, histone deacetylase-, and sequence-specific manner (Tan et al.,

2004). The C-terminal repression domain was shown to be functionally distinct from the amino-terminal KRAB repression domain and includes elements that modulate its DNA-binding activity (Tan et al., 2004). The binding of *BRCA1* to this C-terminal repression domain (CTRD) of ZBRK1 was found to be necessary but not sufficient for CTRD repression activity (Tan et al., 2004). Additionally, an alternative *BRCA1*-independent mode of GADD45a induction following DNA damage has been proposed (Yun and Lee, 2003). GADD45 is also regulated in a *p53* independent manner, dependent on a functional *BRCA1* transactivation domain (Jin et al., 2000). *BRCA1* was also found to physically associate with transcription factor Oct-1 and NF-YA, which directly bind to the CT-1 and CAAT motifs in the GADD45 promoter (Fan et al., 2002b). These reports suggest that *BRCA1* coordinates the *p53*-independent induction of GADD45 following DNA damage by derepression of ZBRK1 and stimulation of transcription through its association with specific transcription factors (Mullan et al., 2006).

FUTURE PROSPECTIVES

BRCA1 and Error-Prone Repair Linked

The pathway determining malignant cellular transformation, which depends upon mutation of the BRCA1 tumor suppressor gene, is poorly defined. Published data suggest that promotion of DNA DSB repair by homologous recombination (HR) may be the means by which *BRCA1* maintains genomic stability, while a role of *BRCA1* in error-prone nonhomologous recombination (NHR) or NHEJ processes has begun to be elucidated (Zhang et al., 2004). As the prevention of *CHK2*-mediated phosphorylation via mutation of serine 988 residue of *BRCA1* disrupts both *BRCA1* dependent promotion of HR and the suppression of NHR, a functional link between recombination control and breast cancer predisposition in carriers of *CHK2* and *BRCA1* germline mutations has been speculated. This suggests that *BRCA1* phosphorylation status "controls the selectivity of repair events dictated by HR and error-prone NHR" (Zhang et al., 2004). Accumulating evidence implicated *BRCA1* in the regulation of NHEJ, which may involve precise relegation of the DSB ends if they are compatible (i.e. error-free repair) or sequence alteration upon rejoining (i.e., error-prone or mutagenic repair) (Zhuang et al., 2006a). The differential control of NHEJ subprocesses by *BRCA1*, in concert with *CHK2*, reduces the mutagenic potential of NHEJ, thereby contributing to the prevention of familial breast cancers (Zhuang et al., 2006a). *ATM* and *CHK2* are believed to act jointly in this regulation of *BRCA1* in controlling the fidelity of DNA end-joining by precise NHEJ (Wang et al., 2006).

As discussed previously, *BRCA1* and BARD1 play a vital role in the cellular response to DNA damage; how though is poorly understood. Following exposure to genotoxic stress, DNA damage-specific interactions were observed between *BRCA1*/BARD1 and the DNA damage-response proteins, TopBP1 and *MRE11/RAD50/NBS1*: two distinct damage-dependent super complexes emerged. Their activation was dependent in part on the actions of specific checkpoint kinases, and each super complex contributed to a distinctive aspect of the DNA damage response. Thus, a multifactorial model has emerged that describes how genotoxic stress enables *BRCA1* to "execute a diverse set of DNA damage-response functions" (Greenberg et al., 2006). "Subclassification of DSB" regulators, according to their residence sites, provides a useful framework for understanding their involvement in diverse processes of genome surveillance (Bekker-Jensen et al., 2006).

In 2005, Huber and Chodosh (2005) found that the majority of *BRCA1* and *BRCA2* proteins (in mice) were found to interact tightly with the nuclear matrix. They suggested that the proteins may perform their DNA repair-related functions from positions that are anchored to the nuclear matrix. These data are consistent with proposed models that suggest that components of specific repair complexes residing on the nuclear matrix function to "recruit" damaged DNA, perhaps "specified by lesion type" (Bove et al., 2002). The primary role of *BRCA2* in maintaining genomic integrity is in HR, specifically to deliver *RAD51* to ssDNA (Saeki et al., 2006).

Translesion Synthesis—A Link?

DNA lesions that have escaped DNA repair are tolerated via translesion synthesis (TLS) of DNA or translesion replication (TLR) or error-prone repair, an error-prone DNA repair process that involves DNA synthesis across DNA lesions and is carried out by specialized error-prone DNA polymerases (Goodman, 2000; Livneh, 2001; Prakash and Prakash, 2002). A number of "error-prone DNA polymerases" are found among eukaryotes from yeasts to mammals including humans that act in backup to error-free polymerases. These DNA polymerases are characterized by the probability of base substitutions or frame shifts of 10(–3) to 7.5 × 10(–1) on DNA injuries, whereas the probability of spontaneous mutagenesis per replicated nucleotide accounts 10(–10)–10(–12) (Krutyakov, 2006). Both misinsertion and misalignment mechanisms are used. Inaccurate DNA polymerases are terminal deoxynucleotidyl transferase (TdT): beta, zeta, kappa, eta, iota, gimel, mu, and Rev1. All are deprived of the corrective 3′-5′ exonucleolytic activity. The ability of TLS polymerases to insert nucleotides opposite a hydrocarbon chain, despite the lack of any similarity to DNA, suggests that they may act via a mode of transient and local template-independent polymerase activity and highlights the robustness of the TLS system in human cells (Adar and Livneh, 2006). Error-prone DNA polymerases are not found in all tissues though some of them are essential for an organism survival. The biological significance of TLS is indicated by the hereditary disease xeroderma pigmentosum variant (XP-V), where the absence of an active TLS polymerase, DNA polymerase n (pol n), causes sunlight sensitivity and predisposition to skin cancer (Johnson et al., 1999; Masutani et al., 1999; Washington et al., 2001; McCulloch et al., 2004).

After bypass it is necessary as soon as possible to switch catalysis of the DNA synthesis from the specialized polymerases to the relatively accurate DNA polymerases 6 and F (fidelity) of 10(–5)–10(–6) (Krutyakov, 2006). The mechanism of regulation of TLS, and polymerase switch, is largely unknown. While translesion bypass is thought to be a process involving polymerase switching that operates mainly during S phase to rescue stalled replication forks, Waters et al., have reported that in yeast, error-prone polymerase Rev1 is subject to pronounced cell cycle control in which the levels of Rev1 protein are approximately 50-fold higher in G2 and throughout mitosis than during G1 and much of S phase (Waters and Walker, 2006). Interestingly *BRCA1* has been documented to regulate the G2/M transition by multiple mechanisms as discussed above as well as the more commonly known function at stalled replication forks at S. *BRCA1* may, as suggested in a previous model, be an error-free complex component that effects or is involved in proper polymerase switch during and after TLS (Bove et al., 2002). *BRCA1* has been documented to interact with other complex members, among them *p53*, *p21*, PCNA, and GADD45 all already associated with TLS.

PCNA and *p53*—Another Link?

So a special challenge presents to regulate mutation rates is the presence of these multiple mutagenic DNA polymerases in mammals. Ubiquitination of PCNA, the DNA sliding clamp that interacts with TLS polymerases (Goodman, 2000; Livneh, 2001; Prakash and Prakash, 2002), appears to be involved in the process, most likely by recruiting TLS polymerases (Hoege et al., 2002; Stelter and Ulrich, 2003; Kannouche et al., 2004; Watanabe et al., 2004). It has been proposed that in mammalian cells TLS is controlled by the tumor suppressor *p53*, and by the cell cycle inhibitor *p21* via its PCNA-interacting domain, to maintain a low mutagenic load at the price of reduced repair efficiency. This regulation may be mediated by binding of *p21* to PCNA and via DNA damage-induced ubiquitination of PCNA, which is stimulated by *p53* and *p21*. Loss of this regulation by inactivation of *p53* or *p21* caused an out of control lesion-bypass activity, which increased the mutational load and might therefore play a role in pathogenic processes caused by genetic instability (Avkin et al., 2006).

The associations that *BRCA1* has with PCNA and *p53* may define another critical link between the breast cancer gene and error-prone repair, and breast cancer etiology. The *BRCA1* containing complex named BASC (Wang et al., 2000) includes tumor suppressors, DNA damage sensors and signal transducers, including the MRN complex, the mismatch repair proteins MSH2, MSH6 and MLH1, the Bloom syndrome helicase BLM, the *ATM* kinase, DNA replication factor C (RFC) and PCNA. As has been discussed, *BRCA1* stabilizes *p53* by facilitating phosphorylation (Fabbro et al., 2004) in response to DNA damage, an event critical for G1/S arrest in response to gamma-irradiation through induction of *p21*cip1/WAF1. BRCA1-stabilized *p53* was found to specifically regulate the transcription of genes involved in DNA repair and growth arrest rather than proapoptotic genes (MacLachlan et al., 2002). The *p53* in turn acts to downregulate *BRCA1* levels in a negative feedback loop (MacLachlan et al., 2000). *BRCA1* (aa 224–500) was shown to interact with the C-terminus of *p53* and in doing so alters the transcriptional activity of *p53* (Zhang et al., 1998).

Evidence is growing that supports our previous prediction that the breast cancer gene(s) play critical roles in the error-free and backup error-prone DNA repair processes (Bove et al., 2002), and that the success or failure or choice of these repair processes contribute to the development of breast cancer. One of the most intriguing findings recently is that the pathways associated with different cellular processes are functionally coordinated through *BRCA1* in disease-free cells (Wen et al., 2006), including several DNA repair systems (Table 10). This lends credibility that *BRCA1* has a role in choosing or subclassifying the appropriate repair event, in recruiting specific DNA damage lesions or DNA polymerases appropriate for specific mechanisms of repair, and/or in effecting the timely switch of polymerases and repair methods through its involvement with ubiquitination enzymes and the ubiquitination process (Table 11).

Repair, NMD, and Tissue Specificity

Participation in one or all of these roles may explain the long puzzling tissue specificity of *BRCA1/2* associated disease as well. A natural or environmental exposure to a possible cancer causing agent or metabolite may be organ specific, like oxidative damage exposure to the breast or ovary (Malins and Haimanot, 1991; Malins et al., 1993). Improper function of the *BRCA* proteins in response to this oxidative damage would selectively cause cancer in

Table 10 *BRCA1* Interacting Proteins

Biological functions	Interacting proteins
Damage response/repair	MSH2, MSH6, MLH1, *ATM*, BLM and the *RAD50/MRE11/NBS1*, DNA replication factor C, *RAD51*, Fanconi anemia proteins, PCNA, H2AX, c-Abl, MDC1
Tumor suppressors	*ATM, ATR, p53, BRCA2*, RB, BARD1, *BACH1*
Oncogenes	*c-Myc*, casein kinase II, E2F1, E2F4, *STK15*, AKT
Transcription	RNA polymerase II holoenzyme (RNA helicase A, RPB2, RPB10α), CBP/p300, HDC and CtIP, estrogen receptor α, androgen receptor, ZBRK1, ATF1, *STAT1*, Smad3, BRCT-repeat inhibitor of hTERT expression (*BRIT1*)
Cell cycle related	Aylin A, Cyclin D1, CDC2, Cdk2, Cdk4, γ-tubulin, *p21*, p27
Stress response	MEKK3, IFI16, X-linked inhibitor of apoptosis protein (XIAP)
Others	BAP1, BIP1, BRAP2, importin α

Source: From Deng (2006).

these susceptible organs. Additionally, the mechanism by which transcripts containing mutations, especially protein truncation mutations, are detected and degraded within cells has been called "nonsense-mediated mRNA decay" (NMD) (Gonzalez et al., 2001; Lykke-Andersen, 2001; Wilusz et al., 2001; Byers, 2002; Perrin-Vidoz et al., 2002). Because of NMD, mutant transcripts do not always lead to the synthesis of truncated proteins, which could have a dominant negative effect (Perrin-Vidoz et al., 2002). A heterozygous alteration of *BRCA1/2* can therefore affect total titer of protein available for repair function because of NMD, leading to the switch to uncontrolled error-prone pathways that allow mutations to accumulate in previously normal cells (Bove et al., 2002). These deleterious effects of titer would be likely seen in response to organ specific initiated damage, as oxidative damage to the breast and ovary.

DNA Repair and Therapeutic Intervention

Cells lacking *BRCA1* or *BRCA2* repair lesions no longer by homologous recombination but by more error-prone mechanisms. In *BRCA2* deficiency, SSA is upregulated (Moynahan et al., 2001; Tutt et al., 2001; Stark et al., 2004); in *BRCA1* deficiency, error-prone NHEJ is used (Moynahan et al., 1999; Stark et al., 2004; Wang et al., 2006; Zhuang et al., 2006a). Because of these forced changes in the choice of repair pathways in response to damage, *BRCA1/2* deficient cells have elevated sensitivity to DNA damaging agents that cross-link DNA such as mitomycin C (MMC) and to the platinum drugs cisplatin and carboplatin (Bhattacharyya et al., 2000; Yu et al., 2000; Tutt et al., 2001; Fedier et al., 2003). This increased sensitivity can be exploited for treatment of *BRCA* cancers. Selective polymerase inhibitors have already been identified (Mizushina et al., 2006).

Another therapeutic approach involves inhibiting the DNA repair protein PARP, poly(ADP-ribose)polymerase-1, to generate specific lesions that require *BRCA1* or *BRCA2* for their removal (Gudmundsdottir and Ashworth, 2006). PARP-1 deficiency causes the failure of repair of single-stranded breaks, creating DSBs (Dantzer et al., 2000; Hoeijmakers, 2001) that require repair by error-free *BRCA* processes. PARP-1 inhibitors have been shown to be selectively lethal to cells deficient in *BRCA1* or *BRCA2* (Bryant et al., 2005; Farmer et al., 2005; McCabe et al., 2005; Wang et al., 2007). No toxicity was evident in *BRCA* heterozygous cells as functional *BRCA* is present. Bentle et al. (2006) have identified a novel anti-tumor agent, beta-lapachone, which blocks transformation by modulating PARP-1.

Homologous recombination, translesion DNA synthesis, and de novo reinitiation of DNA synthesis ensure robust replication by navigating the replication complex passed damaged DNA (Eppink et al., 2006). The *BRCA* genes and their multitude of repair protein partners provide a lush landscape for possible therapeutic intervention in the event of mishap in these processes. As shown with the PARP inhibitors, targeting will have to be specific as DNA repair is universal and necessary to maintain genome integrity in cells throughout the organism. It has been published recently that in addition to the accumulation of genomic instability in the cancer cell, genomic instability accumulates in the cancer stroma as well

Table 11 Possible Roles for *BRCA1* in Error Prone Repair

Phosphorylated *BRCA1* controls the selection of repair events: HR or error-prone NHR/NHEJ
BRCA1/BARD1 attract complexes to subclassify
DSB*BRCA1* complexes in nuclear matrix recruit damaged DNA specified by lesion type
BRCA1, in BASC complex, recruits/switches TLS polymerases

perhaps providing a microenvironment user-friendly to the development of cancer (Weber et al., 2006). So, it is possible that repair-related therapies may be effective before tumor formation becomes apparent lending to novel preventative therapeutic approaches. As defects in genes are identified in a range of cancers, therapies designed to target the DNA repair defects in *BRCA*-deficient cells may be more widely applicable (Turner et al., 2004) (Table 10).

DEDICATION

In light of recent research developments with regard to *BRCA1/2* and DNA repair, this chapter is dedicated to Nat L. Sternberg (1942–1995), a molecular biologist ahead of his time posing an educated judgment that proper or improper functioning error-prone repair systems and other DNA repair systems would be the root of all cancer (personal communication, 1995; Lin et al., 1984, 1990). The topic was of particular significance for Nat who lost a long and debilitating battle with cancer on September 26, 1995.

REFERENCES

Anglian Breast Cancer Study Group (ABCSG). Prevalence and penetrance of BRCA1 and BRCA2 mutations in a population-based series of breast cancer cases. Br J Cancer 2000; 10:1301–1308.

Abeliovich D, Kadwi L, Lerer I, Weinberg N, Amir G, Sagi M, Zlotogora J, Heching N, Peretz T. The founder mutations 185delAG and 5382insC in BRCA1 and 6174delT in BRCA2 appear in 60% of ovarian cancer and 30% of early-onset breast cancer patients among Ashkenazi women. Am J Hum Genet 1997; 60:505–514.

Abkevich V, Zharkikh A, Deffenbaugh AM, Frank D, Chen Y, Shattuck D, Skolnick MH, Gutin A, Tavtigian SV. Analysis of missense variation in human BRCA1 in the context of interspecific sequence variation. J Med Genet 2004; 41(7):492–507.

Adar S, Livneh Z. Translesion DNA synthesis across non-DNA segments in cultured human cells. DNA Repair (Amst) 2006; 5(4):479–490.

Agata S, Viel A, Della Puppa L, Cortesi L, Fersini G, Callegaro M, Dalla Palma M, Dolcetti R, Federico M, Venuta S, Miolo G, D'Andrea E, Montagna M. Prevalence of BRCA1 genomic rearrangements in a large cohort of Italian breast and breast/ovarian cancer families without detectable BRCA1 and BRCA2 point mutations. Genes Chromosomes Cancer 2006; 45(9):791–797.

Agrawal S, Eng C. Differential expression of novel naturally occurring splice variants of PTEN and their functional consequences in Cowden syndrome and sporadic breast cancer. Hum Mol Genet 2006; 15(5):777–787.

Ahmed M, Rahman N. ATM and breast cancer susceptibility. Oncogene 2006; 25(43):5906–5911.

Aiyar SE, Sun JL, Blair AL, Moskaluk CA, Lu YZ, Ye QN, Yamaguchi Y, Mukherjee A, Ren DM, Handa H, Li R. Attenuation of estrogen receptor alpha-mediated transcription through estrogen-stimulated recruitment of a negative elongation factor. Genes Dev 2004; 18(17):2134–2146.

Allinen M, Huusko P, Mantyniemi S, Launonen V, Winqvist R. Mutation analysis of the CHK2 gene in families with hereditary breast cancer. Br J Cancer 2001; 85(2):209–212.

Andersen T, Borresen A, Moller P. A common *BRCA1* mutation in Norwegian breast and ovarian cancer families. Am J Hum Genet 1996; 59:486–487.

Andersen TI. Genetic heterogeneity in breast cancer susceptibility. Acta Oncol 1996; 35(4):407–410.

Anderson S, Schlegel B, Nakajima T, Wolpin E, Parvin J. BRCA1 protein is linked to the RNA polymerase II holoenzyme complex via RNA helicase A. Nature Genet 1998; 19:254–256.

Andrews HN, Mullan PB, McWilliams S, Sebelova S, Quinn JE, Gilmore PM, McCabe N, Pace A, Koller B, Johnston PG, Haber DA, Harkin DP. BRCA1 regulates the interferon gamma-mediated apoptotic response. J Biol Chem 2002; 277(29):26225–26232.

Andrieu N, Goldgar DE, Easton DF, Rookus M, Brohet R, Antoniou AC, Peock S, Evans G, Eccles D, Douglas F, Nogues C, Gauthier-Villars M, Chompret A, Van Leeuwen FE, Kluijt I, Benitez J, Arver B, Olah E, Chang-Claude J. Pregnancies, breast-feeding, and breast cancer risk in the International BRCA1/2 Carrier Cohort Study (IBCCS). J Natl Cancer Inst 2006; 98(8):535–544.

Anton-Culver H, Cohen PF, Gildea ME, Ziogas A. Characteristics of BRCA1 mutations in a population-based case series of breast and ovarian cancer. Eur J Cancer 2000; 36(10): 1200–1208.

Antoniou A, Pharoah PD, Narod S, Risch HA, Eyfjord JE, Hopper JL, Loman N, Olsson H, Johannsson O, Borg A, Pasini B, Radice P, Manoukian S, Eccles DM, Tang N, Olah E, Anton-Culver H, Warner E, Lubinski J, Gronwald J, Gorski B, Tulinius H, Thorlacius S, Eerola H, Nevanlinna H, Syrjakoski K, Kallioniemi OP, Thompson D, Evans C, Peto J, Lalloo F, Evans DG, Easton DF. Average risks of breast and ovarian cancer associated with BRCA1 or BRCA2 mutations detected in case Series unselected for family history: a combined analysis of 22 studies. Am J Hum Genet 2003; 72(5):1117–1130.

Antoniou AC, Durocher F, Smith P, Simard J, Easton DF. BRCA1 and BRCA2 mutation predictions using the BOADICEA and BRCAPRO models and penetrance estimation in high-risk French-Canadian families. Breast Cancer Res 2006; 8(1):R3.

Antoniou AC, Easton DF. Models of genetic susceptibility to breast cancer. Oncogene 2006; 25(43):5898–5905.

Antoniou AC, Pharoah PD, McMullan G, Day NE, Stratton MR, Peto J, Ponder BJ, Easton DF. A comprehensive model for familial breast cancer incorporating BRCA1, BRCA2 and other genes. Br J Cancer 2002; 86(1):76–83.

Antoniou AC, Pharoah PP, Smith P, Easton DF. The BOADICEA model of genetic susceptibility to breast and ovarian cancer. Br J Cancer 2004; 91(8):1580–1590.

Armaou S, Konstantopoulou I, Anagnostopoulos T, Razis E, Boukovinas I, Xenidis N, Fountzilas G, Yannoukakos D. Novel genomic rearrangements in the BRCA1 gene detected in greek breast/ovarian cancer patients. Eur J Cancer 2007; 43(2):443–453.

Armes JE, Egan AJ, Southey MC, Dite GS, McCredie MR, Giles GG, Hopper JL, Venter DJ. The histologic phenotypes of breast carcinoma occurring before age 40 years in women with and without BRCA1 or BRCA2 germline mutations: a population-based study. Cancer 1998; 83(11):2335–2345.

Armes JE, Trute L, White D, Southey MC, Hammet F, Tesoriero A, Hutchins AM, Dite GS, McCredie MR, Giles GG, Hopper JL, Venter DJ. Distinct molecular pathogeneses of early-onset breast cancers in BRCA1 and BRCA2 mutation carriers: a population-based study. Cancer Res 1999; 59(8): 2011–2017.

Armstrong K, Micco E, Carney A, Stopfer J, Putt M. Racial differences in the use of BRCA1/2 testing among women with a family history of breast or ovarian cancer. JAMA 2005; 293(14):1729–1736.

Arnes JB, Brunet JS, Stefansson I, Begin LR, Wong N, Chappuis PO, Akslen LA, Foulkes WD. Placental cadherin and the basal epithelial phenotype of BRCA1-related breast cancer. Clin Cancer Res 2005; 11(11):4003–4011.

Arnold K, Kim MK, Frerk K, Edler L, Savelyeva L, Schmezer P, Wiedemeyer R. Lower level of BRCA2 protein in heterozygous mutation carriers is correlated with an increase in DNA double strand breaks and an impaired DSB repair. Cancer Lett 2006; 243(1):90–100.

Avkin S, Sevilya Z, Toube L, Geacintov N, Chaney SG, Oren M, Livneh Z. p53 and p21 regulate error-prone DNA repair to yield a lower mutation load. Mol Cell 2006; 22(3):407–413.

Aziz H, Hussain F, Sohn C, Mediavillo R, Saitta A, Hussain A, Brandys M, Homel P, Rotman M. Early onset of breast carcinoma in African American women with poor prognostic factors. Am J Clin Oncol 1999; 22(5):436–440.

Aziz S, Kuperstein G, Rosen B, Cole D, Nedelcu R, McLaughlin J, Narod SA. A genetic epidemiological study of carcinoma of the fallopian tube. Gynecol Oncol 2001; (3):341–345.

Baer R. With the ends in sight: images from the BRCA1 tumor suppressor. Nat Struct Biol 2001; 8(10):822–824.

Baldeyron C, Jacquemin E, Smith J, Jacquemont C, De Oliveira I, Gad S, Feunteun J, Stoppa-Lyonnet D, Papadopoulo D. A single mutated BRCA1 allele leads to impaired fidelity of double strand break end-joining. Oncogene 2002; 21(9):1401–1410.

Barcenas CH, Hosain GM, Arun B, Zong J, Zhou X, Chen J, Cortada JM, Mills GB, Tomlinson GE, Miller AR, Strong LC, Amos CI. Assessing BRCA carrier probabilities in extended families. J Clin Oncol 2006; 24(3):354–360.

Barroso E, Milne RL, Fernandez LP, Zamora P, Arias JI, Benitez J, Ribas G. FANCD2 associated with sporadic breast cancer risk. Carcinogenesis 2006; 27(9):1930–1937.

Bartek J, Bartkova J, Vojtesek B, Staskova Z, Rejthar A, Koverik J, Lane DP. Patterns of expressions of the p53 tumor suppressor in human breast tissues and tumors in situ and in vitro. Int J Cancer 1990; 46:839–844.

Bean GR, Ibarra Drendall C, Goldenberg VK, Baker JC, Jr., Troch MM, Paisie C, Wilke LG, Yee L, Marcom PK, Kimler BF, Fabian CJ, Zalles CM, Broadwater G, Scott V, Seewaldt VL. Hypermethylation of the breast cancer-associated gene 1 promoter does not predict cytologic atypia or correlate with surrogate end points of breast cancer risk. Cancer Epidemiol Biomarkers Prev 2007; 16(1):50–56.

Bekker-Jensen S, Lukas C, Kitagawa R, Melander F, Kastan MB, Bartek J, Lukas J. Spatial organization of the mammalian genome surveillance machinery in response to DNA strand breaks. J Cell Biol 2006; 173(2):195–206.

Belgrader P, Marino M, Lubin M, Barany F. A multiplex PCR-ligase detection reaction assay for human identity testing. Genome Sci Technol 1996; 1:77–87.

Bell DW, Varley JM, Szydlo TE, Kang DH, Wahrer DC, Shannon KE, Lubratovich M, Verselis SJ, Isselbacher KJ, Fraumeni JF, Birch JM, Li FP, Garber JE, Haber DA. Heterozygous germ line *hCHK2* mutations in Li-Fraumeni syndrome. Science 1999; 286(54499):2528–2531.

Bentle MS, Bey EA, Dong Y, Reinicke KE, Boothman DA. New tricks for old drugs: the anticarcinogenic potential of DNA repair inhibitors. J Mol Histol 2006; 37(5–7):203–218.

Berman D, Wagner-Costalas J, Schultz D, Lynch H, Daly M, Godwin A. Two distinct origins of a common BRCA1 mutation in breast-ovarian cancer families: A genetic study of 15 185delAG-mutation kindreds. Am J Hum Genet 1996b; 58:1166–1176.

Berman DB, Costalas J, Schultz DC, Grana G, Daly M, Godwin AK. A common mutation in BRCA2 that predisposes to a variety of cancers is found in both Jewish Ashkenazi and non-Jewish individuals. Cancer Res 1996a; 56:3409–3414.

Bernard-Gallon DJ, Dechelotte PJ, Le Corre L, Vissac-Sabatier C, Favy DA, Cravello L, De Latour MP, Bignon YJ. Expression of BRCA1 and BRCA2 in male breast cancers and gynecomastias. Anticancer Res 2003; 23(1B):661–667.

Berry DA, Iversen ES, Jr., Gudbjartsson DF, Hiller EH, Garber JE, Peshkin BN, Lerman C, Watson P, Lynch HT, Hilsenbeck SG, Rubinstein WS, Hughes KS, Parmigiani G. BRCAPRO validation, sensitivity of genetic testing of BRCA1/BRCA2, and prevalence of other breast cancer susceptibility genes. J Clin Oncol 2002; 20(11):2701–2712.

Bhattacharyya A, Ear US, Koller BH, Weichselbaum RR, Bishop DK. The breast cancer susceptibility gene BRCA1 is required for subnuclear assembly of Rad51 and survival following treatment with the DNA cross-linking agent cisplatin. J Biol Chem 2000; 275(31):23899–23903.

Bignell G, Micklem G, Stratton MR, Ashworth A, Wooster R. The BRC repeats are conserved in mammalian BRCA2 proteins. Hum Mol Genet 1997; 6(1):53–58.

Birch J, Heighway J, Teare M, Kelsey A, Hartley AL, Tricker K, Crowther D, Lane D, Santibanex-Koref M. Linkage studies in a Li-Fraumeni family with increased expression of p53 protein but no germline mutation in p53. Br J Cancer 1994; 70:1176–1181.

Birgisdottir V, Stefansson OA, Bodvarsdottir SK, Hilmarsdottir H, Jonasson JG, Eyfjord JE. Epigenetic silencing and deletion of the BRCA1 gene in sporadic breast cancer. Breast Cancer Res 2006; 8(4):R38.

Bochar D, Wang L, Beniya H, Kinwv A, Xue Y, Lane W, Wang W, Kashanchi F, Shiekhattar R. BRCA1 is associated with a human SWI/SNF-related complex: linking chromatin remodeling to breast cancer. Cell 2000; 102:257–265.

Bogdanova N, Enssen-Dubrowinskaja N, Feshchenko S, Lazjuk GI, Rogov YI, Dammann O, Bremer M, Karstens JH, Sohn C, Dork T. Association of two mutations in the CHEK2 gene with breast cancer. Int J Cancer 2005; 116(2):263–266.

Bork P, Hofmann K, Bucher P, Neuwald AF, Altschul SF, Koonin EV. A superfamily of conserved domains in DNA damage-responsive cell cycle checkpoint proteins. FASEB J 1997; 11(1):68–76.

Borressen AL, Andersen TI, Garber J, Barbier-Piraux N, Thorlacius S, Eyfjord J, Ottestad L, Smith-Sorensen B, Hovig E, Malkin D, Friend H. Screening for germ line TP53 mutations in breast cancer patients. Cancer Res 1992; 52:3234–3236.

Bose S, Chandran S, Mirocha JM, Bose N. The Akt pathway in human breast cancer: a tissue-array-based analysis. Mod Pathol 2006; 19(2):238–245.

Botuyan MV, Nomine Y, Yu X, Juranic N, Macura S, Chen J, Mer G. Structural basis of BACH1 phosphopeptide recognition by BRCA1 tandem BRCT domains. Structure 2004; 12(7):1137–1146.

Bougeard G, Limacher JM, Martin C, Charbonnier F, Killian A, Delattre O, Longy M, Jonveaux P, Fricker JP, Stoppa-Lyonnet D, Flaman JM, Frebourg T. Detection of 11 germline inactivating TP53 mutations and absence of TP63 and HCHK2 mutations in 17 French families with Li-Fraumeni or Li-Fraumeni-like syndrome. J Med Genet 2001; 38(4):253–257.

Bove BA, Roland L. Dunbrack J, Godwin AK. BRCA1, BRCA2, and hereditary breast cancer. Breast Cancer: Prognosis, Treatment, and Prevention, Pasqualini JR (ed.), Marcel Dekker, Inc., New York, 2002, 555–624.

Bowcock A. Breast cancer genes. Breast 1997; 3(suppl 3):1–6.

BRCA1 Exon 13 Duplication Screening Group. Theexon 13 duplication in the BRCA1 gene is a founder mutation present in geographically diverse populations. Am J Hum Genet 2000b; 67:207–212.

Breast Cancer Association Consortium. Commonly studied single-nucleotide polymorphisms and breast cancer: results from the Breast Cancer Association Consortium. J Natl Cancer Inst 2006; 98(19):1382–1396.

Breast Cancer Information Core (BIC). An open access on-line breast cancer mutation data base: BIC database. Available at: http://www.nhgri.nih.gov/Intramural_research/Lab_transfer/Bic/index.html (2007)

Breast Cancer Linkage Consortium (BCLC). Cancer risks in BRCA2 mutation carriers. J Natl Cancer Inst 1999; 91(15):1310–1316.

Breast Cancer Linkage Consortium (BCLC). Cancer risks in BRCA2 mutation carriers. J Natl Cancer Inst 2000; 91:1310–1316.

Brekelmans CT, Seynaeve C, Bartels CC, Tilanus-Linthorst MM, Meijers-Heijboer EJ, Crepin CM, van Geel AA, Menke M, Verhoog LC, van den Ouweland A, Obdeijn IM, Klijn JG. Effectiveness of breast cancer surveillance in BRCA1/2 gene mutation carriers and women with high familial risk. J Clin Oncol 2001; 19(4):924–930.

Brenner B, Fried G, Levitzki P, Rakowsky E, Lurie H, Idelevich E, Neuman A, Kaufman B, Sulkes J, Sulkes A. /*Cancer 2002; 94(8):2128–2133.

Brinkman H, Barwell J, Rose S, Tinworth L, Sodha N, Langman C, Brooks L, Payne S, Fisher S, Rowan A, Tomlinson I, Hodgson S. Evidence against a major genetic basis for combined breast and colorectal cancer susceptibility. Clin Genet 2006; 70(6):526–529.

Brody LC, Biesecker BB. Breast cancer susceptibility genes. BRCA1 and BRCA2. Medicine (Baltimore) 1998; 77(3):208–226.

Brose MS, Rebbeck TR, Calzone KA, Stopfer JE, Nathanson KL, Weber BL. Cancer risk estimates for BRCA1 mutation carriers identified in a risk evaluation program. J Natl Cancer Inst 2002; 94(18):1365–1372.

Brunet JS, Ghadirian P, Rebbeck TR, Lerman C, Garber J, Tonin PN, Abrahamson J, Foulkes WD, Daly M, Wagner-Costalas J, Godwin AK, Olopade F, Moslehi R, Liede A, Futreal PA, Weber B, Lenoir GM, Lynch HT, Narod SA. The effect of smoking on breast cancer incidence in BRCA1 and BRCA2 carriers. J Natl Cancer Inst 1998; 90:761–766.

Bryant HE, Schultz N, Thomas HD, Parker KM, Flower D, Lopez E, Kyle S, Meuth M, Curtin NJ, Helleday T. Specific killing of BRCA2-deficient tumours with inhibitors of poly(ADP-ribose) polymerase. Nature 2005; 434 (7035):913–917.

Brzovic PS, Meza J, King M-C, Klevit RE. The cancer-predisposing mutation C61G disrupts homodimer formation in the NH_2-terminal BRCA1 RING finger domain. J Biol Chem 1998; 273:7795–7799.

Brzovic PS, Rajagopal P, Hoyt DW, King MC, Klevit RE. Structure of a BRCA1-BARD1 heterodimeric RING-RING complex. Nat Struct Biol 2001; 8(10):833–837.

Burke W, Daly M, Garber J, Botkin J, Kahn M, Lunch P, McTiernan A, Offit K, Perlman J, Petersen G, Thomson E, Varricchio C. Recommendations for follow-up care of individuals with an inherited predisposition to cancer. II. *BRCA1* and *BRCA2*. Cancer Genetics Studies Consortium. JAMA 1997; 277:997–1003.

Byers PH. Killing the messenger: new insights into nonsense-mediated mRNA decay. J Clin Invest 2002; 109(1):3–6.

Cabart P, Chew HK, Murphy S. BRCA1 cooperates with NUFIP and P-TEFb to activate transcription by RNA polymerase II. Oncogene 2004; 23(31):5316–5329.

Caligo M, Ghimenti C, Cipollini G, Ricci S, Brunetti I, Marchetti V, Olsen R, Neuhausen S, Shattuck-Eidens D, Conte P, Skolnick M, Bevilacqua G. *BRCA1* germline mutational spectrum in Italian families from Tuscany: a high frequency of novel mutations. Oncogene 1996; 13:1483–1488.

Campbell IG, Baxter SW, Eccles DM, Choong DY. Methylenetetrahydrofolate reductase polymorphism and susceptibility to breast cancer. Breast Cancer Res 2002; 4(6):R14.

Cantor SB, Andreassen PR. Assessing the link between BACH1 and BRCA1 in the FA pathway. Cell Cycle 2006; 5(2): 164–167.

Cantor SB, Bell DW, Ganesan S, Kass EM, Drapkin R, Grossman S, Wahrer DC, Sgroi DC, Lane WS, Haber DA, Livingston DM. BACH1, a novel helicase-like protein, interacts directly with BRCA1 and contributes to its DNA repair function. Cell 2001; 105(1):149–160.

Carcangiu ML, Radice P, Manoukian S, Spatti G, Gobbo M, Pensotti V, Crucianelli R, Pasini B. Atypical epithelial proliferation in fallopian tubes in prophylactic salpingo-oophorectomy specimens from BRCA1 and BRCA2 germline mutation carriers. Int J Gynecol Pathol 2004; 23(1):35–40.

Carvalho MA, Marsillac SM, Karchin R, Manoukian S, Grist S, Swaby RF, Urmenyi TP, Rondinelli E, Silva R, Gayol L, Baumbach L, Sutphen R, Pickard-Brzosowicz JL, Nathanson KL, Sali A, Goldgar D, Couch FJ, Radice P, Monteiro AN. Determination of cancer risk associated with germ line BRCA1 missense variants by functional analysis. Cancer Res 2007; 67(4):1494–1501.

Casey MJ, Synder C, Bewtra C, Narod SA, Watson P, Lynch HT. Intra-abdominal carcinomatosis after prophylactic oophorectomy in women of hereditary breast ovarian cancer syndrome kindreds associated with BRCA1 and BRCA2 mutations. Gynecol Oncol 2005; 97(2):457–467.

Casilli F, Tournier I, Sinilnikova OM, Coulet F, Soubrier F, Houdayer C, Hardouin A, Berthet P, Sobol H, Bourdon V, Muller D, Fricker JP, Capoulade-Metay C, Chompret A, Nogues C, Mazoyer S, Chappuis P, Maillet P, Philippe C, Lortholary A, Gesta P, Bezieau S, Toulas C, Gladieff L, Maugard CM, Provencher DM, Dugast C, Delvincourt C, Nguyen TD, Faivre L, Bonadona V, Frebourg T, Lidereau R, Stoppa-Lyonnet D, Tosi M. The contribution of germline rearrangements to the spectrum of BRCA2 mutations. J Med Genet 2006; 43(9):e49.

Chai YL, Cui J, Shao N, Shyam E, Reddy P, Rao VN. The second BRCT domain of BRCA1 proteins interacts with p53 and stimulates transcription from the p21WAF1/CIP1 promoter. Oncogene 1999; 18(1):263–268.

Chamberlain J, Boehnke M, Frank TS, Kiousis S, Xu J, Guo S, Hauser E, Norum R, Helmbold E, Markel D, Keshavarzi S, Jackso C, Calzone K, Garber J, Collins F, Weber B. BRCA1 maps proximal to D17S579 on chromosome 17q21 by genetic analysis. Am J Hum Genet 1993; 52:792–798.

Chang JC, Wooten EC, Tsimelzon A, Hilsenbeck SG, Gutierrez MC, Elledge R, Mohsin S, Osborne CK, Chamness GC, Allred DC, O'Connell P. Gene expression profiling for the prediction of therapeutic response to docetaxel in patients with breast cancer. Lancet 2003; 362(9381):362–369.

Chang-Claude J, Becher H, Eby N, Bastert G, Wahrendorf J, Hamann U. Modifying effect of reproductive risk factors on the age at onset of breast cancer for German BRCA1 mutation carriers. J Cancer Res Clin Oncol 1997; 123(5): 272–279.

Chappuis PO, Donato E, Goffin JR, Wong N, Begin LR, Kapusta LR, Brunet JS, Porter P, Foulkes WD. Cyclin E expression in breast cancer: predicting germline BRCA1 mutations, prognosis and response to treatment. Ann Oncol 2005; 16(5):735–742.

Chehab N, Malikzay A, Appe M, Halazonetis T. Chk2/hCds1 functions as a DNA damage checkpoint in G(1) by stabilizing p53. Genes Dev 2000; 14:278–288.

Chen GC, Guan LS, Yu JH, Li GC, Choi Kim HR, Wang ZY. Rb-associated protein 46 (RbAp46) inhibits transcriptional transactivation mediated by BRCA1. Biochem Biophys Res Commun 2001; 284(2):507–514.

Chen J, Silver DP, Walpita D, Canton SB, Gazdar AF, Tomlinson G, Couch FJ, Weber BL, Ashley T, Livingston DM, Scully R. Stable interaction between the products of the BRCA1 and BRCA2 tumor suppressor genes in mitotic and meiotic cells. Mol Cell 1998; 2:317–328.

Chen P, Chen U, Bookstein R, Lee W. Genetic mechanisms of tumor suppression by the human p53 gene. Science 1990; 250:1576–1580.

Chenevix-Trench G, Healey S, Lakhani S, Waring P, Cummings M, Brinkworth R, Deffenbaugh AM, Burbidge LA, Pruss D, Judkins T, Scholl T, Bekessy A, Marsh A, Lovelock P, Wong M, Tesoriero A, Renard H, Southey M, Hopper JL, Yannoukakos K, Brown M, Easton D, Tavtigian SV, Goldgar D, Spurdle AB. Genetic and histopathologic evaluation of BRCA1 and BRCA2 DNA sequence variants of unknown clinical significance. Cancer Res 2006; 66(4): 2019–2027.

Cheung AM, Elia A, Tsao MS, Done S, Wagner KU, Hennighausen L, Hakem R, Mak TW. Brca2 deficiency does not impair mammary epithelium development but promotes mammary adenocarcinoma formation in p53(+/−) mutant mice. Cancer Res 2004; 64(6):1959–1965.

Claes K, Machackova E, DeVos M, Poppe B, DePaepe A, Messiaen L. Mutation analysis of the BRCA1 and BRCA2 genes in the Belgian patient population and identification of a Belgian founder mutation BRCA1 IVS5+3A>G. Dis Markers 1999; 15:69–73.

Clapperton JA, Manke IA, Lowery DM, Ho T, Haire LF, Yaffe MB, Smerdon SJ. Structure and mechanism of BRCA1 BRCT domain recognition of phosphorylated BACH1 with implications for cancer. Nat Struct Mol Biol 2004; 11(6):512–518.

Claus E, Risch N, Thompson W. Autosomal dominant inheritance of early-onset breast cancer: implications for risk prediction. Cancer 1994; 73:643–651.

Colgan TJ, Murphy J, Cole DE, Narod S, Rosen B. Occult carcinoma in prophylactic oophorectomy specimens: prevalence and association with BRCA germline mutation status. Am J Surg Pathol 2001; 25(10):1283–1289.

Colilla S, Kantoff PW, Neuhausen SL, Godwin AK, Daly MB, Narod SA, Garber JE, Lynch HT, Brown M, Weber BL, Rebbeck TR. The joint effect of smoking and AIB1 on breast cancer risk in BRCA1 mutation carriers. Carcinogenesis 2006; 27(3):599–605.

Collins FS. *BRCA1*—lots of mutations, lots of dilemmas. N Engl J Med 1996; 334:186–188.

Collins N, Wooster R, Stratton MR. Absence of methylation of CpG dinucleotides within the promoter of the breast cancer susceptibility gene BRCA2 in normal tissues and in breast and ovarian cancers. Br J Cancer 1997; 76(9):1150–1156.

Consortium BCL. Cancer risks in BRCA2 mutation carriers. J Natl Cancer Inst 1999; 91:1310–1316.

Cortez D, Wang Y, Qin J, Elledge S. Requirement of ATM-dependent phosphorylation of brca1 in the DNA damage response to double-strand breaks. Science 1999; 286: 1162–1166.

Cotton RGH. Current methods of mutation detection. Mutat Res 1993; 285:125–144.

Cotton RGH (ed.). Mutation Detection: A Practical Approach. Oxford, UK: Oxford University Press. 1997.

Couch FJ, DeShano ML, Blackwood MA, Calzone K, Stopfer J, Campeau L, Ganguly A, Rebbeck T, Weber BL. *BRCA1* mutations in women attending clinics that evaluate the risk of breast cancer. N Engl J Med 1997; 336:1409–1415.

Couch FJ, Farid LM, DeShano ML, Tavtigian SV, Calzone K, Campeau L, Peng Y, Bogden B, Chen Q, Neuhausen S, Shattuck-Eidens D, Godwin AK, Daly M, Radford DM, Sedlacek S, Rommens J, Simard J, Garber J, Merajver S, Weber BL. BRCA2 germline mutations in male breast cancer cases and breast cancer families. Nat Genet 1996; 13:123–125.

Coutelle C, Hohn B, Benesova M, Oneta CM, Quattrochi P, Roth HJ, Schmidt-Gayk H, Schneeweiss A, Bastert G, Seitz HK. Risk factors in alcohol associated breast cancer: alcohol dehydrogenase polymorphism and estrogens. Int J Oncol 2004; 25(4):1127–1132.

Cox A, Dunning AM, Garcia-Closas M, Balasubramanian S, Reed MW, Pooley KA, Scollen S, Baynes C, Ponder BA, Chanock S, Lissowska J, Brinton L, Peplonska B, Southey MC, Hopper JL, McCredie MR, Giles GG, Fletcher O, Johnson N, Dos Santos Silva I, Gibson L, Bojesen SE, Nordestgaard BG, Axelsson CK, Torres D, Hamann U, Justenhoven C, Brauch H, Chang-Claude J, Kropp S, Risch A, Wang-Gohrke S, Schurmann P, Bogdanova N, Dork T, Fagerholm R, Aaltonen K, Blomqvist C, Nevanlinna H, Seal S, Renwick A, Stratton MR, Rahman N, Sangrajrang S, Hughes D, Odefrey F, Brennan P, Spurdle AB, Chenevix-Trench G, Beesley J, Mannermaa A, Hartikainen J, Kataja V, Kosma VM, Couch FJ, Olson JE, Goode EL, Broeks A, Schmidt MK, Hogervorst FB, Veer LJ, Kang D, Yoo KY, Noh DY, Ahn SH, Wedren S, Hall P, Low YL, Liu J, Milne RL, Ribas G, Gonzalez-Neira A, Benitez J, Sigurdson AJ, Stredrick DL, Alexander BH, Struewing JP, Pharoah PD, Easton DF. A common coding variant in CASP8 is associated with breast cancer risk. Nat Genet 2007; 39(3): 352–358.

Coyne RS, McDonald HB, Edgemon K, Brody LC. Functional characterization of BRCA1 sequence variants using a yeast small colony phenotype assay. Cancer Biol Ther 2004; 3(5):453–457.

Crackower MA, Scherer SW, Rommens JM, Hui CC, Poorkaj P, Soder S, Cobben JM, Hudgins L, Evans JP, Tsui LC. Characterization of the split hand/split foot malformation locus SHFM1 at 7q21.3-q22.1 and analysis of a candidate gene for its expression during limb development. Hum Mol Genet 1996; 5(5):571–579.

Cui J, Antoniou AC, Dite GS, Southey MC, Venter DJ, Easton DF, Giles GG, McCredie MR, Hopper JL. After BRCA1 and BRCA2-what next? Multifactorial segregation analyses of three-generation, population-based Australian families affected by female breast cancer. Am J Hum Genet 2001; 68(2):420–431.

Cummings S, Eckert S, Krueger K, Grady D, Powles T, Cauley J, Norton L, Nickelsen T, Bjarnason N, Morrow M, Lippman M, Black D, Glusman J, Costa A, Jordan V. The effect of raloxifene on risk of breast cancer in postmenopausal women: results from the MORE randomized trial. Multiple Outcomes of Raloxifene Evaluation. JAMA 1999; 281:2189–2197.

Cybulski C, Gorski B, Huzarski T, Masojc B, Mierzejewski M, Debniak T, Teodorczyk U, Byrski T, Gronwald J, Matyjasik J, Zlowocka E, Lenner M, Grabowska E, Nej K, Castaneda J, Medrek K, Szymanska A, Szymanska J, Kurzawski G, Suchy J, Oszurek O, Witek A, Narod SA, Lubinski J. CHEK2 is a multiorgan cancer susceptibility gene. Am J Hum Genet 2004; 75(6):1131–1135.

Cybulski C, Wokolorczyk D, Huzarski T, Byrski T, Gronwald J, Gorski B, Debniak T, Masoje B, Jakubowska A, van de Wetering T, Narod SA, Lubinski J. A deletion in CHEK2 of 5,395 bp predisposes to breast cancer in Poland. Breast Cancer Res Treat 2007; 102:119–122.

Damin AP, Frazzon AP, Damin DC, Roehe A, Hermes V, Zettler C, Alexandre CO. Evidence for an association of TP53 codon 72 polymorphism with breast cancer risk. Cancer Detect Prev 2006; 30(6):523–529.

Daniels MJ, Wang Y, Lee M, Venkitaraman AR. Abnormal cytokinesis in cells deficient in the breast cancer susceptibility protein BRCA2. Science 2004; 306(5697):876–879.

Dantzer F, de La Rubia G, Menissier-De Murcia J, Hostomsky Z, de Murcia G, Schreiber V. Base excision repair is impaired in mammalian cells lacking Poly(ADP-ribose) polymerase-1. Biochemistry 2000; 39(25):7559–7569.

Davies AA, Masson JY, McIlwraith MJ, Stasiak AZ, Stasiak A, Venkitaraman AR, West SC. Role of BRCA2 in control of the RAD51 recombination and DNA repair protein. Mol Cell 2001; 7(2):273–282.

de Jong MM, Nolte IM, te Meerman GJ, van der Graaf WT, Oosterwijk JC, Kleibeuker JH, Schaapveld M, de Vries EG. Genes other than BRCA1 and BRCA2 involved in breast cancer susceptibility. J Med Genet 2002; 39(4):225–242.

de la Hoya M, Diez O, Perez-Segura P, Godino J, Fernandez JM, Sanz J, Alonso C, Baiget M, Diaz-Rubio E, Caldes T. Pre-test prediction models of BRCA1 or BRCA2 mutation in breast/ovarian families attending familial cancer clinics. J Med Genet 2003; 40(7):503–510.

de la Hoya M, Gutierrez-Enriquez S, Velasco E, Osorio A, Sanchez de Abajo A, Vega A, Salazar R, Esteban E, Llort G, Gonzalez-Sarmiento R, Carracedo A, Benitez J, Miner C, Diez O, Diaz-Rubio E, Caldes T. Genomic rearrangements at the BRCA1 locus in Spanish families with breast/ovarian cancer. Clin Chem 2006; 52(8): 1480–1485.

Del Tito B, Poff H, Novotny M, Cartledge D, Walker R, Earl C, Bailey A. Automated fluorescent analysis procedure for enzymatic mutation detection. Clinical Chem 1998; 44:731–739.

Deng C, Scott F. Role of the tumor suppressor gene Brca1 in genetic stability and mammary gland tumor formation. Oncogene 2000; 19:1059–1064.

Deng CX. BRCA1: cell cycle checkpoint, genetic instability, DNA damage response and cancer evolution. Nucleic Acids Res 2006; 34(5):1416–1426.

Devilee P. BRCA1 and BRCA2 testing: Weighing the demand against the benefits. Am J Hum Genet 1999; 64:943–948.

Domchek SM, Friebel TM, Neuhausen SL, Wagner T, Evans G, Isaacs C, Garber JE, Daly MB, Eeles R, Matloff E, Tomlinson GE, Van't Veer L, Lynch HT, Olopade OI, Weber BL, Rebbeck TR. Mortality after bilateral salpingo-oophorectomy in BRCA1 and BRCA2 mutation carriers: a prospective cohort study. Lancet Oncol 2006; 7(3):223–229.

Domchek SM, Weber BL. Clinical management of BRCA1 and BRCA2 mutation carriers. Oncogene 2006; 25(43): 5825–5831.

Dong JT. Prevalent mutations in prostate cancer. J Cell Biochem 2006; 97(3):433–447.

Dong Y, Hakimi MA, Chen X, Kumaraswamy E, Cooch NS, Godwin AK, Shiekhattar R. Regulation of BRCC, a holoenzyme complex containing BRCA1 and BRCA2, by a signalosome-like subunit and its role in DNA repair. Mol Cell 2003; 12(5):1087–1099.

Drucker L, Stackievitz R, Shpitz B, Yarkoni S. Incidence of BRCA1 and BRCA2 mutations in Ashkenazi colorectal cancer patients: preliminary study. Anticancer Res 2000; 20:559–561.

Duell EJ, Millikan RC, Pittman GS, Winkel S, Lunn RM, Tse CK, Eaton A, Mohrenweiser HW, Newman B, Bell DA. Polymorphisms in the DNA repair gene XRCC1 and breast cancer. Cancer Epidemiol Biomarkers Prev 2001; 10(3):217–222.

Dufault MR, Betz B, Wappenschmidt B, Hofmann W, Bandick K, Golla A, Pietschmann A, Nestle-Kramling C, Rhiem K, Huttner C, von Lindern C, Dall P, Kiechle M, Untch M, Jonat W, Meindl A, Scherneck S, Niederacher D, Schmutzler RK, Arnold N. Limited relevance of the CHEK2 gene in hereditary breast cancer. Int J Cancer 2004; 110(3):320–325.

Dumitrescu RG, Cotarla I. Understanding breast cancer risk: where do we stand in 2005? J Cell Mol Med 2005; 9(1):208–221.

Easton D, Ford D, Bishop D. Breast and ovarian cancer incidence in BRCA1-mutation carriers. Breast Cancer Linkage Consortium. Am J Hum Genet 1995; 56:265–271.

Easton DF, Steele L, Fields P, Ormiston W, Averill D, Daly PA, McManus R, Neuhausen SL, Ford D, Wooster R, Cannon-Albright LA, Stratton MR, Goldgar DE. Cancer Risks in two large breast cancer families linked to BRCA2 on chromosome 13q12-13. Am J Hum Genet 1997; 61:120–128.

Edwards SM, Kote-Jarai Z, Meitz J, Hamoudi R, Hope Q, Osin P, Jackson R, Southgate C, Singh R, Falconer A, Dearnaley DP, Ardern-Jones A, Murkin A, Dowe A, Kelly J, Williams S, Oram R, Stevens M, Teare DM, Ponder BA, Gayther SA, Easton DF, Eeles RA. Two percent of men with early-onset prostate cancer harbor germline mutations in the BRCA2 gene. Am J Hum Genet 2003; 72(1):1–12.

Eerola H, Heikkila P, Tamminen A, Aittomaki K, Blomqvist C, Nevanlinna H. Histopathological features of breast tumours in BRCA1, BRCA2 and mutation-negative breast cancer families. Breast Cancer Res 2005a; 7(1):R93–R100.

Eerola H, Heikkila P, Tamminen A, Aittomaki K, Blomqvist C, Nevanlinna H. Relationship of patients' age to histopathological features of breast tumours in BRCA1 and BRCA2 and mutation-negative breast cancer families. Breast Cancer Res 2005b; 7(4):R465–R469.

Egan KM, Newcomb PA, Longnecker MP, Trentham-Dietz A, Baron JA, Trichopoulos D, Stampfer MJ, Willett WC. Jewish religion and risk of breast cancer. Lancet 1996; 347:1645–1646.

Ekblad CM, Wilkinson HR, Schymkowitz JW, Rousseau F, Freund SM, Itzhaki LS. Characterisation of the BRCT domains of the breast cancer susceptibility gene product BRCA1. J Mol Biol 2002; 320(3):431–442.

El-Deiry WS, Harper JW, O'Conner PM, Velculescu VE, Canman CE, Jackman J, Peintenpol JA, Burrell M, Hill DE, Wang Y, Wilman KG, Mercer WE, Kastan MB, Konh KW, Elledge SJ, Kinzler KW, Vogelstein B. WAF1/CIP1 is induced in p53-mediated G1 arrest and apoptosis. Cancer Res 1994; 54:1169–1174.

Ellis D, Patel Y, Yau SC, Hodgson SV, Abbs, SJ. Low prevalence of *BRCA1* exon rearrangements in familial and young sporadic breast cancer patients. Fam Cancer 2006; 5(4): 323–326. Epub 2006 May 25.

Elmore JG, Moceri VM, Carter D, Larson EB. Breast carcinoma tumor characteristics in black and white women. Cancer 1998; 83(12):2509–2515.

ElShamy WM, Livingston DM. Identification of BRCA1-IRIS, a BRCA1 locus product. Nat Cell Biol 2004; 6(10):954–967.

Eng C, Brody LC, Wagner TM, Devilee P, Vijg J, Szabo C, Tavtigian SV, Nathanson KL, Ostrander E, Frank TS. Interpreting epidemiological research: blinded comparison of methods used to estimate the prevalence of inherited mutations in BRCA1. J Med Genet 2001; 38(12):824–833.

Engin H, Baltali E, Guler N, Guler G, Tekuzman G, Uner A. Expression of PTEN, cyclin D1, P27/KIP1 in invasive ductal carcinomas of the breast and correlation with clinicopathological parameters. Bull Cancer 2006; 93(2):E21–E26.

Eppink B, Wyman C, Kanaar R. Multiple interlinked mechanisms to circumvent DNA replication roadblocks. Exp Cell Res 2006; 312(14):2660–2665.

Ergul E, Sazci A, Utkan Z, Canturk NZ. Polymorphisms in the MTHFR gene are associated with breast cancer. Tumour Biol 2003; 24(6):286–290.

Erkko H, Xia B, Nikkila J, Schleutker J, Syrjakoski K, Mannermaa A, Kallioniemi A, Pylkas K, Karppinen SM, Rapakko K, Miron A, Sheng Q, Li G, Mattila H, Bell DW, Haber DA, Grip M, Reiman M, Jukkola-Vuorinen A, Mustonen A, Kere J, Aaltonen LA, Kosma VM, Kataja V, Soini Y, Drapkin RI, Livingston DM, Winqvist R. A recurrent mutation in PALB2 in Finnish cancer families. Nature 2007; 446(7133):316–319.

Esashi F, Christ N, Gannon J, Liu Y, Hunt T, Jasin M, West SC. CDK-dependent phosphorylation of BRCA2 as a regulatory mechanism for recombinational repair. Nature 2005; 434 (7033):598–604.

Esteban-Cardenosa E, Duran M, Infante M, Velasco E, Miner C. High-throughput mutation detection method to scan BRCA1 and BRCA2 based on heteroduplex analysis by capillary array electrophoresis. Clin Chem 2004; 50(2):313–320.

Esteller M. Epigenetic lesions causing genetic lesions in human cancer, promoter hypermethylation of DNA repair genes. Eur J Cancer 2000; 36:2294–2300.

Esteller M, Corn PG, Baylin SB, Herman JG. A gene hypermethylation profile of human cancer. Cancer Res 2001; 61(8):3225–3229.

Euhus DM, Smith KC, Robinson L, Stucky A, Olopade OI, Cummings S, Garber JE, Chittenden A, Mills GB, Rieger P, Esserman L, Crawford B, Hughes KS, Roche CA, Ganz PA,

Seldon J, Fabian CJ, Klemp J, Tomlinson G. Pretest prediction of BRCA1 or BRCA2 mutation by risk counselors and the computer model BRCAPRO. J Natl Cancer Inst 2002; 94(11):844–851.

Evans DG, Eccles DM, Rahman N, Young K, Bulman M, Amir E, Shenton A, Howell A, Lalloo F. A new scoring system for the chances of identifying a BRCA1/2 mutation outperforms existing models including BRCAPRO. J Med Genet 2004; 41(6):474–480.

Eyfjord JE, Bodvarsdottir SK. Genomic instability and cancer: networks involved in response to DNA damage. Mutation Res 2005; 592:18–28.

Fabbro M, Savage K, Hobson K, Deans AJ, Powell SN, McArthur GA, Khanna KK. BRCA1-BARD1 complexes are required for p53Ser-15 phosphorylation and a G1/S arrest following ionizing radiation-induced DNA damage. J Biol Chem 2004; 279(30):31251–31258.

Fan S, Ma YX, Wang C, Yuan RQ, Meng Q, Wang JA, Erdos M, Goldberg ID, Webb P, Kushner PJ, Pestell RG, Rosen EM. p300 Modulates the BRCA1 inhibition of estrogen receptor activity. Cancer Res 2002a; 62(1):141–151.

Fan S, Wang J, Yuan R, Ma Y, Meng Q, Erdos M, Pestell R, Yuan F, Auborn K, Goldberg I, Rosen E. BRCA1 inhibition of estrogen receptor signaling in transfected cells. Science 1999; 284:1354–1356.

Fan W, Jin S, Tong T, Zhao H, Fan F, Antinore MJ, Rajasekaran B, Wu M, Zhan Q. BRCA1 regulates GADD45 through its interactions with the OCT-1 and CAAT motifs. J Biol Chem 2002b; 277(10):8061–8067.

Fanconi G. Familial constitutional panmyelocytopathy, Fanconi's anemia (F.A.). I. Clinical aspects. Semin Hematol 1967; 4(3):233–240.

Farmer H, McCabe N, Lord CJ, Tutt AN, Johnson DA, Richardson TB, Santarosa M, Dillon KJ, Hickson I, Knights C, Martin NM, Jackson SP, Smith GC, Ashworth A. Targeting the DNA repair defect in BRCA mutant cells as a therapeutic strategy. Nature 2005; 434(7035):917–921.

Favis R, Day J, Gerry N, Phelan C, Narod S, Barany F. Universal DNA array detection of small insertions and deletions in BRCA1 and BRCA2. Nat Biotechnol 2000; 18:561–564.

Fedier A, Steiner RA, Schwarz VA, Lenherr L, Haller U, Fink D. The effect of loss of Brca1 on the sensitivity to anticancer agents in p53-deficient cells. Int J Oncol 2003; 22(5): 1169–1173.

Feng Z, Kachnic L, Zhang J, Powell SN, Xia F. DNA damage induces p53-dependent BRCA1 nuclear export. J Biol Chem 2004; 279(27):28574–28584.

Fenton H, Carlile B, Montgomery EA, Carraway H, Herman J, Sahin F, Su GH, Argani P. LKB1 protein expression in human breast cancer. Appl Immunohistochem Mol Morphol 2006; 14(2):146–153.

Feunteun J, Lenoir GM. *BRCA1*, a gene involved in inherited predisposition to breast and ovarian cancer. Biochim Biophys Acta 1996; 1242:177–180.

Fisher B, Costantino JP, Wickerham DL, Redmond CK, Kavanah M, Cronin WM, Vogel V, Robidoux A, Dimitrov N, Atkins J, Daly M, Wieand S, Tan-Chiu E, Ford L, Wolmark N. Tamoxifen for prevention of breast cancer: report of the National Surgical Adjuvant Breast and Bowel Project P-1 Study. J Natl Cancer Inst 1998; 90(18): 1371–1388.

FitzGerald M, MacDonald D, Krainer M, Hoover I, O'Neil E, Unsal H, Silva-Arrieto S, Findelstein D, Beer-Romero P, Englert C, Sgroi D, Smith B, Younger J, Garter J, Duda R, Mayzel K, Isselbacher K, Friend S, Haber D. Germ-line BRCA1 mutations in Jewish and non-Jewish women with early-onset breast cancer. N Engl J Med 1996; 334:143–149.

Fleming MA, Potter JD, Ramirez CJ, Ostrander GK, Ostrander EA. Understanding missense mutations in the BRCA1 gene: an evolutionary approach. Proc Natl Acad Sci U S A 2003; 100(3):1151–1156.

Fodde R, Losekoot M. Mutation detection by denaturing gradient gel electrophoreses (DGGE). Hum Mutat 1994; 3:83–94.

Fodor FH, Weston A, Bleiweiss IJ, McCurdy LD, Walsh MM, Tartter PI, Brower ST, Eng CM. Frequency and carrier risk associated with common BRCA1 and BRCA2 mutations in Ashkenazi Jewish breast cancer patients. Am J Hum Genet 1998; 63:45–51.

Foray N, Marot D, Gabriel A, Randrianarison V, Carr AM, Perricaudet M, Ashworth A, Jeggo P. A subset of ATM- and ATR-dependent phosphorylation events requires the BRCA1 protein. Embo J 2003; 22(11):2860–2871.

Ford D, Easton D, Bishop D, Narod S, Goldgar D. Risks of cancer in BRCA1-mutation carriers. Breast cancer linkage consortium. Lancet 1994; 343:692–695.

Ford D, Easton D, Peto J. Estimate of the gene frequency of BRCA1 and its contribution to breast and ovarian cancer incidence. Am J Hum Genet 1995; 57:1457–1462.

Ford D, Easton D, Stratton M, Narod S, Goldgar D, Devilee P, DT B, Weber B, Lenoir G, Chang-Claude J, Sobol H, Teare M, Struewing J, Arason A, Scherneck S, Peto J, Rebbeck T, Tonin P, Newhausen S, Barkardottir R, Eyfjord J, Lynch H, Ponder A, Gayther S, Birch J, Lindblom A, Stoppa-Lyonnet D, Bignon Y, Borg A, Hamann U, Haites N, Scott R, Maugard C, Vasen H, Seitz S, Cannon-Albright L, Schofield A, Zelada-Hedman M, Consortium BCL. Genetic heterogeneity and penetrance analysis of the BRCA1 and BRCA2 genes in breast cancer families. Am J Hum Genet 1998; 62:676–689.

Fortin J, Moisan AM, Dumont M, Leblanc G, Labrie Y, Durocher F, Bessette P, Bridge P, Chiquette J, Laframboise R, Lepine J, Lesperance B, Pichette R, Plante M, Provencher L, Voyer P, Simard J. A new alternative splice variant of BRCA1 containing an additional in-frame exon. Biochim Biophys Acta 2005; 1731(1):57–65.

Foulkes WD, Brunet JS, Stefansson IM, Straume O, Chappuis PO, Begin LR, Hamel N, Goffin JR, Wong N, Trudel M, Kapusta L, Porter P, Akslen LA. The prognostic implication of the basal-like (cyclin E high/*p27* low/p53+/glomeruloid-microvascular-proliferation+) phenotype of BRCA1-related breast cancer. Cancer Res 2004a; 64(3):830–835.

Foulkes WD, Metcalfe K, Sun P, Hanna WM, Lynch HT, Ghadirian P, Tung N, Olopade OI, Weber BL, McLennan J, Olivotto IA, Begin LR, Narod SA. Estrogen receptor status in BRCA1- and BRCA2-related breast cancer: the influence of age, grade, and histological type. Clin Cancer Res 2004b; 10(6):2029–2034.

Foulkes WD, Stefansson IM, Chappuis PO, Begin LR, Goffin JR, Wong N, Trudel M, Akslen LA. Germline BRCA1 mutations and a basal epithelial phenotype in breast cancer. J Natl Cancer Inst 2003; 95(19):1482–1485.

Frank TS, Deffenbaugh AM, Reid JE, Hulick M, Ward BE, Lingenfelter B, Gumpper KL, Scholl T, Tavtigian SV, Pruss DR, Critchfield GC. Clinical characteristics of individuals with germline mutations in BRCA1 and BRCA2: analysis of 10,000 individuals. J Clin Oncol 2002; 20(6):1480–1490.

Frank TS, Manley SA, Olopade OI, Cummings S, Garber JE, Bernhardt B, Antman K, Russo D, Wood ME, Mullineau L, Isaacs C, Peshkin B, Buys S, Venne V, Rowley PT, Loader S, Offit K, Robson M, Hampel H, Brener D, Winer EP, Clark S, Weber B, Strong LC, Thomas A, et al., Sequence analysis of BRCA1 and BRCA2: correlation of mutations with family history and ovarian cancer risk. J Clin Oncol 1998; 16(7):2417–2425.

Frebourg T, Barbier N, Yan Y, Garber J, Dreyfus M, Fraumeni J, Li F, Friend S. Germ-line p53 mutations in 15 families with Li-Fraumeni syndrome. Am J Hum Genet 1995; 56: 608–615.

Freneaux P, Stoppa-Lyonnet D, Mouret E, Kambouchner M, Nicolas A, Zafrani B, Vincent-Salomon A, Fourquet A, Magdelenat H, Sastre-Garau X. Low expression of bcl-2 in Brca1-associated breast cancers. Br J Cancer 2000; 83 (10):1318–1322.

Freudenheim JL, Ambrosone CB, Moysich KB, Vena JE, Graham S, Marshall JR, Muti P, Laughlin R, Nemoto T, Harty LC, Crits GA, Chan AW, Shields PG. Alcohol dehydrogenase 3 genotype modification of the association of alcohol consumption with breast cancer risk. Cancer Causes Control 1999; 10(5):369–377.

Friedenson B. BRCA1 and BRCA2 pathways and the risk of cancers other than breast or ovarian. MedGenMed 2005; 7(2):60.

Frolov A, Prowse AH, Vanderveer L, Bove B, Wu H, Godwin AK. DNA array-based method for detection of large rearrangements in the BRCA1 gene. Genes Chromosomes Cancer 2002; 35(3):232–241.

Funakoshi M, Li X, Velichutina I, Hochstrasser M, Kobayashi H. Sem1, the yeast ortholog of a human BRCA2-binding protein, is a component of the proteasome regulatory particle that enhances proteasome stability. J Cell Sci 2004; 117(pt 26):6447–6454.

Futamura M, Arakawa H, Matsuda K, Katagiri T, Saji S, Miki Y, Nakamura Y. Potential role of BRCA2 in a mitotic checkpoint after phosphorylation by hBUBR1. Cancer Res 2000; 60(6):1531–1535.

Futreal PA, Liu Q, Shattuck-Eidens D, Cochran C, Harchman K, Tavtigian S, Bennett LM, Haugen-Strano A, Swensen J, Miki Y, Eddington K, McClure M, Frye C, Weaver-Feldhaus J, Ding W, Gholami Z, Soderkvist P, Terry L, Jhanwar S, Berchuck A, Inglehart J, Marks J, Ballinger G, Barrett J, Skolnick M, Kamb A, Wiseman R. BRCA1 mutations in primary breast and ovarian carcinomas. Science 1994; 266:120–122.

Gad S, Caux-Moncoutier V, Pages-Berhouet S, Gauthier-Villars M, Coupier I, Pujol P, Frenay M, Gilbert B, Maugard C, Bignon YJ, Chevrier A, Rossi A, Fricker JP, Nguyen TD, Demange L, Aurias A, Bensimon A, Stoppa-Lyonnet D. Significant contribution of large BRCA1 gene rearrangements in 120 French breast and ovarian cancer families. Oncogene 2002; 21(44):6841–6847.

Gail M, Brinton L, Byar D, Corle D, Green S, Schairer C, Mulvihill J. Projecting individualized probabilities of developing breast cancer for white females who are being examined annually. J Natl Cancer Inst 1989; 81:1879–1886.

Gaiser OJ, Ball LJ, Schmieder P, Leitner D, Strauss H, Wahl M, Kuhne R, Oschkinat H, Heinemann U. Solution structure, backbone dynamics, and association behavior of the C-terminal BRCT domain from the breast cancer-associated protein BRCA1. Biochemistry 2004; 43(51): 15983–15995.

Galkin VE, Esashi F, Yu X, Yang S, West SC, Egelman EH. BRCA2 BRC motifs bind RAD51-DNA filaments. Proc Natl Acad Sci U S A 2005; 102(24):8537–8542.

Gao Q, Neuhausen S, Cummings S, Luce M, Olopade OI. Recurrent germ-line BRCA1 mutations in extended African American families with early-onset breast cancer. Am J Hum Genet 1997a; 60(5):1233–1236.

Gao Q, Neuhausen S, Cummings S, Luce MC, Olopade F. Recurrent germline BRCA1 mutations in extended African American families with early-onset breast cancer. Am J Hum Genet 1997b; 60:1233–1236.

Gapstur SM, Dupuis J, Gann P, Collila S, Winchester DP. Hormone receptor status of breast tumors in black, Hispanic, and non-Hispanic white women. An analysis of 13,239 cases. Cancer 1996; 77(8):1465–1471.

Gatei M, Scott SP, Filippovitch I, Soronika N, Lavin MF, Weber B, Khanna KK. Role for ATM in DNA damage-induced phosphorylation of BRCA1. Cancer Res 2000; 60(12): 3299–3304.

Gatei M, Zhou BB, Hobson K, Scott S, Young D, Khanna KK. Ataxia telangiectasia mutated (ATM) kinase and ATM and Rad3 related kinase mediate phosphorylation of Brca1 at distinct and overlapping sites. In vivo assessment using phospho-specific antibodies. J Biol Chem 2001; 276(20): 17276–17280.

Gatti RA, Berkel I, Boder E, Braedt G, Charmley P, Concannon P, Ersoy F, Foroud T, Jaspers NG, Lange K, et al., Localization of an ataxia-telangiectasia gene to chromosome 11q22-23. Nature 1988; 336(6199):577–580.

Gatti RA, Tward A, Concannon P. Cancer risk in ATM heterozygotes: a model of phenotypic and mechanistic differences between missense and truncating mutations. Mol Genet Metab 1999; 68(4):419–423.

Gayther S, Mangion J, Russell P, Seal S, Barfoot R, Ponder B, Stratton M, Easton D. Variation of risks of breast and ovarian cancer associated with different germline mutations of the BRCA2 gene. Nat Genet 1997; 15:103–105.

Gayther S, Warren W, Mazoyer S, Russell P, Harrington P, Chiano M, Seal S, Hamoudi R,van Rensburg E, Dunning A, Love R, Evans G, Easton D, Clayton D, Stratton M, Ponder B. Germline mutations of the BRCA1 gene in breast/ovarian cancer families: evidence for a genotype/phenotype correlation. Nat Genet 1995; 11:428–433.

Gerry N, Witowski N, Day J, Hammer R, Barany G, Barany F. Universal DNA microarray method for multiplex detection of low abundance point mutations. J Mol Biol 1999; 292:251–262.

Giordano SH, Buzdar AU, Hortobagyi GN. Breast cancer in men. Ann Intern Med 2002; 137(8):678–687.

Glavac D, Dean M. Optimization of the single-strand conformation polymorphism (SSCP) technique for detection of point mutations. Hum Mutat 1993; 2:404–414.

Glover JN, Williams RS, Lee MS. Interactions between BRCT repeats and phosphoproteins: tangled up in two. Trends Biochem Sci 2004; 29(11):579–585.

Godard J, Dodds W, Phillips J, Scanlon G. Peutz-Jeghers syndrome: clinical and roentgenographic features. Am J Roentgenol Radium Ther Nucl Med 1971; 113:316–324.

Goggins M, Hruban R, Kern S. BRCA2 is inactivated late in the development of pancreatic intraepithelial neoplasia: evidence and implications. Am J Pathol 2000; 156:1767–1771.

Goldgar DE, Easton DF, Deffenbaugh AM, Monteiro AN, Tavtigian SV, Couch FJ. Integrated evaluation of DNA sequence variants of unknown clinical significance: application to BRCA1 and BRCA2. Am J Hum Genet 2004; 75(4):535–544.

Gonzalez CI, Bhattacharya A, Wang W, Peltz SW. Nonsense-mediated mRNA decay in Saccharomyces cerevisiae. Gene 2001; 274(1–2):15–25.

Goode EL, Ulrich CM, Potter JD. Polymorphisms in DNA repair genes and associations with cancer risk. Cancer Epidemiol Biomarkers Prev 2002; 11(12):1513–1530.

Goodman MF. Coping with replication 'train wrecks' in Escherichia coli using Pol V, Pol II and RecA proteins. Trends Biochem Sci 2000; 25(4):189–195.

Gorski B, Byrski T, Huzarski T, Jakubowska A, Menkiszak J, Gronwald J, Pluzanska A, Bebenek M, Fischer-Maliszewska L, Grzybowska E, Narod S, Lubinski J. Founder mutations in the BRCA1 gene in Polish families with breast-ovarian cancer. Am J Hum Genet 2000; 66:1963–1968.

Gowen LC, Avrutskaya AV, Latour AM, Koller BH, Leadon SA. BRCA1 required for transcription-coupled repair of oxidative DNA damage. Science 1998; 281(5379):1009–1012.

Greenberg RA, Sobhian B, Pathania S, Cantor SB, Nakatani Y, Livingston DM. Multifactorial contributions to an acute DNA damage response by BRCA1/BARD1-containing complexes. Genes Dev 2006; 20(1):34–46.

Greer JB, Whitcomb DC. Role of BRCA1/2 mutations in pancreatic cancer. Gut 2007; 56(5):601–605. Epub 2006 Sep 14.

Gronwald J, Tung N, Foulkes WD, Offit K, Gershoni R, Daly M, Kim-Sing C, Olsson H, Ainsworth P, Eisen A, Saal H, Friedman E, Olopade O, Osborne M, Weitzel J, Lynch H, Ghadirian P, Lubinski J, Sun P, Narod SA. Tamoxifen and contralateral breast cancer in BRCA1 and BRCA2 carriers: an update. Int J Cancer 2006; 118(9):2281–2284.

Gudmundsdottir K, Ashworth A. The roles of BRCA1 and BRCA2 and associated proteins in the maintenance of genomic stability. Oncogene 2006; 25(43):5864–5874.

Gudmundsdottir K, Lord CJ, Witt E, Tutt AN, Ashworth A. DSS1 is required for RAD51 focus formation and genomic stability in mammalian cells. EMBO Rep 2004; 5(10): 989–993.

Haffty BG, Harrold E, Khan AJ, Pathare P, Smith TE, Turner BC, Glazer PM, Ward B, Carter D, Matloff E, Bale AE, Alvarez-Franco M. Outcome of conservatively managed early-onset breast cancer by BRCA1/2 status. Lancet 2002; 359(9316):1471–1477.

Haffty BG, Silber A, Matloff E, Chung J, Lannin D. Racial differences in the incidence of BRCA1 and BRCA2 mutations in a cohort of early onset breast cancer patients: African American compared to white women. J Med Genet 2006; 43(2):133–137.

Haiman CA, Stram DO, Cheng I, Giorgi EE, Pooler L, Penney K, Le Marchand L, Henderson BE, Freedman ML. Common genetic variation at PTEN and risk of sporadic breast and prostate cancer. Cancer Epidemiol Biomarkers Prev 2006; 15(5):1021–1025.

Halbert CH, Kessler LJ, Mitchell E. Genetic testing for inherited breast cancer risk in African Americans. Cancer Invest 2005; 23(4):285–295.

Hall JM, Lee MK, Newman B, Morrow JE, Anderson LA, Huey B, King MC. Linkage of early-onset familial breast cancer to chromosome 17q21. Science 1990; 250:1684–1689.

Hall M, Olopade OI. Confronting genetic testing disparities: knowledge is power. JAMA 2005; 293(14):1783–1785.

Hall MJ, Li L, Wiernik PH, Olopade OI. BRCA2 mutation and the risk of hematologic malignancy. Leuk Lymphoma 2006; 47(4):765–767.

Hanssen AMN, Fryns JP. Cowden syndrome. J Med Genet 1995; 32:117–119.

Harkin DP, Bean JM, Miklos D, Song YH, Truong VB, Englert C, Christians FC, Ellisen LW, Maheswaran S, Oliner JD, Haber DA. Induction of GADD45 and JNK/SAPK-dependent apoptosis following inducible expression of BRCA1. Cell 1999; 97(5):575–586.

Hartge P, Struewing JP, Wacholder S, Brody LC, Tucker MA. The prevalence of common BRCA1 and BRCA2 mutations among Ashkenazi Jews. Am J Hum Genet 1999; 64:963–970.

Hartman AR, Ford JM. BRCA1 induces DNA damage recognition factors and enhances nucleotide excision repair. Nat Genet 2002; 32(1):180–184.

Hartmann L, Schaid D, Woods J, Crotty T, Myers J, Arnold P, Petty P, Sellers T, Johnson J, McDonnell S, Frost M, Jenkins R. Efficacy of bilateral prophylactic mastectomy in women with a family history of breast cancer. N Engl J Med 1999; 340:77–84.

Hartmann LC, Sellers TA, Schaid DJ, Frank TS, Soderberg CL, Sitta DL, Frost MH, Grant CS, Donohue JH, Woods JE, McDonnell SK, Vockley CW, Deffenbaugh A, Couch FJ, Jenkins RB. Efficacy of bilateral prophylactic mastectomy in BRCA1 and BRCA2 gene mutation carriers. J Natl Cancer Inst 2001; 93(21):1633–1637.

Hashizume R, Fukuda M, Maeda I, Nishikawa H, Oyake D, Yabuki Y, Ogata H, Ohta T. The RING heterodimer BRCA1-BARD1 is a ubiquitin ligase inactivated by a breast cancer-derived mutation. J Biol Chem 2001; 276 (18):14537–14540.

Hearle N, Schumacher V, Menko FH, Olschwang S, Boardman LA, Gille JJ, Keller JJ, Westerman AM, Scott RJ, Lim W, Trimbath JD, Giardiello FM, Gruber SB, Offerhaus GJ, de Rooij FW, Wilson JH, Hansmann A, Moslein G, Royer-Pokora B, Vogel T, Phillips RK, Spigelman AD, Houlston

RS. Frequency and spectrum of cancers in the Peutz-Jeghers syndrome. Clin Cancer Res 2006; 12(10):3209–3215.

Hedenfalk I, Duggan D, Chen Y, Radmacher M, Bittner M, Simon R, Meltzer P, Gusterson B, Esteller M, Kallioniemi OP, Wilfond B, Borg A, Trent J, Raffeld M, Yakhini Z, Ben-Dor A, Dougherty E, Kononen J, Bubendorf L, Fehrle W, Pittaluga S, Gruvberger S, Loman N, Johannsson O, Olsson H, Sauter G. Gene-expression profiles in hereditary breast cancer. N Engl J Med 2001; 344(8):539–548.

Heikkinen K, Rapakko K, Karppinen SM, Erkko H, Knuutila S, Lundan T, Mannermaa A, Borresen-Dale AL, Borg A, Barkardottir RB, Petrini J, Winqvist R. RAD50 and NBS1 are breast cancer susceptibility genes associated with genomic instability. Carcinogenesis 2006; 27(8): 1593–1599.

Hellmold H, Rylander T, Magnusson M, Reihner E, Warner M, Gustafsson JA. Characterization of cytochrome P450 enzymes in human breast tissue from reduction mammaplasties. J Clin Endocrinol Metab 1998; 83(3):886–895.

Hemminki A, Markie D, Tomlinson I, Avizienyte E, Roth S, Loukola A, Bignell G, Warren W, Aminoff M, Hoglund P, Jarvinen H, Kristo P, Pelin K, Ridanpaa M, Salovaara R, Toro T, Bodmer W, Olschwang S, Olsen A, Stratton M, de la Chapelle A, Aaltonen L. A serine/threonine kinase gene defective in Peutz-Jeghers syndrome. Nature 1998; 391:184–187.

Hendrickson BC, Judkins T, Ward BD, Eliason K, Deffenbaugh AE, Burbidge LA, Pyne K, Leclair B, Ward BE, Scholl T. Prevalence of five previously reported and recurrent BRCA1 genetic rearrangement mutations in 20,000 patients from hereditary breast/ovarian cancer families. Genes Chromosomes Cancer 2005; 43(3):309–313.

Hengartner MO. The biochemistry of apoptosis. Nature 2000; 407(6805):770–776.

Herman JG, Baylin SB. Gene silencing in cancer in association with promoter hypermethylation. N Engl J Med 2003; 349(21):2042–2054.

Hilton JL, Geisler JP, Rathe JA, Hattermann-Zogg MA, DeYoung B, Buller RE. Inactivation of BRCA1 and BRCA2 in ovarian cancer. J Natl Cancer Inst 2002; 94(18):1396–1406.

Hoege C, Pfander B, Moldovan GL, Pyrowolakis G, Jentsch S. RAD6-dependent DNA repair is linked to modification of PCNA by ubiquitin and SUMO. Nature 2002; 419 (6903):135–141.

Hoeijmakers JH. Genome maintenance mechanisms for preventing cancer. Nature 2001; 411(6835):366–374.

Hofmann W, Gorgens H, John A, Horn D, Huttner C, Arnold N, Scherneck S, Schackert HK. Screening for large rearrangements of the BRCA1 gene in German breast or ovarian cancer families using semi-quantitative multiplex PCR method. Hum Mutat 2003; 22(1):103–104.

Hogervorst FB, Nederlof PM, Gille JJ, McElgunn CJ, Grippeling M, Pruntel R, Regnerus R, van Welsem T, van Spaendonk R, Menko FH, Kluijt I, Dommering C, Verhoef S, Schouten JP, van't Veer LJ, Pals G. Large genomic deletions and duplications in the BRCA1 gene identified by a novel quantitative method. Cancer Res 2003; 63(7):1449–1453.

Honrado E, Osorio A, Palacios J, Benitez J. Pathology and gene expression of hereditary breast tumors associated with BRCA1, BRCA2 and CHEK2 gene mutations. Oncogene 2006; 25(43):5837–5845.

Honrado E, Osorio A, Palacios J, Milne RL, Sanchez L, Diez O, Cazorla A, Syrjakoski K, Huntsman D, Heikkila P, Lerma E, Kallioniemi A, Rivas C, Foulkes WD, Nevanlinna H, Benitez J. Immunohistochemical expression of DNA repair proteins in familial breast cancer differentiate BRCA2-associated tumors. J Clin Oncol 2005; 23(30): 7503–7511.

Hopper JL, Carlin JB. Familial aggregation of a disease consequent upon correlation between relatives in a risk factor measured on a continuous scale. Am J Epidemiol 1992; 136(9):1138–1147.

Hosking L, Trowsdale J, Nicolai H, Solomon E, Foulkes W, Stamp G, Signer E, Jeffreys A. A somatic *BRCA1* mutation in an ovarian tumour. Nat Genet 1995; 9:343–344.

Houlston R, Damato B. Genetic predisposition to ocular melanoma. Eye 1999; 13:43–46.

Howlett NG, Taniguchi T, Olson S, Cox B, Waisfisz Q, De Die-Smulders C, Persky N, Grompe M, Joenje H, Pals G, Ikeda H, Fox EA, D'Andrea AD. Biallelic inactivation of BRCA2 in Fanconi anemia. Science 2002; 297 (5581):606–609.

Huber LJ, Chodosh LA. Dynamics of DNA repair suggested by the subcellular localization of Brca1 and Brca2 proteins. J Cell Biochem 2005; 96(1):47–55.

Hubert A, Peretz T, Manor O, Kadwi L, Wienberg N, Lerer I, Sagi M, Abeliovich D. The Jewish Ashkenazi founder mutations in the BRCA1/BRCA2 genes are not found at an increased frequency in Ashkenazi patients with prostate cancer. Am J Hum Genet 1999; 65:921–924.

Hughes TA. Regulation of gene expression by alternative untranslated regions. Trends Genet 2006; 22(3):119–122.

Humphrey JS, Salim A, Erdos MR, Collins FS, Brody LC, Klausner RD. Human BRCA1 inhibits growth in yeast: potential use in diagnostic testing. Proc Natl Acad Sci U S A 1997; 94(11):5820–5825.

Hussain S, Wilson JB, Blom E, Thompson LH, Sung P, Gordon SM, Kupfer GM, Joenje H, Mathew CG, Jones NJ. Tetratricopeptide-motif-mediated interaction of FANCG with recombination proteins XRCC3 and BRCA2. DNA Repair (Amst) 2006; 5(5):629–640.

Huusko P, Paakkonen K, Launonen V, Poyhonen M, Blanco G, Kauppila A, Puistola U, Kiviniemi H, Kujala M, Leisti J, Winqvist R. Evidence of founder mutations in Finnish BRCA1 and BRCA2 families. Am J Hum Genet 1998; 62:1544–1548.

Inoue R, Fukutomi T, Ushijima T, Matsumoto Y, Sugimura T, Nagao M. Germline mutation of BRCA1 in Japanese breast cancer families. Cancer Res 1995; 55: 3521–3524.

Jacquemier J, Padovani L, Rabayrol L, Lakhani SR, Penault-Llorca F, Denoux Y, Fiche M, Figueiro P, Maisongrosse V, Ledoussal V, Martinez Penuela J, Udvarhely N, El Makdissi G, Ginestier C, Geneix J, Charafe-Jauffret E, Xerri L, Eisinger F, Birnbaum D, Sobol H. Typical medullary breast carcinomas have a basal/myoepithelial phenotype. J Pathol 2005; 207(3):260–268.

Jakubowska A, Gronwald J, Menkiszak J, Gorski B, Huzarski T, Byrski T, Edler L, Lubinski J, Scott RJ, Hamann U. Integrin {beta}3 Leu33Pro polymorphism increases BRCA1-associated ovarian cancer risk. J Med Genet 2007.

Jakubowska A, Narod SA, Goldgar DE, Mierzejewski M, Masojc B, Nej K, Huzarska J, Byrski T, Gorski B, Lubinski J. Breast cancer risk reduction associated with the RAD51 polymorphism among carriers of the BRCA1 5382insC mutation in Poland. Cancer Epidemiol Biomarkers Prev 2003; 12(5):457–459.

James PA, Doherty R, Harris M, Mukesh BN, Milner A, Young MA, Scott C. Optimal selection of individuals for BRCA mutation testing: a comparison of available methods. J Clin Oncol 2006; 24(4):707–715.

Jekimovs CR, Chen X, Arnold J, Gatei M, Richard DJ, Spurdle AB, Khanna KK, Chenevix-Trench G. Low frequency of CHEK2 1100delC allele in Australian multiple-case breast cancer families: functional analysis in heterozygous individuals. Br J Cancer 2005; 92(4):784–790.

Jenne D, Reimann H, Nexu J, Friedel W, Loff S, Jeschke R, Muller O, Back W, Zimmer M. Peutz-Heghers syndrome is caused by mutations in a novel serine threonine kinase. Nat Genet 1998; 18:38–43.

Jernstrom H, Lubinski J, Lynch HT, Ghadirian P, Neuhausen S, Isaacs C, Weber BL, Horsman D, Rosen B, Foulkes WD, Friedman E, Gershoni-Baruch R, Ainsworth P, Daly M, Garber J, Olsson H, Sun P, Narod SA. Breast-feeding and the risk of breast cancer in BRCA1 and BRCA2 mutation carriers. J Natl Cancer Inst 2004; 96(14):1094–1098.

Jin S, Zhao H, Fan F, Blanck P, Fan W, Colchagie A, Fornace A, Zhan Q. BRCA1 activation of the GADD45 promoter. Oncogene 2000; 19:4050–4057.

Jin Y, Zu ZL, Yang M-CW, Wei F, Ayi T-C, Bowcock AM, Baer R. Cell cycle-dependent colocalization of BARD1 and BRCA1 proteins in discrete nuclear domains. Proc Natl Acad Sci U S A 1997; 94:12075–12080.

Johannsson O, Ostermeyer E, Hakansson S, Friedman L, Johansson U, Selberg G, Brondum-Nielsen K, Sele V, Olsson H, King M, Borg A. Founding BRCA1 mutations in hereditary breast and ovarian cancer in southern Sweden. Am J Hum Genet 1996; 58:441–450.

Johnson RE, Kondratick CM, Prakash S, Prakash L. hRAD30 mutations in the variant form of xeroderma pigmentosum. Science 1999; 285(5425):263–265.

Jonsson G, Bendahl PO, Sandberg T, Kurbasic A, Staaf J, Sunde L, Cruger DG, Ingvar C, Olsson H, Borg A. Mapping of a novel ocular and cutaneous malignant melanoma susceptibility locus to chromosome 9q21.32. J Natl Cancer Inst 2005; 97(18):1377–1382.

Joo WS, Jeffrey PD, Cantor SB, Finnin MS, Livingston DM, Pavletich NP. Structure of the 53BP1 BRCT region bound to p53 and its comparison to the Brca1 BRCT structure. Genes Dev 2002; 16(5):583–593.

Josse L, Harley ME, Pires IM, Hughes DA. Fission yeast Dss1 associates with the proteasome and is required for efficient ubiquitin-dependent proteolysis. Biochem J 2006; 393(Pt 1): 303–309.

Judkins T, Hendrickson BC, Deffenbaugh AM, Eliason K, Leclair B, Norton MJ, Ward BE, Pruss D, Scholl T. Application of embryonic lethal or other obvious phenotypes to characterize the clinical significance of genetic variants found in trans with known deleterious mutations. Cancer Res 2005; 65(21):10096–10103.

Kadam S, McAlpine GS, Phelan ML, Kingston RE, Jones KA, Emerson BM. Functional selectivity of recombinant mammalian SWI/SNF subunits. Genes Dev 2000; 14(19): 2441–2451.

Kadouri L, Hubert A, Rotenberg Y, Hamburger T, Sagi M, Nechushtan C, Abeliovich D, Peretz T. Cancer risks in carriers of the BRCA1/2 Ashkenazi founder mutations. J Med Genet 2007; 44(7):467–471.

Kadouri L, Kote-Jarai Z, Hubert A, Durocher F, Abeliovich D, Glaser B, Hamburger T, Eeles RA, Peretz T. A single-nucleotide polymorphism in the RAD51 gene modifies breast cancer risk in BRCA2 carriers, but not in BRCA1 carriers or noncarriers. Br J Cancer 2004; 90(10): 2002–2005.

Kang HH, Williams R, Leary J, Ringland C, Kirk J, Ward R. Evaluation of models to predict BRCA germline mutations. Br J Cancer 2006; 95(7):914–920.

Kannouche PL, Wing J, Lehmann AR. Interaction of human DNA polymerase eta with monoubiquitinated PCNA: a possible mechanism for the polymerase switch in response to DNA damage. Mol Cell 2004; 14(4):491–500.

Karhu R, Laurila E, Kallioniemi A, Syrjakoski K. Large genomic BRCA2 rearrangements and male breast cancer. Cancer Detect Prev 2006; 30(6):530–534.

Karlsson CT, Malmer B, Wiklund F, Gronberg H. Breast cancer as a second primary in patients with prostate cancer–estrogen treatment or association with family history of cancer? J Urol 2006; 176(2):538–543.

Karppinen SM, Vuosku J, Heikkinen K, Allinen M, Winqvist R. No evidence of involvement of germline BACH1 mutations in Finnish breast and ovarian cancer families. Eur J Cancer 2003; 39(3):366–371.

Kashuk CS, Stone EA, Grice EA, Portnoy ME, Green ED, Sidow A, Chakravarti A, McCallion AS. Phenotype-genotype correlation in Hirschsprung disease is illuminated by comparative analysis of the RET protein sequence. Proc Natl Acad Sci U S A 2005; 102(25):8949–8954.

Kauff ND, Domchek S, Friebel T, Lee JB, Roth R, Robson ME, Barakat RR, Norton L, Offit K, Rebbeck TR, Group PS. Multi-center prospective analysis of risk-reducing salpingo-oophorectomy to prevent BRCA-associated breast and ovarian cancer. J Clin Oncol 2006 ASCO Annual Meeting Proceedings Part I 2006; 24(18S):1003.

Kauff ND, Perez-Segura P, Robson ME, Scheuer L, Siegel B, Schluger A, Rapaport B, Frank TS, Nafa K, Ellis NA, Parmigiani G, Offit K. Incidence of non-founder BRCA1 and BRCA2 mutations in high risk Ashkenazi breast and ovarian cancer families. J Med Genet 2002a; 39(8): 611–614.

Kauff ND, Satagopan JM, Robson ME, Scheuer L, Hensley M, Hudis CA, Ellis NA, Boyd J, Borgen PI, Barakat RR, Norton L, Castiel M, Nafa K, Offit K. Risk-reducing salpingo-oophorectomy in women with a BRCA1 or

BRCA2 mutation. N Engl J Med 2002b; 346(21): 1609–1615.

Kawai H, Li H, Chun P, Avraham S, Avraham HK. Direct interaction between BRCA1 and the estrogen receptor regulates vascular endothelial growth factor (VEGF) transcription and secretion in breast cancer cells. Oncogene 2002; 21(50):7730–7739.

Kennedy RD, Gorski JJ, Quinn JE, Stewart GE, James CR, Moore S, Mulligan K, Emberley ED, Lioe TF, Morrison PJ, Mullan PB, Reid G, Johnston PG, Watson PH, Harkin DP. BRCA1 and c-Myc associate to transcriptionally repress psoriasin, a DNA damage-inducible gene. Cancer Res 2005; 65(22):10265–10272.

Kennedy RD, Quinn JE, Mullan PB, Johnston PG, Harkin DP. The role of BRCA1 in the cellular response to chemotherapy. J Natl Cancer Inst 2004; 96(22):1659–1668.

Kerangueven F, Essioux L, Dib A, Noguchi T, Allione F, Geneix J, Longy M, Lidereau R, Eisinger F, Pebusque M, Jacquemier J, Bonaiti-Pellie C, Sobol H, Birnbaum D. Loss of hererozygosity and linkage analysis in breast carcinoma: indication for a putative third susceptibility gene on the short arm of chromosome 8. Oncogene 1995; 10: 1023–1026.

Khanna M, Park P, Zirvi M, Cao W, Picon A, Day J, Paty P, Barany F. Multiplex PCR/LDR for detection of K-ras mutations in primary colon tumors. Oncogene 1999; 18:27–38.

Khoo U-S, Ozcelik H, Cheung ANY, Chow LWC, Ngan HYS, Done SJ, Liang ACT, Chan VWY, Au GKH, Ng W-F, Poon CSP, Leung Y-F, Loong F, Ip P, Chan GSW, Andrulis IL, Lu J, Ho FCS. Somatic mutations in the BRCA1 gene in Chinese sporadic breast and ovarian cancer. Oncogene 1999; 18:4643–4646.

Kilpivaara O, Bartkova J, Eerola H, Syrjakoski K, Vahteristo P, Lukas J, Blomqvist C, Holli K, Heikkila P, Sauter G, Kallioniemi OP, Bartek J, Nevanlinna H. Correlation of CHEK2 protein expression and c.1100delC mutation status with tumor characteristics among unselected breast cancer patients. Int J Cancer 2005; 113(4):575–580.

King MC, Marks JH, Mandell JB. Breast and ovarian cancer risks due to inherited mutations in BRCA1 and BRCA2. Science 2003; 302(5645):643–646.

King MC, Wieand S, Hale K, Lee M, Walsh T, Owens K, Tait J, Ford L, Dunn BK, Costantino J, Wickerham L, Wolmark N, Fisher B. Tamoxifen and breast cancer incidence among women with inherited mutations in BRCA1 and BRCA2: National Surgical Adjuvant Breast and Bowel Project (NSABP-P1) Breast Cancer Prevention Trial. JAMA 2001; 286(18):2251–2256.

Kirchhoff T, Kauff ND, Mitra N, Nafa K, Huang H, Palmer C, Gulati T, Wadsworth E, Donat S, Robson ME, Ellis NA, Offit K. BRCA mutations and risk of prostate cancer in Ashkenazi Jews. Clin Cancer Res 2004; 10(9):2918–2921.

Kitao H, Yamamoto K, Matsushita N, Ohzeki M, Ishiai M, Takata M. Functional interplay between BRCA2/FancD1 and FancC in DNA repair. J Biol Chem 2006; 281(30): 21312–21320.

Kleihues P, Schauble B, zur Hausen A, Esteve J, Ohgaki H. Tumors associated with p53 germline mutations: a synopsis of 91 families. Am J Pathol 1997; 150:1–13.

Kleiman FE, Wu-Baer F, Fonseca D, Kaneko S, Baer R, Manley JL. BRCA1/BARD1 inhibition of mRNA 3′ processing involves targeted degradation of RNA polymerase II. Genes Dev 2005; 19(10):1227–1237.

Ko LJ, Prives C. P53: puzzle and paradigm. Genes Dev 1996; 10:96–99.

Kojic M, Yang H, Kostrub CF, Pavletich NP, Holloman WK. The BRCA2-interacting protein DSS1 is vital for DNA repair, recombination, and genome stability in Ustilago maydis. Mol Cell 2003; 12(4):1043–1049.

Kojic M, Zhou Q, Lisby M, Holloman WK. Brh2-Dss1 interplay enables properly controlled recombination in Ustilago maydis. Mol Cell Biol 2005; 25(7):2547–2557.

Kote-Jarai Z, Williams RD, Cattini N, Copeland M, Giddings I, Wooster R, tePoele RH, Workman P, Gusterson B, Peacock J, Gui G, Campbell C, Eeles R. Gene expression profiling after radiation-induced DNA damage is strongly predictive of BRCA1 mutation carrier status. Clin Cancer Res 2004; 10(3):958–963.

Kowalska E, Narod SA, Huzarski T, Zajaczek S, Huzarska J, Gorski B, Lubinski J. Increased rates of chromosome breakage in BRCA1 carriers are normalized by oral selenium supplementation. Cancer Epidemiol Biomarkers Prev 2005; 14(5):1302–1306.

Kramer JL, Velazquez IA, Chen BE, Rosenberg PS, Struewing JP, Greene MH. Prophylactic oophorectomy reduces breast cancer penetrance during prospective, long-term follow-up of BRCA1 mutation carriers. J Clin Oncol 2005; 23(34): 8629–8635.

Kriege M, Brekelmans CT, Boetes C, Besnard PE, Zonderland HM, Obdeijn IM, Manoliu RA, Kok T, Peterse H, Tilanus-Linthorst MM, Muller SH, Meijer S, Oosterwijk JC, Beex LV, Tollenaar RA, de Koning HJ, Rutgers EJ, Klijn JG. Efficacy of MRI and mammography for breast-cancer screening in women with a familial or genetic predisposition. N Engl J Med 2004; 351(5): 427–437.

Krogan NJ, Lam MH, Fillingham J, Keogh MC, Gebbia M, Li J, Datta N, Cagney G, Buratowski S, Emili A, Greenblatt JF. Proteasome involvement in the repair of DNA double-strand breaks. Mol Cell 2004; 16(6):1027–1034.

Krum SA, Miranda GA, Lin C, Lane TF. BRCA1 associates with processive RNA polymerase II. J Biol Chem 2003; 278(52): 52012–52020.

Krutyakov VM. Eukaryotic error-prone DNA polymerases: Suggested roles in replication, repair and mutagenesis. Mol Biol 2006; 40(1):3–11.

Kulinski J, Besack D, Oleykowski CA, Godwin AK, Yeung AT. CEL I enzymatic mutation detection assay. Biotechniques 2000; 29:44–48.

Kuperstein G, Jack E, Narod SA. A fluorescent multiplex-DGGE screening test for mutations in the BRCA1 gene. Genet Test 2006; 10(1):1–7.

Kyndi M, Alsner J, Hansen LL, Sorensen FB, Overgaard J. LOH rather than genotypes of TP53 codon 72 is associated with disease-free survival in primary breast cancer. Acta Oncol 2006; 45(5):602–609.

Lakhani S, Easton D, Stratton M, and BCLC. Pathology of familial breast cancer: differences between breast cancers in carriers of *BRCA1* or *BRCA2* mutations and sporadic cases. Lancet 1997; 349:1505–1510.

Lakhani S, Gusterson B, Jacquemier J, Sloane J, Anderson T, van de Vijver M, Venter D, Freeman A, Antoniou A, McGuffog L, Smyth E, Steel C, Haites N, Scott R, Goldgar D, Neuhausen S, Day P, Ormiston W, McManus R, Scherneck S, Ponder B, Futreal P, Peto J, Stoppa-Lyonnet D, Bignon Y, Struewing J, Bishop D, Klijn J, Devilee P, Cornelisse C, Lasset C, Lenoir G, Barkardottir R, Egilsson V, Hamann U, Chang-Claude J, Sobol H, Weber B, Easton D, Stratton M. The pathology of familial breast cancer: histological features of cancers in families not attributable to mutations in *BRCA1* or *BRCA2*. Clin Cancer Res 2000; 6:782–789.

Lakhani S, Jacquemier J, Sloane J, Gusterson B, Anderson T, van deVijver M, Farid L, Venter D, Antoniou A, Storfer-Isser A, Smyth E, Steel C, Haiter N, Scott R, Godger D, Heuhausen S, Day P, Ormisoton W, McManus R, Scherneck S, Ponder B, Ford D, Peto J, Stoppa-Lyonnet D, Bignon Y, Streuwing J, Spurr N, Biship D, Lkijn J, Devilee P, Cornelisse C, Lasset C, Lenoir G, Bardardottir R, Egilsson V, Hamann U, Chang-Claude J, Sobol H, Weber B, Stratton M, Easton D. Multifactorial analysis of differences between sporadic breast cancers and cancers involving *BRCA1* and *BRCA2* mutations. J Natl Cancer Inst 1998; 90:1138–1145.

Lakhani SR, Chaggar R, Davies S, Jones C, Collins N, Odel C, Stratton MR, O'Hare MJ. Genetic alterations in 'normal' luminal and myoepithelial cells of the breast. J Pathol 1999; 189(4):496–503.

Lakhani SR, Reis-Filho JS, Fulford L, Penault-Llorca F, van der Vijver M, Parry S, Bishop T, Benitez J, Rivas C, Bignon YJ, Chang-Claude J, Hamann U, Cornelisse CJ, Devilee P, Beckmann MW, Nestle-Kramling C, Daly PA, Haites N, Varley J, Lalloo F, Evans G, Maugard C, Meijers-Heijboer H, Klijn JG, Olah E, Gusterson BA, Pilotti S, Radice P, Scherneck S, Sobol H, Jacquemier J, Wagner T, Peto J, Stratton MR, McGuffog L, Easton DF. Prediction of BRCA1 status in patients with breast cancer using estrogen receptor and basal phenotype. Clin Cancer Res 2005; 11 (14):5175–5180.

Lakhani SR, Van De Vijver MJ, Jacquemier J, Anderson TJ, Osin PP, McGuffog L, Easton DF. The pathology of familial breast cancer: predictive value of immunohistochemical markers estrogen receptor, progesterone receptor, HER-2, and p53 in patients with mutations in BRCA1 and BRCA2. J Clin Oncol 2002; 20(9):2310–2318.

Lal G, Liu G, Shmocker B, Kaurah P, Ozcelik H, Narod S, Redston M, Gallinger S. Inherited predisposition to pancreatic adenocarcinoma: role of family history and germline p16, BRCA1, and BRCA2 mutations. Cancer Res 2000; 60:409–416.

Lane TF, Deng C, Elson A, Lyu MS, Kozak CA, Leder P. Expression of BRCA1 is associated with terminal differentiation of ectodermally and mesodermally derived tissues in mice. Genes Dev 1995; 9:2712–2722.

Langston AA, Stanford JL, Wicklund KG, Thompson JD, Blazej RG, Ostrander EA. Germ-line BRCA1 mutations in selected men with prostate cancer. Am J Hum Genet 1996; 58: 881–885.

Leach MO, Boggis CR, Dixon AK, Easton DF, Eeles RA, Evans DG, Gilbert FJ, Griebsch I, Hoff RJ, Kessar P, Lakhani SR, Moss SM, Nerurkar A, Padhani AR, Pointon LJ, Thompson D, Warren RM. Screening with magnetic resonance imaging and mammography of a UK population at high familial risk of breast cancer: a prospective multicentre cohort study (MARIBS). Lancet 2005; 365(9473):1769–1778.

Lee J-S, Collins KM, Brown AL, Lee C-H, Chung JH. hCds1-mediated phosphorylation of BRCA1 regulates the DNA damage response. Nature 2000; 404:201–204.

Lee M, Daniels MJ, Venkitaraman AR. Phosphorylation of BRCA2 by the Polo-like kinase Plk1 is regulated by DNA damage and mitotic progression. Oncogene 2004; 23(4): 865–872.

Lee SB, Kim SH, Bell DW, Wahrer DC, Schiripo TA, Jorczak MM, Sgroi DC, Garber JE, Li FP, Nichols KE, Varley JM, Godwin AK, Shannon KM, Harlow E, Haber DA. Destabilization of CHK2 by a missense mutation associated with Li-Fraumeni Syndrome. Cancer Res 2001; 61 (22):8062–8067.

Lehrer S, Fodor F, Stock RG, Stone NN, Eng C, Song HK, McGovern M. Absence of 185delAG mutation of the BRCA1 gene and 6174delT mutation of the BRCA2 gene in Ashkenazi Jewish men with prostate cancer. Br J Cancer 1998; 78:771–773.

Lewis AG, Flanagan J, Marsh A, Pupo GM, Mann G, Spurdle AB, Lindeman GJ, Visvader JE, Brown MA, Chenevix-Trench G. Mutation analysis of FANCD2, BRIP1/BACH1, LMO4 and SFN in familial breast cancer. Breast Cancer Res 2005; 7(6):R1005–R1016.

Li H, Lee TH, Avraham H. A novel tricomplex of BRCA1, Nmi, and c-Myc inhibits c-Myc-induced human telomerase reverse transcriptase gene (hTERT) promoter activity in breast cancer. J Biol Chem 2002; 277(23):20965–20973.

Li J, Yen C, Liaw D, Podsypanina K, Bose S, Wang SI, Puc J, Miliaresis C, Rodgers L, CmCombie R, Bigner SH, Giovanella BC, Ittmann M, Tycko B, Hibshoosh H, Wigler MH, Parsons R. PTEN, a putative protein tyrosine phosphatase gene mutated in human brain, breast, and prostate cancer. Science 1997; 13:1943–1947.

Li J, Zou C, Bai Y, Wazer DE, Band V, Gao Q. DSS1 is required for the stability of BRCA2. Oncogene 2006; 25(8):1186–1194.

Li RP, Fraumeni JF, Mulvihill JJ, Blattner WA, Dreyfus MG, Tucker MA, Miller RW. A cancer family syndrome in twenty-four kindreds. Cancer Res 1988; 48:5358–5362.

Li S, Chen PL, Subramanian T, Chinnadurai G, Tomlinson G, Osborne CK, Sharp ZD, Lee WH. Binding of CtIP to the BRCT repeats of BRCA1 involved in the transcription regulation of p21 is disrupted upon DNA damage. J Biol Chem 1999; 274(16):11334–11338.

Li S, Ting NS, Zheng L, Chen PL, Ziv Y, Shiloh Y, Lee EY, Lee WH. Functional link of BRCA1 and ataxia telangiectasia gene product in DNA damage response. Nature 2000; 406(6792):210–215.

Lichtenstein P, Holm NV, Verkasalo PK, Iliadou A, Kaprio J, Koskenvuo M, Pukkala E, Skytthe A, Hemminki K. Environmental and heritable factors in the causation of cancer–analyses of cohorts of twins from Sweden, Denmark, and Finland. N Engl J Med 2000; 343(2):78–85.

Liede A, Cohen B, Black D, Davidson R, Renwidk A, Hoodfar E, Olopade O, Micek M, Anderson V, DeMey R, Fordyce A, Warner E, Dann JL, King MC, Weber B, Narod S, Steel C. Evidence of a founder BRCA1 mutation in Scotland. Br J Cancer 2000a; 82:705–711.

Liede A, Karlan BY, Narod SA. Cancer risks for male carriers of germline mutations in BRCA1 or BRCA2: a review of the literature. J Clin Oncol 2004; 22(4):735–742.

Liede A, Malik IA, Aziz Z, Rios Pd Pde L, Kwan E, Narod SA. Contribution of BRCA1 and BRCA2 mutations to breast and ovarian cancer in Pakistan. Am J Hum Genet 2002; 71(3):595–606.

Liede A, Metcalfe K, Hanna D, Hoodfar E, Snyder C, Durham C, Lynch HT, Narod SA. Evaluation of the needs of male carriers of mutations in BRCA1 or BRCA2 who have undergone genetic counseling. Am J Hum Genet 2000b; 67(6):1494–1504.

Lin FL, Sperle K, Sternberg N. Model for homologous recombination during transfer of DNA into mouse L cells: role for DNA ends in the recombination process. Mol Cell Biol 1984; 4(6):1020–1034.

Lin FL, Sperle K, Sternberg N. Intermolecular recombination between DNAs introduced into mouse L cells is mediated by a nonconservative pathway that leads to crossover products. Mol Cell Biol 1990; 10(1):103–112.

Lin HR, Ting NS, Qin J, Lee WH. M phase-specific phosphorylation of BRCA2 by Polo-like kinase 1 correlates with the dissociation of the BRCA2-P/CAF complex. J Biol Chem 2003; 278(38):35979–35987.

Linke SP, Bremer TM, Herold CD, Sauter G, Diamond C. A multimarker model to predict outcome in tamoxifen-treated breast cancer patients. Clin Cancer Res 2006; 12(4): 1175–1183.

Lipshutz R, Fodor S, Gingeras T, Lockhart D. High density synthetic ologonucleotide arrays. Nat Genet Suppl 1999; 21:20–24.

Livneh Z. DNA damage control by novel DNA polymerases: translesion replication and mutagenesis. J Biol Chem 2001; 276(28):25639–25642.

Lomonosov M, Anand S, Sangrithi M, Davies R, Venkitaraman AR. Stabilization of stalled DNA replication forks by the BRCA2 breast cancer susceptibility protein. Genes Dev 2003; 17(24):3017–3022.

Lu KH, Garber JE, Cramer DW, Welch WR, Niloff J, Schrag D, Berkowitz RS, Muto MG. Occult ovarian tumors in women with BRCA1 or BRCA2 mutations undergoing prophylactic oophorectomy. J Clin Oncol 2000; 18(14):2728–2732.

Lubinski J, Phelan CM, Ghadirian P, Lynch HT, Garber J, Weber B, Tung N, Horsman D, Isaacs C, Monteiro AN, Sun P, Narod SA. Cancer variation associated with the position of the mutation in the BRCA2 gene. Fam Cancer 2004; 3(1):1–10.

Luo L, Lei H, Du Q, von Wachenfeldt A, Kockum I, Luthman H, Vorechovsky I, Lindblom A. No mutations in the BACH1 gene in BRCA1 and BRCA2 negative breast-cancer families linked to 17q22. Int J Cancer 2002; 98(4):638–639.

Lykke-Andersen J. mRNA quality control: Marking the message for life or death. Curr Biol 2001; 11(3):R88–R91.

Lynch HT, Watson P, Narod SA. The genetic epidemiology of male breast carcinoma. Cancer 1999; 86(5):744–746.

Mack TM, Hamilton AS, Press MF, Diep A, Rappaport EB. Heritable breast cancer in twins. Br J Cancer 2002; 87(3): 294–300.

MacLachlan TK, Dash BC, Dicker DT, El-Deiry WS. Repression of BRCA1 through a feedback loop involving p53. J Biol Chem 2000; 275(41):31869–31875.

MacLachlan TK, Takimoto R, El-Deiry WS. BRCA1 directs a selective p53-dependent transcriptional response towards growth arrest and DNA repair targets. Mol Cell Biol 2002; 22(12):4280–4292.

Malins D, Haimanot R. Major alterations in the nucleotide structure of DNA in cancer of the female breast. Cancer Res 1991; 51:5430–5432.

Malins D, Holmes E, Polissar N, Gunselman S. The etiology of breast cancer. Characteristic alteration in hydroxyl radical-induced DNA base lesions during oncogenesis with potential for evaluating incidence risk. Cancer 1993; 71:3036–3043.

Malkin D, Li F, Strong L, Fraumeni J, Nelson C, Kim D, Kassel J, Gryka M, Bisehoff F, Tainsky M, Friend S. Germ line p53 mutations in a familial syndrome of breast cancer, sarcomas, and other neoplasms. Science 1990; 250: 1233–1238.

Malone K, Daling J, Neal CL, Suter N, O'Brien C, Cushing-Haugen K, Jonasdottir T, Thompson JD, Ostrander EA. Frequency of BRCA1/BRCA2 mutations in a population-based sample of young breast carcinoma cases. Cancer 2000; 88:1393–1402.

Malone KE, Daling JR, Doody DR, Hsu L, Bernstein L, Coates RJ, Marchbanks PA, Simon MS, McDonald JA, Norman SA, Strom BL, Burkman RT, Ursin G, Deapen D, Weiss LK, Folger S, Madeoy JJ, Friedrichsen DM, Suter NM, Humphrey MC, Spirtas R, Ostrander EA. Prevalence and Predictors of BRCA1 and BRCA2 Mutations in a Population-Based Study of Breast Cancer in White and Black American Women Ages 35 to 64 Years. Cancer Res 2006; 66(16):8297–8308.

Manke IA, Lowery DM, Nguyen A, Yaffe MB. BRCT repeats as phosphopeptide-binding modules involved in protein targeting. Science 2003; 302(5645):636–639.

Marie I, Durbin JE, Levy DE. Differential viral induction of distinct interferon-alpha genes by positive feedback through interferon regulatory factor-7. Embo J 1998; 17 (22):6660–6669.

Markoff A, Savov A, Vladimirov V, Bogdanaova N, Kremensky I, Ganev V. Optimization of single-strand conformation polymorphism analysis in the presence of polyethylene glycol. Clin Chem 1997; 43:30–33.

Markoff A, Sormbroen H, Bogdanova N, Preisler-Adams S, Ganev V, Dworniczak B, Horst J. Comparison of conformation-sensitive gel electrophoresis and single-strand conformation polymorphism analysis for detection of mutations in the *BRCA1* gene using optimized conformation analysis protocols. Eur J Hum Genet 1998; 6:145–150.

Marmorstein LY, Kinev AV, Chan GK, Bochar DA, Beniya H, Epstein JA, Yen TJ, Shiekhattar R. A human BRCA2 complex containing a structural DNA binding component influences cell cycle progression. Cell 2001; 104(2): 247–257.

Marroni F, Aretini P, D'Andrea E, Caligo MA, Cortesi L, Viel A, Ricevuto E, Montagna M, Cipollini G, Ferrari S, Santarosa M, Bisegna R, Bailey-Wilson JE, Bevilacqua G, Parmigiani G, Presciuttini S. Evaluation of widely used models for predicting BRCA1 and BRCA2 mutations. J Med Genet 2004; 41(4):278–285.

Marston NJ, Richards WJ, Hughes D, Bertwistle D, Marshall CJ, Ashworth A. Interaction between the product of the breast cancer susceptibility gene BRCA2 and DSS1, a protein functionally conserved from yeast to mammals. Mol Cell Biol 1999; 19(7):4633–4642.

Masutani C, Kusumoto R, Yamada A, Dohmae N, Yokoi M, Yuasa M, Araki M, Iwai S, Takio K, Hanaoka F. The XPV (xeroderma pigmentosum variant) gene encodes human DNA polymerase eta. Nature 1999; 399(6737):700–704.

Mathew CG. Fanconi anaemia genes and susceptibility to cancer. Oncogene 2006; 25(43):5875–5884.

Matros E, Wang ZC, Lodeiro G, Miron A, Iglehart JD, Richardson AL. BRCA1 promoter methylation in sporadic breast tumors: relationship to gene expression profiles. Breast Cancer Res Treat 2005; 91(2):179–186.

Mazoyer S. Genomic rearrangements in the BRCA1 and BRCA2 genes. Hum Mutat 2005; 25(5):415–422.

McCabe N, Lord CJ, Tutt AN, Martin NM, Smith GC, Ashworth A. BRCA2-deficient CAPAN-1 cells are extremely sensitive to the inhibition of Poly (ADP-Ribose) polymerase: an issue of potency. Cancer Biol Ther 2005; 4(9):934–936.

McCulloch SD, Kokoska RJ, Masutani C, Iwai S, Hanaoka F, Kunkel TA. Preferential cis-syn thymine dimer bypass by DNA polymerase eta occurs with biased fidelity. Nature 2004; 428(6978):97–100.

McEwen AR, McConnell DT, Kenwright DN, Gaskell DJ, Cherry A, Kidd AM. Occult cancer of the fallopian tube in a BRCA2 germline mutation carrier at prophylactic salpingo-oophorectomy. Gynecol Oncol 2004; 92(3):992–994.

Meetei AR, Levitus M, Xue Y, Medhurst AL, Zwaan M, Ling C, Rooimans MA, Bier P, Hoatlin M, Pals G, de Winter JP, Wang W, Joenje H. X-linked inheritance of Fanconi anemia complementation group B. Nat Genet 2004; 36(11): 1219–1224.

Mefford HC, Baumbach L, Panguluri RC, Whitfield-Broome C, Szabo C, Smith S, King MC, Dunston G, Stoppa-Lyonnet D, Arena F. Evidence for a BRCA1 founder mutation in families of West African ancestry. Am J Hum Genet 1999; 65(2):575–578.

Mehenni H, Resta N, Park JG, Miyaki M, Guanti G, Costanza MC. Cancer risks in LKB1 germline mutation carriers. Gut 2006; 55(7):984–990.

Meijers-Heijboer H, van Geel B, van Putten WL, Henzen-Logmans SC, Seynaeve C, Menke-Pluymers MB, Bartels CC, Verhoog LC, van den Ouweland AM, Niermeijer MF, Brekelmans CT, Klijn JG. Breast cancer after prophylactic bilateral mastectomy in women with a BRCA1 or BRCA2 mutation. N Engl J Med 2001; 345(3):159–164.

Merajver SD, Pham TM, Caduff RF, Chen M, Poy EL, Cooney KA, Weber BL, Collins FS, Johnston C, Frank TS. Somatic mutations in the BRCA1 gene in sporadic ovarian tumours. Nat Genet 1995; 9:439–443.

Miki Y, Swensen J, Shattuck-Eidens D, Futreal P, Harshman K, Tavtigian S, Liu Q, Cochran C, Bennett L, Ding W, Bell R, Rosenthal J, Hussey C, Tran T, McClure M, Frye C, Hattlier T, Phelps R, Haugen-Strano A, Katcher H, Yakumo K, Gholami Z, Shaffer D, Stone S, Bayer S, Wray C, Bogden R, Dayananth P, Wark J, Tonin P, Narod S, Bristow P, Norris F, Helvering L, Morrison P, Rosteck P, Lai M, Barrett J, Lewis C, Neuhausen S, Cannon-Albright L, Goldgar D, Wiseman R, Kamb A, Skolnick M. A strong candidate for the breast and ovarian cancer susceptibility gene *BRCA1*. Science 1994; 266:66–71.

Milne RL, Knight JA, John EM, Dite GS, Balbuena R, Ziogas A, Andrulis IL, West DW, Li FP, Southey MC, Giles GG, McCredie MR, Hopper JL, Whittemore AS. Oral contraceptive use and risk of early-onset breast cancer in carriers and noncarriers of BRCA1 and BRCA2 mutations. Cancer Epidemiol Biomarkers Prev 2005; 14(2):350–356.

Mirkovic N, Marti-Renom MA, Weber BL, Sali A, Monteiro AN. Structure-based assessment of missense mutations in human BRCA1: implications for breast and ovarian cancer predisposition. Cancer Res 2004; 64(11):3790–3797.

Mizushina Y, Yagita E, Kuramochi K, Kuriyama I, Shimazaki N, Koiwai O, Uchiyama Y, Yomezawa Y, Sugawara F, Kobayashi S, Sakaguchi K, Yoshida H. 5-(Hydroxymethyl)-2-furfural: a selective inhibitor of DNA polymerase lambda and terminal deoxynucleotidyltransferase. Arch Biochem Biophys 2006; 446(1):69–76.

Modan B, Hartge P, Hirsh-Yechezkel G, Chetrit A, Lubin F, Beller U, Ben-Baruch G, Fishman A, Menczer J, Ebbers SM, Tucker MA, Wacholder S, Struewing JP, Friedman E, Piura B. Parity, oral contraceptives, and the risk of ovarian cancer among carriers and noncarriers of a BRCA1 or BRCA2 mutation. N Engl J Med 2001; 345(4):235–240.

Moisan A, Gaudreau L. The BRCA1 COOH-terminal region acts as an RNA polymerase II carboxyl-terminal domain kinase inhibitor that modulates p21WAF1/CIP1 expression. J Biol Chem 2006; 281(30):21119–21130.

Moisan A, Larochelle C, Guillemette B, Gaudreau L. BRCA1 can modulate RNA polymerase II carboxy-terminal domain phosphorylation levels. Mol Cell Biol 2004; 24(16): 6947–6956.

Monteiro AN, August A, Hanafusa H. Evidence for a transcriptional activation function of BRCA1 C-terminal region. Proc Natl Acad Sci U S A 1996; 93:13595–13599.

Monteiro AN, Couch FJ. Cancer risk assessment at the atomic level. Cancer Res 2006; 66(4):1897–1899.

Morrell D, Cromartie E, Swift M. Mortality and cancer incidence in 263 patients with ataxia-telangiectasia. J Natl Cancer Inst 1986; 77(1):89–92.

Morris JR, Pangon L, Boutell C, Katagiri T, Keep NH, Solomon E. Genetic analysis of BRCA1 ubiquitin ligase activity and its relationship to breast cancer susceptibility. Hum Mol Genet 2006; 15(4):599–606.

Moyano JV, Evans JR, Chen F, Lu M, Werner ME, Yehiely F, Diaz LK, Turbin D, Karaca G, Wiley E, Nielsen TO, Perou CM, Cryns VL. AlphaB-crystallin is a novel oncoprotein that predicts poor clinical outcome in breast cancer. J Clin Invest 2006; 116(1):261–270.

Moynahan M, Chiu J, Koller B, Jasin M. Brca1 controls homology-directed DNA repair. Mol Cell 1999; 4:511–518.

Moynahan ME, Pierce AJ, Jasin M. BRCA2 is required for homology-directed repair of chromosomal breaks. Mol Cell 2001; 7(2):263–272.

Mullan PB, Hosey AM, Buckley NE, Quinn JE, Kennedy RD, Johnston PG, Harkin DP. The 2,5 oligoadenylate synthetase/RNaseL pathway is a novel effector of BRCA1- and interferon-gamma-mediated apoptosis. Oncogene 2005; 24(35):5492–5501.

Mullan PB, Quinn JE, Gilmore PM, McWilliams S, Andrews H, Gervin C, McCabe N, McKenna S, White P, Song YH, Maheswaran S, Liu E, Haber DA, Johnston PG, Harkin DP. BRCA1 and GADD45 mediated G2/M cell cycle arrest in response to antimicrotubule agents. Oncogene 2001; 20 (43):6123–6131.

Mullan PB, Quinn JE, Harkin DP. The role of BRCA1 in transcriptional regulation and cell cycle control. Oncogene 2006; 25(43):5854–5863.

Myriad. Mutation prevalence tables for BRCA1/2 genes. 2004. Available at: http://www.myriadtests.com/provider/brca_mutation_prevalence.htm

Nanda R, Schumm LP, Cummings S, Fackenthal JD, Sveen L, Ademuyiwa F, Cobleigh M, Esserman L, Lindor NM, Neuhausen SL, Olopade OI. Genetic testing in an ethnically diverse cohort of high-risk women: a comparative analysis of BRCA1 and BRCA2 mutations in American families of European and African ancestry. JAMA 2005; 294 (15):1925–1933.

Narayan G, Arias-Pulido H, Nandula SV, Basso K, Sugirtharaj DD, Vargas H, Mansukhani M, Villella J, Meyer L, Schneider A, Gissmann L, Durst M, Pothuri B, Murty VV. Promoter hypermethylation of FANCF: disruption of Fanconi Anemia-BRCA pathway in cervical cancer. Cancer Res 2004; 64(9):2994–2997.

Narod S, Feunteun J, Lynch H, Watson P, Conway T, Lynch J, Lenoir G. Familial breast-ovarian cancer locus on chromosome 17q12-q23. Lancet 1991; 338:82–83.

Narod SA. Modifiers of risk of hereditary breast cancer. Oncogene 2006; 25(43):5832–5836.

Narod SA, Brunet JS, Ghadirian P, Robson M, Heimdal K, Neuhausen SL, Stoppa-Lyonnet D, Lerman C, Pasini B, de los Rios P, Weber B, Lynch H. Tamoxifen and risk of contralateral breast cancer in BRCA1 and BRCA2 mutation carriers: a case-control study. Hereditary Breast Cancer Clinical Study Group. Lancet 2000; 356(9245):1876–1881.

Narod SA, Dube MP, Klijn J, Lubinski J, Lynch HT, Ghadirian P, Provencher D, Heimdal K, Moller P, Robson M, Offit K, Isaacs C, Weber B, Friedman E, Gershoni-Baruch R, Rennert G, Pasini B, Wagner T, Daly M, Garber JE, Neuhausen SL, Ainsworth P, Olsson H, Evans G, Osborne M, Couch F, Foulkes WD, Warner E, Kim-Sing C, Olopade O, Tung N, Saal HM, Weitzel J, Merajver S, Gauthier-Villars M, Jernstrom H, Sun P, Brunet JS. Oral contraceptives and the risk of breast cancer in BRCA1 and BRCA2 mutation carriers. J Natl Cancer Inst 2002; 94(23):1773–1779.

Narod SA, Goldgar D, Cannon-Albright L, Weber B, Moslehi R, Ives E, Lenoir G, Lynch H. Risk modifiers in carriers of BRCA1 mutations. Int J Cancer 1995; 64(6):394–398.

Narod SA, Lubinski J, Ghadirian P, Lynch HT, Moller P, Foulkes WD, Rosen B, Kim-Sing C, Isaacs C, Domchek S, Sun P. Screening mammography and risk of breast cancer in BRCA1 and BRCA2 mutation carriers: a case-control study. Lancet Oncol 2006; 7(5):402–406.

Narod SA, Lynch HT. CHEK2 mutation and hereditary breast cancer. J Clin Oncol 2007; 25(1):6–7.

Narod SA, Risch H, Moslehi R, Dorum A, Neuhausen S, Olsson H, Provencher D, Radice P, Evans G, Bishop S, Burnet JS, Ponder A, Oral contraceptives and the risk of hereditary ovarian cancer. Hereditary Ovarian Cancer Clinical Study Group N Engl J Med 1998; 339:424–428.

Nelen MR, van Staveren WC, Peeters EA, Hassel MB, Gorlin RJ, Hamm H, Lindboe CF, Fryns JP, Sijmons RH, Woods DG, Mariman EC, Padberg GW, Kremet H. Germline mutations in the PTEN/MMAC1 gene in patients with Cowden disease. Hum Mol Genet 1997; 6:1383–1387.

Nelson HD, Huffman LH, Fu R, Harris EL. Genetic risk assessment and BRCA mutation testing for breast and ovarian cancer susceptibility: systematic evidence review for the U.S. Preventive Services Task Force. Ann Intern Med 2005; 143(5):362–379.

Neuhausen S, Gilewski T, Norton L, Tran T, McGuire P, Swensen J, Hampel H, Borgen P, Brown K, Skolnick M, Shattuck-Eidens D, Jhanwar S, Goldgar D, Offit K. Recurrent BRCA2 6147delT mutations in Ashkenazi Jewish women affected by breast cancer. Nat Genet 1996; 13: 126–128.

Nevanlinna H, Bartek J. The CHEK2 gene and inherited breast cancer susceptibility. Oncogene 2006; 25(43):5912–5919.

Newill V. Distribution of cancer mortality among ethnic subgroups of the white population of New York City, 1953-58. J Natl Cancer Inst 1961; 26:405–417.

Newman B, Mu H, Butler LM, Millikan RC, Moorman PG, King M-C. Frequency of breast cancer attributable to BRCA1 in a population-based series of American women. JAMA 1998; 2779:915–921.

Nielsen TO, Andrews HN, Cheang M, Kucab JE, Hsu FD, Ragaz J, Gilks CB, Makretsov N, Bajdik CD, Brookes C, Neckers LM, Evdokimova V, Huntsman DG, Dunn SE. Expression of the insulin-like growth factor I receptor and urokinase plasminogen activator in breast cancer is associated with poor survival: potential for intervention with 17-allylamino geldanamycin. Cancer Res 2004; 64(1):286–291.

Nkondjock A, Ghadirian P, Kotsopoulos J, Lubinski J, Lynch H, Kim-Sing C, Horsman D, Rosen B, Isaacs C, Weber B, Foulkes W, Ainsworth P, Tung N, Eisen A, Friedman E, Eng C, Sun P, Narod SA. Coffee consumption and breast cancer risk among BRCA1 and BRCA2 mutation carriers. Int J Cancer 2006; 118(1):103–107.

Oddoux C, Struewing JP, Clayton CM, S. N, Brody LC, Kaback M, Haas B, Norton L, Borgen P, Jhanwar S, Goldgar D, Ostrer H, Offit K. The carrier frequency of the BRCA2 617delT mutation among Ashkenazi Jewish individuals is approximately 1%. Nat Genet 1996; 14:188–190.

Oefner P, Underhill P. Comparative DNA sequencing by denaturing high-performance liquid chromatography (DHPLC). Am J Hum Genet 1995; 57:A266.

Offit K, Pierce H, Kirchhoff T, Kolachana P, Rapaport B, Gregersen P, Johnson S, Yossepowitch O, Huang H, Satagopan J, Robson M, Scheuer L, Nafa K, Ellis N. Frequency of CHEK2*1100delC in New York breast cancer cases and controls. BMC Med Genet 2003; 4:1.

Oishi H, Kitagawa H, Wada O, Takezawa S, Tora L, Kouzu-Fujita M, Takada I, Yano T, Yanagisawa J, Kato S. An hGCN5/TRRAP histone acetyltransferase complex co-activates BRCA1 transactivation function through histone modification. J Biol Chem 2006; 281(1):20–26.

Okada S, Ouchi T. Cell cycle differences in DNA damage-induced BRCA1 phosphorylation affect its subcellular localization. J Biol Chem 2003; 278(3):2015–2020.

Oldenburg RA, Kroeze-Jansema K, Meijers-Heijboer H, van Asperen CJ, Hoogerbrugge N, van Leeuwen I, Vasen HF, Cleton-Jansen AM, Kraan J, Houwing-Duistermaat JJ, Morreau H, Cornelisse CJ, Devilee P. Characterization of familial non-BRCA1/2 breast tumors by loss of heterozygosity and immunophenotyping. Clin Cancer Res 2006; 12(6):1693–1700.

Oleykowski C, Bronson Mullins C, Godwin A, Yeung A. Mutation detection using a novel plant endonuclease. Nucleic Acids Res 1998; 26:4597–4602.

Olivier M, Langerod A, Carrieri P, Bergh J, Klaar S, Eyfjord J, Theillet C, Rodriguez C, Lidereau R, Bieche I, Varley J, Bignon Y, Uhrhammer N, Winqvist R, Jukkola-Vuorinen A, Niederacher D, Kato S, Ishioka C, Hainaut P, Borresen-Dale AL. The clinical value of somatic TP53 gene mutations in 1,794 patients with breast cancer. Clin Cancer Res 2006; 12(4):1157–1167.

Olopade OI, Fackenthal JD, Dunston G, Tainsky MA, Collins F, Whitfield-Broome C. Breast cancer genetics in African Americans. Cancer 2003; 97(1 Suppl):236–245.

Ongusaha PP, Ouchi T, Kim KT, Nytko E, Kwak JC, Duda RB, Deng CX, Lee SW. BRCA1 shifts p53-mediated cellular outcomes towards irreversible growth arrest. Oncogene 2003; 22(24):3749–3758.

Osorio A, Rodriguez-Lopez R, Diez O, de la Hoya M, Ignacio Martinez J, Vega A, Esteban-Cardenosa E, Alonso C, Caldes T, Benitez J. The breast cancer low-penetrance allele 1100delC in the CHEK2 gene is not present in Spanish familial breast cancer population. Int J Cancer 2004; 108(1):54–56.

Ouchi T, Lee SW, Ouchi M, Aaronson SA, Horvath CM. Collaboration of signal transducer and activator of transcription 1 (STAT1) and BRCA1 in differential regulation of IFN-gamma target genes. Proc Natl Acad Sci U S A 2000; 97(10):5208–5213.

Ouchi T, Monteiro ANA, August A, Aaronson SA, Hanafusa H. BRCA1 regulates p53-dependent gene expression. Proc Natl Acad Sci USA 1998; 95:2302–2306.

Palacios J, Honrado E, Osorio A, Cazorla A, Sarrio D, Barroso A, Rodriguez S, Cigudosa JC, Diez O, Alonso C, Lerma E, Dopazo J, Rivas C, Benitez J. Phenotypic characterization of BRCA1 and BRCA2 tumors based in a tissue microarray study with 37 immunohistochemical markers. Breast Cancer Res Treat 2005; 90(1):5–14.

Palacios J, Honrado E, Osorio A, Cazorla A, Sarrio D, Barroso A, Rodriguez S, Cigudosa JC, Diez O, Alonso C, Lerma E, Sanchez L, Rivas C, Benitez J. Immunohistochemical characteristics defined by tissue microarray of hereditary breast cancer not attributable to BRCA1 or BRCA2 mutations: differences from breast carcinomas arising in BRCA1 and BRCA2 mutation carriers. Clin Cancer Res 2003; 9(10 Pt 1):3606–3614.

Palacios J, Honrado E, Osorio A, Diez O, Rivas C, Benitez J. Re: Germline BRCA1 mutations and a basal epithelial phenotype in breast cancer. J Natl Cancer Inst 2004; 96(9):712–714; author reply 714.

Pao GM, Janknecht R, Ruffner H, Hunter T, Verma IM. CBP/p300 interact with and function as transcriptional coactivators of BRCA1. Proc Natl Acad Sci U S A 2000; 97(3):1020–1025.

Parkin D, Iscovich J. Risk of cancer in migrants and their descendants in Israel: II carcinomas and germ-cell tumours. Int J Cancer 1997; 70:654–660.

Parmigiani G, Berry DA, Aguilar O. Determining carrier probabilities for breast cancer-susceptibility genes BRCA1 and BRCA2. Am J Hum Genet 1998; 62:145–158.

Patel K, Yu V, Lee H, Corcoran A, Thistlethwaite F, Evans M, Colledge W, Friedman L, Ponder B, Venkitaraman A. Involvement of Brca2 in DNA repair. Mol Cell 1998; 1:347–357.

Patel KJ. Fanconi anemia and breast cancer susceptibility. Nat Genet 2007; 39(2):142–143.

Paterson JWE. BRCA1: A review of structure and putative functions. Disease Markers 1998; 13:261–274.

Paull TT, Cortez D, Bowers B, Elledge SJ, Gellert M. Direct DNA binding by Brca1. Proc Natl Acad Sci U S A 2001; 98(11):6086–6091.

Peelen T, van Vliet M, Petrij-Bosch A, Mieremet R, Szabo C, van den Ouweland AMW, Hogervorst F, Brohet R, Ligtenberg MJL, Teugels E, van der Luijt R, van der Hout AH, Gille JJP, Pals G, Jedema I, Olmer R, van Leeuwen I, Newman B, Plandsoen M, van der Est M, Brink G, Hageman S, Arts PJW, Bakker MM, Willems HW, van der Looij E, Neyns B, Bonduelle M, Jansen R, Oosterwijk JC, Sijmons R, Smeets HJM, van Asperen CJ, Meijers-Heijboer H, Klijn JGM, de Greve J, King M-C, Menko FH, Brunner HG, Halley D, van Ommen G-JB, Vasen HFA, Cornelisse CJ, van't Veer LJ, de Knijff P, Bakker E, Devilee P. A high proportion of novel mutations in BRCA1 with strong founder effects among Dutch and Belgian hereditary breast and ovarian cancer families. Am J Hum Genet 1997; 60:1041–1049.

Perou CM, Sorlie T, Eisen MB, van de Rijn M, Jeffrey SS, Rees CA, Pollack JR, Ross DT, Johnsen H, Akslen LA, Fluge O, Pergamenschikov A, Williams C, Zhu SX, Lonning PE, Borresen-Dale AL, Brown PO, Botstein D. Molecular portraits of human breast tumours. Nature 2000; 406 (6797):747–752.

Perrin-Vidoz L, Sinilnikova OM, Stoppa-Lyonnet D, Lenoir GM, Mazoyer S. The nonsense-mediated mRNA decay pathway triggers degradation of most BRCA1 mRNAs bearing premature termination codons. Hum Mol Genet 2002; 11(23):2805–2814.

Peto J, Collins N, Barfoot R, Seal S, Warren W, Rahman N, Easton D, Evans C, Deacon J, Stratton M. Prevalence of

BRCA1 and BRCA2 gene mutations in patients with early-onset breast cancer. J Natl Cancer Inst 1999; 91:943–949.

Peto J, Mack TM. High constant incidence in twins and other relatives of women with breast cancer. Nat Genet 2000; 26 (4):411–414.

Petrij-Bosch A, Peelen T, van Vliet M, van Eijk R, Olmer R, Drusedau M, Hogervorst FFL, Hageman S, Arts PJW, Ligtenberg MJL, Meijers-Heijboer H, Klijn JGM, Vasen HFA, Cornelisse CJ, van't Veer LJ, Bakker E, van Ommen G-JB, Devilee P. BRCA1 genomic deletions are major founder mutations in Dutch breast cancer patients. Nat Genet 1997; 17:341–345.

Pharoah PD, Antoniou A, Bobrow M, Zimmern RL, Easton DF, Ponder BA. Polygenic susceptibility to breast cancer and implications for prevention. Nat Genet 2002; 31(1):33–36.

Pharoah PD, Dunning AM, Ponder BA, Easton DF. Association studies for finding cancer-susceptibility genetic variants. Nat Rev Cancer 2004; 4(11):850–860.

Phelan C, Rebbeck R, Weber B, Devilee P, Ruttledge M, Lynch H, Lemoir G, Statton M, Easton D, Ponder B, Cannon-Albright L, Larsson C, Goldgar D, Narod S. Ovarian cancer risk in *BRCA1* carriers is modified by the HRAS1 variable number of tandem repeat (ANTR) locus. Nat Genet 1996; 12:309–311.

Phelan CM, Dapic V, Tice B, Favis R, Kwan E, Barany F, Manoukian S, Radice P, van der Luijt RB, van Nesselrooij BP, Chenevix-Trench G, kConFab, Caldes T, de la Hoya M, Lindquist S, Tavtigian SV, Goldgar D, Borg A, Narod SA, Monteiro AN. Classification of BRCA1 missense variants of unknown clinical significance. J Med Genet 2005; 42 (2):138–146.

Pich A, Margaria E, Chiusa L. Oncogenes and male breast carcinoma: c-erbB-2 and p53 coexpression predicts a poor survival. J Clin Oncol 2000; 18(16):2948–2956.

Piekarski JH, Biernat W. Clinical significance of CK5/6 and PTEN protein expression in patients with bilateral breast carcinoma. Histopathology 2006; 49(3):248–255.

Pierce LJ, Levin AM, Rebbeck TR, Ben-David MA, Friedman E, Solin LJ, Harris EE, Gaffney DK, Haffty BG, Dawson LA, Narod SA, Olivotto IA, Eisen A, Whelan TJ, Olopade OI, Isaacs C, Merajver SD, Wong JS, Garber JE, Weber BL. Ten-year multi-institutional results of breast-conserving surgery and radiotherapy in BRCA1/2-associated stage I/II breast cancer. J Clin Oncol 2006; 24(16):2437–2443.

Pierce LJ, Strawderman M, Narod SA, Oliviotto I, Eisen A, Dawson L, Gaffney D, Solin LJ, Nixon A, Garber J, Berg C, Isaacs C, Heimann R, Olopade OI, Haffty B, Weber BL. Effect of radiotherapy after breast-conserving treatment in women with breast cancer and germline BRCA1/2 mutations. J Clin Oncol 2000; 18(19):3360–3369.

Pietschmann A, Mehdipour P, Mehdipour P, Atri M, Hofmann W, Hosseini-Asl SS, Scherneck S, Mundlos S, Peters H. Mutation analysis of BRCA1 and BRCA2 genes in Iranian high risk breast cancer families. J Cancer Res Clin Oncol 2005; 131(8):552–558.

Pinilla SM, Honrado E, Hardisson D, Benitez J, Palacios J. Caveolin-1 expression is associated with a basal-like phenotype in sporadic and hereditary breast cancer. Breast Cancer Res Treat 2006; 99(1):85–90.

Pisano M, Cossu A, Persico I, Palmieri G, Angius A, Casu G, Palomba G, Sarobba M, Rocca P, Dedola M, Olmeo N, Pasca A, Budroni M, Marras V, Pisano A, Pfarris A, Massarelli G, Pirastur M, Tanda F. Identification of a founder *BRCA2* mutation in Sardinia. Br J Cancer 2000; 82:553–559.

Piver M, Jishi M, Rsudada Y, Nava G. Primaty peritoneal carcinoma after prophylactic oophorectomy in women with a family history of ovarian cancer A report of the Gilda Radner Familial Ovarian Cancer Registry. Cancer 1993; 71:2751–2755.

Powell CB, Kenley E, Chen LM, Crawford B, McLennan J, Zaloudek C, Komaromy M, Beattie M, Ziegler J. Risk-reducing salpingo-oophorectomy in BRCA mutation carriers: role of serial sectioning in the detection of occult malignancy. J Clin Oncol 2005; 23(1):127–132.

Prakash S, Prakash L. Translesion DNA synthesis in eukaryotes: a one- or two-polymerase affair. Genes Dev 2002; 16(15): 1872–1883.

Preisler-Adams S, Schonbuchner I, Fiebig B, Welling B, Dworniczak B, Weber BH. Gross rearrangements in BRCA1 but not BRCA2 play a notable role in predisposition to breast and ovarian cancer in high-risk families of German origin. Cancer Genet Cytogenet 2006; 168(1): 44–49.

Presneau N, La Place-Marieze V, Sylvain V, Lortholary A, Hardouin A, Bernard-Gallon D, Bignon YJ. Mutation by deletion-insertion in *BRCA-1* gene in three unrelated French breast/ovarian cancer families: possible implication of a mobile element (in French). Bull Cancer 1999; 86:385–390.

Puget N, Gad S, Perrin-Vidoz L, Sinilnikova OM, Stoppa-Lyonnet D, Lenoir GM, Mazoyer S. Distinct BRCA1 rearrangements involving the BRCA1 pseudogene suggest the existence of a recombination hot spot. Am J Hum Genet 2002; 70(4):858–865.

Puget N, Stoppa-Lyonnet D, Sinilnikova OM, Pages S, Lynch HT, Lenoir GM, Mazoyer S. Screening for germ-line rearrangements and regulatory mutations in BRCA1 led to the identification of four new deletions. Cancer Res 1999; 59:455–461.

Puget N, Torchard D, Serova-Sinilnikova OM, Lynch HT, Feunteun J, Lenoir GM, Mazoyer S. A 1-kb Alu-mediated germ-line deletion removing BRCA1 exon 17. Cancer Res 1997; 57:828–831.

Radford DM, Zehnbauer BA. Inherited breast cancer. Surg Clin North Am 1996; 76:205–220.

Rahman N, Seal S, Thompson D, Kelly P, Renwick A, Elliott A, Reid S, Spanova K, Barfoot R, Chagtai T, Jayatilake H, McGuffog L, Hanks S, Evans DG, Eccles D, Easton DF, Stratton MR. PALB2, which encodes a BRCA2-interacting protein, is a breast cancer susceptibility gene. Nat Genet 2007; 39(2):165–167.

Ramus S, Friedman L, Gayther S, Ponder B, Bobrow L, van der Looji M, Papp J, Olah E. A breast/ovarian cancer patient with germline mutations in both BRCA1 and BRCA2. Nat Genet 1997; 15:14–15.

Rashid MU, Jakubowska A, Justenhoven C, Harth V, Pesch B, Baisch C, Pierl CB, Bruning T, Ko Y, Benner A, Wichmann HE, Brauch H, Hamann U. German populations with infrequent CHEK2*1100delC and minor associations with early-onset and familial breast cancer. Eur J Cancer 2005; 41(18):2896–2903.

Ravnik-Glavac D, Dean M. Sensitivity of single-strand conformation polymorphism and heteroduplex method for mutation detection in the cystic fibrosis gene. Hum Mol Genet 1994; 3:801–807.

Razandi M, Pedram A, Rosen EM, Levin ER. BRCA1 inhibits membrane estrogen and growth factor receptor signaling to cell proliferation in breast cancer. Mol Cell Biol 2004; 24 (13):5900–5913.

Rebbeck TR, Friebel T, Lynch HT, Neuhausen SL, van 't Veer L, Garber JE, Evans GR, Narod SA, Isaacs C, Matloff E, Daly MB, Olopade OI, Weber BL. Bilateral prophylactic mastectomy reduces breast cancer risk in BRCA1 and BRCA2 mutation carriers: the PROSE Study Group. J Clin Oncol 2004; 22(6):1055–1062.

Rebbeck TR, Friebel T, Wagner T, Lynch HT, Garber JE, Daly MB, Isaacs C, Olopade OI, Neuhausen SL, van 't Veer L, Eeles R, Evans DG, Tomlinson G, Matloff E, Narod SA, Eisen A, Domchek S, Armstrong K, Weber BL. Effect of short-term hormone replacement therapy on breast cancer risk reduction after bilateral prophylactic oophorectomy in BRCA1 and BRCA2 mutation carriers: the PROSE Study Group. J Clin Oncol 2005; 23(31):7804–7810.

Rebbeck TR, Levin AM, Eisen A, Snyder C, Watson P, Cannon-Albright L, Isaacs C, Olopade O, Garber JE, Godwin AK, Daly MB, Narod SA, Neuhausen SL, Lynch HT, Weber BL. Breast cancer risk after bilateral prophylactic oophorectomy in BRCA1 mutation carriers. J Natl Cancer Inst 1999; 91:1475–1479.

Rebbeck TR, Lynch HT, Neuhausen SL, Narod SA, Van't Veer L, Garber JE, Evans G, Isaacs C, Daly MB, Matloff E, Olopade OI, Weber BL. Prophylactic oophorectomy in carriers of BRCA1 or BRCA2 mutations. N Engl J Med 2002; 346(21):1616–1622.

Rebbeck TR, Wang Y, Kantoff PW, Krithivas K, Neuhausen SL, Godwin AK, Daly MB, Narod SA, Brunet JS, Vesprini D, Garber JE, Lynch HT, Weber BL, Brown M. Modification of BRCA1- and BRCA2-associated breast cancer risk by AIB1 genotype and reproductive history. Cancer Res 2001; 61(14):5420–5424.

Reid S, Schindler D, Hanenberg H, Barker K, Hanks S, Kalb R, Neveling K, Kelly P, Seal S, Freund M, Wurm M, Batish SD, Lach FP, Yetgin S, Neitzel H, Ariffin H, Tischkowitz M, Mathew CG, Auerbach AD, Rahman N. Biallelic mutations in PALB2 cause Fanconi anemia subtype FA-N and predispose to childhood cancer. Nat Genet 2007; 39 (2):162–164.

Reis-Filho JS, Steele D, Di Palma S, Jones RL, Savage K, James M, Milanezi F, Schmitt FC, Ashworth A. Distribution and significance of nerve growth factor receptor (*NGFR*/p75NTR) in normal, benign and malignant breast tissue. Mod Pathol 2006; 19(2):307–319.

Renwick A, Thompson D, Seal S, Kelly P, Chagtai T, Ahmed M, North B, Jayatilake H, Barfoot R, Spanova K, McGuffog L, Evans DG, Eccles D, Easton DF, Stratton MR, Rahman N. ATM mutations that cause ataxia-telangiectasia are breast cancer susceptibility alleles. Nat Genet 2006; 38(8):873–875.

Rhei E, Kang L, Bogomolniy F, Federici MG, Borgen PI, Boyd J. Mutation analysis of the putative tumor suppressor gene PTEN/MMAC1 in primary breast carcinomas. Cancer Res 1997; 57:3657–3659.

Richter S, Seth A. One step direct detection of recurrent mutations in the breast cancer susceptibility gene *BRCA1*. Int J Oncol 1998; 12:1263–1267.

Ries L, Kosary C, Hankey B, Harras A, Miller B, Edwards B, eds. SEER Cancer Statistics Reviews 1973–1993. Tables and Graphs. Bethesda, MD: U.S. National Cancer Institute; 1996.

Risch HA, McLaughlin JR, Cole DE, Rosen B, Bradley L, Fan I, Tang J, Li S, Zhang S, Shaw PA, Narod SA. Population BRCA1 and BRCA2 mutation frequencies and cancer penetrances: a kin-cohort study in Ontario, Canada. J Natl Cancer Inst 2006; 98(23):1694–1706.

Risch HA, McLaughlin JR, Cole DE, Rosen B, Bradley L, Kwan E, Jack E, Vesprini DJ, Kuperstein G, Abrahamson JL, Fan I, Wong B, Narod SA. Prevalence and penetrance of germline BRCA1 and BRCA2 mutations in a population series of 649 women with ovarian cancer. Am J Hum Genet 2001; 68(3):700–710.

Roa B, Boyd A, Volcik K, Richards C. Ashkenazi Jewish population frequencies for common mutations in *BRCA1* and *BRCA2*. Nat Genet 1996; 14:185–187.

Robson ME, Chappuis PO, Satagopan J, Wong N, Boyd J, Goffin JR, Hudis C, Roberge D, Norton L, Begin LR, Offit K, Foulkes WD. A combined analysis of outcome following breast cancer: differences in survival based on BRCA1/BRCA2 mutation status and administration of adjuvant treatment. Breast Cancer Res 2004; 6(1):R8–R17.

Rodriguez H, Jaruga P, Leber D, Nyaga SG, Evans MK, Dizdaroglu M. Lymphoblasts of Women with BRCA1 Mutations Are Deficient in Cellular Repair of 8,5′-Cyclopurine-2'-deoxynucleosides and 8-Hydroxy-2'-deoxyguanosine. Biochemistry 2007; 46(9):2488–2496.

Rodriguez-Pinilla SM, Sarrio D, Honrado E, Hardisson D, Calero F, Benitez J, Palacios J. Prognostic significance of basal-like phenotype and fascin expression in node-negative invasive breast carcinomas. Clin Cancer Res 2006; 12 (5):1533–1539.

Rubinstein WS. Hereditary breast cancer in Jews. Fam Cancer 2004; 3(3–4):249–257.

Rubinstein WS, O'Neill SM, Peters JA, Rittmeyer LJ, Stadler MP. Mathematical modeling for breast cancer risk assessment. State of the art and role in medicine. Oncology (Williston Park) 2002; 16(8):1082–1094; discussion 1094, 1097–1089.

Ruffner H, Joazeiro CA, Hemmati D, Hunter T, Verma IM. Cancer-predisposing mutations within the RING domain of BRCA1: loss of ubiquitin protein ligase activity and protection from radiation hypersensitivity. Proc Natl Acad Sci U S A 2001; 98(9):5134–5139.

Ruiz C, Seibt S, Al Kuraya K, Siraj AK, Mirlacher M, Schraml P, Maurer R, Spichtin H, Torhorst J, Popovska S, Simon R, Sauter G. Tissue microarrays for comparing molecular features with proliferation activity in breast cancer. Int J Cancer 2006; 118(9):2190–2194.

Rumbaut R. Immigrants from Latin America and the Caribbean: a socioeconomic profile. JSRI Statistical Brief No. 6/Cifras Breves No. 6. East Lansing, MI: The Julián Samora Research Institute, Michigan State University. April, 1995.

Ruparel H, Ulz ME, Kim S, Ju J. Digital detection of genetic mutations using SPC-sequencing. Genome Res 2004; 14(2): 296–300.

Rutter JL, Chatterjee N, Wacholder S, Struewing J. The HER2 I655V polymorphism and breast cancer risk in Ashkenazim. Epidemiology 2003a; 14(6):694–700.

Rutter JL, Smith AM, Davila MR, Sigurdson AJ, Giusti RM, Pineda MA, Doody MM, Tucker MA, Greene MH, Zhang J, Struewing JP. Mutational analysis of the BRCA1-interacting genes ZNF350/ZBRK1 and BRIP1/BACH1 among BRCA1 and BRCA2-negative probands from breast-ovarian cancer families and among early-onset breast cancer cases and reference individuals. Hum Mutat 2003b; 22(2):121–128.

Sabate JM, Gomez A, Torrubia S, Blancas C, Sanchez G, Alonso MC, Lerma E. Evaluation of breast involvement in relation to Cowden syndrome: a radiological and clinicopathological study of patients with PTEN germ-line mutations. Eur Radiol 2006; 16(3):702–706.

Saeki H, Siaud N, Christ N, Wiegant WW, van Buul PP, Han M, Zdzienicka MZ, Stark JM, Jasin M. Suppression of the DNA repair defects of BRCA2-deficient cells with heterologous protein fusions. Proc Natl Acad Sci U S A 2006; 103(23):8768–8773.

Sakorafas GH, Tsiotou AG. Genetic predisposition to breast cancer: a surgical perspective. Br J Surg 2000; 87:149–162.

Salazar H, Godwin AK, Daly MB, Laub PB, Hogan WM, Rosenblum N, Boente MP, Lynch HT, Hamilton TC. Microscopic benign and invasive malignant neoplasms and a cancer-prone phenotype in prophylactic oophorectomies. J Natl Cancer Inst 1996; 88(24):1810–1820.

Salber E, Trichopulos D, MacMahon B. Lactation and reproductive histories of breast cancer patients in Boston, 1965-66. J Natl Cancer Inst 1969; 43:1013–1024.

Sasco AJ, Lowenfels AB, Pasker-de Jong P. Review article: epidemiology of male breast cancer. A meta-analysis of published case-control studies and discussion of selected aetiological factors. Int J Cancer 1993; 53(4):538–549.

Savitsky K, Bar-Shira A, Gilad S, Rotman G, Ziv Y, Vanagaite L, Tagle DA, Smith S, Uziel T, Sfez S, et al., A single ataxia telangiectasia gene with a product similar to PI-3 kinase. Science 1995; 268(5218):1749–1753.

Schutte M, Seal S, Barfoot R, Meijers-Heijboer H, Wasielewski M, Evans DG, Eccles D, Meijers C, Lohman F, Klijn J, van den Ouweland A, Futreal PA, Nathanson KL, Weber BL, Easton DF, Stratton MR, Rahman N. Variants in CHEK2 other than 1100delC do not make a major contribution to breast cancer susceptibility. Am J Hum Genet 2003; 72 (4):1023–1028.

Scully R, Anderson SF, Chao DM, Wei W, Ye L, Young RA, Livingston DM, Parvin JD. BRCA1 is a component of the RNA polymerase II holoenzyme. Proc Natl Acad Sci U S A 1997a; 94:5605–5610.

Scully R, Chen J, Ochs RL, Keegan K, Hoekstra M, Feunteun J, Livingston DM. Dynamic changes of BRCA1 subnuclear location and phosphorylation state are initiated by DNA damage. Cell 1997b; 90:425–435.

Scully R, Chen J, Plug A, Xiao Y, Weaver D, Feunteun J, Ashley T, Livingston DM. Association of BRCA1 with Rad51 in mitotic and meiotic cells. Cell 1997c; 88:265–275.

Scully R, Livingston D. In search of the tumour-suppressor functions of BRCA1 and BRCA2. Nature 2000; 408: 429–432.

Seal S, Barfoot R, Jayatilake H, Smith P, Renwick A, Bascombe L, McGuffog L, Evans DG, Eccles D, Easton DF, Stratton MR, Rahman N. Evaluation of Fanconi Anemia genes in familial breast cancer predisposition. Cancer Res 2003; 63(24):8596–8599.

Seal S, Thompson D, Renwick A, Elliott A, Kelly P, Barfoot R, Chagtai T, Jayatilake H, Ahmed M, Spanova K, North B, McGuffog L, Evans DG, Eccles D, Easton DF, Stratton MR, Rahman N. Truncating mutations in the Fanconi anemia J gene BRIP1 are low-penetrance breast cancer susceptibility alleles. Nat Genet 2006; 38(11):1239–1241.

Seitz S, Rohde K, Bender E, Nothnagel A, Pidde H, Ullrich O, El-Zehairy A, Haensch W, Jandrig B, Kilble K, Schlag P, Scherneck S. Deletion mapping and linkage analysis provide strong indication for the involvement of the human chromosome region 8p12-22 in breast carcinogenesis Br J Cancer 1997; 76:983–991.

Shaag A, Walsh T, Renbaum P, Kirchhoff T, Nafa K, Shiovitz S, Mandell JB, Welcsh P, Lee MK, Ellis N, Offit K, Levy-Lahad E, King MC. Functional and genomic approaches reveal an ancient CHEK2 allele associated with breast cancer in the Ashkenazi Jewish population. Hum Mol Genet 2005; 14(4):555–563.

Sharan SK, Morimatsu M, Albrecht U, Lim D-S, Regel E, Dinh C, Sands A, Eichele G, Hasty P, Bradley A. Embryonic lethality and radiation hypersensitivity mediated by Rad51 in mice lacking BRCA2. Nature 1997; 386:804–810.

Shattuck-Eidens D, McClure M, Simard J, Labrie F, Narod S, Couch F, Hoskins K, Weber B, Castilla L, Erdos M, Brody L, Friedman L, Ostermeyer E, Szabo C, King M-C, Jhanwar S, Offit K, Norton L, Gilewski T, Lubin M, Osborne M, Black D, Boyd M, Steel M, Ingles S, Haile R, Lindblom A, Olsson H, Borg A, Bishop DT, Solomon E, Radice P, Spatti G, Gayther S, Ponder B, Warren W, Stratton M, Liu Q, Fujimura F, Lewis C, Skolnick MH, Goldgar DE. A collaborative survey of 80 mutations in the BRCA1 breast and ovarian cancer susceptibility gene. JAMA 1995; 273:535–541.

Shattuck-Eidens D, Oliphant A, McClure M, McBride C, Gupte J, Rubano T, Pruss D, Tavtigian SV, Teng DH, Adey N, Staebell M, Gumpper K, Lundstrom R, Hulick M, Kelly M, Holmen J, Lingenfelter B, Manley S, Fujimura F, Luce M, Ward B, Cannon-Albright L, Steele L, Offit K, Thomas A, et al., BRCA1 sequence analysis in women at high risk for susceptibility mutations. Risk factor analysis and implications for genetic testing. JAMA 1997; 278 (15):1242–1250.

Shen D, Wu Y, Subbarao M, Bhat H, Chillar R, Vadgama J. Mutation analysis of BRCA1gene in African-American patients with breast cancer. J Natl Med Assoc 2000; 92: 29–35.

Shieh S, Ahn J, Tamai K, Taya Y, Prives C. The human homologs of checkpoint kinases Chk1 and Cds1 (Chk2) prosphorylate p53 at multiple DNA damage-inducible sites. Genes Dev 2000; 14:289–300.

Shih H, Nathanson KL, Seal S, Collins N, Stratton M, Rebbeck T, Weber B. BRCA1 and BRCA2 mutations in breast cancer families with multiple primary cancers. Clin Cancer Res 2000; 6:4259–4264.

Shiozaki EN, Gu L, Yan N, Shi Y. Structure of the BRCT repeats of BRCA1 bound to a BACH1 phosphopeptide: implications for signaling. Mol Cell 2004; 14(3):405–412.

Shivji MK, Davies OR, Savill JM, Bates DL, Pellegrini L, Venkitaraman AR. A region of human BRCA2 containing multiple BRC repeats promotes RAD51-mediated strand exchange. Nucleic Acids Res 2006; 34(14):4000–4011.

Siddiqui R, Onel K, Facio F, Nafa K, Diaz LR, Kauff N, Huang H, Robson M, Ellis N, Offit K. The TP53 mutational spectrum and frequency of CHEK2*1100delC in Li-Fraumeni-like kindreds. Fam Cancer 2005; 4(2):177–181.

Sidransky D, Tokino T, Helzlsoure K, Zehnbauer B, Rausch G, Shelton B, Prestigiacomo L, Bogelstein B, Davidson N. Inherited p53 gene mutations in breast cancer. Cancer Res 1992; 52:2984–2986.

Signoretti S, Di Marcotullio L, Richardson A, Ramaswamy S, Isaac B, Rue M, Monti F, Loda M, Pagano M. Oncogenic role of the ubiquitin ligase subunit Skp2 in human breast cancer. J Clin Invest 2002; 110(5):633–641.

Simard J, Tonin P, Durocher F, Morgan K, Rommens J, Gingras S, Samson C, Leblanc JF, Belanger C, Dion F, Liu Q, Skolnick M, Goldgar D, Shattuch-Eidens D, Labrie F, Narod SA. Common origins of BRCA1 mutations in Canadian breast and ovarian cancer families. Nat Genet 1994; 8:392–398.

Sinclair CS, Berry R, Schaid D, Thibodeau SN, Couch FJ. BRCA1 and BRCA2 have a limited role in familial prostate cancer. Cancer Res 2000; 60(5):1371–1375.

Sinilnikova OM, Egan KM, Quinn J, Boutrand L, Lenoir G, Stoppa-Lyonnet D, Desjardins L, Levy C, Goldgar D, Gragoudas E. Germline brca2 sequence variants in patients with ocular melanoma. Int J Cancer 1999; 82:325–328.

Smith P, McGuffog L, Easton DF, Mann GJ, Pupo GM, Newman B, Chenevix-Trench G, Szabo C, Southey M, Renard H, Odefrey F, Lynch H, Stoppa-Lyonnet D, Couch F, Hopper JL, Giles GG, McCredie MR, Buys S, Andrulis I, Senie R, Goldgar DE, Oldenburg R, Kroeze-Jansema K, Kraan J, Meijers-Heijboer H, Klijn JG, van Asperen C, van Leeuwen I, Vasen HF, Cornelisse CJ, Devilee P, Baskcomb L, Seal S, Barfoot R, Mangion J, Hall A, Edkins S, Rapley E, Wooster R, Chang-Claude J, Eccles D, Evans DG, Futreal PA, Nathanson KL, Weber BL, Rahman N, Stratton MR. A genome wide linkage search for breast cancer susceptibility genes. Genes Chromosomes Cancer 2006; 45(7):646–655.

Smith TM, Lee MK, Szabo CI, Jerome N, McEuen M, Taylor M, Hood L, King MC. Complete genomic sequence and analysis of 117 kb of human DNA containing the gene BRCA1. Genome Res 1996; 6(11):1029–1049.

Smith TR, Levine EA, Perrier ND, Miller MS, Freimanis RI, Lohman K, Case LD, Xu J, Mohrenweiser HW, Hu JJ. DNA-repair genetic polymorphisms and breast cancer risk. Cancer Epidemiol Biomarkers Prev 2003; 12(11 Pt 1): 1200–1204.

Sobczak K, Krzyzosiak WJ. Structural determinants of BRCA1 translational regulation. J Biol Chem 2002; 277(19): 17349–17358.

Sodha N, Houlston RS, Bullock S, Yuille MA, Chu C, Turner G, Eeles RA. Increasing evidence that germline mutations in CHEK2 do not cause Li-Fraumeni syndrome. Hum Mutat 2002; 20(6):460–462.

Somasundaram K, MacLachlan TK, Burns TF, Sgagias M, Cowan KH, Weber BL, el-Deiry WS. BRCA1 signals ARF-dependent stabilization and coactivation of p53. Oncogene 1999; 18(47):6605–6614.

Somasundaram K, Zharn H, Zeng Y, Houvras Y, Peng Y, Zhang H, Wu G, Licht J, Weber B, El-Diery W. Arrest of the cell cycle by the tumour-suppressor *BRCA1* requires the CDK-inhibitor *p21*WAF1/CiP1. Nature 1997; 389:187–190.

Sone T, Saeki Y, Toh-e A, Yokosawa H. Sem1p is a novel subunit of the 26 S proteasome from Saccharomyces cerevisiae. J Biol Chem 2004; 279(27):28807–28816.

Sorlie T, Perou CM, Tibshirani R, Aas T, Geisler S, Johnsen H, Hastie T, Eisen MB, van de Rijn M, Jeffrey SS, Thorsen T, Quist H, Matese JC, Brown PO, Botstein D, Eystein Lonning P, Borresen-Dale AL. Gene expression patterns of breast carcinomas distinguish tumor subclasses with clinical implications. Proc Natl Acad Sci U S A 2001; 98 (19):10869–10874.

Sorlie T, Tibshirani R, Parker J, Hastie T, Marron JS, Nobel A, Deng S, Johnsen H, Pesich R, Geisler S, Demeter J, Perou CM, Lonning PE, Brown PO, Borresen-Dale AL, Botstein D. Repeated observation of breast tumor subtypes in independent gene expression data sets. Proc Natl Acad Sci U S A 2003; 100(14):8418–8423.

Sotiriou C, Neo SY, McShane LM, Korn EL, Long PM, Jazaeri A, Martiat P, Fox SB, Harris AL, Liu ET. Breast cancer classification and prognosis based on gene expression profiles from a population-based study. Proc Natl Acad Sci U S A 2003; 100(18):10393–10398.

Southern E. DNA chips: Analysing sequence by hybridization to oligonucleotides on a large scale. Trends Genet 1996; 12:110–115.

Spain BH, Larson CJ, Shihabuddin LS, Gage FH, Verma IM. Truncated BRCA2 is cytoplasmic: implications for cancer-linked mutations. Proc Natl Acad Sci U S A 1999; 96(24):13920–13925.

Starita LM, Horwitz AA, Keogh MC, Ishioka C, Parvin JD, Chiba N. BRCA1/BARD1 ubiquitinate phosphorylated RNA polymerase II. J Biol Chem 2005; 280(26): 24498–24505.

Stark JM, Pierce AJ, Oh J, Pastink A, Jasin M. Genetic steps of mammalian homologous repair with distinct mutagenic consequences. Mol Cell Biol 2004; 24(21):9305–9316.

Steck PA, Pershouse MA, Jasser SA, Yung WK, Lin H, Ligon AH, Langford LA, Baumgard ML, Hattier T, Davis T, Frye C, Hu R, Swedlund B, Teng DH, Tavtigian SV. Identification of a candidate tumour suppressor gene, MMAC1, at chromosome 10q23.3 that is mutated in multiple advanced cancers. Nat Genet 1997; 15:356–362.

Steffen J, Nowakowska D, Niwinska A, Czapczak D, Kluska A, Piatkowska M, Wisniewska A, Paszko Z. Germline mutations 657del5 of the NBS1 gene contribute significantly to the incidence of breast cancer in Central Poland. Int J Cancer 2006; 119(2):472–475.

Steinitz R, Katz L, Ben-Hur M. Male breast cancer in Israel: selected epidemiological aspects. Isr J Med Sci 1981; 17(9–10):816–821.

Stelter P, Ulrich HD. Control of spontaneous and damage-induced mutagenesis by SUMO and ubiquitin conjugation. Nature 2003; 425(6954):188–191.

Struewing J, Abeliovish D, Peretz T, Avishai N, Kaback M, Collins F, Brody L. The carrier frequency of the *BRCA1* 185delAG mutation is approximately 1 percent in Ashkenazi Jewish individuals. Nat Genet 1995a; 11:198–200.

Struewing J, Hartge P, Wacholder S, Baker S, Berlin M, McAdams M, Timmerman M, Brody L, Tucker M. The risk of cancer associated with specific mutations of BRCA1 and BRCA2 among Ashkenazi Jews. N Engl J Med 1997; 336:1401–1408.

Struewing J, Tarone R, Broday L, Li F, Boice J. BRCA1 mutations in young women with breast cancer. Lancet 1996; 347:1493.

Struewing JP, Brody LC, Erdos MR, Kase RG, Giambarresi TR, Smith SA, Collins FS, Tucker MA. Detection of eight BRCA1 mutations in 10 breast/ovarian cancer families, including 1 family with male breast cancer. Am J Hum Genet 1995b; 57(1):1–7.

Struewing JP, Coriaty ZM, Ron E, Livoff A, Konichezky M, Cohen P, Resnick MB, Lifzchiz-Mercerl B, Lew S, Iscovich J. Founder BRCA1/2 mutations among male patients with breast cancer in Israel. Am J Hum Genet 1999; 65(6): 1800–1802.

Swensen J, Hoffman M, Skolnick MH, Neuhausen SL. Identification of a 14 kb deletion involving the promoter region of BRCA1 in a breast cancer family. Hum Mol Genet 1997; 6:1513–1517.

Swift M, Morrell D, Cromartie E, Chamberlin AR, Skolnick MH, Bishop DT. The incidence and gene frequency of ataxia-telangiectasia in the United States. Am J Hum Genet 1986; 39(5):573–583.

Swift M, Reitnauer PJ, Morrell D, Chase CL. Breast and other cancers in families with ataxia-telangiectasia. N Engl J Med 1987; 316(21):1289–1294.

Syrjakoski K, Kuukasjarvi T, Waltering K, Haraldsson K, Auvinen A, Borg A, Kainu T, Kallioniemi OP, Koivisto PA. BRCA2 mutations in 154 Finnish male breast cancer patients. Neoplasia 2004; 6(5):541–545.

Tan W, Zheng L, Lee WH, Boyer TG. Functional dissection of transcription factor ZBRK1 reveals zinc fingers with dual roles in DNA-binding and BRCA1-dependent transcriptional repression. J Biol Chem 2004; 279(8):6576–6587.

Taniguchi T, D'Andrea AD. Molecular pathogenesis of Fanconi anemia: recent progress. Blood 2006; 107 (11):4223–4233.

Taniguchi T, Tischkowitz M, Ameziane N, Hodgson SV, Mathew CG, Joenje H, Mok SC, D'Andrea AD. Disruption of the Fanconi anemia-BRCA pathway in cisplatin-sensitive ovarian tumors. Nat Med 2003; 9(5):568–574.

Tarsounas M, Davies D, West SC. BRCA2-dependent and independent formation of RAD51 nuclear foci. Oncogene 2003; 22(8):1115–1123.

Tavitigian S, Rommens J, Couch F, Shattuck-Eidens D, Neuhausen S, Merajver S, Thorlacius S, Offit K, Stoppa-Lyonnet D, Belanger C, Bell R, Berry S, Bogden R, Chen Q, Davis T, Dumont M, Frye C, Hattier T, Jammulapati S, Janecki T, Jiang P, Kehrer R, Leblanc J, Mitchell J, McArthur-Morrison J, Nguyen K, Peng Y, Samson C, Schroeder M, Snyder S, Steele L, Stringfellow M, Stroup C, Swedlund B, Swensen J, Teng D, Thomas A, Tran T, Tran T, Tranchant M, Weaver-Feldhans J, Wond AKC, Shizuya H, Eyfjord J, Cannon-Albright L, Labrie F, Skolnick M, Weer B, Kamb A, Goldgar D. The complete *BRCA2* gene and mutations in chromosomes 13q-linked kindreds. Nat Genet 1996; 12:333–337.

Tavtigian SV, Deffenbaugh AM, Yin L, Judkins T, Scholl T, Samollow PB, de Silva D, Zharkikh A, Thomas A. Comprehensive statistical study of 452 BRCA1 missense substitutions with classification of eight recurrent substitutions as neutral. J Med Genet 2006; 43(4):295–305.

Thakur S, Zhang H, Peng Y, Le H, Carroll B, Ward T, Yao J, Farid L, Couch F, Wilson R, Wever B. Localization of BRCA1 and a splice variant identifies the nuclear localization signal. Mol Cell Biol 1997; 17:444–452.

Thompson D, Duedal S, Kirner J, McGuffog L, Last J, Reiman A, Byrd P, Taylor M, Easton DF. Cancer risks and mortality in heterozygous ATM mutation carriers. J Natl Cancer Inst 2005; 97(11):813–822.

Thompson D, Easton D. Variation in cancer risks, by mutation position, in BRCA2 mutation carriers. Am J Hum Genet 2001; 68(2):410–419.

Thompson D, Easton DF. Cancer Incidence in BRCA1 mutation carriers. J Natl Cancer Inst 2002; 94(18):1358–1365.

Thompson D, Easton DF, Goldgar DE. A full-likelihood method for the evaluation of causality of sequence variants from family data. Am J Hum Genet 2003; 73(3):652–655.

Thorlacius S, Olafsdottir GH, Tryggvadottir L, Neuhausen S, Jonasson JG, Tavtigian S. A single mutation in the BRCA2 gene in male and female breat cancer families with varied cancer phenotypes. Nat Genet 1996; 13:117–119.

Thorlacius S, Sigurdsson S, Bjarnadottir H, Olarsdottir G, Jonasson JG, Tryggvadottir L, Tulinius H, Eyfjord JE. Study of a single BRCA2 mutation with high carrier frequency in a small population. Am J Hum Genet 1997; 60:1079–1084.

Thorlacius S, Struewing J, Hartge P, Olafsdottir G, Sigvaldason H, Tryggvadottir L, Wacholder S, Tulinius H, Eyfjord J. Population-based study of risk of breast cancer in carriers of BRCA2 mutation. The Lancet 1998; 352:1337–1339.

Thorlacius S, Tryggvadottir L, Olafsdottir GH, Jonasson JG, Ogmundsdottir HM, Tulinius H, Eyfjord JE. Linkage to BRCA2 region in hereditary male breast cancer. Lancet 1995; 346(8974):544–545.

Tibbetts R. Functional interactions between BRCA1 and the checkpoint kinase ATR during genotoxic stress. Genes Dev 2000; 14(23):2989–3002.

Tominaga K, Morisaki H, Kaneko Y, Fujimoto A, Tanaka T, Ohtsubo M, Hirai M, H O, Ikeda K, Nakanishi M. Role of human Cds1 (Chk2) kinase in DNA damage checkpoint and its regulation by p53. J Biol Chem 1999; 274:1463–1467.

Tomlinson I, Houlston R. Peutz-Heghers syndrome. J Med Genet 1997; 34:1007–1011.

Tonin P. Genes implicated in hereditary breast cancer syndromes. Semin Surg Oncol 2000; 18:281–286.

Tonin P, Moslehi R, Green R, Rosen B, Cole D, Boyd N, Cutler C, Margolese R, Carter R, McGillivray B, Ives E, Labrie F, Gilchrist D, Morgan D, Simard J, Narod S. Linkage analysis of 26 Canadian breast and breast-ovarian cancer families. Hum Genet 1995a; 95:545–550.

Tonin P, Weber B, Offit K, Couch F, Rebeck T, Neuhausen S, Godwin AK, Daly M, Costalas J, Berman D, Grana G, Fox E, Kane MF, Kolodner RD, Haber D, Struewing J, Warner E, Rosen B, Foulkes W, Lerman C, Pechkin B, Serova O, Lynch HT, Lenoir GM, Narod SA, Garber JE. A high frequency of BRCA1 and BRCA2 mutations in 222 Ashkenazi Jewish breast cancer families. Nat Med 1996; 2:1179–1183.

Tonin PN, Mes-Masson AM, Futreal PA, Morgan K, Mahon M, Foulkes WD, Cole DE, Provencher D, Ghadirian P, Narod SA. Founder BRCA1 and BRCA2 mutations in French Canadian breast and ovarian cancer families. Am J Hum Genet 1998; 63(5):1341–1351.

Tonin R, Serova O, Lenoir G, Lynch H, Durocher F, Simard J, Morgen K, Narod S. BRCA1 mutations in Ashkenazi Jewish women. Am J Hum Genet 1995b; 57:189.

Torres D, Rashid MU, Gil F, Umana A, Ramelli G, Robledo JF, Tawil M, Torregrosa L, Briceno I, Hamann U. High proportion of BRCA1/2 founder mutations in Hispanic breast/ovarian cancer families from Colombia. Breast Cancer Res Treat 2006.

Tournier I, Paillerets BB, Sobol H, Stoppa-Lyonnet D, Lidereau R, Barrois M, Mazoyer S, Coulet F, Hardouin A, Chompret A, Lortholary A, Chappuis P, Bourdon V, Bonadona V, Maugard C, Gilbert B, Nogues C, Frebourg T, Tosi M. Significant contribution of germline BRCA2 rearrangements in male breast cancer families. Cancer Res 2004; 64(22):8143–8147.

Tsutsui S, Inoue H, Yasuda K, Suzuki K, Higashi H, Era S, Mori M. Reduced expression of PTEN protein and its prognostic implications in invasive ductal carcinoma of the breast. Oncology 2005a; 68(4–6):398–404.

Tsutsui S, Inoue H, Yasuda K, Suzuki K, Tahara K, Higashi H, Era S, Mori M. Inactivation of PTEN is associated with a low p27Kip1 protein expression in breast carcinoma. Cancer 2005b; 104(10):2048–2053.

Tulinius H, Olafsdottir G, Sigvaldason H, Tryggvadottir L, Bjarnadottir K. Neoplastic diseases in families of breast cancer patients. J Med Genet 1994; 31:618–621.

Tulinius H, Olafsdottir GH, Sigvaldason H, Arason A, Barkardottir RB, Egilsson V, Ogmundsdottir HM, Tryggvadottir L, Gudlaugsdottir S, Eyfjord JE. The effect of a single BRCA2 mutation on cancer in Iceland. J Med Genet 2002; 39(7):457–462.

Turner N, Tutt A, Ashworth A. Hallmarks of 'BRCAness' in sporadic cancers. Nat Rev Cancer 2004; 4(10):814–819.

Turner NC, Reis-Filho JS. Basal-like breast cancer and the BRCA1 phenotype. Oncogene 2006; 25(43):5846–5853.

Tutt A, Bertwistle D, Valentine J, Gabriel A, Swift S, Ross G, Griffin C, Thacker J, Ashworth A. Mutation in Brca2 stimulates error-prone homology-directed repair of DNA double-strand breaks occurring between repeated sequences. Embo J 2001; 20(17):4704–4716.

Tyrer J, Duffy SW, Cuzick J. A breast cancer prediction model incorporating familial and personal risk factors. Stat Med 2004; 23(7):1111–1130.

Underhill P, Jin L, Lin A, Mehdi S, Jankins T, Vollrath D, Davis R, Cavalli-Sforza L, Oefner P. Detection of numerous Y chromosome biallelic polymorphisms by denaturing high-performance liquid chromatography. Genome Res 1997; 7:996–1005.

Vahteristo P, Tamminen A, Karvinen P, Eerola H, Eklund C, Aaltonen LA, Blomqvist C, Aittomaki K, Nevanlinna H. p53, CHK2, and CHK1 genes in Finnish families with Li-Fraumeni syndrome: further evidence of CHK2 in inherited cancer predisposition. Cancer Res 2001; 61(15):5718–5722.

Vahteristo P, Yliannala K, Tamminen A, Eerola H, Blomqvist C, Nevanlinna H. BACH1 Ser919Pro variant and breast cancer risk. BMC Cancer 2006; 6:19.

Vallon-Christersson J, Cayanan C, Haraldsson K, Loman N, Bergthorsson JT, Brondum-Nielsen K, Gerdes AM, Moller P, Kristoffersson U, Olsson H, Borg A, Monteiro AN. Functional analysis of BRCA1 C-terminal missense mutations identified in breast and ovarian cancer families. Hum Mol Genet 2001; 10(4):353–360.

van 't Veer LJ, Dai H, van de Vijver MJ, He YD, Hart AA, Mao M, Peterse HL, van der Kooy K, Marton MJ, Witteveen AT, Schreiber GJ, Kerkhoven RM, Roberts C, Linsley PS, Bernards R, Friend SH. Gene expression profiling predicts clinical outcome of breast cancer. Nature 2002; 415 (6871):530–536.

van de Vijver MJ, He YD, van't Veer LJ, Dai H, Hart AA, Voskuil DW, Schreiber GJ, Peterse JL, Roberts C, Marton MJ, Parrish M, Atsma D, Witteveen A, Glas A, Delahaye L, van der Velde T, Bartelink H, Rodenhuis S, Rutgers ET, Friend SH, Bernards R. A gene-expression signature as a predictor of survival in breast cancer. N Engl J Med 2002; 347(25):1999–2009.

van der Groep P, Bouter A, van der Zanden R, Menko FH, Buerger H, Verheijen RH, van der Wall E, van Diest PJ. Re: Germline BRCA1 mutations and a basal epithelial phenotype in breast cancer. J Natl Cancer Inst 2004; 96(9): 712–713; (author reply 714).

van der Looij M, Cleton-Jansen AM, van Eijk R, Morreau H, van Vliet M, Kuipers-Dijkshoorn N, Olah E, Cornelisse CJ, Devilee P. A sporadic breast tumor with a somatically acquired complex genomic rearrangement in BRCA1. Genes Chromsomes Cancer 2000; 27:295–302.

Varley J, Evans DG, Birch J. Li-Fraumeni syndrome - a molecular and clinical review. Br J Cancer 1997; 76:1–14.

Velasco E, Infante M, Duran M, Esteban-Cardenosa E, Lastra E, Garcia-Giron C, Miner C. Rapid mutation detection in complex genes by heteroduplex analysis with capillary array electrophoresis. Electrophoresis 2005; 26(13): 2539–2552.

Venkitaraman AR. Cancer susceptibility and the functions of BRCA1 and BRCA2. Cell 2002; 108(2):171–182.

Wada O, Oishi H, Takada I, Yanagisawa J, Yano T, Kato S. BRCA1 function mediates a TRAP/DRIP complex through direct interaction with TRAP220. Oncogene 2004; 23(35): 6000–6005.

Wallace R. DNA on a chip: serving up the genome for diagnostics and research. Mol Med Today 1997; 55:569–574.

Walsh T, Casadei S, Coats KH, Swisher E, Stray SM, Higgins J, Roach KC, Mandell J, Lee MK, Ciernikova S, Foretova L, Soucek P, King MC. Spectrum of mutations in BRCA1, BRCA2, CHEK2, and TP53 in families at high risk of breast cancer. JAMA 2006; 295(12):1379–1388.

Walsh T, King MC. Ten genes for inherited breast cancer. Cancer Cell 2007; 11(2):103–105.

Wang C, Fan S, Li Z, Fu M, Rao M, Ma Y, Lisanti MP, Albanese C, Katzenellenbogen BS, Kushner PJ, Weber B, Rosen EM, Pestell RG. Cyclin D1 antagonizes BRCA1 repression of estrogen receptor alpha activity. Cancer Res 2005; 65(15): 6557–6567.

Wang HC, Chou WC, Shieh SY, Shen CY. Ataxia telangiectasia mutated and checkpoint kinase 2 regulate BRCA1 to promote the fidelity of DNA end-joining. Cancer Res 2006; 66(3):1391–1400.

Wang Q, Zhang H, Kajino K, Greene MI. BRCA1 binds c-Myc and inhibits its transcriptional and transforming activity in cells. Oncogene 1998; 17(15):1939–1948.

Wang X, Liu L, Montagna C, Ried T, Deng CX. Haploinsufficiency of Parp1 accelerates Brca1-associated centrosome amplification, telomere shortening, genetic instability, apoptosis, and embryonic lethality. Cell Death Differ 2007; 14(5):924–931.

Wang Y, Cortez D, Yazdi P, Neff N, Elledge SJ, Qin J. BASC, a super complex of BRCA1-associated proteins involved in the recognition and repair of aberrant DNA structures. Genes Dev 2000; 14(8):927–939.

Wang Z-J, Churchman M, Campbell I, Zu W-H, Yan Z-Y, McCluggage W, Foulkes W, Tomlinson I. Allele loss and mutation screen at the Peutz-Jeghers (LKB1) locus (19p13.3) in sporadic ovarian tumours. Br J Cancer 1999; 80:70–72.

Wardrop SL, Brown MA. Identification of two evolutionarily conserved and functional regulatory elements in intron 2 of the human BRCA1 gene. Genomics 2005; 86(3):316–328.

Warner E, Foulkes W, Goodwin P, Meschino W, Blondal J, Paterson C, Ozcelik H, Goss P, Allingham-Hawkins D, Hamel N, DiProspero L, Contiga V, Serruya C, Klein M, Moslehi R, Honeyford J, Liede A, Glendon G, Brunet J-S, Narod S. Prevalence and penetrance of BRCA1 and BRCA2 gene mutations in unselected Ashkenazi Jewish women with breast cancer. J Natl Cancer Inst 1999; 91:1241–1247.

Warner E, Plewes DB, Hill KA, Causer PA, Zubovits JT, Jong RA, Cutrara MR, DeBoer G, Yaffe MJ, Messner SJ, Meschino WS, Piron CA, Narod SA. Surveillance of BRCA1 and BRCA2 mutation carriers with magnetic resonance imaging, ultrasound, mammography, and clinical breast examination. JAMA 2004; 292(11):1317–1325.

Warren M, Lord CJ, Masabanda J, Griffin D, Ashworth A. Phenotypic effects of heterozygosity for a BRCA2 mutation. Hum Mol Genet 2003; 12(20):2645–2656.

Washington MT, Johnson RE, Prakash L, Prakash S. Accuracy of lesion bypass by yeast and human DNA polymerase eta. Proc Natl Acad Sci U S A 2001; 98(15):8355–8360.

Watanabe K, Tateishi S, Kawasuji M, Tsurimoto T, Inoue H, Yamaizumi M. Rad18 guides poleta to replication stalling sites through physical interaction and PCNA monoubiquitination. Embo J 2004; 23(19):3886–3896.

Waters LS, Walker GC. The critical mutagenic translesion DNA polymerase Rev1 is highly expressed during G(2)/M phase rather than S phase. Proc Natl Acad Sci U S A 2006; 103 (24):8971–8976.

Weber B. Familial breast cancer. Recent Results Cancer Res 1996; 140:5–16.

Weber F, Fukino K, Sawada T, Williams N, Sweet K, Brena RM, Plass C, Caldes T, Mutter GL, Villalona-Calero MA, Eng C. Variability in organ-specific *EGFR* mutational spectra in tumour epithelium and stroma may be the biological basis for differential responses to tyrosine kinase inhibitors. Br J Cancer 2005; 92(10):1922–1926.

Weber F, Shen L, Fukino K, Patocs A, Mutter GL, Caldes T, Eng C. Total-genome analysis of BRCA1/2-related invasive carcinomas of the breast identifies tumor stroma as potential landscaper for neoplastic initiation. Am J Hum Genet 2006; 78(6):961–972.

Weber J, Barbier V, Pages-Berhouet S, Caux-Moncoutier V, Stoppa-Lyonnet D, Viovy JL. A high-throughput mutation detection method based on heteroduplex analysis using graft copolymer matrixes: application to Brca1 and Brca2 analysis. Anal Chem 2004; 76(16):4839–4848.

Wei M, Grushko TA, Dignam J, Hagos F, Nanda R, Sveen L, Xu J, Fackenthal J, Tretiakova M, Das S, Olopade OI. BRCA1 promoter methylation in sporadic breast cancer is associated with reduced BRCA1 copy number and chromosome 17 aneusomy. Cancer Res 2005; 65(23):10692–10699.

Weitzel JN, Lagos V, Blazer KR, Nelson R, Ricker C, Herzog J, McGuire C, Neuhausen S. Prevalence of BRCA mutations and founder effect in high-risk Hispanic families. Cancer Epidemiol Biomarkers Prev 2005; 14(7):1666–1671.

Wen L, Li W, Sobel M, Feng JA. Computational exploration of the activated pathways associated with DNA damage response in breast cancer. Proteins 2006; 65(1):103–110.

Wen W, Bernstein L, Lescallett J, Beazer-Barclay Y, Sullivan-Halley J, White M, Press M. Comparison of TP53 mutations identified by oligonucleotide microarray and convertional DNA sequence analysis. Cancer Res 2000; 60:2716–2722.

Westermark UK, Reyngold M, Olshen AB, Baer R, Jasin M, Moynahan ME. BARD1 participates with BRCA1 in homology-directed repair of chromosome breaks. Mol Cell Biol 2003; 23(21):7926–7936.

Whittemore A, Gong G, Iitnyre J. Prevalence and contribution of *BRCA1* mutations in breast cancer and ovarian cancer: results from three US population-based case-control studies of ovarian cancer. Am J Hum Genet 1997; 60:496–504.

Whittemore AS, Balise RR, Pharoah PD, Dicioccio RA, Oakley-Girvan I, Ramus SJ, Daly M, Usinowicz MB, Garlinghouse-Jones K, Ponder BA, Buys S, Senie R, Andrulis I, John E, Hopper JL, Piver MS. Oral contraceptive use and ovarian cancer risk among carriers of BRCA1 or BRCA2 mutations. Br J Cancer 2004a; 91(11):1911–1915.

Whittemore AS, Gong G, John EM, McGuire V, Li FP, Ostrow KL, Dicioccio R, Felberg A, West DW. Prevalence of BRCA1 mutation carriers among U.S. non-Hispanic Whites. Cancer Epidemiol Biomarkers Prev 2004b; 13(12): 2078–2083.

Williams RS, Glover JN. Structural consequences of a cancer-causing BRCA1-BRCT missense mutation. J Biol Chem 2003; 278(4):2630–2635.

Williams RS, Green R, Glover JN. Crystal structure of the BRCT repeat region from the breast cancer-associated protein BRCA1. Nat Struct Biol 2001; 8(10):838–842.

Williams RS, Lee MS, Hau DD, Glover JN. Structural basis of phosphopeptide recognition by the BRCT domain of BRCA1. Nat Struct Mol Biol 2004; 11(6):519–525.

Wilson CA, Payton MN, Elliott GS, Buaas FW, Cajulis EE, Grosshans D, Ramos L, Reese DM, Slamon DJ, Calzone FJ. Differential subcellular localization, expression and biological toxicity of BRCA1 and the splice variant BRCA1-delta11b. Oncogene 1997; 14(1):1–16.

Wilusz CJ, Wang W, Peltz SW. Curbing the nonsense: the activation and regulation of mRNA surveillance. Genes Dev 2001; 15(21):2781–2785.

Wolpert N, Warner E, Seminsky MF, Futreal A, Narod SA. Prevalence of BRCA1 and BRCA2 mutations in male breast cancer patients in Canada. Clin Breast Cancer 2000; 1(1): 57–63; (discussion 64–55).

Wong A, Pero R, Ormonde P, Tavigian S, Bartel P. Rad51 interacts with the evolutionarily conserved BRC motifs in the human breast cancer susceptibility gene *BRCA2*. J Biol Chem 1997; 272:31941–31944.

Woodward AM, Davis TA, Silva AG, Kirk JA, Leary JA. Large genomic rearrangements of both BRCA2 and BRCA1 are a feature of the inherited breast/ovarian cancer phenotype in selected families. J Med Genet 2005; 42(5):e31.

Wooster R, Bignell G, Lancaster J. Identification of the breast cancer susceptibility gene BRCA2. Nature 1995; 378:789–792.

Wooster R, Newhausen S, Mangion J, Quirk Y, Ford D, Collins N, Nguyen K, Seal S, Tran T, Averill D, Fields P, Marchall G, Narod S, Lenoir G, Lynch H, Frunteun J, Devilee P, Cornelisse C, Menko F, Daly PA, Ormiston W, McManus R, Pye C, Lewis C, Cannon-Albright L, Peto J, Ponder B, Skolnick M, Easton D, Goldgar D, Stratton M. Localization of a breast cancer susceptibility gene, *BRCA2*, to chromosome 13q12-13. Science 1994; 265:2088–2090.

Wooster R, Weber BL. Breast and ovarian cancer. N Engl J Med 2003; 348(23):2339–2347.

Wu LC, Wang Z, Tsan J, Spillman M, Phung A, Zu X, Yang M, Hwang MC, Bowcock A, Baer R. Identification of a RING protein that can interact in vivo with the *BRCA1* gene product. Nat Genet 1996; 14:430–440.

Wu-Baer F, Baer R. Effect of DNA damage on a BRCA1 complex. Nature 2001; 414(6859):36.

Xia B, Dorsman JC, Ameziane N, de Vries Y, Rooimans MA, Sheng Q, Pals G, Errami A, Gluckman E, Llera J, Wang W, Livingston DM, Joenje H, de Winter JP. Fanconi anemia is associated with a defect in the BRCA2 partner PALB2. Nat Genet 2007; 39(2):159–161.

Xia B, Sheng Q, Nakanishi K, Ohashi A, Wu J, Christ N, Liu X, Jasin M, Couch FJ, Livingston DM. Control of BRCA2 cellular and clinical functions by a nuclear partner, PALB2. Mol Cell 2006; 22(6):719–729.

Xiong J, Fan S, Meng Q, Schramm L, Wang C, Bouzahza B, Zhou J, Zafonte B, Goldberg ID, Haddad BR, Pestell RG, Rosen EM. BRCA1 inhibition of telomerase activity in cultured cells. Mol Cell Biol 2003; 23(23):8668–8690.

Xu B, Kim S, Kastan MB. Involvement of Brca1 in S-phase and G(2)-phase checkpoints after ionizing irradiation. Mol Cell Biol 2001a; 21(10):3445–3450.

Xu C, Chambers J, Brown M, Jujeirat Y, Mohammed S, Hodgson S, Kelsell D, Surr N, Bishop D, Solomon E. Mutations and alternative splicing of the *BRCA1* gene in U.D. breast/ovarian cancer families. Genes Chromosomes Cancer 1997; 18:102–110.

Xu J, Fan S, Rosen EM. Regulation of the estrogen-inducible gene expression profile by the breast cancer susceptibility gene BRCA1. Endocrinology 2005; 146(4):2031–2047.

Xu X, Qiao W, Linke SP, Cao L, Li WM, Furth PA, Harris CC, Deng CX. Genetic interactions between tumor suppressors Brca1 and p53 in apoptosis, cell cycle and tumorigenesis. Nat Genet 2001b; 28(3):266–271.

Xu X, Weaver Z, Linke SP, Li C, Gotay J, Wang X-W, Harris CC, Ried T, Deng C-X. Centrosome amplification and a defective G_2-M cell cycle checkpoint induce genetic instability in BRCA1 exon 11 isoform-deficient cells. Mol Cell 1999; 3:389–395.

Yang H, Jeffrey PD, Miller J, Kinnucan E, Sun Y, Thoma NH, Zheng N, Chen PL, Lee WH, Pavletich NP. BRCA2 function in DNA binding and recombination from a BRCA2-DSS1-ssDNA structure. Science 2002; 297 (5588):1837–1848.

Yang WW, Wang ZH, Zhu Y, Yang HT. E2F6 negatively regulates ultraviolet-induced apoptosis via modulation of BRCA1. Cell Death Differ 2007; 14(4):807–817.

Yang YG, Herceg Z, Nakanishi K, Demuth I, Piccoli C, Michelon J, Hildebrand G, Jasin M, Digweed M, Wang ZQ. The Fanconi anemia group A protein modulates homologous repair of DNA double-strand breaks in mammalian cells. Carcinogenesis 2005; 26(10):1731–1740.

Yarden RI, Brody LC. BRCA1 interacts with components of the histone deacetylase complex. Proc Natl Acad Sci U S A 1999; 96:4983–4988.

Yarden RI, Pardo-Reoyo S, Sgagias M, Cowan KH, Brody LC. BRCA1 regulates the G2/M checkpoint by activating Chk1 kinase upon DNA damage. Nat Genet 2002; 30(3):285–289.

Ye Q, Hu YF, Zhong H, Nye AC, Belmont AS, Li R. BRCA1-induced large-scale chromatin unfolding and allele-specific effects of cancer-predisposing mutations. J Cell Biol 2001; 155(6):911–921.

Yim SC, Park HG, Chang HN, Cho DY. Array-based mutation detection of BRCA1 using direct probe/target hybridization. Anal Biochem 2005; 337(2):332–337.

Yu VP, Koehler M, Steinlein C, Schmid M, Hanakahi LA, van Gool AJ, West SC, Venkitaraman AR. Gross chromosomal rearrangements and genetic exchange between nonhomologous chromosomes following BRCA2 inactivation. Genes Dev 2000; 14(11):1400–1406.

Yu X, Baer R. Nuclear localization and cell cycle-specific expression of CtIP, a protein that associates with the

BRCA1 tumor suppressor. J Biol Chem 2000; 275 (24):18541–18549.

Yun J, Lee WH. Degradation of transcription repressor ZBRK1 through the ubiquitin-proteasome pathway relieves repression of Gadd45a upon DNA damage. Mol Cell Biol 2003; 23(20):7305–7314.

Zhang H, Somasundaram K, Peng Y, Tian H, Zhang H, Bi D, Weber BL, El-Deiry WS. BRCA1 physically associates with p53 and stimulates its transcriptional activity. Oncogene 1998; 16(13):1713–1721.

Zhang J, Willers H, Feng Z, Ghosh JC, Kim S, Weaver DT, Chung JH, Powell SN, Xia F. Chk2 phosphorylation of BRCA1 regulates DNA double-strand break repair. Mol Cell Biol 2004; 24(2):708–718.

Zhang X, Krutchinsky A, Fukuda A, Chen W, Yamamura S, Chait BT, Roeder RG. MED1/TRAP220 exists predominantly in a TRAP/Mediator subpopulation enriched in RNA polymerase II and is required for ER-mediated transcription. Mol Cell 2005; 19(1):89–100.

Zheng L, Annab LA, Afshari CA, Lee WH, Boyer TG. BRCA1 mediates ligand-independent transcriptional repression of the estrogen receptor. Proc Natl Acad Sci U S A 2001; 98(17):9587–9592.

Zheng L, Pan H, Li S, Flesken-Nikitin A, Chen PL, Boyer TG, Lee WH. Sequence-specific transcriptional corepressor function for BRCA1 through a novel zinc finger protein, ZBRK1. Mol Cell 2000; 6(4):757–768.

Zhong Q, Boyer TG, Chen PL, Lee WH. Deficient nonhomologous end-joining activity in cell-free extracts from Brca1-null fibroblasts. Cancer Res 2002; 62(14):3966–3970.

Zhong Q, Chen C, Li S, Chen Y, Wang C, Xiao J, Chen P, Sharp Z, Lee W. Association of BRCA1 with the hRad50-hMre11-p95 complex and the DNA damage response. Science 1999; 285:747–750.

Zhu W, Dutta A. An ATR- and BRCA1-mediated Fanconi anemia pathway is required for activating the G2/M checkpoint and DNA damage repair upon rereplication. Mol Cell Biol 2006; 26(12):4601–4611.

Zhuang J, Zhang J, Willers H, Wang H, Chung JH, van Gent DC, Hallahan DE, Powell SN, Xia F. Checkpoint kinase 2-mediated phosphorylation of BRCA1 regulates the fidelity of nonhomologous end-joining. Cancer Res 2006a; 66(3):1401–1408.

Zhuang ZG, Di GH, Shen ZZ, Ding J, Shao ZM. Enhanced expression of LKB1 in breast cancer cells attenuates angiogenesis, invasion, and metastatic potential. Mol Cancer Res 2006b; 4(11):843–849.

Index